Volume 1

ANESTHESIA

SECOND EDITION

Volume 1

ANESTHESIA
SECOND EDITION

Edited by

Ronald D. Miller, M.D.

Professor and Chairman of Anesthesia
Professor of Pharmacology
Department of Anesthesia
University of California, San Francisco
School of Medicine
San Francisco, California

CHURCHILL LIVINGSTONE
New York, Edinburgh, London, Melbourne 1986

Acquisitions editor: *Toni M. Tracy*
Copy editor: *Michael Kelley*
Production designer: *Rosalie Marcus*
Production supervisor: *Sharon Tuder*
Compositor: *Progressive Typographers, Inc.*
Printer/Binder: *The Maple-Vail Book Manufacturing Group*

Accurate indications, adverse reactions, and dosage schedules for drugs are provided in this book, but it is possible that they may change. The reader is urged to review the package information data of the manufacturers of the medications mentioned.

Distributed in the United Kingdom by Churchill Livingstone, Robert Stevenson House, 1–3 Baxter's Place, Leith Walk, Edinburgh EH1 3AF and by associated companies, branches and representatives throughout the world.

First published in 1986

Printed in U.S.A.

ISBN 0-443-08328-2

9 8 7 6

Library of Congress Cataloging-in-Publication Data
Main entry under title:

Anesthesia.

    Includes bibliographies and index.
    1. Anesthesia. I. Miller, Ronald D., date.
[DNLM: 1. Anesthesia. WO 200 A573]
RD81.A54   1986   617'.96   85-17446
ISBN 0-443-08328-2

Manufactured in the United States of America

CONTRIBUTORS

David D. Alfery, M.D.
Member, Anesthesiology Consultants of Nashville, P.C.; Staff Anesthesiologist, St. Thomas Hospital and Parkview Hospital, Nashville, Tennessee

Hassan H. Ali, M.D.
Associate Professor of Anesthesia, Harvard Medical School; Associate Anesthetist, Department of Anesthesia, Massachusetts General Hospital, Boston, Massachusetts

Jeffrey M. Baden, M.B., B.S., F.F.A.R.C.S.
Associate Professor of Anesthesia, Stanford University School of Medicine, Stanford, California; Staff Anesthesiologist, Department of Anesthesia, Veterans Administration Medical Center, Palo Alto, California

Peter L. Bailey, M.D.
Assistant Professor, Department of Anesthesiology, University of Utah School of Medicine, Salt Lake City, Utah

Robert F. Bedford, M.D.
Associate Professor, Departments of Anesthesiology and Neurological Surgery, University of Virginia School of Medicine, Charlottesville, Virginia

Jonathan L. Benumof, M.D.
Professor of Anesthesia, University of California, San Diego, School of Medicine, La Jolla, California

Julien F. Biebuyck, M.D., D.Phil.
Eric A. Walker Professor and Chairman, Department of Anesthesia, Pennsylvania State University College of Medicine, The Milton S. Hershey Medical Center, Hershey, Pennsylvania

Stephen M. Brzica, Jr., M.D.
Director of Anesthesia, St. Paul's Surgical Center, St. Paul, Minnesota; Assistant Professor of Anesthesia, University of Minnesota Medical School, Minneapolis, Minnesota

Norman J. Clark, M.D.
Fellow in Anesthesiology, Department of Anesthesiology, University of Utah School of Medicine, Salt Lake City, Utah

Benjamin G. Covino, M.D., Ph.D.
Chairman, Department of Anesthesiology, Brigham and Women's Hospital, Boston, Massachusetts

Robert K. Crone, M.D.
Director, Multidisciplinary Intensive Care Unit, The Children's Hospital, Boston Massachusetts

David J. Cullen, M.D.
Associate Professor of Anesthesia, Harvard Medical School; Anesthetist, Department of Anesthesia, Massachusetts General Hospital, Boston, Massachusetts

Norbert P. DeBruijn, M.D.
Assistant Professor of Anesthesia and Surgery, Department of Anesthesia, Duke University School of Medicine, Durham, North Carolina

Judith H. Donegan, M.D., Ph.D.
Professor of Anesthesia, Director of Clinical Neuroanesthesia, Department of Anesthesia, University of California, San Francisco, School of Medicine, San Francisco, California

John V. Donlon, Jr., M.D.
Assistant Clinical Director of Anesthesia, Massachusetts Eye & Ear Infirmary; Assistant Clinical Professor of Anesthesia, Harvard Medical School, Boston, Massachusetts

Charles G. Durbin, Jr., M.D.
Associate Professor, Department of Anesthesiology, University of Virginia School of Medicine, Charlottesville, Virginia

Lawrence D. Egbert, M.D., M.P.H.
Professor of Anesthesiology, University of Texas Southwestern Medical School at Dallas, Dallas, Texas

Edmond I. Eger II, M.D.
Professor of Anesthesia and Vice Chairman for Research, Department of Anesthesia, University of California, San Francisco, School of Medicine, San Francisco, California

Thomas W. Feeley, M.D.
Associate Professor of Anesthesia, Associate Medical Director, Intensive Care Unit, Department of Anesthesia, Stanford University School of Medicine, Stanford, California

Dennis M. Fisher, M.D.
Assistant Professor of Anesthesia and Pediatrics, Department of Anesthesia, University of California, San Francisco, School of Medicine, San Francisco, California

Thomas J. Gal, M.D.
Associate Professor of Anesthesia, Department of Anesthesiology, University of Virginia School of Medicine, Charlottesville, Virginia

Charles P. Gibbs, M.D.
Professor of Anesthesiology and Obstetrics & Gynecology, Assistant Dean for Curriculum, University of Florida College of Medicine, Gainesville, Florida

Adolph H. Giesecke, Jr., M.D.
Jenkins Professor and Chairman, Department of Anesthesiology, University of Texas Southwestern Medical School at Dallas, Dallas, Texas

George A. Gregory, M.D.
Professor of Anesthesia and Pediatrics, Department of Anesthesia, University of California, San Francisco, School of Medicine, San Francisco, California

Gerald A. Gronert, M.D.
Professor of Anesthesiology, Mayo Medical School, Rochester, Minnesota

Robert F. Hickey, M.D.
Professor and Vice Chairman, Department of Anesthesia, University of California, San Francisco, School of Medicine; Chief, Anesthesia Service, Veterans Administration Medical Center, San Francisco, California

Thomas F. Hornbein, M.D.
Professor and Chairman, Department of Anesthesiology, University of Washington School of Medicine, Seattle, Washington

Carl C. Hug, Jr., M.D., Ph.D.
Professor of Anesthesiology and Pharmacology, Department of Anesthesiology, Emory University School of Medicine; Director, Cardiothoracic Anesthesia, The Emory Clinic, Atlanta, Georgia

Joel A. Kaplan, M.D.
Professor and Chairman, Department of Anesthesia, Mount Sinai School of Medicine of the City University of New York, New York, New York

Robert R. Kirby, M.D.
Chairman, Department of Anesthesiology, Wilford Hall, USAF Medical Center, Lackland AFB, Texas

Richard J. Kitz, M.D.
Anesthetist-in-Chief, Department of Anesthesia, Massachusetts General Hospital; Henry Isaiah Dorr Professor, Harvard Medical School, Boston, Massachusetts

Donald D. Koblin, M.D., Ph.D.
Resident in Anesthesia, Department of Anesthesia, Pennsylvania State University College of Medicine, The Milton S. Hershey Medical Center, Hershey, Pennsylvania

John B. Leslie, M.D.
Assistant Professor of Anesthesiology, Duke University School of Medicine, Durham, North Carolina

Gershon Levinson, M.D.
Associate Professor of Anesthesia and Obstetrics, Gynecology, and Reproductive Sciences, Department of Anesthesia, University of California, San Francisco, School of Medicine; Attending Anesthesiologist, Anesthesia Service, San Francisco General Hospital, San Francisco, California

Lawrence Litt, M.D., Ph.D.
Assistant Professor of Anesthesia and Radiology, Department of Anesthesia, University of California, San Francisco, School of Medicine, San Francisco, California

Mervyn Maze, M.B., Ch.B., M.R.C.P. (U.K.)
Assistant Professor of Anesthesia, Stanford University School of Medicine, Stanford, California; Staff Physician, Anesthesiology Service, Veterans Administration Medical Center, Palo Alto, California

Richard I. Mazze, M.D.
Professor of Anesthesia, Stanford University Medical Center, Stanford, California; Chief, Anesthesiology Service, Veterans Administration Medical Center, Palo Alto, California

Robert G. Merin, M.D.
Professor of Anesthesiology, University of Texas Medical School at Houston, Houston, Texas

Edward D. Miller, Jr., M.D.
Professor of Anesthesiology and Surgery, Medical Director, Surgical Intensive Care Unit, Department of Anesthesiology, University of Virginia School of Medicine, Charlottesville, Virginia

Ronald D. Miller, M.D.
Professor and Chairman of Anesthesia, Professor of Pharmacology, Department of Anesthesia, University of California, San Francisco, School of Medicine, San Francisco, California

Jerome H. Modell, M.D.
Professor and Chairman, Department of Anesthesiology, University of Florida College of Medicine, Gainesville, Florida

Terence M. Murphy, M.B., Ch.B., F.F.A.R.C.S.
Professor of Anesthesia and Clinical Pain Services, Department of Anesthesiology, University of Washington School of Medicine, Seattle, Washington

Edward V. Norton, J.D.
Attorney at Law, College Park, Maryland

Martin L. Norton, M.D., J.D.
Professor of Anesthesiology and In-House Counsel, Department of Anesthesiology, University of Michigan Hospital, Ann Arbor, Michigan

Fredrick K. Orkin, M.D.
Associate Professor of Anesthesia, University of California, San Francisco, School of Medicine, San Francisco, California

P. Pearl O'Rourke, M.D.
Associate Director, Multidisciplinary Intensive Care Unit, The Children's Hospital, Boston, Massachusetts

David A. Paulus, M.D.
Assistant Professor, Department of Anesthesiology, College of Medicine; Department of Mechanical Engineering, College of Engineering, University of Florida, Gainesville, Florida

Edward G. Pavlin, M.D.
Associate Professor, Department of Anesthesia, University of Washington School of Medicine; Department of Anesthesiology, Harborview Medical Center, Seattle, Washington

Ira J. Rampil, M.D.
Resident in Anesthesia, Department of Anesthesia, University of California, San Francisco, School of Medicine, San Francisco, California

Susan A. Rice, Ph.D.
Assistant Professor of Pharmacology and Toxicology in Anesthesia, Stanford University School of Medicine, Stanford, California; Pharmacologist, Veterans Administration Medical Center, Palo Alto, California

Sandra L. Roberts, M.D.
Fellow in Anesthesia, Department of Anesthesiology, University of Iowa College of Medicine, Iowa City, Iowa

Mark C. Rogers, M.D.
Professor and Chairman, Department of Anesthesiology and Critical Care Medicine, The Johns Hopkins University School of Medicine, Baltimore, Maryland

Michael F. Roizen, M.D.
Professor and Chairman, Department of Anesthesiology, University of Chicago, The Pritzker School of Medicine, Chicago, Illinois

Stephen M. Rupp, M.D.
Assistant Professor of Anesthesia and Neurosurgery, Department of Anesthesia, University of California, San Francisco, School of Medicine, San Francisco, California

John J. Savarese, M.D.
Associate Professor of Anesthesia, Harvard Medical School; Anesthetist, Department of Anesthesia, Massachusetts General Hospital, Boston, Massachusetts

John W. Severinghaus, M.D.
Professor of Anesthesia, University of California, San Francisco, School of Medicine, San Francisco, California

Barry A. Shapiro, M.D.
Professor of Clinical Anesthesia and Director, Division of Respiratory/Critical Care, Department of Anesthesia, Northwestern University Medical School, Northwestern Memorial Hospital, Chicago, Illinois

Harvey M. Shapiro, M.D.
Professor of Anesthesia and Neurosurgery, Department of Anesthesia, University of California, San Diego, School of Medicine; Attending Anesthesiologist, Anesthesia Service, Veterans Administration Medical Center, La Jolla, California

Sol M. Shnider, M.D.
Professor of Anesthesia and Obstetrics, Gynecology, and Reproductive Sciences, Department of Anesthesia, University of California, San Francisco, School of Medicine, San Francisco, California

Robert A. Smith, M.S., R.R.T.
Director, Critical Care Medicine Animal Research Laboratory, Memorial Medical Center, Jacksonville, Florida

Frank G. Standaert, M.D.
Professor and Chairman, Department of Pharmacology, Georgetown University Schools of Medicine and Dentistry, Washington, D.C.

Theodore H. Stanley, M.D.
Professor of Anesthesiology and Research Professor of Surgery, Department of Anesthesiology, University of Utah School of Medicine, Salt Lake City, Utah

Robert K. Stoelting, M.D.
Professor and Chairman, Department of Anesthesia, Indiana University School of Medicine, Indianapolis, Indiana

Daniel M. Thys, M.D.
Assistant Professor of Clinical Anesthesiology, Department of Anesthesia, Mount Sinai School of Medicine of the City University of New York, New York, New York

John H. Tinker, M.D.
Professor and Head, Department of Anesthesia, University of Iowa College of Medicine, Iowa City, Iowa

Anthony J. Trevor, Ph.D.
Professor of Pharmacology, University of California, San Francisco, School of Medicine, San Francisco, California

Leroy D. Vandam, M.D.
Professor of Anesthesia, Emeritus, Harvard Medical School; Department of Anesthesiology, Brigham and Women's Hospital, Boston, Massachusetts

W. David Watkins, M.D., Ph.D.
Professor and Chairman, Department of Anesthesiology, Duke University School of Medicine, Durham, North Carolina

Walter L. Way, M.D.
Professor of Anesthesia and Pharmacology, Department of Anesthesia, University of California, San Francisco, School of Medicine, San Francisco, California

Paul F. White, M.D., Ph.D.
Assistant Professor of Anesthesia and Chief, Outpatient Anesthesia Service, Department of Anesthesia, Stanford University School of Medicine, Stanford, California

PREFACE

Since its publication in 1981, the first edition of *Anesthesia* has become a standard text for the specialty of anesthesia nationally and internationally. My original intent was to focus on the major areas of new development in anesthesia that had occurred over the last 20 years. Despite the very gratifying success of the first edition, the contributors and I recognized that the addition of new material and radical revision would be necessary to retain *Anesthesia*'s position as a standard reference textbook. As a result, the second edition is expanded to provide a broad foundation to the science and clinical practice of our specialty. In addition to the complete revision and updating of the original 46 chapters, 22 new chapters have been added to provide a more in-depth and detailed dissertation on the various subspecialties, and on the physiologic, pharmacologic, and clinical situations associated with anesthesia, making this new edition a truly comprehensive reference text.

The first seven chapters, six of which are new additions, provide the historical, legal, and scientific basis of anesthesia. Five of the last seven chapters are also new and provide an overview of critical care medicine. Other new chapters are sprinkled throughout the text to provide a comprehensive view of the physiology, pharmacology, and clinical principles of anesthesia.

As in the first edition, each contributor was asked to provide a scholarly analysis of the specific topic. Each chapter was written in sufficient depth to provide the fundamental scientific and/or clinical basis of anesthesia for the trainee as well as the practicing clinician. Although no absolute limit on the number of references was imposed, each reference was chosen to allow the reader to further investigate an issue in a more in-depth manner. Because each chapter represents a complete dissertation of a given topic, duplication of specific issues (e.g., preoperative evaluation of hypertension, or succinylcholine and intraocular pressure) often occurs. Because a uniform point of view was not imposed, contributors often present varying or opposing opinions on a given topic. These differences of opinion will provide the reader with a more realistic and complete review of controversial topics.

The contributors were chosen because of their acknowledged expertise in the particular areas. Despite their very busy schedules, the contributors provided their unqualified commitment to this project, which has allowed the second edition to be published in a timely, yet scholarly manner. Without their commitment, the second edition would not exist. They have my deepest gratitude.

Churchill Livingstone, especially Toni Tracy, Donna Balopole, Michael Kelley, and Rosalie Marcus, provided constant support, encouragement, and flexibility during the entire project. Although he has since moved to another publisher, Lewis Reines has been an inspirational force since he originally proposed this project in 1978.

All my colleagues at the University of California, San Francisco, were very patient and supportive, for which I am most appreciative. A special thank you to Susan M.S. Ishida is in order. Her organizational and editorial efforts were a significant factor in the successful completion of the second edition. Last, but not least, I am grateful to my family and friends for their patience during the preparation of *Anesthesia*. Their encouragement and understanding were a continuing source of strength.

Ronald D. Miller, M.D.

CONTENTS

SECTION III. Preparation of the Patient/Use of Anesthetic Agents: Preoperative

SECTION IV.   Preparation of the Patient/Use of Anesthetic Agents: Intraoperative

VOLUME 2

SECTION V.   Preparation of the Patient/Use of Anesthetic Agents: Regional Anesthesia

SECTION VI.   Physiological Functions During Anesthesia

VOLUME 3

SECTION VIII.   Specific Anesthetic Problems and/or Techniques

APPENDIX

INDEX

SECTION I

INTRODUCTION

A History and the Scope of Anesthetic Practice

Richard J. Kitz, M.D.
Leroy D. Vandam, M.D.

A BRIEF HISTORY OF ANESTHETIC PRACTICE

INTRODUCTION

Anesthesia is considered an American invention, although anyone who examines history will understand that innovations of such significance can hardly have arisen spontaneously. Eternally, mankind has suffered pain of various kinds, but the individual's well-being was not genuinely considered until the need for surgical treatment of disease arose; attempts at relieving pain were hitherto sporadic. True, operations had been performed over the centuries but always for the superficial malady —a fracture, amputation, cataract extraction, trephination of the skull, or removal of bladder calculus. To these ends, the anesthetic properties of hypnosis and trance, pressure over peripheral nerves and blood vessels, application of cold, alcohol intoxication, or ingestion of herbal concoctions were in vogue. A more influential approach to illness had been the Galenical concept of disease wherein an imbalance among four cardinal body humors was said to exist: blood, phlegm, and yellow and black bile. Well into the present century did the remedies survive: purging, blood-letting, leaching, and counterirritation.

ANTECEDENTS OF MODERN ANESTHESIA

Insofar as the development of anesthesia is concerned, the gastrointestinal tract long remained the only avenue for medicinal therapy. The inhalation of vapors became an alternative approach. With techniques of anesthetic administration more or less divided into schools, the choice now lies among inhalation, intravenous or regional techniques, or combinations thereof. But the seeds of all three methodologies were implanted during the middle ages. Although this chapter mainly considers subsequent developments and the birth of a new medical specialty, anesthesiology, it is worthwhile to look to the antecedents.

INHALATION ANESTHESIA

Around 1540, one Paracelsus, a Swiss physician and alchemist, sweetened the feed of fowl with sweet oil of vitriol, a substance earlier prepared by Valerius Cordus, then named Aether by Frobenius—the familiar diethyl ether that would later be inhaled by most surgical patients over a span of 100 years or more. Paracelsus was led to exclaim, "and besides, it has associated with it such sweetness that it is taken even by chickens and they fall asleep from it for a while but awaken later without harm."

LOCAL ANESTHESIA

In parallel, insofar as cocaine and local anesthesia are concerned, the coca leaf was believed to be a gift to the Incas from Manco Capac, son of the sun god, as a token of esteem and sympathy for their suffering. Initially used narrowly for religious and political purposes, the leaves achieved a more ominous significance with destruction of the Incan civilization in the sixteenth century by Francisco Pizarro's conquistadores. The lower classes and slaves were paid off in coca leaves, an effective method of increasing and prolonging their productivity—low-cost, high-output labor. Customarily, coca leaves bound into a ball (cocada) with guano and cornstarch were chewed with lime or alkaline ash to release the active alkaloid. Anthropologic documentation of that era indicates that the procedure of trephination was successful as the would-be operator permitted cocaine-drenched saliva to drip from the mouth onto the wound, thereby providing creditable local anesthesia.

INTRAVENOUS ANESTHESIA

Also, insofar as intravenous anesthesia is viewed, one can construe that Harvey's studies of the circulation enabled both Percival Christopher Wren and Daniel Johann Major (Fig. 1-1) to conceive the idea of injection of medicinals into the bloodstream. Consequently, in 1665, Wren wrote that he could

> **easily contrive a way to convey any liquid thing immediately into the circulating mass of blood; thus, in pretty big and lean dogs, by making ligatures on the veins and then opening them on the side of the ligature towards the heart; and by putting into them slender syringes or quills, fastened to bladders containing the matter to be injected . . . whereof the success was that opium, being soon circulated into the brain did within a short time stupefy, though not kill the dog: but a large dose of the crocus metallorum, made another dog vomit up life and all.**

The dried crocus or saffron was at the time employed as a stimulant, antispasmodic, and emmenagogue.

THE RISE OF INHALATION ANESTHESIA

Primary observations on the physiology of the circulation and respiration eventually led to the discovery of gases and vapors and their experimental inhalation. In the mid-seventeenth century, a Belgian, J.B. van Helmont, recognized a group of gases different from those of the atmosphere and attempted to classify them, while Harvey during his studies on the circulation noticed a difference in color, from dark to florid, when blood passed through the lungs. Robert Hooke opened the chest of a dog while sustaining lung inflation with a bellows, thereby proving that their rhythmic expansion is not immediately necessary for survival. A related conclusion was that some part of the atmosphere must enter the lungs, an essential ingredient named phlogiston by Stahl. Concurrently, Robert Boyle in exhausting air from a bell jar containing a lighted taper and a living

◄◗§ (2) §◖►
Delineatio Inſtrumenti Infuſorii,
cum Applicatione Ejus in Brachio Humano.

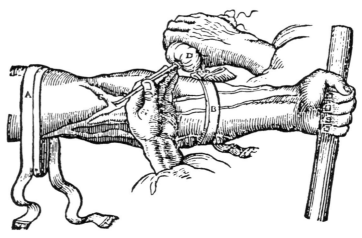

FIG. 1-1 A wood engraving illustrating the intravenous injection of medicinals, employing a quill and bladder and two tourniquets. (Major DJ: Chirurgia Infusoria placidis CL: Virorium Dubiis impugnata, cum modesta, ad Eadem, Responsione. Kiloni, 1667.)

A. *Ligatura prima.* *B. ſecunda.*
C. *Locus applicandi Inſtrumenti.*
D. *Veſica liquorem vena Infundendum conti-
nens, Inſtrumenti orificio majori appenſa &
alligata.*

bird, extinguished the life of both. In 1774, in the process of heating mercuric oxide, Joseph Priestley liberated oxygen, a gas with a "goodness" that sustained life, perhaps identical with the phlogiston of Becher and his pupil Stahl. Incidentally, Priestley also obtained nitrous oxide from nitric oxide. However, Antoine Lavoisier recognized phlogiston as the oxygen we breathe in the atmosphere and arrived at the conclusion that only a smaller share of it was concerned in respiration, the larger share being irrespirable (nitrogen). He also observed that exhaled air precipitated lime water, and concluded that it must also contain chalky air or carbon dioxide. Thus, the bare outlines of external respiration were delineated, so necessary for the concept of inhalation therapy, then anesthesia.

These revelations were mainly of British and continental origin, but a more immediate forerunner in the last decade of the eighteenth century was the establishment in Birmingham, England, of a center for the pneumatic treatment of disease. Joseph Priestley, James Watt, Josiah Wedgewood, and Dr. Richard Pearson and Dr. Thomas Beddoes were among the founders. Ether could be inhaled by a sufferer via funnel to alleviate congestion and phlegm. Beddoes wrote that the medicinal use of these factitious airs was beneficial in the cure of bladder calculus, sea scurvy, and catarrhal fever. Realizing that more intensive experimentation was required, this coterie of people with little knowledge of the causes of disease established a Pneumatic Institute at Clifton, Bristol, and providentially appointed Humphry Davy, the youthful, brilliant chemist and physiologist, as superintendent. First, Davy disproved the theory proposed by the American, Samuel Latham Mitchell, that nitrous oxide was the contagium of disease. While himself breathing nitrous oxide for the relief of headache and the pain of an erupting third molar tooth, Davy experienced a "thrilling and an uneasiness swallowed up in pleasure." Thus originated his seminal pronouncement: "As nitrous oxide in its extensive operation appears capable of destroying pain, it may probably be used with advantage during surgical operations in which no great effusion of blood takes place." Not a surgeon, Davy failed to pursue the idea, but Henry Hill Hickman of Shifnal in Shropshire did so, a practitioner and surgeon who lamented that, "something had not been thought of whereby the fears [of a patient] may be tranquilized and suffering relieved." Having partially asphyxiated to a state of insensibility several animal species with carbon dioxide, Hickman in 1824 addressed his famous message to the Royal Society: "Letter on Suspended Animation—with the view of Ascertaining its Probable Utility in Surgical Operations on Human Subjects." Unfortunately and sadly Hickman came the closest of all to the concept of surgical anesthesia, but utilizing an unlikely agent.

Davy's subjective experiences were duplicated among friends and visitors to the Institute, soon to be taken up by the adventurous public in the form of frolics, not unlike some of the bizarre antics of students of all eras. In the United States, Crawford W. Long, while a student at the University of Pennsylvania in the late 1830s, could very well have observed and participated in such fantasies. Sometime after his return to Jefferson, Georgia, as a general practitioner, Long probably not only introduced such frolics but surely persuaded a young man, James Venable, to inhale ether while a growth was excised from the nape of his neck. Even though this venture was to be repeated several times, the matter was kept secret until the first report appeared in 1848, in the *Southern Medical and Surgical Journal*, several years delayed by influential physicians who were utilizing mesmerism for surgical operations.

Within two years of this first clandestine surgical anesthesia,* on December 10, 1844, Gardner Quincy Colton took his itinerant medicine show to Hartford, Connecticut, where an audience could experience the exhilarating effects of nitrous oxide inhalation. So intoxicated, Samuel A. Cooley did not notice at first

that he had injured a leg in the melee, but in the audience Horace Wells, dentist, was quick to pick up the significance of this suggestion of analgesia. The next day, Wells had one of his own carious teeth painlessly extracted by a fellow dentist, while Colton administered the anesthetic. As the anguish of dental pain could now be assuaged, Wells set about to tell the world of his discovery. Circumstantially, a one-time student of Wells, William Thomas Green Morton, now in practice in Boston and enrolled in a course of lectures at Harvard Medical School, arranged for a demonstration by Wells. Thus, in January 1845, before a group of medical students, the nitrous oxide demonstration proved a failure, as a student screamed out in pain as his tooth came out, even though later admitting to no recollection of pain. No doubt the time of induction was too brief and the gas reservoir too small to provide a surgical plane of anesthesia.

W.T.G. Morton, probably a witness to this abortive demonstration, also yearned to relieve pain, for a dental prosthesis of his invention could only be applied after the rotted roots of teeth were extirpated, an experience few patients would venture to endure. As a domiciliary student with Charles T. Jackson, eccentric geologist and chemist, Morton learned from him that pure ether applied to the gums would through evaporation yield a degree of cold anesthesia. Following experiments with inhalation of the vapor of ether in several animal species, Morton went a step further and on September 30, 1846 in his Boston office, painlessly removed a tooth from the mouth of Eben H. Frost, a merchant of that city. When notice of the operation appeared in a newspaper the next day, Henry Jacob Bigelow, a surgeon at the Massachusetts General Hospital, arranged to observe several additional anesthesias of the kind given by Morton. Suitably impressed and convinced of its surgical utility, Bigelow arranged for a trial of anesthesia at the hospital with John Collins Warren, a renowned surgeon, one-time dean of Harvard Medical School and founder of the hospital in 1821 with several others. Warren was also a progenitor of the *Boston Medical and Surgical Journal*, now the *New England Journal of Medicine*. On October 16, 1846, using a hastily devised glass reservoir incorporating the drawover principle of vapor-

---

* Sometime before 1842, William E. Clark of Rochester, N.Y. gave ether to a Miss Hobbie, as a carious tooth was removed by dentist Elijah Pope.

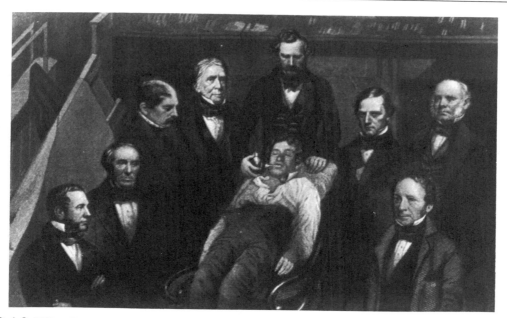

FIG. 1-2 William Thomas Green Morton giving the first public demonstration of etherization at the Massachusetts General Hospital, Boston, October 16, 1846. Physicians around Edward Gilbert Abbott, patient, are from left to right: H.J. Bigelow, A.A. Gould, J. Mason Warren, J. Collins Warren, Morton, Samuel Parkman, George Hayward, and S.D. Townsend. (From a steel engraving in Rice N.P.: Trials of a Public Benefactor, 1859.)

ization, Morton anesthetized Edward Gilbert Abbott, a young printer, while Warren deftly ligated a congenital venous malformation from the left cervical triangle. This feat culminated in J.C. Warren's memorable remark to the assembled gallery, "Gentlemen, this is no humbug" (Fig. 1-2).

The Massachusetts General Hospital has, to this day, designated the incident as the first public demonstration, rather than discovery, while Oliver Wendell Holmes, professor of anatomy and literateur extraordinary, chose the Greek-derived noun, anaesthesia, to characterize the process. He had also considered "neurolepsis," a term employed today to describe the drugs used in one variety of balanced anesthesia. With a medical discovery of universal significance, it was only natural that a prolonged period of controversy would ensue as to who might be given the credit. Fortunately such an outcome did not impede further application of the method, enhanced by the prestige of the hospital and its Harvard-affiliated physicians, who knowledgeably reported on the pharmacology and physiology of the phenomenon.

According to historical accounts, a long list of names might be compiled of those who contributed to the introduction of surgical anesthesia. In a situation of multiple discoveries as recounted here, sociologists of science would assert that the concept was "in the air," merely awaiting the appropriately receptive mind and social circumstance. Perhaps the Americans succeeded because of their pioneering spirit and lack of authoritative medical institutions. In England, on the brink of the industrial revolution, a medical hierarchy had already existed, made up of hospitals and societies, with public health a new concern and the general practitioner the dominant figure—here a revolutionary therapy might not be adopted so readily.

W. Stanley Sykes in an essay on "The

Seven Foundation Stones, in Order of Merit" ranked the contenders for recognition in descending order of importance. First was Hickman who "above all others had the idea of anaesthesia most deeply and spontaneously engrained in him." Second was Horace Wells, who "given the stimulus and the sight of a man partly under the influence of gas failing to notice an injury . . . saw the possibility of it at once, as no one else had done." Third would be W.T.G. Morton "to whom belongs the undoubted credit of introducing successful anaesthesia with sufficient publicity to ensure that it immediately achieved world-wide acceptance." Fourth, "Humphry Davy discovered the analgesic properties of nitrous oxide by inhaling it and made his famous suggestion that it could be used for surgical operations." In fifth place is Crawford W. Long, "another pioneer who could easily have held a much higher place and had only himself to blame." "Long's place in the ranking order is low simply because of his extraordinary reticence." "There was no originality about James Young Simpson," and Charles T. Jackson, the last of the pioneers, "really does not deserve to be in the list at all. He did not have the idea of anaesthesia in the first place. All he did was to try and cash in upon it when it proved to be successful."

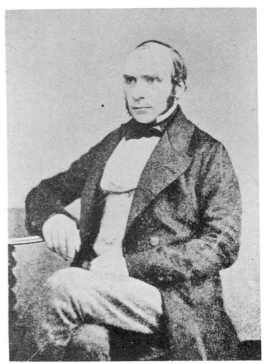

FIG. 1-3 John Snow (1813–1858). Physician, epidemiologist, and first specialist in anesthesia. (Reproduced from the Asclepiad, 1887, vol. 4.)

PROFESSIONAL ANESTHESIA IN ENGLAND: APPLICATION TO OBSTETRICS

After some delay in transmission to England of the news of the demonstration, John Snow, general practitioner, clinical investigator, and epidemiologist (who halted a cholera epidemic in London) became the first of a long line of physician anesthetists, in contrast to America, where that species was to blossom only around the turn of the century (Fig. 1-3). In 1847, within several months, Snow's text on *The Inhalation of the Vapour of Ether* appeared, containing case reports and an elaborate description of the traditional signs and stages of ether anesthesia. An earlier tract on ether written by Robinson, a dentist, had appeared, as

well as an account by Plomley of the stages of anesthesia, but Snow's pronouncements were definitive. Likewise in Great Britain toward the end of 1847, James Young Simpson, obstetrician, who had first utilized ether to relieve the pain of labor, adopted chloroform for the purpose, as suggested to him by David Waldie. The compound had been independently synthesized by Samuel Guthrie of Sackett's Harbor, N.Y., Eugène Soubeiran of France, and Justus von Liebig of Germany. Although the clergy as well as other physicians opposed the concept of relieving pain during childbirth, the method took hold and achieved lasting status after Queen Victoria gave birth to Prince Leopold while given chloroform at the hands of John Snow; dubbed anesthesie à la reine. To further strengthen the principle of obstetric anesthesia, Walter Channing, Professor of Obstetrics and Medical Jurisprudence at Harvard, in 1847, wrote a *Treatise on Etherization in Childbirth* the results of a survey to settle the important issue of safety. Although there is question about the validity of the study, Channing cited the use of morphine during labor and also included cases in which chloroform had been employed. Because of its less objectionable properties, more pleasant odor, as well as rapid induction and emergence, chloroform superseded ether in Great Britain. And, in 1858, a second text by Snow was published, *On Chloroform and Other Anaesthetics,* completed posthumously, with a biography added by Benjamin Ward Richardson, Snow's successor.

DEVELOPMENTS IN SURGERY

Surprisingly, the initial usage of both ether and chloroform led to little alteration in surgical practice, which remained largely of an external nature: trephining the skull, tapping the chest for fluid removal, relief of strangulated hernia, bladder calculus extraction, fracture reduction, and amputation of extremities. Surgical writings and lectures then given by the leaders pertained mostly to anatomy. Moreover, with an increase in the numbers of hospitals both in America and abroad and their consequent utilization rather than the home to treat illness, a new problem arose, that of infection, which came to be known as hospitalism. The initial solution, Listerism, or surgical antisepsis utilizing carbolic acid, was not widely practiced until 1879, when it was acclaimed at an international conference. Then arose steam sterilization and true antisepsis.

Siegrist observed that the introduction of anesthesia was not the first attempt to render patients insensible to pain. Why then did surgery not have its great development before the middle nineteenth century, coincident with rather than resulting from anesthesia? The answer lies in studies of the development of concepts of disease, "for surgery is only one method of treatment and like any other method is largely determined by the concept of disease prevailing at the time." As noted in the introduction to this chapter,

For over 2000 years disease was considered to be the result of a disturbed balance of the cardinal humors of the body which enjoyed

health when in balance but showed symptoms of disease when upset.

Then in the 18th and 19th centuries with Morgagni describing the results of large numbers of autopsies, it was learned that organic lesions were responsible for disease. It seemed, then, that if an organ were abnormal its function would also be abnormal. Consequently it became the purpose of diagnostics to perceive anatomic changes in the living patient, by the use of percussion and auscultation and the use of bulbs and mirrors to look into the body cavities. Roentgenology was the ultimate triumph in this direction. The surgeon by draining an abscess or excising an ulcer or tumor was removing the disease and correcting the organ. But without doubt surgery could not develop freely before the two bonds had been removed that enslaved it — pain and infection.

LOCAL ANESTHESIA

Cocaine began to receive attention in Europe and America in mid-19th century. Around 1860, Albert Niemann, a pupil of Friedrich Wöhler, isolated the alkaloid in crystalline form. Twenty years later, von Anrep wrote an extensive review on the physiologic and pharmacologic properties of cocaine, clearly citing the locally numbing effect on the tongue and dilation of the pupil, the former leading him to suggest that some day it might become of medical importance. Later, Sigmund Freud of Vienna began to study the properties of the drug when given samples for trial by the Merck Company. As a result of reviewing The Index Catalogue of the Library of the Surgeon General's Office of the United States Army which referenced some 25 papers and 10 monographs under the heading, Erythroxylin Coca, Freud, in 1884, wrote his classic paper, "Über Coca." Believing coca to be a worthy substitute for morphine, Freud first attempted to eliminate the morphine addiction of a close friend, Ernst von Fleischl-Marxow, who had long suffered from a painful posttraumatic thenar neuroma. von Marxow developed a new addiction as a consequence, as would many a cocaine user later on, but Freud himself never seemed to go down that path.

FREUD AND KOLLER

Freud and Karl Koller, an intern in the Department of Ophthalmology at the Allgemeinen Krankenhaus in Vienna, using a dynamometer to study the effect of coca on muscle strength, both noticed the numbing effect on the tongue as they swallowed the experimental drug. On the other hand, Koller had a burning desire to anesthetize the cornea and conjunctiva for opthalmologic operations and had already tried morphine and chloral bromide. In Freud's absence, he and Joseph Gaertner dissolved a trace of the white powder in distilled water and instilled the solution into the conjunctival sac of a frog. After a minute or so, "the frog allowed his cornea to be touched and he also bore injury to the cornea without a trace of reflex action or defense." Koller wrote, "one more step had yet to be taken. We trickled the solution under each other's lifted eyelids. Then we placed a mirror before us, took pins, and with the head tried to touch the cornea. Almost simultaneously we were able to state jubilantly: 'I can't feel anything.'" A communication describing this finding, dated early September 1884, was read and a practical demonstration given by Joseph Brettauer at the Ophthalmological Congress at Heidelberg on September 15 of that year. Koller did not have the means to travel there. Koller gave full credit to Freud for the inspiration. Despite the latter's disappointment at not coming in first with the discovery, Freud is considered by many to be the founder of psychopharmacology because of his initial use of cocaine, the forerunner of mescaline, LSD, and the amphetamines to modify behavior and subsequently to relieve mental illness.

JAMES LEONARD CORNING

After Koller, James Leonard Corning deserves citation for his analytic approach to local anesthesia in humans based on laboratory experimentation. Having learned of Koller's report, Corning recalled the experiment in which when strychnine is injected subcutaneously in the frog, the animal is thrown into violent spasms as a result of an effect on the spinal cord. Since, following laminectomy, a much smaller quantity of strychnine injected beneath the membranes is equally effective, he assumed that the poison must act via vascular absorption. Cognizant of the presence of the many small veins, venae spinosum, about the spinal column and cord, Corning reasoned that it might be possible to utilize cocaine therapeutically. Accordingly, in a young dog about 20 minims of a 2 percent solution of cocaine was injected between the spinous processes of the dorsal vertebrae. After some minutes, incoordination of the posterior extremities developed, followed by insensibility. These results were almost immediately applied to a patient, a man suffering from spinal weakness and seminal incontinence. "To this end, I injected 30 minims of a 3 percent solution of the hydrochloride of cocaine into the space situated between the spinous processes of the 11th and 12th dorsal vertebrae." After a lapse of 6 to 8 minutes, when nothing happened, the injection was repeated. Finally, 10 minutes later, anesthesia began to appear in the lower extremities, and a sound could be passed through the urethra without pain. Corning concluded his report with the statement, "Whether the method will ever find application as a substitute for etherization in genito-urinary or other branches of surgery, further experience alone can show." This conclusion follows the pattern of statements made by Wren, Davy, and von Anrep in relation to intravenous, inhalation, and local anesthesia, respectively, thereby further confirming the evolutionary aspects of science. Corning's textbook on local anesthesia, published in 1886, was the first devoted to the subject.

REGIONAL ANESTHESIA TECHNIQUES AND AGENTS: PROCAINE AND EPINEPHRINE

In juxtaposition to inhalation anesthesia, and because of toxicologic problems with chloroform, a high anesthetic mortality, and lack of trained personnel to give general anesthesia, local anesthesia became highly popular wih surgeons, especially in France and Germany, and to some extent in the United States. After a trial on himself that resulted in the first-known development of a lumbar puncture headache, August Bier of Germany began to give spinal anesthesia in 1898, followed by Matas in America and Tuffier in France. Then, because of the evident toxicity and tendency toward addiction of cocaine, a number of ester substitutes were synthesized, procaine (Novocain) by Einhorn becoming the more lasting of the group. As a result of pharmacologist John J. Abel's efforts at Johns Hopkins Medical School, epinephrine was isolated from the capsule of the suprarenal gland in 1897, ultimately crystallized by Takamine. Heinrich Braun, a German surgeon, advocated the use of cocaine in conjunction with epinephrine, when, in 1903, he reported on its practical importance in inducing anemia of the mucosa in rhinolaryngologic and urologic surgery, thereby permitting the concentration of cocaine to be lowered and diminishing the dangers of intoxication.

Most currently used techniques of regional anesthesia were devised during that first decade: brachial plexus block, axillary and supraclavicular approaches; intravenous regional anesthesia (Bier); celiac plexus block; caudal anesthesia; hyperbaric and hypobaric techniques of spinal anesthesia; and all the presently employed nerve blocks about the head and neck as applied in dentistry and plastic surgery. Thereafter, aside from technical innovation and understanding of some of the physiologic and toxicologic responses to local anesthetics, the great impetus to regional anesthesia was to come in the synthesis of the amide local anesthetics and in an understanding of their pharmacodynamic and especially pharmacokinetic properties.

INTRAVENOUS ANESTHESIA

We have cited the primitive experiments of Wren and Major in introducing medicinals into the circulation, quick upon Harvey's description of the circulation. Around the 1850s, the hypodermic hollow needle and glass and metal syringes were introduced via the inventions of Francis Rynd (Scotsman, 1845), his countryman, Alexander Wood (1855), and

Charles Gabriel Pravaz (1853). Although these improvements over the quill and bladder were to herald both intravenous and regional anesthesia, Rynd and Wood were making injections into the vicinity of nerves for the relief of neuralgia, while Pravez injected ferric chloride via trocar into arterial aneurysms in an attempt to induce thrombosis.

PIERRE CYPRIEN ORÉ

W. Stanley Sykes, in a posthumously published essay, cited Pierre Cyprien Oré as the true pioneer of intravenous anesthesia. Employing chloral hydrate for the purpose, his first report on the method was addressed, in 1872, to the Surgical Society of Paris. Utilizing a modification of the Pravaz syringe and needle, as he had found the latter likely to transfix the vein and cause the solution to be injected perivenously, Oré claimed that chloral hydrate was the most powerful of all anesthetics. As usual, opposition arose as critics raised the possibility of development of phlebitis and clotting. In a monograph published with a detailed account of 36 cases, some 18 for cataract surgery, others in treating tetanus, Oré claimed not to have encountered a single instance of clotting or phlebitis. Cardiac arrest occurred in one patient, an otherwise healthy, middle-aged man undergoing cataract extraction. The heart was unresponsive to electrical rheophore stimulation to the epigastrium and over the course of the vagus and phrenic nerves.

ANOCI-ASSOCIATION

Early in the 1900s, an essential concept was proposed toward the development of balanced anesthesia in which intravenous anesthesia is a major component. This was the anoci-association theory of George W. Crile, who in 1901 stated, "In conscious individuals, all noxious stimuli reach the brain. During general anesthesia only the traumatic stimuli are perceived centrally while with complete anoci-association all stimuli are blocked." Enlarged upon by Harvey Cushing in 1902, the idea of anoci-association became the basis for the use of opioids intravenously, so prominent in practice today. Incidentally, George Crile at the Cleveland Clinic and the Mayo Brothers of Rochester were the first to employ nurse anesthetists in their surgical practices. Cushing had a number of "firsts" relative to the development of anesthesia: coinage of the term "regional anesthesia"; keeping of anesthesia records; the first in the United States to employ the Riva-Rocci technique for measurement of blood pressure intraoperatively; first user of a precordial stethoscope during operation; and a surgeon who first appointed a physician in charge of anesthesia at his clinic in Boston, Walter M. Boothby.

THE BARBITURATES

To be sure, the major impetus for the subsequent development of intravenous anesthesia lay in the synthesis of the short-acting, water-soluble barbiturates. In 1903, long after von Baeyer had synthesized barbituric acid or malonylurea (1864), Fischer and von Mering prepared the first sedative barbiturate, diethyl barbiturate, or barbital, a long-lasting hypnotic soon to be succeeded by the sodium salt of phenobarbital. Then, as other soluble compounds were devised, a number of barbiturates of short, medium, and long duration became available. Pernoston, a shorter-acting agent, was first given intravenously in 1927, in 10 percent aqueous solution, while in 1928 John S. Lundy began to supplement inhalation anesthesia with amytal, then pentobarbital intravenously, a procedure he designated balanced anesthesia. As by current standards both drugs provide only a relatively slow onset of action, the advent of hexobarbital, or Evipal, in 1932 (Weese) resulted in the first rapidly acting intravenous anesthetic to receive wide usage. Ultimately, a sulfur derivative of barbituric acid yielded the necessary qualities with the result that thiopental, a derivative of pentobarbital, was adopted both by Lundy at the Mayo Clinic and by Waters at Wisconsin. Dundee noted how remarkable it is that this drug has survived and withstood the challenge of so many others. As in every intravenously given compound, no matter the therapeutic ends, the lasting nature of such drugs is dependent on specific pharmacodynamic and pharmacokinetic properties, as first shown by Brodie and colleagues around 1950.

Concurrently, then, as cardiac surgical procedures made their appearance and deliberate induction of total body hypothermia was used to protect the brain during cardiotomy, Laborit and Huguenard of France devised a pharmacologic method for inducing "artificial hibernation," an intravenous combination of drugs consisting of chlorpromazine (Thorazine) (L'Argactil), one of the shorter-acting barbiturates, and the opioid, meperidine. This "lytic cocktail" as it was called, yielded a moderate degree of hypothermia, complete CNS dissociation, and purportedly antagonism against development of circulatory shock, as experienced during the French–Indochina war. The components of the lytic cocktail were gradually replaced: haloperidol for chlorpromazine, a butyrophenone, then droperidol; phenoperidine instead of meperidine, in turn supplanted by fentanyl (Sublimaze). Anesthesiologists today know of the rapid introduction to practice of extremely potent opioids with unique pharmacokinetics to fit every occasion. So rapid have the developments been, that it is possible these days to use only intravenous agents for operation, particularly on the heart, even foregoing the use of nitrous oxide for analgesia but retaining neuromuscular blocking agents.

THE EVOLUTION OF PROFESSIONALISM IN AMERICA

We have seen how the British were indeed fortunate in having physicians, beginning with John Snow, who specialized in anesthesia, a circumstance that eventually led in the 1890s to the formation of societies and publication of articles in such journals as the *Lancet, British Medical Journal*, then the *Proceedings of the Royal Society of Medicine*, in which the subject of anesthesia had its own section. By definition, professionalism is a calling in which one professes to have acquired some special knowledge used by way of instructing, guiding, or advising others, or in serving them in some art.

THE MILIEU

In America at the time of the first public demonstration, medicine was in a period of frontier expansion, in contrast to Great Britain. The general practitioner did all the work and although the Easterners began to loom as specialists and leaders, a good deal of emphasis was placed on practice as a business, with medical education at a low level. The only medium for scientific publication in the first part of the nineteenth century was the Transactions of the Royal Society. Soon the veil began to lift, so that at the turn of the century we begin to see the emergence of a class of physicians clearly identified with anesthesia. Interestingly, the primordial group was made up mostly of Middle Westerners and Canadians, who may have had as peculiar characteristics, "their pioneering traditions, their common purpose, devotion to equality and their struggle for success." Of the pioneers, Ralph Waters was to remark in a reflective mood that, "the development of a specialty could be traced in terms of men, publications and organizations." Three figures stand out in this regard, Waters among them.

FRANCIS HOEFFER McMECHAN

F.H. McMechan, born in Cincinnati, son of a physician, excelled in college in oratory and dramatics and became a newspaper reporter upon graduation, before matriculation at the Cincinnati Medical School. There, as would be the custom for many a decade, he was required to administer anesthetics, for his father as well, so that he became a devotee of the method. Over the years 1903–1910 he combined anesthesia with general practice, but progressively crippling arthritis forced abandonment of practice and his subsequent preoccupation with organization of anesthesia and medical editing.

In 1912, in conjunction with Bainbridge, a surgeon, Yandell Henderson, a physiologist, and James T. Gwathmey, an anesthetist, Mc-

Mechan founded the American Association of Anesthetists. As a result of his persuasion, the *American Journal of Surgery* began in 1914 to publish a *Quarterly Supplement on Anesthesia* (Fig. 1-4), which survived until 1926, with McMechan as editor; he also served as editor of a *Year Book on Anesthesia and Analgesia*. His formation of one group after another in the United States and Canada led ultimately to the National Anesthesia Research Society, then an International Society whose medium of reporting in 1922 became *Current Researches in Anesthesia and Analgesia*, the first publication devoted solely to those subjects. Assisted in these endeavors by his wife, McMechan, who died in 1939, would have been gratified to know that the International Society and its publication, *Anesthesia and Analgesia*, now a monthly, survive today.

ELMER I. McKESSON

The second of the trio was an innovator, teacher, and inventor, E.I. McKesson, born in 1881 in Walkerton, Indiana. A teacher at first, McKesson was graduated from Rush Medical School and while an intern in Toledo became attracted to anesthesia. Later, he would found the University of Toledo, where he served as associate professor of physiology and physiological chemistry. McKesson invented and developed many a piece of apparatus: gas-oxygen machines, suction apparatus, metabolism measuring devices, intermittent and demand gas flow valves, oxygen tents, and other instruments, all manufactured by the Toledo Technical Appliance Company. The Nargraf apparatus and the McKesson gas machine remained standard equipment until well into the 1950s.

RALPH M. WATERS

Third, we return to R.M. Waters, who left his mark on several generations of anesthetists by way of far-reaching vision, combining in no small measure all the stellar attributes of the other early American anesthetists. Born in 1883 in Bloomfield, Ohio, he was graduated

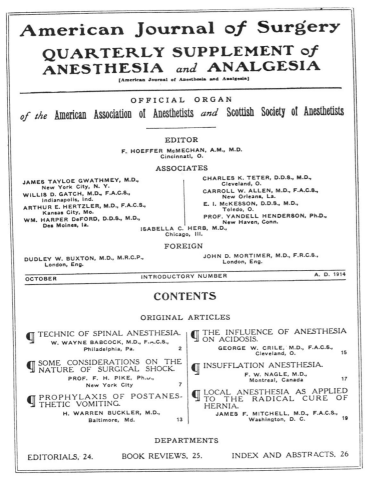

FIG. 1-4 Quarterly Supplement of Anesthesia and Analgesia, Introductory Number, October 1914, edited by F. Hoeffer McMechan, as it appeared in the American Journal of Surgery.

from Western Reserve University Medical School, served as an intern in Cleveland, then practiced privately in Sioux City, Iowa, with obstetrics as a chief interest. After awhile he began to give anesthesia for operations performed by the other practitioners, although some of them employed nurses for that purpose. Self-trained and with only a few specialized writings at his disposal—*Proceedings of the Royal Society,* McMechan's *Quarterly,* and Gwathmey's and Baskerville's *American Text Book of Anesthesia*—Waters in 1919 wrote an article, "Why The Professional Anesthetist." Such was his growing reputation that by 1927 he was invited to a post on the faculty of the University of Wisconsin as assistant professor of surgery in charge of anesthesia, one of a group of luminaries in surgery, physiology, and pharmacology. For the first time ever he established a resident training program in anesthesia coupled with an investigative effort that entailed among other things the examination of hydrocarbon–epinephrine cardiac dysrhythmias, the pharmacology of cyclopropane, and a reexamination of the toxicology of chloroform. Many a piece of apparatus arose from this clinical-investigative milieu, some rediscovered, others new: cuffed endotracheal tubes, laryngoscopic blades and pharyngeal airways, carbon dioxide absorption canisters, and precision-controlled, liquid anesthetic vaporizers.

True, there were other outstanding innovators in American anesthesia, among them Arthur A. Guedel, John Silas Lundy, and a later generation of chairman-university professors, including E.A. Rovenstine (New York University), R.M. Tovell (Hartford Hospital), H.K. Beecher (Harvard), S.C. Cullen (Iowa and San Francisco), John Adriani (Tulane), R.D. Dripps (Pennsylvania), E.M. Papper (Columbia-Presbyterian Hospital), P.P. Volpitto (Georgia), and L.D. Vandam (Harvard).

manpower; affiliation with the World Federation of Societies of Anesthesiologists; and consideration of problems common to all kinds of medical practice. All these matters continue to progress with an eye toward discerning trends and future developments.

THE AMERICAN SOCIETY OF ANESTHESIOLOGISTS

In 1905, a group of physicians, with Adolf F. Erdman as the catalyst, formed the Long Island Society of Anesthetists, "to promote the art and science of anesthesia." As the membership grew in numbers the name of the organization was, in 1911, changed to the New York Society of Anesthetists, then augmented by out-of-state anesthetists so that by 1916, 60 members were enrolled. On the 25th anniversary (1930) of the founding of the Society, a two-day scientific program was convened in New York City. In 1936 the name was once again changed to describe its breadth and character, The American Society of Anesthetists, Incorporated, with 484 adherents.

Over succeeding years all the attributes of a specialty society were fulfilled, and the designation anesthesiologist replaced the nondescript term, to indicate that anesthesiologists are physicians who have received formal training in anesthesia. A certification committee was appointed that led in 1940 to the acceptance of a section on anesthesiology into the hierarchy of the American Medical Association. The preceding year marked the initial publication of its official journal, *Anesthesiology*. The stature of the Society was enhanced by incorporation of the Wood Library–Museum of Anesthesiology in 1950; to accommodate its multiple activities, a society headquarters was erected in Park Ridge, Illinois, in 1962, with an addition two years later to house the Library–Museum. The ASA has dedicated itself to the following goals and endeavors: standards for equipment and patient care; education; repeated self-analysis via survey to crystallize the state and objectives of the Society; issues of

THE SCOPE OF ANESTHETIC PRACTICE

A DEFINITION OF MODERN ANESTHESIA

What is anesthesiology—its content—and what are its boundaries? Wherein are its current opportunities, and what lies in the future? Some answers to these questions comprise the purposes of this section. Although the practice of anesthesiology is constantly changing and inevitably expanding its unique role and special mission, a working definition is essential. We shall first depict the domain of knowledge and practice which are unique to the specialty. The American Board of Anesthesiology (ABA) defines anesthesiology as a practice of medicine dealing with, but not limited to:

a. the provision of insensibility to pain during surgical, obstetrical, therapeutic and diagnostic procedures, and the management of patients so affected,
b. the monitoring and restoration of homeostasis during the perioperative period, as well as homeostasis in the critically ill, injured, or otherwise seriously ill patient,
c. the diagnosis and treatment of painful syndromes,
d. the clinical management and teaching of cardiac and pulmonary resuscitation,
e. the evaluation of respiratory function and application of respiratory therapy in all of its forms,
f. the supervision, teaching, and evaluation of performance of both medical and paramedical personnel involved in anesthesia, respiratory and critical care,

g. the conduct of research at the clinical and basic science levels to explain and improve the care of patients insofar as physiologic function and response to drugs are concerned,

h. the administrative involvement in hospitals, medical schools, and outpatient facilities necessary to implement these responsibilities.

As the Board notes, "these criteria evolved largely from a chimera of the certified specialists created by successive generations of Board Directors." In an important and thought-provoking special article published by the Board entitled "Quality Anesthesia Care: A Model of Future Practice of Anesthesiology," the direction and content of anesthesia practice was predicted for the second millenium. This was done for the Board's own guidance in planning both educational requirements and the evaluating and certifying processes, recognizing that its decisions may profoundly influence both the conduct of training programs and ultimately the nature of their product—the practitioner. This planning document clearly describes the likelihood of an increasing use of a team approach toward the delivery of anesthesia care. The description then proceeds to detail training requirements essential for the anesthesiologist's performing as a consultant on the medical commons. Furthermore, the Board recognized that the model described will be "continuously modified in the light of general medical developments." Indeed, the ABA has recently mandated a full 4-year clinical program for all trainees beginning after May 1986.

From this description of the anesthesiologist as a consultant, we shall describe, in some cases to justify, and in others predict, those aspects of anesthetic practice and associated science disciplines in which consultant anesthesiologists can or should make contribution because of their special qualifications. The universe of anesthesiology is thus bounded at the interface where an anesthesiologist's unique qualifications are superseded by those of other medical practitioners. If ours is a narrow technical practice restricted to operating rooms, then the scope of the specialty we practice is limited. If, on the other hand, we have prepared well and acquired the habits of continuing scholarship, then we have evolved in our specialty to head a health care team able to provide all anesthetic and anesthesia-related services to the ill people of our institutions. We function as consultants among our peers, providing expert advice on diagnostic and therapeutic measures in those areas in which we are uniquely qualified. Because we are committed to this broad definition of the implications of anesthetic practice, this treatise describes only our impressions of an anesthesiologist in the expanded role of consultant.

OPERATING ROOM

That the scope of anesthesia involves ministering to the anesthetic needs of surgical patients in operating rooms is indubitable. And yet the concept as to how an anesthesiologist functions in that arena has been somewhat obfuscated by an historical tenet and a more recent attempt to define an anesthesiologist's role. That all surgeons function as "captain of the ship" in the operating room is a tradition that assigned to them authority and responsibility for all aspects of the surgical experience, including those where they might have little knowledge and surely lesser training. Anesthesia was a prime example. Recognizing that the care of a patient in an operating room is best rendered by a highly skilled team rather than a non-omniscient surgeon, the courts have relieved the surgeon of responsibility for the conduct of anesthesia when conducted or supervised by an anesthesiologist.

That an anesthesiologist is the "internist of the operating room" was perhaps an unfortunate definition, as it seemed to compare us with a group having a different gestalt and who seldom frequent the operating theater. In addition, this suggested to surgeons that we are incapable of handling some of the more fundamental medical aspects of surgical care. Perhaps as a reaction to this philosophy, many anesthesiologists now see themselves as primarily responsible for the "noncutting" aspects of a patient's surgical experience. This aligns us more appropriately with our surgical colleagues.

Fortunately, what has emerged from the brie of debate that accompanied the definition is the concept that an anesthesiologist is just that — an anesthesiologist possessing neither medical nor surgical genes. Truly, we are unique in keeping the patient alive by manipulating vital functions to provide the conditions essential for our colleagues to treat surgical disease. And it is the continual practice of vital organ management that equips us so well to manage critically ill surgical patients in an associated arena, the intensive care unit.

In addition to direct provision of anesthesia services to surgical patients, most anesthesiologists assume responsibility for the efficient management of the operating room complex. Increasingly, anesthesiologists are responsible for preparation of the surgical schedule. Because they must orchestrate services for all surgical subspecialties and because they spend more time in the operating room theater than any other physician, it is rational that anesthesiologists assume the responsibility of allocating operating room resources. This requires that anesthesiologists in charge possess diplomatic skills and see clearly the universality of their duties, which transcend specialty allegiances, while enjoying the support and respect of colleagues from all services. These management characteristics equip the anesthesiologist to conceptualize, plan, build, and supervise hospital units and free-standing surgical clinics as well. As we shall see, the scope of anesthesia practice is approaching the boundaries of our skills, but the operating theater will always remain the corpus of our practice and the principal source of our talents, now so useful in other arenas.

RECOVERY ROOM

Although it can be argued that little good ultimately results from a world at war, it is now quite clear that the shock and resuscitation units organized during World War II, as well as the Korean and Vietnam conflicts, resulted in the most efficient care of the sick and wounded. Many studies revealed a reduction in morbidity and mortality in the care of those patients. Recovery rooms had their genesis in these experiences. Surgeons and anesthesiologists returning from World War II insisted that civilians enjoy similar standards of care. By the 1960s all hospitals in the United States had specialized areas usually adjacent to operating theaters, for the immediate postoperative recovery phase of the patient's surgical treatment. Initially, there was no medical director of the recovery room, which was administered by the nursing service. The nurse would call the surgeon or anesthesiologist as appropriate. It was more natural and efficient for the nurses to ask the help of anesthesiologists in urgent situations requiring therapy because they were readily available, while the surgeon might not be. But the superior skills of anesthesiologists in expeditiously diagnosing and treating such potentially lethal conditions as respiratory insufficiency, hypotension, dysrhythmias, and coma played a pivotal role. Because some of these complications may evolve from the anesthetic, it was also natural for the anesthesiologist to take a keen interest in this kind of postoperative care. Later, when the Joint Commission on Accreditation of Hospitals required appointment of a medical director, virtually all hospitals turned to anesthesiology. Although a team effort involving surgeons, anesthesiologists, and nurses in the care of patients will always be the preferred model, the anesthesiologist is specially qualified to be the medical administrator responsible for establishing criteria for admission and discharge, general care of patients, and prime responsibility for emergency care, equipment, triage, teaching, and those studies required to ensure the highest quality of care. No one argues that the recovery room is not the proper domain for the anesthesiologist.

CARE OF THE CRITICALLY ILL PATIENT

THE RESPIRATORY CARE UNIT

During the mid-1950s, the poliomyelitis epidemic that had started in Europe had reached America. In many European countries, Denmark in particular, physicians and those in training were mobilized over several years to help support patients' vital functions. Simultaneously with the outbreak of bulbar poliomyelitis in New England, the major hospitals adopted the Danish model to deploy their resources and organize treatment protocols for patients with respiratory insufficiency. It is not surprising that the first respiratory intensive care unit in the United States was established under the aegis of an anesthesia department. Soon respiratory physiotherapists were recruited from abroad and supporting laboratories were established. This type of multifold unit became a mecca for training others, leading to the role of anesthesia in the care of critically ill patients.

Perhaps there has been no more worthy development over the past 20 years than the involvement of the anesthesiologist in the care of those who are dangerously ill. The most seriously ill patients in hospitals are the anesthetized sick. All are intoxicated with drugs and often unconscious, apneic, and with manipulated cardiovascular and respiratory systems —all well monitored and modulated from minute to minute. If the degree of a critical illness is measured by vital function impairment, then anesthetized patients are indeed critically ill. It seems logical that only anesthesiologists, perhaps by virtue of their training and daily practice, are uniquely qualified to care for critically ill surgical patients. Likewise it would seem that those patients with major physiologic impairment not in the realm of surgery are probably better cared for by cardiologists, pulmonary physicians, and others.

Although the anesthesiologist's principal role in a surgical intensive care unit entails the support of vital functions, a team approach is clearly required and surely must include surgeons, nurses, medical consultants, administrators, and the clergy. In their role as consultants in the therapy of multiorgan failure, anesthesiologists properly find themselves concerned at the center of therapeutic measures. In general they are given and accept the role of consultant in an ICU role by invitation from a patient's surgeon or primary physician. At the moment that the patient meets discharge criteria, the anesthesiologist's responsibilities cease, as they do not have the time, expertise, or authority to carry on during the patient's convalescence.

Increasingly, anesthesiologists are being asked to participate as members of a team organized to transport the very ill from the community or far-off locations to a tertiary referral center for the reasons cited above. Except under unusual circumstances, it is the emergency medical technician who will assume that responsibility while relinquishing that role to the anesthesiologist to orchestrate the care after the patient has arrived at the hospital.

RESUSCITATION

In many a hospital over the past 20 years, anesthesiologists have often become solely responsible for organizing resuscitation teams in order to respond to emergencies. The medical community recognizes the appropriateness of anesthesiologists' involvement in this activity. The anesthesiologist is often a member of a team organized by the American Heart Association, which sponsors programs to teach cardiopulmonary resuscitation to other physicians, other hospital personnel, and the community as well. This is one of the few instances in which an anesthesiologist accepts a highly visible community responsibility. Few are more qualified.

EMERGENCY ROOM

The portal of entry for the seriously ill who are transported to a tertiary referral hospital is the emergency room. An argument might be made for the anesthesiologist likewise to be in charge of this facility. This, too, might be appropriate if all the patients were indeed seriously ill but, as they are not, an anesthesiologist is perhaps not the best choice. Nevertheless, the consultant role in the management of vital organ failure is clear. Often the management of the very ill and traumatized patient can best be effected by a team of experts, usually under the direction of surgeons or an emergency medicine physician. Once vital organ function is stabilized via proper monitoring and life-support systems, the patient is usually triaged to an operating room or intensive care unit, where "anesthetic" care may continue until the patient once again becomes self-sufficient or succumbs. In this arena, too, the essential role of the anesthesiologist lies in the care of the very ill surgical patient.

TRAUMA CENTERS

Under both national and state legislation, specific hospital complexes are being designated as trauma centers because they offer all the necessary ingredients in terms of manpower, equipment, and program resources essential to the efficient management of the traumatized patient. To reiterate, the role of the consultant anesthesiologist as a member of the trauma team emerges with the principal responsibility for vital organ stabilization in those patients in whom subsequent surgical intervention is required. Although not yet widely replicated, free-standing trauma centers have been established in some communities by commercial interests. Some are managed by anesthesiologists, and all have anesthesia personnel as key members of the trauma team. The relationship of these centers to the local hospital has not yet been clearly defined but will evolve as their appropriate position in the panoply of health care facilities is secured. Wherever that position is finally established, anesthesiologists will always be involved in those aspects of patient management appropriate to the scope of anesthesia practice.

PAIN AND ITS TREATMENT

Ever since the era of Long, Wells, and Morton, anesthesiologists have of necessity been involved in the control of pain. No one argues that this is not an appropriate mission for our specialty; nevertheless, too few anesthesiolo-gists have developed pain-control programs within their institutions or among the 156 residency programs in the United States. This failure may well stem from inadequate training during the residency, the overriding demands of our operating rooms and special care units, the marginal economic incentives that pertain, and perhaps lethargy. But whatever the reason, too few pain-control programs have been established. We believe that there is dereliction in not providing this service to patients.

Where trained personnel are at hand, every hospital with an anesthesia department should offer an organized program of pain control that may range from a mere consultant role in diagnostic and therapeutic nerve blocks, to a formalized pain clinic with regular hours, geographic site, and supporting staff, under the aegis of a pain management team, made up of neurosurgeons, neurologists, radiologists, psychologists, and psychiatrists. The team concept is clearly a community resource that, except for a few outstanding exceptions, has not been replicated throughout the country. A pain consultation service or a more formal pain clinic should be established in all our institutions, as it is so clearly within the scope of anesthesiology. Failure to do so narrows the realm of our specialty.

CLINICAL PHARMACOLOGY

Of the three basic disciplines — bioengineering, pathophysiology, and pharmacology — on which our clinical abilities depend, pharmacology is logically the most cogent. Anesthesia had its beginnings in the use of drugs (opioids, alcohol, coca, ether, chloroform) to produce the desired effects. Although an increasing number of anesthesiologists hold joint appointments in departments of pharmacology, it is somewhat odd that the most appropriate branch of pharmacology, clinical pharmacology, is seldom identified with our discipline. Defined as the "study of drugs in man," clinical pharmacology incorporates a body of knowledge that includes molecular mechanisms; biochemical alterations; interaction of drugs with receptors; the nature of the dose – response relationship; quantitating pharmacodynamic effects of drugs; molecular mechanisms of drug absorption, distribution, metabolism, and excretion; pharmacokinetics; the design, implementation, and interpretation of clinical trials; analytical methodology for quantitating drugs in body compartments; and the epidemiology of adverse drug reactions. Within this broad context, it would seem that all anesthesiologists are by definition clinical pharmacologists. However, a publication, *Clinical Pharmacology: A Guide to Training Programs* (5th edition, 1982), lists 34 established programs in university centers with 297 faculty of whom only 9 (3 percent) are anesthesiologists. Providing more food for thought are 22 new and developing programs with 138 faculty that include only one anesthesiologist.

Why are we not aligned with this endeavor, and what does this portend for the future of our specialty? Whereas anesthesia had its beginnings in the operating room, obstetric suites, and dental establishments, having as its principal mission the attenuation of pain, clinical pharmacology has evolved principally from the efforts of a coterie of internists in the United States in studying cardiovascular drugs. More than 90 percent of the faculty of clinical pharmacology departments are affiliated with departments of medicine and pharmacology. Nevertheless, every anesthetization comprises an exercise in pharmacokinetics and dynamics, meeting all the desiderata listed above. A perusal of any of the anesthesia journals indicates that most of the papers can be classified in the sphere of clinical pharmacology. The time must soon arrive for us to share the results of our research on patients given potent drugs and monitored as they are in operating room and critical care situations with our clinical pharmacology colleagues whose origins, studies, and concepts too often exclude our knowledge. We must begin to expand the image of anesthesiology by attendance at the established clinical pharmacology meetings by giving papers at those forums, by publishing in appropriate journals, and through participation in the activities of the clinical pharmacology divisions. Furthermore, and most importantly, we must seek research training opportunities in clinical pharmacology for our better, young investigators. In that way, perhaps a more general consensus will arise that the scope of anesthesiology justifiably embraces the discipline of clinical pharmacology.

BIOENGINEERING

That our specialty is now technology dependent is obvious in view of the equipment required in modern operating rooms, intensive care units, and pain clinics. It is no longer possible to care for the very ill appropriately without instrumentation on which we, as well as our patients, have become dependent. Furthermore, it is clear that many of the anticipated advances in our specialty will come from our colleagues in bioengineering. But the traditional and currently most common relations between hospitals and engineering schools, that of relative isolation, will prove insufficient to meet requirements. Rather, those specialties dependent on technology, for example, anesthesiology, cardiology, radiation therapy, and radiology, should integrate engineering skills into departmental structure. Engineers must abide with us to sense the most appropriate strategies to help solve our problems. Several of this country's anesthesiology departments can boast of clinical engineering services as well as bioengineering research groups as integral parts of their organizations. Logically, bioengineering that deals principally with clinical interface technology and life-support systems is well within the scope of anesthesiology. The rigor with which our more quantitatively trained engineering colleagues have approached our designated problems has been of immense help in defining the issues and identifying remedial strategies. The next step lies in educating our residents in their roles as leaders of the anesthesiology health care team to work closely with engineers in the provision of expert care. Predictably, the anesthesiologist-gadgeteer of the past will be replaced by the anesthesiologist-engineer in the near term. Defining issues in quantitative terms and the development of solution-oriented strategies, are the hallmark of the kind of engineering on which the future of our specialty now finds itself utterly dependent. Indeed, the scope of anesthesiology putatively includes bioengineering.

EDUCATION

The old adage that knowledge is power remains incontrovertible — the power to do good, to reduce the morbidity and mortality that attend anesthetic processes, and thereby to increase the quality of care. Fortunately, the intellectual context of our practice undergoes a constant process of revision as revealed in the Content Outline prepared by the ABA–ASA (American Society of Anesthesiologists) Joint Council on In-training Examinations for residents. This document is available to all and certainly is the principal focus in identifying a body of anesthetic information appropriate for the medical community at large, for students of anesthesia at all levels, and for graduates' continuing education.

Three organizations are entrusted with the responsibility for providing the educational and training requirements for those entering our specialty and continuing educational programs for practicing anesthesiologists. The American Board of Anesthesiology has listed as its purposes:

1. To maintain the highest standards of the practice of anesthesiology by fostering educational facilities and training in anesthesiology.
2. To establish and maintain criteria for the designation of a consultant in anesthesiology.
3. To advise the Accreditation Council for Graduate Medical Education (ACGME) concerning the training requirement of individuals seeking certification as such requirements relate to residency training programs in anesthesiology.
4. To establish and conduct those processes by which the Board may judge whether physicians who voluntarily apply, should be issued certificates indicating that they have met the required standards for certification as a consultant in anesthesiology. A consultant anesthesiologist possesses adequate measures of knowledge, judgement, clinical, and character skills and personality suitable for assuming independent responsibility for patient care and for serving as the leader of the anesthesia care team.
5. To serve the public, medical profession, hospitals and medical schools, by preparing lists for publication of physicians certified by the Board.

Operationally, the Board establishes criteria for gaining entrance to its examination system, conducts both written and oral examinations and certifies those who satisfy those training and examination requirements. It is clear that the American Board of Anesthesiology controls the very center of the specialty's educational process.

The Board is allied in this mission with the Residency Review Committee (RRC) for Anesthesiology. This tripartite group with representatives from the ABA, ASA, and AMA prescribe the General Requirements for residency training and write the Special Requirements for anesthesiology promulgated by the Accreditation Council for Graduate Medical Education (ACGME). These documents describe the organizational arrangements and resources necessary to mount a residency training program. It does not describe program content, conduct examinations, or certify specialists — the purview of the Board. It does, however, conduct periodic site inspections of all training programs to ascertain the extent to which they meet the General and Special Requirements. The RRC has the power to recommend approval, disapproval, or a probationary status for residencies.

The American Society of Anesthesiologists (ASA) also plays a vital role in the educational process, that of providing an organizational framework for meeting the political and continuing educational needs of its members. The Society addresses the latter commitment in many ways including provision for the Scientific Program and Refresher Courses in its Annual Meeting, conducting Regional Refresher Courses nationwide and distributing a continually updated, Self-Assessment Examination for all practitioners including those unable to attend other continuing education functions.

We must all attempt to acquire the habit of continuing our education by a program of self-education if we are to fulfill the role so long sought and so recently acquired — as consultant anesthesiologists. The scope of anesthesiology is only as narrow or as broad as the knowledge, judgment, and skills that anesthesiologists apply to the ill people under their care.

RESEARCH

The mission of an academic department differs from that in the community hospital setting: the latter must strive to provide the highest quality of care to patients, while the former assumes an additional burden of constantly monitoring, revising, and improving that care. This obligation is discharged through education in residency programs and the identification and implementation of better means to care for the anesthetized ill. Herein is the domain of research. The best academic anesthesia departments offer an ingrained cultural outlook wherein an inquiring mind does exercise, where solutions to problems in anesthesia are anticipated, and where the discovery of a new law of nature is a joy.

A quarter of a century ago, William T. Salter, Professor of Pharmacology at Yale, editorially issued a challenge to our specialty in "The Leaven of the Profession."* For its sagacity, we quote the editorial in its entirety:

> It is true for Anesthesiology as for any other profession that *service* must be leavened with progressive thought. Every profession has its corps of hewers of wood and drawers of water. It must also have its sprinkling of investigators to guide and lead it on its path forward. Without vision, the profession dies. At the present moment the progress of Anesthesia is limited almost exclusively by a lack of knowledge of the basic action of drugs as applied to human organisms which are abnormal. Greater strides must be made in elucidating the pathological pharmacology of such drugs as curare. The relative impor-

tance of analgesia as contrasted with relaxation must be reviewed on the basis of careful physiological measurement made at the bedside with modern methods. Who is to do such essential studies of Applied Pharmacology?

> Obviously, a considerable knowledge of pathological human physiology is involved. In this day and age there is a tendency for the routine anesthetist to "pass the buck" to the professor of physiology or the professor of pharmacology, in the vain hope that the answers can be learned from mice or monkeys. The respective professors named are usually only too eager to cooperate and interested in fostering the development of applied studies on man. They realize all too well, however, that such studies must be made by an applied pharmacologist, appointed by the Department of Anesthesiology. Such a man should be familiar with the everyday problems of the practicing Anesthesiologist. He should have basic training in the fundamental departments mentioned. He would do well perhaps to commence his work with experiments on animals performed under the aegis of the preclinical departments. Ultimately, however, the problem must be taken into the clinic and the definitive answers resolved there.

> To this end, there must be trained a group of so-called "academic Anesthesiologists." These individuals must have the special training and sufficient leisure to advance the basic concepts of applied science. In their earlier years they must be supported by adequate fellowships. In their mature years they must receive adequate recognition in the form of staff appointments and university affiliation. They must not be run ragged with routine asignments, but must be protected from the irate surgeon who demands *service now* in the name of all humanity and the Trustees. At the present time the fellowships and funds available for this purpose are pitifully meager.

> Part of the fault for this lack of opportunity lies in the diffidence of the routine anesthesiologist. The conscientious and overworked anesthetist, while rendering invaluable service to the community, fails to appreciate that his ultimate professional status cannot be guaranteed by *service* alone. Without vision and research, the professions die. It behooves every practicing member of the profession to exert his influence both in his local medical group and in his society of specialists to see to it that opportunities exist for progress.

---

* Reprinted with permission from Salter, W.J.: The leaven of the profession, Anesthesiology 11:374, 1950.

Have we met that challenge? Surely we have come a long way. Especially over the past decade, it is obvious that many of the principal advances in anesthetic practice and knowledge have come from within the specialty. But we are not yet at the knee of the curve leading to self-sufficiency. The paucity of long-term research funding and requirements for increased efficiencies in hospitals have virtually combined to preclude the kind of idyllic scholarliness envisioned by Salter. And until we reach the plateau of self-sufficiency in meeting the needs of our specialty, we cannot begin to mount an assault on the more generic issues and problems—those that have broad scientific and social implications and those that transcend our specialty. Studies on the nature of consciousness, of memory, of central nervous system communication, of methods of measuring the quality of medical practice, and of identifying just means for allocating limited medical resources, to mention just a few. So, although research and education germane to our specialty are clearly within grasp, we will have fully matured only when our vision and accomplishments exceed that scope.

MANPOWER IN ANESTHESIA TODAY

One may ask, Why a section on Manpower in a chapter dealing with the history and scope of anesthesiology? The answer lies in the fact that the history of our specialty is one of accomplishments of people, while the scope of anesthesiology ultimately is defined by the practice patterns and contributions of its practitioners. One wonders where our specialty would be positioned today if its discoverers had been leading surgeons rather than itinerant dentists. In England, it became a physician's specialty only perhaps because the requirements for anesthesia services had not outstripped the capabilities of the medical school establishment to train more practitioners. In the United States, its burgeoning population far exceeded the capabilities of medical schools to meet the demands for any physician services, much less anesthesiology. Hence, it is not surprising that in the early years the conduct of anesthesia was assigned to medical students and junior surgical house officers. Somewhat later, they in turn were replaced by nurse anesthetists usually working under the aegis of the hospital or surgeons, but later under the supervision of anesthesiologists. The number of physicians entering our specialty has held relatively constant at 3 to 4 percent of graduating medical students. Together, nurse anesthetists and anesthesiologists were unable to meet the demands for anesthesia service in operating rooms. Simultaneously, this failure impaired the specialty's ability to respond to needs in other appropriate arenas, such as pain clinics, intensive care units, recovery rooms, and others that fall within the natural scope of our specialty.

For a 30-year period representing the 1950s, 1960s, and 1970s, this vacuum was partially filled by an influx of graduates from foreign medical schools—a phenomenon true for most specialty practices, but perhaps not to the extent as in anesthesiology. But over the past decade, two major events have combined to signal an end to manpower shortages in anesthesia. One such event has been a steadily decreasing birth rate plus zero population growth. The other was a doubling of the number of medical schools in the United States and an increase in student enrollment. Because of these trends, manpower in some specialties now exceeds the need and in most others is close to equilibrium; for a few such as anesthesiology, it can be predicted with some confidence that we will be close to meeting the needs for anesthesia services by the American people by 1990. In a recent study by the ASA's Committee on Manpower, it was clear that more than 90 percent of all anesthetics in the United States are given by anesthesiologists directly or by nurses under supervision of anesthesiologists. The remainder are given by obstetricians, independent nurse anesthetists, surgeons, general practitioners, and dentists.

A related and just as important an issue is the quality of anesthesia manpower. It is gratifying to realize that our specialty is now attracting an increasingly large number of the very best medical students and physicians with training in other specialties, particularly internal medicine and pediatrics. Others gravitating to anesthesiology in increasing numbers are physicians with graduate science degrees who see in our specialty many a challenging research opportunity. So it is with some confidence that we approach 1990 realizing that we will, for the first time, meet manpower needs with the very best of practitioners. In turn, this should create the opportunity for us to move with more vigor into those other areas in which anesthesiologists are especially equipped to preside.

FUTURE

We have assayed to review briefly the history of our specialty and to define the scope of anesthesiology; our specialty seems secure, but not yet mature and fully differentiated. The final step, and one essential for an endowed chair at the high table of established medical practice, forms the challenge for this century. It can be met if we implement the complete scope of anesthesia services in all hospitals, while developing the role of the consultant anesthesiologist and leader of the health care team to the fullest extent possible and by research in those areas germane to anesthetic practices and to society in general. It is on research and education that so much depends — the improvement of the quality of anesthetic care, the advancement of our specialty.

SUGGESTED READINGS

THE HISTORY

Bonner TN: The social and political attitudes of midwestern physicians, 1840–1940. J Hist Med 8:133, 1953

Byck R. (ed): Cocaine Papers. Sigmund Freud. New American Library, New York, 1974

Cartwright FF: The English Pioneers of Anaesthesia. Bristol, John Wright and Sons, 1952

Caws P: The structure of discovery: Scientific discovery is no less logical than deduction. Science 166:1375, 1969

Channing W: A Treatise on Etherization in Childbirth. Boston, William D. Ticknor, 1848

Duncum B: The Development of Inhalation Anaesthesia. Oxford University Press, London, 1947

Faulconer A, Keys TE: Foundations of Anesthesiology. Springfield, Ill, Charles C. Thomas, 1965

Keys TE: The History of Surgical Anesthesia. Schumans, New York, 1945

Laborit H, Huguenard P: Practique de l'hibernotherapie, En Chirurgie et en Medicine. Paris, Masson, 1954

Merton RK: Singletons and multiples in scientific discovery. A chapter in the sociology of science. Proc Am Phil Soc 105:470, 1961

Mortimer WG: History of Coca, "The Divine Plant" of the Incas. And/Or Press, San Francisco, 1974

Oré PC: Etudes, cliniques sur l'anesthesie chirurgicale par la methode des injections de chloral dans les veines. Paris, JB Baillière et Fils, 1875

Siegrist HE: Surgery before anesthesia. Bull School Med U Maryland 31:116, 1947

Smith WDA: Under the influence. A History of Nitrous Oxide and Oxygen Anaesthesia. London, Macmillan, 1982

Snow J: On the Inhalation of the Vapour of Ether. London, John Churchill, 1847

Snow J: On Chloroform and Other Anaesthetics. John Churchill, London, 1858

Sykes WS: Essays on the First Hundred Years of Anaesthesia, Edinburgh, Churchill Livingstone. Vol I, 1960, Vol II, 1960, Vol III, 1982

THE SCOPE

American Board of Anesthesiology: Booklet of Information. Hartford, ABA, 1984

American Board of Anesthesiology: Quality anesthesia care: A model of future practice of anesthesiology. Anesthesiology 47:488, 1977

ASA Committee on Manpower: Who provides anesthesia care in the United States? JAMA (in press)

ASA Subcommittee on Academic Anesthesia Manpower: A survey of academic anesthesiology. Anesthesiology 47:53, 1977

Bunker JP, Barnes BH, Mosteller F (eds): Costs, Risks and Benefits of Surgery. New York, Oxford University Press, 1977

Burroughs Wellcome Foundation: Clinical Pharmacology: A Guide to Training Programs, 5th ed. Research Triangle Park, NC, 1982

Cooper JB: Anesthesiology and the engineer. Eng Med Biol 1:17, 1982

Cooper JB, Newbower RS, Moore JW, et al: A new anesthesia delivery system. Anesthesiology 49:310, 1978

Pontoppidan H, Geffin B, Lowenstein E: Acute respiratory failure in the adult. N Engl J Med 287:690, 1972

Safar P (ed): Advances in Cardiopulmonary Resuscitation. New York, Springer-Verlag, 1977

Salter WJ: The leaven of the profession. Anesthesiology 11:374, 1950

Starr P: The Social Transformation of American Medicine. New York, Basic Books, 1982

Vesell ES, Biebuyck JF: New approaches to assessment of drug disposition in the surgical patient. Anesthesiology 60:529, 1984

2

Legal Aspects of Anesthesia Practice

Martin L. Norton, M.D., J.D.
Edward V. Norton, J.D.

INTRODUCTION

No area of the practice of medicine is as emotion laden as the topic of this chapter — the social, ethical, and legal aspects of anesthesia practice. In reality, we have had guidelines from time immemorial. The Hippocratic Oath[1] and its formal predecessors, the Code of Maimonides[2] and the Code of Hammurabi,[3] are no less familiar than more contemporary codes of ethics (i.e., American Medical Association Principles of Medical Ethics and Current Opinions of the Judicial Council of the American Medical Association) and rules regarding human experimentation[4] and Code of Helsinki,[5] expressing social concern. These guidelines are the expression of the expectations and fears of the citizenry, and are often a reflection of our failure in public relations or action.

The law, whether expressed by statute or judicial interpretation, is a further manifestation of this same process. We see this in the spate of medical negligence actions based on the failure to abide by the well-known admonition, *primum no nocere* (i.e., above all do no harm).

The past 10 years have added a new dimension to the public concern, that of cost containment, as demonstrated by cost-oriented legislation.[6] The physician now functions in a structural practice format (e.g., professional associations), formerly not thought possible.[7] The anesthesiologist has even more concerns as a hospital-based practitioner, for example, issues regarding medical staff law and bylaws[8] and antitrust aspects of exclusive contracts.[9]

The more salient concerns of the practice of anesthesiology will be briefly described in this chapter. Excellent texts are available that can be consulted for further details.[10]

THE PHYSICIAN-PATIENT INTERFACE

INTRODUCTION TO THE PATIENT

Common practice is for the surgeon to schedule surgery electively with a booking office. The anesthesiologist-in-charge then assigns the cases to colleagues and other practitioners. This results in a sterile approach to the doctor–patient relationship and is dictated more by administrative convenience than by patient care considerations.

The introduction of the anesthesiologist to the patient should begin in the surgeon's office at the time surgery is first being considered and when the surgical procedure is discussed. This, as well as an expression of confidence in available anesthesiologic expertise, sets the psychological atmosphere for the proper patient-anesthesiologist relationships. It tells the patient that the surgeon is supportive of his or her colleague as a coprofessional, interested even at this early stage of surgical management in the patient's welfare. A brief memorandum of introduction, highlighting problems extant or anticipated, completes the cycle and allows for appropriate assignment of anesthesia personnel. Thus the anesthesiologist visiting the patient the night before will not be greeting a stranger. More importantly, the patient will be receptive to the visit of the anesthesiologist. This approach will also avoid that most distressing experience, when the patient expresses surprise, first, that of surgery being necessary, and second, that this stranger — the anesthesiologist — is coming to discuss it.

CONSULTATION AND REFERRAL

Where there is a particular problem, pathologic, psychological, or for any other reason, consultation or referral should be considered by the physician.[11] The distinction between consultation and referral is a subtle but important difference.[12] Consultation is a request for evaluation and for an opinion as to the status of the patient and/or recommended medicosurgical therapeutic approach. Referral can and should be limited to the area of expertise of the physician. It is a request to take over the management of a certain aspect of the patient's care. In the first instance, that is, consultation, the referring physician is asking for an opinion. This opinion may or may not be used in the treatment plan. The burden is solely on the referring physician either to justify the course of action that the consultant suggests or to reject the opinion. Where care of the patient has been referred, meaning "take care of that aspect of my patient," each physician bears an independent although cooperative burden (i.e., "joint and several responsibility"). Failure to refer has the legal and ethical implication of expertise in all the necessary areas of that patient's care. That is to say, you purport to be an expert in all areas of patient care.

There is another aspect to the anesthesiologic situation that requires consideration. A continuing series of cases emphasizes the duty of the physician and/or hospital to provide patient care and personnel who are competent to fulfill the special duties they are assigned to. Thus the surgeon does have an obligation to insist on competent assistants (instrument nurse, tableside physician assistants, anesthesiologists, and the like). Obviously, the teaching program is a variant on the theme. The hospital similarly has a responsibility with regard to personnel assignments, exemplified in the agency relationships of administrative supervision.

CONTRACT RELATIONSHIPS

The direct interaction between anesthesiologist and patient is formalized at the time of the preoperative visit. This is the period when an oral contract is established supported by the indicia of a formal contract — offer, acceptance, consideration, and action taken in reliance based on mutual consent.[13] Thus, we have a combination of implied and express consent.

There is no legal obligation to accept any patient. However, the realities of medical staff privileges mandate that the patient receive such care as needed. The hospital environment and governmental restraints mandate that no patient be denied care based on any consideration other than actual medical needs. Acceptance of the patient may be demonstrated by the preoperative anesthetic preparation, obtaining of specific consent, and ordering of preanesthetic medication.

The patient indicates acceptance of the anesthesiologist by consenting to the anesthetic plan, accepting the potential hazards, and granting to the physician the privilege of practicing their profession on the very body of the patient. Voluntary appearance of the patient in the operating suite indicates reliance on the anesthesiologist's presentation of his skills and competency to manage the anesthesiologic situation.

In exchange, the patient agrees to cooperate and to pay the requisite fee. This represents the requirement of consideration and completes the legal requirements of a contract.

Specific mention must be made of the occasion in which a question arises as to consent or to any other issue in the purview of the anesthesiologist. We may hear the surgeon comment, "Don't worry, I'll take care of it", or "I'll take full responsibility—let's go ahead", or some other similar statement. The relationships, obligations, and duties of the surgeon and the anesthesiologist are in many ways "joint and several." They are "joint" in that they may be shared; they are "several" in that they are also individual. These duties are contractual (expressly or implicitly) between the patient and the individual professional health care providers. Once entered upon, they can only be abrogated by the express consent of the patient, and not by the surgeon or any other third party.[14]

INFORMED CONSENT

This concept, expressed in the landmark cases of *Canterbury* v. *Spence* and *Wilkinson* v. *Vesey*,[15] is still in flux. It implies a discussion of the recommended anesthetic plan, alternatives and potential complications. A recent interpretation further extends this concept to an obligation to discuss even totally unacceptable approaches to medical management.[16] This follows the concept that the patient must be provided with whatever he "needs to know" to make a decision. This is the difference from the British system which states that the standard of sufficiency is that which is rightly accepted as proper by a body of skilled and experienced medical men.[17]

Only recently did the Commonwealth of Massachusetts in *Harnish* v. *Children's Hospital Medical Center*[18] accept the "reasonable patient" standard. It requires a determination of the "materiality" of information. The physician must present the various risks, consequences, and alternatives from the perspective of the medically unsophisticated patient. In fact, it is wise to err on the side of overdisclosure.

Some state supreme courts have expressed the need for presentation of alternatives, to wit: where a doctor did not tell a patient about an "alternative treatment," liability for malpractice exists even though the "alternative" is more dangerous than the procedure actually used and is generally not advisable.[19] The court stated that a patient should be able to make an intelligent choice about treatment. A physician who does not have to reveal more dangerous choices is only required to reveal the one alternative that is the least dangerous, and this means the patient has no choice at all. This court adopted the "lay person" test for disclosure. The Connecticut Supreme Court held that a physician must disclose all information that is reasonably related to a patient's decision (unlike the "professional" test, which states that the standard of disclosure is the common practice of professionals). Thus, the conclusion is reached that we must present the anesthetic plan, alternatives to the recommended plan, and the potential problems or risks of each.

Most courts recognize, however, that there may be instances in which sound medical judgment requires withholding of medical information from a patient. This privilege is strictly limited to two areas: (1) where the physician has reason to believe that the patient already has knowledge of specific risks inherent in the procedure, and (2) where disclosure would complicate a patient's condition. These exceptions to the rule are construed very narrowly by the courts, and the burden of proof weighs heavily on the physician. Adequate documentation on the chart will have significant evidentiary weight. In order for a patient's decision to be meaningful, the risks of both accepting and rejecting a proposed treatment or procedure and also of the alternatives must be known.

Where the patient speaks a foreign language, an interpreter should be the intermediary and should sign the consent form as such. It may also be advisable to have a close family member involved in this communication and to cosign the consent form.

SIGNING THE CONSENT FORM

The consent form is merely one piece of evidence indicating an attempt of the physician to communicate with the patient. This can be strengthened by requesting the patient to countersign the preanesthesia evaluation note (on the medical chart progress record) *after reading it* or having it read to him or her. The last sentence of the note should paraphrase the concept that "the patient has been informed of the above and signifies an understanding and agreement to the prepared anesthetic plan and acceptance of its inherent potential complications, by signature below." This approach is specifically taken when there are noted material medical complications discovered in the preanesthetic evaluation visit or consultation. Although such notes made on the chart are rarely signed by the patient, there is no doubt that the signature constitutes recognition that the patient has been informed.

The duty to warn patients about newly discovered dangers in previously initiated treatment is now drawing increased attention by the advocate. It represents a further extension of the informed consent concept in a post facto arena of patient care. Thus, the duration of the patient–doctor relationship would be implicitly extended beyond the usual period of immediate medical need (as long as the patient's condition requires attention).[20] This extension could be for a matter of many years after the physician and the patient have discontinued direct professional contact, as in the estrogen-pregnancy cases.[21] This is usually not a problem in anesthesia.

COMPLICATIONS AND THE PATIENT'S RIGHT TO BE INFORMED

Every anesthesiologist at some time will have a complication relative to his or her conduct of anesthesia. What should be noted on the chart? What should the patient be told?

First, the very basis of the physician–patient relationship is that of mutual trust and reliance. Without this absolutely requisite consideration supported by respect for confidentiality, medical judgment cannot be applied for the patient's benefit. Next, both patient and physician must appreciate the fallibility of our profession in relation to the responsibilities we bear. This is partly expressed under the concept of informed consent.

The physician has the ethical and legal obligation to clearly record the events of medical management on the patient's chart. This confidential document memorializes the patient's problems for two purposes:

1. To provide a visual consecutive record and thus indicate to reviewers (or the court) the course and trends of the current therapeutic process.
2. To provide a similar chart for subsequent health care providers. As such, it is mandatory to provide all pertinent *facts* including the facts of adverse responses to therapeutic management (sometimes euphemistically called therapeutic misadventures). What is required is a factual description of the events not a judgmental recantation. A statement of sequential events with basis for original decision making and the response to the therapeutic approach contributes most to this memorialization.

The physician should never modify the record in a post hoc fashion to justify action

to
has
itu-
heir
epts
licy,
they
here-
ofes-
eight

spital
edical
ature,
f laws
es by
ide of
t care,
e, and
our re-

is con-
il prac-
institu-
assume
w with
ed by a
ument"
, every
ulations
ral man-
munica-
establish
patient.
hat both
they are
ie public
e of their

ials are
is. Viola-
ie prima
y (one of
and the
from the

worded
ompetent
ated pre-
terms to
t and ac-
to ensure

sequent knowledge. It is a contem-
cord. If corrections are required,
be done in the form of an adden-
y dated, timed, signed, and with
n of the reason for the addition.
n must be made during the writ-
rd, only a single line should be
the incorrect word or phrase,
ls should be imprinted. At the
pace an appended notation, as
, should be attached.

do we tell the patient?[22] The
me—the facts! The physician
responsibility to the patient,
this situation. This clearly
hysician's duty to the patient
ity to himself or herself. This
iship manifestly applies for
patient to whom the physi-
lationship of trust and a high
lity. Judgmental opinions as
t, self-serving exculpatory
ressions of assumed "guilt"
the welfare of the patient,
ie profession.

CARE AND EXPERT NESSES

efines the "standard of
equally qualified physi-
e for a specific patient
stances. This definition
lelines for the physician
uities. Medically, it at-
evel of care that is up to
ly at the pinnacle of med-
uggest that anything less
dge and practice" would
late. It further suggests a
tics, which is often con-
.

t of the legal process, the
etermined by the testi-
itness." This individual
e a physician anesthesi-
rney firms usually have
ysician as an employee
edical implications. As-

suming this screening personage suggests a negligent act (duty, failure of duty, proximate relationship between that failure and subsequent injury), the attorney seeks outside testimony of an "expert witness." The expert may be a carefully nurtured friend, social acquaintance, medical school professor, or prominent community physician. There are many individual career witnesses or organizations composed of panels of professional witnesses of varying background. The final acceptance of a witness categorized as an "expert" lies in the judgment of the trial court (judge) based on a *voir dire* (examination by the attorneys as to competence to testify as an expert witness). This individual reviews the written record only and, on the basis of his knowledge and experience, expresses an opinion as to what probably occurred, what was the failure of duty leading to the injury, and thereby indicates what should have been done. Invariably, the opposing attorney will bring out in court the facts that (1) the expert was not present at time of surgery and/or (2) the expert never examined the patient, and (3) significant payment was made related to the provision of the expert testimony. What ultimately develops is a battle of the experts, with the jury being swayed by the most persuasive.

The areas most often addressed under this topic are preanesthesia evaluation and preparation (correction of pathophysiologic conditions, e.g., stabilization of diabetic status), monitoring during surgery, specific errors in management (e.g., overdosage), and failure to supervise and administer follow-up care in the operating room, in the recovery room, and postoperatively. The latter includes the problem of postoperative management of complications.

Previously, the definition of standard of care also included the concept of the "locality rule." This incorporated the practices of physicians in their region or locality. With the advent of mass communication media, this was extended to include practices in "similar communities." The locality rule has almost vanished from consideration. One of the last holdouts to discard this outdated concept is South Carolina,[23] which held that the definition of the standard of care that a medical doctor must meet is no longer limited to the practice or custom of particular locality or geographic area.

Thus, in a medical malpractice action, the plaintiff's medical expert must be allowed to testify regarding a national standard of care for anesthesiologists.

Of particular note in this discussion is the burden of demonstrating the standard of care in this country. Modern medicine has seen a great deal of mobility of medical practitioners. This includes movement of physicians from other countries to the United States. While these physicians are required to be licensed in the states of their practice, such licensure does not ordinarily establish knowledge of or compliance with standards of care in this country. While basic anatomy, physiology, and pharmacology are the same anywhere in the world, specific clinical practices and levels of care are not. Thus, practices that may be acceptable in foreign countries are often not acceptable in the United States.[24] The burden of proof for the foreign-trained physician is subtly shifted to demonstrate the knowledge of the standard of care in this country and compliance therewith.

It is also interesting to note that lesser trained persons (e.g., nurse anesthetists) can testify as to their knowledge of the standard of care of a board certified M.D. anesthesiologist while being required themselves only to abide by the lesser (non-board-certified M.D.) standards of care of the paraprofessional.

One beneficial aspect is the implied requirement that all professionals maintain their status by being up to date on the current and changing philosophies of medical practice. Indeed, most states have statutory requirements for continuing medical education, as recommended by the American Medical Association and the various specialty accreditation organizations.

STANDARDS

In addition to the concept of "standard of care," another kind of standard has grown in evidentiary importance. Organizations such as the Joint Committee on Accreditation of Hospitals and the American Society of Anesthesiologists, as well as hospitals and departments, promulgate standards and procedural manuals

or directives. Their significance is related the fact that it is the profession itself that established the criteria. Furthermore, inst tions and individuals functioning under t aegis are expected to comply with the cond presented. Similarly, if a hospital has a po it must make sure it is enforced.[25] In fact, establish the parameters of practice and t fore the standard of care expected of the pr sion. Thus, they have great evidentiary w in the eyes of a judge or jury.

Every physician practicing in a ho environment must be a member of the m staff. As such, we agree (by conduct, sign or inference) to abide by the medical sta and bylaws. These are the general ru which we function and cover a multit areas including but not limited to patien due process rights, insurance coverag peer review.[26] We accept limitations on search activities and clinical practices.[2]

These bylaws, rules, and regulatio stitute a contract between the individu titioner, his or her department, and the tion in which we function. As such, we contractual obligation enforceable at la consequent liability for damages incur violation of the "four corners of the doc (contractual provisions). Furthermore department establishes procedural reg either formally or informally. Procedu uals, written directives, and oral com tions of expected conduct of practice self-regulative standards of care for the

The public is aware of the fact t categories of standards do exist, even i not aware of the specific provisions. T relies on these rules as being protectiv interests as patients.

Increasingly, procedural man being considered as binding obligatio tion of the provisions thereof becor facie evidence of a violation of a du the elements of a negligence action burden of proof therefore may shift plaintiff to the alleged tortfeasor.

Procedural manuals should be with great care and reviewed by a c attorney. The provisions must be st cisely but in the broadest possible allow flexibility of medical judgmer tion. Specific attention must be given not only that contemporary practices are established, but also that provisions for changing practices will be incorporated by reference. Periodic review and modifications should be provided and entered into with due consideration of the implications. We must take great care to ensure that these provisions meet national standards of practice and are not merely limited to local community conditions. Keep in mind that the "locality rule" as a measure of standard of care has largely been replaced by the concept of national standards or at least the comparable community concept. University and teaching hospitals are expected to provide a level of care that is at the leading edge of the professional practice. However, every new development in medical knowledge need not be mandated until general acceptance by the wider medical community is demonstrated by clinical practices.

To this point, we have discussed contract and negligence in an interrelated fashion. As theories of law, however, they are distinguished. An action in contract may have a differing time element for its institution (statute of limitation) than a negligence action (especially in a "discovery rule" jurisdiction). The mode of relief in courts of equity or law will be different. More than one law suit may be possible on the various theories of law between different parties even if based on the same or similar facts.

The question of minimum versus optimum medical practice, current standards versus ideal practice, is addressed by the legal profession, but is not answered. The phrase "what the *reasonable* physician would do" gives no help. The obligation of the medical profession is to provide the best care possible under the totality of circumstances extant. (Note that we do not address here the issues of establishing standards for departmental or medical staff admission.)

The process of writing standards in anesthesiology should include due process concepts. There must be openness and representation of interests. Consideration of negative comments must be included. Clarity of writing should lead to clarity in subsequent interpretation of standards. There must be an appeals mechanism. Lastly, the standards should be submitted to both departmental and institutional review. This latter review should include participation by competent in-house legal counsel and, in case of conflict, invited outside counsel. The use of these standards must be enforced within the institution.

What all this means is that institutional and departmental standards must be viewed as having widespread implications, in similar fashion to the failure to promulgate these guidelines of practice.

PRIVACY AND CONFIDENTIALITY

The conduct of medical practice has always relied on principles of trust. Essential to this is the patient's reliance on the physician's keeping all information "in confidence." This is often confused with the patient's right of privacy. At law these are distinct issues, although in fact they may become entangled.

Black's Law Dictionary describes the right of privacy as a "generic term encompassing various rights recognized to be inherent." It includes the "right of an individual . . . to withhold himself . . . from public scrutiny."[28] Technically this can be based on intrusion, consisting of violating the plaintiff's solitude or seclusion.[29] It can also be based on public disclosure of private facts, wherein an action would exist for defamation.[30]

Another view of this problem is presented by the definition of invasion of privacy. This is the "unwarranted appropriation . . . of one's private affairs with which the public has no legitimate concern or the wrongful intrusion into one's private activities, in such a manner as to cause mental suffering, shame, or humiliation to a person of ordinary sensibilities."[31] In essence, this provides for one to be left alone and unnoticed if he so chooses. It is very important to recognize that the party involved (the patient) need not be aware that his or her privacy is being violated. The fact of violation is prima facie to the tort. The classic situation here is the unconsented-to presence during surgery of individuals not specifically required for the accomplishment of that surgery.

The reader will note the similarity of the category "public disclosure of private facts" to the lay concept of confidentiality. Confidential information is that intended to be held in confidence or kept secret. From these descriptions it is evident that privacy is the broader term including physical acts (e.g., unwarranted presence in the operating room, photography during surgery), whereas confidentiality is a subgroup relating more to information whether spoken or written.

Photography is of special sensitivity. Surgeons, particularly, rely on the purported lack of identifiability of the patient from the photograph. In fact, the law does not support this contention. The key elements to the wrong are (1) unwarranted intrusion, (2) lack of consent of the patient, and (3) communication to a third party who has no legally supportable right to that communication. Again, note that the patient's contemporaneous awareness of this communication is not required.

Where does the anesthesiologist become involved? First, any information communicated by the patient must be assumed to be of a confidential nature, that is, entrusted for the sole and specific purpose of aiding in medical judgment making. Second, the anesthesiologist, as one of the indicia of his function, clouds the sensorium of the patient. Thus, the patient cannot protest invasions of privacy relative to observers in the operating room or to unapproved photography. The anesthesiologist therefore becomes a significant contributory party to the tortious act.

FOLLOW-UP AND ABANDONMENT

The anesthesiologist's duties in general management of the patient begin with meeting the patient but by no means end when the patient leaves the operating room. Yet, most patients (ASA I category) do not require extensive postoperative management (e.g., airway, cardiorespiratory, intravascular fluid, electrolyte, endocrinologic). Some patients must be followed to and through the specialized intensive care units and to their individual room locations. The key is the need of the patient. Although the patient originally contracted with the surgeon, there is a subsequent contract with the anesthesiologist. This results in joint

and several responsibilities in the care of the patient. The anesthesiologist has altered the patient's pharmacophysiologic state in order to effectuate needed surgery. Management of the consequences of these alterations must continue. To do less would constitute abandonment.[32]

We have discussed the need for continuing care through the postanesthesia period. Here we also pay particular attention to the recovery room and to the sometimes conflicting interests of anesthesiologist and surgeon. In the recovery room context we are dealing with complications from the intraoperative surgicoanesthetic period as well as complications postoperatively as the anesthesia wears off and the patient becomes semiconscious.[33]

The basic and absolute principle underlying tort law is that the wrongdoer (tortfeasor) is responsible (liable) for the consequences of his acts. This means that our professional duties include continuing in professional attendance as long as is necessary to manage the consequences or complications of the anesthetic period. Note that the term consequences need not imply a complication. It does include any event that may flow from the administration of pharmacologic agents or procedures and instrumentation (e.g., insertion of Swan-Ganz or arterial cannulae, epidural catheters). Thus, failure to continue in attendance is abandonment.

The ASA has, in committee, established the guidelines for the continuing postanesthesia recovery room care of the patient[34]: "(4) that the individual responsible for administering anesthesia remain with the patient as long as his presence appears necessary," and "(7) management of related anesthesia complications."

The anesthesiologist should be prepared to respond to at least four categories of postanesthesia problems: respiratory, cardiovascular, metabolic, and postoperative pain and delirium.[35] This is the standard of care to which the anesthesiologist is held.

Ascher[33] specified the conditions under which the physician may withdraw from the patient–doctor relationship, to wit:

The jury is instructed that once a physician enters into a professional relationship with a patient, he is not at liberty to terminate that relationship at will. That relationship will continue until it is ended by one of the following circumstances: (1) the patient's lack of need for further care; or (2) *the withdrawing physician being replaced by an equally qualified physician.* Withdrawal from the case under any other circumstances constitutes a wrongful abandonment of the patient, and if the patient suffers any injury as a proximate result of such wrongful abandonment, the physician is liable for it." (Emphasis supplied.)

The key factors are the needs of patients and, furthermore, that substitution of another physician is not adequate unless that other doctor is an "equally qualified professional." The surgeon who assumes this responsibility (i.e., control of the recovery room patient to the implied exclusion of the anesthesiologist) assumes at law the liability of one who purports to be skilled in all aspects of postoperative anesthesia management (i.e., during the recovery period).

The next factor that must be considered is that of availability. Post-anesthetic management requires constant and immediate availability of properly qualified personnel—the surgeon who must return to the operating room for further surgery, or go to his office for the usual office hours (not always in the hospital) or the anesthesiologist who must start another anesthetic do not meet these criteria. A physician should not unnecessarily leave the hospital or otherwise fail to attend the patient, if he or she wishes to avoid liability.[36] The immediate availability of the anesthesiologist or colleague as a hospital-based specialist does provide for the continuum of medical care required.

MALPRACTICE

Malpractice is "professional misconduct or unreasonable lack of skill. This term is . . . applied to such conduct . . . [for] failure of one rendering professional services to exercise that degree of skill and learning commonly applied under all the circumstances in the community by the average prudent reputable member of the profession with the result of injury, loss or damage to the recipient of those

services or to those entitled to rely upon them."[37]

In the medical context, the predominant theory of liability is that of negligence. The elements of negligence[38] required for recovery are as follows:

1. A duty or responsibility based on the existence of the physician–patient relationship
2. The violation of an applicable professional standard of care
3. A compensable injury
4. A causal connection between violation of the applicable standard of care and the injury complained of

Note that intent to do harm is not an element in this tort. Therefore, the intent to do good is not a legally acceptable defense. This latter principle is most confusing for the layman (physician, in contradistinction to attorney). The confusion arises from the criminal law concepts of mens rea and mea culpa (guilty knowledge and willfullness).[39] However, this principle does not apply to the field of civil law which is predominantly concerned with civil or private rights and remedies.

DAMAGES IN MALPRACTICE

The emotions evoked in a discussion of malpractice are exceeded only by a consideration of consequent damages. We can usually appreciate specific related health care costs, loss of income, recompense for pain and suffering, and costs of occupational retraining. There are, however, other allowable damages, namely loss of consortium, loss of comfort, care of children, and loss of parental guidance as examples. Often, experts such as actuaries may be called upon to determine the values of these factors.

In the past, lump sum payments have been made. Under the principles enunciated in the landmark case,[40] payments for health care or income loss provided from other sources (e.g., insurance companies) are usually not considered. The exact wording of the reference case is very important: "If an injured party received some compensation for his injuries from a source wholly independent of the tortfeasor, such payment should not be deducted from the damages which the plaintiff would otherwise collect from the tortfeasor."

This is the "collateral source" rule of damages. The medical profession considers this rule to be unjust and inequitable particularly as regards to payment of bills related to health care or income loss by insurance companies or services provided by governmental institutions. The concept of the "structured settlement" has developed. This latter approach permits payment of damages over a period of time related to the actuarily determined life circumstances of the injured party. It decreases the immediate impact on the defendant's resources by allowing for purchase of annuities and investments to provide for future payments.

Another source of irritation to our profession is the practice of having the balance of payments awarded the plaintiff go to the estate of the injured party when he dies. Recently proposed statutes that would have the payments cease on the death of the injured party have met with major opposition from such groups as the Association of Trial Lawyers of America.

OTHER PROFESSIONALS AND THE ANESTHESIOLOGIST

SURGEON – ANESTHESIOLOGIST RELATIONSHIPS

The start of the interaction between anesthesiologist and surgeon is established at time of consideration and scheduling of the patient for surgical procedures. Introduction of the anesthesiologist to the patient rightfully starts in the surgeon's office when he or she first informs the patient that surgery is contemplated. It is reinforced when the preanesthesia visit is made. This visit implicitly involves communication of the anesthesiologist with the surgeon. Next, the team concept in the operating room goes into high gear with the induction of anesthesia and skin incision and continues until the postanesthesia recovery phase is completed. But what about conflicts? Who is captain of the ship? Who is master and who is agent?

Most courts expressly reject the captain-of-the-ship concept in regard to the accredited anesthesiologist.[41]

The anesthesiologist is a coequal professional even in those institutions in which the Division or Section of Anesthesia is a subsection of the overall Department of Surgery. Surgeons and anesthesiologists have independent as well as joint and several areas of responsibility towards the patient. Normally, neither controls nor directs the activities of the other.[42] This is the culmination testing the maturity of the professional in interaction with colleagues. It requires a demonstration of growth professionally and emotionally. The resultant judgement as a member of the team can avoid an adversarial relationship. Still, the difficult question remains: what do we do in an unresolvable situation? Before the anesthesia is administered, it might prove advisable to withdraw (with proper notice to the patient and usually referral to another anesthesiologist). Once anesthesia has been administered this choice is no longer available. Teamwork must be more than mere verbiage, but patient safety reigns supreme. If another anesthesiologist is available, a tableside consultation is in order. If not, the anesthesiologist must act in his or her fiduciary capacity, that is, for the sole benefit of the patient. The anesthesiologist should indicate on the medical record the basis for his/her decision, his/her action, and the consequences thereof.

PARAMEDICAL PERSONNEL AND THE NURSE IN AN EXPANDED ROLE

The nurse anesthetists are the foremost paramedical practitioners of the health care industry. There are growing efforts to make hospital privileges available to these "expanded-practice" nurses.[43] It is interesting to note that the federal government is pursuing the encouragement of this trend through its regulatory authority. The rubric of antitrust regulation was recently used.[44] An insurance company decided on a risk management basis not to insure physicians who agree to provide ongoing medical supervision to self-employed nurse midwives, in contrast to those physicians, whom it continues to insure, who employ nurse-midwives. After pressure by the Federal Trade Commission, a consent decree was obtained wherein the company will now assure insurance coverage for physicians supervising but not medically directing the independent midwife as well.[45]

Recent legislation in the District of Columbia[46] giving the paraprofessional, nonphysician, and the anesthesiologist the legal right to hospital and staff appointments as independent "medical" practitioners furthers the objectives of the American Association of Nurse Anesthetists. Up to now the nurse anesthetist has been the clear agent of the physician in charge and of the employer (hospital or anesthesia group). This raises the question as to whether the nurse is in fact to be an independent contractor for liability purposes.

The Joint Commission on Accreditation of Hospitals approved a new medical staff standard on December 10, 1983. Specifically, the standard says that a hospital should have a single organized medical staff to be known as "medical staff" and that this body may "include other licensed individuals permitted by law and the hospital to provide patient care services independently." The key word here is "independently," and the legal inference is that this nonphysician providing patient care services could be held to be an independent contractor.

An independent contractor is defined as the party who contracts to perform a designated task on behalf of another party. However, the manner in which this is accomplished is within the sole control of that independent contractor. This contrasts markedly from the agent concept as we use it herein. An agent is one who performs a task for another party but the specifics of that accomplishment, that is, the manner of conduct, is in the control of the superior party (by virtue of supervision and/or medical direction). The latter concept follows from the principle called "respondeat superior."

The concept of agency is intimately associated with that of control. The nurse anesthetist was initially trained as a registered nurse for general patient care, after a high school education. The trend then progressed to a college program leading to a bachelor of science in nursing, followed by a nurse anesthesia program of 2 years' duration. Most of these programs are not affiliated with or integrated with physician anesthesia residency training programs. To date, the nurse anesthetist has worked under the Nursing Practice Acts of the respective states.[47] Several states license or certify nurse anesthetists.[48] The nurse has in the past usually worked under the supervision and medical direction of a physician (not necessarily limited to a qualified anesthesiologist). This has been in recognition of the great disparity in education between the physician and nurse.

The legal term "agency" is expressed as a relationship wherein one individual is authorized to act on behalf of another, and wherein the manner of such action is under the direction and control of the principal. The trend toward registered nurses functioning in an expanded capacity has accompanied the use of other paramedical personnel, such as the physician's assistant.

Nurse anesthesia started in 1878, when Sister Mary Bernard was called upon to assume the duties of anesthetist at St. Vincent's Hospital in Erie, Pennsylvania.[49] One of the first university-based programs was established at the University of Michigan Hospital during September 1919. This had been preceded by clinical use of nurse anesthetists at the Mayo Clinic, Rochester, Minnesota, in the 1890s. Other expansions of the nurses function includes nurse clinicians and even physician assistant designation.

A more recent trend has included resurrection of the midwife as a health practitioner. Midwifery is as ancient as the history of medicine itself.[50] With the development of modern medicine and following the Flexner Report,[51] medical specialization came to the fore and maternal and infant mortality rates fell drastically.

In the current price-conscious climate, the

public demand has been for low-cost medical care. An aspect of this has been renewed interest in midwifery. This change in stance was supported by the American College of Obstetrics and Gynecology ("Statement on Maternity Care As Provided by the Obstetrician/Gynecologist and Nurse-Midwife," list of principles approved by the Executive Board of The American College of Obstetricians and Gynecologists on April 23, 1982 and "Joint Statement of Practice Relationships Between Obstetricians/Gynecologists and Certified Nurse-Midwives", and the American College of Obstetricians and Gynecologists). It is also important to note that the College specifically states for its own members, "No physician shall be compelled to practice with a nonphysician."[52]

The prime forces behind the drive to renewed recognition of midwives are the high cost of medical care and the American College of Nurse-Midwives. Many states and jurisdictions provide legitimacy by statute.[53] Some states also have lay midwives practicing, therein. In other jurisdictions the midwife must practice under the supervision and direction of an obstetrician who is responsible for developing written policies and procedures.

The anesthesiologist is faced with a real dilemma related to professional prerogatives. Questions arise as to extent and area of legal liability, issues of superior knowledge, responsibility for resuscitation of neonates, and ethics and morality of participating in a lesser quality or standard of medical care. We must keep in mind the trend for the physician anesthesiologist to be trained in more than one discipline, including obstetrics. Furthermore, we cannot ignore the legal hazards of charges of an anticompetitive conspiracy under antitrust legislation (*supra*, 15 USC Sec. 1).

The analogy of the midwife with the nurse anesthetist is obvious. The thrust of its proponents[54] is that (1) nurse anesthetists services are purportedly indistinguishable from those provided by anesthesiologists, (2) nurse anesthetists are the least costly competent providers of anesthesia care, and (3) provision of anesthesia care is to be considered a nursing service. Thus, we see that coalitions of nonphysician health care providers are now successfully directing a legal and political effort to gain independent hospital access and direct reimbursement for anesthesiologic services.

Tradition has been followed by law as the basis for paramedical direction and supervision by the physician. In some jurisdictions even the dentist-anesthesiologist must perform professional duties under the medical guidance of the physician-anesthesiologist. Of import in this reasoning was the fact that the physician's training and experience was general, including during his internship and later residency experience in all the then major fields of medicine (medicine, surgery, obstetrics, and gynecology) and the purported subspecialties (anesthesiology, pathology, radiology and psychiatry among others). The question remains as to the supervision and direction of paraprofessionals. The paraprofessional, while anxious for ever-increasing professional independence, has withdrawn behind this shield of medical supervision and direction when liability (therefore dollar financial responsibility) issues arise in malpractice cases.

Some physician-anesthesiologists unilaterally refuse to provide their anesthesiologic services for patients of midwives. This raises interesting potential liability issues in the areas of contract (apparent or ostensible agency vis à vis the hospital and patient), and even abandonment of the patient by a member of the medical staff.

The physician is obligated morally and ethically, if not legally, to render needed medical care. We discuss the concept of medical staff membership as a matter of contract law elsewhere. We must also recognize our obligations to the institution wherein we function. The public, not sophisticated in the multiplicity of relationships of the hospital with its medical staff, quite reasonably assumes that the full services of the hospital are available on admission for professional services. Failure to provide these services could be interpreted as an abandonment of the patient by a lay jury. In addition, the anesthesia group, the medical staff, and the hospital through its board of trustees could be involved in an antitrust action[55] claiming a conspiracy to prevent or limit competition based upon refusal to provide anesthesiologic services for patients of independently practicing paraprofessionals. While no case has presented itself to date, these issues are by no means speculative.

Other institutions have taken a more positive attitude. They recognize that anesthesiologic management imposes stresses in addition to the primary pathophysiology of disease. These more enlightened professionals present the problem to the medical staff (now including representatives of the paraprofessionals). Consideration of the complexity of anesthetic management for both mother and fetus (and neonate) leads one to the recognition of the requirement of obstetrical physician consultation and/or referral during the birthing process wherein anesthesiologic stresses are to be imposed. This concept is of particular importance during a malpractice suit in which the "deepest pocket" is characteristically sought (as among hospital, physician, and paramedical) as punitive recompense for injuries claimed. Thus, in those institutions, if the anesthesiologist is to be in attendance, an obstetrician's consultation is required.

The Tax Equity and Fiscal Responsibility Act[56] and administrative regulations published in the Federal Register specifically differentiate between supervision (administrative) and medical direction.[57] They further specify that application of these concepts in no way changes the classic liability factor of the responsibility of the principal for the acts of the agent.[58]

PERSONNEL

There is also another obligation, that of providing properly trained personnel to operate the equipment. The burden is on the hospital as well as on the physician through the medical staff organization. The hospital must hire and train,[59] and the physician must medically direct. This implies and necessitates great confidence and trust by the patient and a high degree of good faith on the part of the physician.[60] Out of such a relationship the law implies that neither party may exert undue influence or pressure on the other except in the exercise of the utmost good faith and full knowledge and

consent of the other. As such, the physician has a particular obligation to ensure that people caring for his or her patient are adequately trained and skilled, to avoid subjecting the patient to additional risk, and to ensure the patient's safety and care.

THE OPERATING ROOM STAFF

Every clinical anesthesiologist soon learns that among the most crucial people affecting practice are the operating room staff. Their cooperative interaction aids in scheduling, expedites the case performance, and in many other ways contributes to patient care. They assist the anesthesiologist by supportive attitudes toward the patient and by helping during induction of anesthesia and intubation of the trachea in particular. It is their responsibility to obtain drugs and to sterilize instrumentation among other duties. As such, they can be considered under the borrowed-servant doctrine. This latter phrase applies wherein an individual is employed by one party (the hospital) but functions under the direction of a second party (the physician). The problem arises when the physician fails to recognize that the operating room personnel are professionals in their own right. Attitudes towards co-workers reflect themselves in doctor–patient attitudes. In fact, the patient senses these interactions and reacts with confidence, or lack of confidence, as a response. The borrowed servant concept is not intended to be a servile representation but rather a technical allocation of responsibilities and functional administrative chain of command. Mutual respect and consideration benefits the entire operating room team.

It is not clear whether the borrowed-servant concept limits or extends liability. Under this approach there are the agent (OR staff), primary principal (hospital), and borrowing physician. In this area of agency law, the jury must determine whose work was being done, who had the right to control the manner of work and its objective, and who thereby benefited.[61] Respondeat superior and the borrowed-servant doctrine are aspects of this agency law.

We must recognize that the OR personnel have a dual duty: (1) to the employing hospital, and (2) to the directing physician. But neither need negates their duty to their own profession. No physician has the absolute right to mandate actions contrary to accepted/approved procedural standards and policies.[62]

THE HIGH-TECH ERA

INSTRUMENTATION AND TECHNOLOGY

The anesthesiologist bears an obligation to check equipment for availability, safety, and function.[63] The failure to fulfill this obligation to inspect, or the inadequate inspection of that equipment in itself constitutes negligence. This is a form of tort often confused with, but distinct from, "products liability." The latter refers to the manufacturer's responsibility for products produced. In the present context, the duty of the physician has been expanded from mere reliance on the manufacturer's assurances to the obligation to review the equipment or have it independently reviewed by competent outside personnel of his choice. It does not relieve the physician of the duty to be aware of needs and principles of basic concepts such as grounding electrical equipment[64] and other matters pertaining to patient safety.

High-technology anesthesia care presents particular problems of liability. Patients may require renal dialysis, special beds (e.g., electrical, water, Stryker frames), aortic balloon pumps, hyperbaric oxygen units, and various types of ventilators, pacemaker, and automatic infusion sources. We may also expect to find gas chromatography, computed tomography, nuclear magnetic resonance, electrocardiography, cardiac output, Doppler transducers, and other monitors, both invasive and noninvasive. Heat lamps and hypo/hyperthermia blankets are only a few other items.

First we must consider the issue of "standard of care." Modern management of multiple organ system failure situations by definition require state-of-the-art diagnostic and therapeutic modalities. The landmark case of T.J. Hooper[65] stated that someone can be negligent in failing to use the latest technology as well as in using technology negligently. The obligation of the physician in charge, therefore, is to assure the availability of current instrumentation needed for the care of the patient. The institution setting itself before the public and purporting to have proper facilities has a similar duty.

COMPUTERS
(Also See Ch. 6)

There are three areas in which computers can be of value in anesthesiology. First is the ready availability of medical information. Second is the interrelationship of patient monitoring data with anesthesiologic input data (servoanesthesia), and third is the administrative booking process (assignment of anesthesia personnel). The legal concerns related to medical information primarily lie with confidentiality and privacy issues. The development of servoanesthesia raises problems of standards of care. The last process (ministerial) includes the hazard of remoteness in consideration of case assignment, whether of attending anesthesiologist, resident, or nurse and requires a consideration of the competency of the assignee, the potential needs of the patient and surgeon.[66]

NEW TECHNIQUES AND APPLICATION

Recently, the use of epidural and subarachnoid opiates alone or in combination with local anesthetic agents has been demonstrated to provide segmental pain relief.[67] The main advantage of this technique is the production of analgesia with little or no effect on voluntary motor or sympathetic function (also see Chs. 31 & 60). Food and Drug Administration rules related to pharmacologic agents should be consulted and specifically to the concept of new uses of already approved drugs.[68] Specifically, should this technique be used by the clinician when it has not been approved by the FDA? Such approval is not required if a select community of experts supported by scientific evidence and literature sources recognize the drug and/or use as an acceptable one. Note that the "newness" is not relative to age, in relation to other agents, but to a status of recognition among the select community of experts.[69] In addition, both the safety and efficacy must be demonstrated.[70]

However, a drug that is "generally recognized as safe and effective" (GRASE) is by virtue of that legal status outside the statutory definition of a new drug.[71] Familiarity and recognition are the keys to GRASE status.[72]

It is important to keep in mind the ambiguities and medicolegal burdens implicit in the statement of the FDA[73] regarding "Use of Approved Drugs for Unlabeled Indications":

The appropriateness or the legality of prescribing approved drugs for uses not included in their official labeling is sometimes a cause of concern and confusion among practitioners.

Under the Federal Food, Drug, and Cosmetic (FD&C) Act, a drug approved for marketing may be labeled, promoted, and advertised by the manufacturer only for those uses for which the drug's safety and effectiveness have been established and which FDA has approved. These are commonly referred to as "approved uses". This means that adequate and well-controlled clinical trials have documented these uses, and the results of the trials have been reviewed and approved by FDA.

The FD&C Act does not, however, limit the manner in which a physician may use an approved drug. Once a product has been approved for marketing, a physician may prescribe it for uses or in treatment regimens or patient populations that are not included in approved labeling. Such "unapproved" or, more precisely, "unlabeled" uses may be appropriate and rational in certain circumstances, and may, in fact, reflect approaches to drug therapy that have been extensively reported in medical literature.

The term "unapproved uses" is, to some extent, misleading. It includes a variety of situations ranging from unstudied to thoroughly investigated drug uses. Valid new uses for drugs already on the market are often first discovered through serendipitous observations and therapeutic innovations, subsequently confirmed by well-planned and executed clinical investigations. Before such advances can be added to the approved labeling, however, data substantiating the effectiveness of a new use or regimen must be submitted by the manufacturer to FDA for evaluation. This may take time and, without the initiative of the drug manufacturer whose product is involved, may never occur. For that reason, accepted medical practice often includes drug use that is not reflected in approved drug labeling.

With respect to its role in medical practice, the package insert is informational only. FDA tries to assure that prescription drug information in the package insert accurately and fully reflects the data on safety and effectiveness on which drug approval is based.

ADMINISTRATION

RISK MANAGEMENT

There is one area of potential liability that has not yet hit the health care professions. This area is the practice, even a tradition, of working on-call physicians for what may be considered unconscionable hours. Surgical or anesthesia personnel do work 24 hours at a stretch with no time off to rest. Risk management professionals have been decrying this practice to no avail. Despite clear and convincing data demonstrating the decrease in efficiency and even hazardous conduct resulting from sheer exhaustion, the medical profession refuses to face the problem realistically.[74]

Law follows principles of *stare decisus* otherwise called case law precedent. While there are no medically related cases as yet, analogous decisions do exist. One of the more recent cases comes from the Supreme Court of West Virginia.[75]

In this case the employer required the employee to work 27 hours. The employee subsequently injured a third party while driving home. The court allowed the injured party to bring suit against the employer and allowed recovery on the basis of reasonable foreseeability of risk. This important case has recently been cited by both majority and dissenting justices of the Texas Supreme Court[76] in an analogous situation of the employee who is impaired by alcohol (or drugs). The duty of the employer to abstain from causing an unreasonable risk of harm to others (third parties) is being progressively imposed on the basis of the new court ruling:

> When because of an employee's incapacity, an employer exercises (or fails to exercise) control over the employee, the employer has a duty to take such action as a reasonably prudent employer under the same or similar circumstances would take to prevent the employee from causing an unreasonable risk of harm to others.

Here, the court addressed the issue of proximate cause (one of the four prerequisites for liability based on negligence). Their conclusion was that if the company could have "reasonably anticipated" that an accident would result, a jury could find that the employing company's negligence and not the employee's was the "proximate cause" of the accident. As the "duty" owed (another critical criterion of negligence), the court traced the history of tort law and quoted a 100-year-old case suggesting that there was an "original moral duty" to avoid conduct that might cause injury to anyone at all. The question to be answered is only how long it will take for the legal profession to use this expanding concept to hold hospitals responsible for the "therapeutic misadventures" of exhausted house officers and other employees.

ANESTHESIA PRIVILEGES

Hospitals have been held responsible for the quality of medical care since the landmark cases of *Bing* v. *Thunig*[77] and *Darling* v. *Charleston Community Memorial Hospital.*[78] This concept of corporate liability applies no less to the anesthesia department through its administratively approved chairman. The chairman's ministerial duties include specific delineation of anesthesia privileges. This was further outlined as a corporate responsibility in *Johnson* v. *Miseracordia Community Hospital,*[79] in which the court found a duty to screen physicians appointed to the medical staff carefully before appointment and to limit clinical privileges to procedures physician are competent to do. This duty is a continuing responsibility[80] requiring periodic review.

PEER REVIEW

Social responsibility is the recognition of our relationships and interactions with members of our culture. For the professional, this responsibility includes an overview of the work of our coprofessionals. In the terminology of regulative agencies this means peer review. The basic function is to ensure the quality of care that our specialty provides to our patients. This is accomplished by review of the actions of colleagues with regard to continuing education and the application of current and developing concepts to our clinical practice for the benefit of each individual patient as well as society. This latter society includes the profession of medicine.

Many physicians have avoided this responsibility because of the fear of litigation. This fear is not unfounded. We are living in a litigious era in which people sue for not obtaining what one prominent U.S. senator calls "the right to health." This has been most apparent in Good Samaritan legislation[81] of early times and in the current drive for protective peer review statutes.[82]

Our ethical and moral obligation clearly is to provide oversight for the conduct of our profession. Yet, we must be free to conduct our deliberations free of the Damoclean Sword of lawsuits for defamation. "Defamation is that which tends to injure reputation . . . to diminish esteem, respect, goodwill or confidence . . . to excite adverse, derogatory or unpleasant feelings or opinions . . . or to deter persons from associating or dealing."[83] The publication which transmits this result may be by action, oral or written means. This communication is that which the recipient correctly or mistakenly but reasonably understands it was intended to express.[84] In practicality it really does not matter whether the lawsuit is successful. The mere filing of the lawsuit leads to such publicity and emotional reactions as to serve as an inhibition of the willingness of professionals to serve voluntarily on peer review committees. Thus the real purpose of such protective statutes is to encourage top-quality individuals to serve and to discourage punitive or threatening action by the individuals being reviewed.

RECORDS

The professional often looks on record-keeping as an annoyance, inconvenience, and imposition. In fact, anesthesia records perform two major functions. First and foremost, they show the evaluative factors trends and course of the anesthetic period. Second, they serve as a memorialization of the medical considerations, for teaching and research, and for subsequent review if needed. They are legal documents. Who owns the record? Who has a right of access? Is this information admissible as evidence?

Most courts take the view that the medical record is physically the work product of the hospital and its agents (implied or real) and as such belongs to the institution. The hospital requires record keeping under a mandate of the Joint Commission on Accreditation of Hospitals. The format, rules and regulations of record keeping are prescribed by the records committee of the respective medical staff. They are then stored under the aegis of the medical record librarian.

The medical record, to fall under the "business record" exception to the hearsay rule of evidence, must be made during the regular course of business activity. One court[85] stated that medical records are admissible as business records pursuant to the Uniform Business Records Act if the following criteria are met:

1. **It was made contemporaneously with the events it purports to relate**
2. **At the time it was prepared it was impossible to anticipate reasons for making a false entry**
3. **The person responsible for the statements contained in the report is known.**

On the other hand, the information in the medical record is considered to be the property of the patient. It is subject to the legal expectation of confidentiality, and other privacy rights.[86]

SPECIAL PROBLEMS

RELIGIOUS INFLUENCES

Another area of interest encompasses the influence of religious beliefs held by groups such as Jehovah's Witnesses and Christian Scientists. The First Amendment of the Constitution assures all citizens freedom of religious beliefs. The courts have diligently protected this inalienable right in many areas of our society (e.g., medical practice, education, service in the armed forces) to the extent that this is consistent with the public health and welfare. The classic situation is refusal of immunization prior to entry into school,[87] where the court held that the societal interest in protecting the public health outweighed the individual's First Amendment rights.

The Jehovah's Witnesses' (Watchtower Bible and Tract Society) admonition forbidding administration of blood and blood products is of particular concern to the anesthesia practitioner (also see Ch. 39). This admonition is founded on biblical text.[88] Justice Cardozo's decision in *Schloendorff* v. *Society of New York Hospital*[89] and the prior Mohr case,[90] stated the proposition that the patient has the sole right of determination as to what shall be done with his or her own body:

> Under a free government, at least, the free citizen's greatest right, which underlies all others — the right to the inviolability of his person, in other words, the right to his person is subject to universal acquiesence, and this right necessarily forbids a physician or surgeon, however skillful or eminent . . . to violate, without permission, the bodily integrity of his patient. . . .

There are only limited exceptions centered on the State's interest in life or the rights of innocent third parties.[91]

The pediatric patient presents a somewhat different situation. The courts stress the public policy interest in the welfare of children who cannot speak for themselves (i.e., legally) and, on application, will assume jurisdiction in *loco parentis* (charged with a parent's rights, duties, and responsibilities) and provide a substituted judgment (putting the court's judgment in the place and position of the child's). The trend exacerbated by current attention to the battered child syndrome is to consider parents as only guardians of the child, acting in a fiduciary capacity. Thus, on request to the court, orders directing blood transfusion to minors are available.[92] A finding of neglect can also be followed by a court order for custody and treatment.

Two other cases are of note. In one case, the court appointed a guardian to authorize surgery for a severely handicapped newborn who with surgery had a chance for a relatively normal lifespan.[93] In the other case,[94] the court intervened to order chemotherapy for a child whose parents had stated they would not pursue that alternative, even though it only might save the child's life. The courts generally intervene when the life or health of a minor is at stake.

NO CODE AND THE LIVING WILL

Very few areas have produced as much soul searching as that of "no code" orders. The anesthesiologist may be part of this determina-

tion in "last chance" surgical situations. The enigma for the anesthesiologist arises when requested to be responsible for anesthetic management in a patient for whom a "no code" or a "living will" is in effect. To date, the appellate literature has a dearth of cases exactly *en pointe*. Most have been drawn from discontinuation of therapy.

The Dinnerstein case[95] is of such great importance that it must be discussed in depth. Here the attending physician recommended entry of a no code order on a terminally ill patient. The court held that attempts to resuscitate would do nothing to cure or relieve the illnesses "which will have brought the patient to the threshold of death" (Dinnerstein, at 139). Life-saving and life-prolonging treatments are defined by this court (Dinnerstein, at 137–138) as

> Treatments administered for the purpose and with some reasonable expectation, of effecting a permanent or temporary cure of or relief from the illness or condition being treated . . . not . . . a mere suspension of the act of dying, but . . . at the very least, a remission of symptoms enabling a return towards a normal, functioning integrated existence.

The court concluded that this case "presents a question peculiarly within the competence of the medical profession . . . subject to court review only to the extent that it may be contended that he has failed to exercise the degree of care and skill of the average qualified practitioner, *taking into account the advances in the profession*" (emphasis supplied) (Dinnerstein, at 139). Thus, we see judicial recognition of the place of the medical practitioner limited primarily by "taking into account the advances of the profession." This latter clause places on the physician the burden of determining whether those advances provide sufficient hope for "at the very least, a remission of symptoms enabling a return towards a normal functioning, integrated existence" (Dinnerstein, at 138).

The practice of triage similarly raises questions of legal, ethical, and moral deference. Triage as to equipment and bed availability exerts significant if sub rosa influence. Considering the economy and governmental (political) stress on costs of medical care, as well as the sparsity of facilities, the choice of admitting a "no code" patient to a high-technology special care unit may appear to be anachronistic.[96] Yet refusing the patient admission may be a failure of the duty to meet the standard of care required. The patient is also frequently sought after as a potential organ donor. The balance or conflict of interests (ethical, social, moral) raises great concern, yet the courts have skirted this aspect of critical care to date. Since the law addresses primarily the rights of the individual, the standard of care applied may relate only to the best interests of the specific patient. A first-come, first-serve approach meets the standard. It does not consider the cost-effective relationships of triage. When we discuss costs we must include personnel, training time, and study factors. Perhaps we need to extend ICU-type care to the ward or "floor" situations. This would mean a reversal of the concept that floor care is essentially custodial, and a reversion to prior concepts of special duty nursing care. Modern medicine has already taken a step in this direction with the establishment of inter-mediate care units. The legal approach for the individual is that he must receive that level of attention which is responsive to needs of that patient. Morally, triage is questionably acceptable considering the needs of the patient within the context of cost–benefit ratio (the "cost" of providing care counterbalanced against the benefit probability). The moral question addresses the value of one human being's life and health as measured against another's — or that of the group.

The legislature traditionally addresses group interests in statute. Similarly, the judiciary (or, at least, the trial court) protects the individual while considering the public as a whole. An example is the refusal of smallpox immunization on the basis of religion (individual constitutional protection of religious freedom), which the courts have determined as not being absolute when balanced against the constitutional mandate for government to protect the general societal health and welfare.[97] Usually the courts will protect the individual right, as it did in *Kolbeck v. Kramer.*[98]

How do we establish a no code? This decision is no longer in the sole traditional province of the physician. The classic criteria are ex-

pressed in *Orders Not to Resuscitate* by Rabkin, Gillerman, and Rice (see Appendix B).

Of particular note is the view that the same principle would compel physicians to honor the refusal of an incompetent patient to consent to further livesaving care, if such current refusal is consistent with earlier refusals made before the onset of incompetence.[99] In substance, Dinnerstein lays down clear criteria, legally defensible, limited to and consistent with extant medical practice standards. We must emphasize that in most jurisdictions following the decision of the New York Supreme Court in Matter of Eichner,[100] "no code" orders may be written without judicial preapproval in appropriate cases.

The issue still to be decided is the obligation of the physician who in good conscience cannot or will not accept a "no code" order whether based on a living will or other directive. Our experience suggests withdrawing from the case but this is not always possible. However, the respecting of the ethical and especially the moral integrity of the medical profession is not to be discarded lightly. Are we in fact discarding the ultimate duty to prevent suffering and preserve life so long mandated by our codes of ethics (Hammurabi, Hippocrates, Maimonides)? Are we in fact generating a philosophy prostituting our time-honored tradition to unceasingly strive to preserve life, limb, and vital organ?

CONCLUSION

We have presented herein some of the most important medicolegal problems of the time. Our objective has been to indicate areas of potential liability and trends in the law. The reader should be aware of changes in the law — that "the law" is a vibrant constantly developing expression of society's interests, and the implications and inferences to be drawn for the modern practitioner of anesthesia.

REFERENCES

1. Hippocratic Oath—not a single code, found in several books, Greek, 4th–5th century BC
2. Code of Maimonides, Judaic Codex, Moshe ben Maimon 1135–1204 Mishneh Torah
3. Code of Hammurabi—King of Babylon, 20th century BC, found in Persia
4. Protection of Human Subjects, Policies and Procedures HEW, National Institute of Health, 38 CFR 221, Nov. 16, 1973, as amended; see also Nuremberg Code: Trials of War Criminals before the Nuremberg Military Tribunals under Control Council No. 10, vol 2, 1947, pp 181–182
5. Code of Helsinki, 18th World Medical Assembly, Helsinki, Finland, 1964, and as revised by 29th World Medical Assembly, Tokyo, Japan, 1975; Norton ML: When does an experimental innovative procedure become an accepted procedure? Pharos 38:4 161, 1975
6. TEFRA: P.L. 97–248, Tax Equity and Fiscal Responsibility
7. *Linder v. United States*, 268 US 5, 1925
8. Norton ML: Medical staff law and bylaws, Int Soc Barristers 17:4, 401, 1983
9. Thompson MJ: Antitrust and the Health Care Provider. Aspen Systems Corp, 1979, pp 154–157
10. Peters JD, Fineburg KS, Kroll DA, et al: Anesthesiology and the Law. Ann Arbor, Mich, Health Administration Press, 1983)
11. *Lenny v. Munroe, Fla.*, (Broward County Circuit Court, No. 82–1296 CM, June 15, 1983)
12. Higdon JH: Medical/legal status of consultants. J Legal Med 35: 1976; and Holder A: Duty to consult. JAMA 225: 135, 1974
13. Simpson LP: Contracts. 2nd ed West, 1965
14. *Czubinsky v. Doctor's Hospital*, 188 Cal Rptr 685 (Ct App 1983).
15. *Canterbury v. Spence*, 464 F2d (DC Cir), cert denied 409 US 1064 (1972), and *Wilkinson v. Vesey* (110 RI 606 (1972)
16. *Martha Logan v. Greenwich Hospital Association et al.* Connecticut Supreme Court, No. 10969, Sept 6, 1983
17. *Sidaway v. Board of Governors of Bethlem Royal Hospital*, Court of Appeal, The Times Law Reports 24:24, 1984
18. *Harnish v. Childrens Hospital Medical Center*, 439 NE2d 240 (1982) Washington D.C.
19. *Logan v. Greenwich Hospital Association*, Conn. Supreme Court No. 10969, Sept. 6, 1983

20. *De Haan v. Winter*, 258 Mich 293, 241, NW 923 (1932); *Buchanan v. Kull*, 323 Mich 381, 35 NW2d 351 (1949)
21. Caffee BE: What you don't know will hurt you: Physician's duty to warn patients about newly discovered dangers in previously initiated treatment. Cleve State LR 31:649, 1982
22. Id.
23. *Moultrie v. Medical University of South Carolina*, No. 22030, South Carolina Supreme Court, Jan 18, 1984
24. Lunn JN, Mushin WW: Mortality associated with Anaesthesia, London, Nuffield Provincial Hospitals Trust, 1982; MacIntosh RR: Death under anaesthetics. Br J Anaesth 21:107, 1948; Lunn JN: The role of mortality studies, Quality of Care in Anaesthetic Practice. Edited by Lunn JN. Basingstoke; Macmillan, 1983; Lunn JN, Hunter AR, Scott DB: Anesthesia-related surgical mortality. Anaesthesia 38: 1090, 1983; Report on Confidential Enquiries Into Maternal Deaths in England and Wales 1976–1978, Dept. of Health and Social Security, Report on Health and Social Subjects, RHSS26, HMSO
25. *Williams v. St. Clare Medical Center*, 657 SW2d 590 (Ky App 1983)
26. *Supra*, 8
27. Norton ML: When does an experimental/innovative procedure become an accepted procedure? Pharos 38(4): 161, 1975 (and supra, 5)
28. Warren WL, Brandeis L: The right to privacy, Harvey Lect 4: 193, 1890
29. *Bazemore v. Savannah Hosp*, 171 Ga 257, 155 SE 194 (1930); Prosser, W. Handbook of the Law of Torts 139, 802–818 (4th ed. 1971)
30. *Melvin v. Reid*, 112 Cal App 285, 297 P 91 (1931)
31. *Shorter v Retail Co.*, DCSC, 251 F Supp. 329, 330 (1966)
32. *McGulpin v. Bessemer*, 241 Iowa 119, 43 NW2d 121 (1950); *Lee v. Dembre*, 362 SW2d 900 (Tex Civ App 1962); *Ascher v. Guttierrez*, 533 F2d 1235 (DC Cir 1976)
33. *Prack v. U.S. Fidelity and Guaranty Co.*, 1870 So 2d 170 (La App 1966); *Alimchandani v. Goings*, 39 Md App 353, 386 A2d 789 (1978); see also *Ascher v. Guttierrez*, 533 F2d 1235 (DC Cir 1976). This landmark case of blatant abandonment by the anesthesiologist elucidated the key principles of medical abandonment and the method by which a physician may withdraw from a case
34. ASA: Basic Guidelines for Anesthesia Care, American Society of Anesthesiologists Directory of Members, 48th ed, 1983, p 467; see also JCAH Standards, Sec. 7.81
35. Cullen BF, Cullen SC: Postanesthetic complications. Su Clin North Am 55:987 1975

36. *Pederson v. Dumouchel*, 72 Wash2d 73, 431 P2d 973 (1967)
37. Black's Law Dictionary, 5th ed., West, 1979
38. *Kosberg v. Washington Hospital Center, Inc.*, 129 US App DC 322, 394 F2d 947, 949
39. *United States v. Greenbaum*, 138 F2d 437, 438 (1943)
40. *Helfend v. Southern Cal. Rapid Transit Disc. Helfend v. Southern Cal. Rapid Transit Disc.*, 2 Cal3d, 1, 465 P2d 61, 84 Cal Rptr 173 (1970)
41. *Foster v. Englewood Hosp. Assn.*, 19 Ill App3d 1055, 313 NE2d 255 (1974); *Sesselman v. Muhlenberg Hosp.* 124 NJ Super 285, 306 A2d 474 (1973); *Sparger v. Worley Hosp. Inc.*, 547 SW2d 582 (Tex 1977)
42. *Spannans v. Otolaryngology Clinic*, 308 Minn 334, 242 NW2d 594 (1976); *Marvulle v. Elshire*, 27 Cal App 3d 180, 103 Cal Rptr 461 (1972)
43. Comments of the Bureau of Competition, Bureau of Consumer Protection and Bureau of Economics, Federal Trade Commission, to the Board of Licensing Health Care Facilities of the State of Tennessee, FTC. Release, Nov. 19, 1983
44. Sec. 5 of the Federal Trade Commission Act, 15 U.S.C. Sec. 45
45. State Volunteer Mutual Insurance Co., FTC Docket No. C-3115 (Sept. 28, 1983); see also An Analysis of the Revised Medical Staff Standards of the Joint Commission on Accreditation of Hospitals, Office of Legal and Regulatory Affairs and American Academy of Hospital Attorneys; American Hospital Association, March 1984
46. DC Law 5-48, Feb. 28, 1984
47. Colo Rev Stat Sec 12-38-209 (1) (c) (1978); Ariz Rev Stat Ann Sec 32-1602 (Supp. 1980)
48. Ark Stat Ann Sec 72-745 (1979); La Dept of Health and Human Resources Bd of Nursing Rules Sec RN 3.043 (1981); Mich Comp Laws Ann Sec 333-17210, (1980); 244 Code Mass Reg Sec's 4.11 (4), 4.12 (1) (1979)
49. Thatcher VS: History of Anesthesia, With Emphasis on the Nurse Specialist. Philadelphia, JB Lippincott, 1953, p 54
50. Exodus I:15, Pentateuch
51. Flexner A: Medical Education in the U.S. and Canada. Bull No 4. New York, Carnegie Foundation for the Advancement of Teaching, 1910
52. Final Board approved version—Item #4, 4/23/82
53. Cal Bus & Prof Code Sec's. 2746 *et seq* (1980); 16 Cal Admin Code Sec's. 1461 *et seq* (1979); La Dept Health and Human Resources, Bd of Nursing, RN 3.042, Mass GL Ann ch 112 & 80 C&D, Supp 1980, and 244 Code Mass Req & 4.21; 12 NJ Req Sec's 13:35-13:91 *et seq* (1980) Mich C L Ann 333.17210 and 333.17201; Ga Rules, Bd of Nursing, ch.410-12-01
54. American Society of Law and Medicine and the Center for Health Law Studies of the St. Louis University School of Law: Conference on Regulation of, and Hospital Privileges for, Health Care Providers, Nov 10-12, 1983
55. Sherman Anti-Trust Act. Sec. 1
56. P.L. 97-248, Tax Equity and Fiscal Responsibility
57. 48 Fed Register, 42, 8929, Cal 1 & 2 Wed, Mar 2, 1983, Rules and Regulations
58. 48 Fed Register, 42, 8929, Col 2, (shared servant, borrowed servant doctrines) and in section 1801 of the Act "facetiously" forbids interference in the practice of medicine
59. *Elam v. College Park Hosp.*, Ct App, 4th App District, Div One, State of Calif 4 Civ No 24479; June 25, 1982.
60. *Williams v. Griffin*, 35 Mich App 179, 192 NW2d 283, 285 (1971)
61. *Collins v. Haud* 431 Pa 378, 246 A2d 398 (1968); *Grubb v. Albert Einstein Medical Center*, 255 Pa Super Ct 381, 387 A2d 480 (1778)
62. *Czubinsky v. Doctors Hospital*, 188 Cal Rptr 685 (Ct App 1983); see also *Mason v. Lodi Community Hospital, Cal.*, San Joaquin County Superior Court, No. 165743 Aug 24, 1983
63. *Block v. Neal*, cert to US Court of Appeals, 6th Cir, No. 81-1494, March 7, 1983; see also *United Scottish Insurance v. U.S.A.*, No. 81-5062, October 8, 1982, and *Varig Airlines v. U.S.A.*, US Court of Appeals, 9th Circ, No 181-5366, 1982
64. Morrison R: Grounding and Shielding Techniques in Instrumentation. 2nd ed. New York, Wiley, 1977
65. The T.J. Hooper, 60 F2d 737 (2nd Cir) 1932; *cert denied* 287 US 662, 77 L Ed 571, 53 S Ct 220 (1932)
66. Brown ACD: Development of an On-Line Surgeon—Specific Operating Room Time Prediction System, as presented at the Eighth Annual Symposium on Computer Applications in Medical Care., Washington Hilton, Washington, D.C., November 4-7, 1984; Brown ACD: A Computer Generated Aid for Scheduling Operating Rooms, as presented at the American Association For Medical Systems Informatics Congress, May 1984, San Francisco, California; McQuarrie DG: Limits to efficient operating room scheduling. Arch Surg 116:1065, 1981; Brown ACD: Computer management of operating room time information with proposed standards definitions for the measurement of utilization. 6th Annual Symposium on Computer Applications in Medical Care, Blum BL (ed). Computer Soc. Press, 1982
67. Lanz E, Theiss D, Riess W, et al: Epidural morphine for postoperative analgesia: A double-

bind study. Anesth Analg 61:236, 1982; Knill RL, Clement JL, Thompson WR: Epidural morphine causes delayed and prolonged ventilatory depression. Can Anaesth Soc J 28:537, 1981; Gustafsson LL, Schildt B, Jacobsen K: Adverse effects of extradural and intrathecal opiates: Report of a nationwide survey in Sweden. Br J Anaesth 54:479, 1982; Brownridge P: Epidural and intrathecal opiates for postoperative pain relief. Anaesthesia 38:74, 1983; Brownridge P, Wrobel J, Watt-Smith J: Respiratory depression following accidental subarachnoid pethidine. Anaesth Intens Care 11:237, 1983; Cohen SE, Rothblatt AJ, Albright GA: Early respiratory depression with epidural narcotic and intravenous droperidol. Anesthesiology 59:559, 1983

68. Federal Food, Drug and Cosmetic Act, 21 USC Sec 331–337, 371–372, as amended, and 21 U.S.C. 355 (Note: the "newness" may arise from a new use of an old drug.)

69. Generic Drugs: Breaking the Definitional Barriers to FDA Regulations. 76 NW UhL Rev 613 (1981); McConachie: Marketing Generic Drugs without FDA Approval? Pharm Tech 6:76, 1982; see also *U.S. v. Generic Drug Co.*, -US-, 103 S Ct 1298 (1983)

70. 1962 Drug Amendments Publ No. 87-781, 76 Stat 780, 87th Cong 2nd Session (1962); 21 USC Sects 355

71. 21 USC Sec. 321 (p)

72. Food Drug and Cosmetic Act at 1326 (1983) and *Newport Pharmaceutical International Inc.* v. *Schweiber*, Food Drug Cos L Rep (CCH) par 38148 (DDC 1981)

73. FDA Drug Bull 12(1):3–4, 1982

74. Cooper JB: Avoiding Preventable Mishaps, in ASA Annual Refresher Course Lectures 201, 1980; see also Cooper et al: Preventable anesthesia mishaps: A study of human factors. Anesthesiology 49:399, 1978; Cooper, JB, Long CD, Newhower RS, et al: Multi-hospital study of preventable anesthesia mishaps. Anesthesiology 51:S348, 1979

75. *Robertson v. LeMaster*, W Va St Ct No 15543, March 24, 1983; 301 SE2d 563 (1983)

76. *Otis Engineering Corp.* v. *Clark*, Texas Supreme Court, Docket No. C-1227, November 30, 1983

77. *Bing v. Thunig*, 143 NE2d 3 (NY 1957)

78. *Darling* v. *Charleston Community Memorial Hospital*, 211 NE32d 253 (Ill 1965)

79. *Johnson* v. *Miseracordia Community Hospital*, 294 NE2d 501 (Wis App 1980), affd, 301 NW2d 156 (Wis 1981)

80. *Elam v. College Park Hospital*, 183 Rptr 156 (Cal App 1982)

81. Good Samaritan Laws: Mass GLA. 112S 12B and

E; Mich CLA. 691.1501 and .1502; see also Matts in Homsi, 308 NW2d 284, 106 Mich App 563 (1981)

82. *Coburn v. Seda and Kadlec Hospital*, Wash State Sup Ct, No 49549-1, Feb. 23, 1984

83. Black's Law Dictionary, 5th edition; see also *McGowan v. Prentice*, La App, 341 So2d 55, 57 (1977)

84. Restatement, 2nd, Torts, Sec's. 559, 563

85. *Sauro v. Shea*, 257 Pa 66, 390 A2d 259 (1978)

86. *Gaertner v. State of Michigan*, 385 Mich 49, 187 NW2d 429 (1971) *Rabens v. Jackson Park Hosp. Foundations*, 41 Ill App3d. 113, 351 NE2d 276, (1976)

87. *Prince v. Commonwealth*, 321 US 158, 166-167 (1943)

88. Genesis 9:3,4; Leviticus 3:17, 17:10, 17:13, 14, Deuteronomy 12:23–25, I Samuel 14:32, 33 (King James Version)

89. *Schloendorff* v. *Society of New York Hospital*, 211 NY 125, 101 NE 92 (1914)

90. *Mohr v. Williams*, 95 Minn 261, 104 NW 12, 14 (1905)

91. *Superintendent of Belchertown State School* v. *Saikowitz*, 373 Mass 728, 370 NE2d 417 (1977); In Re: Osborn 294 A2d 372 (DC Circ 1972); and *Holmes* v. *Silver Cross Hospital*, 340 F Supp. 125 (ED Ill 1972)

92. In re: Levy 319 So2d 52 (Fla App 1975); *Santos v. Goldstein* 16 AD2d 755, 227 NYS2d 450, *app dismissed* 12 NYS2d 642, 232 NYS2d 465, 185 NE2d 904 (1962); see also Application of Brooklyn Hospital, 45 Misc2d 914, 258, NYS2d 621 (1965). In People ex. rel. *Wallace v. Labrenz*, 411 Ill 618, 104 NE2d 769, *cert denied* 344 US 824, 97 L Ed. 2d 647, 73 S Ct 24 (1952)

93. Application of Cicero 101 Misc2d 699, 421 NYS2d 955 (1979)

94. Custody of a Minor 375 Mass 733, 279 NE2d 1053 (1978); 393 NE2d 836 (Mass 1979). (Chad Green case)

95. In re: Matter of Dinnerstein, 6 Mass App 466, 380 NE2d 134 (1978): criticized as overboard in Matter of Spring, 399 NE2d 493, 497 (1979) rev'd. on other grounds 405 NE2d 115 (1980)

96. Optimum care of hopelessly ill patients. N Engl J Med 295:362, 1976

97. *Supra*, 87

98. *Kolbeck v. Kramer*, 84 NJ Super 569, 202 A2d 889 (1964)

99. In re: Estate of Brooks, 32 Ill2d 361, 205 NE 435 (1965) and In re: Maeda Yetter, 62 PaD and C2d 619 (1973)

100. In Matter of *Eichner v. Dillon*, 73 App Div2d 431, 426 NYS2d 517 (1980); mod (1981) 52 NY2d 363, 438 NYS2d 266, 420 NE2d 64 (1981)

Appendix A
Glossary of Terms

Abandonment: To constitute abandonment by conduct, action . . . must be positive, unequivocal, and inconsistent with the existence of the contract, and implies not only nonperformance, but an intent not to perform which may be inferred from acts which necessarily point to actual abandonment.

> *Lohn* v. *Fletcher Dil Co,* 38 Cal App2d 26, 100 P2d 505, 507, (1940)

Agency: The fiduciary relationship that results from the manifestation of consent by one person to another that the other shall act on his behalf and subject to his control and consent by the other to so act.

> Restatement, Second, Agency Sec. 1.

Agency by estoppel: One created by operation of law and established by proof of such acts of the principal as reasonably leads to the conclusion of its existence.

> Black's Law Dictionary, 5th ed., West, 1979

Burden of proof: Used to mean either the necessity of establishing a fact, that is, the burden of persuasion, or the necessity of making a prima facie showing, that is the burden of going forward.

> *State Farm Life Insurance Co.* v. *Smith,* 29 Ill App3d, 942, 331 NE2d 275, 280 (1975)

Duty: The obligation to conduct oneself in a particular manner at the risk that if he does not do so he becomes subject to liability to another to whom the duty is owed for any injury sustained by such other, of which that actors conduct is a legal cause.

> Restatement, Second, Torts Sec. 4

Guardian: A person lawfully invested with the power, and charged with the duty of taking care of the person . . . and rights of another person, who, for defect of age, understanding or self control, is considered incapable of administering his own affairs.

> Black's Law Dictionary, 5th ed., West, 1979

Hearsay: Evidence not proceeding from the personal knowledge of the witness, but from the mere repetition of what he has heard others say. That which does not derive its value solely from the credit of the witness, but rests mainly on the veracity and competency of other persons; not generally admissable under rules of evidence.

> Black's Law Dictionary, 5th ed., West, 1979

Incompetency: A relative term employed to show lack of physical or intellectual fitness, incapacity, the quality or state of being incapable.

> *Bole* v. *Civil City of Ligonier,* 130 Ind App 362, 161 NE2d 189, 194 (1959)

Independent contractor: One who renders service in the course of independent employment or occupation, and, who follows employer's desires only as to results of work, and not as to means whereby it is to be accomplished.

> *Sparks* v. *L.D. Folsom Co.,* 217 Cal App2d 279, 31 Cal Rptr 640, 643 (1963)
> *Housewright* v. *Pacific Far East Line Inc.,* 229 Cal App2d, 259, 40 Cal Rptr 208, 212 (1964)

Joint and several: A liability is said to be joint and several when the plaintiff may sue one or more of the parties to such liability separately, or all of them together at his option.

> Black's Law Dictionary, 5th ed., West, 1979

Material: That which tends to influence . . . because of its logical connection with the issue . . . and which by itself or in connection with other evidence is determinative of the case.
> *Camurati* v. *Sutton,* 48 Tenn App 54, 342 SW2d 732, 739 (1961)

Ostensible agency: One which exists where the principal intentionally or by want of ordinary care causes a third person to believe another to be his agent who is not really employed by him.
> Black's Law Dictionary, 5th ed., West, 1979

Prima facie: A fact presumed to be true unless disproved by some evidence to the contrary.
> *State* ex rel. *Herbert* v. *Whims,* 69 Ohio App 39, 38 NE2d 596, 599, (1941).

Proximate cause: That which, in a natural and continuous sequence, unbroken by any efficient intervening cause, produces injury, and without which the result would not have occurred.
> *Wisniewski* v. *Great Atlantic & Pac. Tea Co.,* 226 Pa Super 574, 323 A2d 744, 747, 748 (1974)

Publication: To bring before the public, to exhibit, display, disclose or reveal.
> *Tiffany Productions* v. *Dewing,* DC Md, 50 F2d 911, 914 (1931)

Respondeat superior: Let the master answer —master is responsible for want of care on servant's part toward those to whom master owes a duty of care, provided failure of servant to use such care occurred in course of his employment and legitimate scope of authority.
> *Shell Petroleum Corp.* v. *Magnolia Pipe Line Co.,* Tex CV App, 85 SW2d 829, 832 (1935) *Rogers* v. *Town Black Mountain,* 224 NC 119, 29 SE2d, 203, 205 (1944)

Stare Decisus: Doctrine that states that when a court has once laid down a principal of law as applicable to a certain state of facts, it will adhere to that principle and apply to all future cases, where facts are substantially the same.
> *Horne* v. *Moody,* Tex. CV App, 146 SW2d 505, 509 (1940)

Voir dire: The preliminary examination which the court may make of one presented as a witness . . . where his competency, interest, etc., is objected to.
> Black's Law Dictionary, 5th ed., West, 1979

Appendix B
Orders Not to Resuscitate

Rabkin
Gillerman
Rice

Reprinted, by permission of The New England Journal of Medicine, 295: 364, 1976.

1. Both as a standard of medical care and as a statement of philosophy, it is the general policy of hospitals to act affirmatively to preserve the life of all patients, including persons who suffer from irreversible terminal illness. It is essential that all hospital staff understand this policy and act accordingly.

2. As a matter of policy, hospitals also respect the competent patient's informed acceptance or rejection of treatment, including cardiopulmonary resuscitation, and recognize that in certain cases, the unwanted use of heroic measures on a patient irreversibly and irreparably terminally ill might be both medically unsound and so contrary to the patient's wishes or expectations as not to be justified.

3. The initial medical judgement on such question should be made by the primary responsible physician for the patient after discussion with an ad hoc committee consisting not only of the other physicians attending the patient and the nurses and others directly active in the care of the patient, but at least one other senior staff physician not previously involved in the patient's care.

4. Even if a medical judgement is reached that a patient faces with such an illness and imminence of death that resuscitation is medically inappropriate, the decision to withold resuscitation (Orders Not to Resuscitate, "ONTR") will become effective only upon the informed choice of a competent patient or, with an incompetent patient, by strict adherence to the guidelines discussed below, and then only to the extent that all appropriate family members are in agreement with the views of the involved staff.

a. the decision for Orders Not to Resuscitate and its accompanying consent by the competent patient or the appropriate family members should be recorded promptly in the medical chart.

b. a summary of the staff discussion and decision. . . .

c. the disclosures to the patient, which must include the elements of informed consent, the patient's response, the responsible physician's documentation of the patient's competence. . . .

d. the patient's decision to inform appropriate family members and the resulting discussion with them that may then follow.

e. It is the responsibility of the physician to convey the meaning of the Orders Not to Resuscitate to all medical, nursing and other staff as appropriate, and simultaneously, to insist upon being notified immediately if the patient's condition should change so the orders seem no longer applicable.

f. After the issuing of Orders Not to Resuscitate, the patient's course, including continued evaluation of competence and consent, must be reviewed by the responsible physician at least daily, or at more frequent intervals, if appropriate, and documentation made in the medical chart to determine the continued applicability of such orders. If the patient's condition alters in such a way that the orders are no longer deemed applicable, the Orders Not to Resuscitate must be revoked, the revocation communicated without delay.

SECTION II

SCIENTIFIC FOUNDATIONS
OF ANESTHESIA

3

Pharmacologic Principles

W. David Watkins, M.D., Ph.D.
John B. Leslie, M.D.
Norbert P. DeBruijn, M.D.

INTRODUCTION

Anesthesia necessitates the administration of drugs in such a manner as to produce desired effects yet avoid undesirable side effects or toxicity. In addition to analgesia and amnesia, pharmacologic control of the physiologic and pathophysiologic functions of all major organ systems is often required. These broad therapeutic objectives necessitate integration of the principles of physiology and pathophysiology with basic and clinical pharmacology. The resulting knowledge should form a rational basis for the appropriate administration of drugs to humans. In every instance, the therapeutic objective should be to maintain adequate drug concentrations at the desired sites of action to produce a specific effect. The anesthesiologist should, therefore, strive to select and administer drugs by routes and dosage regimens that will ensure tissue and receptor concentration levels between those that pro-

duce unacceptable toxicity and those that fail to provide effective therapy (i.e., within the range that excludes toxic and subtherapeutic doses).

The empirical approach to drug administration consists of adjusting an initial dose in an amount and rate in accordance with the clinical response of an individual patient. The ability of the anesthesiologist to make these adjustments before administering a chosen dose has often been termed the "art" of anesthesia and will continue to reflect, in part, the skill of establishing an individualized dose – response relationship. With continued experience and research in anesthesiology, a variety of guidelines have emerged by which the "science" of anesthesiology will enhance the "art".

This chapter is divided into three basic sections: pharmacologic principles, pharmacokinetic principles, and pharmacodynamic principles. The pharmacologic section defines the fundamental terminology and principles of drug absorption, distribution, metabolism, and elimination. The latter portion of this section addresses the clinical significance of therapeutic monitoring of drug concentrations.

The second major topic in this chapter consists of describing basic pharmacokinetic principles and their clinical application. The clinical applications of pharmacokinetic principles have been avoided by many clinical anesthesiologists for a variety of reasons. The perceived requisite of a profound mathematical background in understanding pharmacokinetics may account for the reluctance of many physicians to review pharmacokinetics. This section simplifies many of the pharmacokinetic principles to the point where their applications in clinical practice will be appreciated further. This discussion is presented with minimal mathematical interjections and referral to more comprehensive reviews as appropriate.

The final section of this chapter centers on pharmacodynamic principles. As stated earlier, the therapeutic objective is to maintain adequate drug concentration at a given site of action. This section of the chapter reviews the basic concepts of drug receptors and drug–receptor interactions, the dose–response relationship, and the importance of individualization of therapy on the basis of important sources of patient variability.

A clear understanding of pharmacologic, pharmacokinetic, and pharmacodynamic principles will provide the anesthesiologist with a background that will substantially enhance the likelihood of achieving the chosen therapeutic objectives. Selection of the drug of choice should be a function of individual patient variation, lengths of surgical procedures, routes of administration, concurrent drug therapies, and other contributing variables.

PHARMACOLOGIC PRINCIPLES

GENERAL

Many factors play a role in determining the magnitude and duration of a specific effect caused by substances administered to a living system. Ultimately the effect is determined by the availability of drug in the "effect compartment," that is, the theoretical space in which drug molecules interact with receptors to produce an effect.

Drug availability is governed by various modes of transport of molecules across biologic membranes and by the extent to which the drug is bound to proteins in the circulation and in the tissues. Availability at the site of action is further influenced by the blood flow to that site. The availability of unchanged drug is influenced by the extent and speed of metabolic processes that may modify the parent compound to products that may or may not possess biologic activity. Finally, elimination of the drug and/or its metabolic products from the plasma and body influences the extent and the duration of the pharmacologic effect.

ABSORPTION

After administration of a drug, only a fraction may be available for absorption; this fraction describes *bioavailability*. The rate of absorption influences the time course of the drug effect and is an important consideration in determining drug dosage. Also the choice of the route by which a drug is administered is frequently influenced by rate and extent of drug absorption.

TYPES OF TRANSPORT

All drugs must cross biologic membranes to reach the intended receptors. Biologic membranes consist of a central lipid bilayer core and a superficial covering consisting of proteins. Because of this combination of polar and nonpolar components in membrane structure, any drug must possess both lipid and water solubility in order to dissolve in, and thereby traverse, these cell boundaries.

In addition to passive membrane transport, there are specialized mechanisms that enable a variety of substances to cross membranes:

Aqueous diffusion: This passive process may also be described as filtration because it involves bulk flow of water that occurs as a result of hydrostatic or osmotic differences across the membrane. This process enables lipid insoluble substances to pass through membrane pores. However, the structural composition of most drugs has a molecular size too large for passage through the pores. Pores in most cell membranes are not larger than 4 Å, permitting only small water-soluble molecules to pass. In general, molecules with molecular weights greater than 100 to 200 will not pass. A notable exception is the passage of large molecules such as albumin through the 40-Å pores of capillary membranes.

Carrier-mediated active transport: This process is responsible for the rapid transfer of many organic substances across membranes. Characteristic features of this mode of transport are saturability, selectivity, and the requirement for energy. Substances may be mobilized by this means against an electrochemical or concentration gradient (uphill transport). Another form of carrier-mediated transport is facilitated diffusion, which does not require energy coupling but also does not transport compounds against a concentration gradient. This form of transport is, however, also saturable and selective.

Pinocytosis: Drugs of high molecular weight may be transported by this process, in which the molecule is enveloped in a small vesicle, and as such crosses the membrane.

PROTEIN BINDING

Since only the "free" unbound portion of a chemical is pharmacologically active, binding properties of drugs to plasma and tissue proteins are of considerable importance. As far as absorption is concerned, binding of a drug may facilitate absorption by reducing the concentration in the aqueous phase of plasma. Binding is generally a reversible process, arriving at an equilibrium according to the law of mass action. The unbound fraction is available for pharmacologic action and metabolism, while the bound fraction functions as a depot from which drug is made available as the equilibrium is reestablished after removal of free drug. (Protein binding is explained in greater detail later in this section, under distribution of drugs.)

MOLECULAR PROPERTIES

Most drugs are either weak acids or weak bases present in solution in both the ionized and unionized forms. The unionized form is usually lipid soluble and will readily cross membranes. By contrast, the ionized fraction is generally hydrophilic and does not easily cross membranes. The distribution of a weak electrolyte is usually determined by its pKa (the pH at which the compound is ionized for 50 percent) and the pH gradient across the membrane. The gastric lumen has a pH of approximately 1, the intestinal lumen a pH of 7 to 8. A weak acid such as acetylsalicylic acid, with a pKa of 4.4, will be readily absorbed across the "gastric membrane," while basic drugs with a pKa of 9 to 10 will not be absorbed in the stomach but will be readily absorbed in the intestinal lumen. This phenomenon leads to the so-called ion-trapping effect because while acetylsalicylic acid is mostly in the unionized form in the acidic gastric environment, as it crosses the membrane and arrives in the neutral tissue environment (pH = 7.4) it exists mainly in the ionized form, which will not readily cross membranes. In reality, the simple premise that the stomach absorbs weakly acidic drugs is modified by the transit time through the stomach and the morphology of the organ (surface area). A second molecular property of chemicals that affects their absorption is solubility. Drugs administered in aqueous solution are more rapidly absorbed than those administered in oily solution, suspension or solid form.

ROUTE OF ADMINISTRATION

Enteral (oral) administration of drugs is the most commonly used route and very often the most appropriate one. The oral route is convenient, economical, and usually safe but requires a cooperative patient. However, drug absorption may be variable and depends on many of the above-discussed factors. For poorly soluble drugs, absorption may be quite unpredictable. By contrast, intravenously administered drugs circumvent absorption and have a much faster onset of action. The intravenous route permits accurate dosage and is suitable for drugs or compounds that need to be given in large volumes or for substances that are irritating to the gastric mucosa. Subcutaneously administered drugs are readily absorbed from aqueous solution, as are intramuscularly injected drugs.

ORAL ADMINISTRATION

Some of the orally administered drugs are absorbed from the stomach, but most are absorbed from the upper part of the small intestine. Drugs with pKa values in the appropriate range for either the stomach or the small intestine will be readily absorbed. The absorbed drug is carried to the liver by the portal venous system, where a considerable fraction may be completely removed or altered by hepatic metabolism. Only a small fraction of the absorbed drug may pass the liver and gain access to the systemic circulation. This phenomenon has been termed first-pass effect. Depending on the magnitude of this effect, oral dosage may have to be many times larger than intravenous dosage in order to produce the same pharmacologic effect. Orally administered drugs must first be dissolved before they can be absorbed. Many influences play a role in the rate of dissolution, including solubility, particle size, crystalline form and salt form of the drug, rate of disintegration of the solid dosage form into the gastrointestinal (GI) lumen, and the GI pH, mobility, and food content.

SUBLINGUAL ADMINISTRATION

A higher blood concentration of a drug may be achieved by permitting the drug to be absorbed in the mouth rather than swallowed and absorbed from a lower part of the GI tract. The first-pass effect can be minimized, and the drug is not subject to destruction by GI secretions.

RECTAL ADMINISTRATION

The rate of absorption from the rectum is rapid; this route may be useful in circumstances in which oral administration is pre-

cluded by vomiting. The first-pass effect is less important in rectally administered drugs.

SUBCUTANEOUS INJECTION

The advantage of subcutaneously administered drug is a relatively even and slow absorption, which can provide a sustained effect. In addition, the rate of absorption may be manipulated by altering the drug form, as is done with insulin. Also, the rate of absorption may be decreased by combining the drug with epinephrine, as is done with local anesthetic agents. Irritants should not be given subcutaneously, as they may produce sloughing of the skin.

INTRAMUSCULAR INJECTION

Slow absorption from an intramuscular injection site occurs when drugs are in solution in oil or in various suspensions. Aqueous solutions of drugs are rapidly and evenly absorbed.

INTRAVENOUS INJECTION

The main advantage of intravenous administration of drugs is the circumvention of the absorption process. Thus, the desired blood concentration is rapidly attained in a relatively accurate manner. This is also the ideal route for drugs that have to be given in large volumes or that are too irritant for intramuscular or subcutaneous injection. Nevertheless, there are dangers to intravenous administration of drugs: once a drug is injected, there is no way back and, in the event of overdose or idiosyncratic reactions, the effects are immediate and often severe.

INTRATHECAL ADMINISTRATION

When local and rapid effects on the CNS are desired, the limiting effects on rate and extent of drug absorption through the blood–brain barrier can be circumvented by intrathecal administration (also see Chs. 29 & 60). However, access for this route requires considerably more skill and expertise than is needed for the oral, sublingual, rectal, subcutaneous, intramuscular, and intravenous routes.

PULMONARY ADMINISTRATION

Because of the large surface area of the alveoli, gases and volatile agents that are inhaled are rapidly absorbed into the circulation (also see Ch. 19). Also, aerosols of sympathomimetic and other drugs are frequently used to relieve bronchospasm.

SKIN

Local effects can be achieved by application of ointments, creams, lotions, liniments, and pastes. The percutaneous absorption of ionized drugs can be enhanced by applying a drug solution to an electrode placed on the skin; a current is applied between the "drug electrode" and a neutral electrode. This is known as iontophoresis.

BIOAVAILABILITY

Bioavailability is an important concept that describes the relative amount of an administered drug that reaches the systemic circulation and the rate at which this occurs.

The form in which a drug is commercially available will affect its bioavailability. For example, differences in crystal form, particle size, disintegration of dosage form, and dissolution of the drug will influence the rate and extent of absorption. When a drug is administered intravenously, it is considered completely available systemically. If it is injected in the form of a derivative (e.g., an ester which must initially undergo hydrolysis before active drug is available), then it may or may not be completely available systemically, depending on the completeness of the hydrolysis. The systemic availability and bioavailability are reflected by the area below the blood concentration vs time curve.

DISTRIBUTION OF DRUGS

After a drug has reached the systemic circulation via absorption or by intravenous injection, it will be distributed throughout the body. This distribution involves movement through lipid membranes, movement through capillary walls, and distribution between binding sites in different parts of the body. The initial distribution is determined by the physicochemical characteristics of the drug (e.g., ion-trapping effect), as well as cardiac output and regional blood flow to various organs. Lipid-soluble drugs are rapidly distributed to heart, brain, kidney, liver, and other extensively perfused organs. Less rapid distribution into muscle and still slower distribution into fat then occurs because these latter organs receive a smaller fraction of the cardiac output.

Drugs may achieve a higher concentration in peripheral tissues than in blood because of ion trapping, tissue binding, and dissolution in fat. Protein binding profoundly affects drug distribution. Of the plasma proteins, albumin is quantitatively the most important; it has a high capacity for binding drugs. This binding is of low specificity. The bound fraction of a drug, unavailable for specific pharmacologic action or metabolism, acts as a depot from which drug is regenerated as the equilibrium is reestablished after removal of the free drug. The position of the equilibrium and the rate at which the free fraction of drug is removed by metabolism and excretion determine the biologic half-life of a drug. Because albumin and the other plasma proteins possess a limited number of binding sites, drugs with affinity for the same binding site compete for binding to this site. This competition may result in redistribution of a drug between plasma and tissue. A drug that displaces another highly plasma albumin-bound drug from its binding sites forces the latter drug to diffuse into tissues, thereby causing the plasma concentration to decline. Components other than plasma proteins may bind drugs as well. Tissue binding of drugs is difficult to measure. Some drugs have a greater affinity for certain tissues. For instance, thiopental has a high lipid–water partition coefficient, hence the tendency to accumulate in fat, although this happens slowly because of the poor blood flow to fat tissue. Thiopental, therefore, provides a good example of distribution and redistribution of a drug after intravenous administration: initially, thiopental crosses lipid membranes rapidly and soon almost undetectably in the plasma pool. High concentrations are reached in the organs of the vessel-rich group (brain, heart, liver, kidney). As the concentration gradient across the cell membranes reverses, thiopental leaves these organs just as quickly for redistribution to the intermediate vessel group (muscle) and finally into fat.

METABOLISM

As many drugs are lipophilic substances that are not easily excreted in the aqueous urine, their removal from the body must be preceded by chemical changes to render them hydrophilic. This process usually leads to inactivation of the drug. Thus, lipophilic substances are bioinactivated by phase I (or functionalization) metabolism (i.e., oxidation, reduction, or hydrolysis), rendering them more polar. These polar metabolites and any other polar compounds are conjugated by phase II (synthetic) metabolism, rendering them hydrophilic. These hydrophilic substances may subsequently be excreted in the urine. We will briefly review the most important metabolic processes.

PHASE I REACTIONS

Phase I metabolism consists of two types of reaction: oxidation and reduction.

OXIDATION

Oxidation can take place within either the microsomal or nonmicrosomal system.

Microsomal
Side-chain oxidation (e.g., pentobarbital): follows the general rule that oxidation of any longer aliphatic side chain takes place near or at the end-carbon

Aromatic hydroxylation: not very important in human metabolism, yet important in the rat — one of the many causes for species differences

N-oxidation: results in nitroso and hydroxylamine compounds that may be highly toxic

Sulfoxidation (e.g., chlorpromazine): has a sulfur atom in the middle ring that may be oxidized

N-dealkylation: splits off a CH_3 group in a side chain that combines with oxygen to form formaldehyde; appears to be important in humans

O-dealkylation (e.g., phenacetin)
S-dealkylation
Deamination
Desulfuration

Nonmicrosomal
Alcohol oxidation
Aromatization
Purine oxidation
Monoaminooxidation

REDUCTION

The following reductions play an important part in metabolic reactions in the GI tract:

N-reduction
Azo-reduction
Alcohol-dehydrogenation

HYDROLYSIS

Hydrolysis is the last of the phase I metabolic reactions; it may be important in plasma as well as in many tissues. An ester group or amide is split off in this type of reaction. Examples are the rapid metabolism of procaine by a multitude of nonspecific esterases.

PHASE II REACTIONS

Phase II metabolism consists of combining polar unchanged or metabolized compounds with a number of small endogenous substances. These reactions are called conjugations. Cofactors are usually involved and energy is used. In humans the most important conjugation is that with glucuronic acid. It takes place in the microsomal system.

ELIMINATION

Elimination is a general term signifying all processes that terminate the presence of a drug in the body. In addition to metabolism, major processes include renal excretion, hepatobiliary excretion, and, especially in anesthesia, pulmonary excretion. Minor routes of elimination are via saliva, sweat, breast milk, and tears.

RENAL EXCRETION

A major route of excretion of chemicals, both changed and unchanged, is by way of the renal system. Under the driving force of the blood pressure, all substances of low molecular weight are filtered from the blood through the membrane of Bowman's capsule. The ultrafiltrate in the lumen of the proximal convoluted tubule contains both lipophilic and hydrophilic molecules. The hydrophilic molecules remain with the tubular lumen, while the lipophilic molecules are reabsorbed back into the blood perfusing the tubule. Some substances are actively secreted from the blood into the proximal tubule by energy-consuming carrier-dependent processes.

As the renal tubular contents become more concentrated, unionized drug molecules are reabsorbed by diffusion across the tubular epithelium. Thus, in reabsorption the passage of the lipophilic molecules back across the tubular membrane depends, as everywhere else, on lipid solubility, degree of ionization, and molecular shape. Thus, weak acids are reabsorbed best from an acidic urine. As the urine pH varies, it can be seen that renal tubular reabsorption may be manipulated. In a patient who has had an overdose of acetylsalicylic acid, alkalinization of the urine will reduce renal tubular reabsorption and thus will enhance excretion of the drug, especially in combination with forced diuresis.

HEPATOBILIARY EXCRETION

Many metabolites of drugs formed in the liver are excreted into the intestinal tract with the bile. Some of these metabolites may be excreted in the feces, but most commonly they are reabsorbed into the blood and are ultimately excreted with the urine. This is called the enterohepatic cycle. A wide variety of organic cations and anions are actively transported into bile by carrier systems. At least three such systems for the transport of poorly lipid-soluble organic compounds have been identified. In these processes the compounds are transported against a large concentration gradient from the plasma into the bile.

Volatile anesthetics and anesthetic gases are in large part excreted through the lung. In this elimination process, the factors that determine uptake operate in a reverse way. Alveolar partial pressure will depend on the amount of agent released into the alveoli by the blood, where insoluble agents will be readily released from blood and removed by alveolar ventilation.

THERAPEUTIC MONITORING

Monitoring of drug concentrations is indicated under a number of circumstances. It may be helpful with drugs, such as antiepileptic agents, that are not readily assessable by clinical observation or by laboratory test. Therapeutic monitoring is especially useful for drugs that show marked interpatient pharmacokinetic variability; it is obligatory for drugs with a narrow therapeutic window, for which the range between subtherapeutic and toxic doses is small. The interpretation of drug concentration must be made within a context of information about the pharmacokinetic characteristics of the agent, interval between sampling time, and last dose. The sensitivity and specificity of the drug assay are important considerations, as is information about whether bound or free drug has been measured. Serial measurements are always more useful than single measurements. For drugs that produce an effect that may be easily assessed by clinical evaluation, plasma drug concentration measurements are most often unnecessary because the drug dose can be filtrated against the desired end point.

PHARMACOKINETIC PRINCIPLES

GENERAL

The science of pharmacokinetics is often considered a purely mathematical approach to the quantitation of drug disposition in the body. The term was first used by Dost in 1953 in an attempt to quantitate the rate of change in drug concentrations in proposed compartments within the body. The mathematical complexity that has developed in pharmacokinetics to project the phases of drug absorption, distribution, and elimination has prevented many clinicians from developing a basic understanding of this science. Many physicians may question the relevance of pharmacokinetics to clinical pharmacology and the practice of anesthesiology. It will become apparent, however, that as anesthesiologists begin to understand some of the basic principles of pharmacokinetics, it becomes possible in many cases to predict the dose–response relationships of anesthetic drugs in a normal or pathophysiologic state. In the simplest terminology, pharmacokinetics attempts to help explain how the body handles an exogenously administered compound. These basic principles can be applied to the great majority of drugs administered by anesthesiologists. A bare minimum of mathematics is included in this presentation in an attempt to review principles rather than specific drugs or pharmacokinetic models. Several excellent in-depth reviews are listed in the references.

PRINCIPLES OF COMPARTMENTAL MODELS

When a drug is administered to a patient, by whatever chosen route, the onset and duration of its pharmacologic effect are dependent on multiple factors, as outlined in the previous section. Included are those factors affecting drug absorption, distribution, and the process of elimination. The various organ systems represent many combinations of perfusion, drug-binding affinity, drug solubility, drug ionization, and rates of metabolism. In physiologic pharmacokinetic modeling, organ systems having similar drug solubility and blood perfusion characteristics are grouped together, and an attempt is made to conceptualize the process of absorption, distribution, and elimination of the drug from these organ systems. These complex models have required extensive computer resources and are difficult to extrapolate to the individual patient. Mathematical models that assume specific pharmacokinetic compartments within the body, rather than specific anatomic organ system compartments, have simplified the mathematics required to understand and apply the models. With each drug it is possible to utilize accessible drug concentration information from blood or urine and other tissues and to define relationships among drug dose, plasma concentration of the drug, and time. The actual pharmacokinetic compartment as defined may have no specific biologic correlation with a defined organ system or group of systems. The changes in drug concentration that take place over time within the conceptual compartments can be used to derive such parameters as half-life, volume of distribution, distribution characteristics, and other characteristics of drug elimination.

ONE-COMPARTMENT MODEL

Some drugs behave as though they are distributed into a single uniform compartment in the body from which a constant proportion of the drug in the body is eliminated within a cho-

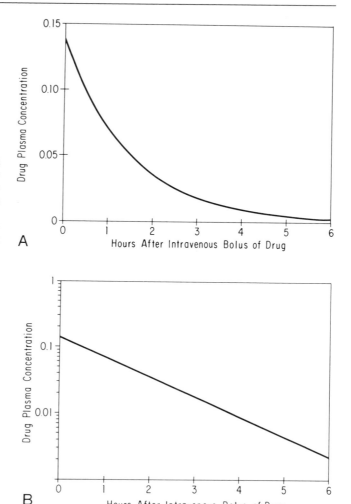

FIG. 3-1 (A) Computer simulation of a drug displaying one-compartment kinetics. The curve generated displays the expected drug:plasma concentration on a linear concentration scale versus time. Ten units of drug was injected intravenously at time 0 and computer input variables were chosen to display an elimination half-life of 1 hour. (B) Computer simulation of the same one-compartment kinetics of the drug concentration versus time plot shown in (A). In this graph, however, the drug:plasma concentration is plotted on a logarithmic scale, thereby producing a straight line because of the single exponential decline of drug level over time.

sen time period (e.g., 1 hour). Figure 3-1 represents a computer simulation of the administration of drug A, distributing into one compartment and eliminated by first-order kinetics. At time 0, an intravenous bolus of 10 units of the drug was administered, and plasma concentrations were determined repeatedly over a 6-hour period. Figure 3-1A compares the decline in plasma concentration on a linear y-axis scale over time on the x-axis. Examination of the drug concentration versus time plot demonstrates that drug concentrations decrease in a constant proportion. At time 0, there was a plasma concentration of 0.14 units. The elimi-

nation half-life ($t\frac{1}{2}$) represents the time taken for the drug concentration to decline to one-half its original value. In this example it can be seen that at the end of 1 hour the concentration was 0.07 units; therefore, one-half the drug was eliminated. Again, between the first and second hour, one-half of the remaining drug was eliminated. The half-life is independent of the amount of drug in the body. Table 3-1 illustrates that five half-lives are required to eliminate 96.9 percent of the administered drug. Elimination half-lives are also useful in selecting drug dosing intervals, in predicting the time required to reach a steady state of drug concen-

TABLE 3-1 Elimination Half-Life

Number of Drug Half-lives	Original Drug Remaining (%)	Original Drug Eliminated (%)
0	100	0
1	50	50
2	25	75
3	12.5	87.5
4	6.25	93.75
5	3.13	96.87
6	1.56	98.44

tration, and in calculating drug accumulation. This will be explained in more detail in the next section.

Mathematically, it has been shown that the elimination half-life

$$t_{\frac{1}{2}} = \ln 2/k = 0.693/k$$

where ln 2 = 0.693 and k represents the first-order rate constant. This elimination rate constant, k, is a proportionality constant that describes the fraction of drug present at any given time that will be eliminated in that time unit. Simple mathematical rearrangement shows $k = 0.693/t_{\frac{1}{2}}$, thus k will have units of reciprocal time, i.e., hr^{-1}. In Figure 3-1, therefore, $t_{\frac{1}{2}} = 1$ hour and $k = 0.693\ hr^{-1}$.

If the same drug plasma concentration – time graph is replotted on a logarithmic concentration scale versus time a straight line results (see Fig. 3-1B). The graphing technique displays the exponential decline as a straight line because of the logarithmic scale. The slope of this line is equal to $-k/2.303$.

TWO-COMPARTMENT MODEL

For most anesthetic drugs, the plot of the decline in the plasma concentration versus time is similar to the computer simulation of Figure 3-2. Figure 3-2A illustrates the decline in the drug plasma concentration on the linear y-axis scale versus time on the x-axis. There appears to be two distinct phases to the decline in plasma concentrations. The first phase in decline represents drug distribution which occurs immediately after injection when a very rapid rate of decline in plasma concentration is

noted. This conceptually represents movement of the drug from the plasma into tissues. The second phase which begins immediately after injection but becomes obvious only after completion of the relatively rapid distribution phase is the slower decline of plasma concentration due to drug elimination from the plasma.

To explain this biphasic behavior, the body is divided conceptually into two compartments: a central compartment of small volume and a peripheral compartment of a larger volume. As stated previously, these defined compartments represent pharmacokinetic compartments (black boxes) not specific organ systems or tissues. Conceptually, the central compartment generally represents the blood or plasma and the highly perfused tissues such as the heart, lungs, kidney, and liver. The peripheral compartment would represent drug present in other tissues.

The drug plasma concentration versus time graph of Figure 3-2A can then be graphed with a logarithmic drug plasma concentration scale for the y-axis. This is illustrated in Figure 3-2B. The biphasic behavior of the drug in the body is again visually apparent. As with the one-compartment model, plotting the drug concentrations on a logarithmic scale permits further conceptualization of the disposition of the drug in the body. For this drug with two-compartment pharmacokinetics, it is apparent from Figure 3-2B that the decline in drug level is a summation of two exponentially declining phases or parameters. These are again the generally shorter distribution phase and the longer elimination phase.

This two-compartment pharmacokinetic model can be defined mathematically by the formula

$$C_p = Ae^{-\alpha t} + Be^{-\beta t}$$

where Cp = drug concentration in plasma at time t, α = rate constant of the distribution phase; β = rate constant of the elimination phase; A = intercept at time 0 of the distribution phase line; B = intercept at time 0 of the elimination phase line, and t = time. Thus, the two-compartment model mathematically represents a biexponential equation in which the first exponential term ($Ae^{-\alpha t}$) summarizes the

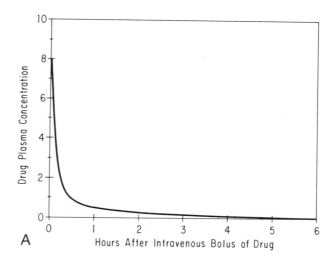

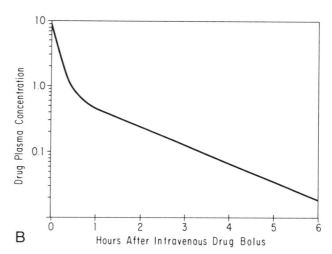

FIG. 3-2 (A) Computer simulation of a drug with two-compartment kinetics. The curve displays the expected drug : plasma concentrations on a linear concentration scale versus time. Two distinct phases of drug plasma concentration changes are visually apparent: the initial rapid decline in drug level during the distribution phase and the slower decline in concentration during the elimination phase. (B) Computer simulation of the same two-compartment kinetics of the drug concentration versus time plot shown in (B). Here the drug : plasma concentration is plotted on a logarithmic scale over time. A combination of two distinctly linear phases is visually apparent because of the biexponential decline of the drug level over time.

distribution phase and the second exponential term $(Be^{-\beta t})$ summarizes the elimination phase. The rate constants α and β can be determined from the slope of the graphs and used to calculate the distribution and elimination half-lives.

OTHER MODELS

Some drug plasma concentration decay curves require three or more exponential terms to characterize the drugs decline from the plasma. A three-compartment model would therefore have three exponential terms and assume one central compartment and two conceptual peripheral compartments. Other techniques of pharmacokinetic analysis beyond the scope of this limited review include blood flow models, rate-limited models, membrane-limited models, nonlinear pharmacokinetic models, and noncompartmental analysis employing statistical moment theory. In practice, a basic understanding of first-order kinetics and one- and two-compartment models is often sufficient.

DERIVED PARAMETERS

Further study of the one- and two-compartment pharmacokinetic models of drug concentration versus time plots demonstrates other valuable clinical pharmacology. These areas are covered briefly in the next four sections.

ABSORPTION

As defined in pharmacokinetics, absorption is the process by which a drug proceeds from the site of administration to a site of measurement, i.e., the plasma or serum. For drugs administered intravenously, the concentration–time plots show an instantaneous peak. For drugs administered by other routes, the peak and time course of the distribution phase will be shifted to the right. A drug that is absorbed slowly may not achieve the desired effect because of a prolonged distribution phase.

ROUTE OF ADMINISTRATION

The route of drug administration will affect the absorption kinetics and the drugs bioavailability. In simple terms, bioavailability refers to the rate and extent of drug absorption. The importance of this time-lag concept is evident in extravascularly-administered compounds and the administration of inhalational anesthetic agents as discussed in the chapter on uptake and distribution of inhalation anesthetics.

RATE OF ADMINISTRATION

Alteration of the rate of administration of a drug may produce dramatic changes in the drug concentration–time plots. Figure 3-3 represents a comparison of 60 units of a drug administered in a one-compartment model either as an intravenous bolus (curve A) or given as a constant infusion over a 6-hour period (curve B). If it is accepted that the drug's effect is dependent on attaining a certain concentration at a site of action then the differences in produced effects by the two different rates of administration is clear. For example, if a plasma concentration of 0.2 units is required for an effect, the intravenous bolus would have been effective for 1½ hours and the constant infusion method would never have produced the desired effect.

Figure 3-4 illustrates the alterations in concentration–time plots that occur when the dosing intervals are altered in relation to the known elimination half-life of a drug. Figure 3-4 represents a computer simulation of a drug that is eliminated by first-order kinetics with

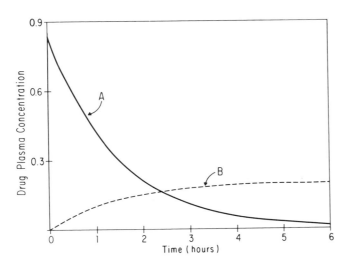

FIG. 3-3 Computer simulation of the differences between administration of 60 units of a drug as an intravenous bolus (curve A) or as a constant infusion of a total of 60 units of drug over a 6-hour period (curve B). Computer input data: A, 1.4 units; B, 0.14 units; α, 6.93; β, 0.693.

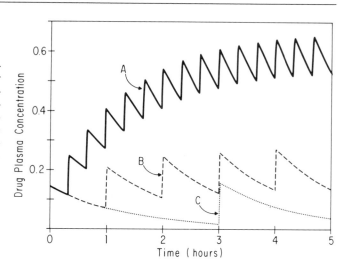

FIG. 3-4 Computer simulation of expected drug : plasma concentrations over time as effected by different dosing intervals relative to the drug elimination half-life. Curve A displays rapid drug accumulation by administration of a chosen dose of drug at intervals less than the elimination half-life of 1 hour. Curve B represents repeated dosing at every drug half-life. Curve C displays the effect of repeating doses every 3 hours, significantly longer than the elimination half-life.

an elimination half-life of 1 hour. Curve A demonstrates that if the same dose is repeated as an intravenous bolus at time intervals of less than the elimination half-life (i.e., every 20 minutes), significant drug accumulation within the plasma will occur. This level of accumulation is significantly higher than the level achieved if the drug is administered as in curve B, every half-life. This is in contrast to curve C, where the drug administration is repeated at three times the half-life, showing that significant accumulation does not appear to occur. It can also be noted that a steady state of plasma concentration has been achieved in both A and B after approximately five drug-elimination half-lives of 1 hour each.

As noted in the previous section, which outlined the factors affecting absorption, any disease process that alters protein binding, ionization, pH, tissue perfusion, blood volume, or other such factors will alter drug absorption, bioavailability, and pharmacokinetic profile.

DISTRIBUTION

In pharmacokinetic terminology, distribution represents the process of reversible transfer of a drug from one compartment to another compartment within the body. Distribution is, therefore, a dynamic process.

VOLUME CONCEPT

It was noted from the example of Figure 3-1 that although 10 units of the drug was administered intravenously, the instantaneous plasma concentration showed a value of 0.14 units. The relationship between a measured plasma concentration and a known administered dosage defines an apparent volume of distribution, V_D. The apparent volume of distribution is a proportionality constant that relates the amount of drug in the body to the concentration in a reference compartment, usually the central compartment. Thus: V_D = total dose/ drug plasma concentration. In the example shown in Figure 3-1 the calculated volume of distribution would be: 10 over 0.14 = 71.4 L. Again, it should be noted that no physiologic or anatomic significance may often be given to V_D. V_D may be as small as a plasma volume or as large as 10,000 times the plasma volume. A large volume of distribution suggests extensive tissue distribution and uptake. There are published tables of apparent volumes of distribution for most drugs. If the plasma concentration of a drug can be measured and the volume of distribution is established, it is simple to calculate the total amount of drug remaining in the body. If a given drug has a large volume of distribution, it may require a larger loading dose to achieve a given plasma level than if a similarly active drug has a smaller volume of distribution. While the concept of an apparent volume of distribution has no specific relationship to organ anatomy, many disease processes can significantly alter the volume of distribution. These alterations may occur in such states as renal failure, hepatic dysfunction, extremes of age, congestive heart failure, shock, and burns. Initiation or termination of cardiopulmonary bypass will also have significant effects on the volume of distribution and therefore on the circulating drug levels. Information about the volume of distribution may be useful in calculating a loading dose and in estimating changes in loading doses where predicted alterations in this volume are known to occur due to disease processes that alter the volume of distribution.

ELIMINATION

In pharmacokinetic terminology, elimination refers to the irreversible loss of drug from the site where the drug is measured. Elimination represents the combination of the processes of metabolism and excretion. The major sites of elimination are kidney, liver, and lung.

ELIMINATION RATE CONSTANTS

The derivation of the elimination rate constant k, as derived in the example of the one-compartment model, represents the fraction of drug that will be eliminated in that time unit. For example, if $k = 0.05$ minute, the plasma concentration will decrease by 5 percent each minute.

ELIMINATION TIME CONSTANTS

The pharmacokinetic parameters of some drugs, especially inhalational agents, are often expressed in time constants: $T_{1/e}$. The time constant estimates the time necessary for the concentration of the agent to change by a factor of $1/e$ and represents a 63 percent change per unit time. The relationship between the time constant and the elimination rate constant is

$T_{1/e} = 1/k$. The time constant can be related to the drug's half-life by the equation:

$$t_{\frac{1}{2}} = 0.693 \, T_{1/e}$$

CLEARANCE CONCEPTS

Total clearance represents that part of the volume of distribution that is cleared of the drug per unit of time. Total clearance is a summation of clearance by the various routes of elimination. Clearance is thus related to the volume of distribution and the rate of elimination from that total volume. Therefore, the units of clearance are volume per time, i.e., milliliters per minute or if corrected for weight, milliliters per minute per kilogram. This is expressed mathematically as follows:

$$\text{Clearance (Cl)} = V_d \times k$$

Conceptually, one may imagine a small box within a large box, where the small box is totally cleared of the drug in the unit time and instantaneously the remainder of the drug will redistribute into the volume of the large box. The small box will then be cleared again in unit time.

Renal

The practical significance of determining renal clearance (Cl$_R$) is to determine that fraction of the dose of the drug that is eliminated through renal mechanisms. This parameter is extremely useful in dosage adjustments in renal failure.

Hepatic

Hepatic clearance (Cl$_H$) represents the fraction of administered drug that is eliminated by the liver. Clearance by any organ is dependent on blood flow through the organ and the amount of drug that is removed with passage through the organ.

Specific organ clearance values can therefore not exceed blood flow. Certain drugs such as propranolol and lidocaine have very high hepatic clearance rates. This results in high presystemic first-pass effect (elimination) if the drug is administered orally. This occurs because the drug absorbed from the gastrointestinal tract must first pass through the liver via the portal vein.

Total Body

Total body clearance is the sum of the clearance rates by renal, hepatic and other routes of elimination. The numerical value of total clearance and the two major components, ClH and ClR, may provide important insight into the elimination processes. As stated, this may be important in anticipating necessary adjustments in dosage regimens with different disease states. A drug with a large ClR value relative to the total clearance in the presence of renal failure will require a greater decrease in dose in the presence of renal failure than is necessary for the dose of a drug that has a larger ClH value. Large values of Cl and ClH often imply significant elimination by the liver; such a drug may, therefore, have a greater systemic effect in patients with liver disease than in normal patients.

PHARMACODYNAMIC PRINCIPLES

GENERAL

It has been stated that the therapeutic objective in anesthesiology is to maintain adequate drug concentration at a site of action to produce a specific effect. The acceptance of this broad therapeutic objective depends on proof of delivery of the drug to the specific site as well as correlation of a resulting effect from the presence of the drug at that site. The changes, or effects, that result from the drug interaction with a specific site of activity encompasses the field of pharmacodynamics. Simply stated, pharmacodynamics attempts to explain what effect the drug has in the body. The following sections attempt to establish a basic concept of receptors and of the nature of drug–receptor interactions.

RECEPTOR CONCEPTS

DEFINITION

In the broadest sense, a receptor is a component of a cell that interacts selectively with an extracellular compound to initiate a biochemical change or a cascade of biochemical alterations that represent the observed effects of the compound. The receptor therefore serves to mediate or amplify the effect of the drug on the biologic system.

The current receptor concept has been well established in the fields of endocrinology, molecular biology, immunology, and pharmacology. The extension of receptor pharmacology to anesthesiology is currently under intense investigation. Many drugs and endogenous circulating compounds have been shown to interact with specific cellular receptors to produce measured effects.

A receptor represents a specific protein or lipoprotein present as membrane-bound components of the normal cell. Many of these receptor proteins have been isolated and well characterized. It is beyond the scope of this review to detail even a list of currently proven receptor proteins. It can be shown, however, that in each instance these receptors function to determine (1) the quantitative relationship between a given dose of a drug and the produced effect, (2) the selectivity of a given drug's activity and effect, and (3) an explanation for the pharmacologic activity of receptor agonists and receptor antagonists.

A compound or drug that behaves as a receptor agonist will produce, when bound to the receptor, a physiologic change that represents a specific induced effect. The pharmacologic structure of a drug will determine which receptor population a given drug may affect. This specific interaction between a compound or drug and the given receptor is predetermined by the configuration of that area of the receptor protein that will bind the drug. The term affinity as related to a given agonist is a measure of the attraction between the given drug and the receptor. A drug with low affinity for a given receptor will tend not to bind to the receptor, hence will produce no effect. A drug that binds avidly to a given receptor will produce the receptor-determined effect at a lower given dose of the receptor agonist. A receptor antagonist is a compound or drug that, when bound to the receptor, either produces a reduction in the expected effect or prevents the expression of that effect. A competitive antagonist can generally be displaced from the receptor complex by the administration of a receptor agonist if given in a large enough concentration and will permit the agonist to produce the expected effect. A noncompetitive antagonist, when bound to the receptor complex, will produce a loss of the expected effect that cannot be reproduced by the concurrent administration of a receptor agonist.

DRUG-RECEPTOR INTERACTION

Classic receptor theory assumes that the compound or drug binds reversibly with the specific receptor site to produce a drug–receptor complex. The generation of this drug–receptor complex represents an intermediate step in producing a specific effect. The effect may cease when there is dissociation of the drug–receptor complex. This process is therefore analogous to the classic model of Michaelis-Menten enzyme kinetics. Mathematically, this may be expressed as

$$[D] + [R] \rightleftharpoons [DR]$$

where $[D] = $ the concentration of drug, $[R] = $ the concentration of receptor, and $[DR]$ represents the concentration of drug–receptor complex. At equilibrium, one can define a KD as the dissociation constant for that given drug. Thus, mathematically

$$KD = \frac{[D] \cdot [R]}{[DR]}$$

When an appropriate concentration of a drug is administered to occupy exactly 50 percent of the receptors, the measured KD will be equal to the administered dose. Under these conditions, the KD will have the dimensions of a concentration. The KD has been determined for many of the drugs currently administered during anesthesia. The reciprocal of KD, the association constant, is therefore a measure of the affinity of the drug for the receptor.

In practice, it is difficult to measure precise drug–receptor occupancy. As stated, it is assumed that the drug–receptor complex represents an intermediate step in the production of a specific effect. It is, therefore, the practice to apply pharmacodynamic theory to compare a given dose of a drug with a resulting effect. An effect can be any biochemical or physiologic parameter that is measurable. A measured effect can be an alteration in a biochemical compound, an enzyme level, a physiologic parameter such as heart rate or blood pressure, or a response to any graded input into the biologic system. For example, in evaluating the pharmacodynamics of muscle relaxants, the measured effect is not a direct measurement of drug–receptor complexes, but rather a response to a neuromuscular stimulus as delivered by a nerve stimulator. It is important that when a given effect is chosen relative to the drug of interest, there should be no measurable effect at zero concentration of the drug and a graded increase in effect to increasing doses of the drug.

From the discussion of pharmacokinetics, it is clear that the delivery of a drug to a given receptor will be time and dose dependent. If the receptor is located within the central compartment, where there may be instantaneous equilibration after an intravenous injection, the peak effect may occur immediately. Even in this example, if the effect is dependent on a drug–receptor complex-induced time-dependent change, the rate of production of an effect will be modified by this variable. If the drug–receptor complex occurs in a peripheral compartment, pharmacokinetic alterations in drug absorption and distribution may further alter the time course of a given drug effect.

To simplify the correlation between drug dose and measured effect, it is often expressed as a comparison of drug dose with the peak effect or equilibrium effect. This will yield a time-independent dose–response relationship. This simplification of expression of the dose–response relationship is the common presentation format for dose–response studies. The actual shape of the dose–response curves is determined by the choice of scales chosen for the two axes. For example, the effect scale can be either in absolute units (i.e., twitch height) or normalized to convert these units to a percentage of the maximum effect (i.e., percent twitch height depression). If the determined pairs (dose and resultant effect) are plotted on scales that are linear both on the x and y axes, the resultant curve will be hyperbolic. If the abscissa is changed to a log scale, the resultant curve, utilizing the same data, will be the classic sigmoid curve.

RECEPTOR AGONISTS

It can be demonstrated that two drugs that presumably act on the same receptor will display parallelism of their log dose–response curves in the presence or absence of antagonists. The log dose–response curve would be superimposed if the two drugs had the same molar affinity constant. The addition of two drugs with varying affinity constants might be predicted to have an effect dependent only on the total amount of drug–receptor complex generated. This would imply a direct linear relationship between receptor–drug complex and a measured effect. It is clear that this is not always the case in biologic systems. For example, in the area of neuromuscular transmission, the measured change in effect on twitch height is not linear when receptor occupancy declines from 100 percent to 90 percent, as compared with the change from 80 percent to 70 percent occupancy.

A further distinction between agonists is based on achievement of the maximum measured pharmacologic response or effect. A full agonist will produce the maximal response at full receptor occupancy. A partial agonist will produce a lower maximal response or effect even at full receptor occupancy. The precise molecular mechanism explaining this blunting of the maximal response of partial agonists is

under investigation. It is possible to imagine that the partial agonist produces a drug–receptor complex configuration that is slightly different from the full agonist drug–receptor complex.

RECEPTOR ANTAGONISTS

The dose–response curve generated from the addition of an agonist in the presence of a competitive antagonist will demonstrate a different effect at every concentration of agonist used until the concentration of agonist is large enough to displace the antagonist from the receptors and will attain full receptor occupancy by agonist. At that concentration, the maximum effect produced by that dose is the same with or without the presence of the competitive antagonist. The dose–response curve generated by the addition of an agonist in the presence of a noncompetitive antagonist will again show failure to attain the same effect with a given dose of agonist, and at no concentration of agonist will the maximal effect be attained. The blockade of effect cannot be reversed.

RECEPTOR DYNAMICS

It is important to conceptualize that receptors are not static entities but are subject to very dynamic regulation by a wide variety of physiologic and pathophysiologic interventions. These dynamic receptor changes have been shown to occur and may account for many altered physiologic or pathophysiologic states. Well-known examples include alterations in diabetes, thyroid disease, adrenal disease, myasthenia, and many other such states. Receptors can also be altered by the administration of agonists and antagonists. For example, the chronic administration of β-adrenergic agonists will cause a decrease in β-receptor number on myocardial tissue. The administration of chronic β-adrenergic antagonists will increase the number of β-adrenergic receptors.

These examples serve to highlight the complexity of a dose–response relationship. The clinician who wishes to produce a given therapeutic effect must therefore consider not only the choice of drug but also the parameters of time, pharmacokinetics, pharmacodynamics, and receptor dynamics.

DOSE-RESPONSE RELATIONSHIP

Several other important parameters of pharmacodynamics can be derived from an understanding of the concepts of efficacy and potency.

EFFICACY

Efficacy refers to a measure of the intrinsic ability of a drug to produce a given effect. It is related to the maximum effect that can be produced by a given drug. Efficacy for a full agonist would be considered to be 1.0, while the efficacy of a pure antagonist is 0. Partial agonists will have efficacies of 0 to 1.0.

POTENCY

The term potency refers to the quantity of drug that must be administered to produce a maximum effect. Two drugs may have the same efficacy, but if one drug produces the maximum effect at 1 mg while the second drug produces the maximum effect only at 100 mg the second drug is less potent.

INDIVIDUALIZATION

The choice of the most rational dosage regimen for safe and effective therapy can only be developed when the time course of pharmacologic effects is quantitatively related to the time course of drug concentrations in the plasma or site of drug-receptor interaction. Individual variation in response can occur due to differences in absorption, distribution, excretion, and dose-response pharmacodynamics. With a greater understanding of these parameters, it becomes possible to make certain predictions in this individual variability of response before administering a chosen dosage regimen. The disease state that will alter any of these parameters forces the clinician to alter the therapeutic regimen. The continuous monitoring of the individual dose-response parameters is an aid to ongoing therapy. Current monitoring techniques attempt to maintain constant input for monitoring of the dose-response relationship. The importance of concurrent drug therapy must always be considered for its effects on the parameters of absorption, distribution, elimination, and the dose-response relationship. The use of computer simulation of projected dose-response curves will prove useful as further definition of this relationship evolves. The measurement of specific alterations in these parameters with specific disease states will be the final aid to the administration of appropriate drug therapy.

SUMMARY

The general area of pharmacology has been reviewed by presentation of relevant principles of pharmacology, pharmacokinetics, pharmacodynamics, and the dose-response relationship. Careful review of these principles will permit the anesthesiologist to conceptualize the movement of a drug from the site of administration through the various body compartments to the site of action for the desired effect. The clinician will be able to individualize the choice of drugs for a patient as personal knowledge of factors affecting each phase of drug movement expands. Hepatic dysfunction, for example, should raise questions of the effects on absorption, protein binding, drug distribution, drug metabolism, and routes of elimination. Consideration must also be given to the possible alterations of the drug-receptor complex relative to production of the desired effect.

The current practice or "art" of administering certain anesthetic agents in given pathophysiologic states can be seen to have an important biologic basis. Further investigation of these practices will demonstrate not only a justification of methods but, more importantly, may suggest more appropriate therapeutic regimens.

The assimilation of drug-specific pharmacokinetic and pharmacodynamic parameters will maximize effective drug therapy. The empirical approach to the administration of many drugs can be replaced by the rational scientific process. This enhancement of the anesthesiologist's understanding of the "science" of anesthesiology will find greatest benefit in the ultimate outcome of optimal patient care.

SUGGESTED READINGS

Bochner F, Carruthers G, Kampmann J, et al: Handbook of Clinical Pharmacology. 2nd Ed. Boston, Little, Brown, 1983

Galeassi RL, Benet LZ, Sheiner LB: Relationship between the pharmacokinetics and pharmacodynamics of procainamide. Clin Pharmacol Ther 25:358, 1979

Gibaldi M, Perrier D: Pharmacokinetics. 2nd Ed. New York, Dekker, 1982

Gibaldi M, Levy G: Pharmacokinetics in clinical practice. 1. Concepts. JAMA 235:1864, 1976

Gibaldi M, Levy G: Pharmacokinetics in clinical practice. 2. Application. JAMA 235:1987, 1976

Gibaldi M, Levy G: Dose-dependent decline of pharmacologic effects of drugs with linear pharmacokinetic characteristics. J Pharmaceut Sci 61:567, 1972

Goodman LS, Gilman A: The Pharmacological Basis of Therapeutics. New York, Macmillan, 6th Edition, 1980

Greenblatt DJ, Koch-Weser J: Drug therapy: Clinical pharmacokinetics. N Eng J Med 293:702, 964, 1975

Holly FO, Ponganis KV, Stanski DR: Effect of cardiopulmonary bypass on the pharmacokinetics of drugs. Clin Pharmacokinet 7:234, 1982

Hug CC Jr.: Pharmacokinetics of drugs administered intravenously. Anesth Analg 57:704, 1978

Hull CJ: Pharmacokinetics and pharmacodynamics. Br J Anaesth 51:579, 1979

La Du BN, Mandel HG, Way EL, (Eds): Fundamentals of drug metabolism and drug disposition, Protein Binding. Baltimore, Williams & Wilkins, 1977

Levy G: Correlation between drug concentration and drug response in man—Pharmacokinetic considerations, pharmacology and the future of man. Proc 5th Int Congr Pharmacol 3:34, 1972

Rowland M, Tozer TN: Clinical Pharmacokinetics: Concepts and Applications. Philadelphia, Lea & Febiger, 1980

Sheiner LB, Stanski DR, Voseh S, et al: Simultaneous modeling of pharmacokinetics and pharmacodynamics: Application to d-tubocurarine. Clin Pharmacol Ther 25:358, 1979

Smith NT, Miller RD, Corbascio AN: Drug Interations in Anesthesia. Philadelphia, Lea & Febiger, 1981

Stanski DR, Watkins WD: Drug Disposition in Anesthesia. New York, Grune & Stratton, 1982

Tiengo M, Cousins MJ (Eds): Pharmacological Basis of Anesthesiology: Clinical Pharmacology of New Analgesics and Anesthetics. New York, Raven, 1983

Wartak J: Clinical Pharmacokinetics: A Modern Approach to Individual Drug Therapy. New York, Praeger, 1983

4

Physics and Anesthesia

Lawrence Litt, M.D., Ph.D.
Ira J. Rampil, M.D.

INTRODUCTION

Although knowledge of modern physics is important to an understanding of the molecular mechanisms of anesthesia (also see Ch. 18), the basic concepts of physics are the fundamental basis of anesthesia. Many fundamental physical processes, such as mass transfer, heat transfer, evaporation, condensation, and mixing take place during routine anesthesia. Physiologic measurements and monitoring have always depended on the detection and measurement of electrical signals, pressure changes, and sound waves. Yet methods of monitoring are constantly evolving (also see Ch. 13), and some of the new equipment seems so complex that its safe use often appears more difficult. Fortunately, much of the new technology has been based on older, familiar principles. This chapter describes some of the important classic physics principles that are relevant

to clinical anesthesia and how they are applied clinically. Many principles of physics not covered in this chapter are explained throughout this book (e.g., mechanisms of anesthesia in Ch. 18 and respiratory care in Ch. 63).

UNITS, STANDARDS, AND DIMENSIONS

The laws of physics are based on experimental measurements. In 1960 a system of units and standards was agreed upon by all scientific communities. The new system is based on the "meter-kilogram-second" (mks) system, known as the Système Internationale (SI). Experiments were carefully described to define the standards, named in parentheses, for six basic units: length (the meter), time (the second), electrical current (the ampere), temperature (degrees Kelvin), and luminous intensity (the candela). A seventh basic unit for mass (the kilogram) was defined in terms of an artifact: a particular platinum–iridium cylinder located at the International Bureau of Weights and Measures near Paris. Many systems of derived units are defined in terms of the basic units.

The mathematical combination of units in a physics formula describes the dimensions of that formula. For example, Newton's law is

$$Force = mass \times acceleration$$

The dimensions of the right-hand side of the equation are mass $\times$ distance/time^2. This combination is used to define derived units of force, such as the newton (SI units), which is 1 kg/m/sec^2; the dyne (cgs units), which is 1g/cm/sec^2; and the pound (U.S. standard units). A newton is 10^5 dynes. Because the acceleration of gravity, g, is measured to be 9.80665 m/sec^2, the force of gravity on a 1-kg mass is 9.80665 newtons.

Pressure is force per unit area, defined in SI units as newtons/m^2, or pascals (Pa). The U.S. standard units of pressure are lb/in^2 (psi). History has burdened us with additional units of pressure. There is the bar, which corresponds to 10^6 dynes/cm^2; mm Hg, which corresponds to the pressure from a 1-mm high column of mercury (density = 13.5951); and, the cm H$_2$O. Consequently, the term 1 standard atmosphere of pressure, defined to mean 760 mm Hg, corresponds to 1,033 g/cm^2, 1.01325 bar, and 14.7 lb/in.^{2}. Anesthesiologists commonly encounter pressure in units of kilopascals (abbreviated kPa); 1 kPa = 1,000 Pa. Because, by definition, 100 kPa = 1 bar, 1 standard atmosphere therefore equals 101.325 kPa. Thus, 1 kPa is very close to 7.50064 mm Hg of pressure, and the pressure of a gas in kilopascals is very nearly equal to its percentage of the total mixture. For example, ambient oxygen at sea level, which is approximately 20.9 percent of the composition of air, has a partial pressure of approximately 20.9 kPa. Pressure in U.S. standard units is occasionally abbreviated PSIA or PSIG. The A and G refer to absolute and gauge pressure, respectively, the latter being the number of pounds per square inch (lb/in.^{2})

above atmospheric pressure. The pressure unit torr, named after Evangelista Torricelli, Professor of Physics at Firenza, inventor of the barometer and the first person to create a sustained vacuum, is not widely used by anesthesiologists. Even the journal, *Anesthesiology*, has stopped using torr, which it has replaced with mm Hg.[1] One torr is very nearly equal to 1 mm Hg.

FORCES, TENSION, AND PRESSURE

The ultimate effect of a force depends on the mass and size of the load being pushed or pulled. For example, premature infants who weigh 0.5 kg and morbidly obese adults who are 400 times heavier exhibit a wide range of force loads. Thus, the clinician rarely refers to total force, but instead expresses quantities in terms of derived units that minimize biovariability.

When an applied external force stretches an object, such as a sheet or a rope, it creates internal forces, called tension, that oppose molecular cohesion and tend to tear the object apart. Suppose that the surface of a fluid-filled cylinder or sphere of radius R experiences a surface tension, T (force per unit length), when the transmural fluid pressure on the walls is P (force per unit area). The law of Laplace, which states that T is proportional to the product $P \times R$, can be explained as follows. In the case of a cylindrical segment of length L (Fig. 4-1), the net upward force exerted by the transmural pressure is just P times the cross-sectional area, or $P \times (2R \times L)$, while the net downward force exerted by the surface tension is just $T \times (2L)$. Equating the two gives Laplace's law for a cylinder: T = PR. A similar calculation can be done for a sphere to get $T = (\frac{1}{2}) \times PR$, as diagrammed in Figure 4-2. In physics, the use of the term tension, or force per unit length, is actually slightly different from the physiologist's and cardiologist's use of the word.[2] Be-

SURFACE TENSION ,T , IN THE WALL OF A CYLINDER

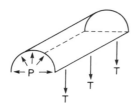

Downward tension x length =
Upward net pressure x cross-sectional surface area

<u>or</u>

T x 2L = P(2RL)

<u>or</u>

T = PR

FIG. 4-1 Laplace's law for a cylinder.

cause the blood vessels and heart chambers can more easily accommodate a larger T when there are more myofibrils in the wall, the medical term wall tension is simply T divided by the wall thickness. In cardiology texts, Laplace's law is often written in the form: wall tension ~ transmural pressure × [(vessel radius)/(wall thickness)]. Laplace's law dictates that a vein can have the same wall tension as an artery, despite its larger radius and thinner wall, because the transmural pressure is smaller. This law also dictates that ventricular hypertrophy reduces wall tension but not T in patients whose left ventricular pressure is pathologically elevated, as in hypertension or aortic stenosis.

SURFACE TENSION ,T , IN THE WALL OF A SPHERE

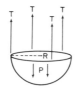

Upward force = Downward pressure force

<u>or</u> $2\pi RT = \pi R^2 P$

<u>or</u> $T = \frac{1}{2}PR$

The above formula is also known as Laplace's Equation

FIG. 4-2 Laplace's law for a sphere.

PRESSURE MANOMETRY

Pressure measurements were first made using open and closed manometers, which are fluid-filled U-shaped tubes. A schematic diagram for an open manometer is sketched in Figure 4-3. An external force pushes down the left side of the tube, forcing fluid to travel up the right side. If a stable equilibrium exists, then the segment of fluid between AA' and CC' is at rest, and the force balancing the left-sided push is just the weight of fluid between BB' and CC'. This is given by Newton's law (F = mass × acceleration) as

Weight = (density × area × height)
        × (gravitational acceleration)

and leads to an expression for the pressure P exerted by the external forces:

$$P = (\text{weight/area}) = \rho \times g \times h$$

Here ρ is the density of the fluid, g is the acceleration of gravity, and h is the height between BB' and CC'. Because ρ and g are kept constant, a manometer is a device that has established a linear relationship between pressure and height. Open manometry is frequently used for monitoring the central venous pressure (CVP). When a manometer is connected to a patient, AA' corresponds to the

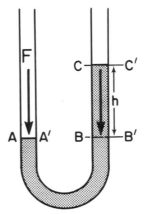

FIG. 4-3 A fluid manometer. An external force, F, pushing down on the left is in equilibrium with the weight of the fluid on the right between BB' and CC'. The height, h, is used to determine the pressure.

height of the right atrium. The zero mark on the manometer, corresponding to BB′, is placed at same height. The CVP, in cm H_2O, corresponds to the height of the column of saline, which is read at the level of CC′. A porous cap on the top of the glass tube prevents dust from entering the CVP line while permitting air to pass.

A clinical example of the physics of pressure is the Pleur-Evac system for chest tube drainage (Fig. 4-4),[3] which is more than 50 years old (also see Ch. 40). Within this three-bottle or two-manometer system, the bottle on the left traps debris that drains from the pleural space. It also protects the pleural space from drawing water into the chest from the waterseal bottle in the middle. When the chest expands during inspiration, intrathoracic pressure falls, and air is drawn from the pharynx into the trachea and the lungs. When a tube penetrates the chest wall, the same decrease in pressure that brings air into the trachea tends to draw air into the chest through the tube.

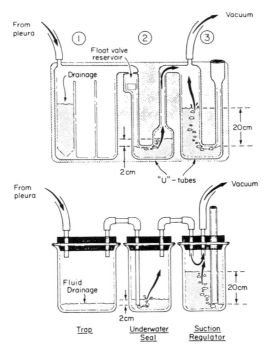

FIG. 4-4 The three-bottle Pleur-Evac circuit. (Fishman NH: Thoracic Drainage—A Manual of Procedures. Copyright © 1983 by Year Book Medical Publishers, Inc., Chicago.)

This is prevented by the waterseal bottle in the middle, which acts as a barrier to air entering the chest tube and as an escape route for air that can be removed from the pleural space by external suction. The waterseal chamber also acts as a manometer. The difference between intrapleural pressure and suction-chamber pressure is determined by the length of tubing below the water surface. That length is normally 2 cm H_2O in the Pleur-Evac system, but it can be greater if more water is put into this chamber. A manometer formation can also be seen at the suction-control chamber connection. As a small amount of vacuum is applied from the wall, air is pulled down the atmospheric vent into the suction-control chamber, and suction is simultaneously transmitted to the waterseal bottle. This suction is then transmitted to the collection chamber and finally, to the pleural cavity. If the strength of the vacuum source is gradually increased, it will reach a point at which the air in the tube to the first bottle is pulled down into it and then pulled out to form a bubble. Application of a constant vacuum to the suction-control bottle results in a steady stream of bubbles and in subatmospheric pressures in the other chambers. The pressure in the suction-control chamber is unchanged if the strength of the wall suction is increased. More bubbles are formed, but ρgh is unchanged. A pressure of -20 cm H_2O occurs in the first-bottle compartment of a Pleur-Evac when it is filled with 415 ml of water. A pressure of -25 cm H_2O results when it is filled with 540 ml of water.

Understanding the operation and function of a Pleur-Evac system is very important following chest closure in thoracotomy procedures (also see Ch. 40). In the operating room there is added breathing difficulty for the thoracotomy patient if spontaneous respirations are permitted before suction is connected to chest tubes in the pleural space. At the end of a case in which a thoracostomy tube is placed, the Pleur-Evac set up should be located so that the chambers are as visible as the other monitors. During closure of the skin, the lungs can be inflated by squeezing the bag on the anesthesia machine to expand the lungs and push air from the pleural space into the chest tube circuit. Bubbles will be seen to copiously traverse the waterseal chamber. When the resulting bubbling is minimized, as much air as possible has been removed, and extubation of the trachea, if indicated, can proceed.

Anesthesiologists frequently visit and transport patients who have a chest tube in place. Checking the functioning of the Pleur-Evac system can frequently benefit the patient. One should examine the waterseal chamber and see whether bubbles are coming through from the collection chamber to the suction chamber. The water level should vary appropriately with respirations. The suction-control chamber should also be checked to see whether water has evaporated. Rates of drainage can be calculated from markings on the collection chamber that indicate the times when accumulation levels were checked. When leaving a patient with a chest tube, the anesthesiologist should also ensure that no dependent loops are in the chest tube circuit. Redundant hose should be properly fixed on the bed. Overhanging loops that become filled with fluid or with clotted blood can decrease the force of suction that reaches the pleural space.

In systems in which the total energy remains constant, the potential and kinetic energies may vary. Steady, smooth flow of an incompressible liquid through a tube of varying cross-sectional diameters constitutes one example (Fig. 4-5). This system was studied by Bernoulli, who recognized that the fluid flow speeds up at the narrow regions and slows down again when the tube widens. He also recognized that the pressure is greatest where the flow is slowest. Energy conservation can be used to understand Bernoulli's observation. The equation for the total energy of a fluid bolus going down the tube may be written as the sum of the internal pressure energy in the fluid, its gravitational potential, and the energy of its motion, or:

Total energy of bolus = internal potential energy + external potential energy + kinetic energy

or

$$\text{Total energy} = PV + \rho(gh)\text{area} + \tfrac{1}{2}mv^2$$

WORK AND ENERGY

By definition, work is the exertion of a force through a distance, or

$$\text{Work} = \text{force} \times \text{distance}$$

When an electric motor pulls an elevator up several floors, it does work against gravity. The work that any system can do, however, is limited by the first and second laws of thermodynamics. The first law states that energy cannot be created or destroyed and that the total energy of a system (kinetic energy plus potential energy) is all that can be made available. Energy conservation does not demand that heat, which is the total kinetic energy of all the molecules in a system, flow only from warm objects to cold ones. Nature's insistence that heat transfer be from warmer objects to colder ones is summarized in the second law of thermodynamics.

BERNOULLI'S LAW –
The pressure is greatest where the velocity is lowest

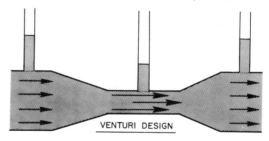

VENTURI DESIGN

Flow is faster through the narrow region. There is no turbulence if the emergence angle is less than ~ 25°

FIG. 4-5 Bernouilli's law and the Venturi effect. Since the total energy of a bolus of fluid remains constant as it flows through this Venturi tube, the increase in the velocity of the fluid (kinetic energy) in the narrow or "throat" region is matched by a drop in the pressure of the fluid (internal potential energy). This Venturi effect forms the basis for atomizers in which the flow of one fluid through a Venturi pulls another fluid into the Venturi throat by the force of the pressure gradient.

where P is pressure, V is volume, ρ is density, g is the gravitational constant, h is the height above baseline, m is the mass and v is the velocity of the fluid.

If the height of the tube is fixed, and the total energy of the bolus of incompressible fluid is constant (no heat loss to walls), then P must drop as v increases, and vice-versa. Venturi realized how complicating factors such as turbulence and compressibility can prevent the fluid from returning to its original speed when the geometry of the tube is restored. He designed a constricted tube for fluid flow that widened out gently, so as to minimize heat loss to the walls and allow for the Venturi effect, which is the nearly complete restoration of pressure after the drop in the high velocity region. The Venturi effect is the basis for nebulization systems and simple air–oxygen dilution systems (also see Ch. 63).

GASES

THE IDEAL GAS LAW AND PARTIAL PRESSURES

The molecules of a gas generally behave like hard spheres colliding with each other and with the walls of the container, according to the laws of classical mechanics. Important properties of a gas include its volume, V; the expansion pressure that it exerts, P; and the average kinetic energy per gas molecule, which is linearly related to the absolute temperature, T. These classic thermodynamic variables are related to the number of molecules in the gas by the ideal gas law

$$PV = NkT$$

N is where the number of molecules, and k is Boltzmann's constant, the average kinetic energy change acquired by one molecule during a temperature increase of 1 degree centigrade.

No gas behaves exactly according to this law, which is why the word "ideal" is used.

The behavior of most gases, however, closely follows the law's predictions. Note that the rest masses of the gas molecules never enter into the formula. Boltzmann's constant, k, is the same for all gas molecules. Thus, the ideal gas law permits only one value of N for a given set of P, V, and T values. This is the statement that at equal volumes, pressures, and temperatures, two gases have the same number of molecules (Avogadro's hypothesis).

The ideal gas law evolved historically from experiments and observations by Robert Boyle (1662), Jaques Charles (1787), Joseph Louis Gay-Lussac (1802), and Amadeo Avogadro (1811). It is also written for n moles of gas as

$$PV = nRT$$

with R, the universal gas constant, having a value of 8.31 joules/(mole/°K) in SI units, which is 62 mm Hg/L/(mole/°K). R is useful for performing classic thermodynamics calculations, and it can be used together with measurements of the specific heat to determine whether a gas is polyatomic or monatomic. Because the ideal gas law follows from the basic principles of statistical mechanics, it does not achieve the same intellectual standing among physicists as Newton's law or Coulomb's law. Nevertheless, it is a very useful law. Anesthesiologists frequently employ the ideal gas law to translate the pressure-gauge reading on a storage cylinder into knowledge of the remaining gas volume.

The ideal gas law is consistent with and complementary to Dalton's law, which states that the total pressure exerted by a gas mixture is the sum of the individual pressures of the constituents. The individual pressures are also called partial pressures. To appreciate how the two laws fit together, consider a mixture of several gases at the same temperature T, in a container of volume V. The ideal gas law can be written separately for each gas:

$$P_i \cdot V = N_i \cdot k \cdot T \qquad (1)$$

According to Dalton's law, however, the sum of the P_i values is just the total pressure P. Summing the equations for each component gas therefore yields

$$P \cdot V = (P_1 + P_2 + \cdots) \cdot V =$$
$$(N_1 + N_2 + \cdots)k \cdot T = N \cdot k \cdot T \quad (2)$$

while division of equation (1) by equation (2) gives

$$P_i/P = N_i/N \quad (3)$$

Thus, the total pressure is the sum of the partial pressures, and any one partial pressure is the total pressure times the fractional concentration of the component of interest.

The anesthetic effect of vapors appears to depend on molecules dissolving into critical hydrophobic regions (also see Chs. 18 & 19). The number of molecules that dissolve into a lipid is directly proportional to the partial pressure of those molecules. Thus, anesthetic effect depends on the partial pressure (i.e., mm Hg) of the anesthetic agent.

This is a very important point if one wants to consider situations of variable barometric pressure, such as hyperbaric anesthesia and anesthesia at high altitude. A change in barometric pressure means that the numerical value of the percentage concentration corresponds to a new numerical value of the partial pressure. For example, at a barometric pressure of one atmosphere (1 atm), a 1 percent concentration corresponds to a partial pressure of 7.60 mm Hg. In a submarine pressurized to 2 atm, a 1 percent concentration corresponds to 15.2 mm Hg. Administering the same anesthetic dose at each of these barometric pressures requires a different percentage concentration.

The independent contributions of a mixture's partial pressures are also exhibited during anesthesia after nitrous oxide diffuses into the balloon cuff of the endotracheal tube. The balloon cuff, initially inflated to a pressure that is approximately 10 mm Hg above barometric pressure, will accept nitrous oxide molecules until the partial pressure of N_2O inside is the same as its partial pressure outside. This tends to raise the total pressure in the balloon cuff and to expand it further. Approximately 5 to 10 cc of nitrous oxide will enter the balloon cuff of a standard endotracheal tube if 70 percent nitrous oxide is administered for 2 hours.[4] The loud bang of a bursting balloon has been known

to surprise unsuspecting anesthetists who are behind in their studies of Dalton's law.

A clinical example that uses some of the above principles is entonox, the commercial name of a single-cylinder gas mixture that is 50 percent O_2 and 50 percent N_2O. Properties of this relatively new product, widely in use in Europe and Canada and not yet in use in the United States,[5,6] are commonly discussed in the context of Dalton's law. Entonox permits medical personnel to provide supplemental oxygen simultaneously with N_2O, an analgesic drug that can quickly be eliminated. The pressure of a full entonox cylinder is 2,200 psi, the same as that of a full oxygen cylinder. According to Dalton's law, the partial pressure of nitrous oxide is therefore 1,100 psi, which is considerably higher than 745 psi, a value that is said to be the maximum possible. Shouldn't the N_2O partial pressure still be 745 psi? Shouldn't there be a puddle of liquid N_2O at the bottom of the entonox cylinder? Will the gas that emerges from the full cylinder really be a 50:50 mixture? Interestingly enough, the 50:50 nature of the mixture is maintained from the first cc until the last, as long as the entonox temperature is kept above $-5.5°C$ (or $22.1°F$). Cooling of the mixture below this temperature can result in condensation of the nitrous oxide, as well as the problems mentioned above.

Two points can be emphasized here. The first is that entonox (when kept warm) does follow Dalton's law. The second is that N_2O behaves differently when mixed with oxygen than it does alone. Cohesive forces between N_2O molecules are not as strong when O_2 is interposed, and condensation does not happen so easily.

Another important clinical example is the mixture of air and oxygen commonly used during the transport and care of neonates. Although the goal—adequate oxygenation without hyperoxia—is usually assured with the aid of one or more monitoring devices, it is important to know the percentage of oxygen that results from choosing the air and oxygen flow rates. It turns out that this is an easy calculation that can be performed as follows:[7] Let f_1 represent the flow rate of air, f_2 the flow rate of oxygen, a the fraction of air that is oxygen (approx 0.21), and A the fraction of the final mixture that is oxygen. The equation for A is

$$A = [af_1 + f_2]/[f_1 + f_2]$$

This can be solved for $[f_1/f_2]$:

(air flow/oxygen flow) $= [f_1/f_2] = (1 - A)/(A - a)$

Thus, a 40 percent O_2 concentration can be achieved in the final mixture (A = 2/5) by having (air/oxygen) $= [f_1/f_2] = (1 - 2/5)/(2/5 - 1/5) = 3/1$. Using the same approximation, a = 1/5, we can calculate that a 33 percent O_2 concentration will result from an air to O_2 flow ratio of 5 : 1.

VAPORS

Atoms and molecules—the building blocks of solid, liquid, and gaseous matter—are constantly in motion. The motion can be very restrained, as in solid substances, so that classical properties like shape and volume are constant. Or, the motion can be wild and random, as in gases, with the molecules darting about and colliding with each other. Because of such unrestrained atomic and molecular motion, the shape and volume of a gas are easily changed. In liquids the molecules are less tightly bound than in solids, so that shape changes occur easily while volume stays constant.

It is easy for the molecules in certain types of liquids, called vapors, to escape into the air through a process known as evaporation. Evaporation happens as a result of random molecular collisions near the liquid's surface. Sufficiently fast molecules can escape and carry away energy. Heat, which is really the total kinetic energy that a substance has due to the atomic and molecular motion within, is lost from the liquid when evaporation occurs. The heat of vaporization is the number of calories required to transform 1 g liquid into a gas. (For water the value is 540 cal/g.) It is possible to vaporize a liquid isothermally, that is, without changing the temperature, or average kinetic energy of the molecules. This requires a constant temperature source, however, which is not usually present. Thus vaporization normally involves both heat transfer and tempera-

ture reduction from the objects in contact with the liquid being vaporized. The swimmer who comes out of the water into a breeze is cooled, as is the surgical patient who has a large abdominal incision and extensive intestinal exposure; as is the isoflurane vaporizer through which there is a high O_2 flow.

Molecular interactions within the liquid phase of a vapor determine how easy it is for molecules to escape into the gas phase. The reverse process, in which molecules go from the gas phase back into the liquid phase, also occurs. This is known as condensation, and it happens when molecules from the gas lose so much energy through collisions that they can no longer resist cohesive intermolecular forces that are trying to restrain their motion. The "fog" that appears in the endotracheal tube during exhalation is an example. However, condensation in a tube simply means that the cavity being ventilated has water vapor within it. The "fog" that appears with exhalation and disappears with inhalation does not guarantee tube placement into the trachea. Condensation can appear in the plastic tube if one is ventilating a stomach containing water.

Temperature changes in a vaporizer are important. Cooling of a vaporizer can occur when vapor is being rapidly consumed due to high flow. Warming of the vaporizer can occur when the operating room is warmed for pediatric cases. The vapor pressure of an anesthetic increases when it is heated and falls when it is cooled, which can result in the delivery of a different anesthetic dose.

The anesthetic dose delivered by a vaporizer can be calculated. Each cc of gas that leaves the vaporizer will have a certain fraction, f, being saturated with anesthetic gas. The partial pressure of the anesthetic gas in the mixture that leaves the vaporizer is V_p, the vapor pressure, and the fraction, f, of molecules that are anesthetic gas is determined by equation (3), which followed Dalton's law.

Let f = (vapor pressure)/(atmospheric pressure) $= V_p/V_{atm}$, let y = [(cc's anesthetic gas formed)/minute], and let z = [(cc/min) of gas flowing into the vaporizer]. Then, f = y/(y + z), which can be rearranged to yield

$$y/z = f/(1 - f) \tag{4}$$

or [cc's anesthetic gas formed)/minute]/[(cc/

minute) of gas flowing into the vaporizer] = f/(1 − f). For the case of halothane and isoflurane, f ≈ (250 mm Hg)/(750 mm Hg) = 1/3, so that f/(1 − f) = [1/3]/[2/3] = 1/2, and 50 cc of halothane or isoflurane emerges from the vaporizer for every 100 cc of O_2 that flows in. Equation (4) permits the computation of anesthetic dose at any barometric pressure. Suppose, for example, that a vaporizer is in a submarine pressurized to 1,500 mm Hg, almost 2 atm. We would then have f = (250)/(2 × 750) = 1/6, so that f/(1 − f) = [1/6]/[5/6] = 1/5. At this hyperbaric pressure, (1,500 mm Hg), 20 cc of halothane or isoflurane would emerge from the vaporizer to accompany every 100 cc of O_2 that enters the vaporizer. Anesthetic effect, however, is determined by partial pressure and not by percentage concentration. A 1 percent, halothane concentration implies a halothane partial pressure of 7.50 mm Hg near sea level and a 15.00 mm Hg partial pressure when the barometric pressure is doubled. To give the sea level anesthetic dose in the pressurized submarine, a 0.5 percent concentration should be chosen. This can be achieved by having a vaporizer flow of 100 cc/min of O_2 (so as to produce 20 cc/min of halothane), together with a total gas flow (vaporizer output + all other gases) of 4 L/min. Note that the final settings for anesthesia delivery at 2 atm are not very different from the settings at sea level, where the total flow is 5 L/min. (Further details of vaporization and vaporizers are discussed in Chapter 5.)

HUMIDITY

The absolute humidity of a gas mixture is the mass of water per unit volume of gas. The relative humidity is the ratio of the amount of water vapor actually present to the maximum that could be present. At any one temperature there is a particular pressure at which evaporation and condensation will occur at the same rate. At that pressure, known as the saturation vapor pressure, as many molecules go from the liquid phase into the gas phase as vice versa. The saturation vapor pressure for water vapor depends on temperature. The dew point is de-

fined as the temperature at which a gas mixture is fully saturated with water. At the dew point, the relative humidity of the water vapor is 100 percent. The presence of additional water molecules in the vapor would result in condensation occurring throughout. The maximum amount of water vapor that air will hold is 17 g/m³ at 20°C and 44 g/m³ at 37°C. If air at 20°C with a relative humidity of 100 percent is warmed to 37°C, the absolute humidity remains unchanged, while the relative humidity falls to approximately 39 percent. The dew point for the air in this example is 20°C.[8]

It was once extremely important to monitor and regulate the humidity of ambient air in the operating suite. Water vapor permits static electric charge to leak to ground. When explosive anesthetics were used, the relative humidity in the operating suite needed to be no less than 60 percent. Of greater clinical importance today is the regulation of the temperature and humidity of the gases used for ventilation.[9-12] If the nose, which warms and humidifies the inspired air, is bypassed by an endotracheal tube or a tracheostomy, cooler air with less moisture will be delivered to the bronchopulmonary tree. This can result in impaired ciliary motility and in thicker secretions that are diffcult to remove,[13-16] in epithelial damage,[13] in decreased lung compliance,[17] and in evaporative fluid loss and heat loss by the patient (see Chs. 63 & 64). Conversely, the delivery of warm, moist inspired gas can be used to help raise and maintain body temperature.[18] A water content of 33 g/m³ (100 percent relative humidity at 35°C) seems adequate to prevent most problems.[8-10] Ultrasonic nebulizers, which produce water droplets whose size is a few microns, can generate water contents of as much as 90 mg/m³, and can cause overhydration and hyperthermia.

AZEOTROPES

The subject of azeotropes commonly arises when the wrong anesthetic is used to fill a half-empty vaporizer. An azeotrope is a mixture of two vapors that evaporates to provide a gas mixture having the agents present in the same ratio that occurs in solution. Azeotropic anesthesia was briefly popular after the introduction of halothane. The idea was to mix it with diethyl ether and to reap the advantages of two agents having counteracting side effects. An azeotropic mixture of halothane with diethyl ether occurs only when the fraction of halothane is 68 percent.

DIFFUSION

GENERAL PRINCIPLES

A localized concentration of a substance tends to spread throughout space and other substances by the process of diffusion. Diffusion refers to the repeated molecular collisions that eventually disperse the starting population. It does not include convection, the background flow or "wind" current that often contributes to transport and mixing. Diffusion is an important mechanism of membrane transport for all substances in pericapillary regions. Oxygen, carbon dioxide, and the anesthetic gases diffuse across the membranes and compartments that separate alveolar gas and the blood in the pulmonary capillaries. Nitrous oxide in the blood will quickly diffuse into any gaseous compartment that is present in the body and cause it to expand. Thus N_2O can expand the volume of gas present in the middle ear, a pneumothorax, a dilated loop of obstructed bowel, or a bubble injected by a surgeon (also see Ch. 19). Nitrous oxide can also diffuse from the inspired gas mixture into the balloon cuff of the endotracheal tube.[4]

The rate of transmembrane diffusion for a substance from one compartment to another depends on (1) the concentration gradient across the membrane, (2) the solubility of the molecules in the membrane and in each compartment, (3) the thickness of the membrane, (4) the molecular size and molecular weight of the substance, and (5) electrical charge. Thus

hydrogen and helium diffuse very quickly, CO_2 diffuses faster than O_2 because of its greater solubility, and injected local anesthetics diffuse very slowly.

The process of diffusion can result in an electrical voltage difference called the diffusion potential. In Figure 4-6 the compartment on the left is shown to have a much more concentrated solution of NaCl than the compartment on the right, and the Na^+ and Cl^- ions are assumed to have different diffusion channels. If changes in the concentrations on both sides of the barrier are negligible and Na^+ ions diffuse more easily, then positive ions will travel to the right side faster than negative ions, and the right side will accumulate a net positive charge. A positive charge will build up along the barrier, and the faster Na^+ ions will be somewhat repelled, while the slower Cl^- ions will be attracted with greater force. A situation will be reached in which the net flow to the right of Na^+ and Cl^- will be the same. The voltage difference that results from the charge buildup is called the diffusion potential, given by the Nernst equation:

$$V(mV) = 58 \frac{u_- - u_+}{u_- + u_+} \log \left[\frac{C_H}{C_L} \right]$$

Symbols u_+ and u_- represent the mobilities of the positive and negative ions in the example, while C_H and C_L represent the high and low concentrations. Setting either u_+ or u_- to 0 gives the more familiar Nernst formula for each ion's equilibrium potential, or the potential that just stops the net diffusion of either species of ion. The equations that describe the physiol-

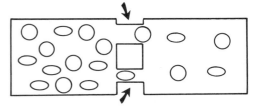

CHLORINE DIFFUSION CHANNEL

SODIUM DIFFUSION CHANNEL

High concentration NaCl   Low concentration NaCl

FIG. 4-6 Model system for studying diffusion potentials.

ogy of transcellular membrane potential are more complex than the Nernst equation.[19]

Intravenous therapy often includes measures aimed at altering membrane potentials, transcellular ion gradients, and the kinetics of transmembrane diffusion and transport. Examples are the administration of KCl and calcium-channel blocking agents such as verapamil (also see Ch. 28).

Diffusion potentials are important in the operation of the glass-sensitive pH electrode. If more hydrogen ion is present on one side of a thin glass strip than on the other, hydrogen will diffuse from the heavily populated side to the other, and a diffusion potential will result. If one side of the glass is kept at a standardized hydrogen ion concentration, a measurement of the voltage difference across the glass can be used to determine the pH on the second side.

BLOOD-GAS ELECTRODES[20,21]
(Also See Ch. 37)

THE pH ELECTRODE

The pH electrode most commonly in use has pH-sensitive glass as the transducing element. The capillary glass pH electrode with a water jacket for temperature control has a standard concentration of hydrogen ion on one side of a film of glass. The solution, typically heparinized blood of which the pH is to be determined, sits on the other side of the glass. The voltage difference across the thin film of glass is measured, and the result is compared with a calibration curve to determine pH. A schematic diagram of the capillary glass pH electrode is shown in Figure 4-7.

The glass film is but one element in the pathway of the complete electrical circuit. The other elements, however, have been chosen so that their circuit properties will be the same for all samples injected through the capillary tube. The side of the glass film maintained at a standard pH has a silver wire electrode that sits in a solution in which AgCl is mixed with 0.1 N HCl. When a metal electrode sits in a solution of one of its own salts, positive metal ions leave

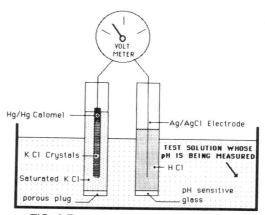

FIG. 4-7 The glass–calomel pH electrode.

the electrode and go into the solution, leaving behind negative charge and creating a voltage difference between the electrode and solution. (This type of potential is called a Galvanic potential, in contrast to a diffusion potential.) The salt solution is saturated with silver, so the galvanic potential is very stable, and the hydrogen ion concentration that results from the complete dissociation of 0.1 N HCl (pH = 1.0) will not be significantly changed by diffusion of hydrogen across the glass to a physiologic sample, or test solution.

The side of the glass that has the test solution whose pH we want to measure also communicates with a reference electrode. The reference electrode usually consists of a platinum wire in contact with mercury that is in contact with a saturated solution of Hg_2Cl_2, or calomel, and an 0.1 N KCl. The KCl solution is separated from the test solution by a porous membrane whose geometry is designed so that the diffusion potential across it is much smaller than that across the glass. This diffusion potential is sometimes referred to as a liquid junction potential. The determination of pH is obtained by monitoring the voltage difference between the two electrode wires. According to the above discussion, changes in this voltage are designed to arise only from changes in the diffusion potential across the pH-sensitive glass. The voltage between the two electrodes is typically 50 mV per pH unit. Two known buffer solutions are used to calibrate the pH meter.

Modern technology has recently made it convenient to use spectrophotometry to determine pH. A pH probe is available that has a sensing region which consists of a dialysis membrane in contact with blood on one side, and either a fluorescent or absorptive, pH-sensitive indicator on the other side. Hydrogen ions can diffuse across the membrane, but blood and the pH indicator cannot. Two thin fiberoptic light guides are in optical contact with the pH indicator. Color changes of the indicator or fluorescence are followed remotely by flashing light into the indicator via one fiberoptic strand and by performing spectrophotometric analysis of the light reflected back on the other strand.

THE CARBON DIOXIDE ELECTRODE[22]

The pH measurement of a bicarbonate solution at fixed concentration permits the determination of PCO_2. The Henderson–Hasselbalch equation connects PCO_2 and pH as follows:

$$pH = pK - \log (PCO_2) + \log [(HCO_3)/S]$$

where S represents the solubility of CO_2 in millimoles per mm Hg, and pK is the apparent dissociation constant. In the Severinghaus electrode, schematically shown in Figure 4-8, a pH-sensitive glass electrode monitors the pH of a thin layer of bicarbonate solution that has its PCO_2 in equilibrium with the PCO_2 of blood. As diagrammed in Figure 4-8, the blood sample being measured is separated from the thin-layered bicarbonate solution by a Teflon layer and a wet spacer soaked with salt, bicarbonate ion, and carbonic anhydrase. The voltage output of the electrode is proportional to the pH; thus it varies as a logarithmic function of PCO_2. A 10-fold change in PCO_2 produces a change of 1.0 pH units. Because the electrode is sensitive to the absolute PCO_2 alone, it responds identically to samples of blood, water, or gas and can be calibrated using compressed gases. Sources of error arise from membrane leaks, insufficiently small samples, gas bubbles in the sampling channel, and temperature instability. The Severinghaus CO_2 electrode, like the O_2 electrode described below, has been adapted for blood-gas machines, ambient air monitor-

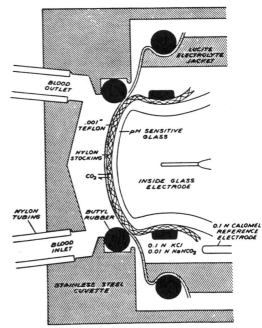

FIG. 4-8 The Severinghaus CO_2 Electrode. (Severinghaus JW: Blood gas concentrations, The Handbook of Physiology, Waverly Press, Baltimore, 1965, pp 1475–1487.)

ing, and transcutaneous, subcutaneous, and intravascular monitoring.

THE OXYGEN ELECTRODE[23]

The polaragraphic oxygen electrode enormously facilitated the measurement of PO_2 in solutions. The term polarography refers to a particular method of electrochemical detection. In this method a constant voltage is maintained between two electrodes in a conducting aqueous medium that contains a reducing substance, or electron acceptor. Oxygen, the great electron acceptor, is the only reductant in the Clark electrode, shown schematically in Figure 4-9, that will release electrons from platinum cathode and permit a current to flow to the silver chloride anode. The geometry and voltage of the system dictate that current flow between the electrodes is proportional to O_2 concentration in the conducting medium. The electrode wires are small, so that oxygen con-

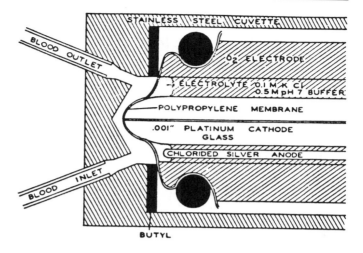

FIG. 4-9 The Clark O_2 electrode. (Clark LC Jr, Bargeron LM Jr, Lyons C, et al: Detection of right-to-left shunts with an arterial potentiometric electrode. Circulation 22:949, 1960. Reprinted by permission of the American Heart Association, Inc.)

sumption by the measurement process does not significantly alter the result.

Selective membrane permeability and polarography are also the basis for electrodes that permit determination of other cations, such as K^+ and Na^+.

FLUID DYNAMICS

VISCOSITY

The molecules of a fluid, which are more strongly attracted to each other than are the molecules of a gas, interact to generate an internal friction, or "stickiness," that causes one region of a fluid to oppose the displacement of a neighboring region. This phenomenon is described by the concept of viscosity. Absolute viscosity is the shearing force per unit area needed to produce a standard velocity difference between different layers of a fluid that are a standard distance apart. The notion that fluid flow can be thought of in terms of sliding adjacent layers is called the concept of laminar flow. Figure 4-10 schematically illustrates the concept of viscosity in the context of laminar flow. Absolute viscosity is most commonly ex-

pressed in terms of the derived unit poise (P), named after Poiseuille. In terms of basic units, the dimensions of Poise are

(shearing force per unit area)/(velocity change per unit thickness)

or

[Force/area]/[(distance/time)/distance]

or

Force × time/area

A liquid that responds to a shearing force of 1 dyne/cm² with a velocity gradient of 1 (cm/

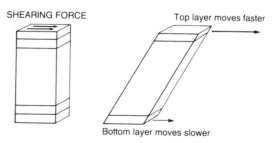

SHEARING FORCE

Top layer moves faster

Bottom layer moves slower

Poise = Dynes × Seconds/cm²
FOR UNIT VELOCITY DIFFERENCE
AND UNIT THICKNESS OF LAYER:
Viscosity = [Shearing Force]/Area

FIG. 4-10 Viscosity. The friction of one layer of fluid moving over another causes a relative slipping from one layer to the next. Fluid layers closest to the walls of a conduit move more slowly than do layers farther away.

sec) per cm thickness of liquid has a dynamic viscosity coefficient, or "viscosity," of 1 Poise (1 P). The unit of viscosity defined in this manner is enormous. In SI units, 1 P = 0.1 (newton · sec)/m². Relative viscosity and specific viscosity are convenient terms that state the viscosity relative to that of water at standard conditions (0.01 P, or 1 cP, at 20°C).

Viscosity, like other frictional forces, increases with temperature and density. For this reason, viscosity is sometimes given in kinematic viscosity units, called stokes (St). The kinematic viscosity is the absolute viscosity divided by the fluid density, with each value being taken at a particular temperature. Liquids of identical temperature and density, however, can have different viscosities. Furthermore, many liquids of complex composition differ from water in that their viscosities seem to vary with the velocity of fluid flow. The viscous properties of such liquids are said to be non-Newtonian, because the equations for viscous flow, originally worked out by Newton, become approximate rather than exact. The application of Newton's equations to studies with blood led to the conclusion that blood has an "apparent viscosity" that is increased at low blood flow, but decreased in vessels with a smaller radius.[24] The "apparent viscosity" of blood increases with the hematocrit, which varies throughout the body, reaching values that are above 80 percent in the spleen and bone marrow and below 20 percent in the medulla of the kidney. The viscosity of blood at 37°C is 0.028 P, while that of water at the same temperature is 0.007 P.

Particle motion within a viscous medium, described by the Navier–Stokes equations, is more complicated than particle motion in free space, where inertial forces and Newton's laws prevail. According to Stokes' law, a sphere of radius A that falls freely in a viscous medium reaches a constant velocity, v, of descent, unlike a particle that falls freely without friction, and accelerates constantly. A little more than 100 years ago, Osborne Reynolds pointed out that the ratio of inertial to viscous forces on the falling sphere of Stokes is given by $Av\rho/n$, or simply by Av/μ, where μ is the kinematic viscosity. This ratio is now called the Reynold's number. When it is very small, viscous forces dominate over classic Newtonian forces. If one considers A to simply be a representative dimension, and v to be a representative velocity, then the given equation can be used to estimate the Reynold's number for many types of situations. The Reynold's number for a man swimming turns out to be approximately 10^4, while that of tropical fish swimming is approximately 10^2. For *Escherichia coli*, which are approximately 1 μm in size, the Reynolds number is 10^{-4} or 10^{-5}. A human could experience physics at this low Reynolds number by putting on a frogman suit, getting into a swimming pool full of molasses, and then never moving any part of the body faster than 1 cm/min.[25]

At high velocities laminar flow does not take place. Fluid flow becomes turbulent. Coulter and Pappenheimer[26] studied the transition to turbulence for blood flow in rigid tubes a few millimeters in diameter. They found that when the Reynolds number is greater than 2,000 turbulence is usually present. In the aorta the Reynold's number exceeds 10,000 during systole. An increase in velocity, an increase in tube diameter, and a decrease in viscosity all raise the Reynold's number and take conditions closer to the threshold for turbulence. Turbulence in blood, however, can also occur at a lower Reynold's number (approximately 1,000) in cases where there is pulsatile flow or abrupt change in geometry. Because laminar flow is silent, turbulence appears responsible for sounds and murmurs from the circulatory system.

Although the Reynold's number is greater for blood vessels with larger radius, there is a limit to how small a vessel can be in order to support laminar blood flow. The composite nature of blood, the pulsatile nature of the driving system, and the collapsibility of thin vessels all add up to the minimum blood vessel diameter for laminar flow being approximately 0.5 mm. In vessels larger than this, then, and at Reynold's numbers below 1,000—which is the case for most of the vascular tree—blood flow is approximately laminar.

In 1846 Hagan and Poiseuille uncovered the pressure–flow relationships that were mathematically derived later from the definition of viscosity. The Hagan–Poiseuille result for laminar fluid flow in a rigid tube of radius r and length L is analogous to Ohm's formula for current flow in an electronic circuit:

$$(P_2 - P_1) = Q \cdot R \qquad \text{(fluids, no turbulence)}$$

Voltage = (electrical current) $\times$ (resistance)
(Ohm's Law — electronics)

where P_1 and P_2 are the pressures at each end of the tube, Q is the flow (volume/time), and R is the resistance. The Hagan–Poiseuille equation is written as follows:

$$Q = (P_2 - P_1)/R$$

where

$$R = \frac{8\eta L}{\pi r^4}$$

Where η = dynamic viscosity.

The principal determinant of resistance to laminar flow in blood vessels and endotracheal tubes, then, is the radius, r, which is raised to the fourth power. When rapid blood transfusions might be important, we should recall from the Hagan–Poiseuille equation that the "standard" 8-inch-long, 16-gauge CVP catheter (1.7 mm diameter) has more than nine times the resistance of a 2-inch long 14-gauge IV catheter (2.1 mm diameter). Furthermore, although the Hagan–Poiseuille law tells us that changes in vascular resistance are primarily due to changes in vessel radius, it says nothing about the origin of the change. For example, when there is a combined increase in vessel diameter and fluid flow, we need more information to be able to say which one resulted from the other. Some vessels can be distended when elevated pressures increase flow. Increased flow can also result from an increased diameter, as in pharmacologically mediated vasodilatation.

The Hagan–Poiseuille law does not apply when the flow is turbulent, since disorderly circular currents are present. If there is turbulence, the doubling of pressure is inadequate to double fluid flow. Turbulent flow, such as that through a stenotic heart valve, increases approximately with the square root of the pressure, the square of the radius, and the reciprocal of the density.

WAVES

A wave is a disturbance that propagates through a medium. Sound waves are density or pressure fluctuations about the equilibrium value, electromagnetic waves are variations in the steady-state values of the electromagnetic fields in space; and fluid waves, like those that rock a sailboat in the ocean, are changes in the height of a fluid as the surface moves up and down.

The motion of a wave must be distinguished from movements made by the medium that transmits the wave. A water wave on the ocean's surface travels in a horizontal direction, while the motion of the water's surface is only up and down. Einstein once described the distinction between wave velocity and motion within a medium by stating that it is possible for a rumor to travel quickly across a distance far greater than that traversed by any of the gossiping parties. His analogy is also true for the circulation, where the periphery senses the blood pressure from a single ventricular contraction of the heart several seconds before receiving the red blood cells that were in the stroke volume.

The velocity of a wave, V, refers to the speed of the disturbance. The frequency of a wave, f, is the rate at which the disturbance is repeated. The length of a wave, or wavelength, L, is the closest distance between identically behaving regions of a wave. These variables are all related by a simple, very important equation:

$$V = f \cdot L$$

The speed of sound is approximately 330 m/sec in air, 1,550 m/sec in soft human tissue, and 4,000 m/sec in skull and bone. Sonic frequencies, those audible by the human ear,

TABLE 4-1. Sound Power Levels in Decibels

Decibels	Stimulus
0	Threshold of hearing
20	Average whisper
50	Office background noise
60	Normal conversation
90	Pneumatic hammer at a few meters
120	Threshold of pain
130	Jet aircraft at 50 meters
200	Saturn rocket at 50 meters

range from about 30 to 20,000 Hz. The intensity of sound is quantified according to the decibel (dB) scale, as listed in Table 4-1. The 0 dB point on the scale has arbitrarily been defined as 10^{-16} watts/cm^2, which is a power level just at the 1,000-Hz hearing threshold in most humans.

Ultrasonic frequencies, arbitrarily defined as those above 150,000 Hz, are required for sonar-style devices that can separate small distances within the human body. We have just noted that sound takes 1 μsec to travel 1.55 mm through soft human tissue. Our formula relating velocity, wavelength, and frequency tells us that a 15.5-MHz ultrasonic transducer will therefore generate wavelengths of 0.1 mm, which is excellent for ultrasonic imaging. Ultrasound is attenuated differently by various parts of the body. Most tissues have attenuation coefficients of 1.3 to 1.7 dB/cm. The lung, however, has an attenuation coefficient of 40 dB/cm, which explains why good echocardiography studies are difficult in patients with oversized lungs that get between the heart and the chest wall. Bone and air have attenuation coefficients close to 10 dB/cm.

Ultrasonic imaging, which is based on the detection of reflected sound waves, involves principles that are very similar to the Navy's use of sonar. A short burst of sound is emitted from a probe at the same time that a clock is started. Reflected waves occur whenever the emitted ultrasound burst encounters a boundary between layers of different acoustical properties. Greater acoustical differences result in larger amplitude reflections. The ultrasonic imager detects the time and amplitude of reflected waves that have bounced straight back to the probe, assumes that the velocity of sound is uniform throughout the tissues, and then uses the formula, distance = velocity × time,

to calculate the distances to reflecting boundaries. These distances are then stored in electronic memory, along with the signal amplitudes that indicated the strength of the reflection. Each burst of ultrasound is used to obtain information about the location and density of matter along a straight line. The automated scanning of several straight lines is used to reconstruct a one or two-dimensional picture of the observations. Ultrasonic probes are available that can be situated in the esophagus, directed at the heart during anesthesia, and used to construct an image of the heart for each cardiac cycle. Beat-to-beat intraoperative monitoring of ventricular distention and cardiac wall motion can be used during vascular surgery to see how a heart responds when an aortic crossclamp is applied, how a heart is performing after the chest has been closed in a coronary revascularization procedure, and whether air emboli are occurring.[27,28]

Reflected ultrasonic waves can be used not only to sense the presence of an object, but also to determine its velocity. This is accomplished by exploiting Doppler's principle, which states that when waves are emitted by a moving source, a stationary observer perceives them at a frequency that is shifted from the one at which they are emitted. People near hospitals commonly experience the Doppler shift when they hear a high-pitched ambulance siren approaching them, and a lower-pitched ambulance siren going away from them. Figure 4-11 illustrates the phenomenon, which comes about because the wave velocity is constant despite the motion of the source. The listener in front of the moving source is seen to receive more sound pulses per second than the listener behind. The formula for the frequency shift is

$$f_{obs} = f_{source} \cdot [1 + (V_{source}/V_{wave})]$$

Doppler blood flow detectors are commonly used by anesthesiologists in pediatric cases as a sensitive detector of the radial pulse and in neurosurgical cases as an early indicator of air embolism (also see Chs. 43 & 49). The successful use of Doppler blood flow detectors requires certain skills. The transmitting and receiving transducers must be properly located so that ultrasound waves will pass through the region of interest; the transducer must be me-

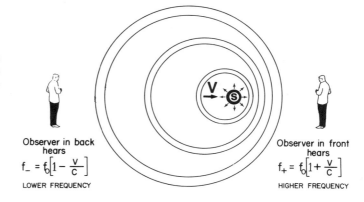

FIG. 4-11 The Doppler effect. The observer ahead of a moving source hears a higher pitch until the source passes him, then the apparent pitch decreases. **S** = source, v = velocity, c = wave velocity, f_0 = frequency heard at zero motion.

Observer in back hears

$$f_- = f_0\left[1 - \frac{v}{c}\right]$$

LOWER FREQUENCY

Observer in front hears

$$f_+ = f_0\left[1 + \frac{v}{c}\right]$$

HIGHER FREQUENCY

chanically secured with tape and acoustically coupled to the skin with proper placement of the appropriate gel, and a human must listen to a loudspeaker and recognize the audio representation of the velocity-induced frequency deviations. Doppler blood flow detectors exist that operate with continuous transmission of ultrasound (CW) and with pulsed transmissions. The Doppler principle is also employed in the Roche Arteriosonde, an automated blood pressure-measuring device that has ultrasonic crystals sensing the transverse motion of the wall of the brachial artery. The wall snaps downward as the rising cuff pressure gets above arterial pressure; it snaps upward when the falling cuff pressure decreases below the arterial pressure.

Because equations can be written for most kinds of waves, wave behavior throughout space and time is often described with mathematically convenient functions, such as sine waves and cosine waves. Because anesthesiologists frequently deal with waves that have complicated space and time variations, they find it useful to employ Fourier's theorem, which states that any wave shape can be expressed as a sum of harmonically related sine and cosine waves. Harmonics are simply integer multiples of an arbitrary fundamental or baseline frequency; thus, the first few harmonics of 15 Hz are 30, 45, 60, and 75 Hz. Fourier's theorem can be mathematically expressed as follows:

The wave = weighted sum of all harmonics

(Weights = A_n)

or

The wave = sum {A_n sine [$2\pi \cdot n \cdot f(t)$]}

The electroencephalographic (EEG) voltage waves observed at one point on the head are commonly expressed as a weighted sum of waves of different frequencies. The mathematical process used to calculate the weight factors A_n is called a Fourier transformation. Automated EEG monitors that are commercially available can record, digitize, and store the measured EEG voltage over a few seconds, do the Fourier transformation to obtain the A_n, and then plot f vs the wave amplitude, A_n, or the wave power, which is usually $(A_n)^2$ or some other function of A_n. The use of Fourier analysis to obtain the distribution of energy across frequency is also sometimes referred to as spectral analysis. The graph that shows EEG power vs frequency is commonly referred to as the compressed spectral array (CSA). A new CSA can be recalculated and drawn every few seconds.

ELECTRICITY AND MAGNETISM

Two very different force laws of electricity and magnetism can be used to define derived units of electric charge. Electrostatic units (esu) of charge, or statcoulombs, are obtained from Coulomb's law, which states that the repulsive electrostatic force between two stationary charges is directly proportional to each charge and inversely proportional to the square of the distance separating them. The dimensions of charge that result from the use of Coulomb's law, then, is as follows:

Charge (esu) = statcoulombs = distance $\sqrt{\text{force}}$

Electromagnetic units (emu) of charge are obtained from the experiments of Ampère, who showed that the attractive magnetic force between two parallel wires carrying current in the same direction is directly proportional to the current in each wire and inversely proportional to the distance separating them. Dimensions of charge result from this relationship:

$$\frac{\text{Force of repulsion}}{\text{per unit length of wire}} = \frac{l_1 \times l_2}{d}$$

as the electrical current, I, has the dimensions of (charge/time). Substitution of (charge/time) for I yields emu of charge (abcoulombs), which has the dimensions of time × $\sqrt{\text{force}}$. An interesting relationship ties together the dimensions of the two sets of units:

$$\frac{\text{charge (esu)}}{\text{charge (emu)}} = \frac{\text{distance} \sqrt{\text{force}}}{\text{time} \sqrt{\text{force}}} =$$

$$\frac{\text{distance}}{\text{time}} = \text{velocity}$$

There is only one possible velocity in nature that could relate electrostatic and electromagnetic phenomena: the velocity of light, c. The ratio of these two impractical sets of units indeed produces this value, which suggests that lots of modern physics lurks in the classical laws of electricity and magnetism. Bovie noise, laser flashes, radio signals, and x-rays are all different types of electromagnetic waves that travel through space at the speed of light.

The laws of Coulomb and Ampère commonly contain multiplicative constants k and μ, as shown in Figures 4-12 and 4-13, so that all quantities can be stated in SI units. The ratio k/μ is exactly equal to c^2.

The force between two electrical currents, expressed by Ampère's law, results from a magnetic interaction. The SI units for magnetic field strength are Tesla. Very high field magnets (approximately 2.0 Tesla) are found inside

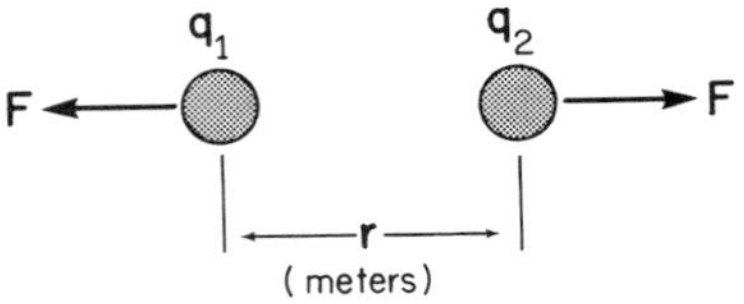

$$F = k \frac{q_1 q_2}{r^2}$$

F(Newtons) is the <u>repulsive</u> force between the two charges(Coulombs)

k = 0.8988 × 10^{10}

FIG. 4-12 Coulomb's law (SI units).

nuclear magnetic resonance imagers (also called NMR and MRI machines), which are becoming increasingly common in hospital radiology departments. Somewhat smaller fields (≈ 0.2 Tesla) are used in the ordinary mass spectrometer, an instrument used in anesthesia departments for the analysis of inspired and exhaled gases.

Magnetic forces act on electric charges moving along a direction that is transverse to the magnetic field. This is diagrammed in Figure 4-14, where the force of the magnetic field, B, on the isolated moving charge, q, is shown to be given by the Lorentz equation:

$$F(\text{newtons}) = qvB$$

A schematic diagram for the mass spectrometer is shown in Figure 4-15. Gas molecules sent to the mass spectrometer are ionized, accelerated through a voltage, and then dispatched on a circular path through a magnetic field. Because the radius of the path is different for each molecular weight, the relative concentrations of different gases in the mixture can be determined.

NUCLEAR MAGNETIC RESONANCE

Advances in electrical engineering and in computer technology have brought NMR into clinical medicine.[29-31] Two physicists, Ed Purcell of Harvard and Felix Bloch of Stanford, shared the 1954 Nobel Prize for physics for discovering the NMR phenomenon, which has since been used in many fields of science to address fundamental questions involving nu-

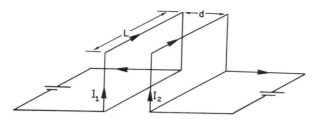

FIG. 4-13 Ampere's law (SI units).

F (Newtons) is the <u>attractive</u> force between two parallel currents (amperes) of length L (meters) and separation d (meters)

$$\frac{F}{L} = \mu \frac{I_1 I_2}{d}$$

where $\mu = 10^{-7}$ newtons/amp²

clear, atomic, and molecular structure. The two primary constituents of atomic nuclei — protons and neutrons — are collectively referred to as nucleons. NMR is based on the fact that there is intrinsic magnetism in those nuclei having an odd number of nucleons. For example, ^{1}H, ^{13}C, ^{19}F, ^{13}Na, ^{31}P, and ^{39}K all have an odd number of nucleons. Each type of nucleus acts like a magnetic dipole, or like a weak compass needle. The nuclear magnetization results in "compass needles" becoming partially aligned or polarized, when the nuclei are placed in a strong magnetic field. Magnetic fields up to 2.0 Tesla are FDA-approved for clinical use. The "compass needles" can be flipped around by high-frequency electromagnetic waves, typically those in the range 10 to 200 MHz. Because extremely high-contrast images of different tissues can be constructed from measurements of the characteristics of the proton flips, the manufacture and installation of NMR body scanners has become very

much in vogue. The NMR technique employs no radioactive substances and is usually performed without the injection of any contrast materials. Neural tissue, cerebrospinal fluid, and small tumors can be carefully studied in vivo, in some cases with as good a resolution as 0.25 mm. Because NMR imaging is becoming such an important diagnostic tool, requests to provide anesthesia for NMR procedures are becoming increasingly common.[31]

NMR techniques can also be used noninvasively in humans to measure intracellular pH and intracellular concentrations of certain

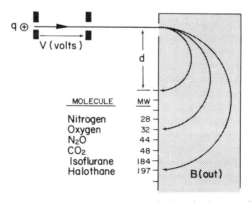

MOLECULE	MW
Nitrogen	28
Oxygen	32
N₂O	44
CO₂	48
Isoflurane	184
Halothane	197

The mass, M, of the charge, q, is given by the equation

$$M = \left[\frac{B^2 q}{8V}\right] d^2$$

FIG. 4-15 The mass spectrometer. A schematic representation of a mass spectrometer. After being ionized, a gas molecule is accelerated by an electrical field of strength V and is then shot into a magnetic field B, where the radius of curvature depends on the mass of the molecule.

$\vec{F}$ (Newtons) $= q\left[\vec{E} + \vec{v} \times \vec{B}\right]$

Units:

$\vec{E}$ (Volts/meter)

$\vec{B}$ (Tesla)

q (Coulombs)

$\vec{v}$ (meters/sec)

FIG. 4-14 The Lorentz force law, for the total force on a charge moving through electrical and magnetic fields.

compounds, such as ATP.[32] The fluorine nucleus associated with halothane, ^{19}F, has been studied in vitro in model membrane systems[33] and in vivo in rabbits.[34] Animal studies suggest that the elimination of fluorinated compounds from neural tissue after halothane and isoflurane anesthesia is considerably slower than expected. Intracellular fluorine is detectable in the brains of rabbits 96 hours after the termination of a 1-hour, 1-MAC anesthetic.[35] The implication of this finding is that come and go patients might experience mild, lingering effects after a vapor anesthetic and that they should not, for example, be allowed to routinely leave the hospital alone.

Anesthesiologists should participate in the design of new diagnostic facilities for NMR procedures. The magnets used for NMR imaging (also called magnetic resonance imaging, or MRI, by radiologists) are commonly superconducting, which means that they have no resistance at all to the flow of electrical currents. Such magnets operate at liquid helium temperatures and are in large rooms with good venting and ventilation. The strong magnetic field is never turned off. It persists so long as the cryostat is filled with liquid helium, which is supposed to be for many years. A typical human-size NMR magnet is a cylinder 8 feet in diameter and 10 feet in length, with a long hole in its center that a human can slide into. Because the extremely strong magnetic field of the magnet can attract metal into its bore with projectile force, and because metal near the magnet will cause small distortions in the field, no magnetic metals can be brought within 30 feet of such magnets. Metal stethoscopes, oxygen tanks, metal manometers, and so forth must all be kept far away. Nonmagnetic metals, such as gold, silver, platinum, and copper, are used when metals must be involved near a superconducting magnet. Electronic monitoring near or inside a magnet is also a problem, because oscilloscope screens will have their tracings distorted, and ECG leads that go into the magnet can act as a radio antenna that will pick up commercially broadcast FM signals. This causes electronic noise and image distortions for the NMR instrument, which is normally inside an electrically isolated and magnetically shielded cage. Despite all these difficulties, low-pass filtering and optical coupling have been used to accomplish successful ECG monitoring inside NMR magnets without compromising the NMR images.[36] Patients have been anesthetized for NMR procedures without compromising the quality of the studies.[31] In addition, animal studies have shown that it is possible to perform NMR spectroscopic studies of the brain while simultaneously recording EEG potentials.

During an NMR scan, the anesthesiologist has some access to the patient. Because there is no radioactivity during the scan, the anesthetist can stand next to the patient, observe and hear the breathing pattern, and palpate the pulse. Plastic stethoscopes should be available, and nonmetallic blood pressure cuff connections should be used. The anesthesia department should ensure that any metal devices that it routinely wants in the room have been firmly bolted to a remote wall and tested for interference in advance by the radiology department. Plans for dealing with trouble during an NMR scan should include the possibility of rapidly removing the patient from the imager and from the room, to an area outside the large magnetic field, where all the familiar resuscitation equipment is available.

MODERN PHYSICS

IONIZING RADIATION: EXPOSURE AND DOSE

Anesthetists frequently find themselves in the vicinity of ionizing radiation that is produced by x-ray machines or radioactive sources. Ionizing particles, defined as those that knock electrons out of stable atomic orbits, can cause cell injury and cell death. Ionized electrons ultimately slow down after many thousands of collisions, during which time they deposit energy that ultimately appears in the form of heat. Several questions about ionizing radiation state only a few of the concerns that have been raised about safety in the operating room: How protective are lead aprons? Should thyroid shields be worn when the C-arm is used? How close and for how long should one stand next to patients with radioactive implants? Will a patient get too large an x-ray dose if one repeats CT scans to recheck the needle position for a celiac plexus block?

The three most commonly encountered ionizing particles are α-rays (helium nuclei), β-rays (electrons), and γ-rays. Gamma particles, which are also called x-rays or high-energy photons, are electromagnetic waves. The activity of radioactive substances, which spontaneously emit such particles, is specified in either Becquerel units (1 Bq = 1 disintegration/sec) or Curies (1 Ci = 3.7×10^{10} disintegrations/sec). As important as activity, however, are exposure and energy absorption. The quantity of x-rays that passes through a region of space can be measured if one is willing to put a small amount of air in the path of the beam and then count how many electrons come flying off. The result, a measure of the exposure, is given in units called Roentgens.[37] One Roentgen (1 R) corresponds to 2.58×10^{-4} coulombs per kg of air, or 8.78×10^{-3} joules/kg of air.

In addition to activity and exposure, absorption and biologic damage are important phenomena that have their own sets of units. Absorbed dose is specified in either rads or Grays (Gy). 1 Gy = 100 rad = 1 joule of absorbed energy per kg. The numbers just given show that a 1-R x-ray exposure, if fully absorbed by tissue, will deposit an absorbed dose of approximately 0.9 rad.

A measure of biologic tissue damage has been defined as the dose equivalent. It can be specified in either Sieverts (Sv) or rem (an abbreviation that comes from roentgen-equivalent-man). 1 Sv = 100 rem, and the number of Sv (or rem) for a particular type of biologic tissue is the number of Grays (or rads) times the quality factor, Q, for the situation. Q depends on the type of radiation. Alpha particles have a Q near 20, while β- and γ-rays have a Q near 1.[38]

Radiation occurs in nature, and the average annual whole-body absorbed dose ranges throughout the world from 40 to 400 mrem. (The average in the United States is approximately 80 mrem.) The lungs receive 10 mrem from inhaled natural radioactivity, mostly

from radon and its decay products.[39] By comparison, a single chest roentgenogram shot at 120 keV, provides a patient with an absorbed dose of approximately 25 mrem.[40] The patient who refuses to submit to a preoperative chest roentgenogram because of worries regarding radiation is concerned about the smallest dose obtainable in the x-ray suite. By contrast, a skull series or an upper gastrointestinal (GI) series provides a dose that ranges from 1 to 2 rem, as does a single "slice" of a computed tomography (CT) scan. This dose range corresponds to more than 10 to 40 years' worth of natural radiation. Note also that the term absorbed dose is really somewhat of a misnomer, because it is defined as the energy absorption per kilogram of tissue. A CT scan that does 20 different slices gives the patient an absorbed dose of about 1 rem, which is the same dose, according to official definitions, as that from only one slice. If a CT slice must be redone because it does not look good, the patient's absorbed dose is doubled by having the second exposure.

A map showing exposure levels usually accompanies patients having radioactive implants for antitumor therapy. On the ward this map is usually prominently displayed, with the radiation levels given in millirems per hour. In the operating suite one finds instead a note on the chart stating what the radiation levels are at different distances from the source that will be implanted. Values are usually stated for the levels with and without shielding. The anesthetist should inquire of the radiation safety officer of his hospital as to whether there are any doubts about the dangers implied by these numbers. However, one can roughly evaluate the maximum dose that an unshielded person could sustain by taking the mrem/hr figure provided by the radiation safety officer, multiplying it by the number of hours that one will be there, and then comparing the answer with a reasonable set of upper and lower annual limits. There is an 80-mrem/year unavoidable exposure from cosmic rays and the earth. The maximum whole-body occupational dose permitted in the United States is 5 rem (5,000 mrem) per year. By comparison, cancer patients frequently undergo x-ray exposures that range between 5,000 and 9,000 rem. Such exposures, in addition to being cytotoxic to radiosensitive tumor cells, are injurious to normal tissues. The anesthesiologist should be prepared for a greater amount of blood loss when the operative site involves an area that has received extensive radiation therapy.

SHIELDING

A 1-mm-thick sheet of lead will stop 99.8 percent of a 100-keV γ-ray beam. Commercially available shielding aprons used when taking portable roentgenograms contain a layer of lead which is either 0.25 mm or 0.5 mm thick. Because the intensity of scattered background radiation is also inversely proportional to the square of the distance from the source, the anesthetist will minimize x-ray exposure by wearing a lead apron and by stepping as far back from the procedure as the clinical circumstances permit. Backscattered x-rays produce greater exposure than do those scattered forward. Therefore, the anesthetist further minimizes occupational exposure by being on the side of the patient opposite the x-ray gun. Similarly, a vertical C-arm shot will cause less occupational exposure for people in the operating room when the x-ray gun is below the table shooting up than when it is above the table shooting down (Fig. 4-16). Because C-arm x-ray imaging devices employ image intensifiers that require smaller x-ray doses per shot, they also produce less background radiation per image than do portable roentgenograms of the same view. Nevertheless, as is the case for all x-ray procedures in the operating room, lead aprons and thyroid shields should be worn by all personnel who are frequently present for these procedures. Concerns about the cumulative occupational organ dosages you receive should be discussed with the radiation safety physicist in your hospital.

Lead aprons provide excellent protection for all naturally emitted α- and β-particles. They may not provide sufficient shielding, however, for x-rays of more than 200 keV. You should definitely consult with a radiation safety physicist if you are working in such an environment or if you are providing anesthesia in the target area of a particle accelerator.

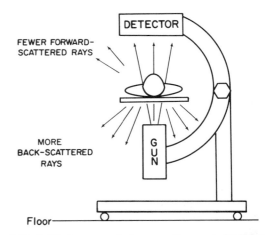

FIG. 4-16 C-arm use in the operating room. (1) Wear lead aprons and thyroid shields; (2) there is more background on the side with the x-ray gun; (3) there is less background if one if farther away.

ELECTROCARDIOGRAPHY

A comprehensive treatise on electronics and monitoring is beyond the scope of this chapter and beyond the instantaneous recall of a busy anesthesiologist in the operating room. The situation is similar in some other professions. For example, airplane pilots and astronauts must often think about their electronic equipment as interconnected black-box modules. This means that input–output characteristics are precisely known for the items being linked together but the user does not need to be aware of all internal details. When an amplifier goes bad during the maneuvers of an orbiting satellite, an astronaut has no time to get out the voltmeter and soldering iron and attack the problem by starting from first principles. Instead, the astronaut recognizes and removes the defective module and replaces it with the backup black box. It is important for anesthesiologists to be familiar with the operating details of the black boxes that they choose to use in the operating room: transducers, amplifiers, digitizers, recorders, on-line computers, display devices, and whatever else. We shall therefore focus the remainder of this section on issues that help the practitioner understand and utilize commonly available electronic equipment.

GENESIS OF THE ELECTROCARDIOGRAM

Cardiac muscle in the course of its rhythmic activity generates a detectable electrical potential that is graphically displayed as the electrocardiogram (ECG), which is discussed in detail in Chapters 14 & 15. Although the genesis of this activity is complex, some insight can be provided by considering a simplified physical model — that of an electric dipole (representing the heart) inside a volume conductor (which represents the body). An electric dipole is composed of two equal and opposite electrical charges separated in space. The straight line joining the charges is called the dipole axis. A volume conductor is an object that permits unrestricted three-dimensional current flow throughout its volume.[41,42] The electrical current at any one spot in a volume conductor depends on the direction and strength of the electric field there. At any location the electrical field from a dipole is determined by the length of a straight line drawn from that location to the center of the dipole and by the angle the line makes with the dipole axis (see Fig. 4-17). In general, larger electrical fields occur closer to the dipole and, at a given distance, the largest field occurs on and along the dipole axis. An electrical current is established when a dipole is placed within a volume conductor, such as a saline bath. The current flow tends to neutralize the two charges of the dipole. Depolarized myocardium is electronegative in comparison with repolarized or inactive myocardium. From afar, the heart seems to act as a dipole generator, and electrical fields arising from the heart can be viewed as coming from a spatially structured wave of dipoles that starts at the AV node and moves throughout the heart from endocardium to epicardium. At any particular instant, a single dipole expresses the sum of the structured wave, and its axis, called the electrical axis of the heart, can be determined from the ECG. Pathologic myocardial regions will change the final form of the structured wave of dipoles and alter the electrical axis in ways that suggest its anatomic location. Currents generated in the volume conductor (the body) will produce changes on the order of magnitude of millivolts at the skin surface.

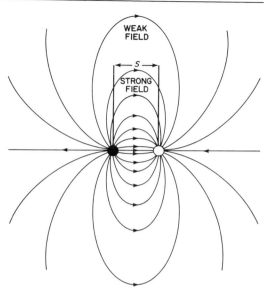

FIG. 4-17 The dipole field is produced by equal and opposite charges. The field direction is indicated by the arrows. The field strength is weaker at large distances.

ELECTRODES

Making an electrical connection between two identical metallic conductors only involves placing them in contact. Making a good electrical connection with the human body is somewhat more complex.[43] The body is like a big electrolyte solution, or volume conductor; when a metal electrode is placed in an electrolyte solution, it chemically reacts with it and forms a junctional dipole layer that is the source of a galvanic potential or junction potential. The junction potential depends entirely on the type of metal and classes of ions in the electrolyte. When two dissimilar metals are placed in the same electrode bath, the difference in their junction potentials makes them capable of driving a current from one metal to the other. This is the basic principle behind the design of household and automobile batteries. The existence of such a potential does not itself present a problem for electrophysiologic measurements. However, statistical fluctuations in the junction potentials do present a problem, because they are generally in the millivolt range, the same range as the biopotentials we are trying to measure.[44] Fortunately, silver and silver chloride can be used to produce a very

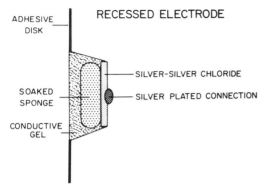

RECESSED ELECTRODE

ADHESIVE DISK

SILVER-SILVER CHLORIDE

SILVER PLATED CONNECTION

SOAKED SPONGE

CONDUCTIVE GEL

FIG. 4-18 The cupped ECG skin electrode.

stable electrode–solute combination.[45] This combination has become the clinical standard for ECG electrodes, which have a cupped design. The silver metal and silver chloride electrolyte are recessed in the cup and separated from the skin by an electrolyte-soaked sponge (Fig. 4-18), so as to prevent mechanical disruption of the junctional dipole layer.

The skin, which is interposed between the silver chloride ECG electrodes and the body volume conductor, also has two important electrical properties.[46] First, the dermis has its own electrical potential gradient; and, second, the skin has electrical resistance, with a large component coming from the stratum corneum. Both the skin resistance and its potential change significantly with the tone of the sympathetic nervous system, forming the basis for the polygraph (or lie detector) test.

Proper attachment of ECG electrodes involves cleansing the skin, gently abrading the stratum corneum, and making sure that there is an adequate gel contact. Furthermore, the wires to the electrodes should not be taut, and the electrodes should be in a location where they will not be mechanically disrupted. In this way, background noise will be minimized as well as motion artifacts due to distortions of the junctional dipole layer and pressure and torsion modifications of the skin potential.

DIFFERENTIAL AMPLIFIERS

The measurement of millivolt potential differences at the body's surface is accomplished with the use of a differential amplifier.

This device magnifies the difference between small electrical signals and generates an output signal large enough to drive an oscilloscope display or chart recorder. Other electrophysiologic monitors used in the operating room, such as the electroencephalograph (EEG) and electromyograph (EMG), employ differential amplifiers as well.

A schematic diagram of a differential amplifier is shown in Figure 4-19. Three lead wires form the input system, whereas only two lead wires form the output. One of the three input lead wires serves an electrical ground, whereas the other two input leads, labeled A and B, carry voltage levels, V_A and V_B, relative to ground. Three leads are needed in order to eliminate unwanted, stray signals known as electrical noise. The body, besides being a volume conductor, also acts like an antenna and picks up electromagnetic waves radiated through space. Most of the radiated noise in the operating room comes from AC power lines in the wall and from AC connections in nearby equipment. Although the detected 60-Hz signal (50 Hz in some parts of the world) is as large as a few volts, which is several hundred times larger than the ECG signal, it is approximately the same throughout the body and is therefore common at any given instant to the three input leads. By having three input leads, a differential amplifier can use two amplifier circuits at its input to generate separate internal signals for (V_A − ground) and (V_B − ground), and to subtract these two signals from each other to get (V_A − V_B). This process, which eliminates the larger noise signal common to the leads, is known as common mode rejection.

If the electrode impedances for the V_A and V_B are not approximately equal, some of the common mode signal can be expected to contaminate the output of the differential amplifier. This explains the frequent appearance of

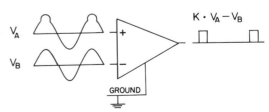

FIG. 4-19 The differential amplifier and common mode signal rejection.

power-line interference in the displayed ECG. Equipment manufacturers ameliorate this problem by making the amplifier impedance much higher than the expected electrode impedance. However, an anesthetist who notices persistent 60-Hz interference should consider reducing and equalizing the skin–electrode impedance by improving the skin preparation with an abrasive.

The quality of common mode rejection can be quantified by measuring the amplifier output that results when the same signal relative to ground is hooked up at both the A and B inputs. This output amplitude, which ideally would be zero but instead is simply small, is then divided into the output amplitude that results from grounding the B lead and connecting the input signal across A and ground. The resulting value, r, is called the common mode rejection ratio. A common mode rejection ratio of 1,000 means that the output generated by a signal difference between A and B is 1,000 times as great as the output that results when the same signal difference simultaneously occurs between grounds and A and B.

FREQUENCY RESPONSE

An ECG amplifier should be capable of amplifying all frequency components of importance in the ECG signal. It should also filter out those frequency components generally considered to be noise. Many ECG monitors have a switch labeled diagnostic/monitor. This switch determines the frequency range being filtered out by circuit elements in the amplifier. When in diagnostic mode, the amplifier will cover a frequency range from approximately 0.05 to 100 Hz, which is very high fidelity for an ECG. One small box on an ECG tracing is 0.04 seconds wide, and a 100-Hz signal could go up and down four times in that period. The monitor setting picks a smaller frequency range, from about 0.50 to 45 Hz,[47] but it minimizes baseline wandering and electrosurgical interference. When set on monitor, the QRS-T morphology can be blurred, and the ST segment can be inaccurate. Cardiac defibrillators that have monitors with a low-frequency cutoff of 0.50 Hz have been shown to produce tracings of nondiagnostic quality with falsely abnormal

readings that could adversely affect patient management.[48]

BLOOD PRESSURE

Blood pressure was first recorded in an intact animal by Stephen Hales in 1733[49] (also see Ch. 13). Routine intraoperative measurement of arterial blood pressure in humans was first performed by medical student Harvey Cushing in 1903. A committee of his professors at the Massachussetts General Hospital, in a report issued in 1904, found no value in this practice. Times have clearly changed. The assurance of adequate organ perfusion presently begins with the measurement of arterial blood pressure, which is generally acknowledged to be one of the most valued physiologic measurements in clinical anesthesia. Application of Bernouilli's equation to measurement of blood pressure details the components of the measured forces:

$$P_{total} = P_{static} + P_{kinetic} + P_{hydrostatic}$$

where P_{static} is the pressure caused by distention of the vascular tree secondary to the ejection of the stroke volume, $P_{kinetic}$ is the pressure caused by converting the kinetic energy of the blood as it "rams" into the transducer/catheter system, and $P_{hydrostatic}$ is caused by disparity in height between site of measurement and site of transducing. The kinetic energy can only be measured by direct intraarterial techniques, and it is usually small compared with the static pressure. However, because $P_{kinetic}$ is proportional to the square of the velocity of blood flow, it may reach significant levels in very high flow vessels such as the aorta during exercise, or even more likely in the vena cava, where the static pressure is low in the face of high flow. The kinetic contribution to blood pressure will be neglected in the remaining discussion. In situations in which the vascular resistance, R, does not substantially change, Ohm's law for fluids provides that blood pressure, P, is proportional to blood flow, Q:

$$P = Q \cdot R$$

Arterial blood pressure is the time varying, cyclic force by the blood per unit area upon the walls of the arterial tree. Continuous measurement of the pressure waveform in a major artery can provide information on myocardial function, vascular distensibility, oxygen balance, peripheral perfusion, and circulatory volume status. The measurement and interpretation of arterial blood pressure are discussed below.

THE ARTERIAL PRESSURE WAVEFORM

The pressure waveform measured by an intravascular catheter in a peripheral artery is shown schematically in Figure 4-20. Physiologically, the blood pressure waveform contains several features of interest, including the systolic and diastolic pressures, the mean arterial pressure (MAP), and the pulse pressure. The systolic pressure is defined as the highest instantaneous pressure in the artery, and the diastolic pressure the lowest. The MAP is the average force per unit area exerted by the fluid on the walls of the vessels. The pulse pressure is the peak-to-peak or systolic-to-diastolic pressure variation generated by the transducer after sensing a pressure wave that traverses the catheter and length of pressure tubing. Hydrostatic pressure, a nonphysiologic component of the measurement, is caused by the column of fluid connecting the site of measurement and the transducer. Hydrostatic pressure is important because it is a background pressure that

must be subtracted at some point in the measurement process in order to obtain physiologic pressures, which are measured relative to the right atrium. Although the hydrostatic contribution can be partly eliminated by placing the pressure transducer at the same height as the heart, one should not forget that it is present, and sometimes even substantial, as is the case when the CVP is being displayed and the surgeon raises the table without moving the transducer. When the transducer is 10 cm below the atria, it generates a reading that is 10 cm H_2O (or 7.35 mm Hg) higher than the true blood pressure. Mean arterial pressure is important because it appears to be a more reliable monitor of perfusion than either systolic or diastolic pressure.[50,51]

Anesthesiologists are familiar with the formula commonly given to calculate mean blood pressure:

$$MAP = 1/3(\text{systolic BP}) + 2/3(\text{diastolic BP})$$

This equation, which assumes that the blood pressure waveform is triangular, is seldom used in clinical settings. Its approximation of the real mean pressure is unfortunately too crude. Fortunately, it has been technically easy to construct automated blood pressure monitoring devices that measure mean arterial blood pressure (MABP) directly. Invasive blood pressure monitors do so by electronically separating the DC (or mean) and AC (or pulsatile) components of the waveform. The electronic determination of mean pressure is relatively immune from problems that plague the mea-

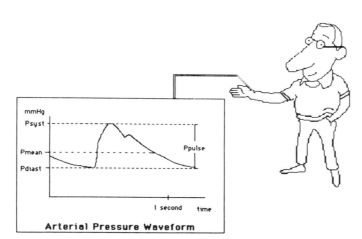

FIG. 4-20 The arterial blood pressure waveform.

surements of systolic and diastolic pressures (e.g., transducer compliance, softness of the catheter tubing, and air bubbles or clots in the line). Continuous monitoring of mean pressure can be a useful adjunct to waveform inspection when advancing a pulmonary artery catheter. The digital display of the mean pressure usually jumps significantly when changing from atrium to ventricle and from ventricle to pulmonary artery. A noninvasive, standard blood pressure cuff can be used to measure the mean pressure if it is connected to an automated device (e.g., the Dinamap.) that employs oscillometric techniques. Although the compliance and response time of a standard blood pressure cuff are very different from those of an intravascular catheter and transducer, they agree quite closely on the measurement of MAP.[52-54]

The systolic pressure is commonly ascribed to be related to the systemic perfusion, but in this regard, the mean pressure is more reliable.[51] The systolic pressure does, however, provide an indication of the myocardial oxygen requirement.[55] The magnitude and duration of diastolic blood pressure are commonly monitored as an index of coronary perfusion.[56] It is curious, given the general availability of invasive and noninvasive blood pressure monitors and the aforementioned importance of mean and diastolic pressure, that so many anesthetic records only have the systolic pressure recorded.

chanical system that is capable of reverberating and absorbing energy from the catheter pulsations. At one particular pulsation frequency, called the resonance frequency, the mechanical system is optimally driven, and oscillations and energy absorption is maximal. If arterial pulsations to the line are suddenly stopped, the mechanical oscillations continue, slowly dissipating, or dampening with time. Transient oscillations that settle down are generally described as being underdamped, overdamped, or critically damped. In an underdamped system, the pressure descends rapidly to its equilibrium value, overshoots it, and oscillates about it for a prolonged period. In an overdamped system, there is no overshoot of the decaying pressure, which takes a very long time to reach its equilibrium value. In a critically damped system, the amplitude returns to its equilibrium value as quickly as possible, without having a single oscillation. Figure 4-21 shows a schematic pressure wave that a hypothetical monitoring system will generate for three damping situations. Curve C represents an overdamped system in which the low-frequency components of the pressure wave (like mean pressure) pass through with little or no attenuation, whereas the higher frequencies are severely attenuated, leading to a transduced pressure waveform that has little more than small undulations about the mean pressure. This case will occur if a small undiscovered air bubble, which has a very high compliance, is in the pressure tubing. Curve A represents an underdamped system. Pressure

DIRECT MEASUREMENT OF BLOOD PRESSURE

Compromises in pressure measurement begin with the impracticality of placing a small pressure transducer directly inside the proximal aorta. The peripheral pressure waveform sensed by a catheter in the distal arterial tree has a greater rate of rise during systole and a wider pulse pressure than the central pressure waveform. Further distortions in the waveform detection process are introduced when the catheter is attached to fluid-filled tubing, stopcocks, and plastic domes, and a pressure transducer. These elements constitute a me-

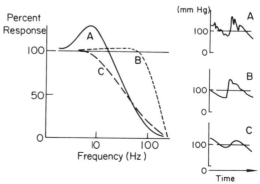

FIG. 4-21 Damping characteristics and frequency dependence.

variations near the resonance frequency (usually approximately 20 Hz) lead to prolonged ringing, an overshot systolic pressure, and an undershot diastolic pressure. Curve B represents a critically damped system, where the transduced waveform is a relatively faithful reproduction of the pressure in the vessel. The resonance frequency and damping characteristics of an arterial pressure line are quantitatively determined by geometry and viscosity. Damped oscillations that occur in a fluid-filled catheter system of length L, compliance $C[= (1/E) = \Delta V/\Delta P]$, radius r, density ρ, and viscosity μ has its damping factor, β, and resonance frequency, f, are described by the following solution[57] to the general wave equation, which describes the behavior of damped harmonic motion:

$$\beta = \frac{4\mu}{r^3} \sqrt{\frac{L}{\pi E}}$$

$$f = \frac{1}{2\pi} \sqrt{\frac{\pi r^2 E}{\rho L}}$$

High viscosity, high compliance, long length, and small radius all add up to a large damping factor, which implies that the observed waveform will be overly smoothed out and that the pulse pressure will be artificially reduced. Low density, short length, and stiff tubing would yield a system with a high resonance frequency. In clinical practice one frequently "fixes" an underdamped tubing system by intentionally introducing a small quantity of air into the dome housing the pressure transducer. This is a suboptimal solution because there can be unrecognized overdamping, as well as a reduction in the resonance frequency that will cause ringing, or voltage oscillations, to appear on the oscilloscope tracing of the pressure waveform. The proper solution to an underdamped system involves using maximally stiff pressure tubing and a minimum length between the catheter and the transducer. Such manuevers will shift the resonance peak to a frequency that is sufficiently higher than significant components of the true pressure waveform, so that the components of the pressure waveform do not excite the resonance. If the resonance frequency of the measuring system is high enough, its damping phe-

nomena will not degrade the pressure tracing. Such a system could be described as having a flat response over the frequency range of interest. The spectrum of frequencies present in a blood pressure waveform varies with heart rate and the condition of the arterial tree but is usually in the range of 0 to 20 Hz.[57] Typical catheter-dome systems resonate at about 10 to 50 Hz,[58,59] thereby explaining the common occurrence of underdamped waveforms. It is also worth remembering that the internal construction of stopcocks renders them vulnerable to the unseen accumulation of air bubbles.

INDIRECT MEASUREMENT OF BLOOD PRESSURE

The most common method of blood pressure measurement involves encircling the arm with a Riva Rocci (air-filled cuff) sphygmomanometer.[60,61] A pressure greater than the systolic value is used to inflate the cuff, which distributes the pressure to an underlying cylinder of tissue, and collapses the brachial artery. A stethoscope is placed over the artery, and the cuff is slowly deflated. As the pressure falls to the systolic pressure, the artery partially opens, and turbulent blood flow begins through the distorted anatomy of the compressed vessel. Turbulent flow is not silent like laminar flow, and is the source of iatrogenic bruits known as Korotkoff sounds,[62] which persist until the cuff pressure drops below intraarterial pressure throughout the entire cardiac cycle. When the cuff pressure is just below the diastolic pressure, the artery remains open, and the Korotkoff sounds become muffled.[63] The muffled sounds persist until the cuff pressure is well below diastolic pressure because of the small amount of vessel constriction and turbulence that are present. The creation of turbulence and hence Korotkoff sounds requires substantial flow through the artery. In cases of low cardiac output or extreme peripheral vasoconstriction, these sounds will not be audible and the technique will fail. The width of the cuff must be appropriate for the size of the limb (about 20 percent wider than the diameter of the limb). For example, if a normal adult arm cuff is used on a massively obese patient, a falsely high blood pressure reading will ensue. This is because a narrow cuff around a thick cylinder of tissue will tend to disperse the constrictive force ineffectively, and so a higher cuff pressure is needed to occlude the artery.

OSCILLOMETERS

Noninvasive blood pressure systems used in the operating room commonly employ oscillometric techniques, which are based on the detection of arterial pulsations transmitted by the cuff. When the cuff pressure is above the systolic pressure, only very small oscillations can be appreciated. If the release valve of the sphygmomanometer is opened slightly, enough to cause a pressure drop of 2 to 3 mm Hg/sec, the indicator needle of the aneroid manometer will appear to pause periodically as it descends the scale of falling cuff pressure. These pauses, synchronous with the heartbeat, are due to small pressure oscillations that increase in amplitude with decreasing cuff pressure. They evolve into obvious upward flicks of the needle and then gradually recede (Fig. 4-22). Although some debate persists as to how the systolic, mean, and diastolic pressure should be obtained from the pattern of oscillations, there is general agreement that the MAP is the lowest pressure in the cuff that will produce maximal oscillations.[52-54] Systolic pressure is the highest cuff pressure at which a large increase in amplitude of oscillations occurs.[64] Diastolic pressure is defined with less assurance as the lowest cuff pressure before the oscillations drop off markedly in amplitude.[65] Automated oscillometers such as the Dinamap (Critikon Medical, Tampa, Florida) and others use the criteria listed above in a consistent, repeatable way. Occasionally the cuff pressure reveals a gradual decline in amplitude, without a clear demarcation between subdiastolic and suprasystolic regions. The blinking digital display of automated devices at such times, indicating that blood pressure was not successfully measured, can frustrate the anesthesiologist. It is useful to have Luer lock or other compatible connections that link the main unit to the tubing from the blood pressure cuff, so that a squeeze bulb and manometer can quickly be substituted and cuff pressure can be measured in a standard way. If the situation permits, trouble shooting of the nonfunctional oscillometer should include checking that the hoses to the cuff are tightly connected and not kinked and that the cuff is properly applied and carefully secured. An adult Dinamap should not be connected to a pediatric patient because the intial inflation pressure can get too high.[66,67] Even adult patients can suffer the consequences of overfrequent cuff inflation.[68] Many automatic oscillometers have a hold feature that permits the anesthetist to stop routinely taking pressures without turning off the main power of the unit. This eliminates the possibility of an inflated cuff interfering with intravenous drug administration and permits the machine to "remember" the previous blood pressure and avoid another high-pressure search. Automated oscillometric devices like the Dinamap are desirable not only because they can ensure regular sampling and documentation of blood pressure, but also because they accurately measure an important parameter, the MAP.

A device known as the Von Recklinghausen oscillotonometer was widely used for oscillometry during the premicroprocessor era.[60] It employed one manometer and a blood pressure cuff with two bladders (see schematic diagram in Fig. 4-23). When a switch on the device is in one position, the manometer reads the blood pressure from the proximal bladder in the standard way. When the switch is thrown into its second position, the distal bladder, which conceptually serves in place of the aus-

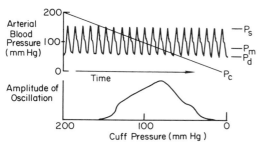

FIG. 4-22 Oscillometry amplitude during the arterial waveform.

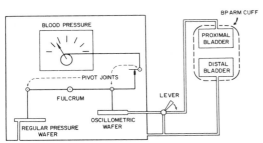

FIG. 4-23 The Von Recklinghausen oscillotonometer.

cultating stethoscope, is connected to a sensitive mechanical amplifier that permits small pressure variations to produce large amplitude swings in the manometer needle. With the switch in the second position, the manometer acts as an oscillometer. Blood pressure is measured with this device in a manner similar to that used with the standard sphygmomanometer. The bulb is squeezed and both bladders inflate above systolic pressure. The valve is then adjusted to permit a slow leak. During deflation, the observer has the switch set for oscillometry and decides by eyeball when the amplitude of oscillations have changed from small to big, hence when systole has been reached. The switch is then flipped to show the pressure reading from the proximal bladder. The decision strategies regarding oscillation amplitudes are the same that were discussed for the automated device. Because of recent technological advances, oscillotonometers have been replaced by automated oscillometers that use consistent objective criteria for each pressure determination.

A disadvantage of oscillometric techniques is that oscillations can become vanishingly small in hypotensive states, and the clinician can be deprived of pressure data when they are most important. The Korotkoff sounds are also well known to disappear with hypotension. A device known as an Arteriosonde (Roche Medical) uses an ultrasonic Doppler signal (see below) to detect the pulsation of the arterial walls under the cuff. This technique permits more consistent sphygmomanometer readings in infants and during hypotension. Besides detecting arterial wall motion, ultrasound can be used to detect blood flow distal to the cuff.

BLOOD FLOW

THE FICK PRINCIPLE, INDICATOR DILUTION, AND CARDIAC OUTPUT (Also See Ch. 13)

In 1870 Adolph Fick described a simplified approach to the measurement of blood flow and cardiac output. He reasoned that, on the average, the amount that an organ extracts each second from 1 cc of its blood flow is equal to the total organ blood flow times its arterial-venous concentration difference. The equation for this, known as the Fick principle, is simply

Quantity removed from blood =

[blood flow] × [arterial content − venous content]

For the case of the lungs, where O_2 is added to the blood and the organ blood flow is assumed to be equal to the cardiac output, the Fick principle becomes

Quantity of O_2 added to blood = [cardiac output] × [(O_2 concentration in pulmonary veins)

− (O_2 concentration in pulmonary artery)]

and it leads to the following equation for the cardiac output (CO):

$$CO \ (L/min) = \frac{\text{oxygen uptake by lungs (ml/min)}}{\text{arterial} - \text{venous oxygen content difference (ml/L)}}$$

For example

$$\frac{250(\text{ml/min O}_2 \text{ uptake})}{200(\text{ml/L arterial}) - 150(\text{ml/L venous})} = 5.0 \text{ L/min}$$

Although O_2 uptake can be measured by using spirometry, and systemic arterial blood analyzed instead of pulmonary venous blood, it is not clinically convenient to use this technique, which requires a 3 to 5-minute collection of exhaled gases, during which time one must assume that the cardiovascular system is stable.[69]

The indicator-dilution technique is a method that permits the cardiac output to be determined from a single stroke volume. It requires a rapid bolus injection into the central venous system and the ability to continuously and accurately monitor an indicator, usually a dye. Indicators that have been successfully used in the past include electrolyte solutions, colored dyes, nonphysiologic gases (i.e., N_2O, H_2), and radioactive tracers. Endogenous potassium and sodium have also been successfully used as indicators. Decreases in serum concentrations were detected after dilution by the injection of water. Currently, the most frequently used method involves the rapid injection of 10 ml of cold saline or dextrose into the CVP port of a pulmonary artery catheter.[70] The indicator, (temperature) is detected by a probe inside the catheter tip in the pulmonary artery. The measurement of flow depends on the instrument's ability to determine the product of the washout time with the mean value of the indicator's concentration. Once this is determined, a computation can be performed, based on two assumptions: (1) that all the washed out indicator is detected by the system, and (2) that there has been uniform mixing of the indicator throughout the unknown blood volume that dilutes it. The equation for blood flow is derived as follows:

Indicator added (mg) = indicator detected (mg)

$$= \int (\text{flow}) \times (\text{concentration}) \times \text{time}$$

or

Indicator added (mg) = [average flow]
$\times$ [average concentration] $\times$ [washout time]

which leads to

[Average flow] = [cardiac output] = CO
$$= \frac{[\text{indicator added (mg)}]}{[(\text{average concentration}) \times (\text{washout time})]}$$

In commonly used clinical equipment, a known quantity of indicator is injected and the denominator of the preceding equation is calculated as an integral.

Figure 4-24 schematically illustrates a system in which a bolus of indicator is injected from an upstream mixing chamber. A steady stream, the flow rate of which must be measured, dilutes the injected indicator, which then appears at the outflow of the mixing chamber. The downstream concentration is shown in Figure 4-25 to be rapidly rising at first, and then slowly tapering down. If the mixing chamber is inside a closed circulation, the indicator will reappear at the detector as a recirculation peak that adds to the normal exponentially falling washout curve (see Fig. 4-25). At any time, t, the quantity of indicator leaving the mixing chamber is the product of the flow out of the chamber times the concentration in the chamber at that instant. The sum over time of the outgoing indicator is assumed to add up to the amount of indicator that was injected.

The rectangle drawn in Figure 4-25 is meant to have the same area as that under the curve for the measured concentration versus time. From such a rectangle one can approximate the cardiac output from the measured tracing. Before the advent of microcomputer-

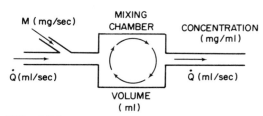

FIG. 4-24 The mixing chamber for the indicator–dilution technique.

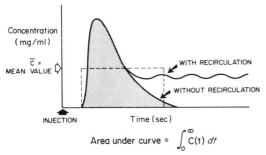

FIG. 4-25 The indicator–dilution curve.

containing instruments, which now quickly calculate the area below the concentration curve, tedious computations and approximations were necessary. Microprocessors also incorporate calibrated correction factors for temperature loss and fluctuations. Indicator dilution techniques are not accurate in low cardiac output situations or in cases of valvular regurgitation.

The indicator dilution technique is routinely used for the measurement of regional blood flow. Cerebral blood flow was first measured this way in 1945 by Kety and Schmidt,[71] and the ability to measure regional cerebral perfusion was pioneered by Lassen and Ingvar in 1961,[72,73] using intracarotid injections of radioactive gas. Intracerebral washin and washout curves of the radioactive gas were measured using large arrays of external scintillation counters.

DOPPLER

The Doppler principle can be used to determine intravascular blood flow. Blood in motion can act as a target for a narrow ultrasonic beam directed along the blood vessel. Ultrasound, the frequency range of which is 1 to 10 MHz, is used because higher frequencies result in larger frequency shifts and because ultrasonic wavelengths are less than 1 mm, which allows for narrow beams.

The schematic diagram for an ultrasonic blood flow detector is given in Figure 4-26. A trigonometric factor is needed when computing frequency shifts, because the ultrasound transmitter and receiver are each aligned at an angle θ with respect to the source. The receiver amplifies the reflected beam and subtracts the original transmitted frequency, leaving the residual frequency-shifted components. These shifted components are actually not a single frequency but rather a collection of frequencies the shift of which is centered about the average velocity in the flow profile of the vessel.

ELECTROMAGNETIC FLOW PROBE

Plasma is an electrolyte solution, that is moderately conductive to electricity. When a conductor moves perpendicular to a magnetic

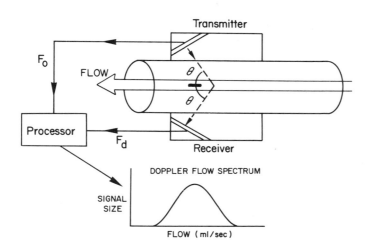

FIG. 4-26 Schematic diagram of an ultrasonic blood flow detector.

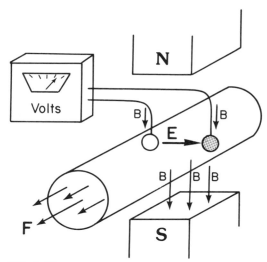

FIG. 4-27 Principle of voltage induction in the electromagnetic flow probe.

field, an electrical field of magnitude $v \cdot B$ (volts/meter) is generated across the conductor, in accordance with the Lorentz force law. This is diagrammed in Figure 4-27. Magnetic blood flow probes are constructed to have a magnetic field, B, resembling that of Figure 4-27. They use an electromagnetic coil instead of a permanent magnetic field, as shown in Figure 4-28. The voltage, V, induced by blood

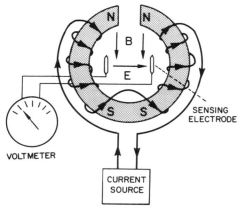

TOROIDAL CUFF EM FLOW PROBE

FIG. 4-28 Schematic diagram of the electromagnetic flow probe. Blood flow is perpendicular to the plane of the figure.

rushing through the magnetic field, is proportional to the velocity through the probe. Because the area through which the blood flows is known, the blood flow through the vessel (ml/sec) can be calculated. Numerous technical problems complicate the operation of the electromagnetic flow probe. Interference from ECG machines and fluctuations in the electrolyte potential have driven manufacturers to higher-frequency AC magnetic fields, typically at approximately 400 Hz. Intravascular (catheter tip) flow probes are also available.[74]

ELECTRICAL SAFETY IN THE OPERATING ROOM

INTRODUCTION

Understanding electrical safety is an important responsibility for anesthesiologists.[75-78] For example, if leakage currents from a pressure transducer were to reach the heart through an arterial or central venous pressure line, they could cause ventricular fibrillation.[79,80] More commonly, electrical malfunctions cause tissue burns, fires and explosions, central and peripheral nerve stimulation and damage, muscle stimulation and contracture, pacemaker interference, and the sudden loss of electrical power to other equipment. Most of these complications are preventable.

ELECTRICAL GROUND

To the clinician, an electrical ground is a wire that connects to the third prong on plugs that are inserted into electrical wall outlets. Specifically, an electrical ground is an object capable of instantaneously supplying or receiving arbitrarily large amounts of electrical charge.

The electrical power supplied in an operating room is isolated from the electrical ground used elsewhere throughout the hospital. Furthermore, many electrical circuits in the operating rooms are *not* connected to any ground. Yet the metal that encases the circuits is always grounded. Contact with electrical ground can be dangerous if it enables large electrical currents to travel through the body. Living organisms tolerate small currents only. Thus, ground should only be touched through a sizable resistance. Operating rooms that have conductive floors use the correct resistive materials; they may not be built of electrical conductors that are as good as metal.

The concept that the electrical ground is the zero point of the electrical potential is important to understand. The voltage at any point in a circuit is the voltage difference between that point and the electrical ground. In other words, the voltage difference between two points in a circuit — *not* the "absolute voltage" at either point — determines the electrical current flow between them. The ground connection in a commercial circuit helps one safely check that circuit against a manual. A connection from the voltmeter can be safely attached to ground, and the voltmeter probe can be used to examine different points in the circuit. Voltage readings can be compared with a manufacturer's table, and problem spots in the circuit can be easily identified. Specifying the location of ground thus helps people communicate standards for circuit performance. The location of ground makes no intellectual difference in the design of a circuit.

ELECTRICAL ISOLATION

Every operating suite has electricity that is isolated from the main power source by an isolation transformer. An isolation transformer has the two hot wire contacts for each power outlet come from the secondary winding of the transformer. The primary circuit of the transformer is attached to ground, but the secondary circuit of the transformer is not. The third contact in all the power outlets, which is for the groundwire in the plug, is connected to the standard hospital ground, and not to the isolation transformer. This is illustrated in Figure 4-29A.

Thus, electrical ground is the same for all operating rooms, and all the electrical equipment is said to be grounded. But what this means is that the external case is grounded, not the powered circuits that constitute the functional part of the equipment. When an electrical device, such as an ECG monitor, is plugged in, neither of the two hot wires from the secondary of the transformer is connected to ground by the ECG circuitry. This is illustrated in the schematic diagram shown in Figure 4-29B for the ECG monitor.

The ECG case is connected to the hospital's electrical ground. The circuitry inside the ECG unit is connected to an isolated power supply. This is an example of a safe system. If any electrical current accidentally gets a chance to leave the circuitry and travel through ground, the path through the third wire, attached to the case, is there to divert current that could pass through the anesthetist. However, thanks to the isolation transformer, electrical current will not leave the circuitry to pass through ground, unless there is a second pathway which will allow the current to return to the circuitry at some other location. The next sche-

SCHEMATIC OF ISOLATION TRANSFORMER

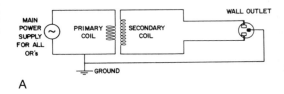

A

SCHEMATIC OF POWER CONNECTION (Outlet to Equipment)

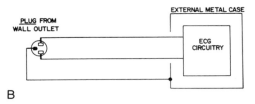

B

FIG. 4-29 Schematic diagrams (A) of an isolation transformer and (B) of electrical grounding for an ECG in the operating room.

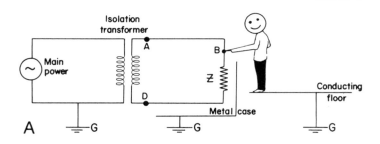

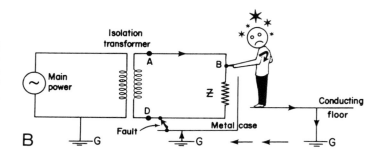

FIG. 4-30 Diagrams showing (A) that *no* electric shock occurs if an isolated power line is touched, (B) that an electric shock *does* occur if a faulted secondary power line is touched, and (C) that a line isolation monitor can watch for a fault.

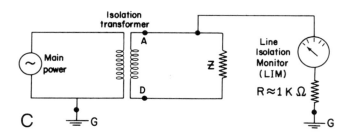

matic diagram (Fig. 4-30A) shows this. If you touch the knob, at B, will you get a shock?

The answer is *no*, because touching the knob at B does not complete a path that leads from the first hot wire at A to the second "hot wire" at D. The only way for electrical current to get from point A to point D is through the impedance Z. Nevertheless, touching the knob at B could be very dangerous. Serious consequences could follow if a short circuit were to occur. For example, if the second hot wire, that is, the one on the D side, were to become grounded, touching knob B would complete a pathway from A to D, and a shock would result, as shown in Figure 4-30B.

It should now be apparent why circuits inside operating room equipment are not grounded. A fault that would enable one to

touch the ungrounded side would also allow a pathway to be completed between the hot wires that would result in a shock. A device has been invented to help avoid problems like the one we have just discussed. It is called the line isolation monitor (LIM), and as its name implies, it monitors the isolation of the transformer in every operating suite. The meter for the LIM is usually very close to the transformer panel. The workings of this meter can be understood from Figure 4-30C, which shows the meter attached to one hot wire, ready to give a large deflection if the other hot wire becomes grounded.

If D were to connect to ground, G, then electrical current would flow from A to B, through the meter to G, and finally back to D. The ammeter so placed thus shows the mil-

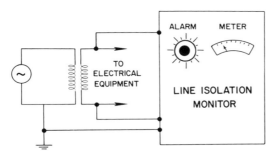

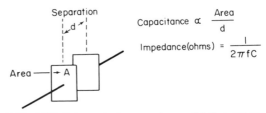

FIG. 4-32 Schematic diagram of a parallel plate capacitor.

FIG. 4-31 Schematic showing complete connections of the line isolation monitor. The alarm sounds impedance if either isolated power line is less than 25,000 ohms or if a fault would draw more than 2 mA.

liampere current that would result if the opposite hot wire were directly connected to ground. Because either hot wire could be grounded, the LIM monitors both isolated power lines and is set to alarm when either side has an impedance to ground that is less than 25,000 Ω, or when the maximum current that a short circuit could cause exceeds 2 mA. The actual connection of the line isolation monitor is shown in Figure 4-31.

If the LIM goes off in the operating room, the piece of equipment that triggered it should immediately be unplugged. There is a region on or inside that piece of equipment that could electrically shock someone. The sounding of the alarm means that one side of the isolation line is grounded, and that this must not be allowed to happen to the other side, especially if you or your patient are part of the connection.

CAPACITIVE COUPLING

The parallel plate capacitor, sketched in Figure 4-32, is a circuit element that permits the passage of alternating current. It does not, however, permit the passage of direct electrical current. Higher-frequency currents traverse a capacitor more easily than lower frequency currents. This is demonstrated by the formula for the impedance to alternating current flow in ohms, which is given in terms of the AC frequency, f, and the capacitance C in farads

$$Z(\Omega) = 1/(2\pi f C)$$

For the parallel plate capacitor C is directly proportional to the area of the capacitor plates, and inversely proportional to the spacing between them. Note that as the AC frequency, f, increases, the impedance to current flow becomes smaller. Because any two conducting objects in a room are a kind of capacitor, the D side of our isolation transformer circuit is always coupled to ground at AC frequencies. The concept of an equivalent capacitor refers to the coupling that would occur if an isolated circuit located in an enormous room far away from all walls and objects had a capacitor added to it that could produce the same coupling that arises from the walls and objects in the small room. Although capacitive coupling can sometimes be significant at frequencies of 60 cycles/sec, it is more commonly a problem during electrosurgery, or use of the Bovie, which occurs at higher frequencies, typically hundreds to thousands of kilocycles/sec.

ELECTRICAL SHOCKS

The passage of electrical current through the body can interfere with the normal functioning of muscles and nerves. Macroshock refers to application of large voltages or currents to the skin or tissue at locations remote from the heart. Microshock refers to the application of very small voltages or currents directly to the heart, as occurs intentionally with pacemaker electrodes, and unintentionally with saline that carries inadvertent currents through a central line.

MACROSHOCK

The response to an electrical current flow through a person's arm depends on the amplitude and frequency of the current. Sensation of a 60-cycle current will occur at approximately 300 mA, and pain will occur near 1 mA. After a certain current is reached, known as the "let go" current, the person is unable to let go of objects.[81] The value of the let-go current varies with frequency and also among individuals. The range of average values is shown in Figure 4-36 as a function of AC frequency. The 50 and 60 cycles/sec have the lowest values, and thus are in the most dangerous range. The frequency dependence of response to electroshock is similar in cardiac muscle.

Electrical current is more important than voltage when issues of electrical safety arise. The range of responses to increasing total body currents is given in the Table 4-2.[75] Ventricular fibrillation can be caused by continuous total body currents in the range of 0.1 to 2.5 A (approximately 10 times the "let go" value). The electrical current generated in one pulse by an implanted cardiac pacemaker ranges from 0.1 to 10 mA. Thus, only a small part of the total body current needs to pass through the heart for cardiac function to be altered. The electrosurgical unit generates so much power that it can induce microshock currents when it is used near implanted pacemaker wires. However, the last convincing report of fibrillation induced by electrosurgery was in 1968 thanks to the safe grounding practice we have described.[82]

MICROSHOCK

Microshock occurs when small amounts of electrical power and electrical energy are delivered to the heart. Your asking for 400 watt-sec (or joules) during closed chest CPR is a request for an energy dose to the body from the defibrillator that approximates that delivered by a large-caliber handgun. (A 0.45-caliber bullet weighs 250 grains and has a muzzle velocity of 860 ft/sec when fired. This corresponds to an energy of approximately 540 watt-sec.) Thus, a very small portion of a defibrillator's energy dose is needed to depolarize the heart.

Electrical current is the variable most convenient for setting safety limits. Because fibrillation in human hearts is alleged to require a minimum of 50 μA,[83-84] the national code sets 10 μA as the maximum permissible leakage current allowed through electrodes or catheters that contact the heart, which is considerably smaller than the peak electrical current generated during a single pulse from an implanted pacemaker (0.1 to 10 mA). Thus, the LIM provides no protection against microshock hazards. (Recall that 2 mA is the warning level.)

Although ECG monitoring electrodes are electrically isolated from the power circuits in the monitor by an isolation transformer in the main unit — a second level of isolation — an anesthesiologist who wishes to perform intravenous or intracardiac ECG monitoring, as in CVP placement, should have the ECG monitor checked for microampere leakage currents by qualified personnel. In some ECG and EEG sys-

---

TABLE 4-2. Average Effects of 60-Hz Currents on Humans Applied at Body Surface and Passing Through the Trunk

Current (mA) (1-sec contact)	Effect
1	Threshold of perception
5	Accepted as maximum harmless current intensity
10–20	"Let-go" value achieved — sustained muscle contraction next
50–100	Pain; possible fainting, exhaustion, mechanical injury; heart and respiratory function continue
100–2,500	Ventricular fibrillation; respiratory center intact
6000 or more	Sustained myocardial contraction followed by normal rhythm; Temporary respiratory paralysis; burns if the current density is high (usually if J > 100 mA/cm²)

tems, the electrode signals from the patient are translated into light by a battery-powered amplifier with a photodiode output, and then optically coupled to the main ECG or EEG unit. (A more thorough second level of isolation.)

ELECTROSURGERY

Most of our concerns with electrical safety in the operating room come from the need to use electrosurgical units—such as the Bovie, which can cause shocks, burns, and explosions, dysrhythmia, and pacemaker interference.[85] Electrosurgical units operate at frequencies of approximately 300,000 to 2,000,000 cycles/sec (300 kHz to 2 MHz), so as to minimize the likelihood of ventricular fibrillation. (See Figure 4-33 in the macroshock section regarding frequency dependence.) Despite the considerable engineering efforts that have gone into making electrosurgical units safe, concerns with electrosurgery alone account for the presence of an isolation transformer in every operating room.

Electrical energy and electrical power determine tissue injury. These clearly depend on the strength and path of the electrical current density. Unipolar electrosurgical devices, the ones most commonly used, generate currents that enter the patient in a small area where an electrode tip is applied, and leave the patient in a large area where a "ground pad" has been applied. The current density is determined to the surgeon's satisfaction by adjustment of the coagulation and cutting controls. The engineering of this device has made it safe for tissue

that is more than a few millimeters away from the electrode tip. The fanning out of the electronic current is illustrated in Figure 4-34.

Skin burns can result if the ground pad is dry or otherwise in poor contact with the patient. The skin resistance to the returning current will be high if much of the conducting gel is gone and the surface area traversed is small. If the resistance is high, the power dissipation in the skin, which is proportional to the square of the current times resistance, or I^2R, will also be high.[86] Electrical burns have been reported at the site of the ECG leads in situations where the grounding pad was defective, and the ECG leads served as an alternate path for the returning high-frequency electrosurgery current.[87,88]

Some locations of the body are never safe for unipolar electrosurgery. Neurosurgeons exclusively employ bipolar devices, which have the electric current spending only a few millimeters in the tissue as it travels from one pencil point electrode to another. Bipolar devices must also be used if electrosurgery is done on the ovary or fallopian tubes. Several cases of fatal bowel injury have been reported following female sterilizations with unipolar devices.[89,90] Patients with implanted pacemakers frequently come to the operating room for procedures that employ electrosurgery. Bipolar devices should always be used in these cases, although pacemaker interference may sometimes nevertheless occur. The avoidance of pacemaker interference depends on the type of pacing electrodes in the patient (i.e., unipolar or bipolar), on how well the pacemaker circuitry is shielded, and on the strength and proximity of the electrosurgical unit's discharge.

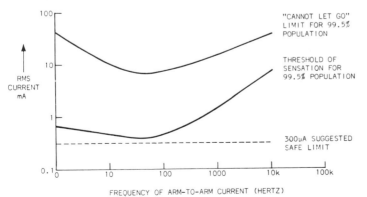

FIG. 4-33 Frequency dependence of the "let-go" and pain-threshold currents.

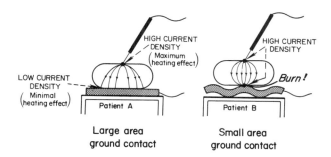

FIG. 4-34 Electrical currents through the body for small- and large-area grounding pads.

SAFE PRACTICE

Because explosive anesthetic agents are no longer used,[91] hospitals are no longer required to regulate the conductivity of the operating room floors and tables. Problems that result from poor electrical grounding might therefore occur more frequently in the future. We list below some general guidelines for safe electrical practice.

1. All electrical equipment in that is used in the OR should be grounded equipment. (Such equipment will contain ungrounded circuits.) If the power plug for the electrical outlet has only two prongs, the equipment should not be there.
2. Do not connect patients to the operating room electrical ground.
3. When electrosurgery is in use, *do* connect patients to the electrosurgery machine's ground. This should be done via a large area well-gelled plate or pad. Inspect this during long cases, and regel or replace if necessary. Place the electrosurgical ground plate as near to the operative site as possible, and as remote from pacemaker wires and ECG wires as possible.
4. If increasing current levels are required for electrosurgery, rule out faulty connection of the electrosurgical grounding pad.
5. If the LIM goes off, immediately unplug the offending piece of equipment. The piece of equipment that caused the alarm to go off has allowed the secondary side of the main isolation transformer to be coupled to ground. You can try unplugging other equipment, and then try replugging in the item that caused the LIM alarm to go off. It is possible

for so many items to be plugged in at once, that their combined capacitance couples the secondary side to ground. If, however, the LIM alarm goes after other equipment has been unplugged, remove the offending item from the operating room. It has an unwanted connection to ground somewhere.

6. Use a bipolar unit when electrosurgery is rquired in patients with an implanted cardiac pacemaker. Understand the type of pacemaker your patient has, and have the appropriate magnets and equipment available for immediate use in case of pacemaker interference or total dysfunction. Know how you would pharmacologically treat complete heart block in any of your pacemaker-dependent patients.
7. Make sure that all electrical equipment is periodically tested by experienced personnel and that proper maintenance is conducted to assure that the standards of performance[92-97] are met.

REFERENCES

1. Michenfelder JD: Who's afraid of Blaise Pascal? Anesthesiology 56:245, 1982
2. Badeer HS: Contractile tension in the myocardium. Am Heart J 66:432, 1963
3. Fishman NH: Thoracic Drainage—A Manual of Procedures. Chicago, Year Book, 1983
4. Bernhard WN, Yost LC, Turndorf H, et al: Physical characteristics of and rates of nitrous oxide

diffusion into tracheal tube cuffs. Anesthesiology 48:413, 1978

5. Warren VN, Crawford AN, Young TM: The use of entonox as a sedation agent for children who have refused operative dentistry. J Dent 11(4): 306, 1983

6. Donen N, Tweed WA, White D, et al: Pre-hospital analgesia with entonox. Can Anaesth Soc J 29(3):275, 1982

7. Priano L, Solanki D, Gloyna DF: A simple method for mixing air and oxygen. Anesthesiology 57:145, 1982

8. Barnes PK: Principles of lung ventilators and humidification, Scientific Foundations of Anaesthesia. Edited by Scurr C, Feldman S. Chicago, Year Book, 1982, pp 533–544

9. Boys JE, Howells TH: Humidification in anesthesia. A review of the present situation. Br J Anaesth 44:879, 1972

10. Chalon J, Ali M, Ramanathan S, et al: The humidification of anaesthetic gases: its importance and control. Can Anaesth Soc J 26:361, 1979

11. Chalon J, Patel C, Ali M, et al: Humidity and the anesthetized patient. Anesthesiology 50:195, 1979

12. Weeks DB: Humidification during anesthesia. NY State J Med 75:1216, 1975

13. Chalon J, Loew DAY, Malebranche J: Effects of dry anesthetic gases on tracheobronchial ciliated epithelium. Anesthesiology 37:338, 1972

14. Forbes AR: Humidification and mucus flow in the intubated trachea. Br J Anaesth 45:874, 1973

15. Forbes AR: Temperature, humidity and mucus flow in the intubated trachea. Br J Anaesth 46:29, 1974

16. Hirsch JA, Tokayer JH, Robinson MJ, et al: Effects of dry gas and subsequent humidification on tracheal mucus velocity in dogs. J Appl Phys 39(2):242, 1975

17. Knudson J, Lomhold N, Wisborg K: Postoperative pulmonary complications using dry and humidified anaesthetic gases. Br J Anaesth 45:363, 1973

18. Stone DR: Humidification and body temperature during anesthesia in adults. Anesthesiology 51(3):S359, 1979

19. DeVoe RD, Maloney PC: Principles of cell homeostasis, Medical Physiology. 14th Ed. Edited by Mountcastle VB. St Louis, CV Mosby, 1980, pp 36–42

20. Severinghaus JW: Methods of measurement of blood and gas CO_2 during anesthesia. Anesthesiology 21:717, 1960

21. Severinghaus JW: Electrodes for blood and gas PCO_2, PO_2, and blood pH. Acta Anaesthesiol Scand (suppl)11:207, 1962

22. Severinghaus JW: Blood gas concentrations, The Handbook of Physiology. Waverly Press, Baltimore, 1965, pp 1475–1487

23. Clark LC Jr, Bargeron LM Jr, Lyons C, et al: Detection of right-to-left shunts with an arterial potentiometric electrode. Circulation 22:949, 1960

24. Fahraeus R, Lindqvist T: The viscosity of the blood in narrow capillary tubes. Am J Physiol 96:562, 1931

25. Purcell EM: Life at low Reynolds number. Am J Phys 45:3, 1977

26. Coulter NA Jr, Pappenheimer JR: Development of turbulence in flowing blood. Am J Physiol 159:401, 1949

27. Macovski A: Medical Imaging Systems. Englewood Cliffs, NJ, Prentice-Hall, 1983, pp 173–224

28. Cahalan MK, Kremer P, Schiller N, et al: Intraoperative monitoring with two-dimensional echocardiography. Anesthesiology 57:A153, 1982

29. Gadian DG: Nuclear Magnetic Resonance and Its Applications to Living Systems. Oxford, Clarendon Press, 1982

30. Margulis AR, Higgins CB, Kaufman L, et al (eds): Clinical Magnetic Resonance Imaging. San Francisco University of California, Radiology Research and Education Foundation, 1983

31. Roth JL, Nugent M, Gray JE, et al: Patient monitoring during magnetic resonance imaging. Anesthesiology 61(3A):A157, 1984

32. James TL, Margulis AR: Biomedical Magnetic Resonance Imaging. San Francisco University of California, Radiology Research and Education Foundation, 1984

33. Trudell JR, Hubbel WL: Localization of molecular halothane in phospholipid bilayer model nerve membranes. Anesthesiology 44:202, 1976

34. Wyrwicz AM, Pszenny MH, Schofield JC, et al: Noninvasive observation of fluorinated anesthetics in rabbit brain by fluorine-19 nuclear magnetic resonance. Science 222:429, 1983

35. Wyrwicz AM, Pszenny MH, Nichols BG, et al: In-vivo ^{19}F NMR Study of halothane and isoflurane elimination from a rabbit brain. Anesthesiology 61(3A):A156, 1984

36. Higgins CB, Lanzer P, Stark D, et al: Imaging by nuclear magnetic resonance in patients with chronic ischemic heart disease. Circulation 69:523, 1984

37. The Radiological Health Handbook. Revised Edition January 1970. US Department of Health, Education and Welfare. US Public Health Service.

38. Aguilar-Benitez M, Cahn RN, Crawford RL, et al: Review of particle properties. Rev Mod Phys 56(2), Part II, 1984

39. Feldman KL (ed): Radiological quality of the environment in the United States, 1977. EPA 520/1-77-009. Washington, DC US Environmental Protection Agency, Office of Radiation Programs

40. Rosenstein M: Organ doses in diagnostic radiology. HEW Publication (FDA) 76-8030, Superin-

tendant of Documents, Washington, DC, US Government Printing Office

41. Brinley FJ Jr: Volume conductor theory, Medical Physiology. 14th Ed. Edited by Mountcastle VB. St Louis, CV Mosby, 1980, pp 290–293

42. Nunez PL: Electric fields of the brain. New York, Oxford University Press, 1981

43. Geddes LA, Baker LE: Electrodes for bioelectric events, Principles of Applied Biomedical Instrumentation. 2nd Ed. New York, Wiley–Interscience, 1975, pp 196–268

44. Geddes LA: Electrodes and the Measurement of Bioelectric Events. New York, Wiley, 1972

45. O'Connell DN, Tursky B, Orne MT: Electrodes for recording skin potential. Arch Gen Psychiatry 3:252, 1960

46. Geddes LA, Baker LE: The electrodermal phenomena, Principles of Applied Biomedical Instrumentation. 2nd Ed. New York, Wiley–Interscience, 1975, pp 489–509

47. Thomas HE: Handbook of Biomedical Instrumentation and Measurement. Reston, Virginia, Reston Publications, 1974, p 108

48. Stein RA, Ben-Zvi S, LaBelle P: The modern monitor defibrillator—A potential source of falsely abnormal ecg recordings. JAMA 246:1697, 1981

49. Hales S: Statistical essays: Containing haemastaticks. Reprint. History of Medicine Series, Vol 22, Library of New York Academy of Medicine. New York, Hafner, 1964

50. Cox RH: Determination of systemic hydraulic power in unanesthetized dogs. Am J Physiol 226:579, 1974

51. Ream AK: Systolic, diastolic, mean or pulse pressure: Which is the best measurement of arterial pressure?, Essential Noninvasive Monitoring. Edited by Gravenstein JS, Newbower RS, Ream AK, Smith NT. New York, Grune & Stratton, 1980, pp 53–74

52. Posey JA, Geddes LA, Williams H, et al: The meaning of the point of maximum oscillations in cuff pressure in the indirect measurement of blood pressure, Part I. Cardiovasc Res Cent Bull 8:15, 1969

53. Yelderman M, Ream AK: Indirect measurement of mean blood pressure in the anesthetized patient. Anesthesiology 50:253, 1979

54. Ramsey M III: Noninvasive automatic determination of mean arterial pressure. Med Biol Eng Comp 17:11, 1979

55. Sarnoff SJ, Braunwald E, Welch GH Jr, et al: Hemodynamic determinates of oxygen consumption of the heart with special reference to the tension–time index. Am J Physiol 192:148, 1958

56. Buckberg GD, Fixler DE, Archie JP, et al: Experimental subendocardial ischemia in dogs with normal coronary arteries. Circ Res 30:67, 1972

57. McDonald DA: Appendix I: The theoretical analysis of manometer behaviour, Blood Flow in Arteries. Baltimore, Williams & Wilkins, 1974

58. Shinozaki T, Deane RS, Mazuzan JE: The dynamic response of liquid filled catheter systems for direct measurement of blood pressure. Anesthesiology 53:498, 1980

59. Gardner R: Direct blood pressure measurement —Dynamic response requirements. Anesthesiology 54:227, 1981

60. Geddes LA: The Direct and Indirect Measurement of Blood Pressure. Chicago, Year Book, 1970

61. Bruner JMR: Handbook of Blood Pressure Monitoring. Littleton, Mass, PSG Publishing, 1978

62. Whitcher C: Blood pressure measurement, Techniques in Clinical Physiology (A Survey of Measurement in Anesthesiology). Toronto, Macmillan, 1969

63. Kirkendall WM, Burton AC, Epstein FH: Recommendations for Human Blood Pressure Determination by Sphygmanometers. New York, American Heart Association, 1967

64. Apple HP: Automated noninvasive blood pressure monitors, Essential Noninvasive Monitoring. Edited by Gravenstein JS, Newbower RS, Ream AK, Smith NT. New York, Grune & Stratton, 1980, pp 7–23

65. Canzoneri J III: Electronic detection of indirect systolic and diastolic blood pressure. Thesis, Department of Electrical Engineering, University of Houston, Texas, 1964, p 7

66. Showman A: Hazard of automatic blood pressure monitoring. (Correspondence.) Anesthesiology 55:717, 1981

67. Kimball KJ, Darnall RA Jr, Yelderman M, et al: An automated oscillometric technique for estimating mean arterial pressure in critically ill newborns. Anesthesiology 54:423, 1981

68. Sy WP: Ulnar nerve palsy possibly related to use of automatically cycled blood pressure cuff. Anesth Analg 60:687, 1981

69. Prys-Roberts C: Measurement of cardiac output and regional blood flow, The Circulation in Anaesthesia. Edited by Prys-Roberts C. Oxford, Blackwell, 1980

70. Forrester JS, et al: Thermodilution cardiac output determination with a single flow-directed catheter. Am Heart J 83:306, 1972

71. Kety SS, Schmidt CF: Determination of cerebral blood flow in man by the use of nitrous oxide in low concentrations. Am J Physiol 143:53, 1945

72. Lassen NA, Ingvar DH: The blood flow of the cerebral cortex determined by radioactive krypton. Experientia 17:42, 1961

73. Hoedt-Rassmussen K, Sveimsdottir E, Lassen NA: Regional cerebral blood flow in man by intra-arterial injection of radioactive gas. Circ Res 18:237, 1966

74. Mills CJ, Shillingford JP: A catheter tip velocity probe and its evaluation. Cardiovasc Res 1:263, 1967

75. Bruner JMR: Hazards of electrical apparatus. Anesthesiology 28:396, 1967

76. Bruner JMR: Common abuses and failures of electrical equipment. Anesth Analg 51(5):810, 1972

77. Bruner JMR: Fundamental concepts of electrical safety. Refresher Courses Anesthesiol 2:11, 1974

78. Ward CS: On electrical safety. Anaesthesia 35(9):921, 1980

79. Atkin DH, Orkin LR: Electrocution in the operating room. Anesthesiology 38:181, 1973

80. Chambers JJ, Saha AK: Electrocution during anaesthesia. Anaesthesia 34:173, 1979

81. Dalziel CF, Lee WR: Lethal electrical currents. IEEE Spectrum 6(2):44, 1969

82. Titel JH, El Etr AA: Fibrillation resulting from pacemaker elctrodes and electrocautery during surgery. Anesthesiology 29:845, 1968

83. Geddes LA, Cabler P, Moore AG, et al: Threshold 60 Hz current required for ventricular fibrillation. Med Instrum 7:158, 1973

84. Roy OZ: 60 Hz ventricular fibrillation and rhythm thresholds and the nonpacing intracardiac catheter. Med Biol Eng 13:228, 1975

85. Aronow S, Bruner JMR: Electrosurgery. Anesthesiology 42:525, 1975

86. Battig CG: Electrosurgical burn injuries and their prevention. JAMA 204:91, 1968

87. Chandra P: Severe skin damage from EKG electrodes. Anesthesiology 56:157, 1982

88. Parker EO: Electrosurgical burn at the site of an esophageal temperature probe. Anesthesiology 61:93, 1984

89. Deaths following female sterilization with unipolar electrocoagulating devices. 30, April 10, 1981

90. Tubal-Sterilization Related Deaths in the US 1977–1981. In Leads from the MMWR 32(19), 1983. JAMA 249:3011, 1983

91. Fineberg HV, Pearlman LA, Gabel RA: The case for abandonment of explosive anesthetic agents. N Engl Med J 303:613, 1980

92. Whelpton D: Safety of electrical equipment: J Med Eng Technol 3(2):62, 1979

93. Whelpton D: Acceptance testing of medical electrical equipment. J Med Eng Technol 8(1):19, 1984

94. Rubinstein ML: Electrical safety standards for electrocardiographic apparatus. Circulation 62(6):1392, 1980

95. Millar K, Oliver GC, Plonsey R, et al: Electrical safety standards for electrocardiographic apparatus. Circulation 61:669, 1980

96. NFPA No 76C: High Frequency Electricity in Health Care Facilities. Boston, National Fire Protection Association, 1975

97. NFPA No 56A: Standard for the use of inhalation anesthetics, 1973

98. McGregor M: Pulsus paradoxus. N Engl J Med 301:480, 1979

SUGGESTED READINGS

Adriani J: The Chemistry and Physics of Anesthesia. 2nd Ed. Springfield, Ill, Charles C Thomas, 1967

Mackintosh R, Mushin MW, Epstein HG: Physics for the Anesthetist, 3rd Ed. Philadelphia, FA Davis, 1963

Mountcastle VB (ed): Medical Physiology. 14th Ed. St Louis, CV Mosby, 1980

Parbrook GD, Davis PD, Parbrook EO: Basic Physics and Measurement in Anaesthesia. London, Camelot Press, Heinemann, 1982

Purcell EM: Electricity and Magnetism. San Francisco, McGraw-Hill, 1965

Scurr C, Feldman S: Scientific Foundations of Anaesthesia. 3rd Ed. Chicago, Heinemann–Year Book Publications, 1982

5

Anesthetic Systems

Fredrick K. Orkin, M.D.

INTRODUCTION

The anesthetic system delivers anesthetic gases from the flowmeters of the anesthetic machine to the mask or tracheal tube. Functionally, the system consists of the anesthetic equipment through which the patient breathes. Properly chosen and used, the anesthetic system is a convenient and efficient way to deliver anesthetic gases (and oxygen) and remove exhaled carbon dioxide. In contrast, a poorly designed or improperly used system prolongs the induction of, and recovery from, anesthesia and risks more serious problems and complications, largely of a respiratory nature.

This chapter presents the principles underlying the safe use of anesthetic systems —sometimes loosely termed anesthetic or breathing circuits—and their components and accessories, such as CO_2 absorbers, volatile anesthetic vaporizers, excess gas scavenging equipment, inspiratory gas monitors, and anesthesia ventilators. Because of limited space and the rapidity with which equipment is modified and replaced, the reader is referred to other sources for discussion of the historical development of this equipment[1] and manufacturer-specific details.[2-6]

EQUIPMENT, HUMAN FACTORS, AND ADVERSE ANESTHETIC OUTCOMES

Between 2 and 10 anesthetic-related deaths occur for every 10,000 operations, depending on definition and other analytic details.[7-10] Although relatively unstudied, anesthetic-related morbidity undoubtedly occurs considerably more frequently (also see Ch. 12). Most important are two very sobering facts. First, anesthesia is rarely therapeutic apart from the surgical procedure and, thus, significant risk is assumed without any hope of improving the patient's condition. Second, 50 to 87 percent of adverse anesthetic outcomes have been deemed preventable.[8-14] The more prominent problems identified are breathing system disconnections and connection errors.[15,16] Associated human factors include inadequate total experience, inadequate familiarity with the equipment, and failure to check equipment properly before use.[16-18] It is the unfortunate confluence of several of these events and factors that often leads to catastrophe (Fig. 5-1).

As anesthesiology continues to mature, fewer adverse outcomes related to gaps in basic medical science should occur. Instead, an increasing portion of the risk of anesthesia will be attributable to preventable factors such as misuse of breathing systems. Herein lies the necessity of becoming knowlegeable about anesthesia systems. In addition to educating staff about equipment and its limitations, other aspects of an effective risk management program include checking equipment before each use (also see Ch. 12), improved clinical supervision, improved human-factors design in equipment, periodic inspection and maintenance of equipment, institution of and action on incident reports, use of additional monitoring devices, and recognition of limitations affecting individual performance.[19-23]

Regulations only very recently approved under the Medical Device Amendments of 1976 (PL 94-295) have empowered the Food and Drug Administration (FDA) to regulate medical equipment for safety and efficacy in much the same fashion that it maintains oversight of pharmaceuticals for adverse responses.[24,25] Under these regulations, manufacturers and distributors of medical equipment must report, by telephone within 5, and in writing within 15 business days, on equipment that has caused death or serious injury, that has a malfunction that could cause death or injury, that may provide inaccurate diagnostic infor-

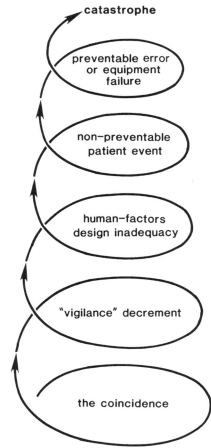

FIG. 5-1 The anesthetic mishap chain through which a coincidence involving a lapse in vigilance couples with an equipment design defect or perhaps a clinical event, leading to catastrophe. (Courtesy of Jeffrey B. Cooper, Ph.D., Massachusetts General Hospital.)

mation that could result in improper treatment, or that is already subject to remedial action by the manufacturer. In addition, a voluntary program has been established under which anesthesiologists are encouraged to report equipment problems directly to the FDA. However, no reporting program will obviate the necessity for each practitioner to become familiar with his or her equipment and to maintain vigilance during its use.

PHYSICAL PRINCIPLES

GAS FLOW AND RESISTANCE

Anesthetic gas flow from the anesthesia machine to the patient in response to a pressure gradient that exists between the gas pressure regulators or reducing valves at the machine (usually about 2600 mm Hg, 345 kPa, or 50 lb/in²) and the patient (atmospheric pressure). The gas flow rate through a straight tube of uniform bore is proportional to the pressure gradient and the fourth power of the radius and is related inversely to the viscosity of the gas and the length of the tube. These relationships are summarized in the Hagen-Poiseuille equation:

$$\dot{Q} = \frac{\pi p r^4}{8\eta l} \tag{1}$$

where $\dot{Q}$ is the flow rate in cubic meters per second, p is the pressure gradient in Newtons per square meter, r is the radius in meters, l is the length of the tube in meters, and η is the viscosity of the gas in Newton-seconds per square meter. Thus, for a given pressure gradient and tube length, the critical determinant of flow rate is the radius of the tube, since this term is present in the Hagen-Poiseuille equation raised to the fourth power. Alternatively, since the pressure gradient required to effect flow is measure of the resistance to flow, resistance is also directly proportional to the flow rate but is inversely related to the fourth power of the radius.

LAMINAR FLOW

The molecules comprising the gas typically move in paths parallel to the sides of the tube; therefore, the flow is termed *laminar*. Laminar flow is characterized by adherence to the Hagen-Poiseuille equation and a parabolic flow pattern in which the highest velocity is at the center of the lumen and least (zero) at the wall of the tube. This pattern of different velocities reflects the underlying differences in shear forces between apposed particle layers that retard particle movement. The shear force is greatest at the periphery because the tubing wall is immobile, and the force is progressively smaller toward the center of the tube (Fig. 5-2a).

TURBULENT FLOW

When the flow rate exceeds a critical velocity, the flow loses its parabolic velocity profile, becomes disorderly, and is termed turbulent (Fig. 5-2b). The critical velocity is itself

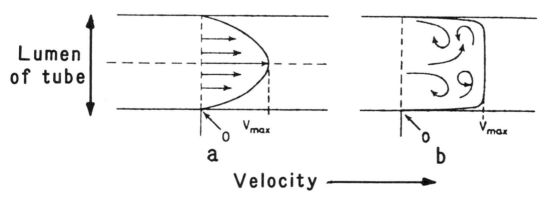

FIG. 5-2 Flow profiles characterizing (a) laminar and (b) turbulent flow. (Modified from Hill DW: Physics Applied to Anaesthesia. 4th Ed. London, Butterworths (Publishers) Ltd. 1980.)

proportional to the viscosity of the gas and is inversely related to the density of the gas and the radius of the tube (Fig. 5-3). These relationships are summarized as follows:

$$v_c = \frac{k\eta}{\rho r} \qquad (2)$$

where v_c is the critical velocity in centimeters per second, k is a constant known as the Reynold's number (approximately 2,000), η is the viscosity in Newtons per square meter, ρ is the density of the gas in grams per cubic centimeter, and r is the radius of the tube in centimeters. Laminar flow can also become turbulent as a result of irregularities in the tube lumen, such as abrupt narrowing, turns, or branching. When turbulent flow exists, the relationship between pressure gradient (or resistance) and flow rate is no longer governed by the Hagen-Poiseuille equation. Instead, the pressure gradient required (or the resistance encountered) during turbulent flow varies as the square of the flow rate. Given the high flow rates present during turbulent flow, this is an inefficient way

to move gas, since a much greater pressure gradient must be generated—or, alternatively, a much greater resistance must be overcome—than during laminar flow.

A special case of turbulence exists when a gas flows through an orifice that may be considered a very unusual tube, the diameter of which is considerably larger than its length. Although flow through an orifice can be laminar at low flow rates, the flow through such an aperture is generally at least partially turbulent. Empirical evidence indicates that the flow rate across an orifice is given by the following expression:

$$\dot{Q} \propto r^2 \sqrt{\frac{p}{\rho}} \qquad (3)$$

where $\dot{Q}$ is the flow rate, r the radius of the orifice, p the pressure gradient, and ρ the density of the gas. Thus, as in the more general case of turbulence, the pressure gradient (or resistance) varies as the square of the flow rate; however, in this special case, the flow rate is dependent on the density rather than the viscosity of the gas.

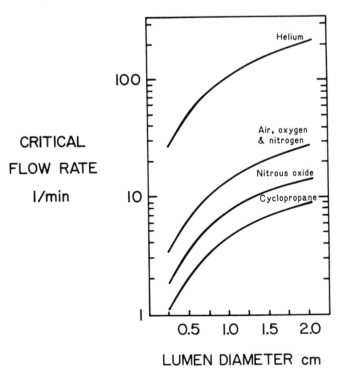

FIG. 5-3 Approximate critical flow rates of helium, air, oxygen, nitrogen, nitrous oxide, and cyclopropane at room temperature through smooth, straight tubes of various internal diameters. For a given diameter, there is a critical flow rate, which is dependent on gas viscosity and density, above which laminar flow becomes turbulent. (Values for air taken from ref. 2; values for other gases calculated.)

CLINICAL IMPORTANCE

Much of the equipment discussed in this chapter constitutes a tubular extension to the patient's upper airway. Because peak inspiratory flows as high as 60 L/min are reached during resting spontaneous ventilation in humans, anesthetic systems can add considerable resistance to respiration.[26-31] The resistance imparted by any system is determined most by those portions having the smallest bore, typically the tracheal tube and connector (Fig. 5-4). For example, the resistance of a Mapleson A breathing system is 0.25 cm H_2O (25 N/m²) at a constant flow rate of 50 L/min; adding a tracheal tube having an internal diameter of 10 mm with a curved connector increases the resistance to 2.5 cm H_2O (250 N/m²); finally, changing the curved connector to a right-angle

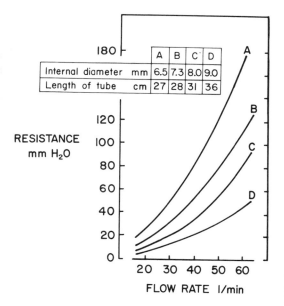

FIG. 5-4 Resistance as a function of tracheal tube internal diameter and flow rate. The relationship between flow rate and resistance is not linear—that is, the flow is not laminar—particularly as the lumen becomes smaller, because most of the flow rates depicted are above the critical velocities. Note also that flow rate must always be specified with values of resistance. (Modified from Macintosh R, Mushin WW, Epstein HG: Physics for the Anaesthetist. 3rd Ed. Oxford, Blackwell Scientific Publications, 1963.)

one increases the pressure drop across the system to 5.0 cm H_2O (500 N/m²).[32]

To counter increased respiratory resistance, the spontaneously breathing patient must generate a greater pressure gradient, which constitutes an increase in the work of breathing, to effect the same exchange of gas, or suffer hypoventilation.[33,34] In response to a mean increase of 241 percent in inspiratory resistance, infants in one study tolerated a mean increase of 205 percent in the work of breathing without CO_2 retention and acidosis.[35] However, these infants lacked cardiorespiratory disease; it should also be emphasized that hypercarbia and acidosis are late signs of respiratory decompensation. Increasing the inspiratory resistance further resulted in extremely variable responses. In unselected adult surgical patients, some of whom had cardiorespiratory disease, the imposition of increased respiratory resistance resulted in an immediate, presumably reflex increase in inspiratory pressure generated to partially counter the added resistance; an increase in minute ventilation occurred during the next few minutes. Breathing through resistors that simulated the resistance of pediatric endotracheal tubes having an external diameter of 24 Fr and 16 Fr (approximately 5.5 mm and 3.5 mm internal diameter, respectively), these adults experienced mean reductions of 7 and 21 percent in minute ventilation, respectively. There was marked scatter in their responses, with some patients maintaining a near-normal minute ventilation inspiring against 17 cm H_2O, whereas one patient became apneic at 12 cm H_2O.[36]

The added respiratory resistance due to anesthesia equipment is somewhat less clinically relevant now that assisted and controlled ventilation have supplanted spontaneous respiration during anesthesia. However, respiratory resistance remains an important consideration in the intensive care unit (ICU), where a patient may breathe spontaneously for a considerable period through a tracheal tube (e.g., T-piece trial, intermittent mandatory ventilation), whose lumen can be encroached upon progressively by inspissated secretions.

Minimizing respiratory resistance requires that components of the anesthetic system have the shortest length and greatest diameter practicable; thus, the corrugated breathing system tubing has a very large bore, and the tracheal tube should be the largest that can be accommodated. Sharp bends and other sudden changes in lumen size should be avoided; similarly, curved tracheal tube connectors (e.g., Magill) are preferable to right-angled ones (e.g., Cobb, Rowbotham). In clinical circumstances that simulate a narrow orifice, such as croup and tracheal stenosis, the use of a gas having a lower density than air, such as helium, as the carrier for oxygen results in improved gas flow (Fig. 5-3). A mixture of 80 percent helium in oxygen in place of air or oxygen augments gas flow rate by approximately 75 percent, thereby decreasing the work of breathing.[37]

CARBON DIOXIDE ELIMINATION

REBREATHING

Carbon dioxide is continuously produced in the body as a result of cellular metabolism and is transported to the lungs for elimination via pulmonary ventilation. An anesthetic breathing system can impair CO_2 elimination because the breathing system — effectively a tubular extension of the patient's upper airway — adds apparatus dead space to the patient's physiologic dead space. The latter includes the anatomic dead space (volume in nonventilating conducting airways) and alveolar dead space (volume in ventilated, nonperfused alveoli). Upon the imposition of the additional dead space, the patient breathes again, or rebreathes, a volume of exhaled gases approximating that of the added dead space.

PHYSIOLOGIC EFFECTS

The effects of rebreathing depend on the volume and composition of the gas that is rebreathed; one cannot predict precisely the physiologic responses in the clinical setting.[38] The volume of rebreathing can differ from that

determined volumetrically because of turbulence and other peculiarities of gas flow; moreover, the patient's anatomic dead space can vary, affecting the volume of total dead space. The composition of the rebreathed gas depends on which portion of the dead space is rebreathed. The composition of the gas in the apparatus dead space varies with the arrangement of components comprising the given breathing system. Gas in the anatomic dead space has a composition resembling that of the inspired concentration but is saturated with water vapor within a few degrees of body temperature. Alveolar gas is also saturated and contains 5 to 6 percent CO_2.

Altered Inspired Concentrations

Rebreathing alveolar gas from which CO_2 has not been removed necessarily results in an increased $PaCO_2$ value. Although an awake, healthy person can tolerate even large increases in dead space by increasing minute ventilation, the anesthetized patient generally cannot compensate for even small amounts of rebreathing (also see Chs. 21 & 32). The increase in the CO_2 concentration in alveolar air, coupled with the uptake of oxygen and nitrogen washout early during anesthesia, results in a decreased inspired concentration of oxygen. Rebreathing also causes a discrepancy between delivered and inspired concentrations of inhaled agents, because the rebreathed gas is a mixture of fresh gas and exhaled gas. Hence, during induction of anesthesia, when the alveolar concentration of anesthetic is lower than the inspired level, rebreathing dilutes the inspired concentration, reducing the alveolar concentration further and prolonging induction of anesthesia. In contrast, rebreathing slows the elimination of anesthetic during emergence by maintaining a higher alveolar concentration of anesthetic.

Heat and Water Retention

Since anesthetic gases are dry and at ambient temperature and exhaled gas is saturated with water vapor at body temperature, rebreathing conserves heat and water.

CARBON DIOXIDE ABSORPTION

Gas warfare during World War I provided the impetus for finding a way to remove exhaled CO_2 from the totally closed breathing system of the gas mask.[39] A general approach resulted that involves chemical neutralization of an acid by a base.[40] The CO_2 combines with water to form carbonic acid, which ionizes readily, releasing hydrogen ion, the acid. The base is the hydroxyl ion, resulting from the ionization of the hydroxide salt of the alkali metals (e.g., potassium, sodium) and of the alkaline earth metals (e.g., barium, calcium). The CO_2 absorbent is actually a mixture of the hydroxide salts, which are fused and then crushed into granular fragments having a large surface area for absorption of the CO_2.

GRANULE SIZE

The size of the granules represents a compromise between absorptive activity and resistance to airflow: absorptive activity increases as granule size decreases because total surface area increases. But the smaller the granules, the smaller the interstices through which gas must flow, hence the greater the resistance. Empirically, the optimal granule size has been found to be 4 to 8 mesh.[41] (A granule size of 4 mesh will pass through a screen having four or fewer wires per linear inch.)

WATER CONTENT

Although a small amount of water may be pesent in the hydrated salt, water is added to the granules by the manufacturer before sealing in an airtight package. Additional water is needed to raise the total water content to a level at which the particular absorbent mixture absorbs optimally: too much water reduces the surface area available for absorption, whereas too little water retards the formation of carbonic acid.[42] (Inadequate moisture is also associated with adsorption of sufficient halothane to prolong the induction of anesthesia.[43]) The water also dissipates some of the heat generated in the exothermic neutralization reaction.

INDICATOR

An indicator is a weak acid or base that forms a salt, the color of which depends on hydrogen ion concentration.[44] When the color change specific for the given indicator becomes apparent through the transparent canister, the absorptive capacity has been reached and the absorbent should be changed. If the absorbent is not changed, the color often reverts during disuse; however, minimal regeneration will have occurred, and, upon reuse, the dye quickly changes color again.[45] Commonly used indicators and their colors are listed in Table 5-1.

CHANNELING

Loose packing of the granules in a CO_2 canister, or poor design of the canister, results in the gas passing preferentially through the canister by way of paths of very low resistance. Such channeling is particularly likely to occur along the sides of the canister[40] and results, in turn, in exhaustion of the granules constituting the low-resistance paths, with passage of CO_2 through the canister if the absorbent is not changed. Shaking the canister gently before use can reduce the likelihood of channeling without substantially increasing resistance to airflow.

ABSORPTIVE CAPACITY

The maximum volume of CO_2 that can be absorbed is approximately 26 L of CO_2 per 100 g of the commonly used absorbents.[46] Consider-

TABLE 5-1. Indicators Used in Carbon Dioxide Absorbents

Indicator	Color When Absorbent	
	Fresh	Exhausted
Phenolphthalein	Colorless	Pink
Ethyl violet	Colorless	Purple
Clayton yellow	Red	Yellow
Ethyl orange	Orange	Yellow
Mimosa Z	Red	Colorless

(Modified from Dorsch JA, Dorsch SE: Understanding Anesthesia Equipment: Construction, Care and Complications. 2nd Ed. © 1984 The Williams & Wilkins Co., Baltimore.)

ably less CO_2 is actually absorbed due to diverse factors such as canister design, moisture content, degree of channeling, and the particular endpoint used to detect exhaustion. For example, only 10 to 15 L of CO_2 per 100 g is absorbed in a single-chambered canister, whereas 18 to 20 L is absorbed in a dual-chambered design. In the latter, the chamber through which the exhaled gas flows first is discarded when the indicator changes color, the second chamber is moved to the position formerly occupied by the first, and a new chamber containing fresh absorbent is added to the canister.

INCOMPATIBILITY WITH TRICHLOROETHYLENE

During 1943 and 1944, some two dozen case reports of cranial nerve injuries following trichloroethylene anesthesia appeared.[47] Patients emerged from anesthesia with an unusual amount of nausea and vomiting, often with concomitant headache. Days later, bilateral facial numbness (cranial nerve V) and weakness (VII), loss of corneal reflexes (V), oculomotor palsy (III), hoarseness (X), weakness of the tongue (XII), diminished hearing (VIII), and constriction of visual fields (II) occurred. Although these signs and symptoms vanished in some patients within a few months, most had permanent facial numbness and weakness, and several died of encephalitis. No effective therapy was found. All affected patients had received trichloroethylene anesthesia via breathing systems containing a CO_2 absorber or had followed patients who had received the agent through the same breathing system. At the same time, trichloroethylene was found to decompose to neurotoxic agents (dichloroacetylene, phosgene) in the presence of alkali and heat—conditions found in the CO_2 absorber.

Although the intentional use of this anesthetic in breathing systems with CO_2 absorbers ended with the publicity that the syndrome attracted, and this agent has been abandoned in the United States, trichloroethylene is still used in other countries on occasion, and this complication may occur. For example, a patient who self-administered trichloroethylene by hand-held vaporizer during obstetric labor may receive general anesthesia soon thereafter for removal of retained placental fragments and exhale residual amounts of the agent into the absorber. Or, this agent may be mistakenly substituted for another volatile agent when filling a vaporizer.[48]

SODA LIME

The most commonly used absorbent today, soda lime, is a mixture the composition of which has evolved over six decades (Table 5-2). The principal component is calcium hydroxide, but smaller amounts of the more active sodium and potassium hydroxides are present as activators. Silica is added to give hardness to the mixture, minimizing the formation of alkaline dust. Such dust can be forced out of the canister into the breathing system and even into the patient's lungs, where it can cause respiratory irritation that can present as bronchospasm.[49,50]

The following reactions describe the absorption of carbon dioxide by soda lime:

$$CO_2 + H_2O \longrightarrow H_2CO_3$$

$$H_2CO_3 + 2\ NaOH\ (and\ KOH) \longrightarrow$$
$$Na_2CO_3\ (and\ K_2CO_3) + 2\ H_2O + heat$$

$$Na_2CO_3\ (and\ K_2CO_3) + Ca(OH)_2 \longrightarrow$$
$$CaCO_3 + 2\ NaOH\ (and\ KOH)$$

Some CO_2 reacts directly, but more slowly, with the calcium hydroxide:

$$CO_2 + Ca(OH)_2 \longrightarrow H_2O + CaCO_3 + heat$$

The heat generated is termed the heat of neutralization and amounts to about 13.7 kcal/mole of CO_2 (22.4 L) absorbed.

TABLE 5-2. Approximate Composition of "Wet" Soda Lime

Ingredient	Percentage of Wet Weight
Sodium hydroxide	4.0
Potassium hydroxide	1.0
Water	14–19
Silica	0.2
Calcium hydroxide	Balance

BARALYME

Baralyme is a newer, but less commonly used, absorbent composed of 80 percent calcium hydroxide and 20 percent barium hydroxide; the latter serves as an activator. Unlike soda lime, baralyme contains moisture as the bound water of crystallization in the octahydrate salt of barium hydroxide. This water binds the absorbent sufficiently so that no silica is necessary. The bound water also accounts for the greater stability of baralyme in water content and, thus, its greater reliability of performance in dry environments, as compared with soda lime.[51] Because optimal activity requires a water content of 11 to 14 percent, additional water is added.

Carbon dioxide absorption proceeds as follows:

$$Ba(OH)_2 \cdot 8H_2O + CO_2 \longrightarrow$$
$$BaCO_3 + 9\ H_2O + heat$$
$$9\ H_2O + 9\ CO_2 \longrightarrow 9\ H_2CO_3$$
$$9\ H_2CO_3 + 9\ Ca(OH)_2 \longrightarrow$$
$$CaCO_3 + 18\ H_2O + heat$$

Heat production is similar to that occurring with soda lime.[52]

VAPORIZATION

All the commonly used potent general anesthetics are volatile liquids at room temperature and atmospheric pressure. These agents must be transformed into the vapor phase for clinical use. The safe use of vaporizers for these agents requires an understanding of vaporization. The concepts reviewed here also explain and suggest preventive measures for the cold stress resulting from the evaporation of water from the airway when the patient breathes dry gas through the anesthetic system.

THE PHENOMENON OF VAPORIZATION

According to the kinetic theory of matter, the molecules comprising matter are in constant, random motion. Motion requires energy, and the velocity with which molecules move and the number of collisions per unit time reflect the amount of energy imparted to the matter. As a form of energy, heat is both a source of energy and a representation of the average kinetic energy of the molecules in the given matter. Thus, a higher temperature connotes a greater number of collisions per unit time and a higher velocity; upon losing energy, the matter has a lower temperature and the constituent molecules are less active.

Consider a closed container in which there is both liquid and air. Within the densely packed array of molecules of which the liquid is composed are two types of motion: the bulk of the molecules move about randomly because intermolecular attractive forces are rather symetrically applied about each molecule, thereby negating each other. An asymmetrical arrangement of intermolecular forces, however, is applied to the small number of molecules at the liquid–air interface. This is because surrounding a given molecule at the surface there are many more molecules within the liquid than in the air above. As a result, there is a net attractive force pulling the surface molecules into the liquid—a force that must be overcome if the surface molecules are to enter the air, where their relatively sparse density constitutes a vapor. Consequently, the transition from the liquid to the vapor phase requires energy. The *heat of vaporization* of a liquid is the number of calories required at a specified temperature to convert 1 g of the liquid into a vapor (Table 5-3). The heat of vaporization is temperature dependent; the colder the liquid, the greater the amount of energy needed to vaporize a given amount of liquid. As a result of the energy expenditure incurred in vaporization, the aggregate energy of the remaining liquid decreases; thus, the temperature of the liquid falls.

Vaporization does not continue indefinitely in this hypothetical closed container, but rather ceases when an equilibrium is reached between the liquid and vapor phases such that the number of molecules in the vapor phase is constant. That is, as many molecules leave the liquid as reenter it per unit time. The molecules in the vapor phase collide with each other and the walls of the container, creating a pressure termed the vapor pressure (or saturated vapor pressure, to emphasize that at equilib-

TABLE 5-3.   Physical Properties of Volatile Anesthetic Agents and Water

	Molecular Weight	Boiling Point (°C, 760 mm Hg)	Vapor Pressure (20°C, 760 mm Hg)	Liquid Density (g/ml, 20°C)	Vapor Density (g/L, 20°C)	Heat of Vaporization (cal/g, 20°C)	Antoine A (kPa/mm Hg)	Equation B	Constants C
Chloroform	119.0	61.2	160	1.50	4.12	64	5.978 / 6.854	1125.05	222.0
Diethyl ether	74.1	34.6	440	0.71	2.55	87	6.151 / 7.027	1109.58	233.2
Divinyl ether	70.0	28.3	550	0.77	2.42	90	6.094 / 6.970	1044.14	227.0
Ethyl chloride	65	12.3	1003	0.90	2.22	92	6.514 / 7.390	1269.62	269.2
Halothane	197	50.2	243	1.86	8.90	35	5.892 / 6.768	1043.70	218.3
Methoxyflurane	165	104.7	23	1.42	6.68	58.6	6.206 / 7.082	1336.58	213.5
Trichloroethylene	131	87.1	60	1.47	4.53	58	5.961 / 6.837	1198.48	216.4
Enflurane	184.5	56.5	175	1.5125*	7.54*	42*	6.112 / 6.988	1107.84	213.1
Isoflurane	184.5	48.5	239	1.5125*	7.54*	41*	4.822 / 5.698	536.46	141.0
Water	18	100	17.5	1.00		540	7.167 / 8.043	1716.98	232.5

* Values at 25°C.

(Modified from Dorsch JA, Dorsch SE: Understanding Anesthetic Equipment: Construction, Care and Complications. © 1975 The Williams & Wilkins Co., Baltimore, except for Antoine constants, which are taken from Rodgers RC, Hill GE: Equations for vapour pressure versus temperature. Br J Anaesth 50:415, 1978.)

rium the vapor phase contains a maximal number of molecules of anesthetic agent per unit space). Like the heat of vaporization, vapor pressure is also temperature dependent; a higher temperature is associated with a greater number of molecules in the vapor phase, hence a higher vapor pressure. The relationship between vapor pressure and temperature is given by the Antoine equation[53]:

$$\log P = A - \frac{B}{t + C} \qquad (4)$$

where P is the pressure, t is the temperature in °C, and A, B, and C are constants derived experimentally. Constants for the volatile anesthetics are listed in Table 5-3, which also includes room temperature values for the vapor pressure. Such an equation facilitates the generation of vapor pressure curves for each agent (Fig. 5-5).

If a hole is made in the container, molecules in the vapor phase can escape and the equilibrium is upset. More molecules leave the liquid than reenter it, resulting in a progressive decrease in the temperature of the remaining liquid.

THE IDEAL ANESTHETIC VAPORIZER

From the foregoing it would seem that a simple vaporizer might consist of an otherwise closed container with oxygen (or a mixture of oxygen and nitrous oxide) flowing through the space above the liquid anesthetic. However, such a laudably simple design would present several problems in clinical use. As vaporization proceeds, as in the case of the closed container with the hole, the temperature of the remaining liquid would decrease with time, and progressively less vaporization would occur. The maximum concentration delivered by this device is given by the quotient of the vapor pressure of the given anesthetic at a specified temperature and atmospheric pressure. For example, for halothane, the vapor pressure at room temperature is 243 mm Hg (Table 5-3), or about one-third of atmospheric pressure (243/760); hence, the gas exiting from this vaporizer under optimal circumstances would be 32 percent halothane, a most certainly lethal concentration. It is very unlikely, however,

FIG. 5-5 Vapor pressure curves for inhaled anesthetics.

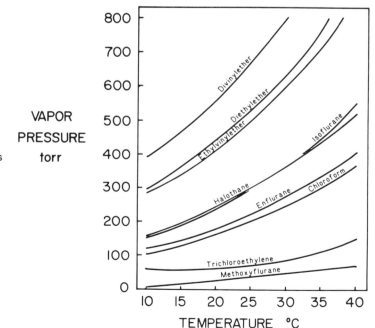

that the carrier gas would have sufficient contact with the halothane vapor to equilibrate completely, so the effluent gas would contain a lower concentration of halothane. Similarly, the higher the flow rate of the carrier gas, the less time afforded for contact, and the lower the concentration of halothane in the effluent gas. The performance of this vaporizer is not only unknown—the output can vary between lethal concentrations of anesthetic and, perhaps, no anesthetic—but is also uncontrollable.

An "ideal anesthetic vaporizer" would satisfy these deficiencies, as well as the attributes listed in Table 5-4. That there are more than a dozen different vaporizer designs should suggest, however, that the "ideal" has not been achieved.

VAPORIZER DESIGN

There are three general approaches to vaporizer design: flow-over, bubble-through, and a combination of both. Because the designs are so numerous, technical, and ever-changing, only a few representative approaches are mentioned here, following some general comments. There are several excellent sources of further information.[3-5]

COMMON FEATURES

Since the vapor pressure of commonly used volatile anesthetics ensures a saturation concentration well above clinical concentrations (recall the saturation vapor pressure of 32 percent for halothane), vaporizer design includes some provision for diluting the vapor generated. Vaporization-induced lowering of the liquid temperature is largely prevented in many designs through the use of copper in the construction of the vaporizer. Copper has a relatively high specific heat (a measure of the amount of heat required to change the temperature of a substance) and a very high thermal conductivity (a measure of the speed with which heat flows through a substance). Thus, copper serves as a reservoir for heat and readily

TABLE 5-4. Attributes of the "Ideal Anesthetic Vaporizer"

Vaporizer performance should be independent of several characteristics:
 Carrier gas flow rate
 Ambient temperature and pressure
 Vaporization-induced temperature decrease
 Pressure fluctuations consequent to mode of respiration

Other vaporizer characteristics
 Low resistance to gas flow
 Minimal servicing requirement
 Corrosion- and solvent-resistant construction
 Light weight
 Small liquid requirement
 Economy and safety in use

(Modified from Schrieber P: Anaesthetic Equipment: Performance, Classification and Safety. Berlin, Springer-Verlag, 1972.)

gives it up to the anesthetic liquid, the temperature of which thereby maintained. Many designs also include a bimetallic strip that functions as a thermostat to counter a decrease in vaporizer temperature by permitting more carrier gas to pass through the vaporizing chamber. An ambient temperature water bath in some designs serves as a heat reservoir, and an electric heater is present in other designs.

Safety is enhanced by designing the vaporizer with the anesthetic liquid-filling port in a relatively low position to prevent overfilling of the vaporizer. This diminishes the possibility that anesthetic *liquid* may be carried into the breathing system and even into the patient's lungs, usually resulting in death.[54-56]

FLOWOVER VAPORIZERS

As the name suggests, in flowover vaporizers the carrier gas flows over the anesthetic liquid, carrying vapor out of the vaporizer. Vaporization is enhanced by increasing the area of contact between carrier gas and anesthetic liquid by means of baffles and/or wicks, as well as by directing the carrier gas as close to the liquid as possible. The saturation concentration is diluted to clinical concentrations through the use of a variable bypass that diverts the major portion of the carrier gas away from the vaporizing chamber (Fig. 5-6).

Assuming equilibration of the carrier gas with the anesthetic vapor, the carrier gas becomes saturated with vapor and the concentration of anesthetic leaving the vaporizing chamber is expressed in the same fashion as in the case of the closed container:

$$\text{\% anesthetic leaving chamber} = \frac{P_a}{P_b} \times 100\% \qquad (5)$$

where P_a is the vapor pressure of the anesthetic and P_b is the barometric pressure. Since the pressure exerted by a mixture of gases is the sum of the partial pressures of the individual gases (Dalton's law of partial pressures), equation (5) may be rewritten as follows:

$$\text{\% anesthetic leaving chamber} = \frac{V_a}{V_a + V_c} \times 100\% \qquad (6)$$

where V_a is the volume of anesthetic vapor and V_c is the volume of carrier gas. Similarly, the concentration of the anesthetic in the gas at the vaporizer's outlet may be expressed as follows:

$$\text{\% anesthetic leaving vaporizer} = \frac{V_a}{V_a + V_b + V_c} \times 100\% \qquad (7)$$

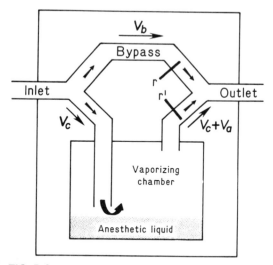

FIG. 5-6 Schematic diagram of flowover vaporizer design. The incoming gas flow is divided between a bypass route and a vaporizing chamber inlet according to the ratio of the resistances (r,r'). The resistance on the outlet is usually calibrated in volume percent. A vaporization-induced decrease in liquid temperature, hence vaporization, results in an increasing flow through the chamber, maintaining the ratio of flow through the two resistance points.

where V_b is the bypass gas flow and the denominator represents the total gas flow. Since V_a is not measured, equations (5) and (6) can be solved for V_a and the result substituted into equation (7) to obtain a more useful expression for the concentration of anesthetic at the outlet:

$$\text{\% anesthetic leaving vaporizer} = \frac{V_c \cdot P_a}{V_b(P_b - P_a) + V_c \cdot P_b} \times 100\% \qquad (8)$$

The Agent-Specific, Calibrated Vaporizer

In the commonly used modern vaporizer, the desired concentration is obtained by turning a knob that alters the ratio of gas flowing through the bypass to that flowing through the vaporizing chamber (Fig. 5-7). Settings of the knob are calibrated directly in volume percent, obviating the need for computation. Temperature- and flow-compensating mechanisms ensure constant output at a given setting—except in low-flow and closed systems, where the gas flows may be below those for which the vaporizer is calibrated. Also, vaporizer output between "off" and the first concentration setting may not be linear.[57] Accuracy of the settings is maintained by returning the vaporizer at least annually to the manufacturer for cleaning and recalibration.

The penalty for this technological progress is the introduction of the possibility of a variety of hazards. The wrong anesthetic agent can be put into an agent-specific vaporizer, resulting in the delivery of an unknown and possibly high concentration. This error is particularly hazardous when a highly volatile agent is used in a vaporizer designed for one of lower volatility, leading to anesthetic overdosage.[58-60] A related error is the addition of the wrong agent to a vaporizer already containing the appropriate anesthetic, a relatively common accident with agent-specific vaporizers having the same external configuration.[61] Unpredictable, threefold to fourfold underdosage and overdosage can result in these circumstances because liq-

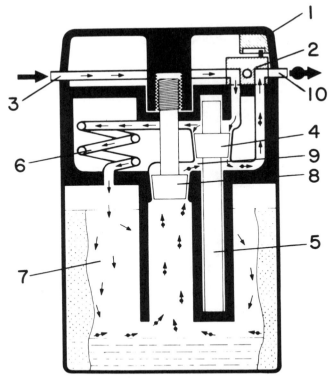

FIG. 5-7 Schematic diagram of Drager Vapor 19.1. This is a modern flow-over, temperature- and flow-compensated, agent-specific vaporizer, with models available for use with halothane, enflurane, and isoflurane. Turning a knob (1) to desired concentration (volume percent) opens a shunt (2) that permits carrier gas (oxygen or an oxygen–nitrous oxide mixture) entering the inlet (3) to reach a cone (4) with a temperature-compensating expansion rod (5), which diverts a small portion of the flow into a long spiral tube (6) that permits compensation for pressure changes in the breathing system (e.g., consequent to different modes of respiration) before reaching the vaporizing chamber (7). Saturated carrier gas leaves the vaporizing chamber at a control cone (8) that regulates the concentration delivered according to the position of the knob (1), mixes with the bypass carrier gas (9), and exits the vaporizer through the outlet (10). (Modified from North American Drager Company brochure, Telford, PA.)

uid halogenated anesthetics do not form ideal mixtures, in which partial pressures are proportional to their molar fractions.[61,62] The likelihood of causing this error is minimized with a pin-indexing system at the filling port, similar to that used for compressed gas tanks at the yokes of the anesthesia machine; yet, this safety feature is present in few vaporizers and is cumbersome where it exists. Vaporizer contamination can also occur when, as is the usual case, two or more vaporizers are arranged in series and more than one is accidentally "on" simultaneously. This results in the deposition of anesthetic agent from the upstream vaporizer into the downstream one, producing

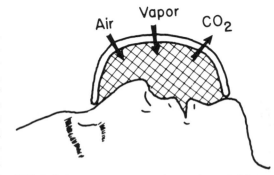

FIG. 5-8 Schematic diagram of open-drop administration using the Schimmelbusch mask with gauze moistened with a highly volatile anesthetic agent. Rebreathing can be diminished by insufflating oxygen beneath the mask.

an unknown and potentially hazardous mixture.[60,63,64] Educating staff to make certain that only one in-series vaporizer is "on" at a time and placing the vaporizer with the agent of lowest vapor pressure upstream will minimize such crosscontamination. The incorporation of a vaporizer interlock device,[65] selector valve, or simple physical disconnection into anesthesia machine design can prevent this problem, but each of these can result in still other problems.[66] In the end, as in other aspects of clinical practice, there is no substitute for increased vigilance.

Open-Drop Administration

In 1847, Simpson administered chloroform by pouring small quantities of the volatile liquid on a handkerchief held over his patient's nose and mouth. Open-drop administration survives in primitive circumstances with a Schimmelbusch mask, a wire frame that supports several layers of gauze (Fig. 5-8). This "vaporizer" is satisfactory only for the more volatile agents, most of which are flammable and, hence, rarely used, and, even then, only with small children. Delivered concentration is unknown and difficult to control, and the mask often becomes so cold (and thereby diminishes subsequent vaporization) that it must be changed frequently to avoid prolonging the induction. This "vaporizer" is discussed further as an example of an open breathing system.

The EMO Inhaler

As portable as open-drop administration but much more controllable, the Epstein-Macintosh-Oxford (EMO) inhaler was developed for use in field conditions, where nitrous oxide, and even oxygen, may not be available.[67] The patient's own inspiratory effort is also the motive force with this device. Air is drawn through a low-resistance, temperature-compensated device whose delivered concentration is set with a calibrated lever. Vaporization-induced changes in anesthetic liquid temperature are minimized by a temperature-compensating mechanism and a water bath. A foot-operated bellows is available for assisted and controlled respiration.

The Ohio No. 8 Bottle

Rarely used, but often found on older anesthesia machines, this flow-over vaporizer deserves passing mention because of its unique location within the circle breathing system. This placement results in the possibility of unintentionally delivering very high concentrations of volatile agent (see discussion of the circle system). Other deficiencies result directly from its very simple design: a glass jar, a wick with a large surface area, and a valve that permits the diversion of some or all the breathing system flow through the vaporizing chamber. Less wasteful of anesthetic than the open-drop mask, it is not calibrated and there is no provision for maintaining the temperature of the liquid anesthetic. Hence, the delivered concentration is unknown and changes unpredictably with use.

BUBBLE-THROUGH VAPORIZERS

In the bubble-through design, efficient vaporization is achieved by increasing the surface area available for vaporization through the use of very small bubbles. The smaller the bubble, the greater the surface:volume ratio of the bubble and, thus, the more likely that the gas within the bubble will become saturated with anesthetic vapor when in contact with anesthetic liquid. Fine bubbles are formed by passing oxygen through a porous plate or sintered bronze disk at the bottom of the liquid-filled vaporizing chamber. Because these vaporizers lack a temperature-compensation mechanism and a dilution bypass, the effluent gas contains a very high concentration of the anesthetic vapor in oxygen, as determined by the vapor pressure of the given anesthetic at the ambient temperature. To make this device clinically useful, the oxygen carrier gas is regulated with a flow meter and the effluent gas is diluted in the manifold of the anesthesia machine with the other gases (e.g., oxygen, nitrous oxide) that are being administered. The concentration of anesthetic delivered to the breathing system can be calculated by using equation 8, with the oxygen flow to the kettle substituted for V_c and the other gas flows substituted for V_b. Although bubble-through vaporizers are less convenient to use because they are not calibrated, clinical "rules of thumb" are quickly learned (e.g., with enflurane, 100 ml oxygen through the kettle at 20°C with other flows totalling 3 L produces a 1 percent concentration). Moreover, these vaporizers can be used with all volatile agents and with all flows, including those used for low-flow and closed-system techniques.

The Copper Kettle

This prototype bubble-through vaporizer is constructed entirely of copper because of this element's high heat capacity and thermal conductivity (Fig. 5-9).[68] Thermal stability is enhanced by its attachment to the metal work surface of the anesthesia machine, although, with prolonged use at high carrier gas flow rates, the temperature of the anesthetic liquid decreases.[69] Nonetheless, this versatile device can be used with all liquid anesthetics to produce a predictable inspired concentration under a wide variety of flow rates, even with a closed-system technique.[69]

Vernitrol

Constructed of bronze, which also has a high heat capacity and thermal conductivity, this vaporizer is an integral part of one brand of anesthesia machine and is functionally identical to the Copper Kettle.

FLOW-OVER, BUBBLE-THROUGH VAPORIZERS

This combination design is not used in the United States, although it is found in Great Britain in the Boyle's Bottle.

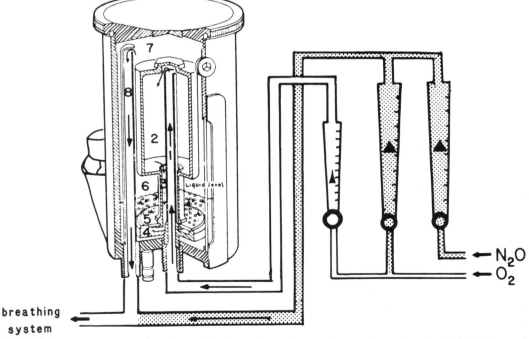

FIG. 5-9 Schematic diagram of the Copper Kettle vaporizer. A metered oxygen flow enters the inlet at the base of the vaporizer, travels up a center tube (1) to the loving cup (2) (which dissipates the effect of sudden surges of gas), turns downward (3), and passes through a sintered bronze disk (5). The resultant bubbles rise through the anesthetic liquid (6) in the vaporizing chamber (7), and the saturated vapor exits through an outlet tube (8), where it is diluted by joining other gases in the manifold of the anesthesia machine en route to the machine gas delivery. (Reproduced by courtesy of Foregger Co. Reprinted, with modification, by permission of the publisher from Hill DW: Physics Applied to Anaesthesia. 4th Ed. London, Butterworths (Publishers) Ltd. 1980.)

HUMIDIFICATION

Humidification—the process of adding moisture (water vapor) to a gas—is merely a subset of vaporization. Humidification assumes special clinical importance because it occurs within the patient who is breathing dry anesthetic gases who then incurs the deleterious side effects of varporization such as heat loss.

Air passing through the nose en route to the lungs is subjected to the air conditioning function of the upper airway, which consists of warming, humidification, and filtering. Before reaching the carina, the air rises to within a few percent of body temperature and of saturation with water vapor. Inhalational anesthesia prevents such air-conditioning when administration is via a tracheal tube that bypasses the upper airway. A more consistent problem, however, is that anesthetic gases are water free because water would otherwise condense and freeze in the pressure-reducing valves of the anesthesia machine's high-pressure system. Anesthetic gases are also generally at room temperature, or even lower if the gas sources are machine-mounted cylinders.

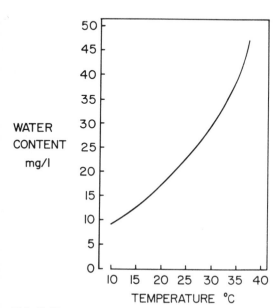

FIG. 5-10 Absolute water content of saturated gas as a function of temperature.

Bypassing the upper airway and using such dry, relatively cold gases leads to cytologic damage to the respiratory ciliated epithelium in as short a period as 1 hour.[70,71] Continued inhalation of dry gas has been associated in dogs with increased pulmonary shunting and reduced compliance.[72] Whether the inhalation of dry gases is associated with an increased incidence of postoperative pulmonary complications is controversial.[73,74] However, breathing dry gas for several hours can result in drying of secretions, crusting, and, when an endotracheal tube is used, even airway obstruction from inspissated secretions. Even more clinically important are the water and heat losses that occur because the respiratory mucosa adds water and warmth so that air is at body temperature and is fully saturated with water in the lungs. Discussion of these losses requires an understanding of the way in which the water content of a gas is quantitated.

HUMIDITY

Two terms are used to express the water content of a gas: the weight of water vapor in a given volume of gas (in mg/L) at a specified temperature is the *absolute humidity*; the ratio of absolute humidity of a gas sample to the absolute humidity of that sample if it were saturated with water at that temperature is termed the *relative humidity*. Because the absolute water content of saturated gas is an exponential function of temperature (Fig. 5-10), the relative humidity of a given sample of gas changes markedly upon entering the body. For example, the relative humidity of gas saturated at room temperature is only 38 percent at body temperature. Generally, however, absolute humidity, expressed in terms of mg/L, is more useful when considering the water and heat loss consequent to humidification.

WATER LOSS

The respiratory moisture loss can be quantitated simply as the product of the minute ventilation and the gradient existing between the water content of the inspired and exhaled air. The minute ventilation may be measured or estimated from a nomogram,[75-77] and the water content of exhaled air (i.e., fully saturated air at 37°C) may be taken as 45 mg/L. Thus, the hourly respiratory water loss can be estimated as follows:

$$\text{Respiratory water loss per hour} = 60 \ \dot{V}_E(45 - A_t) \qquad (9)$$

where A is the water content at temperature t°C. For the 70-kg adult who is breathing air with a relative humidity of 50 percent at room temperature (i.e., a water content of 9 mg/L), the respiratory water loss is approximately 13 g/hr, which agrees reasonably well with empirical observations of 250 to 300 g/day.[78] Even using a nonrebreathing system with dry gases, the respiratory water loss would rise to only about 16 g/hr. Such a loss is small compared with daily fluid requirements and is easily replaced by intravenous fluids, without any special effort. Values in children are proportional to their smaller minute ventilation. Clearly, the magnitude of the respiratory water loss is too small to argue cogently for instituting humidification of anesthetic gases solely to counter water loss.

RESPIRATORY HEAT LOSS

There are two ways in which heat loss via the respiratory tract occurs. The first and quantitatively less important way is the warming of inspired gases to body temperature. The heat expended is dependent on the minute ventilation, the temperature gradient, and the specific heat of the gases and may be estimated as follows:

$$\text{Heat loss due to warming (per min)} = \dot{V}_E(37 - t) \text{ (specific heat)} \qquad (10)$$

where t is the temperature (°C) of the inspired gas. Under particularly adverse circumstances, such as the open-drop administration of ether, the temperature of the inspired gas can drop to 0°C, and the rate of heat expenditure to warm this gas to body temperature approximates 90

cal/min in the adult. However, with currently used breathing systems, the inspired gas is at room temperature, so the heat loss due to warming is less than half as much.

The more important way in which heat is lost via the respiratory tract is vaporization. In addition to having a lower temperature, the inspired air also has a lower water content than that of the exhaled air. Heat is expended to vaporize a sufficient amount of water to saturate the inspired air at body temperature. For each gram of water vaporized, 580 cal must be supplied by the patient. The resultant heat loss constitutes a clinically significant threat to the temperature homeostasis of infants and small children during general anesthesia, which renders the body poikilothermic. In fact, merely supplying anesthetic gases warmed to 37°C and 100 percent humidified maintains the body temperature of patients anesthetized for as long as four hours.[79] Herein lies the principal rationale for the use of a humidifier. In addition to possibly diminishing the incidence of postoperative respiratory complications,[74] humidification also reduces heat loss sufficiently to reduce, in turn, the incidence of postoperative shivering.[80-82]

HUMIDIFIERS

The simplest method of raising the water content of anesthetic gases, merely wetting the lumen of the breathing system tubing, results in a water content of about 22 mg/L.[83] With either the adult circle breathing system[84] or a pediatric semiopen system,[85] a water content as high as 29 mg/L can be obtained by passing inspired gas through the soda lime canister, which is heated by the exothermic reaction that occurs with carbon dioxide absorption; heating enables the gas to hold more water (Fig. 5-10). Respiratory moisture can also be conserved by placing a fine-mesh condenser, the so-called artificial nose, just proximal to the tracheal tube.[82,86,87] Moisture from the warm, moist exhaled gas condenses on the cooler mesh, which is warmed by the gas; cool, otherwise dry inspired gas is warmed and humidified as it passed through the warm, moist mesh. Unfortunately, the condenser effect requires such a fine mesh that considerable respiratory resistance and dead space can result, undesirable characteristics for a device that would find greatest use with infants and small children.

Obtaining a higher water content requires a considerably more complex design that involves heating water in contact with inspired gas and/or nebulizing water to effect supersaturation of the inspired gas. With improved efficiency of humidification comes a variety of potentially serious complications, including nosocomial infection secondary to bacterial contamination,[88-92] particularly in conjunction with the use of mechanical ventilators; water intoxication[93] and increased respiratory resistance[94] from nebulizers, especially in infants; hyperthermia[95] and tracheal "burn" from excessively heated inspired gas; and electrocution, explosion, and other problems related to malfunction of electrical equipment. These hazards, as well as the bulkiness of the devices, explain why humidifiers are used infrequently.

TABLE 5-5. Attributes Desired in an Anesthetic Breathing System

Accuracy and precision in delivery of anesthetics and oxygen
Small dead space
Efficient elimination of expired CO_2
Low respiratory resistance
Conservation of respiratory moisture
Convenience and safety in clinical use

effectiveness in medical care. Although the ideal breathing system is not at hand, the variety of systems available satisfy diverse clinical requirements reasonably well. The anesthesiologist must therefore be sufficiently familiar with the available systems to be able to choose the most appropriate one as well as be aware of potential problems with each.

The systems are described here according to a classification scheme (Table 5-6) based on the presence of a gas reservoir bag, rebreathing of exhaled gases, a carbon dioxide absorber, and unidirectional valves. This scheme is comprehensive yet functionally adequate, although it is only one among many others proposed.[96] Nonetheless, because distinctions between systems are blurred (e.g., a semiclosed system functions as a closed system when all exhaled gases except CO_2 are rebreathed), the plea has been made that the components and fresh gas flow be stated when describing a given system.[97]

BREATHING SYSTEMS

The design of anesthetic breathing systems has been an evolutionary process, albeit a haphazard one. The systems available today possess desirable characteristics, in varying degrees (Table 5-5). New knowledge has prompted modification in available systems, as well as a return to breathing systems abandoned decades ago; an example of the latter is the renewed interest in the closed system when there is greater concern about both anesthetic pollution of the operating room and cost-

OPEN SYSTEMS

Lacking a reservoir bag and rebreathing of exhaled gases, open systems are the simplest and least expensive systems, if not the most primitive systems (Table 5-6). Because they have no physical connection to the patient's airway, open systems do not impose respiratory resistance. Yet, many disadvantages severely limit their use. The lack of physical connection to the airway results necessarily in the spillage of large quantities of anesthetics into the operating room, loss of respiratory moisture, inability to control ventilation, and, when flammable agents are used, an increased risk of explosion. Their major disadvantage is an unstable anesthetic level. During light anesthesia, there is an

TABLE 5-6. Classification of Anesthetic Breathing Systems

Breathing System	Gas Reservoir Bag	Rebreathing of Exhaled Gases	CO$_2$ Absorber	Unidirectional Valves*	Fresh Gas Inflow Rate†
Open					
Insufflation	No	No	No	0,0	Unknown
Open drop	No	No	No	0,0	Unknown
Semiopen					
Nonrebreathing valve	Yes	No	No	1,0	High
Mapleson A, B, C, D	Yes	No‡	No	0,1	High
Bain	Yes	No‡	No	0,1	High
Mapleson E	No	No‡	No	0,1	High
Jackson-Rees	Yes	No‡	No	0,1	High
Semiclosed					
Circle	Yes	Partial	Yes	2,1	Moderate
Closed	Yes	Total	Yes	2,1	Low

  * First value is number of valves through which inspired gases flow; second value is presence of expiratory ("popoff") valve.

  † Low = 0.3 to 0.5 L/min; moderate = 3 to 6 L/min; high = greater than 6 L/min.

  ‡ No rebreathing when fresh gas inflow rate meets or exceeds requirement of given system.

associated large tidal volume whose peak flow rate—instantaneously as high as 50 L/min in the adult and child and 10 L/min in the infant[98]—can exceed that delivered. Consequently, there is increased dilution of the inspired anesthetic concentration with room air, resulting in even lighter levels of anesthesia. In contrast, as the anesthetic level deepens, the patient's tidal volume decreases and less dilution with room air occurs, resulting in an increasing anesthetic concentration and, in turn, a deeper level of anesthesia. Thus, light anesthesia begets lighter anesthesia, and deep anesthesia, deeper.

INSUFFLATION

Insufflation is the delivery of the anesthetic directly from the anesthesia machine's delivery hose or from a mask held above the patient's face. This technique is useful for inducing anesthesia in children ("steal induction") and in bronchoscopy and laryngoscopy.

OPEN-DROP ADMINISTRATION

An inhaled agent with a high vapor pressure and moderate potency (e.g., diethyl ether, halothane) is administered dropwise onto layers of gauze held in a Schimmelbusch mask (Fig. 5-8). Once the mask is lowered onto the face, this technique is no longer strictly nonrebreathing. Elimination of exhaled carbon dioxide is impaired when water condenses and freezes in the gauze mesh as the mask temperature drops consequent to vaporization. The CO$_2$ trapped beneath the mask also dilutes the room air, resulting in hypoxemia. Oxygen insufflation (250 to 500 ml/min) under the mask with an "ether hook" treats both problems but increases the hazard of explosion with flammable agents and decreases inspired anesthetic concentration. However, the condensation of respiratory moisture on the mask results in the inhalation of very dry (and cold) gas. For these reasons, this technique is rarely used, although its portability favors use in disaster and other field circumstances.

SEMIOPEN SYSTEMS WITH NONREBREATHING VALVES

As in the open system, the semiopen system permits no rebreathing; however, the latter does include a reservoir bag (Table 5-6). The addition of a nonrebreathing valve[99]—a device that directs fresh gas into the patient and exhaled gas out of the system—permits a lower

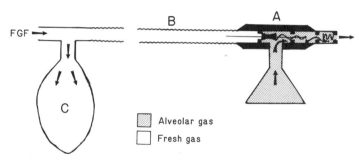

FGF →

B   A

C

▨ Alveolar gas

☐ Fresh gas

FIG. 5-11 Semiclosed breathing system with a Ruben nonrebreathing valve and a reservoir bag.

fresh gas flow to be used, often as low as that equal to the patient's minute ventilation (Fig. 5-11). The principal advantage of the semiopen system is that the composition of the inspired gas approximates that delivered to the system; thus, the concentrations of inspired gases can be changed rapidly. Also, the presence of the reservoir bag enables assisted and controlled ventilation, including tactile assessment of pulmonary compliance.

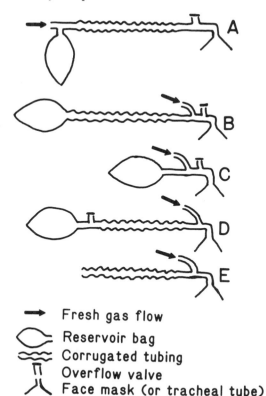

→ Fresh gas flow

Reservoir bag

Corrugated tubing

Overflow valve

Face mask (or tracheal tube)

FIG. 5-12 Semiopen breathing systems, as classified by Mapleson. (Redrawn from Mapleson WW: The elimination of rebreathing in various semiclosed anaesthetic systems. Br J Anaesth 26:323, 1954.)

Numerous disadvantages, however, mostly relating to the nonrebreathing valve, have relegated this system to use in resuscitative equipment: The bulky valve must be located immediately proximal to the patient, a location that may be inconvenient in many circumstances. The valve also adds considerable respiratory resistance, so that its use in infants and, given the high flow rates needed that further increase the resistance, in adults is unwise.[100] In addition, condensation of respiratory moisture makes the valve stick. With the more commonly used valves (e.g., Fink, Stephen-Slater, Ruben), respiratory obstruction occurs when minute ventilation exceeds fresh gas flow. The Steen valve prevents this by permitting ambient gas to enter, preventing a cardiorespiratory catastrophe such as a pneumothorax but dilutes the anesthetic concentration. All nonrebreathing valves are subject to occlusion of the exit port—for example, when excessive fresh gas flow jams the valve in the inspiratory position—unless a pressure-relief device is placed elsewhere in the system. Like the open system, there is no conservation of respiratory moisture.

SEMIOPEN SYSTEMS WITHOUT VALVES

These semiopen systems grossly resemble those with nonrebreathing valves except that an expiratory (relief or "popoff") valve is substituted (Table 5-6). Because this valve is not interposed *between the fresh gas flow and the patient*, these semiopen systems may be regarded as not having valves. These systems generally share the same components, arrangements (Fig. 5-12) of which affect their perform-

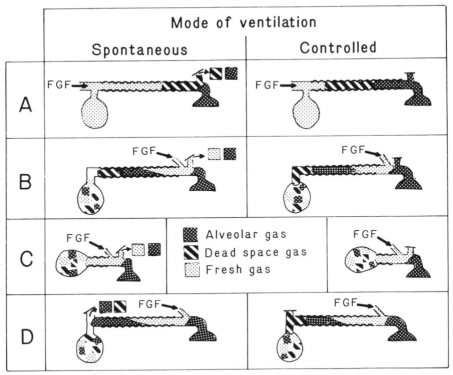

FIG. 5-13 Semiopen breathing systems, as classified by Mapleson, with gas disposition at end-expiration, during spontaneous and controlled ventilation. FGF = fresh gas flow. (Redrawn from Sykes MK: Rebreathing circuits: A review. Br J Anaesth 40:666, 1968.)

ance with respect to the efficiency of exhaled CO_2 elimination (Fig. 5-13). The classification scheme is the one proposed by Mapleson.[101]

THE MAPLESON A SYSTEM

Sometimes called the Magill attachment, the Mapleson A system is particularly efficient in CO_2 elimination during spontaneous ventilation (Figs. 5-12 and 5-13). In fact, rebreathing does not occur with this system until fresh gas flow decreases to a value equal to the patient's alveolar ventilation.[102,103] In clinical usage, however, fresh gas flow should equal or exceed the patient's minute ventilation.[101] This efficiency results from the fact that during exhalation the fresh gas flow flushes exhaled CO_2 out the expiratory valve. During inspiration, the patient inhales fresh gas from both the fresh gas inflow and the reservoir bag, which then col-

lapses. Upon exhalation, dead space gas and then alveolar gas enter the expiratory limb. The reservoir bag fills as the exhaled gases meet the fresh gas flow, and the pressure within the system increases. Later in exhalation, the pressure rises sufficiently to force the expiratory valve to open, and alveolar gas exits. If fresh gas flow is high enough, dead space gas also exits, although whether this occurs is of little physiologic consequence.

During assisted or controlled ventilation, this system is much less efficient.[104] This is because, with closing down of the expiratory valve and squeezing of the bag, gas exits from the system during *inspiration* rather than exhalation. Thus, exhaled gas and some fresh gas collect in the expiratory limb during exhalation and enter the patient during inspiration before the pressure within the system rises sufficiently to force the expiratory valve open. The fresh gas flow required to prevent rebreathing during assisted or controlled ventilation with this system is dependent not on only the fresh gas flow but on the tidal volume, respiratory rate, and rate of pressure rise within the system during inspiration as well. Since this system is so inefficient under these circumstances and the fresh gas flow requirement cannot be estimated easily, this system is generally used only with spontaneous ventilation.

THE MAPLESON B SYSTEM

Moving the fresh gas inflow to the end of the expiratory limb near the patient, just distal to the expiratory valve, results in a Mapleson B system that, although not as efficient as the A system during spontaneous ventilation, is clinically useful and behaves in a similar way for any mode of ventilation (Figs. 5-12 and 5-13). The location of fresh gas inflow allows exhaled gas (and some fresh gas) to collect in the reservoir bag and expiratory limb during exhalation. The bag fills with a mixture of dead space, alveolar, and fresh gas, whereas the corrugated tubing receives alveolar and fresh gas. Once the bag has filled and the pressure in the system has risen sufficiently, the expiratory valve opens, allowing mostly fresh gas to exit. Upon inspiration, with lowering of pressure within the system, the expiratory valve closes, and the patient receives fresh gas, as well as gas from the expiratory limb. The fresh gas flow rate determines the composition of the inspired mixture: with high flows, the mixture consists of fresh gas and some alveolar gas, whereas with lower flows a greater proportion of alveolar gas will be inhaled. A fresh gas flow of at least twice the minute ventilation is needed to minimize rebreathing.[38,104]

THE MAPLESON C SYSTEM

The Mapleson C system is a Mapleson B system the expiratory limb of which has been shortened (Figs. 5-12 and 5-13). As a result, the inspired gas contains more alveolar gas than is the case with the B system, and a fresh gas flow of at least twice the minute ventilation is needed to prevent rebreathing.[38] This system can be used with any mode of ventilation.

THE MAPLESON D SYSTEM

In the Mapleson D system, a commonly used system, the arrangement of components most closely resembles that in the B system except that the expiratory valve is located at the reservoir bag (Figs. 5-12 and 5-13). Not insignificantly, however, exchanging the locations of the fresh gas inflow valve converts a D system to an A system. As a result of this altered configuration and the flushing effect of the fresh gas flow, there is greater efficiency of CO_2 elimination with the Mapleson D system during assisted or controlled ventilation than during spontaneous ventilation.[38] In fact, during assisted or controlled ventilation with the D system, the flushing effect forces alveolar and dead space gas out the expiratory valve, resulting in an inspired mixture of almost solely fresh gas, when using a fresh gas flow as low as twice minute ventilation.[38]

During spontaneous ventilation, the D system is as complicated as the A system is during controlled ventilation: fresh gas and alveolar gas flow down the expiratory limb during expiration. Once the bag has filled and pressure has risen within the system, the expiratory valve opens, thereby permitting some of this mixture to exit. Upon inspiration, the patient inhales fresh gas and gas from the expiratory limb. The latter may be fresh gas or a mixture of fresh gas and alveolar gas, depending upon the duration of the expiratory pause and patient's tidal volume, as well as on the fresh gas flow. A short expiratory pause does not permit much flushing by the fresh gas, regardless of its flow rate; similarly, a tidal volume greater than can be satisfied by the fresh gas flow results in the inhalation of gas containing exhaled CO_2 from farther down the expiratory limb.

THE BAIN SYSTEM

In the Bain system, a modification of the Mapleson D system, fresh gas flows through a narrow tube within the corrugated expiratory limb (Fig. 5-14).[105] Among the claimed advantages of this coaxial configuration are the warming of the fresh gas by the surrounding exhaled gases in the expiratory limb, improved

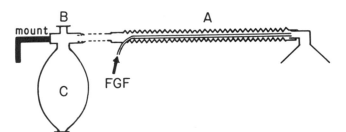

FIG. 5-14 Schematic diagram of a Bain breathing system showing fresh gas flow (FGF) into modified Mapleson D system (A), overflow valve (B), and reservoir bag (C). (Redrawn from Bain JA, Spoerel WE: A streamlined anaesthetic system. Can Anaesth Soc J 19:426, 1972.)

humidification as a result of partial rebreathing at the patient end of the expiratory limb,[106] reduced weight (because they are supplied as disposable, plastic items), sterility (again, because they are single-use items), ease of scavenging waste anesthetic gases from an expiratory valve, and the convenience and safety of having the expiratory valve further from the patient (especially in the case of head and neck surgery).

Sharing the configuration of the Mapleson D system, the same flow considerations apply. However, explicit recommendations regarding fresh gas flow requirements are controversial because additional factors, such as anesthetic agent,[107] respiratory waveform (including drug effects),[107-111] and even geographical location of the patient,[112] influence the requirement. Nonetheless, a clinical range can be specified: During controlled ventilation, a fresh gas flow rate as low as 70 ml/kg body weight will maintain normocarbia, with 100 ml/kg producing mild hyperventilation.[113,114] Although similar flow rates may prove satisfactory during spontaneous ventilation in some patients, a fresh gas flow of 200 to 300 ml/kg is recommended.[115,116] This more conservative recommendation recognizes that the patient may not be able to increase his or her minute ventilation, or at least increase it sufficiently, due to anesthetic-induced respiratory depression, increased CO_2 production secondary to hyperthermia, or increased apparatus or physiologic dead space.

The price paid for the simplicity of this potentially "universal" breathing system[117] is a group of new complications and concerns that include increased respiratory resistance due to a relatively high flow rate through the narrow bore of the inner tube, unrecognized disconnection[118] or misconnection[119] of the inner tube with severe hypercarbia, absence of flow due to unrecognized kinking of the inner tube,[120] and, as might be expected, hypercarbia from an inadequate fresh gas flow during spontaneous ventilation.[121]

THE MAPLESON E SYSTEM

The Mapleson E system consists of an expiratory limb connected to Ayre's T piece (Figs. 5-12, 5-13, 5-15). The later was introduced in 1937 as a means of supplying endotracheal anesthesia for children undergoing cranial surgery and cleft palate repair without cumbersome equipment near the surgical field.[122-124] In its original design, this device consists of a tube, whose internal diameter is 1 cm, that receives fresh gas from a smaller side arm (Fig. 5-15). During exhalation, both exhaled gas and fresh gas flow down the open expiratory limb. During inspiration, varying ratios of fresh gas and exhaled gas can be inhaled, depending on the fresh gas flow rate and the volume of the expiratory limb. With an expiratory limb the volume of which is one-third the patient's tidal volume, a fresh gas flow of about three times minute ventilation avoids rebreathing during spontaneous ventilation. Flow rates as low as twice minute ventilation can prevent rebreathing if the expiratory pause increases and/or the inspiratory flow rate decreases.

Although there is no reservoir bag, respiration can be controlled by intermittent occlusion of the expiratory limb, which forces fresh gas into the trachea. Assisted and controlled ventilation is facilitated by the Jackson-Rees modification of the Ayre's T piece—the addition of a reservoir bag at the end of the expiratory limb, with an adjustable aperture at the open end of the bag.[125] The T piece system has minimal dead space and respiratory resistance

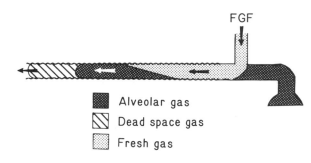

FIG. 5-15 Ayre's T-piece breathing system, with gas disposition at end-expiration shown. FGF = fresh gas flow. (Redrawn from Sykes MK: Rebreathing circuits: A review. Br J Anaesth 40:666, 1968.)

and can be used with a mask or tracheal tube, but this system still wastes large volumes of anesthetics.

OVERVIEW

Comparing the various Mapleson systems during spontaneous ventilation, the most efficient in eliminating carbon dioxide is the A system, followed by the D, C, and B. During controlled ventilation, the most efficient is the D system, followed by the B, C, and A.[126] Although these systems are simple, lightweight, sturdy, and easy to clean and offer low resistance to respiration, the high flow rates needed incur loss of respiratory moisture and pollute the operating room. The Bain system addresses many of these problems but, as noted, introduced some new ones. The high flow, however, does result in the inspired mixture having a composition very similar to that being delivered from the anesthesia machine and, thus, enables rapid changes in the concentrations of gases inspired.

SEMICLOSED SYSTEMS

The semiclosed breathing system is the most commonly used breathing system for adults and larger children. This system includes a reservoir bag and provides partial rebreathing of exhaled gases. Rebreathing is acceptable in this system because a CO_2 absorber is used, resulting in some conservation of respiratory moisture and body heat. Moreover, the fresh gas inflow rate is not of paramount concern and can even be lower than the patient's minute ventilation, thereby reducing pollution of the operating room.

THE CIRCLE SYSTEM

The circle system, the most widely used example of the semiclosed system, is named for the overall arrangement of components and, thus, is a true breathing circuit.

COMPONENTS

To prevent excessive rebreathing, two unidirectional valves are placed in the system so that the gases flow in only one direction, making a pass through the CO_2 absorber each time around (Fig. 5-16). The principal conduit for the circle gases is a wide-bore (22 mm) corrugated hose that offers little resistance. Even the properly filled CO_2 canister adds little resistance, due to its large cross-sectional area. Other components include an expiratory valve to permit the escape of excess gases, a reservoir bag, and a Y connector to attach the mask or tracheal tube to the breathing system. Optional components include bacterial filters, a circulator, and an in-system (e.g., Ohio No. 8) vaporizer. As with the Mapleson systems, the arrangement of these components determines the behavior of the system.

PREVENTION OF CO_2 REBREATHING

To prevent the rebreathing of exhaled CO_2 in the circle system, the arrangement of components must obey three rules: (1) a one-way valve must be located between the patient and

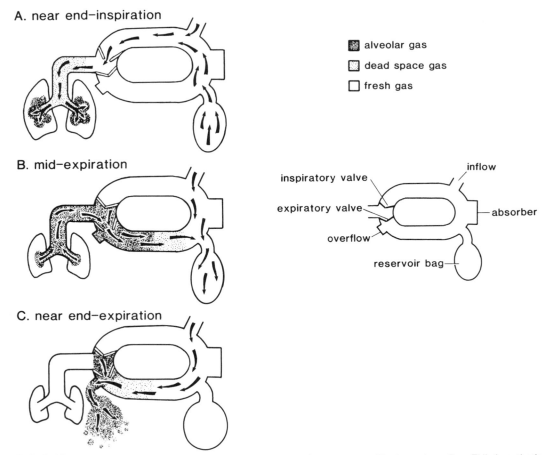

A. near end–inspiration

alveolar gas

dead space gas

fresh gas

B. mid–expiration

inspiratory valve

expiratory valve

overflow

inflow

absorber

reservoir bag

C. near end–expiration

FIG. 5-16 Circle breathing system with optimal arrangement of components. (Redrawn from Eger El II: Anesthetic Uptake and Action. Baltimore, Williams & Wilkins, 1974. © 1974 El Eger II, M.D.)

rebreathing bag on both the inspiratory and expiratory limbs of the circuit; (2) fresh gas inflow must not enter the circuit between the expiratory valve and the patient; and (3) the expiratory valve must not be located between the patient and the inspiratory valve.[127]

CONSERVATION OF FRESH GASES

Avoiding rebreathing of CO_2, however, does not ensure the most efficient use of the fresh gas inflow. In the more efficient arrangements, the expiratory valve is located on the expiratory limb, often near the patient, to vent alveolar gas preferentially. This arrangement results in a higher inspired concentration of an-

esthetic and oxygen, as well as prolongs the life of the absorber.[128]

In the most efficient system for both spontaneous and controlled ventilation (Fig. 5-16), the expiratory valve is close to the patient on the expiratory limb but just distal to the expiratory valve, fresh gas enters the circuit between the absorber and inspiratory valve, and the reservoir bag is located between the absorber and expiratory valve.[129] As in the Mapleson A system, fresh gas flushes alveolar gas preferentially before any dead space gas leaves the circuit. At end-inspiration, fresh gas fills the inspiratory limb. With the beginning of expiration, dead space gas and then alveolar gas flows down the expiratory limb, forcing the fresh gas ahead into the reservoir bag, which simultaneously receives fresh gas in a retrograde fashion. Once the bag has filled, and the pressure within the circuit has risen sufficiently, the expiratory valve opens, allowing the escape of alveolar gas; this escape is hastened by retrograde flow of fresh gas in the expiratory limb. The presence and location of the one-way valves enables the same high efficiency regardless of whether ventilation is spontaneous or controlled. With this arrangement, the inspired concentration is equal to the inflow concentration when the fresh gas inflow is equal to or exceeds the alveolar minute ventilation.[129] Unfortunately, this optimal arrangement is impractical in the clinical setting because the relatively bulky unidirectional and expiratory valves are located near the patient.

A more practical, although somewhat less efficient, arrangement is shown in Figure 5-17. This arrangement is less efficient because moving the expiratory valve down the expiratory limb further from the patient permits mixing of alveolar and dead space gas. Hence, when the expiratory valve opens, dead space gas is lost with alveolar gas.

VAPORIZER LOCATION

A vaporizer may be located proximal to the anesthetic breathing system (out-of-system) or, rarely, within the breathing system (in-system).

Out-of-System Location

The vaporizer receives its inflow directly from the flow meters of the anesthesia machine. Thus, the concentration of volatile anesthetic in the vaporizer effluent is dependent only on considerations such as vaporizer characteristics, vaporizer setting, and ambient temperature. The anesthetic concentration within the circuit is modified by anesthetic uptake, as well as changes in the concentration delivered by the vaporizer. Thus, during induction when uptake is great and ventilation is increased, the anesthetic in the fresh gas inflow is diluted by the gas within the circuit; as a result, inspired concentration is lower than that delivered by the vaporizer. As uptake diminishes, the inspired concentration rises to equal that deliv-

A. mid-expiration

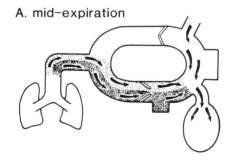

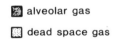

■ alveolar gas

□ dead space gas

□ fresh gas

B. end-expiration

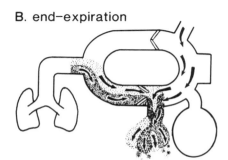

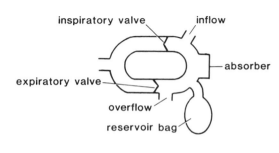

FIG. 5-17 Circle breathing system the components of which are arranged in a less efficient way than the arrangement shown in Figure 5-16. The pairing of dead space gas with alveolar gas indicates complete mixing. (Redrawn from Eger EI II: Anesthetic Uptake and Action. Baltimore, Williams & Wilkins, 1974. © 1974 EI Eger II, M.D.)

ered by the vaporizer. The dilution effect of uptake upon the inspired concentration is countered clinically by increasing the fresh gas flow and the vaporizer setting. At no time, however, is the inspired concentration greater than that delivered by the vaporizer.

In-System Location

The concentration of volatile anesthetic leaving the in-system vaporizer (e.g., Ohio No. 8 Bottle) depends on the same considerations as in the case of the out-of-system vaporizer but is modified by the composition of the gas entering the vaporizer. The vaporizer inflow is a mixture of circuit gas containing exhaled anesthetic and fresh gas (lacking volatile anesthetic) from the anesthesia machine. The concentration of volatile agent in this mixture is particularly sensitive to the relationship between fresh gas inflow and the patient's minute ventilation. With low fresh gas inflow rates and the resultant greater recirculation of circuit gas through this vaporizer, circuit concentration rises. Thus, during controlled respiration, it is all too easy to raise the concentration in the circuit to dangerously high levels. The in-system vaporizer is less hazardous during spontaneous ventilation because the patient's ventilation is the motive force for the recirculation; as anesthesia deepens, anesthetic-induced respiratory depression effectively reduces gas flow through the vaporizer, and the anesthetic concentration within the circuit decreases. Increasing the fresh gas flow decreases the inspired concentration because fresh flow merely dilutes circuit gases; at high inflow rates, the circuit behaves as if it were a nonrebreathing system, and the in-system vaporizer no longer has a concentrating effect.

OVERVIEW

The advantages of the circle system relate principally to the presence of rebreathing: there is relative constancy of inspired concentration, and containment of anesthetic gases so that there is conservation of respiratory moisture and heat, diminished operating room pollution, and less risk of fires and explosions with flammable agents. The price paid includes increased resistance to respiration, increased difficulty in cleaning, greater bulk with loss of portability, and increased opportunity for malfunction of a more complex apparatus. Moisture may collect on the valve leaflets, causing them to stick and thereby increasing respiratory resistance further. Also, as a corollary of the stability of the circle concentration, inspired concentration changes slowly unless the fresh gas inflow (or anesthetic concentration delivered to the circle) is increased. An additional problem is the inability to predict the inspired oxygen concentration when using low flows (i.e., fresh gas inflow below 1.2 L), which necessitates the use of an oxygen analyzer in the circuit.[130]

CLOSED SYSTEMS

The semiclosed system becomes a closed system when the fresh gas inflow is decreased sufficiently so that the expiratory valve remains closed. At that inflow, the closed system just satisfies the patient's metabolic oxygen requirement and the uptake of anesthetic agents.

THE TO-AND-FROM SYSTEM

This system, also called the Water's canister, resembles a Mapleson C system in which a CO_2 absorber is placed just distal to the fresh gas inflow (Fig. 5-18). Without valves between the patient and the fresh gas, there is little resistance to respiration. Simple, sturdy, and easy to assemble and clean, the to-and-fro system conserves respiratory moisture and heat optimally, particularly because of the proximity of the absorbent and its exothermic neutralization reaction. In fact, the canister becomes so hot that the patient can become hyperthermic.[95]

More common problems, however, explain its demise. The proximity of the bulky, hot absorber to the patient is inconvenient and increases the likelihood of inhalation of the caustic dust, especially during assisted or controlled ventilation. Absorbent nearest the pa-

A. END-EXPIRATION WITH FRESH ABSORBER

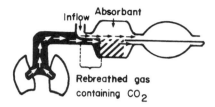

B. END-EXPIRATION WITH PARTIALLY EXHAUSTED ABSORBER

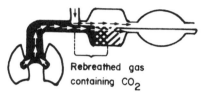

FIG. 5-18 To-and-fro breathing system before (A) and after (B) partial exhaustion of the CO_2 absorbent. (Redrawn from Eger EI II: Anesthetic Uptake and Action. Baltimore, Williams & Wilkins, 1974. © 1974 EI Eger II, M.D.)

tient becomes exhausted earliest, progressively increasing the apparatus dead space; thus, rebreathing results (Fig. 5-18). This is minimized by reversing or changing the absorber periodically. Alternatively, the inflow rate is increased and the expiratory valve is opened, but then the advantages of the closed system (economy of fresh gases, conservation of heat and moisture) are lost. Even with fresh absorbent, the system is inefficient because the alveolar gas is last to leave the patient but first to be inspired.

Popular with cyclopropane, especially in cases of pulmonary infection, this system was used as a semiclosed system during induction to denitrogenate the patient. The flow was then decreased to the metabolic oxygen requirement, with the anesthetic turned off intermittently. Abandonment of flammable agents and availability of bacterial filters and disposable circle systems relegated this system to one of theoretical interest.

THE CLOSED CIRCLE SYSTEM

The closed circle system is merely the circle system with very low flow rates (i.e., 500 to 600 ml/min). All the advantages and disadvantages of the circle system discussed earlier apply here. The challenge imposed by the closed system is principally one of delivering a safe and appropriate inspired mixture.

INSPIRED OXYGEN CONCENTRATION

The unpredictable inspired oxygen concentration when using the circle system with low flows[130] is also a problem with the closed system, especially during induction. It is at this time that the greatest variations in inspired concentrations occur. Anesthetic uptake is maximal; nitrogen is excreted into the lung in large volumes, thereby diluting the available oxygen[131]; and oxygen requirement is somewhat uncertain. The inspired oxygen concentration is particularly precarious when one of the agents is administered in large volumes, such as nitrous oxide, for even small changes in its uptake can have a large effect on the concentrations of other gases in the circle, especially oxygen. Thus, the use of an oxygen analyzer on either limb of the circle system preferably on the inspiratory limb, is mandatory during closed system techniques to ensure that the patient is receiving an adequate inspired oxygen concentration.

ANESTHETIC ADMINISTRATION

The problem posed by the closed system upon the administration of the anesthetics is quite different. We need not know precisely how much we are administering because we closely monitor clinical signs of anesthesia and individual patients vary in their dose requirement. Rather, the problem is *how* to administer the inhaled volatile anesthetic agent safely.

Starting with a Semiclosed System

Clearly, one option is to induce anesthesia with the circle used as a semiclosed system with high flow (i.e., greater than 3 L/min) and to "close" the system after denitrogenation, perhaps 15 minutes later.[132] Thereafter, oxygen is supplied with sufficient nitrous oxide to result in both a desired oxygen concentration (e.g., $F_EO_2 = 0.3$ to 0.4) on the oxygen analyzer and a constant volume in the moderately filled rebreathing bag. Observing the fullness of the rebreathing bag assists in detecting leaks in the breathing system, as well as in maintaining constant circuit volume. Later, when a ventilator is substituted for the rebreathing bag, circuit volume monitoring is accomplished by observing the excursion of the upward-travelling bellows; for this monitoring function, the flow meters should be adjusted so that the bellows falls short of full excursion by a small amount (e.g., 100 ml). Potent inhalation agent is added from induction, as needed, using a vaporizer or by injecting an appropriately calculated amount of liquid anesthetic into the expiratory limb of the breathing system. Anesthetic elimination is facilitated by either resorting to a semiclosed system or by adding a charcoal filter shunt within the closed system.[133]

Starting with a Closed System

The alternative approach is a closed system from the beginning of induction: Again, nitrous oxide, oxygen, and volatile agent are administered as in the semiopen induction; however, alterations in administration will be required more frequently early in the induction. Unless a nitrogen–oxygen mixture is desired, denitrogenation should be accomplished before induction by administering oxygen at a high flow rate (e.g., 10 L/min) through a tight-fitting mask; every 1 to 3 hours the system should be changed to semiclosed in order to waste out additional nitrogen and accumulated volatile metabolites. Other aspects of anesthetic administration are otherwise the same.

Calculating Volatile Agent Dosage

Without resorting to uptake models (Ch. 19), it is readily apparent from daily practice that the amount of anesthetic required to achieve and then maintain a desired anesthetic level decreases as administration continues. An empirical approximation of this observation is that anesthetic uptake varies as the square root of the time,[134] or uptake is constant for the intervals between consecutive "squared" minutes. Thus, the anesthetic uptake (or requirement) in the period between the first and fourth minutes is the same as that between the sixteenth and twenty-fifth minutes. The corollary is that the first dose "lasts" for the first minute, a repeat dose will continue the induction to the fourth minute, then another dose continues the anesthetic to the ninth minute.

Approximate dosage schedules have been prepared based upon the following empirical relationship[134]:

$$\text{Dose (ml vapor)} = 2 \times AD_{95} \times \lambda_B \times \dot{Q}_c \quad (11)$$

where AD_{95} is the anesthetic dose required to anesthetize 95 percent of patients (roughly the product of 1.3 and the minimum alveolar concentration [MAC]), λ_B is the blood-gas solubility coefficient for the volatile anesthetic, and $\dot{Q}_c$ is the cardiac output (in dl/min). The cardiac output, in turn, can be estimated by the following relationship:

$$\text{Cardiac output (dl/min)} = 2 \times kg^{3/4} \quad (12)$$

where $kg^{3/4}$ is an estimation of the patient's metabolically active mass. Other useful physiologic parameters are obtained by multiplying the metabolically active mass by other integers: 10 for oxygen requirement (dl/min), 8 for CO_2 production (dl/min), and 5 for basal water requirement (ml/hr).

OVERVIEW

Beyond the advantages of the semiclosed circle system, the closed circle system adds improved humidification, less pollution, and great economy in the use of anesthetics. The closed system conserves respiratory moisture better than any other but necessarily exhausts the CO_2 absorbent at a faster rate. There is less pollution, yet the need for a program to control waste anesthetics is not obviated; instead, the closed system is but one part of such a program (see section on anesthetic pollution). Because the safe use of the technique is so dependent on both knowledge of uptake and distribution of inhalation agents and close monitoring of anesthetic administration, the closed system also promotes continuing education and perhaps even better care.

THE BREATHING SYSTEM AND NOSOCOMIAL INFECTION

Hospital-acquired respiratory infection is a well-recognized postoperative complication associated with general anesthesia. Yet preventive measures relating to the anesthetic breathing system are highly controversial.[135,136]

CONTAMINATION OF ANESTHETIC EQUIPMENT

Bacterial contamination of the anesthetic breathing system undoubtedly can occur, given the moist surfaces within the equipment and its proximity to the patient's bacteria-laden upper airway. Yet such contamination is very uncommon. Few organisms are actually transmitted during the quiet breathing typical of the anesthetized state. Those organisms liberated during coughing originate from the anterior portion of the oropharynx and rarely contain respiratory pathogens. Moreover, the metallic ions present in breathing system components (copper, brass, chromium, zinc), concentrations of oxygen, and changes in both humidity and temperature are all bactericidal.

CROSS-INFECTION BETWEEN SUSCEPTIBLE PATIENTS

Because the environment within the anesthetic system is not conducive to bacterial survival, infection of and cross-infection between unselected patients is a relevant consideration only in selected clinical situations. Indeed, well-conducted prospective studies have demonstrated that neither the sterile disposable breathing circuit[137] nor the bacterial filter[138] influences the incidence of postoperative respiratory infection associated with the use of a clean breathing system.

However, these studies have not specifically considered patients with impaired host defenses, who might otherwise be more susceptible to nosocomial infection during anesthesia. Examples include patients with immune suppression, either drug induced (e.g., transplant recipient) or disease related (e.g., metastic cancer, severe malnutrition). Similarly, these studies did not consider the special cases of patients having or suspected of having tuberculosis, hepatitis, acquired immune deficiency syndrome (AIDS), or other communicable diseases that may be spread via the respiratory route. The care of such susceptible and infected patients requires the use of as much sterile disposable equipment as is practical. Nondisposable equipment should be disinfected with a method appropriate to the infectious agent.[136]

ANESTHESIA VENTILATORS

Assessment and control of pulmonary ventilation is an integral part of anesthesia practice, given the dose-related respiratory depression that is part of the pharmacology of current inhalation anesthetics (also see Ch. 21). In turn, the anesthesia ventilator has become an important accessory to the anesthetic breathing system, for it enables generally reliable ventilation while freeing the anesthetist to perform other tasks. This equipment is actually a subset of and uses the same principles as the intensive care ventilators (also see Ch. 63).[139]

VENTILATOR DESIGN

The most conspicuous feature of the anesthesia ventilator is its bellows, which functionally replaces the rebreathing bag in the circle system. The motive force for bellows compression is externally applied gas pressure, which is intermittent in pneumatic designs, continuous in fluidic models, or, most commonly, some combination of both designs.[139] Ventilators also differ in the direction that the bellows travels: up ("standing") or down ("falling", "hanging"). A standing bellows is generally preferable because it facilitates detection of small leaks with a closed circle system and disconnection with any breathing system. Regardless of bellows design, however, this equipment should incorporate an alarm that warns of disconnection and other critical circumstances such as an excessive inflating pressure.

Anesthesia ventilators are classified as pressure-cycled, volume-cycled, or time-cycled, in the same manner as the intensive care machines, according to mechanism that terminates the inspiratory phase. However, common models are either time (e.g., Air-Shields) or time and volume (e.g., Drager, Ohio) cycling. Although theoretically a ventilator that is used with adults can be used with children—assuming appropriate settings for tidal volume, inspiratory flow rate, and respiratory rate—pediatric ventilators are often necessary for smaller children. This is because the compression volumes within adult ventilators usually exceed the small child's tidal volume; hence, small changes in pulmonary compliance can result in large changes in ventilation.

CLINICAL USE OF VENTILATORS

Anesthesia ventilators have fewer controls than do their intensive care counterparts. Although tidal volume and ventilatory rate can be specified, they are set directly on some models by determining other ventilatory parameters, such as inspiratory flow rate, inspiratory time, and expiratory pause time. The movement of the bellows along a calibrated scale offers only an approximate measure of tidal volume, because of fresh gas inflow during the inspiratory phase,[140] compliance of the tubing in the breathing system (especially in pediatric circuits[141]), and otherwise inapparent leaks in the system. Typically, a spirometer or respirometer, often used on the inspiratory limb of the breathing system, measures the tidal volume and minute ventilation. An estimate of the required minute ventilation is provided by the Radford nomogram.[75] Many ventilators also permit adding positive end-expiratory pressure (PEEP) (also see Chs. 63 & 64), retarding exhalation, assisting (rather than controlling) ventilation, and limiting the peak inspiratory pressure.

MONITORING THE BREATHING SYSTEM

Although patient monitoring during anesthesia is a well-established activity, monitoring of the anesthetic system itself has attracted attention only relatively recently. Many of the available devices monitor both the patient and the equipment. But a sampling of the more clinically useful "black boxes" available for attachment to the breathing system are mentioned here. For others, as well as further discussion of physical principles, the reader should consult several excellent sources[3,96,142–144] (also see Ch. 3).

MONITORING DEVICES

OXYGEN ANALYZERS

There are a variety of different designs for oxygen analyzers. Monitoring oxygen concentration within the breathing system is as fundamental now as monitoring the patient's blood pressure, as well as being necessary with closed system anesthesia.

Paramagnetic Analyzer

The paramagnetic (Pauling) oxygen analyzer deserves mention if only for its simplicity and reliability when current equipment fails. The underlying physical principle is simple. Whereas most gases found within the breathing system are repelled by a magnetic field (diamagnetism), only oxygen is attracted to a magnetic field (paramagnetism). Within a container are two spheres filled with a weakly diamagnetic gas (N_2) connected and hung by a wire that permits them to rotate in a magnetic field; however, the suspension is arranged so that they tend to remain in the strongest part of the magnetic field. When oxygen enters the container and is attracted to the center of the magnetic field, it displaces the spheres, and they rotate on their wire with a degree of displacement related to the number of oxygen molecules present. Light shining on a mirror attached to the wire deflects the light to a different portion of a translucent screen calibrated in percent oxygen. Its disadvantages are a relatively slow response time (close to 1 minute), need for a pump to draw the sample into the device, and lack of an alarm. Although batteries are required, they are commonly available flashlight batteries.

Electrochemical Analyzers

Current analyzers involve electrochemical processes in one of three types of cells: amperometric, galvanic (e.g., full cell), and polarographic (e.g., Clark Electrode). Although the process differs slightly among the different cells, the oxygen molecules diffuse through a membrane and electrolyte solution to a cathode; electrical current is produced proportional to the partial pressure of the oxygen. The galvanic cell has a life expectancy related inversely to its concentration-hour exposure to oxygen. Equipped with a replaceable battery, the polarographic cell is less costly over its life, but it does require warmup.

CARBON DIOXIDE ANALYZER

Because CO_2 contains two dissimilar atoms, this gas absorbs infrared radiation in a spectral range that is convenient to measure.

The underlying physical principle is quite simple: Radiation from an infrared lamp contains a spectrum of wavelengths. The gas to be analyzed passes through this radiation, absorbing differentially in one or more regions of the spectrum. To facilitate quantitation of the absorption spectrum in the clinical setting, the infrared spectrophotometer has been modified as the capnograph. This device has two gas chambers through which infrared radiation is beamed, one containing the gas sample and the other a reference tube usually filled with air. The unabsorbed radiation passes through the end of each chamber and impinges on heat detectors. Differential heating of the detectors is transduced to a meter calibrated directly in percent CO_2. Because the infrared absorption of nitrous oxide overlaps that of CO_2, either calibration against a known gas mixture or the use of a correction factor is required.

Gas is obtained continuously from a catheter at the distal end of the breathing system, permitting end-tidal samples. Besides immediately detecting disconnection at the tracheal tube connector and a variety of other equipment problems, this device can assist in the diagnosis of a wide variety of metabolic (e.g., malignant hyperthermia), circulatory (e.g., pulmonary embolus), and ventilatory problems in which carbon dioxide excretion is altered. In addition, the capnograph facilitates the ventilatory control of cerebral edema by obviating the need for arterial blood gases.

MASS SPECTROMETER

As its name suggests, the mass spectrometer analyzes the components of a gas mixture according to the spectrum of its molecular mass-to-charge ratios. A small gas sample is drawn into an evacuated ionization chamber in which the molecules are bombarded by electrons. The resultant charged ions diffuse out of the chamber and are attracted to and pass through a negatively charged plate. The ion stream then encounters a magnetic field oriented at a right angle to the ion stream. The ions are deflected differentially by charge (essentially the same for all) and mass, with the lightest ions deflected most, producing a spectrum of mass-to-charge ratios. The analysis is both instantaneous and continuous.

Commercial models analyze the composition of the breathing system gas for all the clinically important gases: oxygen, carbon dioxide, nitrogen, nitrous oxide, halothane, enflurane, and isoflurane. Although too costly for a single operating room (about $40,000 in 1985), this monitoring device can be shared by an entire operating suite (total cost about $90,000), using sequential sampling from long catheters that end distally in each breathing system throughout the suite and remote display of results in each room.[145] Among the benefits of such monitoring are the immediate detection of breathing system disconnection, other breathing system malfunctions,[146] hypoxia due to erroneous gas mixtures, problems related to vaporizers (e.g., improper filling, two simultaneously on, malfunction), malignant hyperthermia (increased CO_2 excretion), air embolism (nitrogen spike and decreased $P_{end\text{-}tidal}$ CO_2), and physiologic gas abnormalities without a blood-gas specimen. In addition to enhancing patient safety, this device facilitates the use of closed system anesthesia (with resultant savings), education, and clinical research.[145]

MONITORING AND OVERALL SYSTEM INTEGRATION

Available breathing system (and patient) monitoring devices exist as discrete accessories to patient care that are unrelated functionally or physically. Although a given device may yield useful clinical information, the data are generally not integrated with data from other devices. As a result, the anesthetist may be bombarded by so much information (only some of which comes from such monitors) as to be unable to use all the information effectively. With increasing complexity of surgery and anesthesia care, this lack of overall integration in the process of anesthesia delivery can be an important element in the chain leading to adverse anesthetic outcomes discussed at the beginning of this chapter (Fig. 5-1).[146,148] Recent advances in microprocessors now permit integration of the various monitoring devices and anesthesia delivery equipment by capturing continuous data from each in electronic form that can be aggregated and analyzed instantaneously.[149] Several prototype microprocessor-controlled anesthesia machines have been developed.[150] Until such equipment becomes commonly available, the anesthetist must continue to perform such integration with his own native computer (Table 5-7).

CONTROLLING EXPOSURE TO WASTE ANESTHETIC GASES

THE PROBLEM

As early as 1920, "ether poisoning," characterized by gastrointestinal and CNS symptoms, occurred among those exposed to ether vapor while making gunpowder during World

TABLE 5-7. Differentiation of Major Breathing System Problems

Equipment or Clinical Circumstance	Breathing System Disconnection	Oxygen Flow Meter Off	Oxygen Source Disconnection
Low pressure alarm on?	Yes	No	No
Ventilator power on?*	Yes	Yes	No
Ventilator bellows full?†	No	Yes	No
Oxygen analyzer alarm on?	No	Yes	No
Anesthetic gas/vapor flow meter(s) on?*	Yes	Yes	No
Breath sounds and chest rising?	No	Yes	No

* Applies to standard anesthesia machines with oxygen-dependent anesthetic flow meters and ventilators.
† Applies to ventilators with upward-traveling bellows.
(Courtesy of Alan T. Suyama, MD, University of California at San Francisco.)

War I.[151] Anecdotal reports during the subsequent decades noted that personnel in poorly ventilated operating rooms experienced headaches, depression, anorexia, excessive fatigue, and memory loss, all of which disappeared with absence from the operating room or the installation of improved room ventilation. Beginning in the late 1960s, however, there was growing concern that chronic exposure to low levels of anesthetic gases constitutes a health hazard to operating room personnel.[152,153] The hazard has been alleged to include an increased incidence of spontaneous abortion, congenital abnormalities, hepatic and renal diseases, and cancer, as well as changes in mood and intellectual function (also see Ch. 22).

Although the validity of these allegations is uncertain due to methodological flaws in the design of many of the surveys,[153-157] it is likely that adverse reproductive outcomes are more common for women chronically exposed to anesthetic gases during pregnancy.[157] Given the problems inherent in studying such health problems, it is doubtful whether the existence of occupational hazards associated with chronic exposure to low levels of anesthetic gases can be proved, at least in the foreseeable future. Yet, even in the absence of unassailable proof, control of excess anesthetic gases ought to be undertaken because (1) these gases do have offensive odors, (2) there are sufficient similarities in the results of the surveys and laboratory studies to encourage a conservative approach, and (3) many persons are at risk — approximately 70,000 in operating rooms, 100,000 in dental operatories, and 50,000 in veterinary settings.[158] Furthermore, regulatory agencies require control measures, even if the available data are inadequate for establishing exposure limits.[159] In particular, the general duty clause of the Occupational Safety and Health Act of 1970 mandates the Secretary of Labor to require each employer to maintain a workplace free from hazards. The National Institute of Occupational Safety and Health (NIOSH) has issued recommendations for control and other aspects of waste anesthetic gases,[158] and Occupational Safety and Health Administration (OSHA) personnel have cited hospitals and anesthesiologists for alleged violations of the general duty clause.

QUANTITATING WASTE ANESTHETIC CONCENTRATIONS

Low concentrations of a gas are expressed on a volume/volume basis as parts per million (ppm). Thus, a sample composed of 100 percent of a gas contains 1,000,000 ppm, and one containing 1 percent, 10,000 ppm.

GAS SAMPLING AND ANALYSIS

There are two major categories of air-monitoring programs.[160] In *area monitoring*, sampling is undertaken in the general workplace, but not necessarily close to where personnel actually experience their typical exposure. More appropriate is *personal monitoring*, in which samples are obtained in the breathing zone of the anesthesia personnel, often during anesthetic administration. Within either program, sampling can be active or passive. In *active dosimetry*, the gas sample is aspirated into a gas syringe, evacuated test tube, or other leak-free container, whereas in *passive dosimetry* the gas is adsorbed selectively by a specific medium, without a special power source or effort.[161]

Similarly, there are two general approaches to the timing of gas sampling,[158,160] the simplest of which is the *instantaneous sample*. This can be repeated later during anesthesia to assess adequacy of excess gas control measures or after some intervention such as changing the room ventilation rate. A *time-weighted* sample is more representative of the average concentration to which personnel are exposed because it is obtained at a constant rate over, perhaps, hours and thereby averages short-term variations.

A variety of analytic methods can be used to determine concentrations of anesthetic gases in the sample, including manometry (e.g., Van Slyke), combustion, gas chromatography, and infrared spectrophotometry.[158,160] Gas chromatography and infrared analysis are most commonly used. Since nitrous oxide is present in a much higher concentration than are other agents, a cogent argument can be made for monitoring nitrous oxide exclusively as a tracer for anesthetic pollution generally.[160]

TYPICAL AMBIENT CONCENTRATIONS

In the absence of specific control measures, the average concentration of nitrous oxide in the operating room is 130 to 6,800 ppm, and that of halothane, from 1 to 85 ppm. Nitrous oxide concentrations in dental operatories are generally considerably higher.[158,160] The higher values are obtained in the breathing zone of the anesthesiologist when nonrebreathing or high-flow circle systems in poorly ventilated rooms are used. With control measures, nitrous oxide concentrations below 180 ppm and halothane below 2 ppm can be achieved.[158,160] However, NIOSH has recommended concentration levels of nitrous oxide of less than 25 ppm and of halogenated agents used simultaneously of less than 0.5 ppm (2 ppm when halogenated agents are used alone).[148] It is doubtful that such low levels can be achieved consistently in the clinical setting.

SOURCES OF WASTE ANESTHETIC GASES

HIGH-PRESSURE SYSTEM LEAKAGE

The high-pressure system extends from the nitrous oxide sources—the tanks (5,180 kN/m, or 750 lb/in.²) attached to the anesthesia machine and the central gas system (345 kN/m or 50 lb/in.²)—to the flowmeters of the anesthesia machine. Even when no anesthesia is being administered, leakage from any portion of this system can give rise to background nitrous oxide concentrations substantially above the NIOSH recommendation of 25 ppm. Moreover, a recirculating room ventilation system can spread the pollution throughout the operating suite. Particularly likely leakage sites are the quick coupler (e.g., Shrader) at the de-

livery end of the flexible hose of the central nitrous oxide system and the tank yokes on the anesthesia machine.

LOW-PRESSURE SYSTEM LEAKAGE

The low-pressure system extends from the flowmeters to the patient. Leakage can be so great that an otherwise effective control program is negated. Although a myriad of leakage sites exist (Table 5-7), one of the most common ones is the gasket seal of the CO_2 canister. The gasket may become worn and cracked, or granules of soda lime may prevent a tight seal.

ANESTHETIC TECHNIQUE

By definition, open-drop and insufflation techniques constitute unopposed spillage of large volumes of anesthetic into the operating room and thereby rapidly lead to concentrations considerably in excess of the NIOSH recommendation. At the other extreme is the closed system technique which, once established, should prevent clinically significant anesthetic spillage. For example, one study found the nitrous oxide concentration in the anesthesiologist's breathing zone to be below 31 ppm with a closed system nitrous oxide flow rate of 500 ml/min, and even less pollution with lower flows. The institution of a control program, including the removal of excess breathing system gases (scavenging), resulted in concentrations below 8 ppm.[162] Other anesthetic techniques result in levels of pollution between these extremes.[158,160]

CONTROL MEASURES

An effective program for the control of excess anesthetic gases requires the elimination of leakage from the anesthetic equipment, alteration of anesthetic technique, and use of equipment to collect and remove excess breathing system gases (scavenging).[158,160,163-165] Such a program must not detract from patient care, which should continue to be the anesthesiologist's principal concern.

IMPROVED MACHINE MAINTENANCE

Periodically, anesthesia machines should be serviced by factory-trained personnel, with particular attention focused on correcting leakage in both the high- and low-pressure systems. Leakage, however, can develop between service visits and can even continue despite such a maintenance program. Anesthesia personnel must therefore be familiar with the rudiments of testing for leakage.

Leakage in the high-pressure system requires disconnecting the anesthesia machine from the central gas supply, closing the flowmeter valves, and opening a tank of nitrous oxide, closing that tank, and noting the pressure. If more than a minimal decrease in pressure occurs within an hour and the leakage site is not found to be the tank yoke or quick coupler, the leak is within the machine and the service representative should be called.

Unlike leakage testing of the high-pressure system, testing the low-pressure system requires the flow of anesthetic gas. The presence and amount of leakage in the commonly used semiclosed circle system can be determined by closing the expiratory valve, occluding the Y piece at the patient end of the system, and noting the oxygen inflow required to maintain a pressure of 30 cm H_2O. Since leakage varies linearly with pressure, and pressure in the breathing system during controlled ventilation averages about 10 cm H_2O, a 150-ml/min leakage rate at 30 cm H_2O represents leakage of about 50 ml/min during controlled ventilation. Although leakage of this magnitude contributes less than 5 ppm to the average operating room, greater leakage requires correction. Monitoring for specific leakage sites can be as simple as applying a 20 percent soap solution in water to components (e.g., gaskets of the CO_2 absorber) of and connections (e.g., quick couplers in the central nitrous oxide supply hose) in the high- and low-pressure systems

and observing for bubbles. Correction of leakage often involves such simple maneuvers as replacing a torn canister gasket or removing a deformed washer on a tank yoke.

SCAVENGING

In an otherwise leak-free breathing system, the only site of spillage of anesthetic gases is the expiratory valve, through which excess gases normally exit. Scavenging is the collection and removal of this effluent. A system that accomplishes this has a gas-capturing assembly, a disposal route, and between them an interface.

THE GAS-CAPTURING ASSEMBLY

The gas-capturing assembly collects gases from the breathing system, broadly defined to include the ventilator and extracorporeal pump oxygenator, and conducts the potential pollutant to the disposal route. Because effluent volumes vary greatly, especially when a ventilator is used, particular attention must be directed to matching a scavenging system of sufficient capacity (e.g., in L/min flow) to the given breathing system. An interface prevents pressure variations in the breathing system, which might otherwise affect system dynamics or delivered gas concentrations, consequent to scavenging. Gas-capturing assemblies are readily available for the expiratory valves of the breathing system and the ventilator, although those for pump oxygenators are still evolving.[166-168]

THE DISPOSAL SYSTEM

Once collected, the waste gases can be directed into the exhaust grill of a nonrecirculating room ventilation system. Airflow into the exhaust grill is sufficient to entrain the waste gases. Because a nonrecirculating system is relatively expensive to operate, especially in very warm or cold climates, a recirculating system is encountered more frequently. If the waste gases do not enter this system distal to the recirculation point, all operating rooms ventilated from a common manifold will be polluted. An alternate disposal route is the central vacuum system; however, National Fire Protective Association regulations prohibit disposal of flammable anesthetic agents into such a system. Another alternate disposal system is an independent ("dedicated") vacuum system that is vented to avoid personnel exposure. Before any vacuum system is used, the hospital engineer should verify that the system has sufficient capacity and is resistant to corrosive materials. Waste gases can also be directed passively through the wall of the operating room. Finally, activated charcoal adsorbers can remove halogenated anesthetic agents but are relatively expensive, have a short life span, and do not absorb nitrous oxide.

THE INTERFACE

Scavenging risks establishing marked pressure differences between the breathing system and the waste gas disposal system. Attaching any of the vacuum systems directly to the expiratory valve of the breathing system threatens removal of substantial gas volumes from the breathing system, unless the fresh gas inflow is greater than the suction rate. The hazard of an excessive rate of suction commonly manifests itself by collapse of the breathing bag and consequent inability to ventilate the patient. With certain ventilator designs, there may also be malfunction of the ventilator alarm.[169] On the other hand, if the disposal route becomes occluded (e.g., stepping on the tubing), the gases that normally exit via the expiratory valve are effectively contained within the breathing system, and the pressure rises within the system, impeding pulmonary ventilation and eventually leading to pulmonary barotrauma. The interface is a pressure-balancing device that thereby prevents the development of negative and positive pressure in the breathing system. Although designs vary, the typical interface consists of two components: a reservoir contains the waste gases that collect, often intermittently, when outflow from the expiratory valve exceeds the disposal rate: a unidirectional valve with a negative pressure-relief mechanism at the expiratory valve permits gases to leave the breathing system pas-

sively when a threshold pressure (e.g., 5 mmHg) is reached, but prevents gas flow into or active removal (i.e., suction) of gas from the breathing system. The negative pressure-relief mechanism in the latter can be as simple as several holes that permit the disposal system to communicate with the atmosphere; thus, room air is entrained, protecting the breathing system (including the patient's lungs) and the anesthesia ventilator from the negative pressure. The holes also permit escape of waste gases into the room should the disposal route be occluded. Thoughtful design notwithstanding, pressure differentials can still be established as a result of malfunction, with potential harm to the patient.[169-176] The addition of a second negative pressure relief mechanism, perhaps having a dissimilar design, has been suggested as a possible remedy.[176]

ALTERATION OF ANESTHETIC TECHNIQUE

Altering anesthetic technique and general work habits is also an important aspect of an effective control program. Poor fit of the face mask, as well as permitting anesthetic gases to flow before application of the mask and during tracheal intubation and suctioning, can result in the spillage of substantial amounts of gases into the room. Administering 100 percent oxygen for as long as practical at the end of an anesthetic can also diminish gas spillage because this washes out the breathing system and the patient's lungs. The use of low-flow or closed-system techniques can also diminish the level of waste gas contamination in the operating room; however, scavenging is not obviated. Particular care should be taken when filling vaporizers, since each milliliter of anesthetic vaporizers to approximately 200 ml of gas (e.g., 212 ml for halothane, 184 ml for enflurane and isoflurane) at room temperature. If halothane spillage is detectable by smell, the level of contamination is likely to be at least 33 ppm.[177] Assuming even gas mixing, spilling just 1 ml of liquid halothane in a box 6 m on a side and 3 m tall, approximately the dimensions of an operating room, results in a concentration of 2 ppm, four times the NIOSH recommended limit for a halogenated agent used with nitrous oxide.

EFFICIENT ROOM VENTILATION

A nonrecirculating ventilation system offers the advantage of providing a simple disposal route for scavenging but requires that all of the air must be heated or cooled, which is costly in cold or warm climates. While having a lower operating cost, the recirculating system can unfortunately redistribute excess anesthetic gases throughout the operating suite, to all rooms served by the same ventilation system. Redistribution, however, tends to lower the excess gas concentrations that might otherwise exist in a room in which anesthesia is being administered. The hospital engineer should determine the efficiency of ventilation (in terms of room air turnovers per hour) in each room periodically; in addition, the ventilation filters should be examined for debris to ensure that the rooms are ventilated evenly.

ENVIRONMENTAL MONITORING

Several times a year excess anesthetic concentrations should be determined in each operating room after it has been out of service for at least eight hours, using either an instantaneous ("grab") sample or infrared analysis. Another sample should be obtained in the breathing zone of the anesthesiologist 30 minutes after induction of anesthesia. There is no firm basis at this time for considering particular concentrations "dangerous" or "toxic." Particularly high concentrations (e.g., nitrous oxide in excess of 180 ppm), however, should alert personnel to search for leaks and consider modifications in the anesthetic technique and work habits.

PERSONNEL INVOLVEMENT

An otherwise excellent control program cannot be effective in reducing the concentrations of excess anesthetic gases without the active participation of all personnel in the anesthesia department. Results of the periodic environmental monitoring can serve as the focus for reminding personnel of the need to check equipment for leaks and modifying techniques and habits to minimize contaminant levels. In addition, periodically all operating room personnel ought to be informed of the status of knowledge regarding the possible hazards resulting from chronic exposure to anesthetics.[178]

REFERENCES

1. Thomas KB: The Development of Anaesthetic Apparatus. Oxford, Blackwell Scientific Publications, 1975
2. Macintosh R, Mushin, WW, Epstein HG: Physics for the Anaesthetist. 3rd Ed. Oxford, Blackwell Scientific Publications, 1963
3. Hill DW: Physics Applied to Anaesthesia. 4th Ed. Butterworths, London, 1980
4. Dorsch JA, Dorsch SE: Understanding Anesthetic Equipment: Construction, Care and Complications. 2nd Ed. Baltimore, Williams & Wilkins, 1984
5. Schreiber P: Anaesthetic Equipment: Performance, Classification and Safety. Berlin, Springer-Verlag, 1972
6. Wyant GM: Mechanical Misadventures in Anaesthesia. Toronto, University of Toronto Press, 1978
7. Phillips O: Historical perspective and results of early studies, Health Care Delivery in Anesthesia. Edited by Hirsh RA, Forrest WH Jr, Orkin FK, Wollman H., Philadelphia, George F. Stickley, 1980, p 5
8. Dripps RD, Lamont A, Eckenhoff JE: The role of anesthesia in surgical mortality. JAMA 178:261, 1961
9. Marx GF, Mateo CV, Orkin LR: Computer analysis of postanesthetic deaths. Anesthesiology 39:54, 1973
10. Lunn JN, Mushin WW: Mortality Associated with Anaesthesia. London, Nuffield Provincial Hospitals Trust, 1982
11. Edwards G, Morton HJV, Pask EA, et al: Deaths associated with anaesthesia: Report on 1000 cases. Anaesthesia 11:194, 1956

12. Clifton BS, Hotten WIT: Deaths associated with anaesthesia. Br J Anaesth 35:250, 1963
13. Wylie WD: There, but for the grace of God. . . . Ann R Coll Surg 56:171, 1975
14. Utting JE, Gray TC, Shelley FC: Human misadventure in anaesthesia. Can Anaesth Soc J 26:472, 1979
15. Taylor G, Larson CP, Prestwich R: Unexpected cardiac arrest during anesthesia and surgery. JAMA 236:2758, 1976
16. Cooper JR, Newbower RD, Long CD, et al: Preventable anesthesia mishaps: A study of human factors. Anesthesiology 49:399, 1978
17. Craig J, Wilson ME: A survey of anaesthetic misadventures. Anaesthesia 36:933, 1981
18. Cooper JB, Long CD, Newbower RS: Human error in anesthesia management, Quality of Care Review in Anesthesia. Edited by Grundy BL, Gravenstein JS. Springfield, IL, Charles C Thomas, 1982, p 114
19. Newbower RS, Cooper JB, Long CD: Learning from anesthesia mishaps: Analysis of critical incidents in anesthesia helps reduce patient risk. QRB 7(3):10, 1981
20. Duberman S, Wald A: An integrated quality control program for anesthesia equipment. QRB 9(11):328, 1983
21. Herr GP: Anesthesia mishaps: Occurrence and prevention. Semin Anesth 2:213, 1983
22. Cooper JB, Newbower RS, Kitz RJ: An analysis of major errors and equipment failures in anesthesia management: Considerations for prevention and detection. Anesthesiology 60:34, 1984
23. Cooper JB: Toward prevention of anesthetic mishaps. Int Anesthesiol Clin 22(2):167, 1984
24. Final rule on medical device reporting. Fed Reg p 36326, September 14, 1984
25. US Congress, Office of Technology Assessment: Federal Policies and the Medical Device Industry. OTA-H-230. Washington, DC, October 1984
26. Orkin LR, Siegel M, Rovenstine EA: Resistance to breathing by apparatus used in anesthesia. Anesth Analg 33:217, 1954
27. Proctor DF: Studies of respiratory air flow. IV. Resistance to air flow through anesthesia apparatus. Bull Johns Hopkins Hosp 96:49, 1955
28. Hinforomi BK: The resistance of air flow of tracheostomy tubes, connections and heat and moisture exchangers. Br J Anaesth 37:454, 1965
29. Brown ES, Hustead RF: Resistance of pediatric breathing systems. Anesth Analg 48:842, 1969
30. Sullivan M, Paliotta J, Saklad M: The endotracheal tube as a factor in the measurement of respiratory mechanics. J Appl Physiol 41:590, 1976
31. Hammond JE, Wright DJ: Comparison of the resistances of double-lumen endobronchial tubes. Br J Anaesth 56:299, 1984
32. Conway CM: Anaesthetic breathing systems, Scientific Foundations of Anaesthesia. 3rd Ed. Edited by Scurr C, Feldman S. London, Heinemann, 1982, p 557
33. Smith WDA: The effects of external resistance to respiration. Part I. General review. Br J Anaesth 33:549, 1961
34. Smith WDA: The effects of external resistance to respiration. Part II. Resistance to respiration due to anaesthetic apparatus. Br J Anaesth 33:610, 1961
35. Graff TD. Sewall K, Lim HS, et al: The ventilatory response of infants to airway resistance. Anesthesiology 27:168, 1966
36. Nunn JF, Ezi-Ashi TI: The respiratory effects of resistance to breathing in anesthetized man. Anesthesiology 22:174, 1961
37. Duncan PG: Efficacy of helium–oxygen mixtures in the management of severe viral and post-intubation croup. Can Anaesth Soc J 26:206, 1979
38. Sykes MK: Rebreathing circuits: A review. Br J Anaesth 40:666, 1968
39. Wilson RE: Soda lime as absorbent for industrial purposes. Ind Eng Chem 12:1000, 1920
40. Adriani J, Rovenstine EA: Experimental studies on carbon dioxide absorption for anesthesia. Anesthesiology 2:1, 1941
41. Adriani J: Disposal of carbon dioxide from devices used for inhalation anesthesia. Anesthesiology 21:742, 1960
42. Brown ES, Bakamjian V, Seniff AM: Performance of absorbents: Effects of moisture. Anesthesiology 20:613, 1959
43. Grodin WK, Epstein RA: Halothane adsorption by soda lime. Anesthesiology 51:S317, 1979
44. Adriani J: Soda lime containing indicators. Anesthesiology 5:45, 1944
45. Ten Pas RH, Brown ES, Elam JO: Carbon dioxide absorption. Anesthesiology 29:231, 1958
46. Brown ES: Performance of absorbents: Continuous flow. Anesthesiology 20:41, 1959
47. Kelley JM: Cranial nerve injury following trichloroethylene, Complications in Anesthesiology. Edited by Orkin FK, Cooperman LH. Philadelphia, JB Lippincott, 1983, p 338
48. Case history No. 39: Accidental use of trichloroethylene (Trilene, Trimar) in a closed system. Anesth Analg 43:740, 1964
49. Debban DG, Bedford RF: Overdistention of the rebreathing bag, a hazardous test for circuit-system integrity. Anesthesiology 42:365, 1975
50. Lauria JI: Soda-lime dust contamination of breathing circuits. Anesthesiology 42:628, 1975
51. Adriani J, Batten DH: The efficacy of mixtures of

barium and calcium hydroxides in the absorption of CO_2 in the rebreathing appliances. Anesthesiology 3:1, 1942

52. Adriani J: Rebreathing in anesthesia. South Med J 35:798, 1942

53. Rogers RC, Hill GE: Equations for vapour pressure versus temperature: Derivation and usage of the Antoine equation on a hand-held programmable calculator. Br J Anaesth 50:415, 1978

54. Munson WM: Cardiac arrest: Hazard of tipping a vaporizer. Anesthesiology 26:235, 1965

55. Mark LC, Marx GF, Erlanger H, et al: Improper filling of kettle-type vaporizers. NY State J Med 65:1151, 1965

56. Kopriva LJ, Lowenstein E: An anesthetic accident: Cardiovascular collapse from liquid halothane delivery. Anesthesiology 30:246, 1969

57. Gartner J, Stoelting RK: A laboratory comparison of Copper Kettle, Fluotec Mark 2, and Pentec vaporizers. Anesth Analg 53:187, 1974

58. Keasling HH, Pittinger CB: Fluotec performance. Anesthesiology 29:682, 1958

59. Munson ES: Hazards of agent-specific vaporizers. Anesthesiology 34:393, 1971

60. Murray WJ, Zsigmond EK, Fleming P: Contamination of in-series vaporizers with halothane-methoxyflurane. Anesthesiology 38:487, 1973

61. Karis JH, Menzel DB: Inadvertent change of volatile anesthetics in anesthesia machines. Anesth Analg 61:53, 1982

62. Bruce BL, Linde HW: Vaporization of mixed anesthetic liquid. Anesthesiology 60:342, 1984

63. Dorsch SE, Dorsch JA: Chemical cross-contamination between vaporizers in series. Anesth Analg 52:176, 1973

64. Wickett RE, Jenkins LC, Root LS: Downstream contamination of in-series vapourizers. Can Anaesth Soc J 21:114, 1974

65. Browne RA, McDonald S: A vapourizer interlocking system. Can Anaesth Soc J 30:653, 1983

66. Dorsch JA, Dorsch SE: Vaporizers. Understanding Anesthetic Equipment: Construction, Care and Complications. 2nd Ed. Baltimore, Williams & Wilkins, 1984, p 213

67. Epstein HG, Macintosh R: An anaesthetic inhaler with automatic thermo-compensation. Anaesthesia 11:83, 1956

68. Morris LE: A new vaporizer for liquid anesthetic agents. Anesthesiology 13:587, 1952

69. Gartner J, Stoelting RK: A laboratory comparison of Copper Kettle, Fluotec Mark 2, and Pentec Vaporizers. Anesth Analg 53:187, 1974

70. Farmati O, Quinn JR, Fennell RM: Exfoliative cytology of the intubated larynx in children. Can Anaesth Soc J 14:321, 1967

71. Chalon J, Loew DAY, Malebranche J: Effect of dry anesthetic gases on tracheobronchial ciliated epithelium. Anesthesiology 37:338, 1972

72. Rashad KF, Wilson K, Hurt HH Jr, et al: Effect of humidification of anesthetic gases on static compliance. Anesth Analg 46:127, 1967

73. Knudsen J, Lomholt N, Wisborg K: Postoperative pulmonary complications using dry and humidified anaesthetic gases. Br J Anaesth 45:636, 1973

74. Chalon J, Patel C, Ali M, et al: Humidity and the anesthetized patient. Anesthesiology 50:195, 1979

75. Radford EP: Ventilation standards for use in artificial respiration. J Appl Physiol 7:451, 1955

76. Nunn JF: Prediction of carbon dioxide tension during anaesthesia. Anaesthesia 15:123, 1960

77. Nunn JF: Predictors for oxygen and carbon dioxide levels during anaesthesia. Anaesthesia 17:182, 1962

78. Dery R: Water balance of the respiratory tract during ventilation with a gas mixture saturated at body temperature. Can Anaesth Soc J 20:719, 1973

79. Stone DR, Downs JB, Paul WL, et al: Adult body temperature and heated humidification of anesthetic gases during general anesthesia. Anesth Analg 60:736, 1981

80. Tausk HC, Miller I, Roberts RB: Maintenance of body temperature by heated humidification. Anesth Analg 55:719, 1976

81. Chalon J, Patel C, Ramanathan S, et al: Humidification of the circle absorber system. Anesthesiology 48:142, 1978

82. Chalon J, Markham JP, Ali M, et al: The Pall Ultipor Breathing Circuit Filter—An efficient heat and moisture exchanger. Anesth Analg 63:566, 1984

83. Chase HF, Trotta R, Kilmore MA: Simple methods for humidifying nonrebreathing anesthesia gas systems. Anesth Analg 41:249, 1962

84. Chalon J, Ramanathan S: Water vaporizer heated by the reaction of neutralization by carbon dioxide. Anesthesiology 41:400, 1974

85. Chalon J, Simon R, Patel C, et al: An infant circuit with a water vaporizer warmed by carbon dioxide neutralization. Anesth Analg 57:307, 1978

86. Mapleson WW, Morgan JG, Hilard EK: Assessment of condenser-humidifiers with special reference to a multiple-gauze model. Br Med J 1:300, 1963

87. Weeks DB, Ramsey FM: Laboratory investigation of six artificial noses during endotracheal anesthesia. Anesth Analg 63:758, 1983

88. Joseph JM: Disease transmission by insufficiently sanitized anesthesiology apparatus. JAMA 149:1196, 1952

89. Stark DCC, Green CA, Pask EA: Anaesthetic machines and cross-infection. Anaesthesia 17:12, 1962

90. Philips I, Spencer G: Pseudomonas aeruginosa cross-infection due to contaminated respiratory apparatus. Lancet 2:1325, 1965

91. Pundit SK, Mehta S, Agarwal SC: Risk of cross-infection from inhalation anaesthesia. Br J Anaesth 39:839, 1967

92. Grieble HG, Colton FR, Bird TJ, et al: Fine-particle humidifiers: Sources of *Pseudomonas aeruginosa* infections in a respiratory-disease unit. N Engl J Med 282:531, 1970

93. Avery ME, Galina M, Nachman R: Mist therapy. Pediatrics 39:160, 1967

94. Cheney FW, Butler J: The effects of ultrasonically produced aerosols on airway resistance in man. Anesthesiology 29:1099, 1968

95. Clark RE, Orkin LR, Rovenstine EA: Body temperature studies in anesthetized man: Effect of environmental temperature, humidity, and anesthesia system. JAMA 154:311, 1954

96. Dorsch JA, Dorsch SE: The breathing system. I. General Considerations. Understanding Anesthesia Equipment: Construction, Care and Complications. 2nd Ed. Baltimore, Williams & Wilkins, 1984, p 172

97. Hamilton WK: Nomenclature of inhalation anesthetic systems. Anesthesiology 25:3, 1964

98. Munson ES, Farnham M, Hamilton WK: Studies of respiratory gas flows. A comparison using different anesthetic agents. Anesthesiology 24:61, 1963

99. Sykes MK: Non-rebreathing valves. Br J Anaesth 31:450, 1959

100. Orkin LR, Siegal M, Rovenstine EA: Resistance to breathing by apparatus used in anesthesia. II. Valves and machines. Anesth Analg 36:19, 1957

101. Mapleson WW: The elimination of rebreathing in various semiclosed anaesthetic systems. Br J Anaesth 26:323, 1954

102. Kain ML, Nunn JF: Fresh gas economies of the Magill circuit. Anesthesiology 29:964, 1968

103. Norman J, Adams AP, Sykes MK: Rebreathing with the Magill attachment. Anaesthesia 23:75, 1968

104. Sykes MK: Rebreathing during controlled respiration with the Magill attachment. Anaesthesia 31:247, 1959

105. Bain JA, Spoerel WE: A streamlined anaesthetic system. Can Anaesth Soc J 19:426, 1972

106. Weeks DB: Provision of endogenous and exogenous humidity for the Bain breathing circuit. Can Anaesth Soc J 23:185, 1976

107. Byrick RJ, Janssen EG: Respiratory waveform and rebreathing in T-piece circuits: A comparison of enflurane and halothane waveforms. Anesthesiology 53:371, 1980

108. Spoerel WE, Aitkieh RR, Bain JA: Spontaneous respiration with the Bain breathing circuit. Can Anaesth Soc J 25:30, 1978

109. Spoerel WE: Rebreathing and end-tidal CO_2 during spontaneous breathing with the Bain circuit. Can Anaesth Soc J 30:148, 1983

110. Dean SE, Keenan RL: Spontaneous breathing with a T-piece circuit: Minimum fresh gas/minute volume ratio which prevents rebreathing. Anesthesiology 56:449, 1982

111. Stenqvist O, Sonander H: Rebreathing characteristics of the Bain Circuit: an experimental and theoretical study. Br J Anaesth 56:303, 1984

112. Bain JA, Dick W, Englesson S, et al: does geographical location influence inflow requirements of the Bain breathing system? Eur J Anaesthesiol 1:37, 1984

113. Bain JA, Spoerel WE: Flow requirements for a modified Mapleson D system during controlled ventilation. Can Anaesth Soc J 20:629, 1973

114. Henville JD, Adams AP: The Bain anaesthetic system: An assessment during controlled ventilation. Anaesthesia 31:247, 1976

115. Ungerer MJ: A comparison between the Bain and Magill anaesthetic systems during spontaneous breathing. Can Anaesth Soc J 25:122, 1978

116. Rose DK, Byrick RJ, Froese AB: Carbon dioxide elimination during spontaneous ventilation with a modified Mapleson D system: Studies in a lung model. Can Anaesth Soc J 25:353, 1978

117. Chu YK, Rah KH, Boyan CP: Is the Bain circuit the future anesthesia system? An evaluation. Anesth Analg 56:84, 1977

118. Hannallah R, Rosales JK: A hazard connected with re-use of the Bain's circuit: A case report. Can Anaesth Soc J 21:511, 1974

119. Paterson JG, Vanhooydonk V: A hazard associated with improper connection of the Bain breathing circuit. Can Anaesth Soc J 22:373, 1975

120. Mansell WH: Bain circuit: "The Hazard of the Hidden Tube." Can Anaesth Soc J 23:227, 1976

121. Mansell WH: Spontaneous breathing with the Bain circuit at low flow rates: A case report. Can Anaesth Soc J 23:432, 1976

122. Ayre P: Anaesthesia for intracranial operation: New technique. Lancet 1:561, 1937

123. Ayre P: Endotracheal anesthesia for babies with special reference to hare-lip and cleft-palate operations. Anesth Analg 16:331, 1937

124. Ayre P: The T-piece technique. Br J Anaesth 28:520, 1956

125. Jackson-Rees G: Anaesthesia in the newborn. Br Med J 2:1419, 1950

126. Waters DJ, Mapleson WW: Rebreathing during controlled respiration with various semiclosed anaesthetic systems. Br J Anaesth 33:374, 1961

127. Eger EI II: Anesthetic systems: Construction and

function, Anesthetic Uptake and Action. Baltimore, Williams & Wilkins, 1974, p 206

128. Brown ES, Seniff AM, Elam JO: Carbon dioxide elimination in semiclosed systems. Anesthesiology 25:31, 1964

129. Eger EI II, Ethans CT: The effects of inflow, overflow and valve placement on economy of the circle system. Anesthesiology 29:93, 1968

130. Smith TC: Nitrous oxide and low inflow circle systems. Anesthesiology 27:266, 1966

131. Hamilton WK, Eastwood DW: A study of denitrogenation with some inhalation anesthetic systems. Anesthesiology 16:864, 1955

132. Gorsky BH, Hall RL, Redford JE: A compromise for closed system anesthesia. Anesth Analg 57:18, 1978

133. Ernst EA: Use of charcoal to rapidly decrease depth of anesthesia while maintaining a closed circuit. Anesthesiology 57:343, 1982

134. Lowe HJ, Ernst EA: The Quantitative Practice of Anesthesia: Use of Closed Circuit. Baltimore, Williams & Wilkins, 1981

135. duMoulin GC, Hedley-Whyte J: Bacterial interactions between anesthesiologists, their patients, and equipment. Anesthesiology 57:37, 1982

136. Dorsch JA, Dorsch SE: Cleaning and sterilization, Understanding Anesthetic Equipment: Construction, Care and Complications. 2nd Ed. Baltimore, Williams & Wilkins, 1984, p 415

137. Feeley TW, Hamilton WK, Xavier B, et al: Sterile anesthesia breathing circuits do not prevent pulmonary infection. Anesthesiology 54:369, 1981

138. Garibaldi RA, Britt MR, Webster C, et al: Failure of bacterial filters to reduce the incidence of pneumonia after inhalation anesthesia. Anesthesiology 54:364, 1981

139. Pietak SP: The anaesthetic ventilator. Can Anaesth Soc J 30:S42, 1983

140. Mushin WW, Rendell-Baker L, Thompson PW, et al: Physical aspects of automatic ventilators: Some application of basic principles, Automatic Ventilation of the Lungs. 3rd Ed. Oxford, Blackwell Scientific Publications, 1980, p 132

141. Cote CJ, Petkau AJ, Ryan JF, et al: Wasted ventilation measured in vitro with eight anesthetic circuits with and without inline humidification. Anesthesiology 59:442, 1983

142. Sykes MK, Vickers MD, Hull CJ: Principles of Clinical Measurement. Oxford, Blackwell Scientific Publications, 1981

143. Hill DW: Methods of analysis in the gaseous and vapour phase, Scientific Foundations of Anaesthesia. Edited by Scurr C, Feldman S. 3rd Ed. London, Heinemann, 1982, p 80

144. Saidman LJ, Smith NT (Eds): Monitoring in Anesthesia. 2nd Ed. Boston, Butterworths, 1984

145. Ozanne GM, Young WG, Mazzei WJ, et al: Multipatient anesthetic mass spectrometry: Rapid analysis of data stored in long catheters. Anesthesiology 55:62, 1981

146. Pyles ST, Berman LS, Modell JH: Expiratory valve dysfunction in a semiclosed circle anesthesia circuit — Verification by analysis of carbon dioxide waveform. Anesth Analg 63:536, 1984

147. Waterson CK: The anesthesia machine: Current design and alternatives. Med Instrum 17:379, 1983

148. Saunders RJ, Jewett WR: System integration — The need in future anesthesia delivery systems. Med Instrum 17:389, 1983

149. Arnell WJ, Schultz DG: Computers in anesthesiology — A look ahead. Med Instrum 17:393, 1983

150. Brown BR, Calkins JM, Saunders RJ (Eds): Future Anesthesia Systems. Philadelphia, FA Davis, 1984

151. Hamilton A, Minot GR: Ether poisoning in the manufacture of smokeless powder. J Indust Hyg 2:41, 1920

152. Cohen EN (Ed): Anesthetic Exposure in the Workplace. Littleton, MA, PSG, 1980

153. Dorsch JA, Dorsch SE: Controlling trace gas levels, Understanding Anesthetic Equipment: Construction, Care and Complications. 2nd Ed. Baltimore, Williams & Wilkins, 1984, p 247

154. Vessey MP: Epidemiological studies of the occupational hazards of anaesthesia — A review. Anaesthesia 33:430, 1978

155. Cohen EN: Inhalation anesthetics may cause genetic defects, abortions, and miscarriages in operating room personnel, Controversy in Anesthesiology. Edited by Eckenhoff JE. Philadelphia, WB Saunders, 1980, p 47

156. Ferstandig LL: Trace concentrations of anesthetic gases. Acta Anaesthesiol Scand (suppl) 75:38, 1982

157. Buring JE, Hennekens CH, Mayrent SL, et al: Health experiences of operating room personnel. Anesthesiology 62:325, 1985

158. National Institute for Occupational Safety and Health: Criteria for a Recommended Standard — Occupational Exposure to Waste Anesthetic Gases and Vapors. DHEW Publ No (NIOSH) 77-140. Cleveland, US Department of Health, Education and Welfare, National Institute for Occupational Safety and Health, 1977

159. Mazze RI: Waste anesthetic gases and the regulatory agencies. Anesthesiology 52:248, 1980

160. Whitcher C: Monitoring occupational exposure to inhalation anesthetics, Monitoring in Anesthesia. 2nd Ed. Edited by Saidman LJ, Smith NT. Boston, Butterworths, 1984, p 367

161. Whitcher C: Clinical evaluation two dosimeters

for monitoring occupational exposure to N_2O. Anesthesiology 61:A169, 1984

162. Virtue RW, Escobar A, Modell J: Nitrous oxide levels in operating room air with various gas flows. Can Anaesth Soc J 26:313, 1979

163. Lecky JH: The mechanical aspects of anesthetic pollution control. Anesth Analg 56:769, 1977

164. Waste Anesthetic Gases in Operating Room Air: A Suggested Program to Reduce Personnel Exposure. Park Ridge, IL, American Society of Anesthesiologists, undated

165. American National Standard for Anesthetic Equipment: Scavenging Systems for Excess Anesthetic Gases. ANSI Z79.11-1982. New York, American National Standards Institute, 1982

166. Miller JD: A device for the removal of waste anesthetic gases from the extracorporeal oxygenator. Anesthesiology 44:181, 1976

167. Annis JP, Carlson DA, Simmons DH: Scavenging system for the Harvey blood oxygenator. Anesthesiology 45:359, 1976

168. Muravchick S: Scavenging enflurane from extracorporeal pump oxygenators. Anesthesiology 47:468, 1977

169. Heard SO, Munson ES: Ventilator alarm nonfunction associated with a scavenging system for waste gases. Anesth Analg 62:230, 1983

170. Sharrock NE, Leith DE: Potential pulmonary barotrauma when venting anesthetic gases to suction. Anesthesiology 46:152, 1977

171. Mor ZF, Stein ED, Orkin LR: A possible hazard in the use of a scavenging system. Anesthesiology 47:302, 1977

172. Hagerdal M, Lecky JH: Anesthetic death of an experimental animal related to a scavenging system malfunction. Anesthesiology 47:522, 1977

173. Tavakoli M, Habeeb A: Two hazards of gas scavenging. Anesth Analg 57:286, 1978

174. Sharrock NE, Gabel RA: Inadvertent anesthetic overdosage obscured by scavenging. Anesthesiology 49:137, 1978

175. Patel KD, Dalal FY: A potential hazard of the Drager scavenging interface system for wall suction. Anesth Analg 58:327, 1979

176. Milliken RA: Hazards of scavenging systems. Anesth Analg 59:162, 1980

177. Flemming DC, Johnstone RE: Recognition thresholds for diethyl ether and halothane. Anesthesiology 46:68, 1977

178. Lecky JH: Anesthetic pollution in the operating room: A notice to operating room personnel. Anesthesiology 52:157, 1980

6

Computers in Anesthesia

David A. Paulus, M.D.

INTRODUCTION

If computers are to be used in anesthesia, they must be able to solve problems. To determine how computers do and might help, could but have not, and might but have not, we shall first define anesthesiologic problems from a historical and a contemporary perspective and from the patient's and the physician's perspectives. Once these problems are defined, the attempted computerized solutions to these problems and new innovations will be reviewed.

HISTORICAL PERSPECTIVE

Apparently, the first anesthetic death occurred in 1848 during chloroform anesthesia for toe surgery.[1] But it was not until 1894 that the anesthesia record was devised, although not retained in the medical records at the Massachusetts General Hospital. Although a present-day description of the anesthetic problems that occur intraoperatively would be easy, a commentary on them as well as an editorial about things new as seen by Dr. Harvey Cushing appears appropriate[2]: "I think we both became much more skillful in our jobs . . . particularly due, I think, to the detailed attention we had to put upon the patient by the careful recording of the pulse rate throughout the operation." Of things new he writes:

I find I have written on my reprint the verse from Dr. Holmes' Stethoscope Song:

Now such as hate new fangled toys
Begin to look extremely glum;
They said that rattles were made for boys
And vowed that his buzzing was all a hum.

I have always felt that this was one of the most interesting illustrations on record, of

the reaction against the introduction of an instrument of precision into clinical use. It is precisely what happened in the case of the thermometer, the stethoscope, X-ray and indeed of the watch itself, if one may regard Floyer's first use of the pendulum for this purpose as a watch. . . .

I still feel that one of the most important elements in the giving of anaesthetic is to have the anaesthetist keep during its administration a detailed chart of pulse, respiration, and blood pressure. At the time of his notable address some years ago on Ether Day, Dr. Keen, who took up this subject, intimated that too elaborate a record of this kind might take the administrator's mind from his primary job. I feel most emphatically that it keeps his mind *on* his job.

Figure 6-1 shows one of Codman's early records. However, it was not until years later that arterial blood pressure was routinely measured and recorded during surgery. From this historical background, problems in current practice can be identified and compared, several of which were alluded to by Dr. Cushing.

CURRENT PERSPECTIVE
(Also See Chs. 5 & 12)

Calkins diagrammed what he calls the anesthesia delivery system.[3] At each point within the system exist many potential problems, ranging from potential problems with the anesthesiologist — for example, are attention to and familiarity with the equipment, the patient, and the surgical procedure sufficient? — to the patient whose life depends on proper functioning of the whole system at all times.

Cooper et al.[4,5] analyzed critical mistakes made during anesthesia that occurred at several hospitals involving personnel of various levels of experience. As a result of these investigations, changes in present practice would improve anesthetic safety. A total of 139 anesthesiologists, residents, and nurse anesthetists from two academic and two nonacademic hospitals participated in one of these studies, which reported a total of 1,089 critical incidents.[5] A critical incident was defined as "a human error or equivalent failure that could

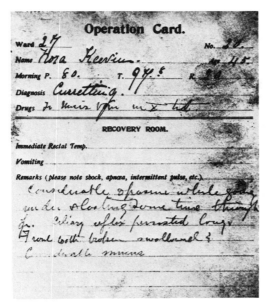 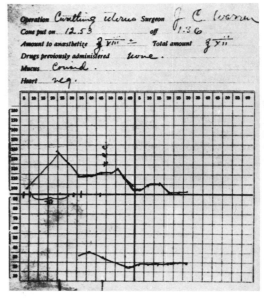

FIG. 6-1 Two sides of an early anesthesia chart, specially designed for this purpose and used for an operation on November 30, 1894, by Dr. E.A. Codman. (Beecher HK: The first anesthesia records [Codman, Cushing]. Surg Gynecol Obstet 71:690, 1940, by permission of Surgery, Gynecology & Obstetrics.)

TABLE 6-1. Distribution of Critical Incidents According to Type of Failure

	Retrospective		Instant Reporting	
	n	%	n	%
Equipment failure	69	11	46	19
Human error	430	70	153	64
Disconnection	80	13	31	13
Other	37	6	9	4
Total coded	616		239	
Nonincidents	541		79	

(Cooper JB, Newbower RS, Kitz RJ: An analysis of major errors and equipment failures in anesthesia management: Considerations for prevention and detection. Anesthesiology 60:35, 1984.)

have led [if not discovered or corrected in time] or did lead to an undesirable outcome, ranging from increased length of hospital stay to death."[5] More than two of every three critical incidents were due to human error and less than one of every five incidents related to equipment failure (Table 6-1). A critical incident that caused death or cardiac arrest or a procedure to be cancelled or that prolonged recovery, intensive care, or hospitalization was defined as having a substantive negative outcome. Only 4 percent of substantive negative outcomes were associated with equipment, while more than 90 percent were associated with human error.

If we are to reduce the risk of anesthesia, we must reduce human error, for which Cooper et al. suggest certain strategies (Table 6-2).

A study of these strategies suggests where computerization may help improve anesthetic care. For example, might computers help in the instruction of practitioners at all levels? Could an "intelligent" terminal provide a second opinion? Since computers provide formats for displaying information, could standard protocols be stored? Would an automated, preanesthetic checklist help stimulate a routine check of equipment? Could some of the checking be done by computer? Can computers help incorporate ergometrics, fluid mechanics, electronics, and other engineering considerations into the design of anesthetic equipment?

The time of critical incidents also contributes to their cause. For instance, Cooper and co-workers reported that critical incidents were distributed over all stages of anesthesia,

TABLE 6-2. Potential Strategies for Prevention or Detection of 70 Incidents with Substantive Negative Outcomes

	Number of Incidents
Additional training	38
Improved supervision/second opinion	20
Specific protocol development	7
Equipment or apparatus inspection	8
More complete preoperative assessment	8
Equipment/human-factors improvements	18
Additional monitoring instrumentation	18
Other specific organization improvements	21
Improved communication	8
Improved personnel selection procedures	5
Unknown (none obvious)	1
Total	152

(Cooper JB, Newbower RS, Kitz RJ: An analysis of major errors and equipment failures in anesthesia management: considerations for prevention and detection. Anesthesiology 60:38, 1984.)

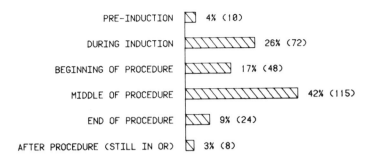

PRE-INDUCTION   4% (10)

DURING INDUCTION   26% (72)

BEGINNING OF PROCEDURE   17% (48)

MIDDLE OF PROCEDURE   42% (115)

END OF PROCEDURE   9% (24)

AFTER PROCEDURE (STILL IN OR)   3% (8)

TOTAL INCIDENTS = 277

FIG. 6-2 Distribution of incidents by stage of anesthesia delivery for induction and in the operating room (OR). (Cooper JB, Newbower RS, Long CD, et al: Preventable anesthesia mishaps: A study of human factors. Anesthesiology 49:404, 1978.)

midway through the surgical procedure being more "dangerous" than anesthetic induction or the end of the procedure (Fig. 6-2).[4] Most of us would think that induction would be the most dangerous time. Consideration must be given to how computers could help alleviate these dangers. Furthermore, at the beginning of the procedure the anesthesiologist has quite a different problem. During this relatively brief period, 26 percent of the preventable mishaps occurred. "This is a stressful time with intense, task oriented procedures requiring tremendous concentration by the anesthesiologist for application of essential manual and mental skills. During this phase of anesthesia, both monitoring and record keeping are severely impeded."[3] So we have two time periods, each with its own character, one of high activity with too much to do in too little time and one of too little to do, when inattention due to boredom may occur.

A time and motion study of anesthesiologists showed that 60 percent of the time they were observing the patient or surgical field and that 40 percent of the time they were looking elsewhere.[6] Also, 72 percent of the time the anesthesiologist was not engaged in manual activity (Fig. 6-3). Writing on the anesthetic record took 6 percent of the anesthetist's time; interestingly, the record was not often used purely for reference.

SUMMARY

There are several problems of medical management in the operating room. Some impinge upon the anesthesiologist, but all of them, in the end, impinge upon the patient.

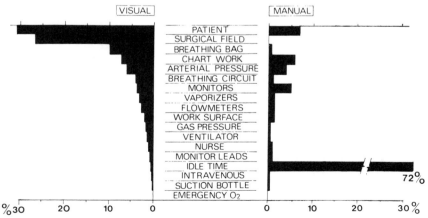

FIG. 6-3 Distribution of anesthesiologists' activities. (Boquet G, Bushman JA, Davenport HT: The anesthetic machine—A study of function and design. Br J Anaesth 52:61, 1980.)

Some of these problems are well suited to computerized solutions:

1. *Repetitive tasks.* The anesthesiologist is asked to remain vigilant to changes in the same parameters throughout the course of anesthesia.
2. *Information overload.* The anesthesiologist must accumulate an enormous amount of data and extract just what is pertinent in a timely fashion.
3. *Complexity.* Although the human body is the most complicated of all "machines," our understanding of it seems quite primitive — we use many fewer instruments to monitor a patient than a pilot uses to monitor an airplane.
4. *Data display.* Data come from different sources with different types of display; the anesthesiologist must therefore gather and integrate information from many sources, some represented by lights, some on meters, some on paper traces.
5. *Equipment control.* The regulation, frequency of measurement, and ranges of normal and alarm settings of many instruments must be coordinated.
6. *Trends.* The anesthesiologist uses the anesthetic record more to record data than to detect trends, but usually the patient's parameters begin to become unsatisfactory over a prolonged period.
7. *Intervention.* The anesthesiologist must continually ask: What parameters can be optimized to improve the patient's condition?
8. *Decision making.* The anesthesiologist must assimilate and assemble data from a multitude of sources in order to reach a proper medical decision.

WHAT IS A COMPUTER?

The definition of a computer has enlarged since the invention of the first electronic digital computer. Initially it was thought of as a device to manipulate numbers and arithmetic. However, any information symbol can be represented in numeric form and can then be manipulated by a computer. A computer then becomes an information processor. As such it may be applied to all human endeavors in which information is used. All we have to do is instruct it ("program" it) properly. By defining a computer as an information processor, descriptive terms such as size and speed become less important.

HOW DOES A COMPUTER WORK?

The electrical elements of all computers have three functions: sensing, judging, and acting. These elements are packaged together to form five logical elements (Fig. 6-4)[7]:

1. *Input.* The input of a computer is the information entered for processing. It may come from physiologic signals (e.g., blood pressure), keyboard, tape, disc, or in some cases voice.
2. *Memory.* Memory is where input, results (intermediate or final), and instructions are stored. Memory may be within the computer or may occur peripherally in tapes or discs.
3. *Arithmetic and logic unit.* This is the site of all calculations — addition, subtraction, division, and multiplication — as well as logic operations.
4. *Control unit.* This unit is controlled by the computer program, which is a series of instructions governing the processing of information and, hence, the overall function of the computer.
5. *Output unit.* The output unit displays the product of the information processing and presents it as instructed by the program. The display may be printed, displayed on a screen, or stored for later display or processing.

Most computers in hospitals are digital computers, defined as "an electronic device capable of manipulating bits of information under the control of sequenced instructions stored within the memory of the device."[7] Basic to the function of the digital computer is the binary system. This system makes use of the fact that an electrical switch is either on or off. If on is represented by a "1" and off by a "0," then information can be coded and deciphered

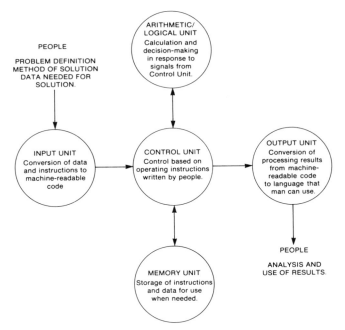

FIG. 6-4 Block diagram of the basic logic elements of a digital computer. (Bronzino JD: Computer Applications for Patient Care. Reading, Mass, Addison-Wesley, 1982, p. 47.)

by a series of 1s and 0s. In our base 10-number system, information is contained by the series of numbers 0 through 9. Compare the representation of values in the binary and decimal system. In the decimal system, the expression "358" is a shorthand way of expressing the following equation:

$$
\begin{array}{rcl}
3 \times 100 & = & 300 \\
5 \times 10 & = & 50 \\
8 \times 1 & = & \underline{8} \\
& & 358
\end{array}
$$

In the binary system, the number 358 is expressed as 101100110, which represents the following equation:

$$
\begin{array}{rcl}
1 \times 2^8 & = & 256 \\
0 \times 2^7 & = & 0 \\
1 \times 2^6 & = & 64 \\
1 \times 2^5 & = & 32 \\
0 \times 2^4 & = & 0 \\
0 \times 2^3 & = & 0 \\
1 \times 2^2 & = & 4 \\
1 \times 2^1 & = & 2 \\
0 \times 2^0 & = & \underline{0} \\
& & 358
\end{array}
$$

The decimal code is a shorter way to express a number but, with the massive storage capacity of digital computers, binary coding is easy. The simple piece of information represented by 0 or 1 is called a bit, while a group of eight bits is called a byte.

Working with long strings of 1s and 0s, the computer, which largely consists of on–off switches, can manipulate information rapidly. The rules, or logic, by which computers work are found in a system of algebra called Boolean logic; three operations called "NOT," "AND," and "OR" are all that are needed for computer calculations. The computer consists of electronic components (hardware) arranged in circuits through which binary information is manipulated and calculated. The instructions (software) for a computer are called a program. The hardware can be considered a system of roads and the software the set of instructions telling us where to turn and how far to drive before we make another turn. Important in all of this is the sequence of instructions, just as the sequence of right and left turns and the mileage intervals are important in driving.

To use a computer, the problem must be defined very precisely and then set up in a step-by-step sequence of operations by which the problem is to be solved. This may be done in a narrative fashion, but a graphic representation of the steps necessary to solve the problem would be more informative. This provides an overview, which allows us to go through a solution element by element. After the problem is defined and the operation sequence drawn on a flow chart, the sequence is reduced to a set of instructions to the computer. This is done by computer programming. To do this, we select a computer language that is known by the user, recognized by the computer, and appropriate to the problem. All of this must be defined exactly for the computer, and each step must occur in an exact sequence; also, ways in which the problem may be altered by an uncommon condition must be taken into account.

Consider the problem, How can the anesthesiologist be warned when the rate–pressure product is too high? Now we must define the problem. First, what is too high? Let us define that as 12,500. To allow more freedom, we may have the physician set the rate–pressure product alarm manually and make 12,500 the default value in case setting the alarm is forgotten. To calculate the rate–pressure product, we must know the systolic blood pressure and the simultaneous heart rate. The frequency at which the calculation is made is also determined. It should be done no more often than the frequency of blood pressure measurements. Usually, the computer is set to calculate the value automatically at fixed intervals (a default setting) or the user can set the frequency.

Thus, we develop a narrative statement of the problem and the operations needed to solve the problem. Unfortunately we cannot easily glance over the narrative or check its logic. A flow chart in which each step in the solution is represented schematically makes such activities much easier (Fig. 6-5). If we were to define our problem and its solution in this way, we could easily alter the sequences. For example, do we always use the default value or only at certain intervals? Do we want to display the product continuously or only when the default value has been reached?

The flow chart can be put into computer language so the problem can be solved by the computer. Different levels of computer language exist and, although many languages are available, we usually think of them in three groups. The first is machine language. This is the working language of the computer. Ma-

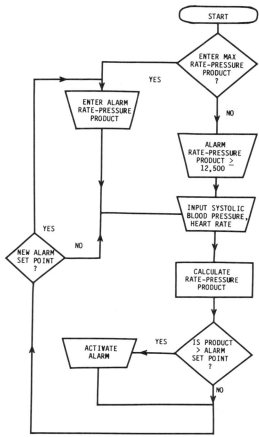

FIG. 6-5 Flow chart for steps necessary to monitor a rate–pressure product.

chine language is difficult to use because it requires that the user know the language and the precise location in computer memory of all the data being manipulated; it is expressed in series of 0s and 1s. It is not used by the novice.

Assembly language is the next level of computer language. Strings of 0s and 1s are replaced by symbolic notation. For example, rather than writing a specified sequence of 1s and 0s to tell the instrument to perform addition, the symbol ADD might be used. This level of sophistication requires a computer for the interpretation of the symbols so they may be reduced to machine language; this is done by an assembler.

At the next level of computer language are

the higher-level languages, which are designed to permit communication with a computer in a more common form of language. This vastly increases the ease of using computers and reduces the level of frustration in programming. The languages are easy to learn, make the creation of a program much easier, and have gained wide acceptance. Because these languages must be interpreted by the computer, they slow the computer and consume much more memory; however, with today's high-speed, large-memory computer, this is of little concern.

INFORMATION MANAGEMENT

Crankshaw suggests that there are four areas of anesthesia in which computers have application.[8] One is auditing records and procedures to establish a medical data base. Another is education, that is, computer-assisted instruction used to present questions and answers to students via an interactive mechanism. Complex systems can be modeled by which students may gain an appreciation of how input interacts to affect outcome.

Manufacturers of medical equipment have made wide use of computers. For example, devices such as automatic blood pressure monitors and infusion pumps, ventilators, gas monitors, and electrocardiographic (ECG) monitors incorporate computers. Processing complex signals such as the electroencephalogram requires a considerable computer program.

A more esoteric area of application is controlling the administration of inhalational or intravenous anesthesia, as well as other drugs such as vasopressors, vasodilators, and insulin. Here a feedback mechanism is used to keep monitored parameters within set limits. Computers are also being used in anesthesia to automate the anesthesia record and in accounting for billing.

AUDITING

Olsson reports on a computer-aided, anesthetic record-keeping system that has been in use for more than 16 years in Sweden.[9] There is a system at the Karolinska Hospital that has computed information from more than 220,000 anesthetic procedures and another system in Stockholm that has computed approximately 100,000 anesthetic procedures per year.[9] The information that is registered includes the following:

Patient's registration number
Patient's name
Date of operation
Clinic or department
Inpatient/outpatient
Elective/emergency surgery
Risk classification (ASA)
Time of starting anesthesia
Time of terminating anesthesia
Operation performed (code)
Anesthetic technique (code)
Hospital
Results, complications, and comments

The results are compiled in an annual record, which has many uses, such as computing complications according to risk classification, which would be useful not only for retrieving information on recent complications during anesthesia, but also for giving administration a sound basis for rational planning and allocation of resources.

COMPUTER-ASSISTED EDUCATION

There have been many attempts at computer-assisted teaching at all levels of education and seemingly in every field. Among some of the earlier attempts in anesthesiology, Attia and co-workers developed a computer program to teach cardiopulmonary resuscitation.[10] These investigators divided first-month anesthesia residents into two groups, which underwent a cognitive evaluation on their first day and on their fifth day. They were provided with reading materials as well as educational objectives. One group was also given computer-assisted instruction. This group showed significantly better learning than the control group. Attia et al. concluded that computer-aided learning was "a highly motivational form of learning." Later Campbell et al.[11] reported that 93 percent of 56 practicing anesthetists who used microcomputers for self-assessment "found the concept of computer assisted self-assessment acceptable." Campbell et al. believed that self-assessment with microcomputers would be a form of peer review acceptable to physicians.

Teaching difficult theoretical concepts is an appealing use of computers in anesthesiology. Heffernan et al.[12,13] reported simulating the pharmacokinetics of halothane and then comparing computer-aided learning, that is, learning with the aid of the simulator, with "traditional" learning, that is, learning without the simulation. The investigators could not distinguish learning engendered by the computer program from that attributable to a tutor but suggested that "the computer simulation . . . stresses principles that cannot easily be demonstrated during clinical anesthesia," and, thus, ipso facto, enhanced the interest of students.

Schmulian et al.[14] used microcomputers for the self-assessment and continuing education of 202 anesthetists who participated in a program in obstetric anesthesia. This study showed that the level of knowledge among anesthetists practicing for a number of years varied significantly. Ninety-one to 100 percent of the participants approved of this method of assessment and continuing education.

McIntyre[15] suggests particular roles for the computer in educating anesthesiologists (Fig. 6-6). He believes that data are insufficient to evaluate computer-assisted learning in anesthesiology but that certain tasks may well be delegated to the computer: "before adopting computer-assisted learning as an instructional system the wise educator will carefully analyze his or her educational problems and the available ways of solving them."

Miller[16] reported in 1983 on a sophisticated computer system that uses techniques of artificial intelligence, known as ATTENDING. This system is designed to work in both a tutorial and a critique mode. In its critique mode the system uses several items as input:

1. A list of a patient's problems
2. The proposed surgical procedure
3. The anesthetic plan, that is, the agents and techniques to be used for the type of anesthesia and for premedication, anesthetic induction, intubation, and maintenance of anesthesia

The system then critiques the plan in terms of risks and benefits. An important differentiation between this system and other medical decision-making systems is that others attempt to simulate decision making. By contrast, ATTENDING acts more to enhance decisions. This system also differs from others in that it deals not with diagnosis but with patient care.

The computer program contains hypothetical cases for educational purposes:

A 34-year-old male with a history of asthma requiring several past hospitalizations comes to surgery after an auto accident for repair of a likely fractured spleen. His blood pressure is 90/50. He recently ate lunch.

The anesthesiologist then outlines the proposed plan. If the plan included (1) induction

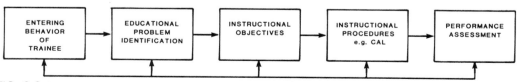

FIG. 6-6 Instructional model for education in anesthesiology. (McIntyre JWR: Computer assisted learning in anesthesiology, Computing in Anesthesia and Intensive Care. Edited by Prakash O. Boston, Martinus Nijhoff, 1983, p. 190.)

with thiopental, (2) rapid sequence intubation with succinylcholine, and (3) maintenance with enflurane, curare, and nitrous oxide in oxygen, the critique would come back as follows:

A number of basic principles are involved in this patient's management. First, in a patient with asthma, one must consider the problem of bronchospasm. Second, in the presence of hypovolemia, one must attempt to prevent hypotension. Third, a patient with a full stomach must be protected from aspiration.

Intubation of this patient is clearly important because of a full stomach. Rapid sequence intubation is a reasonable approach. This does, however, have the possible risk of bronchospasm. An alternative approach, perhaps, to rapid sequence intubation would be intubation after mask induction with cricoid pressure.

In regard to induction, induction using thiopental could have two possible risks. First, in a patient with asthma, there is the conceivable risk of bronchospasm. Second, there is the possible risk of hypotension in the presence of hypovolemia. An alternative approach to induction using thiopental would be induction with ketamine. This has the advantage of helping avoid hypotension, since ketamine is supportive of blood pressure, and of suppressing bronchospasm, since ketamine is a bronchodilator.

From the standpoint of maintenance, inhalational technique has the advantage of preventing bronchospasm by keeping the anesthetic level deep. On the other hand, it could have the risk of hypotension in the presence of hypovolemia. The choice of enflurane involves the conceivable risk of initial bronchospasm resulting from airway irritability. An alternative would be halothane. This has the advantage of helping prevent bronchospasm, since halothane is a bronchodilator. An alternative approach to inhalational technique would be balanced anesthesia. This involves the risk of possible bronchospasm due to light anesthesia. It does, however, have the advantage of maintaining blood pressure.

Looking at other aspects of the proposed plan, there are two considerations worth mentioning: (1) curare would have the conceivable risk of bronchospasm triggered by histamine release, and (2) curare might have the risk of hypotension in the presence of hypovolemia, again, since curare can induce histamine release.

In order to generate such a readable critique, ATTENDING uses artificial intelligence to confront three basic problems: (1) exploring alternative approaches to medical management, (2) evaluating relative risks and benefits of these approaches, and (3) presenting comments and suggestions in readable prose.

To explore alternative approaches, ATTENDING uses augmented decision networks (ADN) to represent a completed anesthetic plan (Fig. 6-7). In this hierarchical system, one starts from an initial state, and a network can be traced by following the arcs from one decision point (circles) to another; for example, two arcs depart and depict general or regional anesthesia. As we traverse the system, networks divide into subnetworks, or subpaths, which divide into more subnetworks to portray a complete anesthesia plan.

RISK ANALYSIS

Miller[16] points out that all anesthetic plans must balance risks. ATTENDING evaluates the risks of each choice by assigning a level of magnitude (low, moderate, high, or extreme) to risks and benefits and then presents a critique in prose (Fig. 6-8). There are several clinical advantages of ATTENDING listed by Miller: (1) the computer becomes an ally rather than a competitor, (2) the physician must evaluate the patient and decisions before seeking computer assistance, and (3) the physician makes the primary decisions.

Among the clinical limitations to ATTENDING are that it deals with a core of anesthetic decisions that excludes other areas, for example, fluids, electrolytes, intraoperative problems, and chronic medications.

SCHEDULING

One of the first uses of computers in anesthesia was for scheduling operations. Ernst and co-workers[17] developed such a schedule in 1977 (Fig. 6-9). Under the function "expand,"

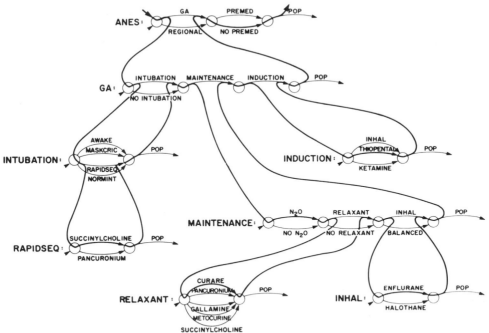

FIG. 6-7 The complete path through the augmented decision networks (ADNs), which corresponds to the sample anesthetic plan (see text). Starting from the initial state (circle) of a network, a path can be traced following one state to another. Such a path ends whenever a POP arc is traversed. GA, general anesthesia. The order of the various decisions in the ADNs is largely arbitrary. (Miller PL: Critiquing anesthetic management: The "ATTENDING" computer system. Anesthesiology 58:366, 1983.)

each surgical request was matched to all the rooms in which it could be performed and to the earliest time the surgeon would be available. The parameters used to limit the "expand" function were as follows:

Operating room information (availability, priority order of services in each operating room, earliest and latest start times)

Procedure information (operating rooms allowed for each procedure, list of procedures according to International Classification of Diseases, Adopted, average degree of difficulty)

Surgical service information (surgeon's priority within each service, surgeon's room preference)

The "order" function was then used to weight requests according to service priority, time, surgeon priority within the surgical service, and room preference. "Sort and assign"

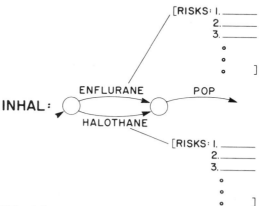

FIG. 6-8 The augmented decision network (ADN) specifying alternative inhalational anesthetics. Each arc has an associated list specifying the possible risks and benefits of using that technique in different circumstances. POP indicates the end of a path from one state to another. (Miller PL: Critiquing anesthetic management: The "ATTENDING" computer system. Anesthesiology 58:366, 1983.)

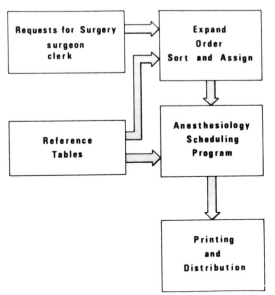

FIG. 6-9 Flow chart for scheduling operating rooms. (Ernst EA, Hoppel CL, Lorig JL, et al: Operating room scheduling by computer. Anesth Analg 56:832, 1977.)

was then used to schedule cases to a particular room at a particular hour, and an anesthesiologist was assigned by an on-line scheduling program. Ernst and colleagues report that the system worked well with "consistently high quality" unaffected by weekends or holidays and minimized problems for the coordinator.

PREANESTHESIA INTERVIEW

Conducting a preanesthesia interview that is thorough, informative to both patient and anesthesiologist, and efficient no matter what the time of day or severity of the disease is not a trivial undertaking. Tompkins et al.[18] reported on a computer-assisted preanesthesia interview that provided rapid and reliable data collection and that conveniently displayed the patient's medical, surgical, and anesthetic histories as well as medications and allergies. To evaluate computer-generated preanesthetic historical summaries, these workers gave the computer-generated summary to one group of anesthesiologists after the preanesthetic visit with a patient and, to another group, before the preoperative visit (Table 6-3). The computer missed fewer findings than did the anesthesiologist; the computer-assisted interview was less variable and more accurate; and the computer summary also appeared to help the anesthesiologist with the interview and to improve the anesthesiologist's retention of pertinent historical information.

MEDICAL EQUIPMENT

Although not widely realized, monitors and other equipment currently used by anesthesiologists in the operating room depend largely on computers.

AUTOMATED BLOOD PRESSURE

Ramsey[19] described the operation of a fully automated electronic blood pressure measuring device that measures blood pressure through oscillometry and noted it is almost identical to the strategy Erlanger developed in 1903. The system operates such that an electronic pump inflates the blood pressure cuff to a pressure above the previous systolic pressure, which is then maintained at a constant level until oscillations and corresponding cuff pressures are received and stored in the memory. The cuff pressure is then decreased incrementally. At each new constant cuff pressure, oscillations are measured and stored. This is repeated until the cuff pressure has decreased five steps below that at which the maximal oscillations occurred. Thus, a table of stored data in the form of the averaged pairs of oscillation amplitudes and the corresponding cuff pressures is accumulated. The mean arterial pressure is that point at which the lowest cuff pressure occurred with maximal oscillation. The systolic and diastolic pressures are defined as when oscillation rapidly increases and rapidly decreases, respectively. The correlation between this method and the invasive method of measuring blood pressure is excellent.[20]

This is a clever use of a small computer that is used for all patients under anesthesia.

TABLE 6-3. Positive Historical Symptoms or Conditions Elicited by Computer and Anesthesiologists

	Positive Symptoms	By Computer		By Anesthesiologist	
		n	%	n	%
Study 1					
Hypertension	4	4	100	3	75
Rheumatic fever	1	1	100	1	100
Congestive heart failure	0	—	—	—	—
Angina	3	4	100	2	67
Other cardiovascular	15	14	93	3	20
Pulmonary/upper respiratory infection	26	24	92	10	38
Renal	5	5	100	2	40
Hepatic	4	4	100	3	75
Endocrine/metabolic	6	5	83	4	67
Central nervous system/ muscular	11	10	91	3	27
Study 2					
Hypertension	4	4	100	3	75
Rheumatic fever	1	1	100	0	0
Congestive heart failure	0	0	—	—	—
Angina	1	1	100	0	0
Other cardiovascular	37	35	95	17	46
Pulmonary/upper respiratory infection	43	40	93	21	49
Renal	16	16	100	4	25
Hepatic	1	0	0	1	100
Endocrine/metabolic	6	6	100	4	67
Central nervous system/ muscular	8	6	75	—	50

(Tompkins BM, Tompkins WJ, Loder E, et al: A computer-assisted preanesthetic interview: Value of a computer-generated summary of patient's historical information in the preanesthesia visit. Anesth Analg 59:9, 1980.)

The computer is automatic, never forgets to measure, knows the alarm limits, and, in short, measures blood pressure as well as a carefully done auscultatory or invasive method.

REAL-TIME OXIMETRY

Among the foremost responsibilities of the anesthesiologist is to ensure that oxygenation is adequate. Along with the observation that arterial blood is "dark" or "the lips look blue," the anesthesiologist must ask: Is it too late? Unfortunately for the patient and the anesthesiologist, changes in heart rate, blood pressure, and cardiac output do not closely parallel oxygenation. Generally, significant desaturation occurs before hypoxia becomes obvious. In the operating room, however, the only other measure of oxygenation is a blood-gas determination. The problem is that a saturation or partial pressure in vitro only indicates the patient's state at a fixed point in time, which, by the time the results are reported to the anesthesiologist, is past.

Hemoglobin saturation and the equations governing the oxygen-carrying capacity of blood have been understood for many years, just as the red color of oxyhemoglobin, which becomes blue when reduced, has also been appreciated for many years. At a given wavelength, light absorption by red oxyhemoglobin differs from that by blue hemoglobin (Fig. 6-10).[21] The Lambert–Beer law is the mathematical expression of this observation

$$I = I_0 \exp(-ECd)$$

where E is the extinction coefficient, C is the concentration of the species sample, d is the

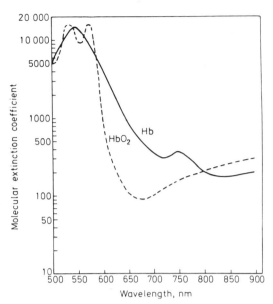

FIG. 6-10 Variation of the molecular extinction coefficients for reduced and oxygenated hemoglobin with light wavelength. (Reprinted by permission of the publisher from Hill DW: Physics Applied to Anaesthesia. 3rd ed. Boston, Butterworths, 1976, p. 338.)

depth of the test chamber, I is the incident light, and I_0 is the light transmitted from the chamber. The application of the Lambert–Beer law and the observation of the relationship between extinction and wavelength allow us to write equations that can determine the oxygen saturation of hemoglobin, for instance, in a finger.

If we wish to look at arterial blood and recognize that arterial blood pulsates whereas venous blood and tissues do not, a convenient location is a fingertip. By subtracting the venous and tissue component of light extinction, we can measure the increase in light absorption with the onset of systole, which is essentially due to arterial blood. The difference in absorption of the nonflow or diastolic baseline from the systolic pulsation reflects the absorption of arterial blood. To solve the equations many times per minute requires a microprocessor. The microprocessor executes an algorithm to determine the pulse amplitude associated with each wavelength. A baseline is established and then, according to Yelderman and Corenman,[22] arterial saturation is calcu-

lated from the ratio of the two wave amplitudes at the two wavelengths. In this fashion, heart rate may also be calculated, which then serves as a check on the system. Arterial saturation then becomes a continuous and current measurement rather than a discontinuous and past measurement.

ELECTROCARDIOGRAPHY AND MYOCARDIAL ISCHEMIA

Although the V_5 chest lead is thought to detect myocardial ischemia early during anesthesia, at least two problems exist: (1) not all episodes of myocardial ischemia result in ST segment shifts at V_5, and (2) continuous observation of the ST segment intraoperatively is impossible without an automated ST trend line. Kotrly et al.[23] have demonstrated a microprocessor devised to determine ST trends. These investigators used an orthogonal lead set, V_5, AVF, and $-V$ (on the back opposite V_1), displayed at four times the normal scale. Using a microcomputer, they sampled the three leads at the J point $+60$ msec, measured the absolute deviation from the isoelectric line, summed the three values, multiplied by four, and displayed the results as a linear trend (Fig. 6-11). With a computer-aided system, leads that are not being displayed can be analyzed automatically and continuously; thus, myocardial ischemia is monitored continuously.

INTRAVENOUS DRUG ADMINISTRATION

Intravenous drug administration in the operating room is done regularly, but frequently the physiologic parameters are inadequately controlled. Precise control of these agents enables excellent medical management of physiologic and neurologic parameters. Another problem is calculating proper dosages.

Skaredoff and Poppers[24] pointed to a study by Lamb et al.[25] in which 10 surgical house officers and 23 experienced critical care nurses were asked to manually compute the rate of dopamine infusion for a particular dose and a

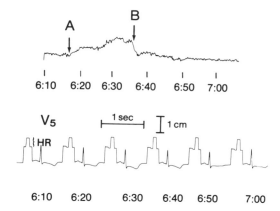

FIG. 6-11 ST trend line (above) and the record of electronically stored V_5 complexes (below). Although the trend line reflects ST segment changes in all three leads that make up the orthogonal set (V_5, AVF, $-V_1$), only the stored V_5 complexes are shown because depression is most obvious in this lead. The generally upward direction of the ST trend line from points A to B indicates the increasing deviation of the ST segment (J point + 60 msec) from the isoelectric line. Point A denotes the time when the patient was put in the head-down position for cannulation of the internal jugular vein. Point B denotes the time when the patient's head was elevated and intravenous nitroglycerin infusion started. To improve clarity, 1-second and 1-cm (1-mV) calibration lines have been substituted for the standard electrocardiographic (ECG) grid lines. Because the electronic markers between stored complexes represent 10 minutes of elapsed time, the 1-second scale may only be used to measure interval times between points on any single ECG complex. The height of the narrow pulse on top of each separating marker preceding the V_5 complexes corresponds to the heart rate (HR), with each millimeter being equal to 10 beats/min. By measuring these pulses, it can be seen that the heart rate increased from approximately 50 to 67 beats/min between 6 : 10 and 6 : 30. (Kotrly KJ, Kotter GS, Mortara D, et al: Intraoperative detection of myocardial ischemia with an ST segment trend monitoring system. Anesth Analg 63:344, 1984.)

patient of a particular weight. Three of the 10 house officers and none of the nurses correctly calculated the rate within 5 minutes. This observation suggests that computer-assisted dose calculation could be quite helpful in this regard.

Sheppard,[26] who has used computer-controlled administration of sodium nitroprusside for many years, showed that blood pressure is better controlled with a computer than without one; a simple feedback mechanism is used (Fig.

6-12).[27] Pace and Westenskow proposed three decision routines for computer-regulated administration of vasoactive drugs.[27] The first is based on waiting until an incremental change in nitroprusside administration has an effect on blood pressure, which dictates the next change in rate administration. This is very similar to manually controlling the infusion pump. The second category is called a proportional-integral-derivative (PID) type. By using a computer, a much tighter control than can be achieved manually is realized. There are three ways to track the difference between the actual and the desired pressure. The first is absolute value, which is a proportional method; the second is rate of change, which is a derivative method; and the third is the accumulated error, which is an integral method. The weighted average of these three measurements is then used to control the infusion rate. Clearly, this degree of sophistication is not possible manually in the clinical setting.

A third category of control uses the adaptive control theory. The patient is described by a mathematical model, and real-time algo-

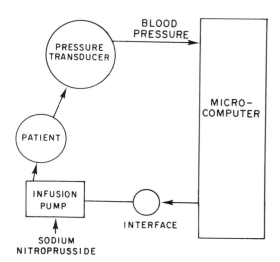

FIG. 6-12 Control system for sodium nitroprusside. The microcomputer uses the difference between the desired blood pressure and the measured blood pressure to adjust drug administration rate. (Pace NL, Westenskow DR: Computer regulated sodium nitroprusside infusion for blood pressure control, Computing in Anesthesia and Intensive Care. Edited by Prakash O. Boston, Martinus Nijhoff, 1983, p. 297.)

rithms are used to control drug administration. With this last method, if a particular patient can be modeled, the control becomes optimal because the coefficients in the mathematical model may be adjusted as experience with the patient is gained. This could be very helpful in avoiding large fluctuations in measured parameters.

IN THE FUTURE

Computers have been used extensively in anesthesia primarily to control monitors as they pertain to one parameter. For example, the microprocessor is used in the automatic oscillometric measurement of blood pressure and has gained wide acceptance. Future efforts will probably revolve around integrating a variety of input for medical and anesthetic management. This will involve feedback loops not dissimilar to those used to control intravenous drug administration. This will require enhanced pattern recognition by computers, smart alarms, voice communication, and an automated anesthesia record.

INHALATIONAL ANESTHESIA

Although there has been discussion for over 100 years of automated anesthesia delivery,[28] few serious efforts have been made. Westenskow and co-workers[29] attempted to computerize the anesthesia machine (Fig. 6-13). The input from the anesthetist includes inspired oxygen concentration, end-tidal anesthetic concentration, circuit volume, and the end-tidal carbon dioxide concentration. In order to operate the system, input analogues are created for the end-tidal CO_2, CO_2 production, airway pressure, tidal volume, volume of the anesthesia circuit, minute volume, inspired oxygen concentration, inspired and

end-tidal inhaled anesthetic concentration, and mean arterial blood pressure.

The computer integrates desired inspired oxygen concentration, end-tidal inhalational agent and CO_2 concentrations, and tidal volume data. Various displays of trends, blood-gas data, and settings are available. Five feedback loops alter ventilation and fresh gas flow. With this system, the worst case of inspired oxygen concentration, considering that oxygen sensors do drift, occurred after 4 hours, inspired oxygen concentration being 4 percent from that desired. The accuracy of oxygen consumption was within 5 percent of its reading.

End-tidal concentration of the inhalational agent was used to control the inspired vapor concentration automatically. Westenskow and co-workers[30] found that they could hold the end-tidal concentration within 0.037 ± 0.067 vol% of the desired concentration. The end-tidal PCO_2 was kept within 0.1 ± 0.17 mm Hg of the desired value even though CO_2 production was variable. The $PaCO_2$ was similarly tightly controlled to within 1.25 mm Hg of that desired.

Using this system in a study of 23 pediatric patients, Westenskow and colleagues[31] observed considerable variability in enflurane uptake (standard deviation greater than 28 percent) among patients but, since the agent was well controlled, variability of end-tidal concentration was less than 0.1 vol% after an 8-minute anesthetic induction. These workers concluded that computer control of fresh gas flows has several advantages: easier use of closed circuit anesthesia, a smoother and more rapid anesthetic induction, and better control of the end-tidal PCO_2.

SPEECH SYNTHESIS AND RECOGNITION

Communication in the operating room between the monitor and the anesthesiologist has historically been visual, ranging from a cathode ray tube to digital displays. The anesthesiologist has usually been alerted to certain measurements, particularly those beyond the normal range, by an audio alarm. The problem with alarms is that there are too many; this

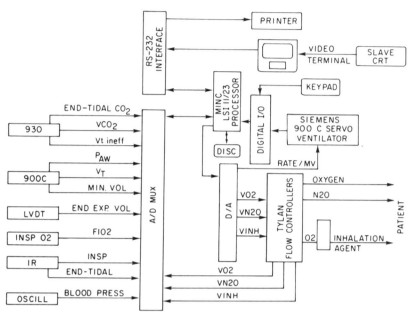

FIG. 6-13 The computer system shown in Figure 6-12 has been added to an anesthesia machine to control the fresh gas flows and to adjust mechanical ventilation. It includes a MINC microcomputer, Tylan mass flow controllers, and a Siemens 900C ServoVentilator. The MINC 11 microcomputer (Digital Equipment Corp, Mynard, Mass.) uses the PDP 11/23 microprocessor with the hardware floating point math package, 64K MOS 16-bit memory, $2\frac{1}{2}$ megabyte disc drives, four programmable clocks, and a graphics terminal. The D/A outputs (12 bit) control the flow of oxygen (0 to 1 L/min) and nitrous oxide (0 to 1 L/min) through mass flow controllers (Tylan Corp, Carson, Calif.). The flow of inhalational agent is controlled by a third Tylan controller, which adjusts the oxygen flow through a copper kettle vaporizer. D/A channels also control the respiratory rate and minute volume of the 900C Servo ventilator (Siemens-Elema, Solna, Sweden) through the ventilator's computer interface. (Westenskow DR, Jordon WL, Hayes JH, et al: Computer control of anesthesia delivery, Computing in Anesthesia and Intensive Care. Edited by Prakash O. Boston, Martinus Nijhoff, 1983, p. 270.)

author recently counted more than 30 in one particular operating room, and their sources can be difficult to locate. Furthermore, the sound of an alarm carries an intimidating, stressful, and even embarrassing connotation.

One potential solution to such problems would be vocal communication. Monitor signals could be relayed to speech synthesizers as well as visual displays. The anesthesiologist could be summoned by a private message through an earpiece that conditions are changing. The message could be toned according to the severity of the situation. For example, a message might be given: "Blood pressure is 120/80, pulse is 75." However, if the blood pressure begins to vary from the normal range, the message might be: "The blood pressure is 155/95 and the heart rate is 100, both are significant increases." As the blood pressure gets

even higher, the messenger, still not panicking, may say: "The blood pressure is 220/120 and the heart rate is 150 beats/min; these values are beyond the alarms you have set and may indicate an emergency." In all these messages the anesthesiologist has received a very private message, one that is graded to the severity of the situation and specific to physiologic parameters that are abnormal.

Vocal communication could also go from the anesthesiologist to the instrumentation, or more specifically to the record keeper. The anesthesiologist is unable, particularly during anesthetic induction, to keep an accurate, detailed record of the patient's condition.[32] Such recording can be done by handwriting or with alphanumeric or special keyboards or bar code readers. According to Sarnat,[33] all these procedures divert the anesthesiologist from the patient. He suggests that data entry by computerized speech recognition would be helpful. In a speech-recognition system, a list of vocabulary words and definitions are programmed, and the user pronounces each word so that the computer learns the word as spoken by the user. Valid sentences can then be constructed. For example, the system may be programmed so that the initial word heard by the computer is the subject of the sentence, followed by the verb. In this fashion sentences can be constructed. So far, computer speech recognition has been found to be 90 percent accurate. The application of speech recognition is still in its infancy in anesthesiology, but in time the vocabulary could include drug names, procedures, drug dosage, and patient's position. Disadvantages of vocal communication include an inflexible response to low volume and offensiveness to the awake patient or distraction to the surgeon.

THE AUTOMATED ANESTHESIA RECORD

Recently several groups have been developing an automated or semiautomated anesthesia record system. Among the current problems of the anesthesia record are a lack of accuracy, legibility, and completeness. An automated anesthesia record could enhance all three aspects. Apple et al.[34] designed and tested a system that records intraoperative physiologic and alphanumeric data. A specially designed key pad with 34 keys and a 32-character alphanumeric display above the key pad is used; a video monitor displays the anesthetic record during the procedure. A data entry key is assigned to each of seven categories: (1) anesthetic gases, (2) intravenous fluids, (3) body fluid losses, (4) blood pressure data, (5) ventilator settings, (6) general patient information, and (7) general events. Drugs are divided into nine categories according to physiologic effect. Data can be entered in real time, in a postentry mode, and in a time-independent mode. When a drug is entered, it is displayed first in a list of choices because drugs are likely to be administered more than once.

Apple and co-workers also developed six video displays that are key-pad controlled, which include a chronological list of all events entered during a case, a list of a specified class of drugs, or four different graphic displays of physiologic data; a printed copy is generated at the end of the case. These workers showed that the key-pad records were more accurate and more legible than handwritten records and that they were usable by administration later on.[31]

Workers at the University of California at San Diego developed what they described as an automated anesthesia record data management and record-keeping system (AADMARKS) with three functions: data acquisition, data processing, and data recording and display. These workers used a multicolor printer plotter to develop the automated anesthesia record.[35] From their experience, Mitchell arrived at several conclusions:

1. Although components are available to generate an automated anesthesia record-keeping system, the cost of high-resolution color graphics and printing devices is a major constraint.
2. User/system interface is necessary.
3. Data selection and raw data display must be autonomous. Processing of data and real-time displays should not have the same format.
4. A commercial application of academic prototypes is slow in development, partly because of a lack of agreement on what an anesthesia record is and should be.
5. The system will only be accepted by anesthesiologists if it reduces their workload and develops a more reliable anesthetic record.

Two new entries into the automatic record-keeping systems produced by commercial enterprises are one developed by Datascope (Fig. 6-14) and another developed by Ohmeda (Fig. 6-15). Although they differ significantly in their approach, neither takes the pen away from the anesthesiologist.

The Datascope™ recorder resembles a clipboard in size and convenience.[36] The left-hand side of the anesthesia record is automatically generated from trends in temperature, blood pressure, heart rate, inspired oxygen concentration, and end-expired CO_2. To the

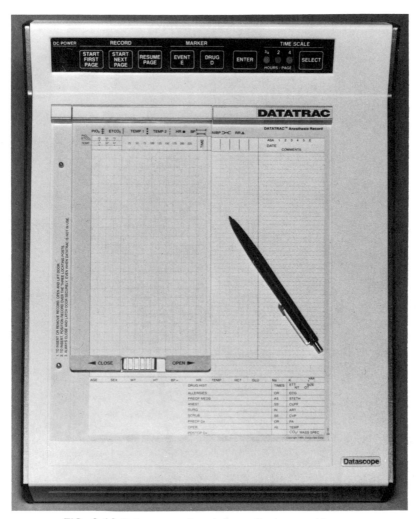

FIG. 6-14 Datascope automated anesthesia record keeper.

right of the automated portion, events and drug notations and special comments can be entered on the record by hand. The system automatically and continuously makes two copies of the record.

The Ohmeda anesthesia record keeper is integral to an Ohmeda anesthesia machine. The record is viewed on the work surface through a plastic cover, which can be lifted to make hand-written entries. Data are transmitted to the record keeper from physiologic monitors and the anesthesia machine and are automatically recorded. The automatic data include heart rate, blood pressure, tempera-

ture, inspired oxygen concentration, and pulse oximetry values. Data are also entered by a menu-driven entry panel; drug names and dosages, fluid type and amount, and demographic data are entered in this way.

Work has also been done at Emory University on automated anesthesia record generation. Workers there recognizing the need, particularly in complex cases, to generate a complete anesthetic record have developed a computer-assisted anesthetic record (CARR), a console that concentrates on optimal data display and standard components including the anesthesia machine, monitoring system, data

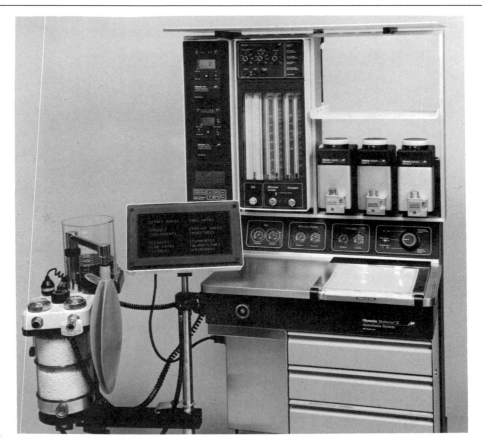

FIG. 6-15 The Ohmeda automated anesthesia record keeper records real-time data from typically employed OR monitors. The information is formatted onto a hard copy record similar to a standard manual anesthesia record. A separate input/display screen is used to enter information not available in electrical signal form. This screen operates as the "key board" using a touch panel approach. The printer is located beneath the table top, and the record is viewable through a plexiglass cover and accessible for hand entries simply by lifting the cover. The data input/display screen is located to the left of the gas machine close to the absorber.

management system, and mass spectrometer. This system allows regeneration of the anesthetic record by a plotter and by hand.[37]

CLINICAL MONITORING

Beneken and Blom[38] suggest that if we are to both increase the number of variables that can be monitored and develop monitoring techniques, we must consider how all these signals are to be processed. These workers developed a matrix (Fig. 6-16). Horizontally there is an increasing number of variables, and vertically the signal processing increases in complexity. If no signal processing occurs, then the number of monitored variables makes them incomprehensible; if one to three variables are monitored, there are not enough data to monitor a patient adequately in all clinical situations. The application of statistics to signals, trend calculation, and comprehensive display

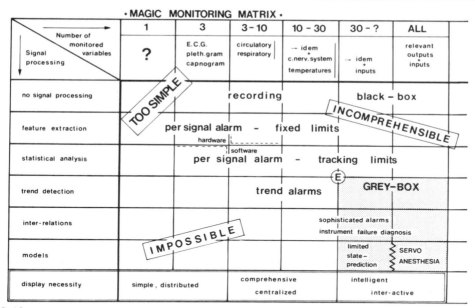

FIG. 6-16 Monitoring in terms of increasing numbers of variables and different levels of signal processing. (Reprinted by permission of the publisher from Beneken JEW, Blom JA: An integrative patient monitoring approach, An Integrated Approach to Monitoring. Edited by Gravenstein JS, Newbower RS, Ream AK, Smith NT. Boston, Butterworths, 1983, p. 127.)

makes monitoring possible. The gray area of the matrix represents when interpretation becomes difficult, that is, information overload.

This approach is quite similar to that of Arnell and Schultz,[39] who represented an information system with a block diagram based on three assumptions. One is that all quantitative variables can be formatted as computer input. Second, the system can be flexible enough that variables not measurable today can be inputted in the future, making flexibility in the type of display important. The third assumption is that many of the data generated in the operating room today are lost. In the proposed information system, we have data acquisition by reliable instruments, which may be numbered in terms of the number of parameters being monitored. Once the data are acquired, they go on to the record keeper, which is automated, and then to the record display.

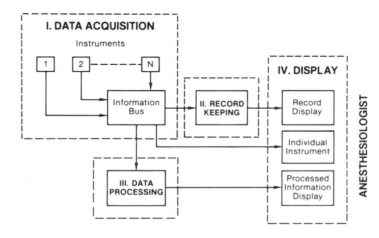

FIG. 6-17 Schematic rendering of the Duke Automatic Monitoring Equipment (DAME) system. (Courtesy of Frank Block.)

THE DAME SYSTEM

The Duke Automatic Monitoring Equipment (DAME) system was developed as a computerized, multichannel, operating room monitoring system.[40] There is an individual unit in each monitoring location, a network that interconnects each unit, a data manager, and a host computer (Fig. 6-17). A single bipolar electroencephalogram (EEG), a single bipolar lead electrocardiogram (ECG), a finger pulsimeter, one thermometer, and one pressure transducer are connected at the front end of a portable monitoring cart; a noninvasive blood pressure monitor is also located on the cart.

Data can be inputted by both keyboard and bar code, the bar code being used to enter drug data and also to modify the screen display and even calibrate the pressure transducer. The input signals are converted to digital form. They are then sent to a computer, which displays information and stores data according to a program for each monitoring package of the data manager, which can also print the anesthetic record.

The DAME system has been used in more than 20,000 cases in 10 operating rooms with good results. Problems include the physical size of the system and the data entry, the keyboard and bar code methods being considered by the system's developers to be inadequate.

CONCLUSION

Computers in anesthesia are being well used and are not, as personal computers have been described, a solution looking for a problem. Our enthusiasm must be tempered so that we do not procure a computer and computer experts at considerable cost and then wonder, as did a department chairman who received a multichannel recorder to replace the previously used smoke drums, "Now that I have this, can you suggest some experiments I can do with it?"

REFERENCES

1. Simpson JY: The alleged case of death from the action of chloroform. Lancet 1:175, 1848
2. Beecher HK: The first anesthesia records (Codman, Cushing). Surg Gynecol Obstet 71:689, 1940
3. Calkins JM: Guest editorial. Med Instrum 17:377, 1983
4. Cooper JB, Newbower RS, Kitz RJ: An analysis of major errors and equipment failures in anesthesia management: Considerations for prevention and detection. Anesthesiology 60:34, 1984
5. Cooper JB, Newbower RS, Long CD, et al: Preventable anesthesia mishaps: A study of human factors. Anesthesiology 49:399, 1978
6. Boquet G, Bushman JA, Davenport HT: The anaesthetic machine — A study of function and design. Br J Anaesth 52:61, 1980
7. Bronzino JD: Computer Applications for Patient Care. Reading, Mass, Addison-Wesley, 1982, p 47
8. Crankshaw DP: Editorial-computer symposium. Anaesth Intensive Care 10:183, 1982
9. Olsson GL: An interactive information system for anaesthesia, Computing in Anesthesia and Intensive Care. Edited by Prakash O. Boston, Martinus Nijhoff, 1983, pp 86–95
10. Attia RR, Miller EV, Kitz RJ: Teaching effectiveness: Evaluation of computer-assisted instruction for cardiopulmonary resuscitation. Anesth Analg 54:308, 1975
11. Campbell D, Kenny GNC, Schmulian C, et al: Computer-assisted self-assessment in anaesthesia: A preliminary study. Anaesthesia 35:998, 1980
12. Heffernan PB, Gibbs JM, McKinnon AE: Teaching the uptake and distribution of halothane. Anaesthesia 37:9, 1982
13. Heffernan PB, Gibbs JM, McKinnon AE: Evaluation of a computer simulation program for teaching halothane uptake and distribution. Anaesthesia 37:43, 1982
14. Schmulian C, Kenny GNC, Campbell D: Use of microcomputers for self-assessment and continuing education in anaesthesia. Br Med J 284:403, 1982

15. McIntyre JWR: Computer assisted learning in anaesthesiology, Computing in Anesthesia and Intensive Care. Edited by Prakash O. Boston, Martinus Nijhoff, 1983, pp 184–192
16. Miller PL: Critiquing anesthetic management: The "ATTENDING" computer system. Anesthesiology 58:362, 1983
17. Ernst EA, Hoppel CL, Lorig JL, et al: Operating room scheduling by computer. Anesth Analg 56:831, 1977
18. Tompkins BM, Tompkins WJ, Loder E, et al: A computer-assisted preanesthesia interview: Value of a computer-generated summary of patient's historical information in the preanesthesia visit. Anesth Analg 59:3, 1980
19. Ramsey M III: Noninvasive blood pressure monitoring methods and validation, Essential Noninvasive Monitoring in Anesthesia. Edited by Gravenstein JS, Newbower RS, Ream AK, Smith NT. New York, Grune & Stratton, 1980, p 44
20. Green M, Paulus DA, Roan VP, et al: Comparison between oscillometric and invasive blood pressure monitoring during cardiac surgery. Int J Clin Monit Comput 1:21, 1984
21. Hill DW: Physics Applied to Anaesthesia. 3rd ed. Boston, Butterworths, 1976, p 338
22. Yelderman M, Corenman J: Real time oximetry, Computing in Anesthesia and Intensive Care. Edited by Prakash O. Boston, Martinus Nijhoff, 1983, pp 328–341
23. Kotrly KJ, Kotter GS, Mortara D, et al: Intraoperative detection of myocardial ischemia with an ST segment trend monitoring system. Anesth Analg 63:343, 1984
24. Skaredoff MN, Poppers PJ: An interactive program for intravenous drug infusion management, Computing in Anesthesia and Intensive Care. Edited by Prakash O. Boston, Martinus Nijhoff, 1983, pp 170–183
25. Lamb J, Rose EA, King TC, et al: A simple, programmable calculator technique for dosage determination and administration of drugs by continuous infusion. Heart Lung 10:72, 1981
26. Sheppard LC: Computer control of the infusion of vasoactive drugs. Ann Biomed Eng 8:431, 1980
27. Pace NL, Westenskow DR: Computer regulated sodium nitroprusside infusion for blood pressure control, Computing in Anesthesia and Intensive Care. Edited by Prakash O. Boston, Martinus Nijhoff, 1983, pp 292–309
28. Clover JS: Remarks on the production of sleep during surgical operations. Br Med J 1:200, 1874
29. Westenskow DR, Jordan WS, Hayes JK, et al: Computer control of anesthesia delivery, Computing in Anesthesia and Intensive Care. Edited by Prakash O. Boston, Martinus Nijhoff, 1983, pp 269–278
30. Westenskow DR, Jordan, WS, Hayes JK: Feedback control of enflurane delivery in dogs—inspired compared to end-tidal control. Anesth Analg 62:836, 1983
31. Westenskow DR, Jordan WS, Hayes JK: Uptake of enflurane: a study of the variability between patients. Br J Anaesth 55:595, 1983
32. Paulus DA, van der Aa JJ, McLaughlin G, et al: A more accurate anesthesia record: the electronic clipboard. (Abstract) Anesthesiology 61: A178, 1984
33. Sarnat AJ: Computerized speech recognition for anesthesia recordkeeping. Med Instrum 17:25, 1983
34. Apple HP, Schneider AJL, Fadel J: Design and evaluation of a semiautomatic anesthesia record system. Med Instrum 16:69, 1982
35. Mitchell MM: Automated anesthesia data management and record keeping. Med Instrum 16:279, 1982
36. Paulus DA, van der Aa JJ, McLaughlin G, et al: A semi-automated anesthesia record keeper, The Automated Anesthesia Record and Alarms. Edited by Gravenstein JS, Newbower R, Ream AK, Smith NT. Stoneham, Butterworths, in press.
37. Frazier WT, Paulsen AW, Harbort RA, et al: Integrated anesthesia delivery monitoring system with computer-assisted anesthesia record generation, 17th Annual Meeting. Arlington, Virginia, Association for the Advancement of Medical Instrumentation, 1982
38. Beneken JEW, Blom JA: An integrative patient monitoring approach, An Integrated Approach to Monitoring. Edited by Gravenstein JS, Newbower RS, Ream AK, Smith NT. Boston, Butterworths, 1983, pp 121–131
39. Arnell WJ, Schultz DG: Computers in anesthesiology—A look ahead. Med Instrum 17:393, 1983
40. Block FE, Burton LW, Rafal MD, et al: Two computer-based anesthetic monitors: the Duke automatic system and the microdame. J Clin Monit 1:30, 1985

7

Statistics in Anesthesia

Dennis M. Fisher, M.D.

INTRODUCTION

As research in pharmacology, physiology, and other scientific disciplines contributes more to the practice of anesthesia, increasingly knowledge will be obtained from scientific literature. The ability to evaluate results from the many journals and textbooks critically depends on the scientific background obtained during medical education and training. In addition, as scientific literature has turned increasingly to statistical analysis to support its conclusions, the clinician must be aware of the techniques of statistics.

Clinicians who are not knowledgeable about the language and techniques of statistics may believe that journal editors will evaluate the appropriateness and accuracy of statistical techniques used in their publications. Unfortunately, this may not be true: several reviews have demonstrated a high incidence of statistical errors in reputable journals.[1,2] In response to these criticisms, one journal, *Circulation Research*, has adopted the policy that articles accepted for publication must undergo review by a statistician.[3] This policy has not been widely accepted, probably because of potential delays in the editorial process, lack of agreement among statisticians themselves, and the additional costs of using a statistical advisor.

The investigator who completes a research project must organize and analyze the data, draw conclusions, and then communicate the results. To embark on this task, he or she should first select the variables to be analyzed. Next, data are summarized so that relationships and contrasts can be examined. After the investigator notes the magnitude and direction of these contrasts, scientific judgment must be applied to determine their importance. Only then should he or she use statistical tools to establish "significance."

In recent decades, emphasis on statistical analysis in research studies has increased.

Readers tend to believe that any conclusion accompanied by the statement "P < 0.05" is true; in turn, all observations not supported by that statement are believed to be untrue. This emphasis on statistical significance has encouraged investigators to focus their analyses on statistical testing rather than actually examining individual data points. When data have been collected, the investigator might call upon one of several resources such as a hand-held calculator, a computer, or even a statistician (many of whom lack expertise in the statistical concerns relating to medicine). The raw data are entered, along with instructions as to which test is desired, and the investigator is "rewarded" with a number of statistical results. For example, when data are analyzed by linear regression, the output from a computer program might state "P < 0.001." If the investigator does not understand terms such as "within-groups variance," "residual mean square," or "standard error of the estimate," the statement "P < 0.001" suggests that the data show a strong statistical association. As we will examine later, for linear regression, the validity of the association is better supported by other statistical statements. However, the uninitiated researcher is usually pleased with the probability associated with this low value and may not devote additional time to interpreting or understanding the results. Of greater importance, he or she may not realize that these results do not ensure that a statistical difference exists, that the correct statistical test was employed, or even that the study was performed in a manner that permits any conclusions to be drawn.[4]

Gaining a thorough knowledge of statistical techniques requires much time and energy. However, most statistical techniques used in medical research are simple. Emerson and Colditz[5] reviewed the statistical tests employed in original articles published in the *New England Journal of Medicine* from 1978 to 1979. They found that seven statistical techniques (descriptive tests, t-tests, contingency tables, nonparametric tests, epidemiologic statistics, Pearson correlation, and simple linear regression) comprised 82 percent of all the tests used in these studies. A compilation of the statistical tests reported in *Pediatrics*[6] articles demonstrates similar findings, as does a review of the two major American anesthesia journals, *Anesthesiology* and *Anesthesia and Analgesia*.

This chapter introduces the reader to the principles governing these simple statistical tests. First, descriptive statistics (how to examine and describe data) and the concept of probability will be discussed. These concepts will then be used to examine the principles of inferential statistics (that is, using statistics to draw conclusions). For each statistical test, the mathematical derivation of that test and examples will be provided. The chapter concludes with a guide to the selection of the appropriate statistical test for a variety of research designs as well as a review of some resources for statistical analysis. This chapter is not a definitive treatise on statistics but rather an introduction to basic principles.

DESCRIPTIVE STATISTICS

The initial step in statistical analyses is to categorize and summarize the data, that is, to apply the techniques of "descriptive statistics."

TYPES OF DATA

The most familiar type of data, *data on a ratio scale*, has two characteristics (Table 7-1). First, the size interval between successive units on the measurement scale is constant. For example, the difference between cardiac outputs of 4 and 5 L/min is the same as the difference between cardiac outputs of 7 and 8 L/min. Second, the measurement scale must have a zero point, and this zero value must have physiologic significance. These characteristics permit statements about the ratio of different values on the measurement scale. For example, a drug effect lasting 30 minutes is twice as long as a drug effect lasting 15 minutes.

Data on an interval scale also have constant intervals but lack a true zero point. For example, most measurements of pressure are referenced to atmospheric pressure (approxi-

TABLE 7-1. Types of Data

Type of Data	Characteristics	Examples
Data on a ratio scale	Measurement scale has constant intervals and a true zero point	Duration of drug effect, cardiac output
Data on an interval scale	Measurement scale has constant intervals, but no true zero point	Airway pressure, body temperature
Data on an ordinal scale	Data are ordered or ranked, not measured	ASA physical status, Apgar scores
Data on a nominal scale	Data are classified not by a numerical measurement but by some quality or attribute	EEG patterns, survival, genotypes of pseudocholinesterase

mately 760 mm Hg) rather than to a true zero point. The pressure represented by 20 cm H_2O (14.7 mm Hg) is not twice as great as the pressure represented by 10 cm H_2O (7.4 mm Hg). To calculate the true ratio, we would have to convert the pressures to absolute measurements by adding the reference zero value, in this case 760 mm Hg. Similarly, the temperature represented by 36°C is not twice the temperature represented by 18°C.

For many physiologic variables, there are known numerical differences between subjects. However, the data may indicate only a relative, rather than a measurable, difference between subjects. For example, a patient whose ASA physical status is III is a greater risk of harm from undergoing anesthesia than is the patient having a physical status of I. However, the difference in terms of degree of illness between patients having a physical status of II and those having a status of III is not necessarily the same as the difference between patients having a status of I and those having a status of II. Similarly, an Apgar score of 8 is better than one of 5; however, the difference between these two scores, in terms of neurobehavioral well-being, is not necessarily the same as the difference between Apgar scores of 5 and 2. These scoring systems are examples of *data on an ordinal scale*. Ordinal scales have arbitrary intervals that describe relative, rather than absolute, relationships between the ranks. They convey less information than data on a ratio or interval scale, because only relative comparisons can be made (e.g., that an Apgar score of 10 is better than a score of 5). In medical literature it is common to see data on an ordinal scale treated as if they were on a ratio or an interval scale. For example, the extent of sensory blockade produced by spinal or epidural anesthesia is often reported in units of dermatomes, although a segment in the sacral region may not be identical, in terms of the amount of anes-

thetic required to produce loss of sensation, to a segment in the thoracic region. The treatment of ordinal data with statistical techniques more appropriately applied to interval or ratio data is so common as to be widely accepted.[7] Nevertheless, special techniques are available that are more appropriate for the analysis of these types of data.

On occasion, we choose to describe, that is, name, a variable in terms of a quality rather than a quantity. Variables described in this fashion are called *data on a nominal scale*. For example, electroencephalographic waveforms can be identified as α, β, θ, or δ. Similarly, genotypes of pseudocholinesterase are identified by names rather than by numerical measurements.[8] To permit mathematical comparisons, we can obtain ratio-scale measurements of pseudocholinesterase activity for each of the genotypes. Using these ratio scale measurements, rather than the nominal-scale measurements, we can make comparisons of the various groups. Finally, some variables have only two possible attributes. For example, after surgery, a patient is either alive or dead.

The investigator must correctly identify the type of data collected. Only then can the appropriate statistical analysis be applied.

SIGNIFICANT DIGITS

For all measurements, there are limits to precision. For example, blood pressure is usually measured to the nearest millimeter of mercury; and arterial oxygen (PaO_2) and carbon dioxide ($PaCO_2$) partial pressures, to the nearest millimeter or, at best, the nearest tenth of a millimeter of mercury. In neuromuscular studies, because the ulnar nerve is usually stimulated less frequently than once every 5 seconds, onset times cannot be measured with a precision of greater than 5 seconds. Whenever data are reported, a greater degree of precision should not be suggested than really exists.

POPULATIONS AND SAMPLES

Inherent in statistical analysis of a measured variable is the desire to draw conclusions about that variable. To accomplish this goal, the investigator could measure the variable for the entire population. For example, if we were interested in knowing $PACO_2$ for all adult patients anesthetized with an end-tidal concentration of halothane of 1.0 percent at the University of California, San Francisco, in 1984, we could measure that variable in all eligible subjects. The values for $PACO_2$ might then be presented in a histogram displaying the number of subjects having each value of $PACO_2$; the histogram might also display the percentage of subjects having each value of $PACO_2$ (Fig. 7-1).

Obtaining measurements for all eligible subjects would be cumbersome and expensive. To simplify the task, we might select a smaller sample of the original population and assume that this sample represents the entire population. Values for $PACO_2$ for a hypothetical sample are shown in Figure 7-2. Note that extreme values (greater than 58 mm Hg and less than 36 mm Hg) are not represented, nor are certain intermediate values (e.g., 42, 44, 45 mm Hg). Using these data, we cannot conclude that $PACO_2$ is always somewhere between 36 and 58 mm Hg during light halothane anesthesia, only that extreme values did not occur in this sample. The values obtained from this sample of 12 subjects suggest that during light halothane anesthesia, $PACO_2$ is frequently between 40 and 52 mm Hg.

Although measurements have been made on 12 subjects, the purpose of our study was to make predictions about a larger group, the entire population of adults undergoing light halothane anesthesia. In order for this prediction to be valid, we must assume that the sample represents the entire population. If this assumption is not true, the results may not apply to the entire population. For example, Stanley and Webster[9] found that fentanyl, in doses of 50 μg/kg, provided sufficient anesthesia for cardiac surgery; however, subsequent studies suggested that larger doses are necessary for most patients. The studies by Stanley and Webster were conducted in Salt Lake City, a community that is predominantly Mormon. Because Mormons abstain from alcohol and other drugs, the low-dose requirement observed by Stanley and Webster may have resulted from the personal habits of the subjects; therefore, this sample may represent the population of Salt Lake City, Utah, but not the population of the United States. Recognizing these types of bias is important. If possible, these biases should be avoided. If they cannot be avoided, they must be stated.

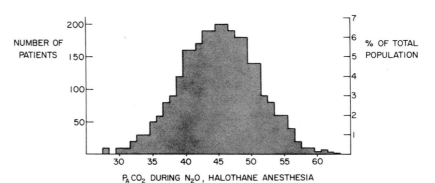

FIG. 7-1 Histogram showing hypothetical values for $PACO_2$ for all patients undergoing light halothane anesthesia at the University of California, San Francisco, during 1984. The *X* axis represents values for $PACO_2$. There are two *Y* axes. The left-hand axis represents the actual number of patients with each value of $PACO_2$. The right-hand axis shows these values as a percentage of the total population.

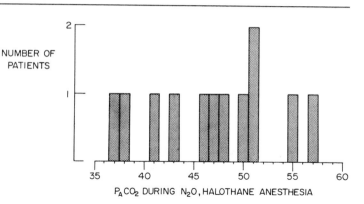

FIG. 7-2 Histogram showing hypothetical values for $PACO_2$ obtained from 12 subjects undergoing light halothane anesthesia. These 12 values represent a sample taken from the values in Figure 7-1.

CENTRAL TENDENCY

After the investigator selects the sample population and obtains measurements, he or she must then describe the results. All the measured values could be displayed as in Figure 7-2 or in other formats such as a table. Although these methods of data presentation permit the reader to make judgments about the individual data points, they limit communication about the general nature of the sample. To describe a variable for the entire population, the investigator would like to be able to select the single value from his or her sample that would represent the "center" of the entire population, a value known as the *index of central tendency*.[10] If all the values in the sample were identical, the investigator would report that single value. However, for most variables, the sample will contain many different values for individual members.

MEAN

The value most widely used to represent the population is the *arithmetic mean*, usually referred to as the mean. The mean is determined by adding all the values of the population and dividing by the number of values in the population. This is described mathematically as population mean = sum of observations/number of observations. When a large number of terms is being summed, a shorthand

way of expressing the process, called "summation notation," is used:

$$\mu = \frac{\sum_{i=1}^{N} X_i}{N} \quad (1)$$

where μ is the population mean, X_i are the individual values, and capital sigma (Σ) means to sum these values. Therefore, this expression is read as follows: μ is equal to the sum of all individual values from X_1 to X_N divided by N. Since we usually sum all the values of the population, it is conventional to omit several of these symbols and write

$$\mu = \frac{\sum X_i}{N} \quad (2)$$

When the investigator is studying a sample rather than the entire population, another term, $\overline{X}$, is used to represent the sample mean. $\overline{X}$ is equal to the sum of all measurements in the sample divided by the number of measurements in the sample. The mean is expressed with the same units as the individual observations.

MEDIAN

Alternatively, central tendency might be expressed with the median or the mode. To determine the median, the individual values are ranked from smallest to largest (or from largest to smallest). The *median* is the "middle" measurement, i.e., the value below which half of the values lie and above which the other half lie. Because the median is based on the rankings of the values rather than the magnitude of the individual values, the median is used infrequently in statistics.

MODE

The *mode* is the value that occurs most frequently. With the small number of observations in many medical studies, there will be no mode if each observed value occurs only once.

The arithmetic mean is a valid description of the location of the population only when ratio or interval data are used; for nominal data, the arithmetic mean has no meaning. For example, the arithmetic mean of 5 is not the appropriate value to describe a sample consisting of subjects having Apgar scores of 0 and 10.[11] Instead, the location of the sample is more accurately described with values such as the median or the mode, or in this case, with individual values.

For many sets of measurements, the arithmetic mean will represent the population accurately. For the measurements of $PaCO_2$ during halothane anesthesia, the arithmetic mean is $(37 + 38 + \cdots + 57)/12$ or 47 mm Hg. Individual values range from 37 to 57 mm Hg and most are between 40 and 52 mm Hg. Thus, the arithmetic mean of 47 mm Hg is "close" to each of the members of the sample and can be considered a fair representative of all the members of the sample.

In contrast, two patients in this small sample had values of 51 mm Hg, making this value the mode. Although the mode is theoretically a measure of central tendency, in this instance it lies near one extreme of the sample and therefore does not represent the population. Since the number of members of this sample is even, no value lies exactly in the middle. In such circumstances, the median is taken to be the average of the two values ranked nearest the middle of the population (47 and 48 mm Hg, respectively), that is, 47.5 mm Hg. Therefore, of the three values describing the location of this population, the mean and median represent the population well, whereas the mode does not. In all statistical analyses, the investigator must examine the values in his or her sample to determine how the central tendency of the sample can best be described.

Finally, just because we have selected a value to represent the sample does not necessarily imply that this value represents the larger population from which the sample was drawn. For example, our sample might have been biased towards, or away from, certain members of the population; or by chance we might have selected highly unusual members of the population. We must always remember that the mean represents the sample, rather than the population. If we extrapolate conclusions to the population, we must also consider our sampling process and the ability of this sampling process to identify the mean of the population.

DATA TRANSFORMATION

Most samples can be well represented by one of these three indicators of central tendency, particularly the arithmetic mean. However, some samples are not well represented by the arithmetic mean. Feinstein[12] determined that the arithmetic mean for four concentrations of hydrogen ion (0.3162×10^{-1}, 0.2512×10^{-3}, 0.1995×10^{-6}, and 0.1259×10^{-8}) was 0.0797×10^{-1}. This value is close to the first member of the sample and far from the other three. Rather than use the arithmetic mean to locate the central tendency of the population, he suggested using another indicator, the geometric mean, which is equal to the nth root of the product of each of the observations. Therefore, the geometric mean of these four concentrations would be $[(0.3162 \times 10^{-1}) \times (0.2512 \times 10^{-3}) \times (0.1995 \times 10^{-6}) \times (0.1259 \times 10^{-8})]^{1/4}$, or 0.6683×10^{-5}. In this instance, the geometric mean, being larger than two of the observations and smaller than the other two, is more representative than is the arithmetic mean. Alternatively, the hydrogen ion concentrations could be converted to pH values of 1.5, 3.6, 6.7, and 8.9, respectively. The arithmetic mean of these pH values is 5.2, which corresponds to a hydrogen ion concentration of 0.6683×10^{-5}. Thus, the central tendency of hydrogen ion concentration is best expressed using the geometric mean, whereas the central tendency for pH is best expressed using the arithmetic mean.

The above example demonstrates how data might be converted to an easier-to-use form ("transformed" or "coded") by applying simple arithmetic processes such as taking the logarithm or square root of each value. Data transformation permits easier manipulation of the data or changes the distribution. Before using a calculator or computer to determine the arithmetic mean, the investigator should examine the data to determine whether the arithmetic mean is representative of the sample and whether transformation may be necessary to improve statistical analysis.

THE NORMAL DISTRIBUTION

The ability of the arithmetic mean to express the central tendency of the population is a function of the distribution of the values within the population. For many variables, such as $PaCO_2$ (shown above), values tend to cluster around a central value, fewer values being located towards the extremes. If one obtains a sufficiently large sample, for many biologic variables the histogram would assume the shape of a bell (Fig. 7-3A). This distribution, known as the "normal" distribution, was first described by de Moivre[13] but is credited to Karl Gauss, being called the Gaussian distribution. Many statistical tests described in this chapter assume that the population under examination is distributed normally. Because medical studies often use a small sample size, the assumption that resulting data have a Gaussian distribution frequently is not tested.

Populations that do not have a Gaussian distribution may assume a number of different shapes (Fig. 7-3B,C). For example, administration of an imaginary drug, histodrenaline, might result in the release of histamine in some individuals and in the release of catecholamines in others. Therefore, if we measured the change in blood pressure after administration of this drug, half the subjects might have an increase in blood pressure while the other half had an equal decrease (Fig. 7-3B). If the

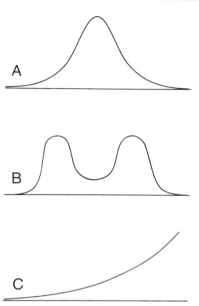

FIG. 7-3 The distribution of values for a population may assume many shapes. One shape frequently encountered in biologic experiments is the normal distribution (A). On occasion, distributions may be bimodal, i.e., humped (B), or J-shaped (C).

mean value were zero, we might be led to believe that histodrenaline had no cardiovascular effects. A more appropriate conclusion would be that the arithmetic mean did not represent the population. The importance of examining the distribution of the data points should now be readily apparent: on occasion, the investigator will find that the arithmetic mean should not be used to describe the population. In that case, alternate methods of describing the results of the study, such as a histogram or table, become essential.

VARIABILITY

Identifying the central location of the sample is not sufficient to describe the population entirely. For example, had all $PaCO_2$ values during halothane anesthesia ranged from 44 to 49 mm Hg, the mean might have been 47 mm Hg. Although the mean for this sample would have been the same as that for the sample described earlier, these two samples probably describe different populations, one having a broad range of $PaCO_2$ values during halothane anesthesia and the other having a narrow range. Thus, in addition to describing the central location of the sample, we need to describe how dispersed the data are, that is, the variability of the sample.

MEAN DEVIATION

One technique used for this purpose is to find the average deviation from the mean. However, because some deviations are positive and others negative, their sum is always zero; therefore, the average deviation has no value as an indicator of dispersion of the data. Alternatively, the investigator could sum the absolute values of these differences from the mean and divide by n, thus producing the *mean absolute deviation*. This technique is mathematically cumbersome and has not become popular.

SUM OF SQUARES

Another approach to the problem of describing how dispersed the data are is to sum the square of the deviations from the mean, a method that eliminates the negative signs and produces positive values. Squaring the deviations has a second effect: it increases ("weights") the contribution of the values according to their distance from the mean. For example, if the deviations from the mean were $-1, -5, +1$, and $+5$, the sum of squared deviations would be 52. A sample containing deviations of $-3, -3, +3$, and $+3$ would produce a smaller sum of squared deviations, 36. Although the mean absolute deviation (3) is the same for both samples [$(1 + 5 + 5 + 1)/4$ or $(3 + 3 + 3 + 3)/4$], the sample containing values more distant from the mean has the larger sum of squares. This sum of the squared deviations from the mean, known as the *sum of squares* (SS), is a fundamental tool used repeatedly in statistics. It is expressed mathematically as

$$SS = \sum (X_i - \bar{X})^2 \qquad (3)$$

Calculating the value of this equation requires two passes through the data: the first pass to sum the individual values to determine the mean value, and the second pass to determine the difference between individual values and the mean. Calculators and computers reduce this to a single step, known as a *machine formula*, which is derived as follows:

$$SS = \sum (X_i^2 - 2X_i\bar{X} + \bar{X}^2) \qquad (4)$$

This can be expanded to

$$SS = \sum X_i^2 - \sum 2X_i\bar{X} + \sum \bar{X}^2 \qquad (5)$$

The second part of this equation can be simplified to $2 \times \bar{X} \times \sum X_i$, which is equal to $(2 \times \sum X_i / N \times \sum X_i)$, or $[2 \times (\sum X_i)^2 / N]$. Similarly, the third part of the equation can be simplified to $(N \times \bar{X}^2)$, or $[N \times (\sum X_i / N)^2]$. Since $(\sum X_i / N)^2$ is equal to $(\sum X_i)^2 / N^2$, the formula can be simplified to

$$SS = \sum X_i^2 - \frac{\left(\sum X_i\right)^2}{N} \qquad (6)$$

Using this machine formula, we can determine the sum of squares in a single pass through the data; this technique greatly simplifies data manipulation.

VARIANCE

Dividing the sum of squares by the sample size yields the average squared deviation from the mean, also known as the *mean squared deviation* or *population variance* (σ^2):

$$\sigma^2 = \frac{\sum (X_i - \mu)^2}{N} \qquad (7)$$

This formula is read as follows: population variance is equal to the sum of the squared differences between individual values and the population mean, divided by the sample size. Usually we are dealing with samples rather than populations, and when we calculate the *sample variance*, we must use the sample mean as an estimate of the population mean. If we represent the difference between the sample mean and the population mean as ϵ, equation (7) could be written as

$$\text{Sample variance} = \frac{\sum [X_i - (\bar{X} + \epsilon)]^2}{N} \qquad (8)$$

As with Equation (3), this can be expanded to

$$\text{Sample variance} = \frac{\sum (X_i - \overline{X})^2 - 2 \sum \epsilon(X_i - \overline{X}) + \sum \epsilon^2}{N} \tag{9}$$

The first term is what we would obtain had we used the sample mean instead of the population mean to estimate the sample variance. The second term always equals zero, because it is equivalent to the sum of the average deviations from the mean. The third term is equal to $N\epsilon^2/N$ or ϵ^2. Thus, the estimates for sample variance differ when it is determined using sample mean rather than population mean, sample variance being underestimated by the amount ϵ^2. Since we usually do not know the population mean, we might use the sample mean to calculate sample variance. This, however, would produce a biased estimate. We correct for this bias by decreasing the denominator by 1. This process produces a better estimate for sample variance (s^2):

$$s^2 = \frac{\sum (X_i - \overline{X})^2}{N - 1} \tag{10}$$

The corrected denominator then represents the *degrees of freedom* (*df*). If there are N values that are squared and summed to determine the sample variance [Equation (10)], after one determines the $N - 1$th value, the remaining difference has been predetermined [the sum of the average deviations from the mean $[\Sigma(X_i - \overline{X})]$ must equal zero]. Thus, the number of independent values used to calculate sample variance differs from the sample size and is known as the "degrees of freedom." A more elaborate proof that using $(N - 1)$ as the denominator yields a less biased estimate is available elsewhere.[14]

STANDARD DEVIATION

Although it is possible to express variability of the sample or the population using the respective variances, this is impractical because the units for variance for a sample are different from those for the population. [Since variance is determined by squaring the differ- ences between individual values and the mean, the units for variance consist of the square of the original units. For example, for $P_{A}CO_2$ values, the units for variance would be $(\text{mm Hg})^2$.] A more common approach is to obtain the square root of the variance, known as the *standard deviation*. As before, the standard deviation for the population (σ) and the standard deviation for the sample (s) differ depending on whether N or $(N - 1)$ is used in the denominator. In most situations, the standard deviation of the sample, rather than of the population, should be used, even though it is a larger number.

Now we have estimated the central tendency and the variability of the sample, two values that describe the location and dispersion of the entire sample. If the population has a Gaussian distribution, most values lie near the mean and only a few values lie far from the mean. That is, approximately 68 percent of the values lie within 1 SD above or below the mean, approximately 95 percent lie within 2 SD above or below the mean, and more than 99 percent of all values lie within 3 SD of the mean.[*]

Returning to the values for $P_{A}CO_2$ during halothane anesthesia, we find that the standard deviation is 6.3 mm Hg. If we examine values ranging from 1 SD below the mean ($47 - 6 = 41$ mm Hg) to 1 SD above the mean ($47 + 6 = 53$ mm Hg), we find that two-thirds of the values in the sample lie in this range and that one-third lies outside this range. The range from 2 SD below the mean to 2 SD above the mean (34 to 60 mm Hg) includes all the values in this sample. If $P_{A}CO_2$ for any subject had been higher than 65 mm Hg or lower than 29 mm Hg, 3 SD below or above the mean would have been necessary to include those values.

---

[*] In a Gaussian distribution, 95 percent of all values are actually found within 1.96 standard deviations of the mean. The range of 2 SD from the mean actually includes 95.44 percent of all values. However, it is common practice to use 2.0, rather than 1.96, standard deviations to describe the variability of populations.

COEFFICIENT OF VARIATION

If the sole information communicated about a sample is that the standard deviation is 6 mm Hg, we cannot assess whether variability is large or small. For a mean arterial pressure of 100 mm Hg, a standard deviation of 6 mm Hg is small; however, for a pulmonary artery pressure of 12 mm Hg, a standard deviation of 6 mm Hg suggests greater variability. The ratio of standard deviation to the sample mean is known as the *coefficient of variation* and is often expressed as a percentage. The coefficient of variation is valuable in describing the variability of the sample. Since the units of the numerator and denominator are the same, the coefficient of variation has no units.

STANDARD ERROR OF THE MEAN

If we were to repeat our measurements of $PaCO_2$ during halothane anesthesia in another 12 subjects, we would probably obtain slightly different results. For example, $PaCO_2$ values might be 34, 36, 40, 41, 44, 44, 47, 48, 48, 49, 54, and 55 mm Hg. The mean of this sample would be 45 mm Hg and the standard deviation 6.5 mm Hg. A third sample of 12 subjects might yield a mean of 44 mm Hg; additional samples might have mean values of 43, 44, 48, and 49 mm Hg. Which of these mean values best represents the population? Had we not divided these patients into six groups, we would have had a single sample containing 72 members. The mean value for such a sample would have been 46 mm Hg. This could be calculated by summing the values for all 72 subjects or by determining the weighted average of the means for the individual groups: $[(12 \times 43) + (12 \times 44) + (12 \times 45) + \cdots + (12 \times 49)]/(12 + 12 + 12 + \cdots)$, or $3,312/72$ or 46 mm Hg. These different techniques yield identical results. Since this new mean value, the mean of mean values (also known as the "grand mean"), was obtained from a larger sample, it better represents the population than each of the other values. As sample size increases, so does the ability of the sample to represent the population from which it came.

Since the sample mean is only an estimate of the mean of the population, we would also like to describe how closely this value approximates the population mean. This is accomplished with the *standard error of the mean* (SEM), also called the *standard error* (SE). The SE is obtained by dividing the standard deviation of the sample (or population, if appropriate) by the square root of the size of the sample. The term "standard error of the mean" is curious, because this value is neither "standard" nor an error. This phrase originated during the Industrial Revolution, at which time reproducibility of measurements was important. If one measured the length of an object repeatedly, successive measurements would differ slightly, and an individual measurement would be unlikely to represent the true length of the object. Repeating the measurement and determining the average of these measurements provides a better estimate. If we then calculate the standard error of the mean value, we determine the "error" with which our measurement was made or how far from the true length the measured values are.

Using our initial set of values for $PaCO_2$ during halothane anesthesia, we find that the standard error is $6.3/12^{1/2}$, or 1.8 mm Hg. Just as approximately 68 percent of the sample lies within 1 SD of the mean, approximately 68 percent of all sample means lies within 1 SE of the population mean. As before, increasing the range to 2 SE above and below the population mean increases to approximately 95 percent the likelihood that the sample mean is included. Expanding the range to 3 SE increases the likelihood to more than 99 percent. Note that doubling the population does not decrease the standard error by a factor of 2; to decrease the standard error by 2, one would have to increase the population by a factor of 4.

CONFIDENCE LIMITS

These ranges, when used to describe the mean, are called *confidence limits*. The 68 percent confidence limits include all values from 1 SE below the mean to 1 SE above the mean (written as "mean ± SE"). More commonly reported are the 95 percent confidence limits, which include all values within 2 SE of the mean (mean ± 2 SE). Since the likelihood is 95 percent that the mean is included in these confidence limits, they are a valuable way to describe both the location and the variability of the mean.

WHAT TO REPORT: STANDARD DEVIATION OR STANDARD ERROR?

When reporting data, investigators must decide whether to report the standard deviation or standard error of the mean. This decision should follow from the purpose of the study, which is, usually, to describe the sample in order to predict values for the population. Because the standard deviation describes the variability of the sample and, hence, is used to estimate values for the population, it seems that standard deviation should always be reported.

Why, then, are standard errors reported with such frequency? The answer to this question lies in the mathematical relationship between the two values, standard error being standard deviation divided by the square root of the sample size. This relationship means that the standard error is always smaller than the standard deviation; the difference between the two increases as the sample size increases. When describing a sample, it is a common practice to provide the mean ± a value describing variability without identifying whether that value is the standard deviation or the standard error.[15] Since the standard error is the smaller of the two values, it suggests less variability than would the standard deviation.

Two solutions might lessen the ambiguity. First, since it is usually more important to describe the variability of the population rather than the variability of the mean (and the standard error can be calculated by the reader if sample size is reported), perhaps investigators should be required to report only standard deviation rather than standard error. A simpler solution would be to require that all values describing the sample be identified as standard deviation or standard error, a practice occurring with increasing frequency. Whenever standard error is reported, the investigator should ensure that the reader can determine the sample size for that value and thus be able to calculate standard deviation.

z TRANSFORMATIONS

If we select a single value from the population, it would be of value to know the location of that value within the population. For example, if we found that 30 minutes after administration of pancuronium, subject A had a serum drug concentration of 150 ng/ml, we might inquire how that subject compared in that regard with other subjects given the same dose. If we knew that the average serum drug concentration for a number of other subjects was 200 ng/ml 30 minutes after drug administration, we could conclude that the value for subject A was lower than the mean. However, without knowing the distribution of data for the other subjects, we would not be able to conclude whether this subject had an unusual response. If we also knew the standard deviation for the other subjects, we would be able to better estimate whether this subject differed from others. If the standard deviation for the sample were 40 ng/ml, the value for subject A would be less than 2 SD from the mean. In contrast, if the standard deviation was 5 ng/ml, the value for subject A would be 10 SD below the mean; such an occurrence would represent an unusual response.

The distance that a value lies from the mean can be expressed mathematically as the difference between that value and the mean divided by the standard deviation. This statistic, known as the z *transformation*, is calculated as

$$z = \frac{X_i - \overline{X}}{\sigma} \qquad (11)$$

If z is large, the new value is far from the mean; if z is small, the value is near to the mean.

PROBABILITY

If we measured $PaCO_2$ in a single subject undergoing light halothane anesthesia, we might obtain a value of 61 mm Hg, a value that occurred infrequently in our other subjects (Fig. 7-1). If the population mean were 46 mm Hg and the standard deviation 6 mm Hg, the z score would be $(61 - 46)/6$ or 2.5, a value that indicates this subject had an unusual response to light halothane anesthesia. If we established that this subject was healthy and that no other obvious reason existed for the greater degree of respiratory depression, we would be able to say that this response is unlikely. However, statistics does not permit us to conclude that the response is abnormal.

The concept of probability attaches a numerical likelihood to the occurrence of an event. Regarding the occurrence of a P_{ACO_2} of 61 mm Hg during light halothane anesthesia, we can conclude from our other measurements that this event occurs in fewer than 2 percent of all anesthetics; this degree of likelihood is expressed as "$P < 0.02$." Is this a "significant" event? Instinct tells us that an event occurring less frequently than once in 50 times is unusual and therefore worthy of notice. Is an event occurring once in 10 times ($P = 0.10$) worthy of notice? By convention, statisticians accept as "significant" any event that occurs less frequently than once in 20 times ($P < 0.05$). However, no biologic or mathematical rationale exists for choosing 5 percent as the level of statistical significance. R. A. Fisher, a noted statistician, observed that "The value for which $P = 0.05$, or 1 in 20, is 1.96 or nearly 2 [standard deviations]; it is convenient to take this point as a limit in judging whether a deviation is to be considered significant or not. Deviations exceeding twice the standard deviation are thus formally regarded as significant."[16] Later he wrote, "It is usual and convenient . . . to take 5 percent as a standard level of significance . . . [and] to ignore all results which fail to reach this standard."[17] Although a probability of 5 percent is the usual standard for statistical significance, one publication, the *Journal of Experimental Psychology*, has encouraged a significance level of 1 percent (i.e., $P < 0.01$).[18]

TYPE I AND TYPE II ERRORS

The level of probability we select as representing "significance," known as α, is also the frequency with which we erroneously conclude that a difference exists when there is no real difference. This is known as a *type I error*, or an "α error." Alternatively, we could ask how often we can afford to be wrong. An investigator who repeats an experiment frequently will eventually select a sample whose mean differs significantly from the population mean. If we select a probability level of 5 percent ($\alpha = 0.05$), we accept a 5 percent chance of being wrong. If the "price" for being wrong is very great, we might select a stricter criterion for statistical significance—for example, $\alpha = 0.01$.

Thus far, we have focused on the issue of erroneously concluding that a difference exists when none exists in reality. A second issue involves whether we can truly state that no difference exists between two populations. For example, if we were to measure recovery of twitch tension 60 minutes after administration of a dose of pancuronium in one group of subjects and 90 minutes after administration of the same dose in another group, instinct would tell us that more recovery would have occurred in the group studied at 90 minutes. If the samples consisted of two patients each, the variability within each of the groups might be great enough to prevent us from detecting a difference. Within samples of 20 subjects or more, we are more likely to detect a difference. The ability of a statistical test to detect a difference, known as its "power," depends on the expected difference between groups, the variability within the groups, and the size of the samples. If the sample size is not sufficiently large, we will not be able to detect real differences between groups. This is known as a *type II error*, or a "β error."

ONE-TAILED VS TWO-TAILED COMPARISONS

Thus far, we have considered the idea that a value located towards either extreme of the probability distribution is unlikely to occur. If α equals 0.05 and the distribution is symmetrical, then the 5 percent of values considered unlikely to occur (and therefore worthy of note) would be found equally at both ends of the distribution. That is, the "left-hand tail" of the curve would contain 2.5 percent of the values, and the "right-hand tail" of the curve would contain 2.5 percent of the values. This is known as *two-tailed comparison,* because we assume that extreme values are located within both "tails" of the distribution.

An investigator often has *a priori* assumptions that he or she is interested in testing. For example, in assessing the relationship between volume status and blood pressure, we would only be interested in assessing whether blood pressure was lower in hypovolemic patients, because we assume that hypovolemia would decrease, rather than increase, blood pressure. If we performed the two-tailed test, we would be able to answer two questions: First, does blood pressure differ between normovolemic and hypovolemic subjects? If so, is blood pressure higher or lower in hypovolemic patients? If we are interested in only one extreme, we can examine the 5 percent located at one end of the distribution, rather than the 2.5 percent located at each end of the distribution. This is known as a *one-tailed comparison.* If the investigator is able to make an *a priori* assessment as to the direction of the relationship between groups and is willing to limit statistical evaluation to that issue, a one-tailed test may be appropriate. The investigator must decide to perform a one-tailed comparison before the data are collected. It is inappropriate to examine the data, observe a difference between groups, and then test the significance of the difference using a one-tailed comparison.

HYPOTHESIS TESTING AND STATISTICS

Statistics does not permit us to conclude whether or not an association is valid, only whether it is likely or unlikely to occur. For example, if we studied three adults with chronic lung disease whose $PACO_2$ values were 54, 57, and 59 mm Hg during halothane anesthesia, we might ask whether these patients differed from the adults whose $PACO_2$s were measured during halothane anesthesia. A statistician would convert this question into a *null hypothesis,* meaning that there is no difference between this sample and the population. The likelihood of this hypothesis would then be tested. If the α were low (e.g., less than 5 per-

cent), the statistician would reject the null hypothesis, stating that there is little probability that the sample was selected from the original population. In turn, we can conclude that there is likely to be a difference between these subjects and the original sample.

Before continuing to a discussion of inferential statistics, we should define certain terms more specifically. The word "statistics" describes not only the name of the discipline that is the subject of this chapter, but also certain numerical entities calculated as part of that discipline. For example, the mean, standard deviation, and variance are all statistics. A "statistic" is an estimate, based on random sampling of the population, of "parameters" of the population. In addition, t, F, and a multitude of other symbols represent statistics. Tests employing these statistics are known as "parametric tests"; such tests are based on the actual magnitude of the values. By contrast, tests based on ranking of the values are known as *nonparametric tests.*

INFERENTIAL STATISTICS

After determining the descriptive statistics and noting differences between groups, the investigator would typically like to draw statistical conclusions regarding these differences. To draw these conclusions, the investigator employs a second area of statistics known as *inferential statistics.*

ONE- AND TWO-SAMPLE *t*-TESTS

The most widely used and misused statistical test is Student's *t*-test, a group of statistical tests designed for the analysis of a single group or the comparison of two groups. The name of this test refers to a pseudonym used by W. L. Gosset. Gosset's employer, the Guinness Brewing Company, did not permit its employees to publish their research. However, because of the importance of this work, Gosset was permitted to publish under the name "Student."[19] Gosset's contribution was to develop the t distribution. The z distribution described earlier is based on an infinite sample size. Gosset recognized that with smaller sample sizes (e.g., less than 30), the distributions differed from the exact bell shape of the Gaussian distribution. In particular, the presence of an extreme value (i.e., one far from the mean) was more likely to occur in a small sample. Gosset examined a variety of distributions of small samples and determined the frequency with which the more extreme values occurred.

Earlier we observed that in a normally distributed sample, 95 percent of all observations fell within 1.96 standard deviations of the mean. Gosset found that with a sample size of 20, a slightly larger range, 2.09 SD were necessary to include the same 95 percent of the observations. As the sample size decreased to 10, 2.26 SD were necessary; with a sample size of 5, an even larger range, 2.78 SD, was necessary to include 95 percent of all observations. These values (e.g., $t = 2.09$ for $\alpha = 0.05$ and $N = 20$) make up the t distribution. Every value in the t distribution is associated with a sample size and a value for α. As the sample size becomes large (e.g., greater than 30), the values for the t distribution are nearly identical for those for the z distribution.

These observations were then used to define three statistical tests: the one-sample, the two-sample, and paired-sample t-tests.

PARAMETRIC *t*-TESTS

ONE-SAMPLE *t*-TESTS

If an investigator measures a variable in a single group of subjects, he or she may be interested in determining whether the mean for this sample differs from zero (or alternatively, from some other specific value). This analysis can be performed using the one-sample t-test.

To examine the association between diuretic drugs and acid–base status, we might identify a group of patients taking diuretic drugs, obtain arterial blood samples, and determine base excess. A hypothetical set of values is shown in Table 7-2. The mean of these values is 3.0, a fact that might suggest an association between diuretic drugs and alkalosis. However, two of the subjects have negative values and two have zero values. Because a quick and informal appraisal of the data cannot determine whether 3.0 differs significantly from zero, we must use statistical analysis—in this case, the one-sample t-test. If we assume that this sample represents the population and that the distribution of these values is normal, we can state with 95 percent confidence that the population mean lies between [mean − (t × SE)] and [mean + (t × SE)]. This statement is similar to an earlier one that the population mean lies between [mean − (1.96 × SE)] and [mean + (1.96 × SE)]. However, the value 1.96 (the z value to include 95 percent of the population) must now be replaced by the value of t appropriate for the sample size (i.e., 2.20). This value can be found on a table of t distribution by locating the row corresponding to the appropriate degrees of freedom (in this case, the value for degrees of freedom is one less than the sample size) and the desired value of α (typically 0.05). Sample values for t distribution are shown in Table 7-3. A more complete listing can be found in any statistical textbook. In this case, the 95 percent confidence limits for the

TABLE 7-2. Hypothetical Set of Values for Base Excess for Subjects Given Diuretic Drugs

Subject	Base Excess (mEq/L)
1	0
2	8
3	1
4	6
5	−3
6	7
7	9
8	2
9	1
10	0
11	−1
12	6
N = 12	
Mean = 3.0	
SD = 3.98	
SE = 1.15	
df = 11	

TABLE 7-3. Critical Values of the t Distribution (Two-Tailed)

(df)	α		
	0.05	0.01	0.001
3	3.18	5.84	12.92
4	2.78	4.60	8.61
5	2.57	4.03	6.87
10	2.23	3.17	4.59
20	2.09	2.84	3.85
50	2.01	2.69	3.50
100	1.98	2.63	3.39
1,000	1.96	2.58	3.30
∞	1.96	2.58	3.29

mean are 0.47 and 5.53; these limits do not include the value zero. To determine the 99 percent confidence limits, we use the t value for $\alpha = 0.01$ and 11 df, 3.11. This results in 99 percent confidence limits of -0.57 and 6.57, a range that does include zero. We can conclude with 95 percent, but not 99 percent, confidence that the use of diuretic drugs is associated with alkalosis.

An alternate approach, more familiar to some readers, is shown in Table 7-4. The division of the mean value by the standard error produces a value for t. This value is compared with a t value appropriate for the desired level of significance (usually $\alpha = 0.05$, or 5 percent) for the appropriate degrees of freedom. If the value for t exceeds the value from the table (known as the "critical value"), the null hypothesis is rejected, and we would conclude that a difference exists (at the α level) between zero and the mean value for this population. In this instance, the value for t is 2.6. The critical value of t for $\alpha = 0.05$ and 11 df is 2.20; the value of t for $\alpha = 0.01$ and 11 df is 3.11. The value for t exceeds the critical value for α of

TABLE 7-4. One-Sample Student's t-Test Applied to Hypothetical Data from Table 7-2

$$t = \frac{\text{Mean}}{\text{SE}} = \frac{3.0}{1.15} = 2.6$$

$$t_{0.05(2),11}{}^* = 2.20$$
$$t_{0.01(2),11}\dagger = 3.11$$

Therefore, $0.01 < P < 0.05$

* Read, "the two-tailed t value when $\alpha = 0.05$ and degrees of freedom $(df) = 11$." Notation taken from Zar.[13]

† Read, "the two-tailed t value when $\alpha = 0.01$ and $df = 11$."

0.05 but not for α of 0.01. This fact also leads us to conclude that the mean for this sample differs from zero, and that the likelihood is between 95 and 99 percent.

The one-sample t-test can also be applied to populations for which mean values are expected to be other than zero. For example, if we were interested in whether 90 mm Hg was the mean PaO_2 of smokers, we would determine the difference between 90 mm Hg and the mean value for the sample population, divide this value by the standard error of the sample to determine the t statistic, and then compare the resulting value with the critical value for t.

TWO-SAMPLE t-TESTS

More commonly, we make measurements on two groups of subjects and compare the responses. Such a comparison requires use of the two-sample t-test. In this form of t-testing, two independent samples are being compared, that is, an individual datum in one sample is not associated with another datum in the second sample. For example, we might want to compare blood pressure in normovolemic and hypovolemic individuals. Hypothetical values are provided in Table 7-5. In this instance, an informal appraisal of the data would establish that a significant difference exists between the mean values. This difference can be confirmed by using the two-sample t-test to evaluate the null hypothesis that there is no difference between these two samples, that is, that they come from the same population.

Computation of the t statistic for the two-sample test is slightly more complicated than for the one-sample test. In the one-sample test, we divided the mean by its standard error. With two samples, each sample has its own standard error; we then determine the standard error of the difference between the means. Although the derivation of the standard error between the means is beyond the scope of this chapter (see Feinstein[20]), the equation is similar to that for the one-sample test:

$$SE_{\bar{X}_1 - \bar{X}_2} = (SE_{\bar{X}_1}{}^2 + SE_{\bar{X}_2}{}^2)^{1/2} \quad (12)$$

Alternate methods are available to calculate the standard error of the difference between means, one of which uses a pooled var-

TABLE 7-5. Application of the One-Tailed, Two-Sample Student's *t*-Test to Hypothetical Sets of Mean Blood Pressure Values for Normovolemic and Hypovolemic Subjects

	Normovolemic Subjects	Hypovolemic Subjects
	77	72
	91	62
	101	51
	81	81
	76	47
	68	74
	72	52
	82	65
N	8	8
Mean	81.0	63.0
SD	10.6	12.3
SE	3.76	4.33

$$SE_{(\bar{x}_1 - \bar{x}_2)} = \left[\frac{10.6^2}{8} + \frac{12.3^2}{8} \right]^{1/2} = 5.74$$

$$t = \frac{\bar{X}_1 - \bar{X}_2}{SE_{(\bar{x}_1 - \bar{x}_2)}} = (81.0 - 63.0)/5.74 = 3.1$$

$$t_{0.05(1),14}{}^* = 1.76$$
$$t_{0.01(1),14}\dagger = 2.62$$

Therefore, $P < 0.01$

* Read, "the one-tailed *t* value when $\alpha = 0.05$ and *df* = 14."

† Read, "the one-tailed *t* value when $\alpha = 0.01$ and *df* = 14."

iance instead of the separate variances of Equation (12) (see Feinstein[20]). Despite the different methods for calculation, the standard errors are similar.

Next, the difference between groups is divided by this standard error; this process produces the now familiar *t* statistic, which is then compared with the critical value from the tables. If the value for *t* exceeds the critical value, the null hypothesis is rejected; if *t* is less than the critical value, the null hypothesis cannot be rejected. An instinctive approach to the comparison between the calculated value for *t* and the critical value is as follows: the numerator is the difference between the mean values, an estimate of the distance between the location of the two samples. The denominator, Equation 12, is the standard error of the difference between means, an estimate of the variability within the samples. The ratio of these values estimates how much of the difference between means can be explained by the variability existing in each of the samples. If the variability within each of the samples is small, only a small difference between mean values

should be sufficient to suggest that a difference exists between the samples. By contrast, if the variability within one or both of the samples is great, the difference between the means of the samples must be larger if the investigator is to have confidence that a difference exists between groups.

Before using a table of *t* values to determine the critical value for this example, we should consider one special aspect. In our hypothetical situation, we have been comparing blood pressure in normovolemic and hypovolemic individuals. Our *a priori* assumption is that blood pressure will be lower, rather than higher, in the hypovolemic group. Therefore, rather than perform a two-tailed comparison that would permit us to assess all possible relationships between the data, it would be appropriate to perform a one-tailed test. Because the critical value for *t* ($\alpha = 0.05$, *df* = 14) is lower for a one-tailed comparison (1.76) than for a two-tailed comparison (2.14), we have increased our chances of detecting a statistically significant difference by using the former.

In this example, the *t* statistic is markedly greater than the critical value; we conclude that it is unlikely ($P < 0.05$) that these two samples were selected from the same population. Therefore, the mean value for blood pressure is lower for these hypovolemic individuals than for normovolemic individuals. Since the *t* statistic is markedly greater than the critical value for $\alpha = 0.05$, we can refer to the table to determine the critical values for higher levels of significance. With 14 *df*, *t* is 2.62 when $\alpha = 0.01$ and 2.98 when $\alpha = 0.005$. Since the *t* statistic exceeds both these values, we can conclude that the likelihood of these samples being from the same population is extremely small, less than 0.005, or 1 in 200.

PAIRED-SAMPLE *t*-TESTS

On occasion, an investigator obtains measurements before and after an intervention and then studies whether this intervention produced a significant effect. Under these circumstances, when the two samples being compared are in some way related to each other ("paired"), a "paired-sample *t*-test," more commonly called a "paired *t*-test," is used. For example, measuring cardiac output before an

TABLE 7-6. Application of the Paired *t*-Test to Hypothetical Values for Cardiac Output (L/min) Before and After Administration of Pancuronium

Subject		Cardiac Output Before Pancuronium (L/min)	Cardiac Output After Pancuronium (L/min)	Change in Cardiac Output (L/min)
1		4.3	5.7	+1.4
2		5.6	5.4	−0.2
3		3.9	4.6	+0.7
4		5.7	7.3	+1.6
5		4.8	6.0	+1.2
6		5.2	5.3	+0.1
	Mean	4.92	5.72	0.80
	SD	0.72	0.91	0.73
	SE	0.29	0.37	0.30

$$t = 0.80/0.30 = 2.69$$
$$t_{0.05(2),5}{}^* = 2.57$$

Therefore, $P < 0.05$

* Read "the two-tailed *t* value when $\alpha = 0.05$ and $df = 5$."

after the administration of pancuronium might produce the values shown in Table 7-6. In this instance, an informal appraisal of the data suggests a strong difference between the "before" and "after" values, since five of six subjects had an increase in cardiac output. The paired *t*-test is used to confirm this observation. A new sample is created whose members are equal to the difference between "before" and "after" values for each subject. This new sample is then analyzed by the one-sample *t*-test. The mean value for this sample is 0.80 L/min, and the standard error is 0.30 L/min. In this case, the *t* statistic is 2.69, a value that exceeds the critical value of 2.57. We would conclude that the "before" and "after" measurements are unlikely to be from the same population. This conclusion suggests that pancuronium increases cardiac output.

An alternate statistical approach to this hypothetical situation would be to use the two-sample *t*-test (Table 7-7). This test produces a *t* value of 1.69, which is less than the critical value of 2.23. Despite the greater degrees of freedom for the two-sample test (10) than for the one-sample test (5), the unpaired test does not support our belief that a difference exists between the "before" and "after" values. This lack of confirmation results because of the variability of the "before" and "after" values.

Had the investigator obtained the "before" measurements in one group of subjects and the "after" measurements in another group, the paired test would not be applicable. For example, a change in cardiac output from 4 to 6 L/min in a subject means something entirely different than would the measurement of 4 L/min in one subject before pancuronium and the measurement of 6 L/min in a different subject after pancuronium.

NONPARAMETRIC *t*-TESTS: THE MANN-WHITNEY *U*-TEST

Data on an ordinal scale require special treatment, since determining means and variances for this kind of data is usually inappropriate. In order to make statistical comparisons on ordinal data, nonparametric tests, which assess the relative ranks rather than the magnitude of the data, are applied. Most parametric tests have a corresponding nonparametric test. Nonparametric tests are also valuable for

TABLE 7-7. Inappropriate Application of the Two-Sample *t*-Test to Hypothetical Analysis of Data of Table 7-6

$$SE_{(\bar{x}_1 - \bar{x}_2)} = \left[\frac{0.72^2}{6} + \frac{0.91^2}{6} \right]^{1/2} = 0.47$$

$$t = \frac{\bar{X}_1 - \bar{X}_2}{SE_{(\bar{x}_1 - \bar{x}_2)}} = (5.72 - 4.92)/0.47 = 1.69$$

$$t_{0.05(2),10}{}^* = 2.23$$

Therefore, $P > 0.05$

* Read, "the two-tailed *t* value when $\alpha = 0.05$ and $df = 10$."

analyzing samples that deviate strongly from the normal distribution. Although parametric tests assume a normal distribution, they are sufficiently powerful (statisticians use the term "robust") to detect differences even when samples are not distributed normally. However, as the samples stray significantly from a normal distribution, parametric tests lose their ability to detect differences.

The nonparametric test corresponding to the two-sample t-test is the Mann-Whitney U-test. With this test, the values in each of the two groups are assigned ranks. The smallest (or largest) value is assigned the rank 1; the next smallest (or next largest), the rank 2. This process continues until the largest (or smallest) value has been assigned the rank equal to the sum of the two sample sizes. If values are tied in rank, they are assigned a value equal to the average of the corresponding ranks. For example, if two samples are tied for ranks 4 and 5, both are assigned rank 4.5. The statistics R_1 and R_2 are equal to the sum of the ranks for groups 1 and 2, respectively. The test statistic, U, is determined by the following equation:

$$U = n_1 n_2 + \frac{n_1(n_1 + 1)}{2} - R_1 \qquad (13)$$

The value for U is then compared with critical values for U obtained from a table. The data comparing the blood pressures of normovole-mic and hypovolemic subjects (Table 7-5) can be analyzed using the Mann-Whitney U-test, as shown in Table 7-8. As with the two-sample t-test, the results of the Mann-Whitney U-test suggest a difference between the two groups ($P < 0.05$). Nonparametric tests such as the Mann-Whitney U-test have not been used frequently in the anesthesia literature; however, because they are valuable for data sets that are not normally distributed, they should probably be used more frequently. The nonparametric version of the paired t-test is the Wilcoxon paired-sample test.

APPROPRIATE USE OF THE t-TEST

The critical values for t are calculated with the assumption that comparisons are being made between only two groups. If the investigator collected data on three groups of subjects, three comparisons would be possible: A vs B, A vs C, and B vs C. If each of these comparisons was made using the two-sample t-test and $\alpha = 0.05$, we would be accepting a 5 percent risk of committing a type I error for each comparison. For three comparisons, the chance of committing a type I error increases to 3×5 percent, or 15 percent, a level that is usually considered unacceptable. As the number of groups

TABLE 7-8. Nonparametric Comparison of Hypothetical Data from Table 7-5 Using the Mann-Whitney U-Test

Blood Pressure		Rank	
Normovolemic	Hypovolemic	Normovolemic	Hypovolemic
77	72	11	7.5
91	62	15	4
101	51	16	2
81	81	12.5	12.5
76	47	10	1
68	74	6	9
72	52	7.5	3
82	65	14	5

$N_1 = 8$ $N_2 = 8$
$R_1 = (11 + 15 + \cdots + 14) = 92$ $R_2 = (7.5 + 4 + \cdots + 5) = 44$
$U = n_1 n_2 + n_1(n_1 + 1)/2 - R_1 = (8 \times 8) + (8 \times 9/2) - 92 = 8$
$U' = n_1 n_2 + n_2(n_2 + 1)/2 - R_2 = (8 \times 8) + (8 \times 9/2) - 44 = 56$
$U_{0.05(2)8,8}{}^* = 51$
$U_{0.01(2)8,8}\dagger = 57$

Therefore, $0.01 < P < 0.05$

* Read, "the two-tailed U value when $\alpha = 0.05$, $N_1 = 8$, and $N_2 = 8$."
† Read, "the two-tailed U value when $\alpha = 0.01$, $N_1 = 8$, and $N_2 = 8$."

increases, the number of possible comparisons increases such that, with enough groups, the investigator will eventually uncover a nonexistent difference.

Thus, the *t*-test is properly used for comparing only two groups. When more than two groups are being compared, other tests, particularly analysis of variance, are more appropriate. If the investigator chooses to use the *t*-test to compare more than two groups, a correction must be made to prevent type I errors. When one such correction, the *Bonferroni inequality*, is applied, the α level for each comparison is divided by the number of comparisons to be performed. For example, if the investigator chooses a value of 0.05 for α and three comparisons are possible, a value of 0.0167 for α should be used for each of the comparisons. Then, the investigator is able to state that, overall, the chance of committing a type I error is less than 5 percent.

If the Bonferroni inequality is used, the investigator must decide in advance which of the comparisons will be made. For example, if there are four groups, the investigator may choose to compare group I with each of the other groups (for example, if subjects in group I were given the placebo and subjects in groups II through IV were given one of three different drugs). In this case, only three of the six possible comparisons will be made. It is inappropriate to examine the data and then decide which comparisons to make.

MULTISAMPLE TESTS: ANALYSIS OF VARIANCE

PARAMETRIC ANALYSIS OF VARIANCE

ONE-WAY ANALYSIS OF VARIANCE

The *t*-test enabled examination of a single group or comparison of two groups. For comparison of three or more groups, another test, *analysis of variance* (also known as "single-factor analysis of variance" or "one-way analysis of variance") is necessary. Analysis of variance

is similar in principle to the two-sample *t*-test. Using analysis of variance, we determine two values, one value describing the variability between groups, and the other describing the variability within the groups. For the two-sample *t*-test, these values consisted of the difference between mean values and the standard error of the difference between the means. For analysis of variance, the square of corresponding values is used. The variability between groups is called the *between-groups variance* (also the "groups variance"); variability within groups is called the *within-groups variance* (also the "error variance"). For the two-sample *t*-test we divided the difference between the mean of each of the groups by the appropriate standard error; similarly, for analysis of variance, we divide the between-groups variance by the within-groups variance. This process produces the statistic *F*. As with the *t*-test, this *F* value is compared with critical values from a table of *F* values: if *F* exceeds the critical value for the desired probability, we conclude that it is unlikely that the difference between the mean values occurred by chance and we reject the null hypothesis.

To determine the between-groups variance, we create a sample consisting of the mean values of the individual groups, determine its sum of squares, and divide by the appropriate degrees of freedom. However, the resulting value estimates the variance of the mean rather than of the population. Since we know that the variance of the mean is equal to the variance of the population divided by sample size (this is equivalent to saying that standard error of the mean is equal to standard deviation divided by the square root of the sample size), we can estimate the between-groups sum of squares by using the following formula:

$$\text{Between-groups SS} = \sum_{i=1}^{k} n_i(\overline{X}_i - \overline{X})^2 \quad (14)$$

where k is the number of groups and n_i is the number of subjects in each group. The between-groups variance (also known as the "between-groups mean square") is then estimated as follows:

$$\text{Between-groups MS} = \frac{\sum_{i=1}^{k} n_i(\overline{X}_i - \overline{X})^2}{k - 1} \quad (15)$$

The within-groups sum of squares is obtained by calculating the sum of squares for each individual group and adding these values. This sum of squares is then divided by the appropriate degrees of freedom (the sum of degrees of freedom of the individual groups, i.e., one less than the size of each group) resulting in the within-groups mean square:

$$\text{Within-groups MS} = \frac{\sum_{i=1}^{k}\left[\sum_{j=1}^{n_i}(X_{ij} - \overline{X}_i)^2\right]}{N - k} \quad (16)$$

where N is the total number of subjects in all groups.

The Σ in brackets represents the sum of squares for each of the groups; the outer Σ means to sum these values. Having estimated the between-groups variance (the between-groups mean square) and the within-groups variance (the within-groups mean square), we calculate their ratio, F:

$$F = \frac{\text{between-groups MS}}{\text{within-groups MS}} \quad (17)$$

We then refer to a table of F values to learn whether this value exceeds the critical value. If F exceeds this value, we conclude that the difference between the mean values of the groups was not likely to occur as a result of the variability within groups. Thus, we can reject the null hypothesis and conclude that a difference exists between the groups.

In Table 7-9, analysis of variance is used to compare volumes of distribution for "histodrenaline" (the imaginary drug causing release of either histamine or epinephrine) in infants, children, and adults. The between-groups variance is 35,060 and the within-groups variance

TABLE 7-9. Use of Single-Factor Analysis of Variance to Compare Hypothetical Values for Volume of Distribution (ml/kg) of "Histodrenaline" in Three Age Groups

Infants	Children	Adults
465	291	192
293	225	212
371	287	270
405	302	251
451	210	290

	Infants	Children	Adults
N	5	5	5
Mean	397	263	243

Grand mean $= (397 + 263 + 243)/3 = 301$

Between-groups SS $= 5(397 - 301)^2 + 5(263 - 301)^2 + 5(243 - 301)^2 = 70,120$
Between-groups $df = 3 - 1 = 2$
Between-groups MS $= 35,060$

$$\text{Infant SS} = (465 - 397)^2 + (293 - 397)^2 + \cdots = 19,096$$
$$\text{Child SS} = (291 - 263)^2 + (225 - 263)^2 + \cdots = 7,134$$
$$\text{Adult SS} = (192 - 243)^2 + (212 - 243)^2 + \cdots = 6,564$$

Within-groups SS $=$ Infant SS $+$ child SS $+$ adult SS $= 32,794$
Within-groups $df = 3(5 - 1) = 12$
Within-groups MS $= 2,732.83$

$$F = \frac{\text{between-groups MS}}{\text{within-groups MS}} = 35,060/2,732.83 = 12.83$$

$$F_{0.05(1),2,12}† = 3.89$$
$$F_{0.0025(1),2,12}‡ = 10.3$$

Therefore, $P < 0.0025$, regarding the possibility that at least one group mean differs from the others.

* An imaginary drug causing release of either histamine or epinephrine.
† Read, "the one-tailed F value when $\alpha = 0.05$, the between-groups $df = 2$, and the within-groups $df = 12$."
‡ Read, "the one-tailed F value when $\alpha = 0.0025$, the between-groups $df = 2$, and the within-groups $df = 12$."

is 2,732.83; the resulting value for F is 12.83. Since this value exceeds the critical value for F for $\alpha = 0.05$ and the appropriate degrees of freedom (note that we must now consider the number of degrees of freedom in both the numerator and the denominator), we can conclude that it is unlikely that the three samples were selected from the same population.

Using analysis of variance, we tested the null hypothesis that there is no difference between the mean value of any of the multiple groups. If we reject the null hypothesis, we can conclude that at least one of the mean values differs from at least one of the other mean values, not that each of the groups is different from each of the other groups. To determine which group means actually differ, additional tests, known as multiple comparison tests (described below) are necessary.

REPEATED-MEASURES (TWO-WAY) ANALYSIS OF VARIANCE

Just as the paired *t*-test may detect differences not found with the two-sample *t*-test, a "paired" test corresponding to analysis of variance, *(repeated-measures analysis of variance)* may detect differences not found with single-factor analysis of variance. If the investigator obtains more than two measurements on each subject (each measurement on a subject will be called a "treatment"), repeated-measures analysis of variance should be employed. Just as the

TABLE 7-10. Application of Repeated-Measures Analysis of Variance to Hypothetical Data for Heart Rate (beats/minute) Before and After the Simultaneous Administration of Neostigmine and Atropine

	Drug Administration:		
Before (beats/min)	1 min After (beats/min)	5 min After (beats/min)	15 min After (beats/min)
67	92	87	68
92	112	94	90
58	71	69	62
61	90	83	66
72	88	71	69
Mean 70	90	81	71
N 5	5	5	5

$$\text{Grand mean} = (70 + 90 + 81 + 71)/4 = 78$$

$$\begin{aligned}\text{Within-subjects SS} = &[(67 - 78.5)^2 + (92 - 78.5)^2 + (87 - 78.5)^2 + (68 - 78.5)^2] \\ &+ [(92 - 97)^2 + (112 - 97)^2 + \cdots] \\ &+ [(58 - 65)^2 + \cdots] \\ &+ [(61 - 75)^2 + \cdots] \\ &+ [(72 - 74.5)^2 + \cdots] = 1{,}634\end{aligned}$$

$$\text{Treatment SS} = 5(70 - 78)^2 + 5(90 - 78)^2 + 5(81 - 78)^2 + 5(71 - 78)^2 = 1{,}330$$
$$\text{Treatment } df = 4 - 1 = 3$$
$$\text{Treatment MS} = 433.33$$

$$\text{Error SS} = \text{Within-subjects SS} - \text{treatment SS} = 1{,}634 - 1{,}330 = 334$$
$$\text{Error } df = 3(5 - 1) = 12$$
$$\text{Error MS} = 25.33$$

$$F = \frac{\text{Treatment MS}}{\text{Error MS}} = (433.33/25.33) = 17.50$$

$$F_{0.05(1),3,12}* = 3.49$$
$$F_{0.0005(1),3,12}\dagger = 12.7$$

Therefore, heart rate at one time interval differs from the heart rate at another time interval. A multiple comparison test (such as the Student–Newman–Keuls test or Dunnett's test) is necessary to determine which of these groups differs from the remainder.

* Read, "the one-tailed F value when $\alpha = 0.05$, the treatment $df = 3$, and the error $df = 12$."
† Read, "the one-tailed F value when $\alpha = 0.0005$, the treatment $df = 3$, and the error $df = 12$."

standard error for the paired *t*-test was calculated in a different manner than for the two-sample *t*-test, the denominator for repeated-measures analysis of variance is calculated differently than for single-factor analysis of variance. The within-subject variability results from two factors, that is, variability inherent to the subject (equivalent to the error variability for single-factor analysis of variance) and the variability resulting from the treatments. This can be stated as

rather than single-factor analysis of variance, should be used whenever two or more measurements are obtained on the same subject. For example, to assess the effects of neostigmine and atropine on heart rate, we might measure heart rate before drug administration and 1, 5, and 15 minutes after drug administration (Table 7-10). When repeated-measures analysis of variance is performed, F is 17.50, a value that exceeds the critical value. In Table 7-11, these same hypothetical data are ana-

$$\text{Within-subject SS} = \text{error SS} + \text{between-treatments SS} \qquad (18)$$

The within-subject sum of squares is determined by calculating the sum of squares for each subject and determining the sum of these values. The between-treatments (treatment) sum of squares (identical to the between-groups sum of squares for analysis of variance) is calculated from the sample of means for the treatments. The difference between the within-subject sum of squares and the treatment sum of squares is the error sum of squares [Equation (18)]. The variances are determined by dividing the sums of squares by the appropriate degrees of freedom; F is the ratio of the treatment variance to the error variance.

Repeated-measures analysis of variance,

lyzed inappropriately using analysis of variance. When this technique is applied, F is 2.83, a value less than the critical value, despite the greater degrees of freedom. This situation is analogous to that shown in Tables 7-5 and 7-6, in which the paired *t*-test suggested differences not supported by the two-sample *t*-test.

As with analysis of variance, repeated-measures analysis of variance permits the conclusion that at least one group differs from the others regarding heart rate and the administration of neostigmine and atropine. In the example shown in Table 7-10, we were able to conclude that at least one of the groups differs from the others. To determine which of the group

TABLE 7-11. Inappropriate Application of One-Way Analysis of Variance to the Hypothetical Data from Table 7-10

Grand mean = 78

Between-groups SS = $5(70 - 78)^2 + 5(90 - 78)^2 \cdots = 1{,}330$
Between-groups *df* = 3 − 1 = 2
Between-groups MS = 433.33

Within-groups SS = $[(67 - 70) + (92 - 70) + (58 - 70) \cdots]$
$+ [(92 - 90) + (112 - 90) + \cdots]$
$+ [(87 - 81) + (94 - 81) + \cdots]$
$+ [(68 - 71) + (90 - 71) + \cdots] = 2{,}510$

Within-groups *df* = 4(5 − 1) = 16
Within-groups MS = 156.88

$$F = \frac{\text{Between-groups MS}}{\text{Within-groups MS}} = 433.33/156.88 = 2.83$$

$$F_{0.05(1),3,16}{}^* = 3.24$$

Therefore, when this inappropriate statistical test is applied, *P* > 0.05.

* Read, "the one-tailed *F* value when $\alpha = 0.05$, the between-groups *df* = 3, and the within-groups *df* = 16."

means differs, we must apply the multiple comparison tests described earlier.

INTRAGROUP COMPARISONS

Analysis of variance, both one-way and repeated-measures, permits the investigator to test the null hypothesis that there is no difference between mean values of any of the multiple groups. If the null hypothesis is accepted, no additional comparisons are necessary; if the null hypothesis is rejected, the investigator must use additional tests to determine which group means differ from the remaining values. For example, in Table 7-9, analysis of variance suggests that at least one group differs from the other groups. Examination of the data shows that the mean value for infants differs from the other mean values, and that no difference appears to exist between children and adults. To verify this observation, we need to apply multiple comparison tests. These tests fall into one of several categories, depending on whether the investigator is interested in all possible comparisons between pairs (the number of possible comparisons is equal to one half the product of the number of groups and the number of groups minus one) or only specific ones.

ALL POSSIBLE COMPARISONS

A number of tests permit multiple comparisons, such as the Newman–Keuls test (also known as the Student–Newman–Keuls test, or SNK), Duncan's test, the least-significant difference test (LSD), Tukey's test, and Scheffé's method. Although there is no consensus regarding the best multiple comparison test, the Student–Newman–Keuls test exemplifies the general procedure and will be described here.

To perform the Student–Newman–Keuls test, the investigator calculates the difference between the largest and smallest group, followed by the next-largest to the smallest, and so on, until all possible differences have been calculated. The standard error is determined in a manner similar to that for the *t*-test, as the square root of the within-groups mean square

divided by the square root of the size of each of the samples.* The between-groups differences are then divided by the appropriate standard error, much as with the two-sample *t*-test. This process produces the Student-Newman-Keuls statistic, q; critical values for q are also obtainable from a table. If we select enough samples from the population, samples having extreme means may show significant differences even though the values were selected from the original sample. Therefore, in evaluating the difference between the extreme means and the less extreme means, we need a correction factor that considers the number of ranks (p) between the means being compared.[21] As a result, the critical values for q are based on the number of means being spanned in the comparison. In Table 7-12, the Student–Newman–Keuls test is applied to the hypothetical data of Table 7-9.

For instructions regarding the use of other multiple comparison tests, the reader is referred to any standard textbook on statistics.

COMPARISON WITH THE CONTROL VALUE

The Student–Newman–Keuls test and other multiple comparison tests are valuable when all possible comparisons must be made. However, the investigator pays a penalty for the opportunity to perform all possible comparisons between pairs, a penalty that may not be acceptable when the investigator is interested in a limited number of comparisons. For example, if subjects were given either placebo or one of four drugs, the investigator may be interested only in the comparison of each of the four drugs with the control state, rather than any comparisons between the four drugs. Although there are 10 (5 × 4/2) possible comparisons between the five groups, the investigator is interested in only four of these comparisons.

When an investigator is interested in only

---

* With the Student–Newman–Keuls test, if sample sizes are unequal, the standard error is calculated as:

$$SE = \left[\frac{s^2}{2} \left(\frac{1}{n_a} + \frac{1}{n_b} \right) \right]^{1/2} \quad (19)$$

where s^2 is the within-groups mean square, and n_a and n_b are the sizes of the two samples. Thus, standard error may differ for each of the comparisons if sample sizes differ.

TABLE 7-12. Application of the Student–Newman–Keuls Test for Multiple Comparisons with the Hypothetical Data from Table 7-9

	Infants	Children	Adults
Mean	397	263	243
N	5	5	5

Error mean square = 2,732.83

$$SE = \left(\frac{2732.83}{5}\right)^{1/2} = 23.4$$

Comparison	Difference	SE	q	p*	$q_{0.05,12}$†	Conclusion
Infants vs adults	154	23.4	6.58	3	3.77	$P < 0.05$
Infants vs children	134	23.4	5.73	2	3.08	$P < 0.05$
Children vs adults	20	23.4	0.85	2	3.08	$P > 0.05$

Therefore, the mean value for infants differs from the mean values for children and adults. No difference exists between the mean values for children and adults.

* The number of mean values across which the comparison is made.
† Read, "the q value when $\alpha = 0.05$ and $df = 12$."

the comparisons between control group and each of the test groups, Dunnett's test is most appropriate. First, the difference between the control mean and the mean of each of the other groups is determined. Then the standard error is determined: $SE = (2s^2/n)^{1/2}$, where s^2 is the within-groups mean square determined by analysis of variance, and n is the size of each of the groups.* The differences between the control value and each of the other means is then divided by the appropriate standard error; the result is the test statistic, q'. As before, these values are compared with the appropriate critical value. Table 7-13 provides an example of how to apply Dunnett's test to compare systolic blood pressure for four hypothetical groups of subjects.

SPECIFIC COMPARISONS

In certain instances, the investigator may desire to make only specific comparisons between groups. For example, in comparing the values for halothane MAC for six ethnic groups (e.g., Chinese, Japanese, German, French, Argentinian, and Peruvian), the investigator may

---

* With Dunnett's test, if group sizes are unequal, standard error is calculated as

$$SE = \left[s^2\left(\frac{1}{n_a} + \frac{1}{n_b}\right)\right]^{1/2} \qquad (20)$$

where n_a and n_b are sizes of each of the samples.

be interested in only three (Chinese vs. Japanese, German vs. French, and Argentinian vs. Peruvian) of the 15 ($6 \times 5/2$) possible comparisons. The multiple-comparison tests described above would be inappropriate for this use. If the investigator is interested in only a small number of comparisons, it is occasionally appropriate to perform multiple t-tests with the Bonferroni correction (Bonferroni inequality). As mentioned earlier, α values are adjusted to the number of comparisons to be performed. If the investigator is interested in performing three comparisons with an overall significance level of 0.05, the significance level is adjusted to 0.05/3 or 0.0167. For each of the comparisons, a level of 0.0167 must be achieved to permit the investigator to claim a difference between any of the groups. As the number of comparisons increases, the level of significance required by each (0.05 divided by the number of comparisons) is difficult to achieve, and the test becomes overly conservative (i.e., the investigator is unlikely to detect a difference even if one exists). To use Bonferroni's t-test (the application of the Bonferroni inequality to the two-sample t-test), the investigator must make an *a priori* decision as to which comparisons will be made. In the example described above, the choice of comparisons was based on geographic considerations. It is not considered acceptable to perform multiple t-tests, make an *a posteriori* decision as to which are the most significant, and then use the Bonferroni inequality based

TABLE 7-13. Application of Dunnett's test to Systolic Blood Pressure Values for Hypothetical Subjects Given a Placebo or Premedications A, B, or C

Group 1 (Placebo)		Group 2 (Premed. A)	Group 3 (Premed. B)	Group 4 (Premed. C)
	131	120	97	134
	127	117	105	147
	110	131	112	122
	125	110	121	138
	147	122	100	129
Mean	128	120	107	134
N	5	5	5	5

Error mean square (determined from analysis of variance) = 104.13
Standard error = $[2(104.13)/5]^{\frac{1}{2}} = 6.45$

Comparison	Difference	SE	q'	p	$q'_{0.05,12}$*	Conclusion
1 vs 3	21	6.45	3.26	3	2.42	$P < 0.05$
1 vs 2	8	6.45	1.24	2	2.12	$P > 0.05$
1 vs 4	6	6.45	0.93	2	2.12	$P > 0.05$

Therefore, compared with the placebo, premedication B (but not premedications A or C) decreases systolic blood pressure.

* Read "the q' value when $\alpha = 0.05$ and $df = 16$."

on the number of comparisons that are likely to be significant.

NONPARAMETRIC ANALYSIS OF VARIANCE: THE KRUSKAL–WALLIS TEST

A nonparametric version of analysis of variance, the Kruskal–Wallis test, can be used for ordinal data or data that are not distributed normally. The test is performed by ranking the values in much the same manner as for the Mann-Whitney U-test. The sums of ranks are determined, and a test statistic, H, is calculated:

$$H = \frac{12}{N(N + 1)} \sum_{i=1}^{k} \frac{R_i^2}{n_i} - 3(N + 1) \qquad (21)$$

where n_i is the number of observations in the kth group, k is the number of groups, N is the total number of observations, and R_i is the sum of ranks in each group.

The H value is then compared with the critical value obtained from a table. Although a nonparametric version of the Student–Newman–Keuls test exists, it unfortunately requires equal sample sizes for each of the groups.

CONTINGENCY TABLES AND χ^2 ANALYSIS

For data on an ordinal or nominal scale, different techniques are available for the presentation and analysis of results. Histograms, which are useful for presentation of ratio or interval data, are of limited value, since ordinal and nominal data can assume only a limited number of values. To present ordinal or nominal data collected for two or more variables simultaneously, the investigator would use a *contingency table*, that is, a table displaying the frequency of occurrence of events or characteristics. Contingency tables are described by the number of rows and columns they contain; for example, a "2 × 4 contingency table" has two rows and four columns. Table 7-14 is an example of a "2 × 2 contingency table" depicting the hypothetical incidences of succinylcholine-induced myalgias with "antisore" (an imaginary defasciculating drug) or placebo. Examination of these data suggests that the incidence of myalgias is markedly lower after administration of "antisore" than after administration of a placebo. Statistical confirmation of this observation requires varying the techniques described previously. This section will describe analysis of ordinal data using a varia-

TABLE 7-14. A "2 × 2" Contingency Table Depicting Hypothetical Incidences of Succinylcholine-Induced Myalgias in Subjects Given "Antisore"* vs Placebo

| | Number of Subjects | | |
	Myalgias	No Myalgias	Total
"Antisore"	8	22	30
Placebo	16	9	25
Total	24	31	55

* An imaginary defasciculating drug.

tion of the z test, followed by an introduction to another variant of the z test, χ^2 analysis.

For the data presented in Table 7-14, the incidence of myalgias in each group can be described as the number of patients having myalgias divided by the total number in that group (N). This ratio, the proportion (p), is analogous to the central location for ratio or interval data. To perform a statistical analysis, we need to determine the standard deviation for these samples. If we assign a value of 1 to subjects having the attribute (in this instance, myalgias), the value zero to subjects not having the attribute, and the mean equal to p, we can use Equation (7) to determine the sample standard deviation:

$$s = \left[\frac{(1 - p)^2 + (1 - p)^2 + \cdots + (0 - p)^2 + (0 - p)^2}{n} \right]^{1/2} \qquad (22)$$

This formula can be simplified to

$$s = [p(1 - p)]^{1/2} \qquad (23)$$

Since standard error of the mean is equal to standard deviation divided by the square root of the sample size, the standard error is calculated as follows:

$$SE = \frac{[p(1 - p)]^{1/2}}{n^{1/2}} \qquad (24)$$

Table 7-15 shows the computation of standard error for each of the hypothetical samples from Table 7-14. Then, to compute the test statistic, we must determine the standard error of the difference between the two proportions:

This equation is similar to that for the two-sample t-test. The test statistic z is then calculated as follows;

$$z = \frac{p_2 - p_1}{[p_1(1 - p_1)/n_1 + p_2(1 - p_2)/n_2]^{1/2}} \qquad (26)$$

This value for z is then compared with the critical value obtained from a table. As before, if the value for z exceeds the critical value, the null hypothesis (that the two samples were drawn from the same population) is rejected, and we conclude that a difference probably exists between the two samples. As with the two-sample t-test, the z statistic can be calculated using a pooled variance.[2]

This approach to determining statistical difference between proportions is mathematically cumbersome, since the investigator must determine several standard deviations and standard errors. An alternate approach, χ^2 square analysis, arrives at identical conclusions using many fewer mathematical calculations. To use χ^2 analysis, the investigator creates a second contingency table (Table 7-16), the values of which correspond to the values expected to occur if no difference existed between the two treatments. For example, of the 55 subjects in Table 7-14, 24 had myalgias, the overall incidence being 43.6 percent. Had there been no difference between treatments, we would expect 13 (13.1) of the 30 subjects given "antisore" and 11 (10.9) of the subjects given a placebo to experience myalgias. The χ^2 statistic is determined as follows:

$$\chi^2 = \sum \frac{(O - E)^2}{E} \qquad (27)$$

where O is the observed frequency and E is the expected frequency. If the observed frequencies are similar to the expected frequencies, the squared differences will be small relative to the expected values, and the value for χ^2 will be small. Conversely, large differences between

$$SE_{(p_2 - p_1)} = [p_1(1 - p_1)/n_1 + p_2(1 - p_2)/n_2]^{1/2} \qquad (25)$$

TABLE 7-15. Calculation of the Standard Error of a Proportion, the Difference between Proportions, and the z Statistic for the Hypothetical Data from Table 7-14

For "Antisore": $P = 8/30$, $N = 30$

$$SE = \frac{[8/30(1 - 8/30)]^{1/2}}{30^{1/2}} = 0.081$$

For placebo: $p = 16/25$, $N = 25$

$$SE = \frac{[16/25(1 - 16/25)]^{1/2}}{25^{1/2}} = 0.096$$

To find the difference between "Antisore" and the placebo:

$$SE = \left[\frac{\frac{8}{30}\left(1 - \frac{8}{30}\right)}{30} + \frac{\frac{16}{25}\left(1 - \frac{16}{25}\right)}{25} \right]^{1/2} = 0.125$$

Calculation of the z statistic:

$$z = \frac{p_2 - p_1}{SE_{(p_2 - p_1)}}$$

$$z = \frac{0.64 - 0.27}{0.125} = 3.0$$

$z_{0.05(2)}\dagger = 1.96$

* An imaginary defasciculating drug.
† Read, "the two-tailed z value when $\alpha = 0.05$."

expected and observed values will result in a large value for χ^2. This value for χ^2 is then compared with the critical value. To determine the critical value, we must first determine the degrees of freedom. Unlike the previously discussed statistical techniques, in which the degrees of freedom were a function of the size of the samples, degrees of freedom for χ^2 analysis is a function of the dimension of the contingency table, the product of the number of rows minus one and the number of columns minus one. This contingency table includes two rows and two columns, resulting in $(2 - 1) \times (2 - 1)$,

TABLE 7-16. A "2 × 2" Contingency Table of Hypothetical Expected Values for Succinylcholine-Induced Myalgias If No Difference Existed Between "Antisore"* and a Placebo

	Number of Subjects		
	Myalgias	No Myalgias	Total
"Antisore"	13.1	16.9	30
Placebo	10.9	14.1	25
Total	24	31	55

* An imaginary defasciculating drug.

or 1 *df*. The critical value for χ^2 is determined from the χ^2 table using the appropriate degrees of freedom. A χ^2 analysis of the data from Table 7-14 is performed in Table 7-17. Note that the value for χ^2, 7.75, approximates the square of the value for z obtained in Table 7-15 (differences are due to rounding errors). This occurrence is owing to the fact that χ^2 analysis is mathematically equivalent to z analysis.

YATE'S CORRECTION

As the population sum of squares underestimates the sample sum of squares, a correction factor, a smaller denominator (usually n − 1 instead of n) must be applied to ensure reliable estimates for various statistics such as t and F. A similar problem exists with χ^2 analysis of 2 × 2 tables. This problem is usually resolved by using the Yate's (continuity) correction. Instead of using Equation (27) to calculate χ^2, the following formula is preferable:

$$\text{Chi-square} = \sum \frac{|O - E| - 0.5)^2}{E} \quad (28)$$

Yate's correction reduces the denominator for each value and produces χ^2 values that are smaller than those obtained with Equation (27). However, these values are less likely to result in a type I error and should always be used to analyze 2 × 2 tables.

LARGER CONTINGENCY TABLES

An investigator will frequently obtain data involving more than two groups or possible outcomes. These data can also be presented in contingency tables and analyzed by χ^2 analysis. Table 7-18 provides a larger contingency table (2 × 4) for hypothetical incidences of vomiting associated with four doses of an imaginary antiemetic drug, "calm." Determination of the χ^2 statistic is performed in a similar manner, by summing the squared differences between the observed and expected values and then dividing this value by the expected values. The resulting value is then compared with the critical value for χ^2 for 3 *df* [(4 − 1) × (2 − 1)].

TABLE 7-17. Calculation of the χ^2 Statistic Using the Hypothetical Data from Table 7-14

$$\chi^2 = \frac{(8 - 13.1)^2}{13.1} + \frac{(16 - 10.9)^2}{10.9} + \frac{(22 - 16.9)^2}{16.9} + \frac{(9 - 14.1)^2}{14.1}$$

$$\chi^2 = 7.75$$
$$\chi^2_{0.05(2),1}{}^* = 3.84$$

Therefore, $P < 0.05$

* Read, "the two-tailed χ^2 value when $\alpha = 0.05$ and $df = 1$."

LIMITS OF χ^2 ANALYSIS

The assumptions of χ^2 analysis are valid only when certain conditions are followed. For 2 × 2 tables, the expected value for each of the "cells" must be at least 5, or the resulting value for χ^2 will be biased (i.e., may suggest that a difference exists when, in fact, it does not). If the expected value for one or more cells is less than 5, the Fisher exact test[13] (a test involving binomial distributions) is recommended. For larger tables, the expected value for each cell should be at least 1.0, and no more than 20 percent of the cells should have expected values less than 5.0. Violating this condition results in biased estimates for χ^2 and should be avoided either by combining columns or rows to form a smaller contingency table or by collecting additional data.

ANALYSIS OF LINEAR REGRESSION AND CORRELATION COEFFICIENT

Earlier in this chapter, statistics was used to compare values for different variables, e.g., blood pressure in hypovolemic vs. normovolemic patients, blood pressure before and after the administration of pancuronium, and the effects of placebo vs those of premedications. In these analyses, the independent variable was divided into discrete groups. In certain instances, dividing the independent variable into discrete groups may be undesirable or impossible. For example, the subjects in Table 7-5 were categorized as either normovolemic or hypovolemic, despite the fact that there are various degrees of hypovolemia, each of which might be associated with differing amounts of hypotension. To investigate the association between

TABLE 7-18. Calculation of the χ^2 Statistic for a "4 × 2" Contingency Table Representing Hypothetical Incidences of Vomiting with "Calm"*

	Observed Frequency		Expected Frequency	
	Vomiting	No Vomiting	Vomiting	No Vomiting
Placebo	9	11	8.5	11.5
"Calm," 1 mg	10	10	8.5	11.5
"Calm," 2 mg	8	12	8.5	11.5
"Calm," 4 mg	7	13	8.5	11.5
Total	34	46	34	46

$$\chi^2 = \frac{(9 - 8.5)^2}{8.5} + \frac{(10 - 8.5)^2}{8.5} + \frac{(8 - 8.5)^2}{8.5} + \frac{(7 - 8.5)^2}{8.5} + \frac{(11 - 11.5)^2}{11.5}$$

$$+ \frac{(10 - 11.5)^2}{11.5} + \frac{(12 - 11.5)^2}{11.5} + \frac{(13 - 11.5)^2}{11.5}$$

$$\chi^2 = 1.02$$
$$\chi^2_{0.05(2),3}\dagger = 7.82$$

Therefore, $P > 0.05$.

* An imaginary antiemetic drug.
† Read, "the two-tailed χ^2 value when $\alpha = 0.05$ and $df = 3$."

the degree of hypovolemia and the extent of hypotension, the investigator might measure systolic blood pressure while inducing various degrees of hypovolemia by removing blood. These values might then be plotted on a scattergram (Fig. 7-4), which is similar to a two-dimensional histogram. The scattergram permits the investigator to examine the relationship between the independent variable (in this case, the amount of blood loss) and the dependent variable (blood pressure). Figure 7-4 shows that larger amounts of volume loss are associated with lower blood pressures.

This relationship also could be analyzed with Student's t-test by dividing the independent variable into two groups, mild hypovolemia ($<$ ml/kg) and severe hypovolemia (10 to 25 ml/kg). The investigator would find that blood pressure was lower during severe blood loss than during mild blood loss. Moreover, several smaller groups could be formed, depending on the amount of blood loss, permitting the use of analysis of variance.

The limitation of these analyses, however, is that they do not describe the apparently linear relationship between blood loss and blood pressure (Fig. 7-4). There is no discrete difference in blood pressure with blood loss of more than or less than 10 ml/kg; rather, the relationship between the two variables is continuous. The slope and Y intercept of the line that best describe that relationship are determined using *analysis of linear regression*. The equation for this line is

$$\hat{Y} = \alpha X + \beta$$

where α is the slope and β the Y intercept of the line ($\hat{Y}$ is read "Y-hat"). The line that fits "best" is one that minimizes the sum of squared differences between the values of Y and $\hat{Y}$. This accounts for the other name for linear regression analysis, *least-squares regression*. The distance between each point and the line is equal to $(Y - \hat{Y})$, or $[Y - (\alpha X + \beta)]$. The sum of squared distances can be written as

$$\text{Sum of squared distances} = \Sigma[Y - (\alpha X + \beta)]^2 \qquad (29)$$

The reader knowledgeable in calculus will realize that when the partial derivatives of the equation with respect to α and β are equal to zero, the sum of squared distance is minimized. These *simultaneous equations* can be solved to yield the following equations for slope and intercept of the least-squares regression line:

$$\alpha = \frac{\Sigma(X_i - \bar{X})(Y_i - \bar{Y})}{\Sigma(X_i - \bar{X})^2} \qquad (30)$$

$$\beta = \bar{Y} - \alpha\bar{X} \qquad (31)$$

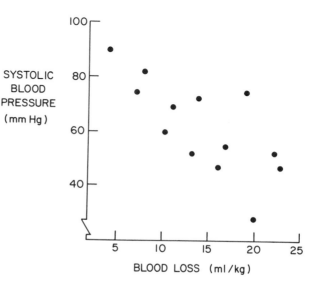

FIG. 7-4 This scattergram results from the plotting of a hypothetical set of values for two variables (in this instance, blood loss and systolic blood pressure) having a linear relationship.

TABLE 7-19. Analysis of Linear Regression for Hypothetical Data Shown in Figure 7-4

$\overline{X} = 14.2$
$\overline{Y} = 61.9$

Slope $= -2.08$
Intercept $= 91.4$

Total sum of squares $= 3520.9$
Regression sum of squares $= 1859.4$
Residual sum of squares $= 1661.5$

Regression mean square $= 1859.4$
Residual mean square $= 151.0$

$F = 1859.4/151.1 = 12.3$
$R^2 = 1859.4/3520.9 = 0.53$
$R = 0.73$

Standard error of the estimate $= (151.0)^{1/2} = 12.3$

Table 7-19 demonstrates analysis of linear regression for the hypothetical data in Figure 7-4. The line produced by this technique (Fig. 7-5) lies close to all the data points. Just as the index of central tendency was a value near the center of the population, the least-squares regression line lies near the center of the values: seven of the data points are above the line and six are on or below.

Using analysis of linear regression, we were able to minimize the sum of squared distances between this sample of points and the regression line. With a second sample, analysis of linear regression would identify a different (although possibly similar) *best-fit* line. Each different sample would result in a different line, eventually resulting in a family of best-fit lines.

Just as the standard error of the mean describes the variability with which the sample mean located the population mean, some statistical techniques assess the variability (*goodness of fit*) of this family of regression lines. The first test, an analysis of variance, evaluates whether the regression analysis suggests a trend between the independent and dependent variables. The investigator first determines the regression sum of squares, which is equal to the variability resulting from the linear regression:

$$\text{Regression sum of squares} = \Sigma(\hat{Y} - \overline{Y})^2 \quad (32)$$

This can be simplified to

$$\text{Regression sum of squares} = (\Sigma xy)^2/\Sigma x^2 \quad (33)$$

where Σxy is another notation for $\Sigma(X_i - \overline{X})(Y_i - \overline{Y})$ and Σx^2 is equivalent to $\Sigma(X_i - \overline{X})^2$, or

Regression sum of squares
$$= \text{slope} \times \Sigma xy \quad (34)$$

which has 1 *df*.

As with analysis of variance, the total sum of squares can be partitioned into two components, the regression sum of squares and the residual sum of squares, which is the variability not accounted for by the regression, that is, the sum of squared distance between Y_i and $\hat{Y}$:

$$\text{Residual sum of squares} = \Sigma(Y_i - \hat{Y})^2 \quad (35)$$

The residual sum of squares has $n - 2$ *df*.

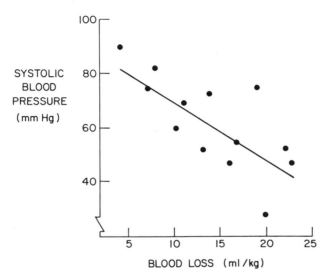

FIG. 7-5 Best-fit curve for hypothetical data in Figure 7-4 using analysis of linear regression.

The ratio between the regression mean square and the residual mean square,

$$F = \frac{\text{Regression mean square}}{\text{Residual mean square}} \qquad (36)$$

is then compared with the critical value for F obtained from a table. If F exceeds the critical value, the regression is significant, that is, a relationship exists between the independent and dependent variables. If F is less than the critical value, the slope does not differ from zero, and the analysis does not support the hypothesis that an association exists between the independent and dependent variables.

The residual mean square (often noted as $s^2_{y \cdot x}$) has a second important role. Its square root, $s_{y \cdot x}$, called the *standard error of the estimate* (or occasionally, the *standard error of the regression*), represents the "average" deviation of y values from the regression line. The standard error of the estimate provides an estimate for regression analysis in a manner similar to the way that standard deviation describes variability of the sample. For the sample described in Figure 7-4, the standard error of the estimate is 12.3, a figure that represents the average distance of the points from the regression line.

The third method of describing fit to the regression line is by determining the correlation coefficient. The variability of the dependent variable, Y, has already been partitioned into two components, the component that is accounted for by the regression line (the regression sum of squares) and the component that is not accounted for by the regression line (the residual sum of squares). The sum of these sums of squares, the total sum of squares, can also be expressed as

$$\text{Total sum of squares} = (Y_i - \bar{Y})^2 \qquad (37)$$

The ratio of the regression sum of squares to the total sum of squares is equal to the percentage of the variability of one variable explained by the variability of the other variable. This ratio, r^2, is known as *the coefficient of determination*. If the regression line "fits" the sample exactly, the error sum of squares is equal to zero and the regression sum of squares is equal to the total sum of squares. This results in a coefficient of determination equal to 1. The greater the distance between the values in the sample and the regression line, the larger the value of the error sum of squares and the smaller the value of r^2.

The value for r^2 always lies between zero and 1, with larger values implying a better fit between the regression line and the sample. More commonly reported than r^2 is its square root, r, known as the *correlation coefficient* or the *product-moment correlation coefficient*. Since r^2 is always between zero and 1, its square root will always lie between -1 and $+1$, and its sign is identical to that of the slope. The advantage of using the coefficient of determination and the correlation coefficient is that they lack units, whereas the slope of the regression line depends on the magnitude of the units used to express the independent and dependent variables.

In addition to these techniques for evaluating the significance and *goodness of fit* of a regression line, a number of techniques compare the slopes and positions of two or more regression lines. These techniques can also be applied to two or more dose–response curves or to other data analyzed by linear regression.

The investigator who uses analysis of linear regression must decide which results to report to the reader. It is often tempting to search a computer output for a statement of probability such as $P = 0.02$. Reporting only this value limits the information provided to the reader, since it provides no information as to the goodness of fit of the regression line. This is particularly important with large samples in which it is possible to obtain significant probabilities for the regression line (e.g., $P = 0.05$), despite large standard errors of the estimate and poor coefficients of determination. The variability of the regression analysis is better described by two statistics, the standard error of the estimate and the coefficient of determination (or the correlation coefficient). The standard error of the estimate describes the average distance of the points from the regression line, whereas the coefficient of determination describes the proportion of the variance that can be accounted for by the regression.

SEQUENTIAL ANALYSIS

To compare the results of two treatments, the investigator first estimates the difference in outcomes for each treatment and uses this difference to estimate how many subjects will be required to demonstrate a statistical difference between treatments. Once the study has commenced, the investigator should not analyze the results until the predetermined number of studies has been performed.[22] In addition, should this number of subjects not yield statistically significant results, the investigator should not increase the number of subjects studied until statistical significance is achieved. These requirements are based on the same rationale as support the prohibition against multiple *t*-tests: the test statistic is based on the assumption that only one comparison is to be made between the two treatments.

In certain instances it is vital to determine rapidly which treatment is more efficacious. For example, if the cost of conducting trials is excessive, or if knowledge of an improved therapy might greatly influence morbidity, the investigator might desire to learn very quickly the difference between treatments. Sequential analysis is particularly suited for this purpose.[23] The investigator uses a chart similar to that shown in Figure 7-6. Paired subjects are given treatments (e.g., one subject is given an antiemetic drug; another subject a placebo), and their scores regarding some predetermined response (e.g., vomiting) are compared. If scores are the same, or "tied," (e.g., vomiting occurred in both trials), the results are ignored. If a difference exists that favors the antiemetic drug, a mark is made one unit upward and to the right; if a difference exists that favors the placebo, a mark is made one unit downward and to the right. Once the mark leaves the enclosed area, the trial is complete. If the resulting line is above the enclosed area, the trial favors the antiemetic drug; if the resulting line is below the enclosed area, the trial favors the placebo. Completion of the trial beyond the right-hand border indicates that no statistical difference exists between the two treatments. Using sequential analysis, Abramowitz et al.[24] demonstrated the antiemetic effect of droperidol using only 11 untied treatment pairs and a total of 42 subjects. By contrast, Cohen et al.[25] found that the incidence of vomiting was lower in subjects given droperidol than in those given a placebo, but these workers were unable to demonstrate a statistical difference using χ^2 analysis.

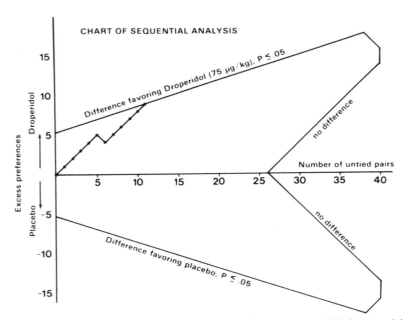

FIG. 7-6 Using sequential analysis, Abramowitz et al.[24] demonstrated that droperidol decreased the incidence of postoperative vomiting. (Abramowitz MD, Oh TH, Epstein BS, et al: The antiemetic effect of droperidol following outpatient strabismus surgery in children. Anesthesiology 59:579, 1983.)

STATISTICAL ERRORS

Many clinicians and investigators distrust statistical analysis. Sometimes this distrust is based, in part, on lack of knowledge of the terms used by the investigator or on the inability of the investigator to communicate thoughts clearly. However, distrust also occurs when the data presented by an investigator appear to contradict the statistical conclusions. For example, one study[26] reported that the elimination half-life of theophylline was 216 minutes in one group and 72 minutes in a second group, a threefold difference that they claimed was not statistically significant. By contrast, the distribution half-lives for the same groups were 2.7 minutes and 3.0 minutes, a 10 percent difference for which the investigators claimed statistical significance ($P < 0.05$). Because neither the individual data points nor the standard deviations was reported, the reader was unable to examine the data and draw his or her own conclusions. Thus, the reader can only be suspicious regarding the conclusion.

Perhaps the most common error is presentation of descriptive data without indicating whether the values for variability represent the standard deviation or the standard error. Since there is no consensus or conventional practice regarding which of these should be reported, investigators may be tempted to report the smaller value (suggesting less variability in the data), the standard error, without identifying it as such. The reader may have insufficient information to determine which value is being reported. This problem occurs less frequently than in past years, probably because of the heightened interest in statistics in recent years.[27,28]

Another error is to use sample sizes that are too small to detect the expected differences. The denominator used in t-tests and analysis of variance is the variability within the groups, a value determined using sample size [see Equations (16) and (17)]. If the sample size is small, the denominator will be large, and the t or F will be smaller than they would be with a large sample size. Thus, the investigator may be unable to detect differences between groups.

An additional reason for obtaining the wrong statistical conclusion is the use of the wrong statistical test. This error occurs most frequently when multiple t-tests are performed without applying the appropriate correction. The resulting type I errors can be avoided by using the appropriate statistical test, such as analysis of variance. Alternately, the investigator might select a test that is inappropriately strict. For example, if three or more measurements were obtained on the same subject, the investigator would be correct in avoiding multiple paired t-tests. Unless the investigator is knowledgeable of statistical techniques such as repeated measures analysis of variance, he or she might erroneously use one-way analysis of variance. One-way analysis of variance ignores the information gained by obtaining repeated measurements on the same subject. Just as the two-sample t-test may be unable to find differences that can be detected with a paired t-test, a one-way analysis of variance may be unable to find differences that can be detected with the repeated-measures test.

SELECTING THE APPROPRIATE STATISTICAL TEST

Most statistics courses focus attention on the techniques necessary to perform statistical analysis and give the student examples of each statistical test. In contrast, when performing research, the investigator must decide which statistical test is appropriate for the data collected. Because statistics courses emphasize performance of the tests rather than study design and how to select the appropriate test, the investigator may have difficulty selecting the appropriate test. Ironically, with the great availability of hand-held calculators, microcomputers, and even "user-friendly" mainframe computers, performing complicated statistical tests is now possible for almost all medical investigators. The greatest difficulty, therefore, lies in selecting the appropriate test.

The first question the investigator should

ask is, "What type of data have I obtained?" If the data are on a nominal scale, the choice of analytic techniques is generally limited to χ^2 analysis. For data on an ordinal scale, the investigator is generally restricted to nonparametric analyses. For data on a ratio or interval scale, a large variety of tests, both parametric and nonparametric, are appropriate. To choose between parametric and nonparametric tests, the investigator should consider the sample size and whether the data are distributed normally. If the data are not distributed normally, a parametric test may not demonstrate statistical significance, because the distribution of critical values is based on the assumption of normality. Because of the small sample size frequently used in many medical studies, nonparametric techniques should probably be used more frequently. The major argument against their use is that, if the data are distributed normally, nonparametric tests are slightly less powerful and may not detect real differences. Typically, the advantage they yield with abnormal distributions significantly outweighs the minor lack of power compared with parametric analyses.

Once the investigator determines the type of data obtained, the data should be displayed in a readily understandable form, such as a histogram or scattergram. Appropriate visual presentation permits the investigator both to learn whether the data are distributed normally and to perform a quick and informal visual analysis. Many analyses can be terminated at this point. If no obvious difference exists between groups, statistical analysis will be fruitless, although an investigator might be able to find an obscure statistical test that produces "significance."

The next step is to determine the descriptive statistics (including the mean, standard deviation, and standard error). These statistics describe the location and variability of the sample; in addition, they are prerequisites for subsequent analyses. Only after completing these preliminary steps should the investigator embark on inferential statistics. The choice of which inferential test to use depends on the nature of the data. If the independent variable consists of only a single or paired measurement on one group, the one-sample *t*-test should be used. For two groups, the two-sample *t*-test

should be used. For more than two groups, analysis of variance is the appropriate statistical test, although an investigator may choose the two-sample *t*-test with the Bonferroni correction. If measurements have been repeated on the same subject, repeated-measures analysis of variance should be used rather than the paired *t*-test. For each of these tests, the investigator must select the parametric or nonparametric version. Finally, if the independent variable is continuous and cannot be divided readily into discrete groups, analysis of linear regression is the appropriate test to apply.

For most of the research reported in the anesthesia literature, these statistical techniques are sufficient. As study design becomes more complicated, more sophisticated techniques may become necessary. Because a more detailed discussion of these tests is beyond the scope of this chapter, the investgator should turn to the resources described below. These resources permit investigators to design their studies for optimal data collection and analysis.

When these guidelines are used, the choice of statistical tests is simple. The most common errors involve the use of multiple *t*-tests when analysis of variance is appropriate, or the use of analysis of variance when repeated-measures analysis of variance is appropriate. Once the investigator understands the importance of type I and type II errors, the importance of selecting the appropriate statistical test will become apparent.

STATISTICAL RESOURCES

The techniques described in this chapter should permit the reader to examine a data set, to determine descriptive statistics, and to perform simple tests such as the one-sample or two-sample *t*-test. More complicated tests such as analysis of variance or linear regression analysis, if done manually, are tedious and require mathematical precision beyond the ability and scope of many investigators. In addition, mathematical errors occur, which, as the number of calculations increases, may be compounded. To avoid these problems, most investigators turn to a variety of resources. The simplest of these, a scientific calculator (such as those produced by Hewlett-Packard, Texas Instruments, or Casio) permits accurate calculation of means, standard deviations, and standard errors. More sophisticated calculators, particularly those that are programmable, can perform analysis of variance and linear regression analysis.

Microcomputers (e.g., Apple, IBM PC) have become commonplace in offices, laboratories, and homes. A variety of statistical packages having various degrees of sophistication are available for these computers. Recently, Carpenter et al.[29] compared 24 statistical software packages for microcomputers. These statistical packages perform complicated analyses with minimal effort.

Users of minicomputers and mainframe computers have additional options for statistical services. Several comprehensive statistical software packages are widely available at university centers. The most popular packages are BMDP (Biomedical Statistical Software, University of California Press), SPSS (Statistical Package for the Social Sciences), and SAS (Statistical Analysis Systems). Although these programs were designed for mainframe computers, they have been adapted for use by minicomputers such as the Digital Equipment Corporation Series 11.

Regardless of the statistical package, the results must be examined by the investigator. I have found errors in two statistical software packages, one produced locally and the other widely available. On occasion, errors are subtle and may escape notice; in some instances, the errors are obvious even to the casual user. Several steps are available to confirm the accuracy of the statistical package. First, the investigator can use a data set analyzed in a standard textbook; differences between the results offered in the textbook and those from the statistical package should alert the investigator to errors. Second, the investigator should always examine the entire output from the statistical package, not just the statistical results. If the mean values, standard deviations, or other results differ from those predicted from the data, the investigator should be suspicious of the results.

Materials are readily available to guide the investigator toward more sophisticated statistical techniques. Glantz has written an excellent monograph, *Primer of Biostatistics*.[30] Textbooks by Zar,[13] Dixon and Massey,[31] and Colton[32] are also valuable resources, particularly if the investigator has selected a particular test and needs guidance through the individual steps.

In addition, the number of statisticians who have biomedical expertise is increasing. These statisticians have knowledge of the particular problems associated with medical research, including small sample sizes and abnormal distributions. Biostatisticians can be useful in directing the medical investigator toward the appropriate statistical test, in performing the analyses, and in interpreting the results.

A word of caution regarding study design. Inexperienced investigators may accumulate a large amount of data before identifying the most appropriate statistical techniques to be used. When an attempt is made to select the appropriate statistical test, the investigator may learn that the data have been collected in a way that prohibits appropriate statistical analysis. This problem can usually be avoided if the investigator considers the issue of statistical analysis before data are collected, particularly if outside advice is necessary. With increasing awareness among anesthesia researchers, these problems should occur less frequently.

OVERVIEW

The aim of this chapter has been to provide an introduction to the techniques used in many statistical analyses. Emphasis has been placed on descriptive statistics, particularly on identifying the location and distribution of data. This focus was chosen because of the increasing tendency of investigators to perform complicated analyses using sophisticated statistical techniques without spending sufficient time examining the data. The chapter also emphasized the more common abuses of statistics: (1) reporting variability of the data without identifying whether standard deviation or standard error is being used, and (2) inappropriate use of multiple *t*-tests. Repeated-measures analysis of variance, a statistical technique that is appropriate for many of the studies performed in anesthesia, has been described, with the hope that it will be used with greater frequency.

Undoubtedly, many investigators will continue to view statistical analysis as a necessary evil in research. Despite increased awareness of the abuses of statistics, errors continue to appear in the anesthesia literature (as in all medical literature). However, with time, with improved editorial vigilance, with the availability of newer statistical resources for investigators, and with education for investigators, we are likely to see improvements in the future.

REFERENCES

1. Gore SM, Jones IG, Rytter EC: Misuse of statistical methods: Critical assessment of articles in BMJ from January to March 1976. Br Med J 1:85, 1977
2. Glantz SA: Biostatistics: How to detect, correct and prevent errors in the medical literature. Circulation 61:1, 1980
3. Rosen MR, Hoffman BF: Statistics, biomedical scientists, and Circulation Research. (Editorial.) Circ Res 42:739, 1978
4. Feinstein AR: Clinical biostatistics. XXXVII. Demeaned errors, confidence games, nonplussed minuses, inefficient coefficients, and other statistical disruptions of scientific communication. Clin Pharmacol Ther 20:617, 1976
5. Emerson JD, Colditz GA: Use of statistical analysis in *The New England Journal of Medicine*. N Engl J Med 309:709, 1983
6. Hayden GF: Biostatistical trends in *Pediatrics*: Implications for the future. Pediatrics 72:84, 1983
7. Feinstein AR: Clinical biostatistics. XLIX. The basic data structures used in quantitative indexes. Clin Pharmacol Ther 26:525, 1979
8. Viby-Mogensen J: Succinylcholine neuromuscular blockade in subjects heterozygous for abnormal plasma cholinesterase. Anesthesiology 55:231, 1981
9. Stanley TH, Webster LR: Anesthetic requirements and cardiovascular effects of fentanyl-oxygen and fentanyl-diazepam-oxygen anesthesia in man. Anesth Analg 57:411, 1978
10. Feinstein AR: Clinical biostatistics. L. On choosing a mean and other quantitative indexes to describe the location and dispersion of univariate data. Clin Pharmacol Ther 27:120, 1980
11. Student: Illegal number crunching. (Correspondence.) Pediatrics 71:864, 1983
12. Feinstein AR: On central tendency and the meaning of mean for pH values (editorial). Anesth Analg 58:1, 1979
13. Zar JH: Biostatistical Analysis. Englewood Cliffs, NJ, Prentice-Hall, 1974, p 70
14. Feinstein AR: Clinical biostatistics. LV. The t test and the basic ethos of parametric statistical inference (Part 1). Clin Pharmacol Ther 29:548, 1981
15. Brown GW: Standard deviation, standard error. Which 'standard' should we use? Am J Dis Child 136:937, 1982
16. Fisher RA: Statistical Methods for Research Workers. 2nd Ed. Oliver and Boyd, Edinburgh, 1928, p 45
17. Fisher RA: The Design of Experiments. 2nd Ed. Oliver and Boyd, Edinburgh, 1937, pp 15–16
18. Melton AW: (Editorial.) J Exp Psychol 64:553, 1962
19. "Student": The probable error of a mean. Biometrika 6:1, 1908
20. Feinstein AR: Clinical biostatistics. LVI. The t test and the basic ethos of parametric statistical inference (Conclusion). Clin Pharmacol Ther 30:133, 1981
21. Schefler WC: Statistics for the Biological Sciences. 2nd Ed. Addison-Wesley, Reading, Mass 1979, pp 136–139
22. McPherson K: Statistics: The problem of examining accumulating data more than once. N Engl J Med 290:501, 1974
23. Armitage P: Sequential Medical Trials. 2nd Ed. Oxford, Blackwell, 1975, pp 23–40
24. Abramowitz MD, Oh TH, Epstein BS, et al: The antiemetic effect of droperidol following outpatient strabismus surgery in children. Anesthesiology 59:579, 1983
25. Cohen SE, Woods WA, Wyner J: Antiemetic efficacy of droperidol and metoclopramide. Anesthesiology 60:67, 1984
26. Berger JM, Stirt JA, Sullivan SF: Enflurane, halothane, and aminophylline—uptake and pharmacokinetics. Anesth Analg 62:733, 1983
27. Longnecker DE: Support versus illumination:

Trends in medical statistics. (Editorial.) Anesthesiology 57:73, 1982

28. Ford I: Can statistics cause brain damage? (Editorial.) J Cereb Blood Flow Metab 3:259, 1983

29. Carpenter J, Deloria D, Morganstein D: Statistical software for microcomputers. Byte 9:234 (April) 1984

30. Glantz SA: Primer of Biostatistics. New York, McGraw-Hill, 1981

31. Dixon WJ, Massey FJ Jr: Introduction to Statistical Analysis. 4th Ed. New York, McGraw-Hill, 1983

32. Colton T: Statistics in Medicine. Boston, Little, Brown, 1974

SECTION III

PREPARATION OF THE PATIENT/USE OF ANESTHETIC AGENTS: PREOPERATIVE

8

Routine Preoperative Evaluation

Michael F. Roizen, M.D.

INTRODUCTION

The preoperative meeting of patient and anesthesiologist fulfills three functions: it educates the patient about anesthesia and thus reduces anxiety (also see Ch. 11); it seeks pertinent information about medical history and physical and mental conditions; and it obtains informed consent. This chapter correlates medical history and physical and mental conditions with the need for preoperative laboratory testing. A major rationale for preoperative medical assessment is reduction in perioperative morbidity by optimizing preoperative status and by planning the perioperative management. Because perioperative mortality and morbidity increase with severity of preexisting disease,[1-7] preoperative evaluation and treatment should reduce perioperative morbidity and mortality (also see Chs. 9 & 10).[3,8,9] Other reasons for preoperative assessment include evaluation of risk for anesthesia and surgery and the determination of baseline function, against which intraoperative and postoperative function can be compared.

Most hospitals and many anesthesia departments have rather arbitrary rules and recommendations as to what questions should be asked and what physical examinations and laboratory tests should be performed prior to elective surgery. In times of increasingly limited resources, the benefit of these rules and recommendations needs to be examined. Therefore, this chapter investigates the effectiveness of the preoperative evaluation and recommends specific preoperative assessments as being more cost effective or beneficial than others. It cannot be stressed too strongly that no amount of laboratory testing can replace history-taking and physical examination.

225

PREOPERATIVE SCREENING FOR SURGERY

RELATIVE IMPORTANCE OF THE MEDICAL HISTORY, PHYSICAL EXAMINATION, AND LABORATORY TESTS

The history and physical examination have always been key ingredients in determining the presence of disease. Although laboratory tests can help improve a patient's preoperative condition once a disease is suspected or diagnosed, laboratory screening examinations have several shortcomings: they frequently fail to uncover pathologic conditions; they detect abnormalities, the discovery of which does not necessarily improve patient care or outcome; and they are inefficient in screening for asymptomatic diseases.[10-26] In addition, most abnormalities discovered on preoperative screening, or even admission screening for nonsurgical purposes, are neither recorded (other than in the laboratory report) nor appropriately pursued; both of which represent potential medicolegal problems[14,15,24-33] (see later section regarding medicolegal considerations and Ch. 2).

The concept that the history and physical examination are the best screen for disease has been confirmed by many groups. Routine laboratory testing in patients who have a normal history and physical examination is of little value and is probably a waste of money. Delahunt and Turnbull[16] retrospectively evaluated patients who were assessed preoperatively for varicose vein stripping or inguinal herniorrhaphy. For 803 patients undergoing 1,972 tests, only 63 abnormalities were uncovered in patients whose history or physical findings had not indicated the need for tests; in no instance did the discovery of these abnormalities influence patient management. Rossello et al.[32] retrospectively evaluated 690 admissions for elective pediatric surgical procedures. The history and physical examination indicated the probable existence of abnormalities in all 12 patients in whom an abnormality was found through laboratory testing. Also, clinical diagnosis, and not laboratory testing, was the apparent basis for any change in operative plans. Leonard et al.[11] reported that biochemical screening tests had no significant value in the preoperative screening of pediatric patients who were expected to be in the hospital for less than 1 week.

Several groups compared outcome for groups of hospitalized patients that did or did not have routine laboratory screening tests performed to supplement the history and physical examination. Wood and Hoekelman[26] found that 28 of 1,924 children examined had changes in preoperative clinical courses (all had surgery postponed) because of abnormal history, physical examination, or laboratory examination results. Three of the laboratory examinations that culminated in the postponement of surgery were not specifically indicated by history or physical examination. Thus, the history or physical examination dictated appropriate laboratory testing for all but 3 of 1,924 patients. The abnormalities discovered for these three patients pertained to their chest roentgenograms. These children were part of a study comparing perioperative outcome at two hospitals—one that required chest roentgenograms as a screening test for elective surgery in children, and one that did not. No differences in anesthetic or perioperative complications were noted between the two groups of patients. Therefore, Wood and Hoekelman[26] recommended that chest roentgenograms not be obtained routinely for apparently healthy children.

Another study also found the value of screening tests to be dubious. Durbridge et al.[12] compared 1,500 patients randomly assigned to undergo or not undergo screening tests on admission. No benefit resulted from the 8,363 tests obtained regarding length of hospital stay or patient outcome. Also total hospital charges (including those for repeating falsely positive tests) were 5 percent higher for patients undergoing screening tests. Thus, history and physical examination, and not laboratory tests, were the measures truly affecting clinical course and management. Even in a referral population, history and physical examination determine more than 90 percent of the clinical course when a patient is referred for consultation for cardiovascular, neurologic, or respiratory diseases.[10]

Other groups have also demonstrated that the history and physical examination accurately indicate all areas in which laboratory testing later proves beneficial to patients. For example, Rabkin and Horne[14,15] examined the records of 165 patients having "new" (i.e., a change from a previous tracing) abnormalities on electrocardiogram (ECG) that were potentially "surgically significant" (i.e., that might affect perioperative management or outcome). In only two instances were the anesthetic or surgical plans altered by the discovery of new abnormalities on ECG. Thus, for these 165 patients, for whom the benefits of a laboratory test should be maximal—that is, when a new abnormality is detected in the course of preoperative assessment—the history or physical examination usually determined case management. Even in one of the two instances of altered case management—a patient having atrial fibrillation—physical examination should have indicated that an ECG should have been obtained. A history or physical examination was not available for the other patient.[14,15] In another study, Korvin et al.[19] reviewed biochemical tests given routinely to 1,000 patients for admission. None of the tests produced a new diagnosis that was unequivocally beneficial to the patient. In an ambitious, controlled trial of multiphasic screening, Olsen and co-workers[20] found no difference in morbidity between control groups and groups having screening tests.

Performing routine laboratory screening tests persists despite their dubious value to asymptomatic patients because of perceived difficulties in logistics. For example, how can one obtain medical histories and perform physical examinations far enough in advance of the patient's operating room time to ensure that the appropriate laboratory tests are obtained? This problem is perceived to be even greater for "come-and-go" or "come-and-stay" patients. How can one avoid delaying schedules (to obtain and interpret tests, to repeat tests having abnormal results, to obtain consultations, and so forth) and the increasing costs associated with screening tests? At least three solutions are possible. All have been or are being tested and appear acceptable to certain practice situations.

First, the surgeon who sees the patient beforehand can obtain the history and perform the physical. Second, a clinic can be set up in the hospital to perform these two tasks sufficiently early to ensure that the appropriate laboratory tests or consultations are indicated.

Third, a questionnaire answered by either the patient or surgeon can be used to indicate appropriate laboratory tests.

Regarding the first approach, one might ask, "Can the appropriate testing be generated easily from the surgeon's preoperative visit"? One study found that it could be. At the University of California, San Francisco (UCSF), Kaplan et al.[24] found that knowing only a few bits of history could convey enough information to indicate correctly all but 22 abnormalities in more than 2,785 preoperative blood tests obtained, counting the complete blood count and simultaneous multichannel analysis of six variables (SMA 6) as one test. Knowing only the admission diagnosis, previous discharge diagnoses, and scheduled operation, and using previously determined indications for laboratory testing (Fig. 8-1), we were able to detect virtually all abnormalities that would have been detected by routine screening. This can also be accomplished by having the patient fill out a health questionnaire. (see below and Fig. 8-2). Cost savings were estimated to exceed 50 percent of current charges (to patients) and costs (to the hospital).[34] (Extrapolating these data to 20 years of testing at UCSF, Kaplan et al. estimated that, at most, one perioperative morbid event might have been associated with this reduction in laboratory costs of more than $6 million, in 1982 dollars.) Of the approximately 60 percent of 2,785 routine tests not indicated by the admission diagnosis, previous discharge diagnoses, or scheduled operation, only four tests revealed abnormalities of potential perioperative significance (Fig. 8-3). Furthermore, on reviewing the charts of these four patients, Kaplan and co-workers found no discernible alterations in patient care. Indeed, in one instance, abnormal results were described in the discharge summary as normal. The following potentially "surgically significant" abnormalities were discovered on routine laboratory testing but were not indicated by admission diagnosis, previous discharge diagnoses, or scheduled operation (based on Kaplan et al[24] with permission of author):

CASE 1 A 15-year-old male with an endocardial cushion defect was admitted for anastomosis of the superior vena cava to a pulmonary artery. His preoperative platelet count was 101,000/mm^3.

(Text continues on page 232)

SKR #2 M.D. Checklist for Ordering Preoperative Laboratory Tests

(Check indication if positive: Only one positive indication is needed per item.)

Patient's Name: _____

Scheduled Operation: _____

Test to Be Obtained	Indication for Ordering Test
Hb/Hct	_____ Potentially bloody operation (blood to be crossmatched preoperatively)
	_____ Known anemia
	_____ Bleeding disorder
	_____ Hematologic malignancy
	_____ Radiation or chemotherapy
	_____ Chronic renal failure
	_____ Severe chronic disease
	_____ Other (specify): _____
WBCs (differential will be automatic if abnormal WBC or Hb)	_____ Infection
	_____ Disease of WBCs
	_____ Radiation or chemotherapy
	_____ Immunosuppressive therapy or steroid therapy
	_____ Hypersplenism
	_____ Aplastic anemia
_____ Check here if you wish differential in any case.	_____ Collagen vascular disease
	_____ Other (specify): _____ _____
PT/PTT	_____ Known or suspected coagulation abnormality
	_____ Anticoagulant therapy or anticipated therapy
	_____ Hemorrhage or anemia
	_____ Thrombosis
	_____ Liver disease
	_____ Malabsorption or poor nutrition
	_____ Other (specify): _____ _____

FIG. 8-1 Sample checklist for determining which preoperative laboratory tests should be obtained. Hb = hemoglobin; Hct = hematocrit; WBC = white blood cells; PT = prothrombin time; PTT = partial thromboplastin time; SMA 6 and SMA 12 = simultaneous multichannel analysis of 6 and 12 blood components, respectively; SIADH = syndrome of inappropriate antidiuretic hormone secretion; and CPK = creatinine phosphokinase.

PLATELETS

————— Known platelet abnormality
————— Hemorrhage or purpura
————— Leukemia
————— Radiation or chemotherapy
————— Hypersplenism
————— Some anemias (aplastic, autoimmune, myelophthisic, pernicious)
————— Transplant rejection
————— Other

SMA 6

————— Age 60 years or older
————— Use of diuretics
————— Renal disease
————— Other fluid or electrolyte abnormality (diarrhea, SIADH, diabetes insipidus, severe liver disease, malabsorption, fever)
————— Other (specify): _____

SMA 12

————— Age 60 years or older
————— Diabetes mellitus
————— Hypoglycemia
————— Pancreatic disease
————— Pituitary disease
————— Adrenal disease, steroid therapy
————— Liver disease or exposure to hepatitis
————— Radiation or chemotherapy
————— Parathyroid disease

ECG

————— Age 40 years or older
————— Known or suspected cardiac abnormality
————— Other (specify): _____

OTHER TESTS DESIRED
(specify indication):

————— Urinalysis
————— Rapid plasma reagin [syphilis screening test]
————— CPK isoenzymes

OTHERS

(Test name and indication):

————————————   ———————————————————————————
————————————   ———————————————————————————
————————————   ———————————————————————————

FIG. 8-1 (Continued)

229

SKR Preoperative Patient Questionnaire

Patient's Name: _____

Age: _____

	Yes	No	Don't Know
1. Do you currently take any of the following medications?			
a. Aspirin (Excedrin, Anacin, Bufferin, Alka-Seltzer)	___	___	___
b. Anticoagulants (blood-thinning medicine)	___	___	___
c. Quinidine or diltiazem, verapamil, nifedipine, propranolol or Inderal (heart rhythm medicines)	___	___	___
d. Diuretics (water pills)	___	___	___
e. Antihypertensive drugs (blood pressure pills)	___	___	___
f. Digitalis (heart pills)	___	___	___
g. Immunosuppressive drugs (e.g., cyclosporin, cyclophosphamide, azathioprine, 6-mercaptopurine)	___	___	___
h. Steroids (e.g., prednisone, prednisolone)	___	___	___
2. Have you ever been treated for cancer with chemotherapy or radiation (x-ray) therapy?	___	___	___
3. Do you currently have any problems with your:			
a. Liver (e.g., cirrhosis, hepatitis, yellow jaundice, malaria)	___	___	___
b. Kidneys (e.g., stones, infection, failure, dialysis)	___	___	___
c. Spleen	___	___	___
d. Blood (e.g., anemia, leukemia, sickle cell disease)	___	___	___
4. Have you or anyone in your family ever had a serious bleeding problem?	___	___	___
5. Have you ever had prolonged or unusual bleeding from nosebleeds, tooth extractions, cuts, or surgery (e.g., tonsillectomy, hernia, hysterectomy)?	___	___	___
6. Do you bleed from your teeth or gums when you brush your teeth?	___	___	___
7. Are your stools sometimes bloody or black and tarry?	___	___	___
8. Have you vomited blood or material that looks like coffee grounds?	___	___	___
9. Have you received a blood transfusion within the last 6 months?	___	___	___

FIG. 8-2 Sample patient questionnaire for determining which preoperative laboratory tests should be obtained.

10. Have you recently had fever or chills, cold, or flu? _____ _____ _____

11. Have you ever been told you have sugar diabetes? _____ _____ _____

12. Do you wake up to urinate more than once a night? _____ _____ _____

13. Do you have muscle cramps or spasms? _____ _____ _____

14. Do you have problems with your heart (e.g., chest pain, skipped heart beats, high blood pressure)? _____ _____ _____

15. Do you have problems with your lungs or chest (e.g., smoke one pack or more per day, shortness of breath, chest pain, emphysema, asthma, bronchitis)? _____ _____ _____

16. Have you recently been exposed to anyone with hepatitis (yellow jaundice)? _____ _____ _____

17. Are you pregnant? _____ _____ _____

18. Is there any possibility that you are pregnant? _____ _____ _____

19. Do you have a cough, or do you cough frequently? _____ _____ _____

20. Do you cough up sputum? _____ _____ _____

21. When you cough up sputum, have you noticed a change in the color or consistency or type of the sputum? _____ _____ _____

22. Do you have epilepsy or suffer from fits or seizures? _____ _____ _____

23. Do you have neck or back problems? _____ _____ _____

24. Have you or any blood relative had problems related to an operation? _____ _____ _____

25. Have you lost weight recently? _____ _____ _____

26. Are you scheduled to have an operation? _____ _____ _____

If so, which one? _____

27. What medicines do you take?

1. _____   4. _____
2. _____   5. _____
3. _____   6. _____
Others: _____
_____

FIG. 8-2 (Continued)

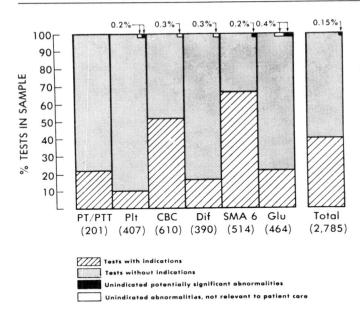

FIG. 8-3 Percentage of preoperative tests by category that are indicated, not indicated, and abnormal. Numbers of patients are provided in parentheses. PT/PTT = prothrombin/partial thromboplastin times; Plt = platelet count, CBC = complete blood count; dif = white blood cell differential; SMA 6 = simultaneous multichannel analyses of sodium, potassium, chloride, bicarbonate, blood urea nitrogen, and creatinine; glu = glucose. (Kaplan EB, Sheiner LB, Boeckmann AJ et al: The usefulness of preoperative laboratory screening. Med Care, in press)

Comment. There was no preoperative note on the chart concerning the abnormality. No platelets were ordered or transfused, and no hemorrhagic complications were noted. Although platelet counts above 100,000/mm³ are considered adequate for hemostasis in major surgery, the quantitative and qualitative effect of cardiopulmonary bypass on platelets may be great enough to increase the risk of intraoperative or postoperative bleeding. Thus, although no interventions or complications were recorded in the chart, this abnormality was considered surgically significant.

CASE 2 A 50-year-old woman was admitted for anal sphincter repair. Preoperative creatinine level was 1.8 mg/dl.

Comment. There was no explicit preoperative acknowledgment of the abnormality, and the particular muscle relaxant used did not require dosage adjustment. Thus, no discernible response to the abnormality was evident. However, as another muscle relaxant might have been used necessitating dosage adjustment due to the marginally decreased renal function, this abnormality was considered surgically significant.

CASE 3 An 81-year-old woman was admitted for metatarsal osteotomy. Plasma glucose concentration was 203 mg/dl. Urinalysis was negative for glucose but was 1+ for ketones.

Comment. There was no notation in the chart about this abnormality. No perioperative complications were reported.

CASE 4 A 34-year-old man having thoracic outlet syndrome was admitted for rib resection. Plasma glucose level was 184 mg/dl; urinalysis was negative for glucose but was 2+ for ketones.

Comment. There was no notation in the chart about this abnormality, and no repeat test was ordered. No perioperative complications were reported. Three months earlier, plasma glucose level had been 86 mg/dl and urinalysis had been 1+ for ketones.

The third approach to the problem of timely history-taking to select appropriate preoperative tests within the confines of normal laboratory work schedules consists of using questionnaires for the surgeon or patient. A current study is in progress (EB Kaplan and MF Roizen, personal communication) to determine whether the responses of patients and surgeons to written questions (Figs. 8-1 and 8-2) can identify prospectively all laboratory tests that will prove to have abnormal results in that patient. After the patient answers the questionnaire (Fig. 8-2), a plastic overlay reveals what tests are indicated. If the patient cannot answer the questions, a standard group of tests is ordered. To date, more than 300 patients have participated; routine perioperative testing has not revealed any significant laboratory abnormalities that could not have been indicated by examining the patient's responses to the questionnaires. Even in a tertiary care hospital that admits very sick patients, more than 60 percent of those laboratory tests now routinely obtained could be eliminated.[24] Also, 93 to 97 percent of the charges billed to patients for these now unnecessary tests could result in cost reductions to the hospital and patient[34] (SN Cohen, personal communication).

Even if unnecessary laboratory tests are eliminated by efficient use of a patient questionnaire, the history and physical examination should still be performed for each patient.

A TYPICAL HISTORY AND PHYSICAL EXAMINATION

Again, the history and physical examination are usually more important than laboratory tests. The following abbreviated approach has been designed especially for preoperative anesthetic evaluation. The questions and physical findings refer to the organ systems that can significantly affect the actions of anesthetics (lungs, liver, kidney), or that can be affected significantly by anesthetics (nervous system, cardiovascular system). In addition, information relevant to anesthesia regarding allergies; previous drug therapy; and social, family, and personal history is sought. If all answers are negative, such an evaluation might proceed as follows:

1. What is the most vigorous thing you have done in the last 2 weeks?
2. Do you vacuum, garden, or carry groceries up stairs?
3. Have you climbed any stairs recently?
4. How many pillows do you sleep on?
5. Have you ever had chest pain?
6. Do you ever wake up short of breath at night?
7. Have you ever had hypertension (high blood pressure)?
8. Have you ever had a heart attack or rheumatic fever or been told you had a heart murmur?
9. Do you smoke? How much?
10. Do you cough every morning?
11. Do you cough some mornings?
12. Have you ever coughed up anything?
13. Have you had a recent cough or cold?
14. Have you ever been hospitalized for pneumonia or bronchitis?
15. Do you drink wine, beer, or hard liquor? How much?
16. Have you ever had hepatitis, yellow jaundice, or malaria? Have you recently been exposed to anyone with those conditions?
17. Have you ever had kidney or renal disease? Do you eat a normal diet? Any bladder infections?
18. Do you get up at night to urinate? How often?
19. Have you ever had a seizure, fit, or convulsion?
20. Have you ever had an arm or leg go dead on you or been paralyzed or numb?
21. Do you have pain anywhere?
22. Have you ever seen double?
23. Do you have headaches frequently?
24. Do you take any medicine or pills or drugs?
25. Are you pregnant, or could you be pregnant?
26. Do you bleed easily?
27. Do you bleed when brushing your teeth?
28. Do you have dentures or false or capped teeth?
29. Do you have any allergies? Have you ever had an operation or anesthesia before?
30. Has any family member ever had a problem after anesthesia or surgery?

Questions 1–9, 18, and 24 search for cardiovascular disease; 1–6, 9–14, and 24, for respiratory disease; 15 and 16, for liver disease; 17 and 18, for renal disease; 19–23, for neurologic disease, and so forth. Positive answers to any of these questions should prompt in-depth questioning. Medical school teaches the physician how to pursue questions that are answered positively and what questions should then be asked. In Chapter 9 abnormalities in these specific organ systems are discussed in detail.

Next, blood pressure values and pulse rates are obtained with the patient lying down and standing; the blood pressure for the other arm is also obtained while the patient is lying down. The teeth and jaw should be examined. The patient should be able to follow the examiner's finger in all six eye-movement positions. The examiner should then palpate the carotid arteries; examine the pulsations of the jugular vein; listen to the lungs, palpate and ausculate the chest for heart sounds, apical impulse, and heaves; and ask the patient to walk 10 feet. These standard procedures superficially evaluate the cardiorespiratory system, central nervous system, and airway. This type of history and physical examination takes about 15 minutes in the "healthy" adult. Therefore, such a routine represents the minimum preoperative evaluation that is appropriate for all patients. Clearly, history-taking is one of, or the best screens for disease.

PREOPERATIVE SCREENING OF HEALTHY INDIVIDUALS FOR ROUTINE SURGERY: WHICH LABORATORY TESTS SHOULD BE PERFORMED?

Prime considerations that guide preoperative test requirements in asymptomatic patients scheduled for peripheral surgery should include (1) the incidence of abnormalities for that test in that age group, (2) the importance of an abnormal test result to perioperative outcome, (3) the cost of the test, (4) the ability to alter perioperative course favorably once an abnormal test result is obtained, (5) other benefits of the test to the patient, and (6) medicolegal issues.

Although the dictum, "there may be minor surgery but there are no minor anesthetics"[8] may be warranted, the various anesthetics clearly differ in complexity. Whereas many anesthetics are used to relieve pain for minor procedures in relatively healthy patients, other anesthetics require manipulation of hemodynamic variables to maintain cardiovascular stability during major vascular procedures. Therefore, preoperative assessment for these two diverse types of anesthesia should, of necessity, differ. This chapter discusses the preoperative assessment of patients believed to be healthy who are undergoing less extensive surgery (i.e., noncardiac). Also, the effectiveness of routinely ordering various laboratory examinations is evaluated. Chapter 9 describes preoperative examinations for specific diseases, intraoperative procedures, and intraoperative hemodynamic manipulations for complex surgical procedures, as well as evaluation of patients having hypertension, scheduled pneumonectomy, or certain familial characteristics (e.g., kidney stones or seizures). The rest of this chapter deals solely with routine screening of the ambulatory patient, that is, the preoperative screening most appropriate for the patient scheduled for inguinal herniorrhaphy, vein stripping, breast biopsy, tonsillectomy, hemorrhoidectomy, etc., who has no other known medical problems.

Prior to the introduction of the multiphasic testing blood screen (the SMA 6, 12, and 21 panels), tests were ordered singly or in small groups to confirm prior clinical impressions. Thus, the results of the history and physical examination dictated what laboratory tests were obtained. Advancing technology and the hope that early presymptomatic diagnosis would lead to longer life and eventually even reduce medical costs led to the widespread use of the screening battery. Even when performed at a cost of about one-twentieth of that in the current hospital laboratory, use of the multiphasic testing screen is difficult to justify for most ambulatory patients.[11,16-22,35-39]

The increasing use of the automated screening battery has magnified two problems that were once rare: which tests (if any) should be required preoperatively, and what should be done with an unexpectedly "abnormal" laboratory result? It seems axiomatic that the more information known about a patient the better. Nevertheless, these additional tests have their disadvantages, including the cost of obtaining and processing the blood, the need for additional tests to rule out false-positive results, the need for additional referrals to other physicians and consultations, the confusion of and delay in operating room schedules, and perhaps most important the anxiety produced in the patient (particularly in the case of false-positive results). In 1984, approximately 6 billion laboratory tests were performed at a cost of $20 billion in the United States.[39] As stated above, in most cases, the 15-minute history and physical examination are probably the best screening tests preparatory to anesthesia.

What conditions that adversely affect surgical outcome or surgical personnel can be detected by laboratory testing? Robbins and Mushlin[40] list 17: anemia, ischemic heart disease, cardiac dysrhythmias, chronic obstructive pulmonary disease, diabetes, nephritis, clotting disorders, thrombocytopenia, nephrotic syndrome, chronic interstitial lung disease, hepatitis, pregnancy, gonorrhea, syphilis, tuberculosis, urinary tract infection, and glaucoma. To this list can be added thyroid disease, pheochromocytoma, Addison's disease, Cushing's disease, inappropriate secretion of antidiuretic hormone, increased intracranial pressure, and congestive heart failure. Clearly, most patients having these conditions are not totally asymptomatic, and the screening history and physical examination will identify the majority of such patients. What, however, is the asymptomatic prevalence of these conditions, and how likely are screening laboratory examinations to detect these abnormalities when asymptomatic?

The central message of the rest of this chapter is that an abnormal test result from an asymptomatic patient may well not indicate disease. In fact, in many cases an abnormal test result in an asymptomatic patient is more likely to reflect health than disease. Because an abnormal test result is not always predictive of disease, the value of performing tests on asymptomatic patients is reduced.

Before answering the question of how preoperative screening may influence the management of anesthesia, what percentage of test results is positive in normal healthy patients needs to be defined. Then, the influence of

these positive results on the management of anesthesia and surgery can be examined. From this analysis, specific preoperative screening procedures will be recommended from both a medical and cost–benefit point of view.

Before this analysis is presented, four points should be emphasized. First, the value of tests in asymptomatic individuals scheduled for peripheral surgery will be assessed. That means that a history and physical examination have not indicated suggestions of disease except in the peripheral area for which surgery is scheduled. Second, the surgical procedure involves only minor blood loss and not major body cavities (e.g., breast biopsy, hernia repair, vein stripping). Third, many assumptions will be used in this analysis, all of which I have chosen to favor the practice of ordering more tests. Fourth, most unexpected abnormal test results are usually ignored preoperatively. This practice results in additional testing and thus may not reduce but actually increase medicolegal liabilities (see the discussion of the medicolegal rationale for laboratory testing below).

The use of the cost-in-dollars method to gauge the usefulness (e.g., saving a life) of a medical procedure is simply one way of comparing the usefulness of that procedure with the usefulness of its alternatives. For instance, one might ask whether it would be more worthwhile, in terms of health, to determine hemoglobin concentrations in asymptomatic individuals under 40 years of age at a cost of $8 per determination, or to monitor a patient having a previous myocardial infarction with a pulmonary artery catheter at a cost of $4,200 per monitoring. Analysis of costs using assumptions stated in Chapter 9 indicate that it costs less than $100,000 to save a year of life using the pulmonary artery catheter in a patient who has had a previous myocardial infarction. In contrast, it costs more than $9 million to save a year of life by determining hemoglobin concentrations in asymptomatic individuals under 40 years of age. Thus, given the two alternatives, I would opt for monitoring with the pulmonary artery catheter. These are required decisions in providing medical care in an environment of finite resources. Although the following cost–benefit analysis clearly ignores the fact that some lives would be saved were resources unlimited, it does not intend to be callous. However, such an analysis does provide a foundation on which to make decisions regarding how best to allocate limited resources.

WHAT DETERMINES THE PREDICTIVE VALUE OF A LABORATORY TEST? WHAT IS AN ABNORMAL LABORATORY TEST RESULT?

To know what an abnormal laboratory test result implies requires an appreciation of how normal values are determined. The normal range is based on the statistical concept of the normal distribution of the Gaussian curve.[39,41] In large groups of "healthy" individuals, 66 percent of values from the population fall within 1 standard deviation of the mean value, and 95 percent of values fall within 2 standard deviations of the mean value. Thus, laboratory results are defined as being outside of the normal range if they are more than 2 standard deviations above or below the mean. Conversely, in a normal population, 5 percent of healthy individuals will have an abnormal result on any one test.[39,41–43] For example, assuming a Gaussian distribution and hemoglobin values of 13.5 to 16.7 g/dl for healthy men, one can expect 5 percent of "normal" healthy men to have a test result outside of that range. If wider limits are used for "normal," fewer patients would have "abnormal" values, and these pa-tients would be more likely to have clinically significant conditions. As a result, you might decide not to change the way you give anesthesia or what you do during anethesia until or unless the hemoglobin was below 9 g/dl or greater than 18.5 g/dl.

Thus, in addition to knowing what percentage of ambulatory patients scheduled for routine surgery have abnormal laboratory test results, knowing what percentage of patients have very abnormal laboratory test results in each age or sex group might be helpful. Of prime importance is knowing what percentage of those abnormal laboratory test values indicates disease. If anesthetic management is altered because of test abnormality, it should indicate a condition that (1) poses a significant risk of perioperative morbidity that can be lessened by perioperative treatment, (2) is undiscoverable through history-taking and physical examination, and (3) is sufficiently prevalent in the population to justify the cost of seeking it. The test should be sensitive enough ("positivity in disease") and specific enough ("negativity in health") to make the test cost efficient (see Table 8-1 for a summary of definitions of terms relating to laboratory testing).

Data regarding the incidence of abnormalities revealed by routine preoperative tests are biased by the sample population from which they were derived. (Later, this bias will be identified for each type of screening test.) Such data are available from three types of sources. The first type is a health maintenance organization, such as Kaiser-Permanente in Oakland, California.[43] These data are biased, however,

TABLE 8-1. Definition of Terms Relating to Laboratory Testing

Term	Definition
Sensitivity	Percentage of tests positive in disease: the percentage of patients who have the suspected disease and an abnormal (or positive) laboratory test result
Specificity	Percentage of tests negative in health: the percentage of healthy patients who have a normal (or negative) laboratory test result
False-positive rate	The percentage of healthy people who have an abnormal test result (100 minus specificity)
Predictive false-positive rate	The percentage of abnormal test results belonging to healthy people: determining this value requires knowledge of sensitivity, specificity, and prevalence of disease

because they pertain to a period when the Kaiser-Permanente population was composed mainly of middle-class working people. Such patients were healthy enough to work and to walk to an ambulatory clinic. A second source is provided by studies that look at specific questions such as, "Are chest roentgenograms worthwhile in individuals under 19 years of age?" or "What is the incidence of abnormalities on routine screening chemistry tests?" Again, this information is biased by the narrowness of the populations studied. The third type of data is the epidemiologic study, such as the Tecumseh[44] and Framingham[67] studies, which examined entire populations and the risk of developing certain diseases. Again, data are biased by the community studied and its environment. For example, only one black family lived in Tecumseh, Michigan, when that study began.[44] Clearly this study group was not a typical population for some hospitals.

Before evaluating the justification for ordering certain laboratory tests, the rationale for routine ordering of tests should be discussed. Although the history and physical examination will provide some basis for deciding which tests to order, patients frequently enter the hospital the evening before elective surgery, often making a thorough examination prior to testing difficult. Let us say, for example, that the patient is admitted at 4 PM and is evaluated by the anesthesiologist at 6 PM. Let us also assume that the evaluation indicates that certain diagnostic tests should be performed. Many hospitals would not be able to perform such tests during the night. A dilemma would arise: Should surgery be delayed until these tests are performed, or should surgery proceed without these tests? This dilemma has led to the arbitrary decision by some to have chest roentgenograms and EKGs obtained routinely before the history is obtained and the physical examination performed. This dilemma also explains why other tests are obtained routinely, in the interest of efficiency (their cost being weighed against the increased cost of prolonged hospitalization) and dependent in part on the evening availability of laboratory services. (Refer to the three solutions to the problem proposed in the earlier section on relative importance of the medical history, physical examination, and laboratory tests.)

LABORATORY TEST ABNORMALITIES IN HEALTHY POPULATIONS

CHEST ROENTGENOGRAMS

The overall valve or a preoperative chest roentgenogram has been evaluated by many authors.[45-57] To illustrate the process of evaluating a laboratory test, the usefulness of the chest roentgenogram will be analyzed on an asymptomatic patient. First, what abnormalities on chest roentgenograms would influence the anesthetic approach? Certainly the existence of tracheal deviation; mediastinal masses; pulmonary nodules; a solitary lung mass; aortic aneurysm; pulmonary edema; pneumonia; atelectasis; new fractures of vertebrae, ribs, or clavicles; dextrocardia; or cardiomegaly may be important to know before proceeding to anesthesia and surgery. However, a chest roentgenogram probably would not detect the degree of chronic lung disease that would alter one's anesthetic technique any better than would the history and physical examination. The conditions that a chest roentgenogram might detect are first discovered by chest roentgenogram in fewer than 1.5 percent of the population under 40 years of age (Table 8-2).

However, not all of these 1.5 percent of the population benefits from that chest roentgenogram. Most of the data in Table 8-2 pertain to studies in which a history was not taken, physical examination was not performed, previous chest roentgenograms were not examined, and false-positive results were not excluded. Almost certainly, the patient with a false-positive result will not benefit from that roentgenogram.

We do not know for certain the exact benefit to the surgical patient of knowing a new positive finding.* Let us assume, however, that by redirecting subsequent anesthetic management into a more appropriate course, such knowledge reduces anesthetic mortality by 50 percent. (I believe that this high a reduction is unlikely. For example, demonstrating that ac-

---

* The following analysis is patterned after that of Neuhauser[58] with permission of the author.

TABLE 8-2. Screening Chest Roentgenograms: Incidence of Abnormal Test Results, the Discovery of Which Might Change Anesthetic Management

Age (years)	Series	Patients Examined (N)	Abnormalities* (%)	New Abnormalities† (%)
0–14	Farnsworth et al.[45]	350	8.9	0.3
0–18	Brill et al.[46]	1,000	1.9	0.7
0–19	Sagal et al.[47]	521	0	0
0–19	Sane et al.[48]	1,500	5.4	2.2
0–19	Wood and Hoekelman[26]	749	4.7	1.2
1–20	Rees et al.[49]	46	0	0
20–29	Sagal et al.[47]	894	1	
21–30	Rees et al.[49]	62	3	
≤30	Loder[50]	437	101	0.2
≥30	Maigaard et al.[51]	1,256	≤4.5	0
30–39	Sagal et al.[47]	942	2.3	
30–69	Loder[50]	515	≤6.0	
31–40	Rees et al.[49]	93	13	
≤40	Catchlove et al.[52]	29	0	0
≤40	Collen et al.[53]	15,978	2.1	
≤40	Sagal et al.[47]	2,357	1.3	1.3
≤40	Combined[45–48,50–52]‡	6,422	4.0	0.8
40–49	Sagal et al.[47]	928	7.1	
40–59	Collen et al.[53]	21,489	7.4	
41–50	Rees et al.[49]	119	19	
≥40	Sagal et al.[47]	3,689	23.9	6.0
>40	Catchlove et al.[52]	50	0	0
≥40	Thomsen et al.[54]	1,823	2.3	0.2
50–59	Sagal et al.[47]	833	20.3	
51–60	Rees et al.[49]	121	40.0	
60–69	Sagal et al.[47]	977	29.7	
>60	Collen et al.[53]	7,196	19.2	
61–70	Rees et al.[49]	134	43.3	
≥69	Loder[50]	48	≤72.9	
≥70	Sagal et al.[47]	832	41.7	
≥70	Törnebrandt and Fletcher[55]	100	37	8.1?
71–80	Rees et al.[49]	76	61.8	
≥81	Rees et al.[49]	16	68.8	
0–90	Delahunt and Turnbull[16]	860		0
0–90?	Petterson and Janower[56]	1,530	9.8	1.3
0–90?	Royal College[57]	3,052	3.8	

* These data constitute an edited summary of the data presented in various articles — edited to select abnormalities that might change anesthetic management.

† Abnormalities not already known by history of physical examination.

‡ Combined studies in under-40 population excluding two studies, Rees et al.[49] and Collen et al.[53]

tive viral pneumonia increases anesthetic risk is so difficult that no evidence exists in the literature. In fact, retrospective evidence indicates that recent upper respiratory infections may not increase anesthetic risk.[22]) Let us also assume that perioperative "anesthetic" mortality in this age group is one death per 5,000 operations.[1–7] We will assume no harm from a false-positive test — that is, no harm caused by additional testing and treatment after a false-positive test report — and that benefits arise largely from reduction in morbidity. However, placing a dollar figure on this analysis (as we are doing) is highly suspect but is biased toward lowering the cost (or overestimating the benefit) of laboratory tests. One can substitute whatever figures one believes is more realistic wherever appropriate. We will assume that these patients have a mean age of 20 years and an expected survival of 60 or more years of life, which public health economists "discount" to the present. Discounting is based on the belief that immediate benefit and distant costs are of greater value than the converse, that is, immediate cost and distant benefit. In this framework, next year is worth more to a person now than a year 20 years in the future is worth to that person now. Although no consensus exists as to what the discount rate should be, the 4 percent discount rate suggested by Neuhauser[58] was used in the following formula to determine future worth:

$$Pn = 1/r[1 - 1/(1 + r)^n]$$

where Pn is the present value measured in years of life, r is the discount rate (0.04), and n is the number of years saved. Therefore, 60 years of life saved yields a present value of 22.6 years of life per current life saved.

Only patients with abnormal test results who actually have disease (true positives) benefit from testing. Therefore, to obtain the number of patients who benefit from testing, the number of people who have abnormal test results but are healthy (i.e., the predictive false-positive results) should be subtracted from the total number of people who have abnormal test results. If a 10 percent predictive false-positive rate is assumed (a low rate for this analysis, as will be discussed below), the number of patients benefiting per 1,000 roentgenograms is [1.5 percent − (1.5 percent × 0.1)] × 1,000 = 13.5 patients (true positives). Therefore, a reduction in operative mortality of 50 percent, or 1 per 10,000 (i.e., 13.5 × 0.5 × 0.0002) gives 0.001350 fewer deaths per 1,000 operations when preoperative chest roentgenograms were obtained. Translating this figure into present value as years of life saved per 1,000 roentgenograms gives 0.001350 × 22.62 = 0.031, the present value in years of life saved. At UCSF, this 0.031 years of life saved would cost $50,000 (an anterior-posterior and lateral chest roentgenogram at UCSF costs $50, not considering fees for consultations, repeated roentgenograms or other laboratory costs; the anxiety to the patient and family and any related costs; or the effects associated with the extra radiation). Therefore, each year of life saved costs about $1,613,000 (i.e., $50,000 ÷ 0.031). However, just as there are other costs, there are other benefits (e.g., treatment of some patients in whom solitary nodules or mediastinal masses

are found may prolong life). Let us arbitrarily assume that these costs and benefits are equal.

Another difficult question to answer is, "What evidence is there that any change in perioperative anesthetic management (based on results from a chest roentgenogram) reduces anesthetic morbidity or mortality?" Little such evidence exists. Then we must ask, "How much cost per year of life saved is too much?" Would a person pay $1,613,000 in 1983 dollars for each additional year of life lived by that person or a family member?

Before these questions can be approached, arbitrary assumptions will be defined that apply to the rest of this chapter. In 1984 dollars $200,000 was chosen as the highest price per year of life saved that would be considered feasible for laboratory testing. It was also assumed that no additional costs would be incurred by additional tests, added length of time involved, effects of radiation, or other biologic risks associated with the tests, worry engendered by incorrect laboratory tests, or benefit other than mortality reductions from the true positive test (for further discussion, see Neuhauser[58] or Bunker et al.[59]). In addition, each true positive for any test was assumed to lead to a 50 percent reduction in perioperative anesthetic morbidity and mortality. A perioperative anesthetic mortality rate of 1 per 5,000 was assumed in the under-40-year-old population, 1 per 2,000 in the population aged 40 to 50, 1 per 1,000 in the population aged 51 to 60, and 5 per 1,000 in the population over 60 years of age. These figures closely approximate the estimates in the literature for elective operations in healthy patients.[1-7] Unless otherwise stated, a predictive false-positive rate of 10 percent was used. These assumptions favor the use of laboratory tests.

Now to the issue of false positives, false negatives, the prevalence of disease in the test population, and the significance of these factors to the abnormal laboratory test result.[39,41] As an example,[41] let us assume that the sensitivity ("positivity in disease") of the test is 95 percent; that is, for 95 of 100 people who actually have pneumonia, the radiologist will record "pneumonia" (or some other significant abnormality) as the diagnosis on the chest roentgenogram report. Let us also assume that the specificity ("negativity in health") of the test is 99 percent; that is, for 99 of 100 people who actually do not have pneumonia, the radiologist will record "without evidence of pneumonia," "normal," or a similar comment on the chest roentgenogram report. Third, let us assume that 1.5 percent of the population about to undergo routine elective surgery has pneumonia. Given the above assumptions, what is the likelihood that a person having a chest roentgenogram report that reads "pneumonia" actually has pneumonia? Among 100,000 people having chest roentgenograms, 1,500 will actually have pneumonia; and 95 of 100 or 1,425 who actually have pneumonia will have a chest roentgenogram report of "pneumonia." On the other hand, 98,500 will not have pneumonia. One per 100 of those who do not have pneumonia (985) will actually have the diagnosis "pneumonia" indicated on the chest roentgenogram report. Thus, 985 or 2,410 patients (40.9 percent) having a roentgenogram reading of pneumonia actually do not have pneumonia.

This discrepancy is what is meant by a "predictive false-positive rate" of 40.0 percent. The predictive false-positive rate is the rate at which abnormal test results indicate that a patient is healthy. Thus, our 10 percent predictive false-positive rate overestimates the usefulness of the laboratory tests and falsely reduces the cost per positive finding. Furthermore, screening laboratory tests should produce significant findings not discernible by history and physical examination. If abnormalities discovered by history or physical examination are subtracted from the true positives and treated as false positives, the cost per unexpected true positive again becomes significantly higher. The cost per positive laboratory test is even greater if more reliable figures are assumed for sensitivity, specificity, and prevalence. Sensitivity (positivity in disease) for chest roentgenograms varies from 58 to 75 percent and specificity (negativity in health) from 97 to 98.7 percent.[60-66]

Data regarding the prevalence of disease in asymptomatic patients are difficult to find. However, by making several assumptions (that again increase the value of laboratory tests), the prevalence of disease can be estimated. To calculate the prevalence of disease, data should be used regarding (1) the incidence of abnormal test results in a specific population, (2) the highest value for sensitivity in the literature, and (3) the highest value for specificity in the literature. For instance, let us assume that 12 percent of chest roentgenograms are abnormal in a population of 10,000 people, that sensitivity is 60 percent, and that specificity is 90 percent. Let us also say that x number of people have "roentgenogram-discoverable disease" and that y number of people are healthy. Then the total population $(x + y)$ equals 10,000, and $0.6x + 0.1y = (0.12)(10,000)$. From these equations we find that the number of people having disease, x, equals 400; and that the number of healthy people, y, equals 9,600. Thus, the prevalence of "roentgenogram-discoverable disease" is calculated to be 4 percent rather than 12 percent, the percentage of abnormal chest roentgenograms. (Calculation of prevalence of most diseases is probably subject to errors of up to 200 percent, but again this is based on the highest values for sensitivity and specificity in the literature, biasing the estimates in favor of the use of screening laboratory testing.)

If the prevalence of pneumonia is assumed to be as high as 0.5 percent in the "healthy" population, and the highest combined figures for sensitivity (75 percent) and specificity (98.3 percent) are used, 1,691 of 2,066 patients (82 percent) with the diagnosis of pneumonia based on chest roentgenogram would be predictive false positives. Thus, it is entirely possible that 82 percent of the chest roentgenograms in otherwise asymptomatic individuals that indicate "infiltrate compatible with pneumonia" actually predict a totally healthy person. If the same rates for sensitivity and specificity are assumed, but using a disease prevalence rate of 2 percent, then 1,666 of 3,166 patients (52.6 percent) having the chest roentgenographic diagnosis of pneumonia would be predictive false positives. If the prevalence of the disease is 10 percent (and test sensitivity and specificity are as good as the best in the literature), 1,530 of 8,030 patients diagnosed as having pneumonia will not have it; in this instance, the predictive false-positive rate would be about 20 percent. Table 8-3 shows how the cost per year of life saved changes as the assumed prevalence of disease changes. This detailed analysis shows

TABLE 8-3. Cost of Benefits Resulting from Screening Chest Roentgenograms: How Do Assumptions Affect Costs?

Assumption	%	%	%	%	%
If sensitivity =	95	75	75	75	75
and specificity =	99	98	98	98	98
and prevalence of disease =	1.5	1.5	0.5	2	10
then the predictive false-positive rate =	41	63	84	56	19
And the cost per year of life saved by screening chest roentgenograms =	$2,500,000	4,097,000*	27,600,000	2,500,000	273,000

* Closest to reality for chest roentgenograms for patients under 40 years of age?

why knowing the sensitivity, specificity, and especially the prevalence of disease in a population group is important in determining the percentage of predictive false positives.

A DIFFERENT COST–BENEFIT ANALYSIS OF THE SAME DATA

Another type of analysis* can be used on these data. Such an analysis is based on the hypothesis that the difference in mortality associated with testing asymptomatic individuals is related to the number of unsuspected abnormalities that are correctly identified. This analysis then makes three assumptions: (1) that the mortality rate of true negatives (MR_{tn}) equals the mortality rate of false positives (MR_{fp}) (i.e., no harm is done by treating a patient with a falsely positive test) ($MR_{tn} = MR_{fp}$); (2) that the mortality of a patient with a known laboratory test abnormality is the same as that for a patient having no abnormality (because of appropriately directed therapy) ($MR_{tp} = MR_{tn}$); and (3) that the patient with an unknown abnormality has twice the mortality rate of a patient with no abnormality ($MR_{fn} = 2MR_{tn}$). Then,

$$D_{+lt} = N_{tn}(MR_{tn}) + N_{tp}(MR_{tp}) + N_{fn}(MR_{fn}) + N_{fp}(MR_{fp})$$

$$D_{-lt} = N_{-lt}(MR_{-lt}) + N_{+lt}(MR_{+lt})$$

where D = the number of deaths, N = the

---

* This analysis was developed in conjunction with E. B. Kaplan.

number of patients, tn = true negative, tp = true positive, fn = false negative, fp = false positive, +lt = with laboratory testing, and −lt = without laboratory testing. Furthermore, $N_{-lt} = N_{tn} + N_{fp}$, $N_{-lt} = N_{tp} + N_{fn}$, $MR_{-lt} = MR_{tn}$, and $MR_{+lt} = MR_{fn}$, and recalling our assumptions that $MR_{tn} = MR_{fp}$, $MR_{tp} = MR_{tn}$, and $MR_{fn} = 2MR_{tn}$, then

$$\begin{aligned} D_{-lt} &= N_{-lt}(MR_{-lt}) + N_{+lt}(MR_{+lt}) \\ &= (N_{tn} + N_{fp})MR_{tn} + (N_{tp} + N_{fn})MR_{fn} \\ &= N_{tn}(MR_{tn}) + N_{fp}(MR_{tn}) + 2N_{tp}MR_{tn} \\ &\quad + 2N_{fn}MR_{tn} \end{aligned}$$

and

$$\begin{aligned} D_{+lt} &= N_{tn}(MR_{tn}) + N_{tp}(MR_{tn}) + 2(N_{fn}MR_{tn}) \\ &\quad + N_{fp}MR_{tn} \end{aligned}$$

or

$$\begin{aligned} \Delta D &= D_{-lt} - D_{+lt} \\ &= N_{tp}(MR_{tn}) \end{aligned}$$

Thus, the difference in death rate with laboratory testing is

$$\begin{aligned} \Delta D &= \text{percentage of true positives} \times MR_{tn} \\ &= (6.5/1,000)(MR_{tn}) \end{aligned}$$

Although the mortality rate of the true-negative patient is not known, it is less than the overall mortality rate (1/5,000). Thus, at most, $\Delta D = (6.5/1,000)(1/5,000)$, or 0.0013 deaths per 1,000 operations. This analysis yields the same results achieved with the other analysis.

Analyzing the efficacy and cost–benefit ratio of chest roentgenograms is a tedious process. However, all laboratory tests should be analyzed in this manner to arrive at logical and valid conclusions regarding their routine use. This analysis shows how difficult such conclusions are to derive. In all other sections, only the essential data and conclusions are given.

Nevertheless, using our assumptions, the data seem to indicate that routine preoperative screening chest roentgenography is not cost effective for patients under 40 years of age. (To reemphasize, by "preoperative screening," we mean looking for disease not already known, not evident, or not suspected by history or physical examination.) Preoperative screening chest roentgenograms are probably not cost effective until the patient is over 60 years of age. The data for ages 40 to 60 years are not explicit enough to allow accurate calculation of the incidence of discovery of new abnormalities on chest roentgenogram. If chest roentgenograms are assumed to be less effective than the history and physical examination in diagnosing significant chronic obstructive pulmonary disease, then, on a cost–benefit basis, they should not be used for patients under 60 years of age.

ELECTROCARDIOGRAMS

The data on the incidence of ECG abnormalities were gathered from studies on either working patient populations (Kaiser[43,53]) or epidemiologic surveys of healthy people (Framingham,[67] Tecumseh[44,68]). The ECG abnormalities that may alter anesthetic management are as follows: atrial flutter or fibrillation; first-, second-, or third-degree atrioventricular block; ST-T changes suggesting myocardial ischemia or recent pulmonary embolism; premature ventricular and atrial contractions; left or right ventricular hypertrophy; short PR interval; Wolff-Parkinson-White syndrome; myocardial infarction; prolonged QT segment; and tall peaked T waves. What is the incidence of finding these abnormalities on a 12-lead preoperative screening ECG at all, and if they were not observed on a standard monitor lead I or MCL$_5$ applied immediately prior to induction of anesthesia in the operating room? Some qualifiers should be mentioned. First, none of the studies on the incidence of electrocardiographic abnormalities excluded patients having histories or physical examinations suggestive of cardiac problems. Second, the studies do not distin-

guish those findings that are evident on monitor leads from those evident only on 6- or 12-lead ECGs.

For the purpose of analysis, 50 percent of abnormalities were assumed to be evident on a monitor lead (premature atrial and ventricular beats, atrioventricular blocks of various degrees, short PR intervals, atrial flutter or fibrillation). Furthermore, 50 percent of the other abnormalities (myocardial infarction, left and right ventricular hypertrophy) were assumed to be discernible by history and physical examination. Recalling the assumption that each unexpected finding results in a 50 percent reduction in morbidity, certain conclusions can be made. When the ECG costs $30 and the data in Table 8-4 are used, it seems justifiable to obtain ECGs for patients over 30 years of age. However, using epidemiologically defined sensitivity, specificity, and prevalence of disease pertaining to electrocardiographic diagnosis,[68–70] preoperative screening ECGs would indicated only for patients over 50 years of age. Even this screening is not justified, however, since reduction in morbidity based on unexpected electrocardiographic findings may not even approximate 50 percent. There are no data to demonstrate that mortality decreases because of routine preoperative electrocardiographic screening.

Why persist in claiming a 50 percent reduction in morbidity for each unexpected finding? Many reports indicate that morbidity and mortality increase in patients who have had recent, as opposed to over 6-month-old, myocardial infarctions[71–77] or that invasive monitoring and treatment of abnormalities at least lessen risk.[78] Also, several studies cite increased morbidity in patients having an electrocardiographic pattern of left ventricular hypertrophy.[69,79] One study reports that more than five premature ventricular contractions per minute represent an increased risk factor.[3] Since at least two of these three findings can cause the anesthesiologist to alter the perioperative course (e.g., postponing surgery for 3 to 6 months, using a pulmonary artery catheter, applying therapy for dysrhythmias, changing the anesthetic technique), the rate of 50 percent reduction in morbidity can be used when unexpected abnormalities are discovered on ECG. Thus, the compromise conclusion is that

TABLE 8-4. Percentage of Patients Having Abnormalities Determined by Screening Electrocardiograms*

Age (years)	Sex	Series	Patients Examined (N)	Total Abnormalities† (%)	LVH	MI	ST-T Changes	AV Block
16–19	M	Ostrander et al.[68]	216	20.3	17.8	0	0.9	1.4
16–19	F	Ostrander et al.[68]	242	5.9	1.3	0	4.2	0.4
20–29	M	Ostrander et al.[68]	452	14.0	7.1	0.2	6.0	0.7
20–29	F	Ostrander et al.[68]	577	11.3	0.2	0.2	9.9	1.0
20–29	M	Collen et al.[53]	3,000	9.6				
20–29	F	Collen et al.[53]	4,000‡	9.3				
>30	Either	Maigaard et al.[51]	1,256	<4.5		0.1		
30–39	M	Ostrander et al.[68]	676		3.0	0	6.9	1.3
30–39	F	Ostrander et al.[68]	699		0.4	0.1	11.6	1.6
30–39	M	Collen et al.[53]	4,000‡	12.1				
30–39	F	Collen et al.[53]	5,000‡	11.7				
35–44	M	Kannel et al.[67,69]			2.9			
35–44	F	Kanel et al.[67,69]			0.9			
40–49	M	Ostrander et al.[68]	468	24*	4.1	1.7	16.1	1.5
40–49	F	Ostrander et al.[68]	474	21‡	0.6	0.8	17.2	0.6
40–49	M	Collen et al.[53]	4,000‡	17.6				
40–49	F	Collen et al.[53]	5,000‡	15.6				
45–54	M	Kannel et al.[67,69]			4.8			
45–54	F	Kannel et al.[67,69]			3.6			
50–59	M	Ostrander et al.[68]	330	30‡	3.3	5.1	20.8	1.2
50–59	F	Ostrander et al.[68]	327	40‡	3.4	0.9	32.4	2.1
50–59	M	Collen et al.[53]	5,000‡	24.9				
50–59	F	Collen et al.[53]	6,000‡	20.7				
55–64	M	Kannel et al.[67,69]			10.1			
55–64	F	Kannel et al.[67,69]			4.1			
<60	Either	Rabkin and Horne[14,15]	309	13.5	2.5	1.6	11.0	1.0
>60	Either	Rabkin and Horne[14,15]	503	24.4	2.2	1.9	13.0	0.6
60–69	M	Ostrander et al.[68]	177		8.4	9.0	37.1	4.5
60–69	F	Ostrander et al.[68]	196		10.2	6.1	42.4	4.1
60–69	M	Collen et al.[53]	2,000‡	35.1				
60–69	F	Collen et al.[53]	3,000‡	29.7				
65–74	M	Kannel et al.[67,69]			7.1			
65–74	F	Kannel et al.[67,69]			9.6			
>70	M	Collen et al.[53]	1,000‡	52.2				
>70	F	Collen et al.[53]	1,000‡	41.2				
70–79	M	Ostrander et al.[68]	100		7.9	9.9	46.5	7.9
70–79	F	Ostrander et al.[68]	119		11.8	2.5	43.8	6.7
>80	M	Ostrander et al.[68]	26		11.5	7.7	46.2	19.2
>80	F	Ostrander et al.[68]	43		16.3	4.7	58.2	9.3

LVH = Left ventricular hypertrophy; MI = myocardial infarction; ST-T changes = ST-T segment changes on electrocardiogram; AV = atrioventricular.

* All studies are 12 lead, except for that of Collen et al.,[53] which is a 6-lead study.

† These data constitute an edited summary of data given in several series — edited to select abnormalities that might change anesthetic management.

‡ Values are approximations that represent "best-guess" numbers from data not explicitly stated in the reports.

screening preoperative ECGs are indicated for patients over 40 years of age, assuming careful observation of the ECG before induction of anesthesia.

How useful is it to repeat ECGs if the patient has had an ECG within the past 2 years? The studies of Rabkin and Horne[14,15] address this question. Data (Table 8-5) indicate that new abnormalities occur with perhaps 25 to 50 percent of the frequency of all abnormalities. Thus, one would be justified in obtaining screening ECGs prior to elective surgery on all patients over 40 years of age, even in those who recently had an ECG.

TABLE 8-5. Number and Percentages of Patients Having a New Abnormality on EKG and a Previous EKG*

	New Abnormality with a Previously Normal EKG		New Abnormality with a Previously Abnormal EKG	
Age (years):	<60	≥60	<60	≥60
No. of patients:				
New abnormality/total no.	18/180	42/192	24/129	81/310
% New abnormality	(10%)	(21.9%)	(18.6%)	(26%)
Abnormality				
T wave	11 (6.1%)	18 (9.4%)	10 (7.8%)	19 (6.1%)
ST-T segment	7 (3.9%)	9 (4.7%)	6 (4.7%)	20 (6.4%)
Dysrhythmias				
SVT or PVCs	3 (1.7%)	7 (3.6%)		8 (2.6%)
Others, including PACs	3 (1.7%)	6 (3.1%)	1 (0.8%)	1 (0.3%)
QRS duration		8 (4.2%)	2 (1.6%)	14 (4.5%)
LVH	3 (1.7%)	4 (2.1%)	5 (3.9%)	7 (2.3%)
Q wave	4 (2.2%)	3 (1.6%)	1 (0.8%)	7 (2.3%)
Ventricular conduction defects	5 (2.6%)	1 (0.8%)	7 (2.3%)	
AV block	2 (1.0%)	3 (2.3%)	1 (0.3%)	

SVT = supraventricular tachycardia; PVCs = premature ventricular contractions; PACs = premature atrial contractions; LVH = left ventricular hypertrophy; AV = atrioventricular.
Abstracted from Rabkin and Horne.[14,15]
* Numbers in parentheses are percentages of patients. Two-thirds of patients had a previous ECG within 2 years of their new ECG.

HEMOGLOBIN, HEMATOCRIT, AND WHITE BLOOD CELL COUNTS

At UCSF, determination of hemoglobin, hematocrit, and white blood cell count costs $8.40; any one of these three tests alone costs $7.40. How abnormal must any of these be before different approaches should be taken perioperatively for supposedly healthy individuals undergoing routine operations involving no major blood loss?

Wasserman and Gilbert[80] found that of 28 patients having uncontrolled polycythemia (hemoglobin greater than 16 g/dl) who underwent major surgery, 22 (79 percent) had complications and 10 (36 percent) died. That group was compared with a group of 53 patients who had controlled polycythemia (hemoglobin ≤16 g/dl) and major surgery; 15 (28 percent) had complications and 3 (5 percent) died. In both groups, most of the complications were related to polycythemia (e.g., hemorrhage or thrombosis). Although the study has deficiencies (e.g., it was a retrospective study, no time frame was given, "minor" surgery was excluded, and it contained no statement as to why polycythemia was controlled preoperatively in

some patients and not in others), its results indicate that knowledge and pretreatment of polycythemia decrease perioperative morbidity and mortality.

No such evidence exists for normovolemic anemia. Rothstein[81] concluded that in patients under 3 months of age, hemoglobin should be over 10 g/dl, whereas in children over 3 months of age hemoglobin of 9 g/dl was adequate. Slogoff[82] concluded that in adults, a hematocrit of 20 percent (hemoglobin of about 7 g/dl) is adequate. However, no data confirm the hypothesis that treatment of moderate or mild normovolemic anemia prior to surgery involving no major blood loss in asymptomatic patients decreases perioperative morbidity or mortality. Similarly, no data exist regarding the possible harm from abnormal white blood cell counts found preoperatively. Therefore, the following ranges of "surgically acceptable values" have been arbitrarily devised: for hematocrit, 29 to 57 percent for men or 27 to 54 percent for women, and for white blood cell count, 2,400 to 16,000/m³ for both men and women.[83] When values fall outside these ranges, an alternative diagnosis is sought before anesthesia is given.[83] How many healthy patients have this degree of abnormality? None was found in the 223 patients for whom tests were not indicated by history.[24] The other limited available data are provided in Table 8-6[84,85]. If we assume that 10 percent of all abnormalities are outside the "surgically acceptable" range,[86] and if the cost–benefit analysis described in the chest roentgenogram section is used, either preoperative hematocrit or hemoglobin levels should be determined for all women and for men over 60 years of age. White blood cell counts appear to be rarely, if ever, indicated.

BLOOD CHEMISTRIES

What blood chemistries would have to be abnormal, and how abnormal would they have to be before perioperative management would have to be altered? Abnormal liver or renal function might change the choice and dose of anesthetic or adjuvant drugs. For example, for the patient in renal failure, pancuronium might be avoided or its dose decreased. Likewise, halothane might be avoided in the patient with active liver disease, although this conclusion is controversial (MK Cahalan, personal communication). About 1 in 700 supposedly healthy patients is actually harboring hepatitis, and 1 in 3 of those will become jaundiced.[87,88]

The available data on screening blood chemistries are presented in Table 8-7[93]. Unexpected abnormalities are reported in 2 to 10 percent of patients screened.[16,24,53,84,86–92,94–97] These abnormalities lead to a great deal of additional studies. In approximately 80 percent of cases, these additional studies lead to conclusions having no significance for the patient.[16–18,24,53,84,86–92,94–98] Unexpected abnormalities that are significant arise in 2 to 5 percent of patients studied. Approximately 70 percent of these findings are related to blood glucose and blood urea nitrogen (BUN) levels.[16–18,24,53,84,86–92,94–97] The 9 or 10 additional tests on the screening SMA 12 panels lead to very few important findings related to anesthesia. In fact, the false-positive rate is so high (i.e., 96.5 percent for calcium[95]) that the cost–benefit value of most of these tests, even when free, is negative.

If a screening test for hepatitis is desired because its incidence is 0.14 percent and because the potential legal problems of postanesthetic jaundice are to be avoided (see section on medicolegal issues, below) the three tests, serum glutamic oxaloacetic transaminase (SGOT), blood glucose, and BUN, seem indicated. At our hospital, these three tests currently cost $20.50, as does the SMA 12, which includes almost all the screening chemistries listed in Table 8-7. However, I recommend the

TABLE 8-6. Abnormalities Discovered by Screening Hemoglobin Tests and White Blood Cell Counts

Age (years)	Sex	Series	Patients Examined (n)	Hemoglobin Abnormalities (%)	WBC Count Abnormalities (%)
<19	Either	Wood and Hoekelman[26]	1,924	0.8	
<40	M	Collen et al.[53]	6,941	1.9	2.6
<40	F	Collen et al.[53]	9,037	12.6	2.6
≥18	Either	Parkerson[27,84]	392	18.8	10.7
40–59	M	Collen et al.[53]	11,832	3.1	2.2
40–59	F	Collen et al.[53]	9,657	10.1	2.2
≥60	M	Collen et al.[53]	4,062	5.6	1.7
≥60	F	Collen et al.[53]	3,134	5.5	1.7
Unspecified	Either	Kaplan et al.[24]	293	0*	0*
Unspecified	Either	Gold and Wolfersberger[85]	3,375	0.33	
Unspecified	Either	Carmalt et al.[86]	278	30.4†	
Unspecified	Either	Huntley et al.[29]	119	23	
Unspecified	Either	Williamson[28]	982	3.2	

* Surgically significant abnormalities.

† Carmalt found that 24.5 percent were new abnormalities; 2 patients had hemoglobin values less than 8 g/dl, 17 had values of 8 to 10 g/dl, and 21 had values of 10 to 12 g/dl.

TABLE 8-7. Screening Blood Chemistries: Percentages of Patients Having Abnormalities

Age (years)	Series	Patients Examined (N)	BUN	Cr	Glucose	SGOT	Uric Acid	Cholesterol	Albumin	Total Protein	Ca	VDRL	Alkaline PTAse	Bilirubin	K+
10-54	Schemel[88]	7,620				0.144									
15-85	Carmalt et al.[86]*	296	1.4	1.0	2.0	0		0.3	0		0.3		0	0	0.3
>18	Parkerson[84]	397		1.2	15.8	2.8	7.9	6.1			2.0			1.2	6.6
>18	Schneiderman et al.[89]	547		9.3	5.0	1.3	4.5						9.7	3.7	
>18	[Thiers, VAMC][90,91]	623	1.1			3.1			1.4	2.4	1.0				4.0
>25	Peery[92]*	1,771	18		21		36	30	0.5	0.5			1.3		3.6
40-59	Collen et al.[53]	21,489		1.4	5.6	4.6	4.8	2.7	0.3	4.4	1.3	1.9			
>40	Collen et al.[53]	15,978		0.8	4.6	3.6	3.4	1.7	0.4	3.5	1.4	0.8			
>60	Collen et al.[53]	7,196		2.7	8.3	4.5	6.0	3.0	0.4	3.9	1.5	2.3			
All	Wataneeyawech and Kelly[87]	6,540				0.234									
All	Bryan et al.[90]	2,846	1.4		5.6				1.4	0.7	0.3				0.3
All	Friedman et al.[93]	8,446	3.4	3.3	5.9	2.7	2.7	3.8	1.5	2.5	5.4		3.9	2.4	1.4
All	Delahunt and Turnbull[16]	332	0	0											0.3
All	Young and Drake[94]*	390	6.4	3.7	7.5						2.0				0
All	Boonstra et al.[95]*	12,000									5.0				
All	Whitehead et al.[96]	2,871	3.4		10.0	1.8	9.2	9.3	2.9		9.2		8.3	6.0	4.7

BUN = blood urea nitrogen; Cr = creatinine; SGOT = serum glutamic oxaloacetic transaminase; Ca = calcium; PTAse = phosphatase; K+ = potassium.
* A high percentage of these findings were analyzed in more depth and found to be clinically unimportant.

three specific tests, as the cost of predictive false positives is so high for the other screening chemistries as to give them a negative cost–benefit ratio even when the first set of screening chemistry results is free. Using the assumptions and method of analysis from the section on chest roentgenogram and assuming the positive rate to be 2 percent and the predictive false-positive rate 10 percent, it can be concluded that all patients should undergo determination of SGOT, BUN, and blood glucose levels. The incidence of significant abnormalities increases with age (e.g., it is 2.5 percent for those under 40 years of age, 5 percent for those aged 40 to 59, and 7.5 percent for those over age years), as indicated by the data collected by Collen et al.[53] If that incidence progression and a predictive false-positive rate of 50 percent are used, then at least from a cost–benefit point of view, only the two screening tests (BUN and blood glucose) are indicated, and only for patients over 40 years of age.

URINALYSIS

Abnormalities are commonly found on urinalysis (Table 8-8).[26,28,29,53,85,98] However, these abnormal results usually do not lead to beneficial changes in management,[17,35,98,99] and most of the abnormal results that do lead to beneficial changes could have been obtained with history or BUN and glucose determinations. Such determinations were already recommended for all patients over 40 years of age. Thus, urinalysis, although initially inexpensive, becomes an expensive test to justify on a cost–benefit basis.

CLOTTING STUDIES

Although measurement of the partial thromboplastin time (PTT) and the prothrombin time (PT) are useful tests to screen patients with a history of bleeding,[100–102] their value as a routine screening test has been questioned. Robbins and Rose[103] examined the PTT values of 1,025 consecutive patients; the times for 143 patients (14 percent) were prolonged. Twenty-three of these patients did not have a known or suspected clotting disorder discernible by history-taking. Nine of those 23 had a repeat test that yielded normal results. The other 14 had surgery without further clotting evaluation and without the occurrence of bleeding complications during surgery. Replying to Robbins and Rose, Baranetsky and Weinstein[104] advocated the continued use of PTT determinations as a screening test. They cited as evidence five patients who had negative bleeding histories and abnormal PTT values (of 2,600 patients screened with the PTT test). Four patients underwent operation without bleeding incidents, the exception being the occurrence of a small hematoma after traumatic insertion of a pacemaker. The fifth patient was given fresh frozen plasma prior to cholecystostomy. This patient had previously undergone herniorrhaphy and laminectomy without prior treatment with fresh frozen plasma. Thus, it is not clear that the 2,600 screening PTT determinations benefited any patient. A. Lorenzi and S. Cohen (personal communication) found that of 578 patients screened with both the PT and PTT tests, 20 had a PT value ≥ 12.5 seconds or a PTT value ≥ 38 seconds. Ten of those patients had minor abnormalities defined as a PT value of 12.5 to

TABLE 8-8. Abnormalities Discovered by Screening Urinalysis

Age (years)	Sex	Series	Patients Examined (N)	Abnormalities (%)	Significant Abnormalities (%)
<19	Either	Wood and Hoekelman[26]	1,859	11.7	0.5
Unspecified	Either	Huntley et al.[29]	119	25	
5–12	F	Cardiff-Oxford[98]	16,800	1.8	
Unspecified	Either	Gold and Wolfersberger[85]	3,375	2.7	
Unspecified	Either	Williamson et al.[28]	982	16.7	
Unspecified	Either	Collen et al.[53]	44,663	14.6	

13 seconds or a PTT value of 38 to 41 seconds. For no patient was there a notation on the chart about this abnormality (perhaps a medicolegal problem if intraoperative bleeding presented a problem); all patients underwent surgery without bleeding problems. Ten patients had a PT value of more than 13 seconds or a PTT value of more than 41 seconds. Four had known bleeding diathesis (one was hemophilic, one had a history of bleeding, as disclosed in the history on admission, and two were receiving warfarin treatment). Five of the remaining six patients underwent surgery without any further evaluation of the PT/PTT abnormalities noted on the chart (a medicolegal cost might have resulted from this neglect) and without the occurrence of unusual bleeding during surgery. The other patient was found to have normal PT and PTT values on repeat study.

We found no benefit to any of the 154 patients who underwent PT or PTT tests that were not indicated by history.[24] Eisenberg et al.[105] found that one patient in 750 might have benefited from PT or PTT determinations as screening tests. In reality, that patient did not benefit; in fact, on reexamination, bleeding was found to be caused by an arterial bleeding site, a circumstance not likely to be mitigated by treatment prompted by an abnormal PT or PTT test. In addition, PT or PTT tests do not predict transfusion requirements during or after major surgery.[106] On the basis of these data, little benefit will be obtained from coagulation tests not indicated by history.

PULMONARY FUNCTION TESTS

The suggested tests for patients having a history of lung disease or smoking are described in Chapters 9, 32, and 59. Pulmonary function tests are not recommended for patients who do not have a history of pulmonary problems. The history, especially the maximum tolerated physical activity without shortness of breath, should be used as a guide.

SUMMARY OF LABORATORY TESTS THAT MIGHT BE ROUTINELY ORDERED

For the asymptomatic "healthy" patient scheduled to undergo operative procedures not involving major blood loss (such as breast biopsy, herniorrhaphy, vein stripping, tonsillectomy, and dilatation and curettage), no laboratory test appears to be indicated if the patient is male and younger than 40 years of age (Table 8-9). For female patients less than 40 years of age, only a hemoglobin test is indicated. For all patients aged 40 to 60, an EKG and determination of BUN and blood glucose levels are indi-

TABLE 8-9.   Screening Studies That Should be Performed on Asymptomatic Healthy Patients Scheduled to Undergo Non-Blood-Loss "Peripheral" Surgical Procedures

Age (years)	Tests Indicated	
	For Men	For Women
Under 40	None	Hemoglobin or hematocrit
40–59	Electrocardiogram BUN/glucose	Hemoglobin or hematocrit Electrocardiogram BUN/glucose
Over 60	Hemoglobin or hematocrit Electrocardiogram Chest roentgenogram BUN/glucose	Hemoglobin or hematocrit Electrocardiogram Chest roentgenogram BUN/glucose

cated; for female patients a determination of hemoglobin or hematocrit should also be made. After 60 years of age, all patients should have an EKG; a chest roentgenogram; and determination of hematocrit or hemoglobin, BUN, and blood glucose levels. It would be even better to select screening tests based on either a physician-generated history and physical examination (Fig. 8-1) or on the patient's answers to a health questionnaire (Fig. 8-2).

OTHER BENEFITS FROM LABORATORY TESTS

Several laboratory screening tests may increase longevity that are not needed preoperatively. A case can be made for routine Papanicolaou smears for detecting cervical cancer, for urine examination (although evidence that microscopic hematuria, as opposed to gross hematuria, as a screening test increases survival is nonexistent), and for urine culture in women over 55 years of age (evidence that treating asymptomatic bacteriuria in patients over 55 years of age lessens disease is also nonexis-

tent).[98,99] Since these tests will not change what the anesthesiologist does for the patient preoperatively, analysis of their yield and cost versus benefit is not discussed in this chapter. Their contribution to life is quite another subject.[107,108]

Benefits other than medical can accrue from testing. For instance, in two studies normal exercise tests in patients having atypical chest pain led to fewer hospital days and more productive life than not testing a matched randomized group of patients.[109,110] These other benefits of testing were assumed to equal other costs in the analysis above. One can substitute an appropriate value and recalculate the analysis if other benefits do not appear to equal other costs.

THE MEDICOLEGAL RATIONALE FOR LABORATORY TESTING

Ordering preoperative laboratory tests for alleged medicolegal protection is not the straightforward matter it may seem. Data sug-

TABLE 8-10. Potential Medicolegal Cost

Series	Type Test	Unexpected Abnormalities (N)	Unexpected Abnormalities Noted Preoperatively (%)
Lorenzi and Cohen*	PT/PTT	20	5
Rabkin and Horne[14,15]	ECG	157	31
Kaplan et al.[24]	CBC/PTT Glucose/SMA 6	12†	17
Robbins and Rose[103]	PT	23	39
Wood and Hoekelman[26]	Hematocrit	15†	27
Parkerson[27,84]‡	Multiple	343	38
	Multiple; > 10% abnormal	63?	60
Williamson et al.[28]‡	Urinalysis	164	17
	FBS	63	32
	Hemoglobin	32	16
Huntley et al.[29]‡	Multiple	343	67
Daughaday et al.[30]	Multiple	167	60
Epstein et al.[31]‡	T4	111	60

PT = prothrombin time; PTT = partial thromboplastin time; CBC = complete blood count; SMA 6 = simultaneous multichannel analyses of sodium, potassium, chloride, bicarbonate, urea nitrogen, and creatinine levels in blood; FBS = fasting blood sugar; and T_4 = thyroxine.

  * Personal communication.

  † Potentially surgically significant abnormalities.

  ‡ Not preoperative.

gest that this practice may actually create a liability, since the total number of false negatives and false positives may exceed the total of true positives. For example, using the highest values for sensitivity and specificity in the literature (75 and 98.3 percent, respectively) and an assumed rate of prevalence of disease in asymptomatic individuals of 1.5 percent, more than 60 percent of chest roentgenograms ordered without indication and reported to be abnormal will be falsely positive. In addition, the rare unexpected positive result does not often alter the decision to proceed with surgery. Documentation in the medical record of justifications for disregarding unexpected abnormal results has been lacking in at least 50 percent of patients in studies of this issue (and, in some studies, is absent on the charts of as many as 95 percent of patients who had unexpected abnormal test results) (Table 8-10). Thus, ordering more tests may not increase medicolegal protection.

The assumptions used to reach the cost–benefit analysis were skewed to overestimate the predictive value of laboratory testing. Thus, for healthy patients, one should probably do less laboratory testing rather than more. We all have a responsibility to provide optimum care within the bounds of finite resources. If we were to limit our laboratory use to that indicated for healthy individuals, perhaps government would allow us to practice optimum medicine (which tends to be more expensive) for the sick who need more laboratory work.

REFERENCES

1. Vacanti CJ, VanHouten RJ, Hill RC: A statistical analysis of the relationship of physical status to postoperative mortality in 68,388 cases. Anesth Analg 49:564, 1970
2. Lewin I, Lerner AG, Green SH, et al: Physical class and physiologic status in the prediction of operative mortality in the aged sick. Ann Surg 174:217, 1971
3. Goldman L, Caldera DL, Nussbaum SR, et al: Multifactorial index of cardiac risk in noncardiac surgical procedures. N Engl J Med 297:845, 1977
4. Marx GF, Mateo CV, Orkin LR: Computer analysis of postanesthetic deaths. Anesthesiology 39:54, 1973
5. Ziffren SE, Hartford CE: Comparative mortality for various surgical operations in older versus younger age groups. J Am Geriatr Soc 20:485, 1972
6. Rehder K: Clinical evaluation of isoflurane. Complications during and after anaesthesia. Can Anaesth Soc J (suppl) 29:S44, 1982
7. Keats AS: The ASA classification of physical status—A recapitulation. Anesthesiology 49:233, 1978
8. Duckett JB: Preoperative assessment of the patient for outpatient anesthesia, Outpatient Anesthesia. Edited by Brown BB Jr. Philadelphia, FA Davis, 1978, pp 21–29.
9. Okelberry CR: Preadmission testing shortens preoperative length of stay. Hospitals 49(Sept 16):71, 1975
10. Sandler G: Costs of unnecessary tests. Br Med J 2:21, 1979
11. Leonard JV, Clayton BE, Colley JRT: Use of biochemical profile in children's hospital: results of two controlled trials. Br Med J 2:662, 1975
12. Durbridge TC, Edwards F, Edwards RG, et al: Evaluation of benefits of screening tests done immediately on admission to hospital. Clin Chem 22:968, 1976
13. North AF Jr: Screening in child care. Am Fam Physician 13:85, 1976
14. Rabkin SW, Horne JM: Preoperative electrocardiography: Effect of new abnormalities on clinical decisions. Can Med Assoc J 128:146, 1983
15. Rabkin SW, Horne JM: Preoperative electrocardiography: Its cost-effectiveness in detecting abnormalities when a previous tracing exists. Can Med Assoc J 121:301, 1979
16. Delahunt B, Turnbull PRG: How cost effective are routine preoperative investigations? NZ Med J 92:431, 1980
17. Fineberg HV: Clinical chemistries: The high cost of low-cost diagnostic tests, Proceedings of the 1977 Sun Valley Forum on National Health. Edited by Altman SH, Blendon R. DHEW publication no. (PHS) 79-3216. Washington DC, US Department of Health, Education, and Welfare, Public Health Service, Office of Health Research, Statistics, and Technology, National Center for Health Services Administration, Bureau of Health Planning, 1979, pp 144–165
18. Bradwell AR, Carmalt MHB, Whitehead TP: Explaining the unexpected abnormal results of

biochemical profile investigations. Lancet 2:1071, 1974

19. Korvin CC, Pearce RH, Stanley J: Admission screening: Clinical benefits. Ann Intern Med 83:197, 1975

20. Olsen DM, Kane RL, Proctor PH: A controlled trial of multiphasic screening. N Engl J Med 294:925, 1976

21. Pless IB: Routine tests in pediatric practice: Things better left undone. Pediatr Dib 21:13, 1979

22. Charap MH: The periodic health examination: Genesis of a myth. Ann Intern Med 95:733, 1981

23. Daniels M, Schroeder SA: Variation among physicians in use of laboratory tests. II. Relation to clinical productivity and outcomes of care. Med Care 15:482, 1977

24. Kaplan EB, Sheiner LB, Boeckmann AJ, et al: The usefulness of preoperative laboratory screening. Med Care (in press)

25. Leonidas JC, Ting W, Binkiewicz A, et al: Mild head trauma in children: when is a roentgenogram necessary. Pediatrics 69:139, 1982

26. Wood RA, Hoekelman RA: Value of the chest x-ray as a screening test for elective surgery in children. Pediatrics 67:477, 1981

27. Parkerson GR Jr: Cost analysis of laboratory tests in ambulatory primary care. J Fam Pract 7:1001, 1978

28. Williamson JW, Alexander M, Miller GE: Continuing education and patient care research. Physician response to screening test results. JAMA 201:118, 1967

29. Huntley RR, Steinhauser R, White KL, et al: The quality of medical care: Techniques and investigation in the outpatient clinic. J Chron Dis 14:630, 1961

30. Daughaday WH, Erickson MM, White W, et al: Evaluation of routine 12-channel chemical profiles on patients admitted to a university general hospital, Multiple Laboratory Screening. Edited by Benson ES, Strandjord PE. New York, Academic Press, 1969, p 181–197

31. Epstein KA, Schneiderman LJ, Bush JW, et al: The "abnormal" screening serum thyroxine (T4): Analysis of physician response, outcome, cost and health effectiveness. J Chron Dis 34:175, 1981

32. Rossello PJ, Cruz AR, Mayol PM: Routine laboratory tests for elective surgery in pediatric patients: Are they necessary? Bull Assoc Med Puerto Rico 72:614, 1980

33. Baker JP, Detsky AS, Wesson DE, et al: A comparison of clinical judgment and objective measurements. N Engl J Med 306:969, 1982

34. Finkler SA: The distinction between cost and charges. Ann Intern Med 96:102, 1982

35. Friedman GD: Effects of MHTS on patients, Multiphasic Health Testing Services. Edited by Collen MF. New York, Wiley, 1978, pp 531–549

36. Dales LG, Friedman GD, Collen MF: Evaluating periodic multiphasic health checkups: A controlled trial. J Chron Dis 32:385, 1979

37. Roberts NJ, Ipsen J, Elsom KO, et al: Mortality among males in periodic-health-examination programs. N Engl J Med 281:20, 1969

38. Kuller L, Tonascia S: Commission on chronic illness follow-up study. Comparison of screened and nonscreened individuals. Arch Environ Health 21:656, 1970

39. Krieg AF, Gambino R, Galen RS: Why are clinical laboratory tests performed? When are they valid? JAMA 233:76, 1975

40. Robbins JA, Mushlin AI: Preoperative evaluation of the healthy patient. Med Clin North Am 63:1145, 1979

41. Gorry GA, Pauker SG, Schwartz WB: The diagnostic importance of the normal finding. N Engl J Med 298:486, 1978

42. Galen RS, Gambino SR: Sensitivity, specificity, prevalence and incidence. Beyond Normality: The Predictive Value and Efficiency of Medical Diagnoses. Edited by Galen RS, Gambino SR. New York, Wiley, 1975, pp 9–14

43. Collen MF (ed): Multiphasic Health Testing Services. New York, Wiley, 1978

44. Napier JA, Johnson BC, Epstein FH: The Tecumseh, Michigan, community health study, Kessler II, Levin ML (eds): The Community as an Epidemiologic Laboratory: A Casebook of Community Studies. Baltimore, Johns Hopkins Press, 1970, pp 25–46

45. Farnsworth PB, Steiner E, Klein RM, SanFilippo JA: The value of routine preoperative chest roentgenograms in infants and children. JAMA 244:582, 1980

46. Brill PW, Ewing ML, Dunn AA: The value(?) of routine chest radiography in children and adolescents. Pediatrics 52:125, 1973

47. Sagal SS, Evens RG, Forrest JV, Bramson RT: Efficacy of routine screening and lateral chest radiographs in a hospital-based population. N Engl J Med 291:1001, 1974

48. Sane SM, Worsing RA Jr, Wiens CW, Sharma RK: Value of preoperative chest x-ray examinations in children. Pediatrics 60:669, 1977

49. Rees AM, Roberts CJ, Bligh AS, Evans KT: Routine preoperative chest radiography in non-cardiopulmonary surgery. Br Med J 1:1333, 1976

50. Loder RE: Routine pre-operative chest radiography. 1977 compared with 1955 at Peterborough District General Hospital. Anaesthesia 33:972, 1978

51. Maigaard S, Elkjaer P, Stefansson T: Vaerdien

af praeoperativ rutinerøntgenundersøgelse af thorax og ekg. (Engl. abstr: Value of routine preoperative radiographic examination of the thorax and ECG). Ugeskr Laeger 140:769, 1978

52. Catchlove BR, Wilson RM, Spring S, Hall J: Routine investigations in elective surgical patients. Their use and cost effectiveness in a teaching hospital. Med J Aust 2:107, 1979

53. Collen MF, Feldman R, Siegelaub AB, Crawford D: Dollar cost per positive test for automated multiphasic screening. N Engl J Med 283:459, 1970

54. Thomsen HS, Gottlieb J, Madsen JK, et al: Rutinemaessig røntgenundersøgelse af thorax inden kirurgiske indgreg i universal anaestesi (Engl abstr: Routine radiographic examination of the thorax prior to surgical intervention under general anaesthesia). Ugeskr Laeger 140:765, 1978

55. Törnebrandt K, Fletcher R: Pre-operative chest X-rays in elderly patients. Anaesthesia 37:901, 1982

56. Petterson SR, Janower ML: Is the routine preoperative chest film of value? Appl Radiol (Jan-Feb):70, 1977

57. Royal College of Radiologists Working Party on the Effective Use of Diagnostic Radiology: Preoperative chest radiology. National study by the Royal College of Radiologists. Lancet 2:83, 1979

58. Neuhauser D: Cost-effective clinical decision making. Pediatrics 60:756, 1977

59. Bunker JP, Barnes BA, Mosteller F (eds): Costs, Risks, and Benefits of Surgery. New York, Oxford University Press, 1977

60. Cochrane AL, Garland LH: Observer error in the interpretation of chest films. An international investigation. Lancet 2:505, 1952

61. Yerushalmy J: The statistical assessment of the variability in observer perception and description of roentgenographic pulmonary shadows. Radiol Clin North Am 7:381, 1969

62. Yerushalmy J: Reliability of chest radiography in the diagnosis of pulmonary lesions. Am J Surg 89:231, 1955

63. Yerushalmy J, Harkness JT, Cope JH, Kennedy BR: The role of dual reading in mass radiography. Am Rev Tuberc 61:443, 1950

64. Newell RR, Chamberlain WE, Rigler L: Descriptive classification of pulmonary shadows. A revelation of unreliability in the roentgenographic diagnosis of tuberculosis. Am Rev Tuberc 69:566, 1954

65. Groth-Petersen E, Løvgreen A, Thillemann J: On the reliability of the reading of photofluorograms and the value of dual reading. Acta Tuberc Scand 26:13, 1952

66. Garland LH: On the scientific evaluation of diagnostic procedures. Presidential address.

Thirty-fourth annual meeting of the Radiological Society of North America. Radiology 52:309, 1949

67. Gordon T, Kannel WB: The Framingham, Massachusetts study twenty years later, The Community as an Epidemiologic Laboratory: A Casebook of Community Studies. Edited by Kessler II, Levin ML. Baltimore, Johns Hopkins Press, 1970, pp 123–146

68. Ostrander LD Jr, Brandt RL, Kjelsberg MO, Epstein FH: Electrocardiographic findings among the adult population of a total natural community, Tecumseh, Michigan. Circulation 31:888, 1965

69. Kannel WB, McGee D, Gordon T: A general cardiovascular risk profile: The Framingham study. Am J Cardiol 38:46, 1976

70. Galen RS, Gambino SR: The electrocardiogram application of the model to a nonlaboratory test. Beyond Normality: The Predictive Value and Efficiency of Medical Diagnoses. Edited by Galen RS, Gambino SR. New York, Wiley, 1975, pp 99–106

71. Tarhan S, Moffitt EA, Taylor WF, et al: Myocardial infarction after general anesthesia. JAMA 220:1451, 1972

72. Fraser JG, Ramachandran PR, Davis HS: Anesthesia and recent myocardial infarction. JAMA 199:318, 1967

73. Arkins R, Smessaert AA, Hicks RG: Mortality and morbidity in surgical patients with coronary artery disease. JAMA 190:485, 1964

74. Topkins MJ, Artusio JF Jr: Myocardial infarction and surgery. A five year study. Anesth Analg 43:716, 1964

75. Goldman L, Caldera DL, Southwick FS, et al: Cardiac risk factors and complications in noncardiac surgery. Medicine (Baltimore) 57:357, 1978

76. Steen PA, Tinker JH, Tarhan S: Myocardial reinfarction after anesthesia and surgery. JAMA 239:2566, 1978

77. Mauney FM Jr, Ebert PA, Sabiston DC Jr: Postoperative myocardial infarction: a study of predisposing factors, diagnosis and mortality in a high risk group of surgical patients. Ann Surg 172:497, 1970

78. Rao TLK, Jacobs KH, El-Etr AA: Reinfarction following anesthesia in patients with myocardial infarction. Anesthesiology 59:499, 1983

79. Ostrander LD Jr: Serial electrocardiographic findings in a prospective epidemiological study. Circulation 34:1069, 1966

80. Wasserman LR, Gilbert HS: Surgical bleeding in polycythemia vera. Ann NY Acad Sci 115:122, 1964

81. Rothstein P: What hemoglobin level is adequate

in pediatric anesthesia? Anesthesiol Update 1:2, 1978

82. Slogoff S: Anesthesia considerations in the anemic patient. Anesthesiol Update 2:7, 1979

83. Kowalyshyn TJ, Prager D, Young J: Review of the present status of preoperative hemoglobin requirements. Anesth Analg 51:75, 1972

84. Parkerson GR Jr: Determinants of physician recognition and follow-up of abnormal laboratory values. J Fam Pract 7:341, 1978

85. Gold BD, Wolfersberger WH: Findings from routine urinalysis and hematocrit on ambulatory oral and maxillofacial surgery patients. J Oral Surg 38:677, 1980

86. Carmalt MHB, Freeman P, Stephens AJH, et al: Value of routine multiple blood tests in patients attending the general practitioner. Br Med J 1:620, 1970

87. Wataneeyawech M, Kelly KA Jr: Hepatic diseases unsuspected before surgery. NY State J Med 75:1278, 1975

88. Schemel WH: Unexpected hepatic dysfunction found by multiple laboratory screening. Anesth Analg 55:810, 1976

89. Schneiderman LJ, DeSalvo L, Baylor S, et al: The "abnormal" screening laboratory results. Its effect on physician and patient. Arch Intern Med 129:88, 1972

90. Bryan DJ, Wearne JL, Viau A, et al: Profile of admission chemical data by multichannel automation: An evaluative experiment. Clin Chem 12:137, 1966

91. Schoen I: Clinical chemistry. A retrospective look at routine screening. Calif Med 108:430, 1968

92. Peery TM: The role of the laboratory in health evaluation, Interim Report No. 77, from the 1964 Technicon International Symposium, New York, NY, as quoted in Schoen I: Clinical chemistry, a retrospective look at routine screening. Calif Med 108:430, 1968

93. Friedman GD, Goldberg M, Ahuja JN, et al: Biochemical screening tests. Effect of panel size on medical care. Arch Intern Med 129:91, 1972

94. Young DM, Drake TGH: Unsolicited laboratory information, presented to the College of American Pathologists, Chicago, 18 Oct 1965, as quoted in Schoen I: Clinical chemistry, a retrospective look at routine screening. Calif Med 108:430, 1968

95. Boonstra CE, Jackson CE: The clinical value of routine serum calcium analysis. Ann Intern Med 57:963, 1962

96. Whitehead TP: Multiple analyses and their use in the investigation of patients. Adv Clin Chem 14:389, 1971

97. Durbridge TC, Edwards F, Edwards RG, Atkinson M: An evaluation of multiphasic screening on admission to hospital. Precis of a report to the National Health and Medical Research Council. Med J Aust 1:703, 1976

98. Cardiff-Oxford Bacteriuria Study Group: Sequelae of covert bacteriuria in schoolgirls. A four-year follow-up study. Lancet 1:889, 1978

99. Nicolle LE, Bjornson J, Harding GKM, et al: Bacteriuria in elderly institutionalized men. N Engl J Med 309:1420, 1983

100. Watson-Williams EJ: Hematologic and hemostatic considerations before surgery. Med Clin North Am 63:1165, 1979

101. Nye SW, Graham JB, Brinkhous KM: The partial thromboplastin time as a screening test for the detection of latent bleeders. Am J Med Sci 243:279, 1962

102. Bowie EJW, Owen CA Jr: The significance of abnormal preoperative hemostatic tests. Prog Hemost Thromb 5:179, 1980

103. Robbins JA, Rose SD: Partial thromboplastin time as a screening test (correspondence). Ann Intern Med 90:796, 1979

104. Baranetsky NG, Weinstein P: Partial thromboplastin time for screening (correspondence). Ann Intern Med 91:498, 1979

105. Eisenberg JM, Clarke JR, Sussman SA: Prothrombin and partial thromboplastin times as preoperative screening tests. Arch Surg 117:48, 1982

106. Ramsey G, Arvan DA, Stewart S, Blumberg N: Do preoperative laboratory tests predict blood transfusion needs in cardiac operations? J Thorac Cardiovasc Surg 85:564, 1983

107. Grogono AW, Woodgate DJ: Index for measuring health. Lancet 2:1024, 1971

108. Grogono AW: Measurement of ill health: A comment. Int J Epidemiol 2:5, 1973

109. Sox HC Jr, Margulies I, Sox CH: Psychologically mediated effects of diagnostic tests. Ann Intern Med 95:680, 1981

110. Faxon DP, McCabe CH, Kreigel DE, et al: Therapeutic and economic value of a normal coronary angiogram. Am J Med 73:500, 1982

9

Anesthetic Implications of Concurrent Diseases

Michael F. Roizen, M.D.

INTRODUCTION

This chapter discusses patients who have conditions requiring special preoperative evaluation and intraoperative management. As with "healthy" patients (also see Ch. 8), it is the history and physical examination of these patients that most accurately predicts not only the associated risks but also the likelihood that a monitoring technique or change in therapy will be beneficial or necessary for survival. Those instances in which specific information should be sought in the history-taking, physical examination, or laboratory evaluations are emphasized. Although controlled studies to confirm that optimizing a patient's preoperative physical condition will result in lower morbidity have not been performed for most diseases, it is logical to assume that such is the case. Studies showing the benefits of optimizing spe-

cific preoperative conditions are highlighted. The fact that such preventive measures would cost less than treating the morbidity that would otherwise occur is an important consideration in a cost-conscious environment. Examples of determining the costs of such benefits can be found in Chapter 8 in the section on preoperative preparation of the patient with cardiovascular disease. Conditions discussed in this chapter are (1) diseases involving the endocrine system and disorders of nutrition; (2) diseases involving the cardiovascular system; (3) disorders of the respiratory and immune systems; (4) diseases of the CNS, neuromuscular diseases, and mental disorders; (5) diseases involving the kidney, infectious diseases, and disorders of electrolytes; (6) diseases involving the gastrointestinal (GI) tract or the liver; (7) diseases involving hematopoiesis and various forms of cancer; and (8) diseases of aging or that occur more commonly in the aged, as well as and chronic and acute medical conditions requiring drug therapy (also see Chs. 47, 48, & 49).

tient's consultants as to what information is needed from the preoperative consultation.

THE ROLE OF THE PRIMARY CARE PHYSICIAN OR CONSULTANT

The role of the primary care physician or consultant is not to select or suggest anesthetic or surgical methods but, rather, to optimize the patient's preoperative status regarding those conditions that increase the morbidity and mortality associated with surgery.

Optimizing a patient's preoperative condition is a cooperative venture between the anesthesiologist and the internist, pediatrician, surgeon, or family physician. If the primary care physician cannot affirm that the patient is in the very best physical state attainable (for that patient) by that physician and his or her consultants, the anesthesiologist and the physician should do what is necessary to optimize that condition. Failure to consult with the primary care physician preoperatively is as risky as not checking the oxygen in the spare tanks. In fact, statements that describe the preoperative physical condition of the patient (e.g., "This patient is in optimum shape," and "I believe the mitral stenosis is more severe than the slight degree of mitral insufficiency") are much more useful to the anesthesiologist than are statements that suggest perioperative procedures ("Avoid hypoxia and hypotension").[1] Internists, pediatricians, and family practitioners usually have little knowledge of the problems, physiologic processes, and drug properties and reactions related to anesthesia.

Although information about the perioperative period is being introduced to physician consultants, such material is currently descriptive, elementary, and incomplete and rarely describes pathophysiologic conditions.[2] Without understanding the physiologic changes that occur perioperatively, it is difficult to prescribe the appropriate therapy. It is therefore part of the anesthesiologist's job to educate the pa-

DISEASES INVOLVING THE ENDOCRINE SYSTEM AND DISORDERS OF NUTRITION

PANCREATIC DISORDERS

PREOPERATIVE DIABETES MELLITUS

This section makes four major points regarding diabetes:

1. Because diabetes represents at least two disease processes, perioperative management may differ between them.
2. A current debate exists as to how closely the blood glucose levels of diabetic patients should be controlled. Chronic "tight" control of type I diabetes probably prevents, retards, or even ameliorates, to some degree, some of the chronic complications of diabetes. However, the debate centers on how great the benefit of tight control is, and what the benefit-risk ratio is. Little evidence indicates that tight perioperative control is a benefit; the benefit–risk ratio of tight perioperative control has not been examined.
3. Different regimens permit almost any degree of perioperative control of blood glucose levels, but the tighter the control desired, the more frequently blood glucose levels must be monitored. Three treatment regimens are outlined.
4. Although the presence of diabetes has long been assumed to increase perioperative risk, results from epidemiologic studies segregating the effects of diabetes per se from those of the organ system, complications of diabetes (e.g., cardiac and vascular disease), and of old age may not support this assumption. Thus, it may be only the end-organ

complications of diabetes and not diabetes itself that increase perioperative risk. Tight perioperative control of glucose levels in diabetic patients may not be as great a benefit as was thought recently.

The 1978 NIH Classification Group divides patients having diabetes mellitus, the most common endocrinopathy, into two main types.[3] Type I, insulin-dependent diabetes mellitus (IDDM), is composed mainly of diabetic persons who are susceptible to ketosis (juvenile-onset diabetics). Type II, non-insulin-dependent diabetes mellitus (NIDDM), consists of diabetic persons who are not prone to ketosis or whose diabetes was induced by drugs or pregnancy. Because diabetes represents at least two (and possibly more) disease processes, perioperative management may differ. Type I diabetes is associated with other autoimmune diseases and has a concordance rate of 25 to 50 percent (i.e., if one monozygotic twin has diabetes, the other twin would have a 25 to 50 percent likelihood of developing the disease as well). Also, the type I patient has insulin deficiency and is susceptible to ketoacidosis if insulin is withheld. By contrast, the type II diabetic patient has a concordance rate of 100 percent (i.e., the genetic material is both necessary and sufficient for the development of type II diabetes), is not susceptible to ketoacidosis in the absence of exogenous insulin, and has peripheral insulin resistance.

Type I and type II diabetes differ in other ways as well. However, age does not firmly differentiate type I from type II diabetes, as was thought formerly, that is, an older person can in fact develop type I diabetes.[4,5] Currently, the IDDM patient is treated by controlling diet and administering insulin (two or four times a day) or by using a continuous subcutaneous insulin infusion pump with home monitoring of blood glucose levels. Previously, the IDDM patient (type II) was treated with diet, weight control, and orally administered drugs, such as acetohexamide (Dymelor), chlorpropamide (Diabinese), tolazamide (Tolinase), tolbutamide (Orinase), or glipizide. Because these drugs might accelerate the atherosclerotic complications of diabetes, they are now used less frequently than before.[6] Data showing that tight control of the type II diabetic patient may decrease the progression of vascular disease may lead to a resurgence in the use of these drugs.[7] Other data do not support this finding.[8] Diabetes is associated with increased atherosclerosis (e.g., coronary and cerebral), microangiopathy (e.g., retinal and renal), infections, and decreased wound-healing tensile strength. The evidence that hyperglycemia itself accelerates these complications, or that tight control of blood sugar levels decreases the rapidity of the progression of microangiopathic disease is very suggestive but not definitive.[9-15] A controversy now exists as to how tightly blood sugar levels should be controlled chronically in diabetic patients. The controversy centers on whether attempts to attain normal blood sugar levels are a greater benefit than risk to diabetic patients.[16]

Increasing evidence indicates that tight control of blood sugar levels can diminish certain functional abnormalities. For example, short-term intensive normalization of blood sugar levels reduces transglomerular escape of albumin and leakiness of retinal capillaries on testing with fluorescein. However, two aspects of insulin therapy do not mimic what happens naturally in the body and thus may somehow prevent correction of the metabolic consequences of hyperglycemia. One difference is that exogenous insulin is injected into the systemic circulation, whereas endogenous insulin enters the portal circulation. The second difference is that all but the genetically engineered commercial exogenous insulins have some degree of antigenicity. Thus, even if hyperglycemia itself were responsible for all the complications of diabetes, intensive treatment regimens might not prove totally effective in preventing these complications until these two aspects of current insulin therapy were taken into consideration.

The perioperative management of the diabetic patient may affect surgical outcome. Physicians advocating tight control of blood glucose levels point to the evidence of increased wound-healing tensile strength and decreased wound infections in animal models of diabetes (type I) under tight control.[17,18] No such evidence exists for type II diabetes. In addition, hyperglycemia may worsen neurologic outcome after intraoperative cerebral ischemia. Thus, the two types of diabetes might require different perioperative management. Type I diabetic patients definitely need insulin and might be considered candidates for tight control of blood glucose levels. Type II diabetic patients have insulin and may not benefit from tight perioperative control.

The key to managing blood glucose levels in diabetic patients perioperatively is to set clear goals and then to monitor blood glucose levels frequently enough to adjust therapy to achieve those goals. Three regimens that afford various degrees of perioperative control of blood glucose levels are listed below.

CLASSIC "NON-TIGHT CONTROL" REGIMEN

Aim:
To avoid hypoglycemia. To avoid ketoacidosis and hyperosmolar states.

Protocol:
1. Day before surgery: Patient should be given nothing by mouth after midnight; glass of orange juice should be at the bedside for emergency use.
2. At 6AM on day of surgery, institute intravenous fluids using plastic cannulae and a solution containing 5 percent dextrose, infusion at the rate of 125 ml/hr per 70-kg body weight.
3. After intravenous infusion is instituted, give one-half the usual morning insulin dose subcutaneously.
4. Continue 5 percent dextrose solutions through operative period, giving at least 125 ml/hr per 70-kg body weight.
5. In recovery room monitor blood glucose concentrations and treat with a sliding scale.

Such a regimen has been found to meet its goals.[19]

"TIGHT CONTROL" REGIMEN 1

Aim:
To keep plasma glucose levels between 79 and 200 mg/100 ml; this practice may improve wound healing and prevent wound infections.

Protocol:
1. Evening before operation, determine preprandial blood glucose level.
2. Through a plastic cannula, begin intrave-

nous infusion of 5 percent dextrose in water at the rate of 50 ml/hr per 70-kg body weight.
3. Next, "piggyback" (Fig. 9-1) to the dextrose infusion an infusion of regular insulin (50 units in 250 ml or 0.9 percent sodium chloride) and an infusion pump. Before attaching this piggyback line to the dextrose infusion, flush the line with 60 ml of infusion mixture and discard the flushing solution. This approach saturates insulin-binding sites of the tubing.[20]
4. Set the infusion rate, using the following equation: Insulin (units/hr) = plasma glucose (mg/100 ml)/150 (*Note:* This denominator should be 100 if patient is taking corticosteroids, e.g., 100 mg of prednisone a day.)
5. Repeat measurements of blood glucose levels every 4 hours as needed and adjust insulin appropriately to obtain blood glucose levels of 100 to 200 mg/100 ml.
6. Day of surgery: Intraoperative fluids and electrolytes are managed by continuing to administer non-dextrose-containing solutions, as described in steps 3 and 4 above.
7. Determine plasma glucose level at the start of operation and every 2 hours for the rest of the 24-hour period. Adjust insulin dosage appropriately.

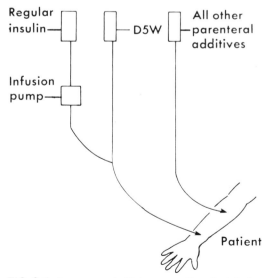

FIG. 9-1 Arrangement of intravenous lines for infusion of regular insulin in a regimen tightly controlling blood glucose levels in diabetic patients undergoing surgery.

Although I have not needed to treat hypoglycemia (i.e., blood glucose levels of less than 50 mg/100 ml), I have been prepared to do so with 15 ml of 50 percent dextrose in water. Under such circumstances, the insulin infusion would be terminated. Such a regimen has been found to accomplish its goals, even in very "brittle" diabetics (i.e., those extremely resistant to treatment) given high doses of steroids.[21]

"TIGHT CONTROL" REGIMEN 2

Aim:
Same as for Tight Control Regimen 1.

Protocol:
1. Obtain a "feedback mechanical pancreas" and set the controls for the desired plasma glucose regimen.
2. Institute appropriate two intravenous lines.

This last regimen may well supersede all others if the cost of a mechanical pancreas can be reduced and if control of hyperglycemia is shown to make a meaningful difference perioperatively.

Despite the fact that hyperglycemic type I diabetic patients have a higher incidence of wound infections, a lower wound-healing tensile strength, and a higher incidence of renal transplant rejections than do normal patients,[22,23] it does not necessarily follow that short-term tight control of blood glucose levels perioperatively would reduce morbidity and mortality. For example, in one study, the incidence of perioperative mortality was 11 times greater for diabetic patients than for asymptomatic healthy patients.[24] However, in two other studies (one involving general surgical procedures[25] and one gallbladder surgery[26]), no increase in wound or systemic infections or in any measure of perioperative morbidity or mortality could be attributable to diabetes itself. Also, when corrections were made for age and end-organ disease (cardiovascular) in those two studies, the increases in morbidity for diabetic patients seemed to disappear.[25,26]

Perhaps only wound healing and rate of infection are important factors during the perioperative period. However, the debate concerns whether control of hyperglycemia itself lowers the incidence of any of the complications associated with diabetes. One editorial implied that tight perioperative control of blood sugar levels would decrease the incidence of infections and increase the quality of wound healing.[27] While many would welcome such a study, no data to support those implications yet exist.

OTHER CONDITIONS ASSOCIATED WITH DIABETES

Diabetes is associated with microangiopathy (in retinal and renal vessels), peripheral neuropathies, autonomic dysfunction, and infection. These abnormalities should be identified and their treatment optimized before surgery is instituted. Perhaps most important, diabetic patients have an increased incidence of atherosclerosis and all its complications. Such patients are particularly susceptible to episodes of painless myocardial ischemia.[28] As with other endocrinopathies, the cardiovascular system should be a focus of the anesthetist's attention for the diabetic patient.

INSULINOMA AND OTHER CAUSES OF HYPOGLYCEMIA

Hypoglycemia can be caused by such diverse entities as a pancreatic islet cell adenoma or carcinoma, large hepatoma, large sarcoma, alcohol ingestion, hypopituitarism, adrenal insufficiency, after gastric surgery, hereditary fructose intolerance, or galactosemia. The last three entities cause postprandial reactive hypoglycemia. Since restriction of oral intake prevents severe hypoglycemia, the practice of giving the patient nothing by mouth and infusing small amounts of a solution containing 5 percent dextrose greatly lessens the possibility of postprandial reactive hypoglycemia. The other causes of hypoglycemia can cause serious problems during the perioperative period.

The symptoms of hypoglycemia fall into two groups: adrenergic excess (tachycardia, palpitations, tremulousness, or diaphoresis), or neuroglycopenia (headache, confusion, mental sluggishness, seizures, or coma). Since all these symptoms may be masked by anesthesia, blood glucose levels should be determined frequently to ensure that hypoglycemia is not present. Because manipulation of an insulinoma can result in massive insulin release, this tumor probably should be operated on only at centers having a mechanical pancreas: such machines have on-line blood glucose analysis and a glucose infusion setup.

A different point of view was expressed by Muir and colleagues,[29] who managed 38 patients undergoing insulinoma resection. Every 15 minutes they noted the plasma glucose concentration in these patients, in whom a mechanical pancreas produced no increase in plasma glucose. Although 9 of the 38 patients became significantly hypoglycemic (i.e., plasma glucose concentrations $<$ 50 mg/dl), in only 4 of 253 measurements before resection did glucose concentration decrease more than 20 mg/dl in any 15-minute period. Muir et al.[29] believe that intermittent sampling of plasma glucose (every 15 minutes) may be satisfactory as long as the plasma glucose concentration is kept at $\geq$ 60 mg/dl. In this series, the absence or presence of a hyperglycemic rebound after tumor resection was not of predictive value in determining completeness of insulinoma resection(s). The other causes of hypoglycemia do not involve release of insulin in such vast quantities (or at all), and therefore less frequent (every 1 to 2 hours) intraoperative blood glucose determinations and continuous dextrose infusion appear to be sufficient.

DISORDERS OF NUTRITION

HYPERLIPIDEMIAS AND HYPOLIPIDEMIAS

Hyperlipidemia may result from obesity, estrogen or corticoid therapy, uremia, diabetes, hypothyroidism, acromegaly, alcohol ingestion, liver disease, inborn errors of metabolism, or pregnancy. Hyperlipidemia may cause premature coronary or peripheral vascular disease or pancreatitis.[30] Hypercholesterolemia, a form of hyperlipidemia, appears to be associated with premature atherosclerosis. Most cholesterol is carried in serum by low-density lipoproteins (LDL), whereas approximately 20 percent of total serum cholesterol is carried by high-density lipoproteins (HDL). High-density-lipoprotein cholesterol is carried in roughly equivalent amounts on two types of HDL: on a less dense HDL_2 subfraction that is negatively associated with coronary artery disease, and on a more dense HDL_3 subfraction that is unrelated to coronary artery disease.[31] In atherosclerosis, LDL, and not HDL, is probably the risk factor. Levels of HDL are 25 percent higher in women than in men; low levels of HDL in women are associated with premature atherosclerosis. Cigarette smoking lowers HDL levels, whereas regular strenuous exercise and small daily intake of alcohol raises HDL levels. However, alcohol increases HDL_3, the HDL subfraction thought to be inert with respect to coronary artery disease[31]; octogenarians have high levels of HDL.

Although controlling diet remains the major treatment modality for all types of hyperlipidemia, clofibrate (Atromid-S), used to treat hypertriglyceridemia, can cause myopathy, especially in patients with hepatic or renal disease; it is also associated with an increased incidence of gallstones. Cholestyramine binds bile acids, as well as oral anticoagulants, digitalis drugs, and thyroid hormones. Nicotinic acid causes peripheral vasodilation and probably should not be continued through the morning of surgery.

Hypolipidemic conditions are rare diseases often associated with neuropathies, anemia, and renal failure. Although anesthetic experience with hypolipidemic conditions has been limited, some specific recommendations can be made: continuation of caloric intake and intravenous administration of protein hydralysates and glucose throughout the perioperative period.

OBESITY

Twenty to 50 percent of adults in the United States weigh more than 20 percent above what is considered the optimum body weight for their height. The pathophysiologic consequences of obesity involve every major organ system. Many of the metabolic, hormonal, and physiologic changes associated with obesity (e.g., insulin resistance, decreased number of insulin receptors, and subsequent diabetes mellitus) can be induced by overfeeding normal subjects and can be reversed by weight reduction. Obesity itself, its complications, and its treatment have significance for the anesthesiologist. Being 30 percent overweight is associated with a 40 percent increase in the chance of dying from heart disease and with a 50 percent increase in the chance of dying from a stroke. Obesity is also associated with higher perioperative morbidity and mortality.[32]

Massively obese individuals with carbon dioxide retention are called pickwickian, alveolar hypoventilation being the hallmark of this condition. Other components of the pickwickian syndrome are somnolence, hypoxemia, failure of the right side of the heart, and secondary polycythemia. These patients often have right ventricular failure (also see Ch. 13 for monitoring considerations).

Although many conditions associated with obesity (diabetes, cholelithiasis, cirrhosis) contribute to morbidity, the main concerns for the anesthesiologist are derangements of the cardiopulmonary system.[33] Cardiac output must increase approximately 0.1 L/min to perfuse each kilogram of adipose tissue. As a result, obese patients often have hypertension, which can cause cardiomegaly and left ventricular failure. Care should be taken to use a blood pressure cuff of correct size when quantitating the degree of hypertension present.

The obese may have limited cardiac reserve and a poor tolerance for stress induced by hypotension, hypertension, tachycardia, or fluid overload associated with the preoperative period. Airway obstruction frequently occurs because of the abundant soft tissue in the upper airway. Functional residual capacity is reduced, as the weight of the torso and abdomen make diaphragmatic excursions more difficult and more position dependent. Thus, preoperative assessment should include not only history-taking and physical examination accentuating cardiopulmonary problems, but also an electrocardiographic (ECG) examination (looking specifically for left or right ventricular hypertrophy, ischemia, and conduction defects). If obesity is severe, arterial blood gases should also be analyzed to quantitate the degree of hy-

poventilation and to aid in assessing the most appropriate time to extubate the trachea. More extensive pulmonary function tests and preoperative treatment of any treatable abnormality (such as infectious and bronchospastic components of pulmonary disease) may be indicated for the obese patient who smokes or has pulmonary symptoms (e.g., a chronic cough, sputum production, wheezing, shortness of breath at rest or on minor exertion).

Other features of obesity are of interest to the anesthesiologist as well. Obese patients have an increased volume and acidity of gastric juices preoperatively, perhaps indicating the wisdom of premedicating such patients with cimetidine, ranitidine, glycopyrrolate, and metoclopramide.[34,35] In addition, obese individuals may metabolize lipophilic drugs to a greater degree (and for longer periods) than their thin counterparts. More fluorine is produced from enflurane given to obese patients than to thin ones.[36] In addition, one would assume that responses to drugs stored in fat (e.g., narcotics, barbiturates, volatile anesthetics) would be prolonged in the obese. However, there is no evidence that use of the more soluble anesthetics delays recovery time in obese subjects.[37]

The anesthesiologist also needs to be aware of conditions caused by remedies to obesity. Drastic dieting can produce acidosis, hypokalemia, and hyperuricemia; protein hydrolysate liquid diets are associated with intractable ventricular dysrhythmias.[38] Metabolic complications of jejunoileal bypass include hypokalemia, hypocalcemia, hypomagnesemia, anemia, renal stones, gout, and liver abnormalities. An attempt to reverse these abnormal conditions should be made prior to anesthesia and may consist of infusing solutions containing amino acids. Because of the high morbidity associated with jejunoileal bypass, this procedure has been supplanted by gastric plication or bypass surgery. However, long-term data about the chronic morbidity of these two procedures are not available.

Drug treatment for obesity also has implications for the anesthesiologist. Amphetamines (and probably mazindol) given acutely increase anesthetic requirements; by contrast, chronically administered amphetamines decrease anesthetic requirements (see section on chronic drug therapy). Amphetamines may interfere with the action of vasoactive drugs given to treat hypotension or hypertension. Fenfluramine (a drug that inhibits the serotinergic system) may decrease both anesthetic requirement and blood pressure.

ANOREXIA NERVOSA, BULIMAREXIA, AND STARVATION

Many endocrine and metabolic abnormalities occur in the patient with anorexia nervosa, a condition of starvation to the point of 40 percent loss of normal weight, hyperactivity, and a psychiatrically distorted body image. Acidosis, hypokalemia, hypocalcemia, hypomagnesemia, hypothermia, diabetes insipidus, and severe endocrine abnormalities mimicking panhypopituitarism need attention prior to anesthesia and surgery. Similar problems occur in bulimarexia, also termed bulimia, a condition that may be present in 50 percent of female college students.[39] As in severe protein deficiency (kwashiorkor), anorexia nervosa and bulimarexia may be accompanied by ECG alterations and cardiomyopathy.[39,40] Total depletion of body potassium makes addition of potassium to glucose solutions useful; however, fluid administration can precipitate pulmonary edema in these patients. Thus, invasive monitoring (radial artery and pulmonary artery catheterization) may be indicated for anorectic, bulimarexic, and malnurtured patients requiring emergency surgery. Elective surgery probably should be delayed until abnormalities are treated.

HYPERALIMENTATION (TOTAL PARENTERAL NUTRITION) (Also See Ch. 67)

For patients receiving hyperalimentation, i.e., total parenteral nutrition (TPN), hypertonic glucose calories are concentrated in the normal daily fluid requirements in solutions containing protein hydrolysates or synthetic amino acids. To diminish the likelihood of essential fatty acid deficiency, Intralipid, a soybean emulsion, can be added to the solution.[41] The major complications of hyperalimentation are sepsis and metabolic abnormalities. The central lines used for TPN require application of an absolutely aseptic technique and should not be used as an intravenous route for drug administration.

Major metabolic complications of TPN relate to deficiencies and to the development of hyperosmolar states. Complications of hypertonic dextrose can develop if the patient has insufficient insulin (diabetes mellitus) to metabolize the sugar or if insulin resistance occurs (e.g., because of uremia, burns, or sepsis).[41]

Gradual decrease in the infusion rate of TPN prevents the hypoglycemia that can occur on abrupt discontinuance. Thus, the infusion rate of TPN should be decreased the night before anesthesia and surgery. The main reason for slowing or discontinuing TPN before anesthesia is to avoid intraoperative hyperosmolarity secondary to accidental rapid infusion of the solution.[42] Hypophosphatemia is a particularly serious complication that results from the administration of phosphate-free or phosphate-depleted solutions for hyperalimentation. The low serum phosphate level causes shifts of the oxygen dissociation curve to the left. Thus, the resulting low 2,3-diphosphoglycerate and ATP levels mean that cardiac output must increase for oxygen delivery to remain the same. Hypophosphatemia of <1.0 mg/dl blood may cause hemolytic anemia, cardiac failure, tachypnea, neurologic symptoms, seizures, and death. In addition, long-term TPN is associated with deficiencies in trace metals such as copper (refractory anemia), zinc (impaired wound healing), and magnesium. For these reasons, I have adopted the following practices.[42] The infusion of TPN is reduced beginning the night before surgery, substituting 5 or 10 percent dextrose solution preoperatively. If serum glucose phosphate and potassium concentrations (measured preoperatively) are abnormal, they are restored to within normal limits. Strict asepsis is maintained. Conversely, one could continue infusing the TPN solution using a pump system, strictly maintaining its normal rate and asepsis, and administering all fluids through a different intravenous site.

ADRENOCORTICAL MALFUNCTION*

Three major classes of hormones—androgens, glucocorticoids, and minerelo-corticoids—are secreted by the adrenal cortex.[43-49] A characteristic clinical syndrome is associated with excess or deficiency of each class. In addition, the widespread use of steroids may result in an inability of the adrenal cortex to respond normally to the demands placed on it by surgical trauma and subsequent healing.[50-69] Although controlled studies comparing perioperative management for individuals having malfunctioning of the adrenal cortex are lacking, reviewing the pathophysiologic changes of, and management techniques for, these diseases should improve care for such patients.[44-49]

PHYSIOLOGIC PROPERTIES OF ADRENOCORTICAL HORMONES

ANDROGENS

Androstenedione and dehydroepiandrosterone, weak androgens arising from the adrenal cortex,[70] constitute major sources of androgens in women. Excess secretion of androgen causes masculinization, pseudopuberty, or female pseudohemaphroditism. With some tumors, androgen is converted to an estrogenic substance, in which case feminization results.[70] No special anesthetic evaluation is needed for such patients. Some congenital enzyme defects that cause androgen abnormalities also result in glucocorticoid and mineralocorticoid abnormalities that should be evaluated prior to surgery.[70]

GLUCOCORTICOIDS

Cortisol is an important regulator of carbohydrate, protein, and lipid metabolism.[44,46] Cortisol is believed to exert its biologic effects

---

* Much of this section of the chapter is taken from reference 43 (see Roizen MF, Lampe GH: Adrenal cortex malfunction: Implications for the anesthetist. *Semin Anest* III(3), 1984).

through a sequence of steps initiated by hormone binding to stereospecific cytoplasmic receptors. This bound complex stimulates nuclear transcription of specific messenger RNAs. These mRNA's are then transcribed to give rise to proteins that mediate the ultimate effects of hormones.

The synthetic glucocorticoids vary in their binding specificity. Those that bind with mineralocorticoid receptor sites cause salt and water retention and loss of potassium and hydrogen ion. Those that do not bind have no mineralocorticoid effect.[46,71] Most cortisol in plasma is bound to corticosterone-binding globulin. It is the relatively small amounts of unbound cortisol that enter cells to induce actions or to be metabolized. Most cortisol is inactivated in the liver and excreted as 17-hydroxycorticosteroids.[44,46,71]

Secretion of glucocorticoids is regulated by pituitary ACTH. ACTH is synthesized from a precursor molecule (preopiomelanocortin) that breaks down to form an endorphin (β-lipotropin) and ACTH.[72,73] (This close relationship between compounds having opioid activity and corticoids is discussed later.) Episodic secretion of ACTH has a diurnal rhythm normally greatest during the early morning hours and is regulated at least in part by light–dark cycles. Its secretion is stimulated by release of corticotropin-releasing hormone from the hypothalamus.[44,46,47,71,73] (An abnormality in the diurnal rhythm of corticoid secretion has been implicated as a cause of "jet lag.") Cortisol and other glucocorticoids exert negative feedback at both pituitary and hypothalamic levels to inhibit secretion of ACTH.[44,46,47,71-73]

MINERALOCORTICOIDS

Aldosterone secreted from the zona glomerulosa of the adrenal cortex causes reabsorption of sodium and secretion of potassium and hydrogen ion, thereby contributing to electrolyte and volume homeostasis.[44,47,74] This action is most prominent in the distal renal tubule but also occurs in salivary and sweat glands. The major regulator of aldosterone secretion is the renin-angiotensin system. Juxtaglomerular cells in the cuff of the renal arterioles are sensitive to decreased renal perfusion pressure or volume and, consequently, secrete renin.[74] Renin splits the precursor angiotensinogen (from the liver) into angiotensin I, which is further converted by a converting enzyme, primarily in lung, to angiotensin II. Mineralocorticoid secretion is increased by increased angiotensin II, increased potassium concentration, and, to a lesser degree, ACTH.[44,47,74]

ADRENOCORTICAL HORMONE EXCESS

GLUCOCORTICOID EXCESS

Excess glucocorticoid secretion (Cushing's syndrome) produces a moon-faced, plethoric individual having a centripetal distribution of fat (trunkal obesity and skinny extremities), thin skin, easy bruising, and striae. These patients often have osteopenia due to decreased formation of bone matrix and impaired absorption of calcium. Fluid retention and hypertension are common, the latter being caused by the mineralocorticoid effects of excess glucocorticoids and by increases in renin substrate and vascular reactivity induced by glucocorticoids. Such patients may also have hyperglycemia and even diabetes mellitus resulting from inhibition of peripheral use of glucose, as well as antiinsulin action and concomitant stimulation of gluconeogenesis.[44,47,48,75]

The most common cause of Cushing's syndrome is administration of glucocorticoids for such conditions as arthritis, asthma, and allergies.[44,46,47] In such conditions, the adrenal glands atrophy and cannot respond to stressful situations (e.g., the perioperative period) by secreting more steriod. Thus, additional glucocorticoids may be required perioperatively (see the section, The Patient Taking Steroids for Other Reasons). Spontaneous Cushing's syndrome may be caused by pituitary production of ACTH (60 to 70 percent of all spontaneous cases), which is usually associated with pituitary microadenoma, or nonendocrine ectopic ACTH production (principally by tumors of the lung, pancreas, or thymus).[44,46,47,75] Ten to 20 percent of cases of spontaneous Cushing's syndrome are caused by an ACTH-independent process, either an adrenal adenoma or carcinoma.

Special preoperative considerations for patients having Cushing's syndrome include regulating diabetes and hypertension and ensuring that intravascular fluid volume and electrolyte concentrations are normal. Ectopic ACTH production may cause marked hypokalemic alkalosis.[44,46,47] In addition, glucocorticoids are lympholytic and immunosuppressive, and therefore increase the patient's susceptibility to infection. Wound-healing tensile strength decreases in the presence of glucocorticoids, an effect at least partially reversed by topically applied vitamin A.[76-80]

In addition to such medical conditions requiring preoperative consideration, specific steps pertain to the surgical approach for each condition. At UCSF, treatment for Cushing's disease and a pituitary microadenoma differs greatly from treatment for pituitary adenomas associated with amenorrhea and galactorrhea.[75] The Cushing's patient tends to bleed more easily and (on the basis of anecdotal evidence) to have higher central venous pressure (CVP). Thus, during transsphenoidal tumor resection in such patients, I routinely monitor CVP to keep it at the low end of the normal range. When Cushing's syndrome is not present, such monitoring is needed only infrequently for transsphenoidal microadenoma resection.

If either unilateral or bilateral adrenal resection is planned, I normally begin administering glucocorticoids at the start of tumor resectioning. Although no definitive studies exist, I normally give 100 mg of hydrocortisone hemisuccinate or hydrocortisone phosphate every 8 to 12 hours IV. I reduce this amount over 3 to 6 days until a maintenance dose is reached. Beginning on day 3, I also give 9α-fluorocortisol (a mineralocorticoid), 0.05 to 0.1 mg/day. In certain patients, both steroids may require several adjustments.[44,46,47] This therapy is continued in the patient who has undergone bilateral resection. In the patient who has undergone unilateral adrenal resection, therapy is individualized according to the status of the remaining adrenal gland. At UCSF, the incidence of pneumothorax in adrenal resection approaches 20 percent; its diagnosis is sought and treatment begun before the wound is closed.

Bilateral adrenalectomy with Cushing's syndrome has a high incidence of postoperative complications and a perioperative mortality of 5 to 10 percent; it often results in permanent mineralocorticoid and glucocorticoid deficiency.[46,81,82] Ten percent of patients with Cushing's syndrome who undergo adrenalectomy will have an undiagnosed pituitary tumor. After reduction of high levels of cortisol by adrenalectomy, the pituitary tumor enlarges.[46,75] These pituitary tumors are potentially invasive and may produce large amounts of ACTH and melanocyte-stimulating hormone (MSH), thereby increasing pigmentation.[44,46,47,75]

Adrenal adenomas do not usually recur after surgical removal, and often the contralateral gland will resume functioning after several months. Frequently, however, the effects of carcinomas are not cured by surgery.[46] In such instances, administration of steroid synthesis inhibitors may ameliorate some symptoms but may not improve survival. These drugs and the aldosterone antagonist spironolactone may aid in reducing symptoms in ectopic ACTH secretion if total excision of the primary tumor proves impossible.[46]

MINERALOCORTICOID EXCESS

Excess mineralocorticoid activity (common with glucocorticoid excess, since most glucocorticoids have some mineralocorticoid properties) leads to potassium depletion, sodium retention, muscle weakness, hypertension, tetany, polyuria, inability to concentrate urine, and hypokalemic alkalosis.[44,83,84] These symptoms constitute hyperaldosteronism, or Conn's syndrome (a cause of low-renin hypertension, as renin secretion is inhibited by the effects of the high levels of aldosterone).

Primary hyperaldosteronism is present in 0.5 to 1 percent of hypertensive patients who do not have other known causes of hypertension.[83,84] Primary hyperaldosteronism most often results from unilateral adenoma, although 25 to 40 percent of patients have been found to have bilateral adrenal hyperplasia. Intravascular fluid volume, electrolyte concentrations, and renal function should be restored to within normal limits preoperatively by administering the aldosterone antagonist spironolactone. The effects of spironolactone are slow in onset and continue to increase for 1 to 2

weeks.[83,84] A patient having a serum potassium level of 2.9 mEq/L may have a deficit of body potassium of as little as 40 mEq or as much as 400 mEq.[85-88] Frequently, at least 24 hours is required to restore potassium equilibrium.[85-88] A normal serum potassium level does not imply correction of a total body deficit of potassium. In addition, these patients have a high incidence of hypertension, and hemodynamic monitoring should be appropriate for the degree of cardiovascular impairment.[89] A retrospective anecdotal study indicated that intraoperative hemodynamic status was more stable when blood pressure and electrolytes were controlled preoperatively with spironolactone than when other antihypertensive drugs were used.[49] Again, the efficacy of optimizing the perioperative status of patients with disorders of glucocorticoid or mineralocorticoid secretion has not been clearly established. Our assumption has been that restoring a normal condition is good medicine and therefore would improve morbidity and mortality.

ADRENOCORTICAL HORMONE DEFICIENCY

GLUCOCORTICOID DEFICIENCY

Withdrawal of steroids or suppression of synthesis by steroid therapy is the leading cause of underproduction of corticosteroids.[46,48] The management of this type of glucocorticoid deficiency is discussed later in this chapter. Other causes of adrenocortical insufficiency include defects in ACTH secretion and destruction of the adrenal gland by cancer, tuberculosis, hemorrhage, or an autoimmune mechanism.[46,48]

Primary adrenal insufficiency (Addison's disease) is caused by a local process within the adrenal gland that leads to destruction of all zones of the cortex and causes both glucocorticoid and mineralocorticoid deficiency if the insufficiency is bilateral. Autoimmune disease is the most common cause of primary (nonexogenous) bilateral ACTH deficiency.

Autoimmune destruction of the adrenals may be associated with other autoimmune disorders, such as Hashimoto's thyroiditis. Enzymatic defects in cortisol synthesis also cause glucocorticoid insufficiency, compensatory elevations of ACTH, and congenital adrenal hyperplasia.[70] Because adrenal insufficiency usually develops slowly, such patients develop marked pigmentation (from excess ACTH trying to stimulate an unproductive adrenal gland) and cardiopenia (apparently secondary to chronic hypotension).[48-48]

Secondary adrenal insufficiency occurs when ACTH secretion is deficient, often because of a pituitary or hypothalamic tumor. Treatment of pituitary tumors by surgery or radiation may result in hypopituitarism and secondary adrenal failure.[45-48]

If not stressed, patients deficient in glucocorticoids usually have no perioperative problems. However, acute adrenal crisis (Addisonian crisis) can occur when even a minor stress (e.g., upper respiratory infection) occurs. Therefore, to prepare such a patient for anesthesia and surgery, hypovolemia, hyperkalemia, and hyponatremia should be treated preoperatively.[45-48] Because these patients are unable to respond to stressful situations, I usually recommend giving a maximum stress dose of glucocorticoids (about 300 mg/70 kg body weight/day of hydrocortisone) preoperatively. However, Symreng and colleagues[54] gave 25 mg of hydrocortisone phosphate IV to adults at the start of the operative procedure, followed by 100 mg IV over the next 24 hours. This therapy produced blood levels closely paralleling the natural cortisol response to major surgery. Because it is desirable to use the minimum drug dose necessary to obtain the appropriate effect, this regimen seems attractive. However, use of such a regimen has not stood the test of time, as have regimens using maximum doses (see under the section, The Patient Taking Steroids for Other Reasons).[44-48,53-55,57,59,90]

MINERALOCORTICOID DEFICIENCY

Hypoaldosteronism, a less common condition,[91] can be congenital or can occur after unilateral adrenalectomy or prolonged administration of heparin. It can also be a consequence of long-standing diabetes. Nonsteroidal inhibitors of prostaglandin synthesis may also inhibit renin release and exacerbate this condition in patients who have renal insufficiency.[91,92]

Plasma renin activity levels are below normal and fail to increase appropriately in response to sodium restriction or diuretic drugs. Most symptoms are caused by hyperkalemic acidosis rather than hypovolemia; in fact, some patients are hypertensive. These patients can have severe hyperkalemia, hyponatremia, and myocardial conduction defects.[91] These defects can be treated successfully by administering mineralocorticoids (9α-fluorocortisol, 0.05 to 0.1 mg/day) preoperatively.[91] Treatment must be carefully titrated and monitored to avoid an increase in hypertension.

THE PATIENT TAKING STEROIDS FOR OTHER REASONS

PERIOPERATIVE STRESS AND THE NEED FOR SUPPLEMENTATION

Many experimental studies and other (mostly anecdotal) reports indicate the following regarding the adrenal responses of normal patients to the perioperative period and the responses of patients taking steroids for diseases other than those just discussed:

1. Perioperative stress relates to the degree of trauma and the depth of anesthesia. Deep general anesthesia or regional anesthesia postpones the usual intraoperative glucocorticoid surge to the postoperative period.[93-101]
2. Few patients who have suppressed adrenal function have perioperative cardiovascular problems if they do not receive supplemental steroids perioperatively.[44,51-69]
3. Although an occasional patient who takes steroids chronically becomes hypotensive perioperatively, only rarely can this event be even possibly attributable to glucocorticoid or mineralocorticoid deficiency.[44,51-69]
4. There is little risk in giving such patients glucocorticoids.[44,51-69,76-80]

The lower dose advocated by Symreng and colleagues[54] might help reduce the risks of supplementation with glucocorticoids (i.e., infection and decreased wound healing). In any case, I never supplement with a dose that is less

TABLE 9-1. The Relative Potency and Equivalent Doses for Commonly Used Glucocorticoids

Steroids	Relative Glucocorticoid Potency*	Equivalent Glucocorticoid Dose (mg)
Short-acting		
Cortisol		
(hydrocortisone)	1	20
Cortisone	0.8	25
Prednisone	4	5
Prednisolone	4	5
Methylprednisolone	5	4
Intermediate-acting		
Triamcinolone	5	4
Long-acting		
Betamethasone	25	0.60
Dexamethasone	30	0.75

* (Based on data in Axelrod L: Glucocorticoid therapy. Medicine (Baltimore) 55:39, 1976.)

than what the patient is already taking (see Table 9-1).[55]

Which patients definitely need supplementation? If in doubt, how can one determine a patient's need for supplementation with glucocorticoids? Because the risk is low, I normally provide supplementation for any patient who has received steroids within a year.[50–69,72] Data indicate that topical application of steroids (even without the use of occlusive dressings) can suppress normal adrenal responses for as long as 9 months to 1 year (Table 9-2).[50,55]

How can one determine when adrenal responsiveness has returned to normal? The morning plasma cortisol level does not reveal whether the adrenal cortex has recovered sufficiently to ensure that cortisol secretion will increase adequately to meet the demands of stress.[102] Inducing hypoglycemia with insulin has been advocated as a sensitive test of pitui-

tary-adrenal competence but is impractical and probably a more dangerous practice than simply administering glucocorticoids.[102] If the plasma cortisol concentration is measured during acute stress, a value of $>25~\mu g/dl$ assuredly (and a value of $>15~\mu g/dl$ probably) indicates normal pituitary-adrenal responsiveness.[58,103]

In another test of pituitary-adrenal sufficiency, the baseline plasma cortisol level is determined. Then, 250 μg of synthetic ACTH (Co-measured 30 to 60 minutes later.[58,59] An increase in plasma cortisol of 6 to 20 $\mu g/dl$ or more is normal.[103] A normal response indicates recovery of pituitary-adrenal axis function. A lesser response usually indicates pituitary-adrenal insufficiency, possibly requiring perioperative supplementation with steroids.

Usually laboratory data defining pituitary-adrenal adequacy are not available before surgery. However, rather than delay surgery or even test most patients, I assume that any patient who has taken steroids within a year has suppressed pituitary-adrenal functioning and will require perioperative supplementation with glucocorticoids.

Under perioperative conditions, the adrenal glands secrete 116 to 185 mg of cortisol daily.[101] Under maximum stress, they may secrete 200 to 500 mg/day.[101] Good correlation exists between the severity and duration of the operation and the response of adrenal gland secretion.[101] Major surgery would be represented by procedures such as colectomy, and minor surgery by procedures such as herniorrhaphy. In one study of 20 patients during major surgery, the mean maximal concentration of cortisol in plasma was 47 $\mu g/dl$ (range 22 to 75 $\mu g/dl$).[53] Values remained above 26 $\mu g/dl$ for a

TABLE 9-2. Recovery of Hypothalamic-Pituitary Adrenal Function After Withdrawal of Steroids

Recovery Time (months)	Plasma 17-Hydroxycorticoid Values	Plasma ACTH Values	Adrenal Response to Exogenous ACTH	Response to Metyrapone
1	Low*	Low	Low	Low
2–5	Low	High†	Low	Low
6–9	Normal	Normal	Low	Low
>9	Normal	Normal	Normal	Normal

* Various subjective manifestations of mild adrenal insufficiency occur during this stage.
† The diurnal rhythm of the plasma concentrations are qualitatively normal during this stage.
(Based on data in Graber AL, Ney RI, Nicholson WE, et al: Natural history of pituitary-adrenal recovery following long-term suppression with corticosteroids. J Clin Endocrinol Metab 25:11, 1965.)

maximum of 72 hours after surgery. During minor surgery, the mean maximal concentration of cortisol in plasma was 28 μg/dl (range 10 to 44 μg/dl).

Although the precise amount required has not been established, I usually administer intravenously the maximum amount of glucocorticoid that the body manufactures in response to a maximal stress, i.e., approximately 300 mg/day of hydrocortisone phosphate per 70 kg of body weight.[53,93-100]

For minor surgical procedures, I usually give hydrocortisone phosphate intravenously, 100 mg/day per 70 kg body weight. Unless infection or some other perioperative complication develops, I decrease this dose by approximately 25 percent a day until oral intake can be resumed. At this point, the usual maintenance dose of glucocorticoids can be resumed. This maximum perioperative stress dose is given to achieve blood levels of glucocorticoids that parallel those normally found after stress.[44,47,51-69,93-99] Recently, however, Symreng and colleagues[54] demonstrated that 25 mg of hydrocortisone phosphate administered intravenously shortly after induction of anesthesia, followed by 100 mg given as a slow infusion drip over the next 24 hours, produced blood levels closely paralleling the natural cortisol response to major surgery.

RISKS OF SUPPLEMENTATION

Rare potential risks of perioperative supplementation with steroids include aggravation of hypertension, fluid retention, inducement of stress ulcers, and psychiatric disturbance. Although data are not available to assess the incidences of these risks, two common complications of short-term perioperative supplementation with glucocorticoids are described in the literature: abnormal wound healing and an increased rate of infections.[51-69,73-80,90,104-106] This evidence is inconclusive, however, as it relates to acute glucocorticoid administration and not to chronic administration and increased acute doses. For example, in a study designed to examine the healing process, Baker and Whitaker[76] inflicted wounds in rats before and after local application of corti-

sone. Cortisone was found to delay formation of granulation tissue and wound closure, to cause thinning of the dermis and atrophy of collagen fibers, and to decrease fibroblasts and proliferation of new blood vessels. Ehrlich and Hunt[78] and Sandberg[77] found that moderate to large doses of steroids exerted their morphologic effects best within 3 days of injury. These workers postulated that the inhibition of the early inflammatory process by steroids after wounding was responsible for delayed healing. Vitamin A was found to protect somewhat against delayed healing, presumably because of its effect on stabilizing lysosomes.[78] Other data give us no better insight into these problems.[51-69,73-79] Such data are not conclusive regarding a short-term increase in supplementation. However, an overall assessment of these results suggests that short-term perioperative supplementation with steroids has a small but definite deleterious effect on wound healing that is perhaps partially reversed by topical administration of vitamin A.[78]

Information regarding the risk of infection from perioperative supplementation with glucocorticoids is also unclear.[79,80,90,104-106] Winstone and Brooke[105] reported four cases of septicemia among 18 surgical patients given perioperative supplementation with glucocorticoids. No similar complications occurred in 17 others who were also taking glucocorticoids but who were not given perioperative supplementation. In a controlled study of 100 patients given perioperative supplementation with glucocorticoids, 11 wound infections occurred in the group treated with steroids, and only one occurred in the control group.[104] Test subjects and controls were not matched for underlying disease. By contrast, Jensen and Elb[106] found no change in the incidence of wound infections or of other infections in an uncontrolled series of 419 patients subjected to surgery and perioperative supplementation with glucocorticoids. Oh and Patterson[90] found only one minor suture abscess in 17 steroid-dependent asthmatic patients undergoing 21 surgical procedures. Thus, although data indicate that the risk of infection to the patient chronically taking steroids is real, such data are inadequate to conclude that perioperative supplementation with steroids increases that risk.

INTERACTION BETWEEN STEROIDS AND OPIOID-LIKE SUBSTANCES

Pituitary ACTH comes from a precursor protein (propiomelanocortin) that is cleaved to form β-lipotropin (an endogenous opioidlike compound) and ACTH. This relationship indicates the close involvement between steroids and opioids. Bilateral adrenalectomy decreases morphine metabolism, which, because of increased bioavailability, enhances the potency of this opiate.[72,73] No other data exist regarding alteration in pharmacokinetics or pharmacodynamics of anesthetic agents by ACTH excess or deficiency without electrolyte abnormalities. This exciting area of research on interactions between opioids and glucocorticoids will undoubtedly reveal important clinical implications for anesthetists in the future.

ADRENAL MEDULLARY SYMPATHETIC HORMONE EXCESS: PHEOCHROMOCYTOMA

Fewer than 0.1 percent of all cases of hypertension are caused by pheochromocytomas, catecholamine-producing tumors derived from chromaffin tissue. Nevertheless, these tumors are clearly important to the anesthetist, since 25 to 50 percent of hospital deaths in patients with pheochromocytomas occur during induction of anesthesia or during operative procedures for other causes.[107] Although usually found in the adrenal medulla, these vascular tumors can occur anywhere, such as in the right atrium, the spleen, the broad ligament of the ovary, or the organs of Zuckerkandl at the bifurcation of the aorta. Malignant spread, which occurs in fewer than 15 percent of pheochromocytomas, usually proceeds to venous and lymphatic channels with a predisposition for the liver. Occasionally the occurrence of this tumor is familial and/or part of the pluriglandular-neoplastic syndrome known as multiple endocrine adenoma-type IIa (consisting of medullary carcinoma of the thyroid, and parathyroid adenoma or hyperplasia

and pheochromocytomas) or type IIb (consisting of medullary carcinoma of the thyroid, marfanoid appearance, mucosal neuromas, and pheochromocytomas) as an autosomal dominant trait. Often bilateral tumors are found in the familial form.

Symptoms and signs that may be solicited preoperatively and that are suggestive of pheochromocytoma are excessive sweating; headache; hypertension; orthostatic hypotension; previous hypertensive or dysrhythmic response to induction of anesthesia or to abdominal examination; paroxysmal attacks of sweating, headache, tachycardia, and hypertension; glucose intolerance; polycythemia; weight loss; and psychological abnormalities. Despite more than 2,000 articles in the literature about pheochromocytomas, little is known about what factors in care affect perioperative morbidity.[108-112]

Although no controlled, randomized, prospective clinical studies have studied the value of preoperative use of adrenergic receptor-blocking drugs, the use of such drugs is generally recommended before surgery. These drugs probably reduce the complications of hypertensive crisis, the wide blood pressure fluctuations during manipulation of the tumor (especially until venous drainage is obliterated), and the myocardial dysfunction that occur perioperatively. The reduction in mortality associated with resection of pheochromocytoma from 40 to 60 percent to the current 0 to 6 percent occurred when α-adrenergic receptor blockade was introduced as preoperative preparatory therapy for such patients (Table 9-3).[111]

α-Adrenergic receptor blockade with prazosin or phenoxybenzamine restores plasma volume by counteracting the vasoconstrictive effects of high levels of catecholamines. This reexpansion of fluid volume is often followed by a decrease in hematocrit. Because some patients may be very sensitive to the effects of phenoxybenzamine, it should initially be given in doses of 20 to 30 mg per 70 kg orally once or twice a day. Most patients usually require 60 to 250 mg/day. Efficacy of therapy should be judged by a reduction in symptoms (especially sweating) and a stabilization of blood pressure. In patients who have carbohydrate intolerance

TABLE 9-3. **Preoperative Mortality Associated with Resectioning of Pheochromocytoma**

Year of Series	Study	Mortality (%)	No Patients in Series
1951	Apgar (review)	45	91
1951	Apgar	33	12
1963	Stackpole	13	100
Earlier than 1960	Mayo Clinic	0–26	101 (?)
Later than 1960	Mayo Clinic	2.9 (?)	44 (?)
Earlier than 1960	Modlin (without α blockade)	18	17
Later than 1967	Modlin (with α blockade)	2	41
1976	Scott	3	33
1976–1983	Roizen	0	36

(Data abstracted from studies discussed in Roizen MF, Hunt TK, Beaupre PN, et al: The effect of alpha-adrenergic blockade on cardiac performance and tissue oxygen delivery during excision of pheochromocytoma. Surgery 94:941, 1983.)

because of inhibition of insulin release mediated by α-adrenergic receptor stimulation, α-adrenergic receptor blockade may reduce fasting blood sugar levels. In patients who exhibit ST-T changes on ECG, long-term preoperative α-adrenergic receptor blockade (1 to 6 months) has been shown to result in ECG and clinical resolution of catecholamine-induced myocarditis.[109,111,112]

β-Adrenergic receptor blockade with propranolol is suggested for patients who have persistent dysrhythmias or tachycardia,[104-112] because these conditions can be precipitated or aggravated by α-adrenergic receptor blockade. β-adrenergic receptor blockade should not be used without concomitant α-adrenergic receptor blockade, lest the vasoconstrictive effects of the latter go unopposed, thereby increasing the risk of dangerous hypertension.

The optimal duration of preoperative therapy with phenoxybenzamine has not been studied. Most patients require 10 to 14 days, as judged by the time needed to stabilize blood pressure and to ameliorate symptoms. On the basis of my experience, this is a minimal period of time.[108,111] Since the tumor spreads slowly, little is lost by waiting until medical therapy has optimized the patient's preoperative condition. Accordingly, the following criteria are recommended:

1. No "inhospital" blood pressure reading higher than 165/90 mm Hg should be evident for 48 hours before surgery.
2. Orthostatic hypotension should be present, but blood pressure on standing should not be lower than 80/45 mm Hg.

3. The ECG should be free of ST-T changes for a period of at least 2 weeks.
4. No more than one premature ventricular contraction should be present every 5 minutes.

Although specific anesthetic drugs have been recommended, I believe that optimal preoperative preparation, a gentle induction of anesthesia, and good communication between surgeon and anesthesiologist are most important. Virtually all anesthetic agents and techniques (including isoflurane, fentanyl, and regional anesthesia) have been used with success. In fact, all agents studied are associated with a high rate of transient intraoperative dysrhythmias (Table 9-4).[109] Because of ease of use, I prefer to give phenylephrine hydrochloride (Neo-Synephrine) or dopamine for hypotension and nitroprusside for hypertension. Phentolamine (Regitine) has too long an onset and duration of action. Once the venous supply is secured, and if intravascular volume is normal (as measured by pulmonary wedge pressure), normal blood pressure usually results. However, some patients become hypotensive, occasionally requiring massive infusions of catecholamines. On rare occasions, patients remain hypertensive intraoperatively. Postoperatively, about 50 percent remain hypertensive for 1 to 3 days—and initially have markedly elevated but declining plasma catecholamine levels—at which time all but 25 percent become normotensive. It is important to interview other family members and perhaps advise them to inform their future anesthetist about the potential for such familial disease.

TABLE 9-4. Incidence of Perioperative Complications in a Randomized Study of Patients Undergoing Resectioning of Pheochromocytoma Under One of Four Anesthetic Techniques

	Anesthetic*			
	Enflurane (6)	Halothane (6)	Droperidol and Fentanyl (7)	Regional (5)
Ventricular tachycardia				
Needing no treatment	5	5	6	5
Needing treatment	0	1	1	0
Vasodilator needed				
Intraoperatively	6	6	7	5
Postoperatively	0	1†	1†	0
Vasopressor needed				
Intraoperatively	0	1	1	0
Postoperatively	0	0	0	0
Myocardial infarction‡	0	0	0	0
Renal failure‡	0	0	0	0
Congestive heart failure‡	0	1	1	1
Stroke‡	0	0	0	0
Death‡	0	0	0	0

* Number of patients shown in parentheses.
† Not all the abnormally secreting tumor tissue was removed from the patient.
‡ Occurring postoperatively.
(Based on data in Roizen MF, Horrigan RW, Koike M, et al: A prospective randomized trial of four anesthetic techniques for resection of pheochromocytoma. Anesthesiology 57:A43, 1982.)

HYPOFUNCTION OR ABERRATION IN FUNCTION OF THE SYMPATHETIC NERVOUS SYSTEM (DYSAUTONOMIA)

Disorders of the sympathetic nervous system include Shy-Drager's syndrome, Riley-Day syndrome, Lesch-Nyhan's syndrome, Gill familia dysautonomia, diabetic dysautonomia, and the dysautonomia of spinal cord transection.

Although individuals can function well without an adrenal medulla,[113] a deficient peripheral sympathetic nervous system poses major problems in almost all facets of life.[113-131] One of the main functions of the sympathetic nervous system appears to be the regulation of blood pressure and of intravascular fluid volume during changing of body position. Common features of all the syndromes of hypofunctioning of the sympathetic nervous system are orthostatic hypotension and decreased beat-to-beat variability in heart rate. These conditions can be caused by deficient intravascular volume, deficient baroreceptor function (as also occurs in carotid artery disease[132]), abnormalities in CNS function (as in Wernicke's or Shy-Drager's syndrome[115]), deficient neuronal

stores of norepinephrine (as in idiopathic orthostatic hypotension[117,118] and diabetes[116]), or deficient release of norepinephrine (as in traumatic spinal cord injury[113,114]). These patients may have an increased number of available adrenergic receptors (a compensatory response) and an exaggerated response to sympathomimetic drugs.[133] In addition to other abnormalities, such as retention of urine or feces and deficient heat exchange, hypofunctioning of the sympathetic nervous system is often accompanied by renal amyloidosis. Thus, electrolyte and intravascular fluid volume status should be evaluated preoperatively. Because many of these patients have cardiac abnormalities, intravascular fluid volume should be assessed preoperatively using a Swan-Ganz catheter rather than by CVP measurement (also see Ch. 13).

Since functioning of the sympathetic nervous system is not predictable in these patients, I usually employ slow gentle induction of anesthesia and treat sympathetic excess or deficiency by infusing, with careful titration, drugs that directly constrict (phenylephrine) or dilate (nitroprusside) blood vessels or that stimulate (isoproterenol) or depress (propranolol) heart rate. I prefer these drugs to agonists or antagonists, which may indirectly release catecholamines. A 20 percent perioperative mortality rate for 2,600 patients with spinal cord transection has been reported,[128] indicating that such patients are difficult to manage and deserve particularly close attention.

After reviewing 300 patients with spinal cord injury, Kendrick et al.[134] concluded that autonomic hyperreflexia syndrome does not develop if the lesion is below spinal dermatome T7. If the lesion is above spinal dermatome T7 (the splanchnic outflow), 60 to 70 percent of the patients experience extreme vascular instability. The trigger to this instability, or mass reflex involving noradrenergic and motor hypertonus,[119] can be a cutaneous, proprioceptive, or visceral stimulus (full bladder is a common initiator). The sensation enters the spinal cord and causes a spinal reflex, which in normal individuals is inhibited from above. Sudden increases in blood pressure are sensed in the pressure receptors of the aorta and carotid sinus. The resulting vagal hyperactivity produces bradycardia, ventricular ectopia, or various degrees of heart block. Reflex vasodilation may occur above the level of the lesion, resulting in flushing of the head and neck.

Depending on the length of time since spinal cord transection, other abnormalities may occur. Acutely (i.e., less than 3 weeks from the time of spinal injury), retention of urine and feces is common and, by elevating the diaphragm, may impair respiration. Disimpaction of the intestine alleviates this respiratory problem. Hyperesthesia is present above the lesion; reflexes and flaccid paralysis are present below the lesion. The intermediate time period (3 days to 6 months) is marked by a hyperkalemic response to depolarizing drugs.[127] The chronic phase is characterized by a return of muscle tone, positive Babinski's sign, and frequently, the occurrence of hyperreflexia syndromes (e.g., mass reflex; see above).

Thus, in addition to meticulous attention to perioperative intravascular volume and electrolyte status, the anesthesiologist should know — by history-taking, physical examination, and laboratory data — the status of the patient's myocardial conduction (as revealed by ECG), the status of renal functioning (by noting the ratio of creatinine to blood urea nitrogen), and the condition of respiratory muscle (by determining the ratio of forced expiratory volume in 1 second to forced vital capacity, (i.e., FEV_1/FVC) (also see Ch. 59). The anesthesiologist must also have obtained a chest roentgenogram if atelectasis or pneumonia was suspected on history-taking or physical examination. Temperature control, the presence of bone fractures or decubitus ulcers, and the normal functioning of urination and defecation systems must be assessed. Confirmation of the last prevents postoperative pneumonia or atelectasis caused by high positioning of the diaphragm.

THYROID DYSFUNCTION

The major thyroid hormones are thyroxine (T_4), a product of the thyroid gland, and the more potent 3,5,3-triiodothyronine (T_3), a product of both the thyroid and the extrathyroidal enzymatic deiodination of thyroxine). Production of thyroid secretions is maintained by secretion of thyroid-stimulating hormone (TSH) in the pituitary, which in turn is regulated by secretion of thyrotropin-releasing hormone (TRH) in the hypothalamus. Secretion of TSH and TRH appears to be negatively regulated by T_4 and T_3. Whether all effects of thyroid hormones are mediated by T_3, or if T_4 has intrinsic biologic activity remains unclear.

Thyroid hormones create their effects through several mechanisms. Binding of T_3 to high-affinity nuclear receptors and the subsequent activation of DNA-directed mRNA synthesis may account for the anabolic, growth, and developmental effects, plus some calorigenic effect, of thyroid hormones. Membrane and mitochondrial effects of T_3 are important to some of the other effects of T_3.

Diagnosis of thyroid disease is confirmed by one of several biochemical measurements: levels of free T_4 or of total serum concentrations of T_4, and by the "free T_4 index." This index is determined by multiplying total T_4 (free and bound) by the T_3 resin uptake. The T_3 resin uptake measures the extra quantity of serum protein binding sites. This measurement is necessary because thyroxine-binding globulin is abnormally high during pregnancy, hepatic disease, and estrogen therapy (all of which would elevate total T_4 levels). In addition, hyperthyroidism can be diagnosed by measuring levels of TSH after administering TRH. Although administering TRH normally increases TSH levels in blood, even a small increase in T_4 or T_3 levels in blood abolishes this response. Thus, a subnormal or absent serum TSH response to TRH is a very sensitive indicator of hyperthyroidism. In hyperthyroidism, cardiac function and responses to stress are abnormal; return of cardiac function to normal parallels the return of TSH levels to normal.

HYPERTHYROIDISM

Although hyperthyroidism is usually caused by the multinodular diffuse enlargement in Graves' disease (also associated with disorders of the skin and/or eyes), it can also be associated with pregnancy,[135] thyroiditis (with or without neck pain), thyroid adenoma, choriocarcinoma, or TSH-secreting pituitary adenoma. Major manifestations of hyperthyroidism are weight loss, diarrhea, warm moist skin, weakness of large muscle groups, menstrual abnormalities, nervousness, jitteriness, intolerance to heat, tachycardia, cardiac dysrhythmias, mitral valve prolapse,[136] and heart failure. When the thyroid is functioning abnormally, the system most threatened is the cardiovascular system. When diarrhea is severe, dehydration should be corrected preoperatively. Mild anemia, thrombocytopenia, increased serum alkaline phosphatase, hypercalcemia, muscle wasting, and bone loss frequently occur in hyperthyroidism. In the apathetic form of hyperthyroidism (seen most commonly in persons over 60 years of age), cardiac effects dominate the clinical picture.[137,138] These signs and symptoms include tachycardia, irregular heart beat, atrial fibrillation, heart failure, and occasionally papillary muscle dysfunction.[136–139]

Although β-adrenergic receptor blockade can control heart rate, its use is fraught with hazard in the patient already in congestive heart failure (CHF). However, decreasing heart rate may improve heart pumping function. Thus, hyperthyroid patients who have fast ventricular rates, who are in congestive heart failure, and who require emergency surgery are given propranolol guided by changes in pulmonary artery wedge pressure and their condition. If slowing the heart rate with a small dose of propranolol (i.e., 0.05 mg) does not aggravate heart failure, I administer more propranolol. The goal, however, is not to impose surgery on any patient having clinically abnormal thyroid functioning. Therefore, I believe only "life-or-death" emergency surgery should preclude making the patient pharmacologically euthyroid, a process that can take 2 to 6 weeks. Antithyroid medications include propylthiouracil or methimazole, both of which decrease synthesis of thyroxine. Propylthiouracil also decreases conversion of thyroxine into the more potent T_3. However, the literature indicates a trend toward preoperative preparation with propranolol and iodides alone.[140,141] This approach is quicker (i.e., 7-14 days vs 2-6 weeks); it shrinks the thyroid gland, as does the more traditional approach; and it treats symptoms, but may not correct abnormalities in left ventricular function.[142] Regardless of approach, antithyroid drugs should be administered chronically and on the morning of surgery. When emergency surgery is necessary before the euthyroid state is achieved, or if hyperthyroidism gets out of control during surgery, intravenous administration of 0.2 to 10 mg of propranolol should be titrated to restore normal heart rate (assuming the absence of CHF) (see above). Also, intravascular fluid volume and electrolyte balance should be restored. However, administering propranolol does not invariably prevent "thyroid storm."[143]

No controlled study has demonstrated clinical advantages of any anesthetic drug over another for surgical patients who are hyperthyroid. Review of cases done at the University of California, San Francisco, from 1968 to 1982 reveals that virtually all techniques and anesthetic agents have been employed without adverse effects being even remotely attributable to agent or technique. Furthermore, although some authors have recommended that anticholinergic drugs (especially atropine) be avoided because they interfere with the sweating mechanism and cause tachycardia, atropine has been given as a test for adequacy of antithyroid treatment. Because patients are now subject to operative procedures only when euthyroid, the traditional "steal" of the heavily premedicated hyperthyroid patient to the operating room has vanished.

The patient having a large goiter and an obstructed airway can be handled in the same way as any other patient having problematic airway management. Preoperative medication should avoid excessive sedation, and an airway should be established, often with the patient awake. A firm armored endotracheal tube is preferable and should be passed beyond the point of extrinsic compression. It is most useful to examine computed tomographic (CT) scans of the neck preoperatively to determine the extent of compression. Maintenance of anesthesia usually presents little difficulty. Postoperatively, extubation should be performed under optimal circumstances for reintubation, in case the tracheal rings have been weakened and the trachea collapses.

Of the many possible postoperative complications (nerve injuries, bleeding, and metabolic abnormalities), "thyroid storm" (discussed below), bilateral recurrent nerve trauma, and hypocalcemic tetany are the most feared. Bilateral recurrent laryngeal nerve injury (by trauma or edema) causes stridor and laryngeal obstruction due to unopposed adduction of the vocal cords and closure of the glottic aperture. Immediate endotracheal intubation is required, usually followed by tracheostomy to ensure an adequate airway. This rare complication occurred only once in over 30,000 thyroid operations at the Lahey Clinic. Unilateral recurrent nerve injury often goes unnoticed because of compensatory overadduction of the uninvolved cord. However, we often test vocal cord function before and after this surgery by asking the patient to say "e" or "moon." Unilateral nerve injury is characterized by hoarseness and bilateral nerve injury by aphonia. Selective injury of adductor fibers of both recurrent laryngeal nerves leaves the abductor muscles relatively unopposed, and pulmonary aspiration is a risk. Selective injury of abductor fibers leaves the adductor muscles relatively unopposed, and airway obstruction can occur. Bullous glottic edema, an additional cause of postoperative respiratory compromise, has no specific cause or known preventive measure.

THYROID STORM

"Thyroid storm" is the name for the clinical diagnosis of a life-threatening illness in a patient whose hyperthyroidism has been severely exacerbated by illness or operation. Thyroid storm is manifested by hyperpyrexia, tachycardia, and striking alterations in consciousness.[144,145] No laboratory tests are diagnostic of thyroid storm, and the precipitating (nonthyroidal) cause is the major determinant of survival. Therapy can include blocking the synthesis of thyroid hormones by administering antithyroid drugs, blocking the release of preformed hormone with iodine, meticulous attention to hydration and supportive therapy, and correcting the precipitating cause. Blocking the sympathetic nervous system with reserpine, guanethidine, or α- and β-receptor antagonists may be exceedingly hazardous and requires skillful management and constant monitoring of the critically ill patient.

HYPOTHYROIDISM

Hypothyroidism is a common disease, occurring in 5 percent of a large adult population in Great Britain, in 3 to 6 percent of a healthy older population in Massachusetts, and in 4.5 percent of a medical clinic population in Switzerland. Usually hypothyroidism is subclinical, serum concentrations of thyroid hormones are in the normal range, and only serum TSH levels are elevated.[146] In such patients, hypothyroidism may have little or no perioperative significance. However, a recent retrospective study of 59 mildly hypothyroid patients found that more hypothyroid patients than control subjects required prolonged postoperative intubation (9/59 vs 4/59) and had significant electrolyte imbalances (3/59 vs 1/59) and bleeding complications (4/59 vs 0/59).[147] Because only a small number of charts were examined, these differences did not reach statistical significance.

In the less frequent occurrences of overt hypothyroidism, relative lack of thyroid hormone results in slow mental functioning, slow movement, dry skin, intolerance to cold, depression of the ventilatory responses to hypoxia and hypercarbia,[148] impaired clearance of free water, slow gastric emptying, and bradycardia. In extreme cases, cardiomegaly, heart failure, and pericardial and pleural effusions manifest as fatigue, dyspnea, and orthopnea.[149] Hypothyroidism is often associated with amyloidosis, which may produce an enlarged tongue, abnormalities of the cardiac conduction system, and renal disease. Hypothyroidism decreases anesthetic requirement slightly.[150]

Ideal preoperative management of hypothyroidism consists of restoring normal thyroid status: I routinely administer the normal dose of T_3 or T_4 the morning of surgery even though these drugs have long half-lives (1.4 to 10 days). For patients with myxedema coma requiring emergency surgery, T_3 can be given intravenously (with fear of precipitating myocardial ischemia, however) while supportive therapy is undertaken to restore normal intravascular fluid volume, body temperature, cardiac function, respiratory function, and electrolyte balance.

Treating hypothyroid patients having symptomatic coronary artery disease poses special problems and may require compromises in the general practice of preoperatively restoring euthyroidism with drugs.[151,152] Although both T_4 and propranolol may be given, adequate amelioration of both ischemic heart disease and hypothyroidism may be difficult to achieve. The need for thyroid therapy must be balanced against the risk of aggravating anginal symptoms. One review suggested early consideration for coronary artery revascularization.[151] It advocated initiating thyroid replacement therapy in the ICU soon after the patient's arrival from the operating room and myocardial revascularization surgery. However, several deaths due to dysrhythmia and CHF as well as cardiogenic shock with infarction have occurred while patients who were not given thyroid therapy were awaiting surgery. Thus, there is need for consideration of true emergency coronary artery revascularization in patients having both severe coronary artery disease and significant hypothyroidism.

In hypothyroidism, respiratory control mechanisms do not function normally.[148] However, the response to hypoxia and hypercarbia and the clearance of free water become normal with thyroid replacement therapy.[148,149] Drug metabolism is anecdotally reported to be slowed, and awakening times from sedatives are reported to be prolonged during hypothyroidism. However, no formal study of the pharmacokinetics and pharmacodynamics of sedatives or anesthetic agents has been published. These concerns disappear when thyroid function is normalized preoperatively. Addison's disease (with its relative steroid deficiency) is more common in hypothyroidism, and some endocrinologists routinely treat noniatrogenic hypothyroid patients with stress doses of steroids perioperatively. The possibility that this steroid deficiency exists should be considered if the patient becomes hypotensive perioperatively.

DISORDERS OF CALCIUM METABOLISM

The three substances that regulate the serum concentrations of calcium, phosphorus, and magnesium — parathyroid hormone, calcitonin, and vitamin D — act on bone, kidney, and gut. Parathyroid hormone stimulates bone resorption and inhibits renal excretion of calcium, two conditions that lead to hypercalcemia. Calcitonin can be considered an antagonist to parathyroid hormone. Through its metabolites, vitamin D aids in absorption of calcium, phosphate, and magnesium from the gut and facilitates the bone resorptive effects of parathyroid hormone.[153]

HYPERCALCEMIA

Regardless of cause, hypercalcemia can present with any of a number of symptoms: anorexia, vomiting, constipation, polyuria, polydipsia, lethargy, confusion, formation of renal calculi, pancreatitis, bone pain, and psychiatric abnormalities. Free intracellular calcium initiates and/or regulates muscle contraction, release of neurotransmitters, secretion of hormones, enzyme action, and energy metabolism. About one-third of all hypercalcemic patients have hypertension that resolves with successful treatment of hypercalcemia.[154] Long-standing hypercalcemia can lead to calcifications in the myocardium, blood vessels, brain (which can manifest as seizures), and kidney (which can manifest as polyuria unresponsive to vasopressin).

Patients with moderate hypercalcemia who have normal renal and cardiovascular function present no special perioperative problem. The ECG should be examined preoperatively and intraoperatively for short P-R or Q-T intervals. Because severe hypercalcemia can result in hypovolemia, normal intravascular volume and electrolyte status should be restored before anesthesia and surgery. In emergency situations, vigorous intravascular volume expansion usually reduces serum calcium concentration to a safe level (less than 14 mg/dl). Also, adminstering saline and furosemide is often helpful. Corticosteroids can be used to inhibit further gastrointestinal absorption of calcium. Mithramycin will lower calcium levels about 2 mg/dl in 36 to 48 hours. It is especially important to know whether hypercalcemia has been chronic, because serious abnormalities in cardiac, renal, or CNS may have resulted.

HYPOCALCEMIA

Hypocalcemia (caused by hypoalbuminemia, hypoparathyroidism, hypomagnesemia, or chronic renal disease) is not usually accompanied by a cardiovascular disorder. The clinical signs of hypocalcemia are clumsiness; convulsions; laryngeal stridor; depression; muscle stiffness; paresthesis (aeral and perioral); Parkinsonism; tetany; Chvostek's sign; dry, scaly skin, brittle nails, and coarse hair; low serum concentrations of calcium; prolonged Q-T intervals; soft tissue calcifications; and Trousseau's sign. Since congestive heart failure improves in patients with coexisting heart disease when calcium and magnesium levels are restored to normal, these ion levels should be normal before surgery. Prolongation of the Q-T interval is a moderately reliable electrocardiographic sign of hypocalcemia.[155] Sudden decreases in blood levels of ionized calcium (as with chelation therapy) can result in severe hypotension.

The intimate involvement of the parathyroid gland with the thyroid gland can result in unintentional hypocalcemia during surgery for diseases of either organ. Because of the affinity of their bones for calcium, this relationship is especially important for patients having advanced osteitis. Internal redistribution of magnesium and/or calcium ions may occur (into "hungry bones") after parathyroidectomy, causing hypomagnesemia and/or hypocalcemia. The most prominent manifestations of acute hypocalcemia are distal paresthesias and muscle spasm (tetany). Potentially fatal complications of severe hypocalcemia include laryngeal spasm and hypocalcemic seizures. Clinical sequelae of magnesium deficiency include cardiac dysrhythmias (principally ventricular tachydysrhythmias), hypocalcemic tetany, and neuromuscular irritability that is independent of hypocalcemia (tremors, twitching, asterixis, and seizures).

In addition to monitoring total serum calcium or ionized calcium postoperatively, one can test for Chvostek's sign and Trousseau's sign. (Note that serum calcium and not ionized calcium is dependent on albumin level, declining about 0.8 mg/dl for each 1 g/dl drop in serum albumin level.) Because Chvostek's sign can be elicited in 10-15 percent of individuals who are not hypocalcemic, an attempt should be made to elicit it preoperatively to ensure its appearance is meaningful. Chvostek's sign is a contracture of the facial muscles produced by tapping the ipsilateral facial nerves at the angle of the jaw. Trousseau's sign is elicited by applying a blood pressure cuff at a level slightly above the systolic level for a few minutes. The resulting carpopedal spasm, with contractions of the fingers and an inability to open the hand, stems from the increased muscle irritability in hypocalcemic states, which is aggravated by ischemia produced by the blood pressure cuff.

PITUITARY ABNORMALITIES

ANTERIOR PITUITARY HYPERSECRETION

The three most common disorders of pituitary hypersecretion are those related to excesses of prolactin (amenorrhea, galactorrhea, and infertility), ACTH (Cushing's disease), or growth hormone (acromegaly). In addition to knowing the pathophysiologic processes of the disease involved, the anesthesiologist must determine whether the patient recently underwent air pneumoencephalography. If so, nitrous oxide should not be used; this practice lessens the risk of intracranial hypertension from gas collection. CT scanning of the sella has largely replaced neuroencephalography. Otherwise, no special preoperative evaluations are required for patients having the microchromophobic adenomas that most commonly cause prolactin excess[156] or for the patients undergoing the transsphenoidal surgery now commonly used for removal of such adenomas.[157] The treatment of microadenomas is currently being reevaluated.[158,159] However, with large prolactin-secreting tumors (macroadenomas), loss of other pituitary function is common, and evaluation of thyroid and adrenocortical status is indicated. Preoperative preparation of patients with Cushing's disease is discussed in the section on adrenocortical hormone excess.

The effects of excessive growth hormone stem from both direct actions of the hormone on tissue and from stimulation of the production of somatomedins. Excessive growth hormone often results in retention of sodium and potassium, inhibition of the peripheral action of insulin (which can result in diabetes mellitus), and the occurrence of premature atherosclerosis (often associated with cardiomegaly). Exertional dyspnea may be either related to heart failure or respiratory insufficiency due to kyphoscoliosis. Cardiac dysrhythmias are common.[160] Preoperative evaluation of the patient with acromegaly might begin by determining whether significant cardiac, hypertensive, pulmonary, or diabetic problems exist. If so, preoperative evaluation should proceed along the lines described in sections discussing those topics. In addition, difficulty with endotracheal intubation should be anticipated in the acromegalic patient; lateral neck films or CT scans of the neck and direct or indirect visualization can identify the patient who has subglottic stenosis or an enlarged tongue, mandibles, epiglottis, or vocal cords.[161,162] If placement of an arterial line is necessary, a brachial or femoral site may be preferable to a radial site.[163]

ANTERIOR PITUITARY HYPOFUNCTION

Anterior pituitary hypofunction results in deficiency of one or more of the following hormones: GH, TSH, ACTH, prolactin, or gonadotropins. Preoperative preparation of those individuals deficient in ACTH and TSH is discussed above. No special preoperative preparation is required for the patient deficient in prolactin or gonadotropins; deficiency in growth hormone can result in atrophy of cardiac muscle, a condition that may require preoperative cardiac evaluation. However, anesthetic problems have not been documented in patients with isolated growth hormone deficiency.

POSTERIOR PITUITARY HORMONE EXCESS AND DEFICIENCY

The secretion of vasopressin, or antidiuretic hormone (ADH) is increased by increased serum osmolality or the presence of hypotension. Inappropriate secretion of vasopressin, without relation to serum osmolality, results in hyponatremia and fluid retention. This inappropriate secretion can result from a variety of CNS lesions; from drugs such as nicotine, narcotics, chlorpropamide, clofibrate, vincristine, vinblastine, and cyclophosphamide; and from pulmonary infections, hypothyroidism, adrenal insufficiency, and ectopic production from tumors. Preoperative treatment of the surgical patient with inappropriate secretion of vasopressin includes appropriate treatment of the causative disorders, and restriction of water. Occasionally, drugs that inhibit the renal response to ADH (e.g., lithium or demeclocycline) should be administered preoperatively to restore normal intravascular volume and electrolyte status.

Lack of ADH which results in diabetes insipidus, is caused by pituitary disease, brain tumors, infiltrative diseases such as sarcoidosis, head trauma, or lack of renal response to ADH. The last can occur with such diverse causes as hypokalemia, hypercalcemia, sickle cell anemia, obstructive uropathy, or renal insufficiency. Preoperative treatment of diabetes insipidus consists of restoring normal intravascular volume by replacing urinary losses and by giving daily fluid requirements intravenously. In severe cases of diabetes insipidus, desmopressin, a vasopressin analogue, is effective for 8 to 24 hours after a single intranasal administration, and appears to be warranted preoperatively.[164]

DISEASES INVOLVING THE CARDIOVASCULAR SYSTEM

HYPERTENSION
(Also See Ch. 10)

Because of the controversy regarding the appropriateness of preoperative treatment of hypertension, the original articles that stimulated this controversy will be evaluated. Smithwick and Thompson[165] and Brown[166] reported overall mortality rates of 2.5 to 3.6 percent, respectively, in hypertensive patients undergoing sympathectomy between 1935 and 1947. These values were five or six times higher than values for normotensive patients undergoing similar operations. Obviously, these patients were not randomly assigned to treatment or nontreatment groups, and no attempt was made to ensure that end-organ disease was equivalent in the two groups. In 1929, Sprague[167] analyzed the records of 75 patients with hypertensive cardiac disease and found that 24 (32 percent) died during or shortly after operations employing general anesthesia.

In the early part of this century, severely ill patients did not do well perioperatively; however, whether preoperative treatment would have improved surgical outcome is still not known. The evolution of drug therapy for hypertension was hampered in the late 1950s and early 1960s by the publication of case reports of severe hypotension and bradycardia in patients receiving antihypertensive drugs before surgery. The tailoring of anesthetic dose to patient condition, and the realization that sympatholytic antihypertensive drugs decreased anesthetic requirement[168] caused such case reports to disappear from the literature. A more recent prospective, controlled, double-blind study by the Veterans Administration (VA) provided a rationale for life-long treatment of hypertension: such treatment decreased the incidence of stroke, CHF, and progression to renal insufficiency and to accelerated (malignant) hypertension.[169,170] Berglund et al.[171] found a decrease in deaths due to myocardial infarction when patients were treated for mild-to-moderate hypertension. Other studies have confirmed the beneficial effect of treating hypertension, even for patients with diastolic pressures of 90 to 104 mm Hg.[172] One study has indicated caution in adding diuretics to therapeutic limits in therapy for the patient with an abnormal ECG whose blood pressure does not decrease after administration of the usual doses of diuretic drugs (see later section on hypokalemia).[173] Other studies in experimental models of hypertension indicate that treatment results in a regression of the cardiac muscle and in autonomic nerve alterations of hypertension.[174] United States government statistics reveal significant decreases (greater than 40 percent) in the death rate from stroke from 1969 to 1983. Deaths related to hypertensive cardiovascular disease and to myocardial infarction have decreased dramatically since 1974, accounting for most of the decrease in cardiovascular death in this time period. This strong evidence from the VA studies and the epidemiologic data have led to the belief that all patients with a diastolic blood pressure above 90 mm Hg should be treated, regardless of age. However, the question is: Should elective surgery be postponed and patient and physician schedules disrupted, so that treatment can be instituted and stabilized? Several schools of thought exist, the two oldest represented by the study conducted by Prys-Roberts et al.[175] in 1971 and by Goldman and Caldera[176] in 1979. Two other studies (Bedford and Feinstein[177] and Assidao et al.[178]) have also been cited. Unfortunately, all four studies have deficiencies that prevent the establishment of a definitive answer to this question.

CRITICAL ANALYSIS OF THE DATA OF PRYS-ROBERTS ET AL.

The followers of Prys-Roberts et al.[175] believe that preoperative treatment of hypertension lowers the incidence of perioperative morbidity and mortality. In this study, three groups were compared: a control group consisting of seven elderly normotensive patients having an average mean arterial blood pressure of 89.5 mm Hg; a group of seven hypertensive patients whose high blood pressure was not treated preoperatively (four were being treated not for high blood pressure but for its complications) who had an average mean arterial blood pressure (MABP) of 129.5 mm Hg; and a group of 15 hypertensive patients whose high blood pressure was treated preoperatively, and who had an average MABP of 129.9 mm Hg. The same doses of thiopental and halothane were given to all groups of patients, and measurements of absolute change in MABP, cardiac dysrhythmias, and ECG evidence of ischemia were performed. Patients with untreated hypertension had the greatest absolute fall in blood pressure and the highest percentage of dysrhythmias and ischemia.

Several flaws in study design create serious doubt as to whether the relationship between preoperative treatment of hypertension and perioperative morbidity has been evaluated objectively in this investigation. First, the wisdom of administering the same dose of anesthetic to both groups of patients should be questioned. If the anesthetic dose had been titrated to the anesthetic needs of the patient, would the results have been different? Second, blood pressure did not differ between the treated and untreated groups. In addition, at least four of the seven hypertensive patients who were not treated for high blood pressure were "sicker" than any of the hypertensive patients who were treated. Why some patients were treated for hypertension and others were not was not explained; selection definitely did not occur on a random basis. Finally, it was not stated whether surgery was similar for all groups.

This study does indicate that patients who are sick preoperatively have more problems perioperatively than do healthy patients. This has been shown many times.[179-182] However, from these data, the efficacy of preoperative treatment of hypertension cannot be established. This study and others by the same group provide useful data regarding the hemodynamic consequences of anesthesia when a standard technique is used on patients who have untreated hypertension.

CRITICAL ANALYSIS OF THE DATA OF GOLDMAN AND CALDERA

The school of thought represented by Goldman and Caldera[176] advocates that preoperative treatment of hypertension does not affect outcome. Goldman and Caldera state that their study is a prospective one. However, the only prospective aspect of their study appears to be that patients were examined preoperatively. These investigators compared surgical outcome for three groups: sick hypertensive patients whose high blood pressure was treated preoperatively; less sick hypertensive patients whose high blood pressure was "undertreated" preoperatively; and less sick, only moderately hypertensive patients who received no treatment preoperatively. No differences in outcome between groups was found.

This study has several flaws in design. Patients were not randomly assigned regarding preoperative treatment, undertreatment, or nontreatment of hypertension. Also, sicker patients were allocated to the treated hyperten-

TABLE 9-5. Analysis of Treatment Groups Used by Goldman and Caldera[176] to Evaluate Effectiveness of Preoperative Treatment of Hypertension in Surgical Patients

Preoperatively Hypertensive Patients	(n)	Preoperatively			
		Diastolic BP >100 mm Hg (n)	BUN >30 mg% (n)	Angina or CHF (%)	TIAs (%)
Treated successfully*	79	0	8	47	13
Treated unsuccessfully	40	34	13	40	18
Not treated	77		1	26	4

Abbreviations used: BP = blood pressure; CHF = congestive heart failure; TIA = transient ischemic attacks.
* These data demonstrate that the patients who were the sickest before surgery were allocated to this group, thereby biasing results toward nontreatment.

sive group (Table 9-5), thus biasing study results toward favoring nontreatment of hypertension.

Other flaws concern statistical methods. Only 34 of the 117 patients who were hypertensive at the time of surgery had diastolic blood pressure of at least 100 mm Hg (Table 9-5). If morbid complications were assumed to be 20 percent in the untreated group, and if treatment was assumed to reduce morbidity 50 percent, then by power analysis,[183] Goldman and Caldera[176] would have had to compare approximately 237 patients to have an 80 percent chance of finding a difference at a confidence level of 0.05 percent. If a lower rate of morbidity in the untreated group (e.g., 15 percent) and a lesser reduction in the rate of morbidity (e.g., 33 percent) were assumed, then even more patients would have to be studied to be 80 percent sure no difference occurred, even at the 0.05 confidence level. For example, if morbid complications were assumed to be 15 percent in the untreated group, and if treatment were assumed to reduce morbidity 33 percent, 764 patients would have had to be studied in each group to be 80 percent certain no difference occurred, the confidence level being 0.05. These major flaws in study design make it impossible to ascertain whether preoperative treatment of hypertension decreased perioperative morbidity.

CRITICAL ANALYSIS OF THE DATA OF BEDFORD AND FEINSTEIN

Bedford and Feinstein[177] and their supporters believe that instability of blood pressure is the condition most frequently predicting morbid perioperative complications. In their study, the responses of three groups to rapid-sequence induction were compared prospectively. Patients were allocated to groups based on the initial admitting room blood pressures (BP) and the average presurgical inhospital blood pressure: Group I (30 patients) had BP less than 140/90 mm Hg during and after admission (normal BP group); group II (12 patients) had BP greater than 140/90 mm Hg on admission but less than 140/90 mm Hg during hospitalization (labile BP group); group III (8 patients) had BP greater than 140/90 mm Hg during and after admission (hypertensive BP group). Whether any of the patients in the labile or hypertensive BP groups were under treatment for hypertension, had end-organ complications of hypertension (such as ischemic heart disease), or were told they were hypertensive was not stated. Patients were given standard (i.e., not tailored to the patient's condition) premedication (morphine, diazepam, and atropine) and a standard rapid-sequence induction (thiopental, 3 to 4 mg/kg IV, succinylcholine, 1.5 mg/kg, IV). After intubation, heart rate and blood pressure increased significantly in all three groups. The increase was greatest in the labile BP group, rising from a mean BP of 102 ± 5 to 152 ± 4 mm Hg. Eight of 12 patients in that group required additional thiopental and/or vasodilating drugs to normalize blood pressure, and 2 of 12 developed transient S-T segment depression in lead II. No patient in either of the other two groups required similar treatment or had S-T segment changes on ECG.

Thus, this study does indicate that patients with labile blood pressure may require more careful titration of anesthetic drugs than those whose blood pressure is either normal or high but stable. However, we do not know whether the results would have been different if the anesthetic had been titrated to the anesthetic needs of the individual patient. Nor do we know whether the groups had equivalent baseline end-organ disease. We do not even know how many patients were being treated for hypertension. Therefore, these data do not shed light on the efficacy of preoperative treatment of hypertension.

CRITICAL ANALYSIS OF THE DATA OF ASSIDAO ET AL.

The study by Assidao et al.[178] is cited by those advocating preoperative treatment of hypertension. In this study, records of 166 cases of unilateral carotid endarterectomy were reviewed to investigate the association of preoperative and intraoperative factors with perioperative complications. The authors found that postoperative hypertension (i.e., systolic blood pressure > 200 mm Hg or diastolic blood pressure > 110 mm Hg) and transient postoperative neurologic deficits occurred more commonly in the 21 patients with poor preoperative control of blood pressure (BP > 170/95 mm Hg) (52 and 23.8 percent, respectively) than in the 79 patients with adequate blood pressure control (BP < 170/95 mm Hg) (35 and 2.5 percent, respectively, or in the 66 normotensive patients (17 and 1.5 percent, respectively). No statistically significant difference was found between the groups regarding permanent neurologic sequelae of surgery or the rate of myocardial ischemia.

The study by Assidao et al. does not tell us whether postoperative hypertension caused the transient neurologic deficits or whether these deficits resulted in a compensation of postoperative hypertension. We also do not know whether the three groups were equivalent in end-organ manifestations of preoperative disease. Nor does the study tell us why blood pressure was not controlled preoperatively in some patients or whether preoperative normalization of high blood pressure would have reduced the rate of postoperative complications. This study does tell us that patients with high blood pressure before surgery are likely to have high blood pressure after surgery.

RECOMMENDATIONS

Although preoperative systolic blood pressure has been found to be a significant predictor of postoperative morbidity,[178,184-186] no data definitively establish whether preoperative treatment of hypertension reduces perioperative risk. Until a definitive study is performed (which is, unfortunately, extremely difficult to conduct), I recommend that preoperative treatment of the patient with hypertension be based on the following beliefs: (1) the patient should be educated as to the importance of the lifelong treatment of hypertension, and (2) perioperative hemodynamic fluctuations are less frequent in treated than in untreated hypertensive patients (as demonstrated by Prys-Roberts et al.[175] and confirmed by Goldman and Caldera[176]) and that hemodynamic fluctuations have some relationship to morbidity.

In addition to deciding whether a hypertensive patient needs treatment and ensuring that none of the complications of antihypertensive drugs is present, preoperative management should include a search for end-organ damage secondary to hypertension, that is, changes in the CNS and coronary arteries, myocardium, aorta, carotid arteries, kidneys, and peripheral blood vessels. Such injury may affect perioperative management. For example, the presence of renal disease may alter the choice and dosage of anesthetic drugs. Similarly, the recent occurrence of myocardial ischemia may warrant a delay in elective surgery. Knowing the location of myocardial ischemia would indicate which ECG lead should be monitored intraoperatively (also see Chs. 14 & 15). Also, to guide intraoperative regulation of blood pressure and to judge the effects of therapy, I obtain multiple blood pressure readings in both arms while the patient is in various positions.

I use such preoperative data to determine the individualized range of values I consider tolerable by a particular patient during and after surgery. That is, if blood pressure is

180/100 mm Hg and heart rate 96 beats/min on admission with no signs or symptoms of myocardial ischemia, I feel confident that the patient can tolerate these levels during surgery. If during the night blood pressure decreases to 80/50 mm Hg and heart rate to 48 beats/min and the patient does not wake with signs of a new cerebral deficit, I believe he or she can tolerate safely such levels during anesthesia. Therefore, from preoperative data, I derive an individualized set of values for each patient. I then try to keep cardiovascular variables within that range and, in fact, plan prior to induction what therapies to use to accomplish that goal (e.g., administration of more/less anesthesia, nitroglycerin or nitroprusside/dopamine, dobutamine, phenylephrine, or propranolol/isoproterenol, atropine) (Fig. 9-2). I believe this sort of planning is especially important in the patient with suspected cardio-

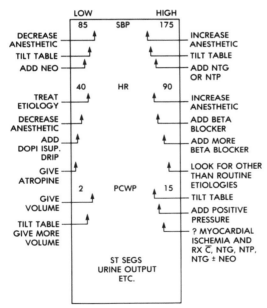

FIG. 9-2 Window of acceptable values. This hypothetical range of "safe" cardiovascular values for one patient illustrates possible therapies that might be employed if actual perioperative values approached the high or low end of that range. The range of safe values, variables treated, and therapies are tailored to the patient and surgical situation. SPB = systemic blood pressure; NTG = nitroglycerin; NTP = nitroprusside; HR = heart rate; PCWP = pulmonary capillary wedge pressure; NEO = neosynephrine; DOPI ISUP = dopamine or isoprel.

vascular disease and relatively unimportant in the totally healthy patient. I do not know for certain that keeping cardiovascular variables within an individualized range of acceptable values improves surgical outcome, but I do believe that such a plan reduces morbidity. For example, in several studies, major intraoperative deviations in blood pressure from the preoperative level have been correlated with the occurrence of myocardial ischemia.[175-177,186]

ISCHEMIC HEART DISEASE

IDENTIFYING ISCHEMIC HEART DISEASE

Any of the following conditions may indicate the presence of ischemic heart disease: a history of viselike chest pain, with or without radiation to the inner arm or neck; dyspnea on exertion, on exposure to cold, with defecation, or after eating; orthopnea; paroxysmal nocturnal dyspnea; nocturnal coughing; nocturia; previous or current peripheral or pulmonary edema; a history of myocardial infarction (MI); a family history of coronary artery disease; diagnosis of MI by ECG or elevated levels of enzymes; and cardiomegaly. Other patients who should be suspected of having ischemic heart disease include those who have diabetes, hypertension (especially if they are cigarette smokers or hyperlipemic[14,15,187]), left ventricular hypertrophy on ECG,[188] peripheral vascular disease,[187-192] carotid bruits,[191-194] asymptomatic carotid artery occlusion,[191-192] or unexplained tachycardia or fatigue.

The more difficult question to answer is: How common is ischemic heart disease in asymptomatic patients or in patients having a normal ECG but predisposing conditions? The history appears to be the best indicator of coronary artery disease. Tomatis et al.[189] recorded coronary angiograms for "nearly all patients" who presented for aortoiliac reconstruction or resection of an abdominal aortic aneurysm. Of those having normal ECGs and histories not suggestive of coronary artery disease, 38 percent had stenosis of at least 50 percent in one or more coronary arteries, and 14 percent had stenosis of at least 75 percent in one or more coronary arteries. The percentages of patients with stenosis were the same for asymptomatic patients having abnormal ECGs. However, a normal ECG was not sensitive in ruling out significant stenosis when vascular disease was present: 44 percent of patients having normal ECGs and peripheral vascular disease had stenosis of at least 50 percent in one or more coronary arteries; and 30 percent had stenosis of at least 75 percent.

Hertzer et al.[190] found that angina and a history of myocardial disease reliably indicated coronary artery disease. These investigators studied 1,000 patients having peripheral vascular disease. Of the 500 patients having normal ECGs and no history of myocardial disease, 37 percent had narrowing of at least 70 percent in one or more coronary arteries. In contrast, of those suspected of coronary artery disease because of history and/or ECG results, 78 percent had narrowing of at least 70 percent in one or more coronary arteries. Also, patients who currently had angina had a 66 percent incidence of either severe correctable or severe inoperable coronary artery disease, whereas those who had peripheral vascular disease but no angina had an incidence of only 22.5 percent.

Several studies of asymptomatic carotid artery disease have shown very high perioperative mortality rates and life risk from associated ischemic heart disease.[191,192,194] Barnes and Marszalek[192] found perioperative mortality rates of 18.2 and 15 percent, respectively, for patients having an asymptomatic carotid bruit or occlusive disease but a rate of only 2.1 percent for patients undergoing similar peripheral vascular procedures who did not have a carotid bruit. Whereas the existence of asymptomatic carotid bruits did not predict the site of stroke or greatly influence the incidence of perioperative stroke, [191-194] it did predict mortality from ischemic heart disease (Table 9-6). Benchimol et al.[188] showed that 15 percent of patients with triple-vessel coronary artery disease have a normal resting ECG.

The important point to remember is that the history is the best indicator of coronary artery disease; in most series, the sensitivity and specificity of the history in indicating such disease range is from 80 to 91 percent[188-190,195-198]

TABLE 9-6. Carotid Artery Bruits and the Risk of Stroke in Elective Surgery

Study	Incidence of Stroke in Patients	
	With Bruits	Without Bruits
Ropper et al.[193]	1/104	4/631
Of those having Vascular surgery	1/37	4/130
Barnes et al.[191]	5/85*	0/364
Perioperative deaths	10.6%	0.3%

* All patients included in this study were undergoing vascular surgery. These 85 patients also had either a bruit or significant carotid artery obstruction, or both.

(also see Ch. 8 for the definition of sensitivity and specificity).

PERIOPERATIVE MORBIDITY

The presence of coronary artery disease, its severity, the time of most recent myocardial tissue death, the arteries affected, and complications and treatment of the disease are important information to the anesthesiologist. These variables influence the manner in which anesthesia is given and, in fact, may determine whether anesthesia and surgery should be postponed.

PREVIOUS MYOCARDIAL INFARCTION

Numerous epidemiologic studies[89,185,199-207] (Table 9-7) have shown that if previous myocardial infarction precedes surgery by less than 6 months, the perioperative reinfarction rate is 5 to 86 percent and mortality 23 to 86 percent. (This 5 to 86 percent value is 1.5 to 10 times higher than the value when previous myocardial infarction and subsequent surgery are separated by more than 6 months.) After 6 months, the perioperative reinfarction rate seems to stabilize at 2 to 6 percent. An investigation by Schoeppel et al.[206] studying a small number of patients produced a 0 percent mortality rate in the first year after infarction but a perioperative reinfarction rate of 16.7 percent and a mortality rate of 67 percent for patients experiencing perioperative reinfarction. Since the in-

TABLE 9-7 Incidence of Perioperative Myocardial Infarction

Time from MI to Operation (months)	Arkins et al.[199] 1963 (Mort.)	Tomkins & Artusio[200] 1959-1963 (Reinf.)	(Mort.)	Fraser et al.[201] 1960-1964 (Mort.)	Tarhan et al.[202] 1975-1976 (Reinf.)	(Mort.)	Sapala et al.[203] 1970-1974 (Reinf.)	(Mort.)	Steen et al.[204] 1980 (Reinf.)	(Mort.)
0-3	40% 11/27	54.5% 12/22	*	38% 19/38	37% 3/8	*	86% 6/7	86% 6/7	27% 2/18	
4-6	*		*	*	16% 3/19	*			11% 2/18	
7-12	*	25.0% 9/36	*	*	5% 2/42	*				
13-18	*	22.4% 11/49	*	*	4% 1/27	*				
19-24	*		*	*	4% 1/21	*	5.7% 9/159	1.9% 3/159	5.4% 30/544	
25-36	*	5.9% 3/51	*	*	5% 11/232	*				
>36	*	1.0% 5/493	*	*		*				
Unknown	*	42.8% 3/7	*	*	5.6% 7/73	*				
Total patients with MI	*	6.5% 43/658	4.7% 31/658	*	6.6% 28/422	3% 15/422	9% 15/166	5.4% 9/166	6.1% 36/587	4.2% 25/587

* Abbreviations used: MI = myocardial infarction; Mort. = mortality; Reinf. = Reinfarction.   *Mortality not stated.

cidence and timing of perioperative reinfarction in the Schoeppel et al. study differ so much from those variables in the other studies listed in Table 9-7, I have put little emphasis on that study. However, for all 10 of the studies listed in Table 9-7, the overall reinfarction rates are similar.[89,185,199-205]

The study of Rao et al.[89] deserves special comment because it proposes to show a vast decrease in perioperative reinfarction rate attributable to the use of modern monitoring techniques. These investigators compared the rates of perioperative reinfarction and mortality at their institution for 364 patients having previous MIs operated on between 1973 and 1976 with the rates for 733 patients having prior MIs operated on between 1976 and 1982. The authors attribute the reduction in overall perioperative reinfarction rate (from 7.7 to 1.9 percent) and in each time period (i.e., from 36 to 5.8 percent when surgery occurs within 3 months of a previous MI) to invasive monitoring and rapid treatment of cardiovascular variables when values deviated from normal values. These two practices apply to both the intraoperative period and the first 72 postoperative hours. (The 72-hour period may be especially important, as virtually all of the 10 studies showed that reinfarction was most likely to occur 24 to 96 hours after surgery.[89,185,199-206]) Most of the reduction in perioperative reinfarction rate was found in patients over 65 years of age.

The editorial evaluating the Rao et al. study stated that the use of historical controls may have biased the conclusions.[208] Also, a different patient mix, improved skills of the sur-geon and anesthetist, and other unidentified or unmeasured changes over time may have contributed to the reduction in reinfarction rate. Other workers have pointed out that certain surgical procedures (such as ophthalmic operations) have low perioperative reinfarction rates,[204-206,209,210] whereas others (such as vascular operations) have high reinfarction rates. The study by Rao et al. does confirm the fact that the perioperative reinfarction rate is higher in the first 6 months after a previous MI. Postponement of surgery for patients who have had an MI less than 6 months earlier should reduce mortality associated with anesthesia. The less severe the coronary artery disease, the more similar the patient's anticipated survival curve to that of patients who do not have coronary artery disease[211] and, probably, the less the perioperative risk.[212,213]

OTHER PREDICTIVE PREOPERATIVE INFORMATION

Treadmill exercise testing, noninvasive imaging, and cardiac catheterization also add information to the history, increasing our knowledge about the likelihood of cardiac disease and perioperative cardiac function.[197,214-217] The electrocardiographic criteria for myocardial ischemia during or after exercise consist of at least 1 mm of J-point depression with downsloping or horizontal S-T segments; slowly upsloping S-T segment depression, defined as being 2 mm of S-T depression measured at 80 msec from the J point; and S-T segment elevation (Fig. 9-3).[197] Other responses to

or Mortality in Patients with Previous Myocardial Infarction

Goldman et al.[205] 1975-1976		Eerola et al.[185] 1970-1974		Schoeppel et al.[206] 1980		Rao et al.[89] 1973-1976		Rao et al.[89] 1976-1982	
(Reinf.)	(Mort.)	(Reinf.)	(Mort.)	(Reinf.)	(Mort.)	(Reinf.)	(Mort.)	(Reinf.)	(Mort.)
4.5% 1/22	23% 5/22	8% 1/12	8% 1/12	0% 0/1	0% 0/1	30% 4/11	*	5.8% 3/52	*
0% 0/13	5.9% 1/12	5.9% 1/17	0% 0/1	0% 0/8	0% 0/8	26% 8/31	*	2.3% 2/36	*
	8% 1/13					5% 6/127	*	1.0% 1/104	*
		4.9% 4/82	12% 1/82	0% 0/10	0% 0/10	5% 6/114	*	1.6% 4/256	*
3.3% 2/66	3.3% 2/66			0% 0/26	0% 0/26	5% 4/81	*	1.7% 4/235	*
	8.9% 9/109			5.7% 3/53	3.8% 2/53	7.7% 28/364	4.1% 15/364	1.9% 14/733	0.7% 5/733

treadmill testing predictive of severe multivessel or of left mainstem coronary artery disease include S-T segment depression exceeding 2.5 mm; serious ventricular dysrhythmias at low heart rates, or early (first 3 minutes) onset of ischemic S-T segment depression; and/or prolonged duration of the ischemic S-T segment depression in the posttest recovery period (>8 minutes).[197]

Nonelectrocardiographic responses to treadmill testing that predict severe coronary artery disease include low achieved heart rates (≤120 beats/min), systolic hypotension (a decrease of >10 mm Hg) in the absence of hypovolemia or antihypertensive medications, a rise in diastolic blood pressure to >110 mm Hg, and the inability to exercise beyond 3 minutes. The treadmill test responses predictive of se-

ECG Patterns indicative of Myocardial Ischemia

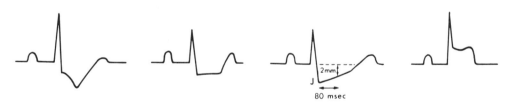

ECG Patterns not indicative of Myocardial Ischemia

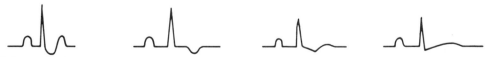

FIG. 9-3 Electrocardiographic criteria for myocardial ischemia consist of at least 1 mm of J point depression with downsloping or horizontal S-T segments; slowly upsloping S-T segment depression, defined as 2 mm of S-T depression measured 80 msec from the J point; and S-T segment elevation. Whereas S-T segment depression indicates nontransmural ischemia, S-T segment elevation often connotes more severe degrees of ischemia reflecting transmural injury. The structure of the S-T segment slope is predictive for the severity of coronary disease shown angiographically, with downsloping S-T depression indicating severe two- and three-vessel coronary artery disease more often than does either horizontal and slowly upsloping S-T depression, and S-T segment elevation indicating high-grade, usually proximal, arterial obstruction in patients without previous myocardial infarction. (Goldschlager N: Use of the treadmill test in the diagnosis of coronary artery disease in patients with chest pain. Ann Intern Med 97:383, 1982.)

TABLE 9-8. Treadmill Test Responses Predictive of Severe Multivessel and/or Left Main Coronary Artery Disease

Electrocardiographic responses
  S-T segment response
    Downsloping
    Elevation
  S-T segment depression exceeding 2.5 mm
  Serious ventricular dysrhythmias occurring at low heart rates (120 to 130 beats/min)
  Early onset (first 3 minutes) of ischemic S-T segment depression or elevation
  Prolonged duration in the post-test recovery period (≥ 8 minutes) of ischemic S-T segment depression
Nonelectrocardiographic criteria
  Low achieved heart rate (≤ 120 beats/min)
  Hypotension* (≥ 10 mm Hg fall in systolic pressure)
  Rise in diastolic blood pressure (≥ 110 to 120 mm Hg)
  Low achieved rate-pressure product (≤ 15,000)
  Inability to exercise beyond 3 minutes

* In the absence of antihypertensive medications or hypovolemia of any cause.
(Modified from Goldschlager N: Use of the treadmill test in the diagnosis of coronary artery disease in patients with chest pain. Ann Intern Med 97:383, 1982.)

vere multivessel and/or left main coronary artery disease are listed in Table 9-8.

Clearly, however, the response to the test must be interpreted in light of the patient's history, and with knowledge that it is more predictive for men than for women (Table 9-9).[197] Ejection fractions of over 50 percent (and normal left ventricular size on plain chest roentgenogram) predict good perioperative cardiac

TABLE 9-9. Electrocardiographic Response to Treadmill Exercise of Angiographically Demonstrated Coronary Disease

Clinical Characteristics	ECG Criteria Alone		
	Prevalence of Coronary Artery Disease (%)	Predictive Accuracy of a Positive Test (%)	Predictive Accuracy of a Negative Test (%)
Asymptomatic	5	10–20	95–100
Noncardiac chest pain	10–25	45–50	80–85
Cardiac chest pain			
Atypical, or probable angina	50–70	80–85	65–70
Typical, or definite, angina	85–95	95–100	50–55

(Modified from Goldschlager N: Use of the treadmill test in the diagnosis of coronary artery disease in patients with chest pain. Ann Intern Med 97:383, 1982.)

function and survival.[213,216] Studies of visual interpretation of the coronary angiogram suggest that the physiologic effects of most coronary artery obstructions cannot be determined accurately by conventional angiographic approaches.[217] Thus, the major signposts of perioperative myocardial function we can obtain before surgery are the history of ischemic pain and its relationship to exercise, and a history of congestive heart failure. The usefulness of this information is enhanced slightly by ECG and non-ECG responses to treadmill exercise, determination of the ejection fraction, and use of an echocardiogram, nuclear imaging, or angiogram.[197,213–217]

RELATIONSHIP TO PREVIOUS CORONARY ARTERY BYPASS GRAFTING

Much of the information upon which altered perioperative anesthetic management for ischemic heart disease is based derives from studies of patients undergoing aortic to coronary artery bypass grafting (CABG) procedures. Although CABG relieves angina and increases exercise tolerance (as did many placebo operations and medications before it),[218] improved survival occurs only for patients having significant left main coronary artery disease[213,219,220] and for those with mild-to-moderate impairment of left ventricular function.[217,221,222] However, a potential additional benefit of CABG surgery has been suggested. Reduced perioperative morbidity during subsequent noncardiac surgical procedures may be an additional benefit of having survived CABG surgery.[190,212,222–225] To provide definitive data for this hypothesis, a randomized, controlled study would be necessary: CABG surgery may constitute a "survival test." That is, CABG surgery may cause reinfarction and/or death in those patients who would have had an MI or who would have died after the noncardiac surgery.[212] This appears to be a likely conclusion, since those patients who do poorly during and after CABG surgery are those with poor left ventricular function and increased left ventricular end-diastolic pressure.[226] Patients with these same cardiovascular conditions also have increased perioperative risk after noncardiac surgery.[190,205,213] Therefore, one proposal to decrease perioperative risk in patients severely disabled with angina (or ischemic heart disease) is to study the coronary arteries and to perform CABG surgery, if the latter is indicated, prior to their noncardiac surgery. Hertzer et al.[190] did just this. Knowing that survival after vascular surgery depends mainly on preserving myocardial function,[227] Hertzer et al. obtained coronary angiograms from, and proposed CABG surgery, when appropriate, to 1,000 consecutive patients needing peripheral vascular surgery (regardless of the degree of suspicion of coronary artery disease prior to angiogram). CABG was believed to be indicated in 251 patients, of whom 226 underwent CABG with 12 (5.13 percent) operative deaths and 130 of whom subsequently underwent peripheral vascular procedures with only one death. Do these figures imply that mortality was decreased or increased by the CABG procedure? Did some patients not undergo their initially indicated vascular procedure because of morbidity associated with CABG? (Why 26 patients who initially were scheduled for peripheral vascular procedures did not have them after their CABG procedure is not revealed in the report.) Thus, the hypothesis that previous CABG surgery decreases the morbidity and mortality in patients undergoing subsequent noncardiac surgery remains just a hypothesis. As stated earlier, this hypothesis deserves to be studied in a randomized clinical trial.

SUMMARY OF PREOPERATIVE AND INTRAOPERATIVE FACTORS THAT CORRELATE WITH PERIOPERATIVE MORBIDITY

To summarize a large number of studies, preoperative findings that correlate with perioperative morbidity and that can be corrected prior to operation are as follows: (1) recent MI (within 6 months),[89,185,199-207] (2) severe CHF (i.e., severe enough to produce rales, an S_3 gallop, or distention of the jugular vein),[89,203,205,213,226] (3) severe angina (see Table 9-10 for classification of severity of angina),[205,213,228] (4) heart rhythm other than sinus,[203,205] (5) premature atrial contractions,[205] (6) more than five premature ventricular con-

TABLE 9-10. New York Heart Association's Classification of Angina

I. *Ordinary physical activity does not cause angina,* such as walking or climbing stairs. Angina with strenuous or rapid prolonged exertion at work or recreation or with sexual relations.

II. *Slight limitation of ordinary activity.* Walking or climbing stairs rapidly, walking uphill, walking or stair climbing after meals, or in cold, or in wind, or under emotional stress, or only during a few hours after awakening. Walking more than two blocks on the level or more than one flight of stairs at a normal pace and in normal conditions.

III. *Marked limitation of ordinary physical activity.* Walking one or two blocks on the level and climbing one flight of stairs in normal conditions and at a normal pace. "Comfortable at rest."

IV. *Inability to carry on any physical activity without discomfort — anginal syndrome may be present at rest.*

tractions per minute,[203,205] and (7) blood urea nitrogen levels higher than 50 mg percent, or potassium levels lower than 3.0 mEq/L.[205]

Preoperative factors that correlate with perioperative risk but that cannot be altered include (1) old age (perioperative risk increases with age),[179-182,205,229-233] (2) significant aortic stenosis,[205] (3) emergency operation,[89,179,199,205,213,232] (4) cardiomegaly,[205,213,216,234] (5) history of CHF,[89,203,205,213] (6) angina (or a history of angina or ischemia) on ECG,[89,197,203,205,213] (7) abnormal S-T segment or inverted or flat T waves on ECG,[205] an abnormal QRS complex on ECG,[205] and (8) significant mitral regurgitant murmur.[205]

Significant introperative factors that may be avoided or altered that correlate with perioperative risk are as follows: (1) unnecessary use of vasopressors,[235] (2) unintentional hypotension[89,186,205,206] (this point is controversial, however, as some investigators have found that unintentional hypotension does not correlate with perioperative morbidity[229,233]), (3) a high rate–pressure product (i.e., if the product of heart rate times systolic blood pressure exceeds 11,000),[236] and (4) long operations.[89,199,204,205,232]

Significant intraoperative factors that correlate with perioperative morbidity and probably cannot be avoided are (1) emergency surgery and (2) thoracic or intraperitoneal surgery, or above-the-knee amputations.[203-205,213,230,231]

Although the evidence for the factors provided above is fairly substantial, virtually none of the data derives from prospective randomized studies indicating that treatment of the above conditions reduces the perioperative risk to patients with ischemic heart disease. Nevertheless, all logic dictates that such treatment does reduce risk. Thus, the goal in giving anesthesia to patients with ischemic heart disease is to have the patient in the best preoperative condition obtainable, by treating those conditions that correlate with perioperative risk. Then one monitors intraoperatively for conditions that correlate with perioperative risk and, by that monitoring and attentiveness to detail, avoids those circumstances that lead to perioperative risk. Although local anesthesia may reduce perioperative risk,[181,203,209] epidemiologic studies do not reveal significant differences in perioperative morbidity for patients with ischemic heart disease who are given local anesthesia as opposed to general anesthesia.

PREOPERATIVE EVALUATION

Preoperative evaluation of the patient with ischemic heart disease should include a review of the clinical course of any previous myocardial infarctions and a review of studies done subsequent to those events. Since the patients most likely to benefit are those who have severe coronary artery disease (i.e., multivessel left mainstem coronary artery disease) and ejection fractions of 21 to 50 percent,[236,237] some strategies have been devised to limit routine exercise and angiographic testing to only such patients (Figs. 9-4 and 9-5).[236,237] Thus, the fact that these studies have been, or are being, performed implies something about the patient's cardiac function.

The preoperative evaluation should also include a review of exercise studies and coronary angiogram, in order to determine which ECG lead to monitor for ischemia. Although, in theory, the ECG lead that first reveals ischemia or best represents the stenosed artery on exercise should be the first to reveal ischemia in the operating room, no study has confirmed this assumption. If no exercise or coronary angiographic study has been performed, precordial lead V_5 is preferred.[238,239]

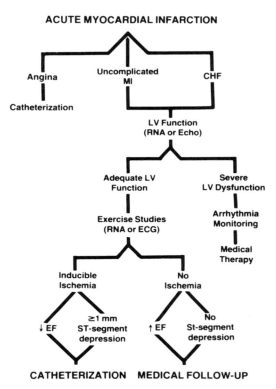

ACUTE MYOCARDIAL INFARCTION

FIG. 9-4 Strategy for identifying patients who should undergo cardiac catheterization after acute myocardial infarction. This strategy is based on clinical assessment, evaluation of left ventricular (LV) function by radionuclide angiography (RNA) or echocardiography, analysis of arrhythmias, and stress testing. MI = acute myocardial infarction; CHF = overt congestive heart failure; EF = ejection fraction. (Epstein SE, Palmeri ST, Patterson SE: Evaluation of patients after acute myocardial infarction. Indications for cardiac catheterization and surgical intervention. N Engl J Med 307:1487, 1982.)

Currently, the only known way to increase oxygen supply to the myocardium of patients with coronary artery stenosis is to maintain diastolic blood pressure, hemoglobin concentration, and oxygen saturation. Therefore, the main goal of anesthesia practice for such patients has been to decrease the determinants of myocardial oxygen demand[1]: heart rate, ventricular wall tension, and contractile performance.[240] Thus, medical management to accomplish the goal of preserving all viable myocardial tissue may include administration of β-adrenergic receptor blocking drugs (propranolol or metoprolol) to decrease contractility and heart rate, and vasodilation [with nitroglycerin

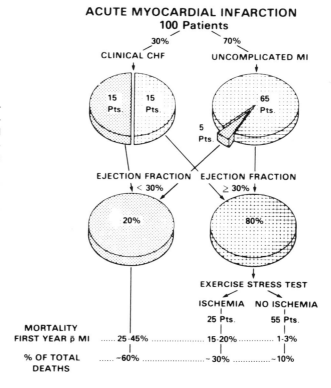

ACUTE MYOCARDIAL INFARCTION
100 Patients

FIG. 9-5 First-year mortality rates for patients with acute myocardial infarction, according to subgroup. MI = acute myocardial infarction; CHF = overt congestive heart failure. Hatched areas represent patients with ejection fractions of more than 30 percent; stipled areas represent patients with ejection fractions of less than 30 percent. (The percentages are, by necessity, rough approximations.) (Epstein SE, Palmeri ST, Patterson SE: Evaluation of patients after acute myocardial infarction. Indications for cardiac catheterization and surgical intervention. N Engl J Med 307:1487, 1982.)

(or its "long-acting" analogues), nitroprusside, hydralazine, or prazosin] to decrease ventricular wall tension. The goal of anesthesia management should be the same, although no prospective controlled studies have documented a decrease in perioperative morbidity by reducing preload or afterload or by decreasing heart rate. However, the goal of keeping cardiovascular variables within an acceptable range and the rate–pressure product below the threshold for angina appears appropriate.[89,227,241,242] The use of Swan-Ganz catheters for this type of patient is described in Chapter 13, and the intraoperative management of ischemic heart disease patients is discussed in further detail in Chapter 41.

Briefly, I believe drugs given chronically (e.g., antihypertensive medications) should be continued through the morning of surgery. The topic of chronic drug therapy is discussed in more detail in the last section of this chapter. Finally, a patient with a subendocardial MI has been assumed to be at less perioperative risk than a patient with a transmural MI. This assumption is now being questioned in medical

circles.[243] Thus, patients with a subendocardial MI should be treated no differently than those with a transmural MI.

VALVULAR HEART DISEASE

Major alterations in the preoperative management of patients with valvular heart disease have been made regarding the use of anticoagulant therapy and based on the causes of disease. Although preoperative and intraoperative management of patients with valvular heart disease are discussed in Chapter 41, a few important points concerning preoperative care are emphasized here. Of prime importance is realizing that stenotic lesions are managed in a fashion exactly opposite that for regurgitant lesions. Therefore, the type of lesion that exists should be determined preoperatively. Although the causes of various forms of valvular heart disease have not changed, the relative frequency has. Rheumatic valvulitis is much less common today than in the 1970s, and syphilitic aortitis has all but disappeared. Now common are congenital bicuspid aortic stenosis, mitral valve prolapse, hypertrophic cardiomyopathy (also called asymmetric septal hypertrophy or subvalvular aortic stenosis), and mitral valve insufficiency due to calcification.

The prognosis and, presumably, the perioperative risk for patients with valvular heart disease depend on the stage of the disease. Although stenotic lesions progress faster than regurgitant lesions, regurgitant lesions secondary to infective endocarditis, rupture of chordae tendineae, or ischemic heart disease can be rapidly fatal. Left ventricular dysfunction is common in the late stage of valvular heart disease.

Preoperative maintenance of drug therapy can be crucial: the patient with aortic stenosis can deteriorate rapidly with the onset of atrial fibrillation or flutter, as the atrial component to left ventricular filling can be critical in maintaining cardiac output. One of the most serious complications of valvular heart surgery and of valvular heart disease prior to surgery are cardiac dysrhythmias. Conduction disorders and chronic therapy with antidysrhythmic and inotropic drugs are discussed elsewhere in this chapter.

MITRAL VALVE PROLAPSE

Mitral valve prolapse, perhaps the most frequent valvular abnormality, occurs in about 6 percent of otherwise healthy people. It is associated with atrioseptal secundum defects,[244-246] thoracic skeletal abnormality (due to time of development of these structures), and, for unknown reasons, migraine anxiety neurosis, and autonomic dysfunction. Hereditary transmission has been proposed as occurring through autosomal dominance with reduced expressivity in humans. Mitral valve prolapse is also associated with Von Willebrand's syndrome, and the presence of one condition requires a search (by at least history and physical examination) for the other. This valvular lesion presents either asymptomatically or with palpitations, dyspnea, atypical chest pain, dizziness, syncope, or sudden death. Supraventricular dysrhythmias (associated with atrioventricular bypass tracts and the preexcitation syndrome) occur in over 50 percent of patients with mitral valve prolapse. Ventricular dysrhythmias (usually in surgery) occur in 45 percent of such patients, bradydysrhythmias in 25 percent, and sudden death in 1.4 percent.[245-248] The frequent occurrence of transient cerebral ischemia has resulted in the chronic use of anticoagulants in patients with mitral valve prolapse, and the potential for endocarditis has led to the recommendation for prophylaxis with antibiotics prior to known bacteremic events.[245-248]

PREOPERATIVE ANTIBIOTIC PROPHYLAXIS FOR ENDOCARDITIS

Patients who have any form of valvular heart disease, as well as those with intracardiac (ventricular septal or atrial septal defects) or intravascular shunt, should be protected against endocarditis at the time of known bacteremic event. Endocarditis has occurred in a sufficiently significant number of patients with cardiomyopathy (subvalvular aortic stenosis, asymmetric septal hypertrophy) and mitral valve prolapse to warrant including such patients in the prophylaxis regimen.

Is endotracheal intubation a bacteremic event? Bacteremia occurs after the following events at these rates: dental extraction, 30 to 80 percent; brushing of teeth, 20 to 24 percent; use of oral irrigation devices, 20 to 24 percent; barium enema, 11 percent; transurethral prostate resection, 10 to 57 percent; upper gastrointestinal endoscopy, 8 percent; nasotracheal intubation, 16 percent (4 of 25 patients); and orotracheal intubation, 0 percent (0 of 25 patients).[249,250] Thus, although bacteremia from orotracheal intubation is rare, I believe that, for patients with valvular heart disease, prophylaxis should be given before instrumentation of the gallbladder, GI tract, oropharynx, or genitourinary tract. The choice of antibiotic for prophylaxis should be aimed at the most commonly occurring (i.e., most numerous) pathogen. Guidelines of the American Heart Association state that all antimicrobial prophylaxis should be started 30 minutes to 1 hour, rather than 24 hours, before a known bacteremic event, so as to reach therapeutic levels without superinfecting the patient with unusual pathogens.[251]

CARDIAC VALVE PROSTHESES AND ANTICOAGULANT THERAPY

Prothrombin time should be within 20 percent of control at the time of operation, or an appreciable risk is incurred.[252] Therefore, to produce a normal prothrombin time on the day of surgery, chronic anticoagulant therapy should be suspended in surgical patients having cardiac valve prostheses. This can be done with safety several days before surgery if the prosthesis is an aortic valve. However, because the risk of thromboembolism is greater with mitral valve prostheses (5 percent) than with aortic valve prostheses (1 to 3 percent), patients having mitral valve prostheses should have rapid reversal of oral anticoagulation with vitamin K the day before surgery. For resumption of anticoagulant therapy after surgery, rapid anticoagulation with heparin 12 hours postoperatively has proved successful in patients with mitral valve prostheses.[253,254] In patients with new aortic valve prostheses, resumption of an-

ticoagulant therapy should start 2 days after surgery. Regional anesthetic techniques probably should be avoided.[255-257]

Another problem that can arise is managing the pregnant patient with a prosthetic valve during delivery. It is recommended that warfarin be replaced by subcutaneous heparin during the peripartum period. During labor and delivery, elective induction is advocated with discontinuance of all anticoagulant therapy, as indicated for the particular valve prosthesis (discussed above).[258]

Auscultation of the prosthetic valve should be performed preoperatively to verify normal functioning (Fig. 9-6).[259] Abnormalities in such sounds warrant preoperative consultation and verification of functioning.

CARDIAC CONDUCTION DISTURBANCES

CARDIAC DYSRHYTHMIAS (Also See Chs. 14 & 15)

Bradydysrhythmias, especially if profound or associated with dizziness or syncope, are generally managed with pacemakers. How-

Prosthesis type	Mitral Prosthesis	Acoustic Characteristics	Aortic Prosthesis	Acoustic Characteristics
Ball Valves	SEM (MC, S₂, MO)	1) A₂–MO interval 0.07–0.11 sec. 2) MO > MC 3) II–III/VI Systolic ejection murmur (SEM) 4) No diastolic murmur	(S₁, S₂, AO, AC)	1) S₁–AO interval 0.07 sec. 2) AO > AC 3) II/VI harsh SEM 4) No diastolic murmur
Disc Valves	SEM, DM (MC, S₂)	1) A₂–MO interval 0.05–0.09 sec. 2) MO is rarely heard 3) II/VI SEM is usually heard 4) I–II/VI diastolic rumble is usually heard	SEM (S₁, P₂, AC)	1) S₁–AO interval 0.04 sec. 2) AO is uncommonly heard, AC is usually heard 3) II/VI SEM is usually heard 4) Occasional diastolic murmur
Porcine Valves	SEM, DM (MC, S₂, MO)	1) A₂–MO interval 0.1 sec. 2) MO is audible 50% 3) I–II/VI apical SEM 50% 4) Diastolic rumble 1/2–2/3	SEM (S₁, P₂, AC)	1) S₁–AO interval 0.03–0.08 sec. 2) AO is uncommonly heard, AC is usually heard 3) II/VI SEM in most 4) No diastolic murmur
Bileaflet Valve (St. Jude)			SEM (S₁, P₂, AO, AC)	1) AO and AC commonly heard 2) A soft SEM is common

FIG. 9-6 Summary of the normal acoustic characteristics of valve prostheses according to type and location. SEM = systolic ejection murmur; DM = diastolic murmur; S_1 = first heart sound; S_2 = second heart sound; P_2 = pulmonary second sound; A_2 = aortic second sound; AO = aortic valve opening sound; AC = aortic valve closure sound; MO = mitral valve opening sound; MC = mitral valve closure sound. (Smith ND, Raizada V, Abrams J: Auscultation of the normally functioning prosthetic valve. Ann Intern Med 95:594, 1981.)

ever, on rare occasion, chronic bifascicular block (right bundle branch block with left anterior or posterior hemiblock, or left bundle branch block with combined left anterior and posterior hemiblocks) even when only first-degree heart block is present, progresses to complete heart block and sudden death perioperatively. But this is a rare occurrence. In five studies, fewer than 2 percent of the approximately 160 patients with bifascicular block progressed to complete heart block perioperatively.[260-264] On the other hand, such patients have a high 5-year mortality (160 of 554 patients, or 35 percent).[265] Most of the deaths were related to tachydysrhythmias or MI—events usually not preventable by pacemakers. Thus, the presence of bifascicular block on ECG should make the anesthesiologist more worried about associated coronary artery disease or left ventricular dysfunction. Nevertheless, these patients rarely have complete heart block perioperatively. Therefore, prophylactic preoperative insertion of temporary pacing wires for bifascicular block does not seem warranted. However, a central route should be established in advance in the event a temporary pacemaker needs to be inserted. The actual pacemaker equipment and appropriate personnel should be immediately available, since symptomatic heart block does occur perioperatively in more than 1 percent of patients.[260-264]

Premature ventricular contractions (PVCs) of more than 5 per minute on preoperative examination correlate with perioperative cardiac morbidity.[205,213] To the classic criteria for treating PVCs (the presence of R-on-T couplets, the occurrence of more than three PVCs per minute, multifocality of PVCs) must be added frequent (>10/hour over a 24-hour period) and repetitive ventricular beats. Electrophysiologic and programmed ventricular stimulation studies are being used to indicate and guide treatment for patients with ischemic heart disease or recurrent dysrhythmias and for survivors of sudden out-of-hospital sudden death.[266-269] Although such patients are often treated with antidysrhythmic therapy, attention to their underlying condition should be a focus of our preoperative management. Chronic antidysrhythmic therapy is discussed in the last section of this chapter.

Premature atrial contractions and cardiac rhythm other than sinus also correlate with perioperative cardiac morbidity.[205] These dysrhythmias may be more a marker of poor cardiovascular reserve than a specific cause of perioperative cardiac complications.

Preexcitation syndrome is the name for supraventricular tachycardias associated with atrioventricular bypass tracts.[270] Successful treatment, which is predicated on an understanding of the clinical and electrophysiologic manifestations of the syndrome, consists of preoperative and intraoperative techniques that avoid release of sympathetic substances and other vasoactive substances, and hence tachydysrhythmias.[270,271]

PACEMAKERS

The types of pacemakers and indications for their use have changed significantly since 1980. More than 90 percent of pacemakers are inserted for bradydysrhythmias, either after tachycardia (brady–tachy syndrome) or by themselves, that is, sick sinus syndrome or atrioventricular conduction disorders. The most common pacemaker for such dysfunction is the ventricular R-wave inhibited (demand) type (VVI) (letter codes are described later and in Table 9-11). More complex pacemakers are

TABLE 9-11. Traditional Five-Letter Code for Pacemaker Systems

1st Letter Chamber Paced	2nd Letter Chamber Sensed	3rd Letter Mode of Response	4th Letter Programmable Features	5th Letter Dysrhythmia Treatment
A = Atrium	A = Atrium	T = Triggered	P = Programmable	B = Burst
V = Ventricle	V = Ventricle	I = Inhibited	M = Multiprogrammable	N = Normal
D = Double	D = Double	D = Double	O = Not programmable	S = Scanning
	0 = None	0 = Not applicable		E = External

now being employed to provide better cardiac output in stressful situations and to decrease myocardial wall stress[272] or to treat ventricular tachydysrhythmias. Lithium batteries now allow a pacemaker to have a 5- to 10-year life span. Programmable pacemakers are adjustable for sensitivity and rate. Atrial pacemakers fired by an outside radiofrequency source now allow termination of reentrant or preexcitation atrial dysrhythmias; similarly, ventricular pacemakers can be used to terminate supraventricular tachycardia and recurrent ventricular tachycardia.[273] Thus, in addition to learning about the patient's underlying disease, current condition, and drug therapy, the anesthesiologist must learn, preoperatively, the following information about any implanted pacemaker[273-275]:

1. The indication for placement of the pacemaker and the default rhythm (i.e., what rhythm is activated if the pacemaker does not capture).
2. The type of pacemaker (demand, fixed, or radiofrequency), the chamber paced, and the chamber sensed. Pacemakers have traditionally been given a five-letter code (Table 9-11). (However, most pacemakers implanted since 1980 have codes consisting of only the first three letters. The *first letter* indicates the chamber paced, i.e., V = ventricle, A = atrium, D = double or both. The *second letter* indicates the chamber sensed, i.e., V = ventricle, A = atrium, O = none. The *third letter* indicates the sensing pattern, i.e., 0 = no sensing, fixed mode; I = inhibited, demand pacer; T = triggered, meaning that the sensing of an electrical impulse triggers a pacemaker spike. For example, a VOO pacemaker paces the ventricle, does not sense, and is in a fixed mode. In other words, it is a fixed-rate ventricular pacemaker. A VVI pacemaker paces the ventricle, senses the ventricle, and is inhibited. It is a ventricular-inhibited demand pacemaker. A DVI pacemaker paces both atrium and ventricle, senses only the ventricle, and is inhibited. Thus, it is a sequential atrioventricular demand pacemaker that fires when it does not sense intrinsic ventricular activity.)

3. How to detect deterioration in battery function (increased rate or decreased rate)
4. How to change the mode or to fire the pacemaker if it is of the radiofrequency type. (These procedures should not only be learned by the anesthesiologist, but also demonstrated to him or her. Also, the magnet and/or programming device must be in the operating room at the time of surgery.)
5. The current rate and sensitivity settings of the pacemaker.
6. If the pacemaker is currently functioning and how well.

Because demand pacemakers can sense electrocautery, which sometimes inhibits pacemaker firing, asystole can occur in the pacemaker-dependent patient. Most pacemakers can be converted to a fixed rate, and the anesthesiologist should do the following: (1) have the cardiologist demonstrate how this is done, and (2) have the necessary magnet and/or programming device available in the operating room. In addition, the ground plate should be as far from the pulse generator and lead as possible, a bipolar form of electrocautery should be used, and, if possible, some measure of blood flow should be monitored, that is, Doppler detector or intraarterial line. The rationale for the latter measure is that electrocautery temporarily affects the accuracy of electrocardiographic results; since asystole could occur during this period, a measure of blood flow is necessary. Currently, at least 12 manufacturers produce a total of more than 50 types of pacemakers, each having a different default program. A default program is the secondary program (i.e., the generator circuit) to which the primary program will revert if it senses problems in the initial circuit. Since default programs differ, pacemaker malfunction will present differently depending on the brand and model. Thus, it is necessary to learn before surgery how problems will manifest with each pacemaker during surgery.[275]

The most common cause of temporary pacemaker malfunction is lack of contact between the electrode wire and the endocardium. Pacemaker spikes continue to exist on the ECG oscilloscope even when no myocardial contractions propel blood. This situation has occurred with muscular exertion, blunt trauma, cardioversion, and positive-pressure ventilation.[276] Treatment consists of advancing the electrode until it captures, administering isoproterenol (if that worked in the past), external pacing, or, failing that, cardiopulmonary resuscitation.

During the preoperative examination, the anesthesiologist must also assess the progression of underlying disease (e.g., CHF, electrolyte disorders, and the condition of all systems related to the underlying disease.[274]

DISORDERS OF THE RESPIRATORY AND IMMUNE SYSTEMS

GENERAL PREOPERATIVE CONSIDERATIONS

The main purpose of preoperative testing is to identify patients at risk of perioperative complications and to institute appropriate perioperative therapy. Also, preoperative assessment should establish baseline function and the feasibility of surgical intervention. Whereas numerous investigators have used pulmonary function tests that define inoperability or high-vs-low-risk groups for pulmonary complications, few have been able to demonstrate that the performance of any specific preoperative or intraoperative measure reliably decreases perioperative pulmonary morbidity or mortality. Since routine preoperative pulmonary testing and care are discussed extensively in Chapters 59 and 64, the current discussion limits itself to assessing the effectiveness of such care.

In fact, only two randomized prospective studies indicate a benefit of preoperative preparation. Stein and Cassara[277] randomly allocated 48 patients to undergo preoperative therapy (cessation of smoking; use of antibiotic treatment for purulent sputum; and use of bronchodilating drugs, postural drainage, chest physiotherapy, and ultrasonic nebulizer) or no preoperative therapy. The no-treatment group

had mortality of 16 percent and morbidity of 60 percent, as opposed to the 0 to 20 percent rates, respectively, for the treatment group. In addition, the treatment group spent an average of 12 postoperative days in the hospital, compared with 24 days for the 21 survivors in the no-treatment group.

Collins et al.[278] prospectively examined the benefits of preoperative antibiotics, perioperative chest physiotherapy and therapy with bronchodilating drugs, and routine postoperative analgesia (morphine) on postoperative respiratory complications in patients with chronic obstructive pulmonary disease (COPD). Of those therapies, only preoperative treatment with antibiotics had a beneficial effect.

Bartlett et al.[279] randomly assigned 150 patients undergoing extensive laparotomy to one of two groups. One group received preoperative instruction in, and postoperative use (10 times/hr) of, incentive spirometry. The other group received similar medical care but no incentive spirometry. Only 7 of 75 patients using incentive spirometry had postoperative pulmonary complications, as opposed to 19 of 75 in the control group. However, other investigators have not shown a benefit for specific treatments, or have been too contaminated with bias to have a clear result emerge. Lyager et al.[280] randomly assigned 103 patients undergoing biliary or gastric surgery to receive either incentive spirometry with preoperative and postoperative chest physiotherapy, or only preoperative and postoperative chest physiotherapy. No difference in postoperative course or pulmonary complications was found between the two groups. Other studies have shown a specific benefit (i.e., above that provided by routine care) for chest physiotherapy and intermittent positive-pressure breathing (IPPB). These studies are usually poorly controlled, not randomized, and/or retrospective in design; these deficiencies probably substantially bias the results.[281-283] Although randomized prospective studies showed no benefit or actual harm from chest physiotherapy and IPPB on the resolution of pneumonia[284,285] or postoperative pulmonary complications,[278,283,285-287] the three studies cited above[277-279] and numerous retrospective studies[281-283] strongly suggest that preoperative evaluation and treatment of patients with pulmonary disease actually decrease perioperative respiratory complications.

TABLE 9-12. Grade of Dyspnea Caused by Respiratory Problems (Assessed in Terms of Walking on the Level at a Normal Pace)

Category	Description
0	No dyspnea while walking on the level at a normal pace
I	"I am able to walk as far as I like provided I take my time"
II	Specific (street) block limitation ("I have to stop for awhile after one or two blocks")
III	Dyspnea on mild exertion ("I have to stop and rest while going from the kitchen to the bathroom")
IV	Dyspnea at rest

(Modified from Boushy SF, Billing DM, North LB, et al: Clinical course related to preoperative pulmonary function in patients with bronchogenic carcinoma. Chest 59:383, 1971.)

The evaluation of dyspnea is especially useful and so warrants discussion here (for a review of the specific pulmonary function tests that identify high-risk groups, see Ch. 59). Boushy et al.[288] found that grades of preoperative dyspnea correlated with postoperative survival. (The grades of respiratory dyspnea are provided in Table 9-12.) Mittman[289] demonstrated an increased risk of death after thoracic surgery from 8 percent in patients without dyspnea to 56 percent in patients who were dyspneic. Similarly, Reichel[290] found that no patients died after pneumonectomy if they were able to complete a preoperative treadmill test for 4 minutes at the rate of 2 mph on level ground. Other studies have found that history and physical examination of the asthmatic subject can also predict the need for hospitalization.[291] Other than dyspnea, what preoperative conditions make postoperative respiratory complications more likely to occur? (also see Ch. 64). The important information and conditions to search for during the history-taking and physical examination are as follows:

1. Dyspnea.
2. Coughing and production of sputum. Sputum, if present, should be Gram stained and cultured, and appropriate antibiotic treatment should be instituted.
3. Recent respiratory infection. Viral respiratory infections affect respiratory function, giving rise to increased airflow obstruction that may persist for as long as 5 weeks.[292,293]

These infections also adversely affect respiratory mechanisms responding to bacteria. However, whether the incidence of complications in normal children is lessened by waiting 5 weeks until the symptoms of respiratory infections have disappeared is open to question.[294]

4. Hemoptysis.
5. Wheezing and prior use of bronchodilating drugs and corticosteroids. Wheezing often suggests potentially reversible airway obstruction but is a notoriously poor indicator of the degree of obstruction. Asthmatics have a fourfold increase in perioperative respiratory complications.
6. Pulmonary complications from previous surgery. Prolonged endotracheal intubation after surgery can be required by many conditions, most probably respiratory and neuromuscular disorders.
7. A history of smoking. The incidence of respiratory complications is higher among tobacco smokers than among nonsmokers.[281,282,295]
8. Age, general history of the patient, and any other significant physical findings. Although other disease conditions probably increase respiratory risk, this hypothesis has not been adequately documented. Old age definitely increases respiratory and cardiac risk.[288,295,296] Cardiovascular history and examinations are obviously important for risk by themselves and especially for signs of pulmonary hypertension, such as right ventricular lift (i.e., lift over the lower sternum), fixed and widely split second heart sound, and S_4 gallop at the left sternal border.
9. Breathing frequency and form. Pursed lips, cyanosis, and use of accessory muscles should be noted.
10. Body habitus:
    a. Abnormalities of the chest wall, trauma, kyphoscoliosis with restrictive lung disease. Development of a barrel chest is a late manifestation of obstructive lung disease.
    b. Obesity. A weight of 30 percent over ideal weight doubles the incidence of respiratory complications.[284,295,297]
11. Adequacy of upper airway, presence of tracheal deviation, ease of face mask application, ease of endotracheal intubation.

12. Presence of rales, rhonchi, wheezing, diaphragmatic excursion, air movement, and rates of expiratory to inspiratory times.
13. Site of proposed surgery. Upper abdominal surgery increases the incidence of perioperative pulmonary complications.[277,282]

Chapters 8 and 59 review the value of the chest roentgenograms and pulmonary function tests in identifying patients with preoperative pulmonary disease as well as which tests should be ordered and for whom. Any patient who will require postoperative ventilatory support should undergo preoperative testing— I conduct such tests on any patient with dyspnea of grade II or higher or on any patient who shows significant abnormalities or risk on the 13 factors listed above.

Despite the lack of definitive data establishing the efficacy of preoperative pulmonary testing and therapy, I recommend the following approach:

1. Eradicate acute infections and suppress chronic infections by using appropriate diagnostic measures and antibiotic treatment.
2. Relieve bronchospasm by using bronchodilating drugs and document such relief with measurements of forced expiratory volume at one second (also see Chs. 59 & 64).
3. Institute measures to improve sputum clearance and to familiarize the patient with respiratory therapy equipment (incentive spirometry) and postural drainage maneuvers. Initiate practice coughing and deep-breathing exercises (also see Chs. 59 & 63).
4. Treat uncompensated right ventricular heart failure with digoxin, diuretics, oxygen, and drugs that decrease pulmonary vascular resistance (e.g., hydralazine).
5. Use low-dose heparin prophylactically to decrease the incidence of venous thrombosis (and pulmonary emboli).
6. Encourage reduction or cessation of smoking. Pulmonary function begins to improve in a few weeks after cessation of smoking.[298,299] Cigarette smoking increases the incidence and severity of influenza.[300] Even young people who smoke only $\frac{1}{2}$ to 1 pack of cigarettes per day exhibit abnormalities in respiratory function.[301]

SPECIFIC DISEASES

PULMONARY VASCULAR DISEASES

Pulmonary vascular diseases include pulmonary hypertension secondary to heart disease (postcapillary disorders), parenchymal lung disease (pulmonary precapillary disorders), pulmonary embolism, and cor pulmonale from chronic obstructive pulmonary disease (COLD).[302] Optimal preoperative management of these conditions requires treatment of the underlying disease.[303-306] Because pulmonary embolism can be especially difficult to diagnose, it is crucial to be especially alert to the possibility of this disease. The clinical findings of pulmonary emboli are not always present or specific for the diagnosis. The history may include tachypnea, dyspnea, palpitations, syncope, chest pain, or hemoptysis. Physical examination can reveal a pleural rub, wheezing, rales, a fixed and split second heart sound, right ventricular lift, or evidence of venous thromboses, none of which is present in most patients. If the ECG shows a S1–Q3 pattern, lung perfusion scans can be obtained to rule out the diagnosis of pulmonary emboli. A high degree of suspicion is necessary to warrant angiography and anticoagulation or fibrinolytic therapy. If possible, the reactivity of the pulmonary vasculature should be determined, for it may be enhanced or decreased by such agents as nifedipine, hydralazine, nitroglycerin, prazosin, tolazoline, and phentolamine.[307,308] Monitoring of pulmonary artery pressure is often required; preoperative measures should be undertaken to ensure that the patient is not exposed to conditions that elevate pulmonary vascular resistance (i.e., hypoxia, hypercarbia, acidosis, lung hyperinflation, COLD)[309] or that decrease blood volume (prolonged restriction of fluid intake) or systemic vascular resistance.

INFECTIOUS DISEASES OF THE LUNG

Preoperative evaluation and treatment should follow the basic guidelines outlined in the introduction to this section; treatment of the underlying disease should be completed before all but emergency surgery is performed. To repeat, viral respiratory infections do affect respiratory function, giving rise to increased airflow obstruction (especially in the small airways) that may persist for at least 5 weeks.[292] Viral respiratory infections also adversely affect respiratory defense mechanisms against bacteria.[293] Within 5 weeks of an upper respiratory tract infection, children may have an increased incidence of perioperative respiratory tract complications.[294]

CHRONIC OBSTRUCTIVE PULMONARY DISEASES

Treatment of COPD (reactive airways) may include the use of β-adrenergic drugs, parasympatholytic agents (especially for exercise-induced asthma), and corticosteroids.[310] There is now a trend toward the use of topically applied steroids, such as beclomethasone dipropionate, which are inactivated after absorption. However, in large doses, these "topical" steroids can suppress adrenal function, and supplemental systemic corticosteroids may be needed at times of stress (see the earlier discussion under the section on adrenocortical malfunction). Preoperative assessment must include knowledge of drug regimens and effects, as these drugs can have dangerous interactions with anesthetic agents (see last section of this chapter). An estimated 10 percent of asthmatic patients exhibit sensitivity to aspirin and may react not only to compounds containing aspirin, but also to tartrazine, yellow dye No. 5, indomethacin, and aminopyrine.[311] Chronic obstructive pulmonary disease takes several forms. Bronchial asthma, which occurs in 3 to 5 percent of the population, is characterized by reversible airway obstruction. When airway obstruction is partially reversible (by steroids or adrenergic mediators), it is often accompanied by chronic bronchitis.[312] Some of these drugs may improve aspects of lung function other than bronchial muscle tone.[312] Chronic bronchitis almost always exists if there is a history of chronic cough and production of sputum on most days for 3 months a year for at least 2 years. These patients are (or almost always have been) smokers, although environmental and occupational or genetic predisposition may contribute to hypertrophy of mucous glands in

major airways, to hyperplasia of goblet cells, and to edema and inflammation of the airways. Hyperinflation of airspaces, abnormal dilatation, and destruction of acinar units distal to the terminal bronchiole define emphysema. Cystic fibrosis is characterized by dilatation and hypertrophy of bronchial glands, mucous plugging of peripheral airways, and often bronchitis, bronchiectasis, and bronchiolectasis. For all these conditions, the measures recommended in the introduction to this section, as well as appropriate hydration to allow for mobilization of secretions, should be followed.

INTERSTITIAL AND IMMUNE LUNG DISEASES

Included in this heterogeneous group of diseases are the hypersensitivity lung diseases, environmental exposure diseases, the inorganic dust diseases, radiation-induced lung disease, sarcoidosis, the collagen-vascular disorders (systemic lupus erythematosus, polymyositis, dermatomyositis, Sjögren's syndrome, rheumatoid arthritis, systemic sclerosis), Goodpasture's syndrome, idiopathic pulmonary hemosiderosis, Wegener's granulomatosis, and the autoimmune diseases.[313,314] The gallium-67 scan localizes pulmonary inflammation and has proved an accurate method of assessing autoimmune pulmonary function disturbance as well as the response to steroid therapy.[315] Many of these disorders affect not only the lungs but the blood vessels, the conduction system of the heart, the myocardium, the joints (including those of the upper airway and larynx), and the renal, hepatic, and/or CNS as well. The reader is referred to a textbook of internal medicine to aid in understanding the pathophysiologic processes and full preoperative assessment of these conditions. Therapy for these conditions includes use of antiinflammatory drugs, corticosteroids, and immunosuppressive drugs.

NEOPLASMS

Solitary nodules consist of tumors that are less than 6 cm in diameter, are surrounded by lung parenchyma, and are *not* associated with adenopathy or pleural effusion. The cure rate for bronchogenic carcinoma presenting as a solitary nodule is 70 percent—much better than the "cure" rate for other presentations.[316] (It should be remembered that tuberculosis can mimic cancer so closely that even surgery has been performed.[317]) Blood studies including calcium and alkaline phosphatase levels and liver function studies help confirm that the neoplasm has not disseminated. If these studies and history and physical examination show no abnormal findings, it is unlikely that bone, brain, or hepatic NMR or CT imaging techniques will indicate metastasis. Surgery need not await the results of these tests, as few patients not found to have metastatic disease by simple blood tests, history, and physical examination will prove to have such disease detected by these scans. Oat cell (small cell) carcinoma of the lung and bronchial adenomas are known for their secretion of endocrinologically active substances, such as ACTH-like hormones. Squamous cell cancers in the superior pulmonary sulcus produce Horner's syndrome as well as a characteristic pain in the areas served by the eighth cervical nerves and first and second thoracic nerves. These tumors are now treated with preoperative radiation; surgical resection leads to an almost 30 percent "cure" rate.[181]

ANAPHYLAXIS, ANAPHYLACTOID RESPONSES, AND ALLERGIC DISORDERS OTHER THAN THOSE RELATED TO LUNG DISEASES AND ASTHMA

ANAPHYLACTIC AND ANAPHYLACTOID REACTIONS

Anaphylaxis is a severe life-threatening allergic reaction. The term "allergic" applies to immunologically mediated reactions, as opposed to those caused by pharmacologic idiosyncrasy, by direct toxicity or drug overdosage, or by drug interaction.[318]

Anaphylaxis is the typical immediate hypersensitivity reaction (type 1). Such reactions are produced by the immunoglobulin E (IgE)-mediated release of pharmacologically active substances. These mediators in turn produce specific end-organ responses in the skin (urti-

caria), the respiratory system (bronchospasm and upper airway edema), and the cardiovascular system (vasodilation, changes in inotropy, and increased capillary permeability). Vasodilation occurs at the level of the capillary and postcapillary venule, leading to erythema, edema, and smooth muscle contraction. This clinical syndrome is called anaphylaxis. By contrast, the term anaphylactoid reaction denotes an identical or very similar clinical response that is not mediated by IgE or (usually) an antigen–antibody process.[319]

In anaphylactic reactions, an injected substance can serve as the allergen itself. Low-molecular-weight agents are believed to act as haptens that form immunologic conjugates with host proteins. The offending substance, whether hapten or not, may be the parent compound, a nonenzymatically generated product or a metabolic product formed in the patient. When an allergen binds immunospecific IgE antibodies on the surface of mast cells and basophils, histamine[320] and eosinophilic chemotactic factors of anaphylaxis (ECF-A) are released from the storage granules in a calcium- and energy-dependent process.[321] Other chemical mediators, including slow-reacting substance of anaphylaxis (SRS-A), which is a combination of three leukotrienes, other leukotrienes,[322,323] kinins, and prostaglandins are rapidly synthesized and subsequently released in response to cellular activation.

The end-organ effects of the mediators produce the clinical syndrome of anaphylaxis. In a sensitized individual, the onset of the signs and symptoms caused by these mediators is usually immediate but may be delayed 2 to 15 minutes or, in rare instances, as long as $2\frac{1}{2}$ hours after the parenteral injection of antigen.[324,325] After oral administration, manifestations may occur at unpredictable times.[321]

In addition, there are multiple effector processes by which biologically active mediators can be generated to produce an anaphylactoid reaction. Activation of the blood coagulation and fibrinolytic systems, of the kinin-generating sequence, or of the complement cascade can produce the same inflammatory substances that result in an anaphylactic reaction. The two mechanisms known to activate the complement system are called classical and alternate. The classical pathway can be initiated through IgG or IgM (transfusion reactions), or plasmin.[326] The alternate pathway can be activated by lipopolysaccharides (endotoxin), drugs (Althesin,[319,327] radiographic contrast media[328,329]), membranes (nylon tricot membranes for bubble oxygenators,[330] cellophane membranes of dialyzers[331]), and perfluorocarbon artificial blood.[332] In addition, histamine can be liberated independent of immunologic reactions.[319] Mast cells and basophils release histamine in response to chemicals or drugs. Most narcotics can release histamine,[333,334] producing an anaphylactoid reaction, as can radiographic contrast media,[328,329] *d*-tubocurarine[335] and thiopental.[336] What makes some patients susceptible to histamine release in response to drugs is unknown, but hereditary and environmental factors may play a role.

CHEMONUCLEOLYSIS: CHYMOPAPAIN

Chymopapain, an agent used to treat herniated nucleus pulposus enzymatically, is associated with a 0.35 to 2 percent incidence of anaphylactic and anaphylactoid reactions. Sensitization of some of the general population occurs because chymopapain or close structural relatives are present in papaya, meat tenderizer, some beers, toothpastes, and cosmetics. However, it is not clearly known whether all vasoactive reactions to chymopapain are anaphylactic: chymopapain may have a direct (nonimmunologic) action on mast cells and thus initiate an anaphylactoid reaction. Women are 3 to 10 times more likely to have anaphylactic or anaphylactoid reactions to chymopapain than are men, the incidence being 0.1 to 0.5 percent for men and 0.7 to 1.5 percent for women. Two of the 1,049 men and 11 of the 536 women in the phase III clinical trials of Chymodiactin (chymopapain) experienced serious anaphylactic reactions after administration of chymopapain.[337] These reactions were manifested by bronchospasm in two subjects, severe hypotension in 13, laryngeal edema in 2, and rash or pilomotor changes in 9. Eleven of the 13 survived.

Since release of Chymodiactin by the Food and Drug Administration (FDA) in November 1982, the incidence of anaphylactic reactions has dropped slightly from that in the phase III trials, the incidence now being approximately 0.3 percent in men and 0.8 percent in women for the first 80,000 patients treated (R. McDermott, personal communication). Two of the anaphylactic reactions were fatal. We believe that the successful outcome for most such reactions has come about through vigilance when administering the drug and pretreatment of the patient with antihistamines and hydration.

Data from these studies indicate that chymopapain administered during anesthesia with local anesthetics may have a lower incidence of reported adverse cardiovascular events than when administered with general anesthesia (R. McDermott, and J. Moss, personal communication).[337-342] It is possible, however, that this lower incidence may merely reflect a misinterpretation of the vasodilation produced by general anesthetics as evidence of an adverse reaction to chymopapain — in that event, there would be no real difference between local and general anesthesia. Nevertheless, since patient and surgeon selection of the type of anesthetic used may influence morbidity of chymopapain injection, a randomized trial of general versus local anesthesia is needed before one can dogmatically prescribe local anesthetics and proscribe general anesthesia when this enzyme is being given.

Intravenous contrast material is probably the most frequently used agent causing anaphylactoid reactions. Since diagnostic (skin and other) tests are helpful only in IgE-mediated reactions, pretesting is not useful in contrast reactions. Pretreatment with diphenhydramine, cimetidine (or ranitidine), and corticosteroids has been reported useful in preventing or ameliorating anaphylactoid reactions due to intravenous contrast material,[343-347] and perhaps to narcotics and chymopapain.[336] Unfortunately, very large doses of steroids (1 g of methyl prednisolone intravenously) may be necessary to obtain a beneficial effect.[348,349] The efficacy of large-dose steroid therapy has not been confirmed. Other common substances associated with anaphylactic or anaphylactoid reactions that might merit preoperative therapy include antibiotics, volume expanders, and blood products (Table 9-13).[318,350-353] The anesthesiologist should be prepared preoperatively to treat an anaphylactic or anaphylactoid response.

Sometimes a patient with a history of ana-

TABLE 9-13. Incidence of Anaphylactic or Anaphylactoid Reactions to Some Common Agents

Agent	Incidence
Plasma protein	
Plasma protein derivative	0.019
Human serum albumin	0.011
Dextran 60/75	0.069
Dextran 40	0.007
Starch	
Hydroxyethyl starch	0.085
Penicillin	0.002*
Chymopapain	0.3–1.5

* Fatal reactions.

(Data from the following sources: Ring J, Messmer K: Incidence and severity of anaphylactoid reactions to colloid volume substitutes. Lancet 1:466, 1977. Levy JH, Roizen MF, Morris JM: Anaphylactic and anaphylactoid reactions: A review. Spine, in press. Moss J, McDermott DJ, Thisted RA, et al: Anaphylactic/anaphylactoid reactions in response to Chymodiactin (chymopapain). Anesth Analg 63:253, 1984.

phylactic or anaphylactoid reaction must receive a substance suspected of producing such a reaction (e.g., iodinated contrast material). Also, some patients have a higher than average likelihood of having a reaction. In such instances, pretreatment and therapy for possible anaphylactic and anaphylactoid reactions should be well planned.[318] Although virtually all evidence on these subjects is merely anecdotal, enough consistent thought recurs through the literature to justify proposing an optimal approach to these problems. First, predisposing factors should be sought; the patient with a history of atopy or allergic rhinitis should be suspected as being at risk. Because anaphylactic and anaphylactoid reactions to chymopapain occur 5 to 10 times more frequently in women, and reactions to contrast media occur 5 to 10 times more frequently in patients with a previously suspected reaction, one might consider giving such patients both H_1- and H_2-receptor antagonists for 16 to 24 hours before exposing them to a suspected allergen.[343,346,354] The H_1-receptor antagonist appears to require this much time to act on the receptor.[346] Volume status should be optimized,[318] and perhaps large doses of steroids (2 g of hydrocortisone) should also be administered before exposing them to agents associated with a high incidence of anaphylactic or ana-

phylactoid reactions.[348,349,355,356] Older patients present a special problem: they are more at risk of having complications from both pretreatment (especially vigorous hydration) and therapy for anaphylactic reactions. Perhaps drugs likely to trigger anaphylactic or anaphylactoid reactions should be avoided, or the treatment protocol altered, for this group.

PRIMARY IMMUNODEFICIENCY DISEASES

The primary immunodeficiency diseases usually present early in life with recurrent infections. Along with survival due to antibiotic and antibody treatment have come new prominent features, cancer, and allergic and autoimmune disorders. Heredity angioneurotic edema is an autosomal dominant genetic disease characterized by episodes of angioneurotic edema involving the subcutaneous tissues and submucosa of the GI tract and the airway and often presenting as abdominal pain. These patients have a functionally impotent inhibitor or a deficiency of an inhibitor to the complement component C1. Treatment of an acute attack is supportive because epinephrine, antihistamines, and corticosteroids often fail to work. Plasma transfusions have been reported to resolve attacks or to make them worse (theoretically by supplying either C1 esterase inhibitor or previously depleted complement components). The severity of attacks can be prevented or decreased by drugs that are either plasmin inhibitors (such as ϵ-aminocaproic acid and tranexamic acid) or androgens (such as danazol). Because trauma can precipitate acute attacks, prophylactic therapy with danazol, intravenous ϵ-aminocaproic acid, plasma, or all three, is recommended prior to elective surgery. Reports have also described the successful use of a partially purified C1-esterase inhibitor in two patients.[357,358]

Most of the 1 in 700 persons who have selective IgA deficiency (i.e., <5 mg/dl) have repeated serious infections or connective tissue disorders.[359] The infections commonly involve the respiratory tract (e.g., sinusitis, otitis) or GI tract (presenting as diarrhea and/or malabsorption). If the patient has rheumatoid arthritis, Sjögren's syndrome, or systemic lupus erythematosus, the anesthetist should consider the possibility of isolated IgA deficiency. However, patients with this disorder can be otherwise healthy. Since patients may develop antibodies to IgA if previously exposed to IgA (as might occur from a previous blood transfusion), subsequent blood transfusions can cause anaphylaxis even when they contain washed erythrocytes. Transfusion should therefore consist of blood donated by another IgA-deficient patient.

DISEASES OF THE CNS, NEUROMUSCULAR DISEASES, AND PSYCHIATRIC DISORDERS

Taking the history and performing the physical examination suggested in Chapter 8 should help identify almost all patients with significant neurologic or mental disease. Historical information warranting further investigation includes the previous need for postoperative ventilation in a patient without inordinate lung disease (indicating the possibility of metabolic neurologic disorders such as porphyria, alcoholic myopathy, other myopathies, neuropathies, and neuromuscular disorders such as myasthenia gravis) and the use of drug therapy (steroids; guanidine; anticonvulsant, anticoagulant, and antiplatelet drugs; lithium; tricyclic antidepressant drugs; phenothiazines; butyrophenones). Although preoperative treatment of most neurologic disorders has not been reported to lessen perioperative morbidity, knowledge of the pathophysiologic characteristics of these disorders is important in planning intraoperative and postoperative management. Thus, preoperative knowledge about these disorders and their associated conditions (such as cardiac dysrhythmias with Duchenne muscular dystrophy or respiratory and cardiac muscle weakness in dermatomyositis) may reduce perioperative morbidity. A major

goal of neurologic evaluation is to determine the site of the lesion in the nervous system. Such localization is essential for accurate diagnosis and appropriate management. (Disorders accompanied by increased intracranial pressure and cerebrovascular disorders are discussed in Chs. 43 & 67, respectively.)

COMA

Little is known about anesthesia for the comatose patient but, like all other conditions, it is imperative to know the cause of the coma, so that drugs can be avoided that might worsen the condition or that might not be metabolized because of organ dysfunction. First the patient should be observed. Yawning, swallowing, or licking of the lips implies a "light" coma with major brainstem function intact. If consciousness is depressed but respiration, pupillary reactivity to light, and eye movements are normal and no focal motor signs are present, metabolic depression is likely. Abnormal pupillary responses may indicate hypoxia, hypothermia, local eye disease, or drug intoxication with belladonna alkaloids, narcotics, or glutethemide; pupillary responses may also be abnormal, however, after use of eye drops. Other metabolic causes of coma include uremia, hypoglycemia, hepatic coma, alcohol ingestion, hypophosphatemia, myxedema, and hyperosmolar nonketotic coma. Except in extreme emergencies, such as uncontrolled bleeding or perforated viscus, care should be taken to render the patient as metabolically normal as possible before surgery. This practice lessens any confusion regarding the cause of intraoperative and postoperative problems. However, too rapid correction of uremia or hyperosmolar nonketotic coma can lead to cerebral edema — a shift of water into the brain due to a reverse osmotic effect caused by the dysequilibrium of urea concentration. The physical examination can be extremely helpful preoperatively in assessing the prognosis.[360-362] Arms flexed at the elbow (decorticate posture) imply bilateral hemisphere dysfunction but intact brainstem, whereas extension of legs and arms (bilateral decerebrate posture) implies bilateral damage to structures at the upper brainstem or deep hemisphere level. Seizures are often seen in uremia and in other metabolic encephalopathies. Hyperreflexia and upward-pointing toes suggest a structural CNS lesion or uremia, hypoglycemia, or hepatic coma; hyporeflexia and downward-pointing toes with no hemiplegia generally indicate no structural CNS lesion.

EPILEPTIC SEIZURES

Epileptic seizures result from paroxysmal neuronal discharges of abnormally excitable neurons. Seizures can be generalized (arising from deep midline structures in the brainstem or thalamus, usually without aura or focal features during the seizure), partial focal motor, or sensory seizures (the initial discharge comes from a focal unilateral area of brain, often preceded by an aura). As with cerebrovascular accidents (CVAs) and coma, knowing the origin may be crucial to understanding the pathophysiologic processes of the disease and to managing the intraoperative and postoperative course. Epileptic seizures can arise from discontinuation of sedative hypnotic drugs or alcohol, use of narcotics, uremia, traumatic injury, neoplasms, infection, congenital malformation, birth injury, drug usage (amphetamines), hypercalcemia or hypocalcemia, and vascular disease and vascular accidents.[362] Thirty percent of epileptic seizures have no known cause. Most partial seizures are caused by structural brain abnormalities (secondary to tumor, trauma, stroke, infection, and other causes). The epileptic patient requires no special anesthetic management other than that for the underlying disease. Anticonvulsant medications should be given in the therapeutic range[363-366] and continued through the morning of surgery; they should also be given postoperatively. Appropriate treatment of status epilepticus may include general anesthesia.[365] High concentrations of enflurane (especially with hyperventilation) can be associated with EEG evidence of epileptic activity and tonic–clonic movements.[367-371] These seizures, however, do not appear to have serious sequelae.[371] Enflurane anesthesia does not appear to in-crease seizure activity in patients with a history of convulsive disorders; it even suppresses seizures induced by electroshock, pentylene-tetrazole, strychnine, picrotoxin, or beme-gride.[369-372] Thus, other than the use of current drug therapy and heeding precautions taken for the underlying disease, no known changes in perioperative management seem indicated.

INFECTIOUS DISEASES OF THE CNS, DEGENERATIVE DISORDERS OF THE CNS, AND HEADACHE

Many of the degenerative CNS disorders have been traced to slowly developing viral diseases. No special perioperative anesthetic considerations appear to apply for infectious disorders of the CNS other than those for increased intracranial pressure (also see Chs. 43 & 66). What prophylactic measures to take if one comes into contact with meningococcal disease or other infectious CNS disease is not well established.[373]

Parkinson's disease is a degenerative disorder of the CNS that may or may not be caused by a virus. Clinically, Parkinson's disease, chronic manganese intoxication, phenothiazine or butyrophenone toxicity, Wilson's disease, Huntington's chorea, traumatic boxing injury, and carbon monoxide encephalopathy all present with similar features: bradykinesia, muscular rigidity, and tremor. The substantia nigra degenerates, and the clinical signs presumably result from decreased production of dopamine in the neurons of the basal ganglia leading to the putamen and caudate nucleus. The effects of this dopaminergic deficiency may be compounded by the unopposed effects of cholinergic neurons bordering the basal ganglia. Therapy is thus directed either at increasing the neuronal release of dopamine or the receptor's response to dopamine, or the direct stimulation of the receptor by bromocryptine and lergotrile, or at decreasing cholinergic activity. Anticholinergic agents are the initial drugs of choice; they decrease tremor more than muscle rigidity. Since dopamine does not pass the blood–brain barrier (BBB), its precursor, L-dopa (levodopa), is used. Unfortunately, L-dopa is decarboxylated to dopamine in the periphery and can cause nausea, vomiting, and dysrhythmia. These side effects are diminished by administration of α-methylhydrazine (Carbidopa), a decarboxylase inhibitor that does not pass the BBB. Refractoriness to L-dopa develops, and the drug is now used only when symptoms cannot be controlled with other anticholinergic medications. "Drug holidays" have been suggested as one way of restoring the effectiveness of these compounds, but cessation of such therapy may result in a marked deterioration of function and the need for hospitalization.[374] Therapy for Parkinson's disease should be continued through the morning of surgery; such treatment seems to decrease drooling, the potential for aspiration, and ventilatory weakness.[374-376] Reinstituting therapy promptly after surgery is important,[374-376] as is avoiding such drugs as phenothiazines and butyrophenones (droperidol) that compete with dopamine at the receptor.[377]

Dementia, a progressive decline in intellectual function, can be caused by treatable infections (e.g., syphilis, cryptococcosis, coccidioidomycosis, tuberculosis), myxedema, vitamin B_{12} deficiency, chronic drug or alcohol intoxication, metabolic causes (liver and renal failure), neoplasms, untreatable infections (Creutzfeldt-Jakob syndrome), or a decrease of acetylcholine in the cerebral cortex (Alzheimer's disease). This last condition occurs in 0.5 percent of Americans.[378] Although such patients are often given cholinergic agonists, controlled trials of these drugs have not shown benefit as yet.[378] Creutzfeldt-Jakob disease has been transmitted inadvertently by surgical instruments and corneal transplants; the causative virus is not inactivated by heat, disinfectants, or formaldehyde.

More than 90 percent of patients with chronic recurring headaches are diagnosed as having migraine, tension, or cluster headaches. The mechanism of tension or cluster headaches may not differ qualitatively from that for migraine headaches; all may be manifestations of labile vasomotor regulation.[379] The treatment for cluster and migraine headaches centers around ergotamine and its derivatives. Other drugs and therapies that may be effective are propranolol, calcium channel inhibitors,

cyproheptadine, prednisone, antihistamines, tricyclic antidepressant drugs, phenytoin, diuretic drugs, and biofeedback.[380] Giant cell arteritis and glaucoma are other causes of headache that might benefit from treatment before surgery. No other special treatment is indicated preoperatively for the patient who has a well-delineated cause for headaches. Acute migraine attacks can sometimes be terminated by ergotamine tartrate aerosol or by injection of dihydroergotamine mesylate intravenously; general anesthesia has also been used. I normally continue all prophylactic headache medicines, except aspirin (because of the potential for bleeding), through the morning of surgery.

BACK PAIN, NECK PAIN, AND SPINAL CANAL SYNDROMES

Acute spinal cord injury is discussed earlier in the section on autonomic dysfunction. Little is written about the anesthetic management of syndromes related to herniated disk, spondylosis (usually of advancing age), and the congenital narrowing of the cervical and lumbar canal that gives rise to symptoms of nerve-root compression.[380-382] One report suggests the use of awake intubation, a fiberoptic bronchoscope, and evoked potential monitoring.[381] The preoperative management of the patient about to undergo chemonucleolysis is discussed earlier under the section on anaphylaxis. Other than the commonsense approach of seeking neurosurgical consultation or, if necessary, using awake positioning of patients in a comfortable position prior to emergency root-decompressing procedures, no special procedures appear to be necessary.

DEMYELINATING DISEASES

This is a diffuse group of diseases ranging from those with no known cause (such as multiple sclerosis) to those that follow infection or vaccination (such as Guillain-Barré syndrome) or antimetabolite treatment of cancer. Therefore, demyelinating diseases can present with very diverse symptoms. Apparently, there is a risk of relapse of these diseases immediately after surgery.[383] Thus far, no mode of treatment has been shown to alter these disease processes, although ACTH and steroids may ameliorate or abbreviate a relapse, especially of multiple sclerosis. Such an effect might suggest an immunologic disorder as the cause of these diseases.

METABOLIC DISEASES

Included in this category is nervous system dysfunction secondary to porphyrias, alcoholism, uremia, hepatic failure, and vitamin B_{12} deficiency. The periodic paralysis that can accompany thyroid disease is discussed under neuromuscular disorders, following this section.

Alcoholism or heavy alcohol intake is associated with acute alcoholic hepatitis (also see Ch. 46) (the activity of which declines as alcohol is withdrawn), myopathy and cardiomyopathy that can be severe, and withdrawal syndromes. Within 6 to 8 hours of withdrawal, the patient may become tremulous, a state that usually subsides within days or weeks. Alcoholic hallucinosis and withdrawal seizures generally occur within 24 to 36 hours. These seizures are generalized grand mal attacks; when focal seizures are manifest, other causes should be sought. Delirium tremens usually appears within 72 hours of withdrawal and is often preceded by tremulousness, hallucinations, or seizures. These three occurrences combined with perceptual distortions, insomnia, psychomotor disturbances, autonomic hyperactivity, and, in a large percentage of cases, another potentially fatal illness (such as bowel infarction or subdural hematoma) comprise delirium tremens. This syndrome is now treated with benzodiazepines. Nutritional disorders of alcoholism include alcoholic hypoglycemia and hypothermia, alcoholic polyneuropathy, Wernicke-Korsakoff syndrome, and cerebellar degeneration. In alcoholic patients (i.e., those who drink at least 2 six-packs

of beer or 1 pint of whiskey per day, or the equivalent), emergency surgery and anesthesia (despite alcoholic hepatitis) is not associated with worsening abnormalities of liver enzymes (S. Zinn, personal communication regarding a randomized study of 26 patients at San Francisco General Hospital given spinal, enflurane, or narcotic-nitrous oxide anesthesia for emergency orthopedic surgery). In addition, about 20 percent of alcoholic patients also have COPD. Thus, the patient who gives a history of alcohol abuse warrants careful examination of many systems to quantify his or her preoperative physical status.

Although hepatic failure can lead to coma with high-output cardiac failure, unlike uremia, it does not lead to chronic polyneuropathy. Uremic polyneuropathy is a distal symmetric sensorimotor polyneuropathy that may be improved by dialysis. The use of depolarizing muscle relaxants has been questioned in polyneuropathies (also see Ch. 27). I believe that patients who have a neuropathy associated with uremia should not be given succinylcholine because of a possible exaggerated hyperkalemic response.

Pernicious anemia caused by vitamin B_{12} deficiency may result in subacute combined degeneration of the spinal cord, its signs being similar to those of chronic nitrous oxide toxicity. Both pernicious anemia and N_2O toxicity are associated with peripheral neuropathy and disorders of the pyramidal tract and posterior column (which governs fine motor skills and the sense of body position). Combined system disease can also occur without anemia, as can N_2O toxicity in dentists and N_2O abusers. Patients with B_{12} deficiency and anemia, if treated with folate, improve hematologically but progress to dementia and severe neuropathy. Thus, intramuscular administration of 100 μg of vitamin B_{12} before giving folate to the patient who has signs of combined system degeneration may be prudent.

The porphyrias are a constellation of metabolic diseases resulting from an autosomally inherited lack of functional enzymes active in the synthesis of hemoglobin. Figure 9-7 schematically depicts the abnormalities resulting from these enzyme deficits. It is important to note that types 1, 3, and 4 can cause life-threatening neurologic abnormalities. These types of

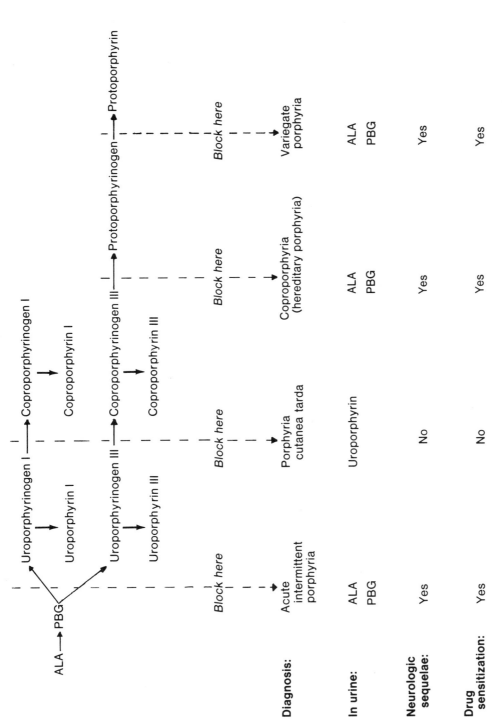

FIG. 9-7 Scheme depicting functional enzyme deficits for some of the porphyrias. ALA = aminolevulinic acid; PBG = porphobilinogen.

porphyrias are characterized by the presence of aminolevulinic acid (ALA) and/or porphobilinogen (PBG) in urine, whereas porphyria cutanea tarda, which is not associated with neurologic sequelae, is not.[384,385] In acute intermittent porphyria, the typical pattern consists of acute attacks of colicky pain, nausea, vomiting, severe constipation, psychiatric disorders, and lesions of the lower motor neuron, which can progress to bulbar paralysis. Certain drugs can induce the enzyme ALA synthetase, exacerbating the disease process.[384-388] These sensitizing drugs include barbiturates, meprobamate, chlordiazepoxide, glutethimide, diazepam, hydroxydione, phenytoin, imipramine, pentazocine, birth control pills, ethyl alcohol, sulfonamides, griseofulvin, and ergot preparations. Patients often have attacks at times of infection, fasting, or menstruation. Administration of glucose suppresses ALA synthetase activity and prevents or ablates acute attacks. Drugs used in anesthetic management that are reported to be safe for patients with porphyria include neostigmine (Prostigmin), atropine, gallamine, succinylcholine, *d*-tubocurarine, pancuronium, nitrous oxide, procaine, propanidid, etomidate, meperidine, fentanyl, morphine, droperidol, promazine, promethazine, and chlorpromazine.[385-388] Although ketamine has been used,[387] postoperative psychoses attributable to the disease may be difficult to distinguish from those possibly caused by ketamine.

NEUROMUSCULAR DISORDERS

This category includes disorders affecting all major components of the motor unit: motor neuron, peripheral nerve, neuromuscular junction, and muscle. Neuropathies may involve all components of the nerve, producing sensory, motor, and autonomic dysfunction, or may preferentially involve one or the other component. Myopathies may involve proximal or distal muscles, or both.

Myasthenia gravis (also see Ch. 27) is a disorder of the muscular system caused by partial blockade or destruction of nicotinic acetylcholine receptors by IgG antibodies. This syndrome is characterized by fluctuating ophthalmoplegia; ptosis; and bulbar, respiratory, or limb weakness and confirmed by a beneficial response to cholinergic drugs.[389,390]

The severity of the disease correlates with the ability of the antibodies to decrease the number of available acetylcholine receptors.[391] Treatment of myasthenia is usually begun with anticholinesterase agents but, in moderate and severe disease, progresses to steroids and thymectomy.[390] Immunosuppressive drugs and plasmapheresis are begun if these more conservative measures fail.[390] One major problem for the anesthesiologist involves the use of muscle relaxants and their reversal.[392] Since much of the care of myasthenia gravis patients involves tailoring the amount of anticholinesterase medication to the maximal muscle strength of the patient, derangement of the course of the disease during surgery could necessitate reassessment of the drug dosage. For that reason, several researchers recommend withholding all anticholinergic drugs for 6 hours before surgery and reinstituting medicine postoperatively with exreme caution, because the sensitivity of these patients to such drugs may have changed. Small doses of succinylcholine can be used to facilitate endotracheal intubation, and tiny doses of nondepolarizing drugs can be used for intraoperative relaxation not obtained by regional anesthesia or volatile agents. Controlled ventilation is usually required for 24 to 48 or more hours postoperatively.[393-395] This practice is especially important for patients who have had myasthenia gravis for more than 6 years, for those who have COLD, for those having a daily pyridostigmine requirement of 750 mg or more, and for those whose vital capacity is less than 40 ml/kg.[396]

The Eaton-Lambert syndrome (myasthenic syndrome) is characterized by proximal limb muscle weakness. Strength or reflexes may increase with repetitive effort. These patients have a decreased release of acetylcholine at the neuromuscular junction. Guanidine therapy enhances the release of acetylcholine from nerve terminals and improves strength. Most men who have this syndrome also have small cell carcinoma of the lung or other malignancy, whereas women often have malignancy, sarcoidosis, thyroiditis, or a collagen-related vascular disease. In addition, these patients have increased sensitivity to both depolarizing and nondepolarizing muscle relaxants.[393,397]

Dermatomyositis and polymyositis are characterized by proximal limb muscle weakness with dysphagia. These conditions are associated with malignancy or collagen-related vascular disease, often involving respiratory and cardiac muscle.

Periodic paralysis is another disease in which sensitivity to muscle relaxants increases. Periodic weakness starts in childhood or adolescence and is precipitated by rest after exercise, sleep, cold, surgery, or pregnancy. Hypokalemic and hyperkalemic forms exist and are associated with cardiac dysrhythmias. Like thyrotoxic periodic paralysis, these hypokalemic and hyperkalemic forms usually spare the respiratory muscles. Anesthetic management consists of minimizing stress and maintaining normal fluid and electrolyte states and body temperature.[397]

Muscular dystrophy patients now survive into their late twenties. Complicating their disease are respiratory infections, kyphoscoliosis, muscle contractions, and cardiac abnormalities. Duchenne muscular dystrophy is a sex-linked recessive disease, the most common of the muscular dystrophies. It occurs after 5 years of age, at which time patients experience a rapid progression of muscle disease that leads to incapacity in their teens. Cardiac involvement is common when the disease affects proximal and pelvic muscles, and respiratory failure is a common cause of death. Limb-girdle muscular dystrophy is not as severe as Duchenne muscular dystrophy; it occurs later in life, has cardiac involvement, and is transmitted as an autosomal recessive trait. Facioscapulohumeral muscular dystrophy (FSHMD) is a disease of autosomal dominant inheritance that has a mild clinical form in adolescence. Patients with FSHMD have a normal lifespan without an increased risk of cardiac complications; however, postoperative respiratory deaths have been recorded. Myotonic dystrophy is a disease in which continued active contraction of the muscles persists after voluntary effort or stimulation has ceased. This autosomal dominant inherited disease begins at 20 to 40 years of age and is associated with cardiomyopathy, baldness, testicular atrophy, cataracts, intellectual and emotional abnormalities, and premature death in the 50- to 60-year age range. The facial, sternocleidomastoidal, distal, and pharyngeal muscles become weak and atrophy. Since the disease involves the muscles themselves, and not their innervation, conduction anesthesia cannot produce adequate relaxation of tonic muscles. Gastric dilatation has also been reported to be a problem, as has malignant hyperthermia. As with the other forms of muscular dystrophies, most problems in myotonic dystrophy arise from cardiac dysrhythmias and inadequacies of the respiratory muscles. With all the forms of muscular dystrophy, as with all the neuropathies (discussed earlier), problems related to exaggerated serum potassium release following administration of depolarizing muscle relaxants have been reported (also see Ch. 27).[398]

Malignant hyperthermia (MH) (also see Ch. 56) in the patient or in a relative of the patient merits careful history-taking and at least consideration of performing a test for susceptibility to MH. Prophylaxis with intravenous dantrolene sodium (Dantrium) may also be warranted (also see Ch. 56). In a minority of cases, MH has been associated with recognizable musculoskeletal abnormalities such as strabismus, ptosis, myotonic dystrophy, hernias, kyphoscoliosis, muscular dystrophy, central core disease, and marfanoid syndrome. Malignant hyperthermia occurs most frequently among children and adolescents, the incidence being 1 in 14,000 anesthetic administrations. The incidence increases to 1 in 2,500 among patients requiring squint surgery.[399] Questions to ask the parents during preoperative evaluation include: Does your child get rigid when upset? Does your child sweat profusely when upset? However, the sensitivity and specificity of such questions in predicting malignant hyperthermia are not confirmed. The reader is referred to Chapter 56 for a complete discussion of the screening procedure to use.

DOWN'S SYNDROME

Down's syndrome (trisomy 21) occurs 1.5 times in 1,000 live births. It is associated with congenital cardiac lesions, such as endocardial cushion defects (40 percent), ventricular septal defects (27 percent), patent ductus arteriosus (12 percent), and tetralogy of Fallot (8 percent), necessitating prophylactic antibiotics prior to predictable bactemic events; with upper respiratory infections; with atlantooccipital instability and laxity of other joints; with thyroid hypofunction (50 percent); with an increased incidence of subglottic stenosis; and with enlargement of the tongue.[400] No abnormal responses to anesthetics or anesthetic adjuvants have been substantiated. A reported sensitivity to atropine has been disproved, although administration of atropine to any patient given digoxin for atrial fibrillation should be done with extreme care.[400] Examination for these conditions should precede surgery.

PREDICTING PREOPERATIVELY WHICH NEUROLOGIC PATIENTS WILL HAVE INCREASED INTRACRANIAL PRESSURE DURING SURGERY

Symptoms and signs of increased intracranial pressure include morning headache or headache made worse by coughing, nausea, vomiting, disturbances of consciousness, a history of large tumors, tumors involving the brainstem, neck rigidity, and papilledema. Patients having these signs, large ventricles as seen on roentgenograms or images of the brain, or edema surrounding supratentorial tumors should be considered at risk of intraoperative intracranial hypertension. Such patients may benefit from preoperative treatment or anesthetic management that assumes this possibility (also see Ch. 43).[401]

Other preoperative considerations in patients with neurologic disease that can cause intracranial hypertension are the associated hypoventilation and hypoxia in patients who have severe hemiplegia and the presence of subarachnoid bleeding or other forms of intracranial hemorrhage (especially likely in women given heparin who have two or more cerebral infarcts on CT scan).[402,403] The drugs used to prevent cerebral arterial spasm[404]—calcium-channel blockers—are discussed in the last section of this chapter.

MENTAL DISORDERS

Perhaps the most important preoperative consideration for patients with mental disorders, in addition to developing rapport with them, is understanding their drug therapy and its effects and side effects. Lithium, tricyclic antidepressants, phenothiazines, butyrophenones, and monoamine oxidase (MAO) inhibitors are used in these patients.[405] These drugs have potent effects and side effects that are discussed in the last section of this chapter.

RENAL DISEASE, INFECTIOUS DISEASES, AND ELECTROLYTE DISORDERS

One may ask why preoperative preparation of the patient with renal disease is discussed in the same section as preoperative preparation of the patient with an infectious disease. Although it is commonly recommended that no surgery except emergency or curative (e.g., drainage of an abscess) be done in patients with infectious disease, it has become evident that renal insufficiency can be caused by antimicrobial agents[406] and that sepsis, not shock, is probably the leading cause of acute postoperative renal failure.[407] The linking of renal failure to electrolyte disorders is more obvious—the kidney is the primary organ for regulating body osmolality and fluid volume and has a major role in the excretion of the end products of metabolism. In performing these functions, the kidney becomes intimately involved in the excretion of electrolytes.

The patient with renal insufficiency whose own kidneys are still functioning is distinct not only from the patient with end-stage renal disease whose renal functions are provided by a dialysis machine, but also from the patient who has a transplanted kidney. These three groups of patients require quite different preoperative preparation. In addition, acute changes in renal function present quite a different problem than do chronic alterations in function. Certain renal diseases require different preoperative preparation than others, but generally renal disease of any origin presents the same preoperative problems (also see Chapters 35 & 45).

RENAL DISEASE

CAUSES AND SYSTEMIC EFFECTS OF RENAL DISORDERS

The nephrotic syndrome may develop in patients with glomerular diseases without disturbing tubular function. The soundness of tubular function is an important consideration, as tubular dysfunction with attendant uremia presents quite different problems than does glomerular disease with only the nephrotic syndrome. This is not to minimize the adverse effects of glomerular disease; the nephrotic syndrome consists of massive proteinuria and consequent hypoalbuminemia. The resulting reduction in plasma oncotic pressure diminishes plasma volume; this calls forth compensatory mechanisms that result in retention of sodium and water. As a result, a common clinical finding in nephrotic syndrome is edema. Thus, patients with the nephrotic syndrome may have excess total body water and decreased intravascular volume. In addition, diuretic drugs are often given in attempts to decrease edema. Thus, the estimation of intravascular volume status is an essential preoperative consideration in patients with the nephrotic syndrome and diminished tubular renal function who do not yet require hemodialysis.

However, in patients with the nephrotic syndrome in whom renal tubular function has been preserved, hypovolemia appears to be a significant cause of deteriorating tubular renal function.[408-413] Consequently, I advocate the same intense preoperative, intraoperative, and postoperative fluid management for patients with the nephrotic syndrome as I do for patients with diminished tubular function. Admittedly, no randomized study shows that close control of intravascular volume status in these groups of patients preserves renal tubular function (or any other measure of perioperative morbidity) to a greater degree than does less rigid control.

Uremia, the end result of renal tubular failure (i.e., failure of the concentrating, diluting, acidifying, and filtering functions) presents in many ways. Changes occur in the cardiovascular, immunologic, hematologic, neuromuscular, pulmonary, and endocrine systems, as well as in bone. These alterations are ascribed either to the toxic end products of protein metabolism or to an imbalance in the functioning of the kidney. As the number of functioning nephrons diminishes, the still-functioning nephrons attempt to increase some solute and body composition preservation functions at the expense of other functions, such as the excretion of phosphate. The accumulation of phosphate increases parathormone levels, which in turn produces osteodystrophy. Osteodystrophy can be managed by restricting dietary phosphate, by administration of gels (such as aluminum hydroxide or carbonate) that bind with intestinal phosphate, by giving supplemental calcium, or by parathyroidectomy.[414,415]

Certain alterations in uremia, such as neuropathy, are most logically attributed to an accumulation of toxic metabolites.[416] Peripheral neuropathy is most often sensory and of the lower extremities but may also be motor; peripheral neuropathies are often improved with hemodialysis and can be dramatically reversed with transplantation.[416] The use of depolarizing muscle relaxants in patients with peripheral neuropathy is controversial; it is discussed in the section on neuropathies (also see Ch. 27). Along with the altered volume states and cardiac complications in uremic patients, autonomic neuropathy may contribute to hypotension during anesthesia. Atherosclerosis is often accelerated in uremic patients; hypertension, with its attendant consequences, is very common.

Cardiac failure (especially episodic) occurs frequently in uremic patients because of the presence of many adverse conditions—anemia with increasing myocardial work, hypertension, atherosclerosis, and altered volume states. Pericarditis can present with pericardial rub alone or with pain (with or without hemorrhage). Cardiac tamponade should be ruled out on the basis of clinical features and by echocardiography if this diagnosis is seriously suspected preoperatively. Also, cardiac tamponade should be treated or planned for preoperatively.

If anemia exists, its severity generally parallels the degree of uremia; chronically uremic patients seem to adapt well to anemia. No hard data substantiate the need to give a preoperative blood transfusion to a chronically uremic patient, even when preoperative hematocrit is as low as 16 or 18 vol percent. One of the major reasons not to transfuse blood in patients having end-stage renal disease has recently been disproved: data show that the more blood transfusions a transplant recipient receives before transplant, the greater the chance that the transplant will function successfully.[417,418] In uremic patients, coagulation and platelet adhesiveness may be abnormal and Factor III activity decreased. Even those uremic patients not given corticosteroids or immunosuppressive drugs may demonstrate abnormal immunity, perhaps meriting increased attention regarding the procedures that lessen patient cross-contamination.

Uremic patients exhibit a wide variety of metabolic and endocrinologic disorders[414,419] including impaired carbohydrate tolerance, insulin resistance, type IV hyperlipoproteinemia, hyperparathyroidism, autonomic insufficiency, hyperkalemia, and anion gap acidosis (caused by the inability of the kidneys to reabsorb filtered bicarbonate and to excrete sufficient ammonium into the urine[419,420]). Also, the excretion and pharmacokinetics of drugs is different in uremic patients than in normal patients. In addition, the complications of hemodialysis include hepatitis B (and persistent hepatitis B antigenemia), nutritional deficiencies, electrolyte and fluid imbalances, and mental disorders. Because these conditions can

however, substantiate the hypothesis that preoperative optimization of these metabolic and endocrinologic disorders reduces perioperative risk in the uremic patient.

As with uremic patients, preoperative optimization of volume status is paramount in patients with kidney stones. Seventy-five percent of all kidney stones are composed of calcium oxalate. Patients with these stones often take diuretic drugs, avoid calcium-rich foods, or restrict their intake of salt. Prevention of dehydration by institution of intravenous fluid therapy at the same time that oral intake is restricted may be as important for these patients as it is for patients with struvate or uric acid stones. Struvate stones often result from urinary infection. Uric acid stones can be prevented by treatment with allopurinol, by preoperative hydration, or by alkalization of the urine. Acidosis may contribute to stone formation. Thus, again, optimization of volume status is important in preventing stones and preserving renal function. More thorough discussion of renal function and physiology is discussed in Chapter 35. Chapter 45 deals with the complexities of managing patients for renal surgery and other urologic procedures.

Creatinine clearance appears to be the most accurate means of quantifying, for pharmacokinetic purposes, the degree of decreased renal function. In the patient with stable renal function, this can be approximated by noting the serum creatinine levels: a doubling of creatinine level represents a halving of glomerular filtration rate (GFR). Thus, a patient with a stable serum creatinine level of 2 mg/dl would have a GFR of approximately 60 ml/min. A stable serum creatinine level of 4 mg/dl would accompany a GFR of approximately 30 ml/min, and a stable serum creatinine of 8 mg/dl would accompany a GFR of 15 ml/min or less. When pregnancy and considerable edema are not present and the serum creatinine level is stable, the following formula can be used to estimate creatinine clearance[419,421]:

$$\text{Creatinine clearance} = \frac{[140 - \text{age (yr)}] \times [\text{body weight (kg)}]}{72 \times \text{serum creatinine (mg/dl)}}$$

lead to serious perioperative morbidity, they should be evaluated before surgery. No data,

Note that renal function must be *stable*. Unstable renal function often is associated with changes in serum creatinine levels that lag by several days. Although knowing the serum creatinine level is more useful than knowing the blood urea nitrogen level, the latter provides some information, as discussed in the next section.

THE PATIENT WITH INSUFFICIENT BUT FUNCTIONING KIDNEYS

I believe that the greatest challenge for the anesthesiologist is presented by those patients whose insufficient renal function needs to be preserved during surgery. The many uremic symptoms and great perioperative morbidity associated with uremia can probably be avoided by attention to detail in the preoperative and perioperative management of patients with insufficient but still functioning kidneys.[407-413,422-429] First, studies demonstrate that acute postoperative renal failure is associated with an extremely high mortality rate. Moreover, acute perioperative renal failure is most likely to occur in patients who had renal insufficiency before surgery. Proper hydration before surgery probably decreases mortality following acute renal failure due to radiocontrast agents.[412,413,422-424] Clues as to the presence of hypovolemia or hypervolemia should be sought from the history and physical examination (e.g., weight loss or gain, thirst, edema, orthostatic hypotension and tachycardia, flat neck veins, dry mucous membranes, decreased skin turgor). In seriously ill patients, insertion of a pulmonary arterial catheter will permit more precise monitoring of intravascular fluid volume. To preserve normal renal function, infusion of saline, mannitol, or furosemide has been recommended. This should be done cautiously, however, because saline infusions and mannitol can lead to fluid overload and myocardial damage; also, diuretic drugs given intraoperatively can produce postoperative hypovolemia, which worsens renal function. Maintaining normal intravascular fluid volume can be guided by pulmonary capillary wedge pressure. At UCSF maintaining normal intravascular fluid volume prevented impairment of renal function after abdominal aortic reconstruction, even when urinary volumes were low.[429] Other causes of deterioration in

function in chronic renal insufficiency are low cardiac output or low renal blood flow (in prerenal azotemia, whether because of cardiac failure or because of fluid depletion from diuretic drugs, BUN often increases disproportionately to increases in creatinine), urinary tract infection, use of nephrotoxic drugs, hypercalcemia, and hyperuricemia. These conditions and drugs should be avoided; if any of these conditions exist, they should be treated preoperatively.

THE PATIENT UNDERGOING DIALYSIS

Because the patient undergoing dialysis has already lost natural renal functioning, the emphasis in preoperative assessment shifts toward protecting other organ systems and toward optimally maintaining vascular access sites for cannulation. Usually this does not require invasive monitoring. Emphasis is placed on intravascular fluid volume and electrolyte status, which can be ascertained by knowing when the patient last underwent dialysis, how much weight was normally gained or lost with dialysis and whether fluid loss was peritoneal or intravascular, and what electrolyte composition the blood was dialyzed against. Although preoperative dialysis may benefit patients who have hyperkalemia, hypercalcemia, acidosis, neuropathy, and fluid overload, the resulting dysequilibrium between fluid and electrolytes can cause problems. Because hypovolemia induced by dialysis can lead to intraoperative hypotension, at our institution, we carefully avoid weight and fluid reduction when giving preoperative dialysis. Also, hypopnea has been found to occur during and after dialysis when the dialysate contained acetate.[430] Avoiding an acetate bathing solution may prevent this cause of hypoventilation.

THE PATIENT WHO HAS HAD A RENAL TRANSPLANT

More than 45,000 patients have received renal transplants (compared with 50,000 currently undergoing dialysis in the United

States). Approximately 70 percent are still alive, although one-third must undergo dialysis.[418,431] When such patients have subsequent surgery, the state of their renal function must be determined (i.e., whether they have normal renal function, insufficient but still functioning kidneys, or end-stage renal disease requiring hemodialysis). Descriptions of side effects from immunosuppressive drugs should also be sought. Because renal transplant places patients at much higher risk of infection, all effort at avoiding invasive monitoring and at preventing patient cross-contamination should be taken.

DRUGS IN RENAL FAILURE

Patients with renal azotemia have a three-fold or greater risk of an adverse drug reaction than do those with normal renal function.[432-434] Risk is increased by either excessive pharmacologic effects (secondary to high blood levels of a drug or its metabolite, such as the metabolite of meperidine), to physiologic changes in target tissues induced by the uremic state (such as excessive sedation in the uremic patient having standard blood levels of sedative hypnotic drugs), or to excessive administration of electrolytes with drugs (e.g., penicillin standardly has 1.7 mEq of potassium per 1 million units).[432-434] Administration of standard doses of drugs dependent on renal excretion for their elimination can result in drug accumulation and enhanced pharmacologic effect. Dosing guidelines about many drugs used by anesthesiologists for patients with and without renal failure were provided by Bennett et al.[432]

INFECTIOUS DISEASE

Since it is commonly recommended that no surgery except emergency or essential (e.g., drainage of an abscess) be done in patients with infectious disease, and since renal insufficiency is known possibly to be caused by antimicrobial agents,[406,412] renal function and organ damage due to renal insufficiency should be assessed preoperatively in the patient with infectious disease. Guidelines for prophylactic antibiotics, summarized elsewhere, help prevent sepsis from bacteremic interventions.[435-438] Sepsis has become a leading cause of postoperative morbidity,[407] probably through a decrease in systemic vascular resistance related to activation of the complement system. Thus, attention to the effects of antibiotic drugs must be supplemented by attention to intravascular volume status.[412,436,439] The degree of impairment of the infected organ and its effect on anesthesia should be assessed. For instance, endocarditis merits examination of volume status, antibiotic and other drug therapy and side effects,[440] myocardial function, and renal, pulmonary, neurologic, and hepatic function —those organ systems that endocarditis can affect.

At least two other considerations merit preoperative consideration—patient isolation to avoid contamination, and patient infectivity to the physician. Both concerns are real. Nosocomial infection is a major source of postsurgical morbidity.[441-446] Acquired immunodeficiency syndrome (AIDS)[447] and many forms of hepatitis (A, B, non-A, and non-B) appear to be due to viral infections but require direct contact with blood or body fluids. Whether screening for specific viruses or for the chronic end-organ effects of these viruses[448] would reduce the risk of infection to both recipients and health care personnel during blood transfusions has not been determined. Usual precautions appear to be effective.[449] These two considerations are the focus of at least two published volumes.[450,451]

ELECTROLYTE DISORDERS
(Also See Chs. 14 & 15)

Disorders of calcium, magnesium, and phosphate balance were discussed in the section on diseases involving the endocrine system and disorders of nutrition.

HYPONATREMIA
AND HYPERNATREMIA

Electrolyte disorders are usually detected by determining the levels of electrolytes in serum. These concentrations reflect the balance between water and electrolytes. Thus, hyponatremia reflects a relative excess of free water and can occur when total body sodium increases (as in edematous disorders), when total body sodium is normal (as in excesses of free water because of inappropriate secretion of antidiuretic hormone), or when total body sodium decreases (as occurs with too-aggressive use of diuretic drugs). Definition of the cause defines treatment. The anesthesiologist is faced with the question: What levels of electrolytes require treatment prior to anesthesia? Although slowly developing hyponatremia usually produces few symptoms, the patient may be lethargic and apathetic. Chronic hyponatremia is better tolerated than acute hyponatremia because of mechanisms regulating intracellular fluid volume that alleviate brain edema; the loss of other solutes from the cell decreases the osmotic movement of water into cells. Despite this, severe chronic hyponatremia (i.e., serum sodium levels <123 mEq/L) can cause brain edema.[452] By contrast, acute hyponatremia may manifest with severe symptoms requiring emergency treatment: profound cerebral edema with obtundation, coma, convulsions, and disordered reflexes and thermoregulatory control.[452] Depending on the cause and relative total sodium and water content, treatment can range from administering hypertonic saline or mannitol (with or without diuretic drugs) to restricting fluids or administering other drugs.[452-455] In hyponatremic patients who have excess total body water secondary to inappropriate secretion of antidiuretic hormone (SIADH), serum levels can be corrected by giving furosemide, 1 mg/kg, and hypertonic saline to replace loss of electrolytes in urine.[454]

In neither acute nor chronic hyponatremia is it necessary to restore serum sodium levels to their normal levels; brain swelling usually disappears at a serum sodium level of 130 mEq/L. This leaves us with the question: What levels of serum sodium make anesthesia more risky? Since no data exist to answer this question, to allow for some error in caring for patients, I have arbitrarily chosen a flexible 131 mEq/L concentration as the lower sodium limit for elective surgery. A discussion of intraoperative hyponatremia in patients undergoing transurethral prostatectomy can be found in Chapter 45.

Hypernatremia occurs much less commonly than hyponatremia. It is often iatrogenic in origin (e.g., can be caused by failure to provide sufficient free water to the patient who is unconscious or who has had a recent stroke-induced deficit of the thirst mechanism) and can occur in the presence of low, normal, or excess total body sodium. The primary symptoms of hypernatremia relate to brain cell shrinking. Because too rapid correction of hypernatremia can lead to cerebral edema and convulsions, correction should be made gradually. Again, with no data to support this stance, I believe that all patients undergoing surgery should have serum sodium concentrations of less than 150 mEq/L prior to anesthesia.

HYPOKALEMIA AND HYPERKALEMIA

Hypokalemia and hyperkalemia are also discussed in Chapters 14 & 15. The relationship between the measured potassium concentration in serum and the total body potassium stores can best be described using a scattergram.[85,456] Only 2 percent of total body potassium is stored in plasma. In normal individuals, 75 percent of the 50 to 60 mEq/L of total body potassium is stored in skeletal muscle, 6 percent in red blood cells, and 5 percent in the liver. Thus, a 20 to 25 percent change in potassium levels in plasma could represent a change in total body potassium of 1,000 mEq or more, if the change were chronic, or as little as 10 to 20 MEq if the change were acute.

As with serum sodium levels,[452] acute changes in serum potassium levels appear to be less well tolerated than chronic changes. Chronic changes are relatively well tolerated because of the equilibration of serum and intracellular stores that takes place over time to return the resting membrane potential of excitable cells to near normal.

Hyperkalemia can result from fictitious elevation of potassium (as in red blood cell hemolysis); excessive exogenous potassium from sources such as salt substitutes, or in large amounts, bananas; cellular shifts in potassium (owing to metabolic acidosis, tissue and muscle damage after burns, use of depolarizing muscle relaxants, or intense catabolism of protein), and decreased renal excretion (as occurs in renal failure, renal insufficiency with trauma, therapy with potassium-sparing diuretic drugs[453] or mineralocorticoid deficiency). The major danger in anesthetizing patients who have disorders of potassium balance appears to be abnormal cardiac function, that is, both electrical disturbances[457-459] and poor cardiac contractility.[458,459] Hyperkalemia lowers the resting membrane potential of excitable cardiac cells and decreases the duration of the myocardial action potential and upstroke velocity. This decreased rate of ventricular depolarization, plus the beginning of repolarization in some areas of the myocardium while other areas are still being depolarized, produces a progressively widening QRS complex that merges with the T wave into a sine wave on ECG. Above a potassium level of 6.7 mEq/L,[457] the degree of hyperkalemia and the duration of the QRS complex correlate well. This correlation is even better than the correlation between the serum potassium level and changes in the T wave. Nevertheless, the earliest manifestations of hyperkalemia are narrowing and peaking of the T wave. Although not diagnostic of hyperkalemia, T waves are almost invariably peaked and narrow when serum potassium levels are 7 to 9 mEq/L. When serum potassium levels exceed 7 mEq/L, atrial conduction disturbances appear as manifested by a decrease in P-wave amplitude and by an increase in the P-R interval. Supraventricular tachycardia, atrial fibrillation, premature ventricular contractions, ventricular tachycardia, ventricular fibrillation, or sinus arrest may all occur. The ECG and cardiac alterations of hyperkalemia are potentiated by low serum levels of calcium and sodium. Intravenous administration of saline, bicarbonate, glucose with insulin (1 unit per 2 g of glucose), and calcium can reverse these changes by shifting some extracellular potassium into the cell. Kayexalate (sodium polystyrene sulfonate) enemas can be given to bind potassium in the gut in exchange for sodium. Dialysis against a hypokalemic solution will also decrease serum potassium levels. However, in the hyperkalemic patient, hypoventilation can be dangerous during anesthesia,[457-460] because each 0.1 pH unit change can produce a 0.4 to 1.5 mEq/L change in serum potassium levels in the opposite direction. For example, if pH decreases from 7.4 to 7.3, serum potassium levels could increase from 5.5 to 6.5 mEq/L.[459,460]

Hypokalemia can be caused by inadequate intake of potassium, excessive GI losses (through diarrhea, vomiting, nasopharyngeal suctioning; chronic use of laxatives, or ingestion of cation-exchange resins, as occur in certain wines), excessive renal losses (because of use of diuretic drugs, renal tubular acidosis, chronic chloride deficiency, metabolic alkalosis, mineralocorticoid excess, excessive ingestion of licorice, use of antibiotics, ureterosigmoidoscomy and diabetic ketoacidosis), and shifts of potassium from extracellular to intracellular compartments (as occur in alkalosis, insulin administration, barium poisoning, and periodic paralysis). As with hyperkalemia, knowledge of the cause of potassium deficiency and its appropriate preoperative evaluation and treatment may be as important as treatment of the deficiency itself. Also like hyperkalemia, hypokalemia may reflect small or vast changes in total body potassium. Acute hypokalemia may be much less well tolerated than chronic hypokalemia. The major worrisome manifestations of hypokalemia pertain to the circulatory system, both the cardiac and peripheral components. In addition, however, chronic hypokalemia results in muscle weakness, hypoperistalsis, and nephropathy.

The cardiovascular manifestations of hypokalemia include autonomic neuropathy (which results in orthostatic hypotension and decreased sympathetic reserve), impaired myocardial contractility, and electrical conduction abnormalities that can result in sinus tachycardia, atrial and ventricular dysrhythmias, and disturbances of intraventricular conduction that can progress to ventricular fibrillation. That these are real concerns for the hypokalemic patient has been attested too many times.[457-459,461-464] In addition to dysrhythmias, the ECG reveals widening of the QRS complex, S-T segment abnormalities, progressive diminution of the T-wave amplitude, and progressive increase in the U-wave amplitude.[465] Surawicz[457] found these changes to be present invariably when serum potassium levels decreased to below 2.3 mEq/L. Although U waves are not specific to hypokalemia, they are sensitive indicators of the condition. Replenishing the total body potassium deficit for a depletion reflected by a serum deficit of 1 mEq/L (e.g., from 3.3 to 4.3 mEq/L) may require 1,000 mEq of potassium. Even if this amount could be given instantaneously (and it should not be replenished at a rate exceeding 250 mEq/day), it would take 24 to 48 hours to equilibrate in all tissues.[87,88] The potassium-depleted myocardium is unusually sensitive to digoxin, calcium, and, most important, potassium. Rapid potassium infusion can produce as severe dysrhythmias in the hypokalemic patient as does hypokalemia itself.[88,466-468]

Thus, the decision about proceeding with surgery and anesthesia in the face of acute or chronic depletions or excesses of potassium depends on many factors.[469] One must know the cause and treatment of the underlying condition creating the electrolyte imbalance and the effect of that imbalance on perioperative risk and physiologic processes. The urgency of the operation, the degree of electrolyte abnormality, the medications given, the acid-base balance, and the suddenness or persistence of the electrolyte disturbance are all considerations.

Retrospective epidemiologic studies attribute significant risk to administration of potassium (even chronic oral administration).[47] In one study, 1,910 of 16,048 consecutive hospitalized patients were given oral potassium supplements. Of these, hyperkalemia contributed to death in seven, making the incidence of complications of potassium therapy one in 250 patients. Armed with such data, many internists do not prescribe oral potassium therapy for patients given diuretic drugs. Yet such patients frequently become moderately hypokalemic.[471-474] Modest hypokalemia occurs in 10 to 50 percent of patients given diuretic drugs. Should surgery be delayed to subject such patients to the risks of potassium therapy?

Two studies investigated whether modest hypokalemia was a problem by prospectively seeking dysrhythmias on ECG in patients with various preoperative potassium levels.[459,475] No difference in the incidence of dysrhythmias was found among 25 normokalemic (K $>$ 3.4 mEq/L) patients, 25 moderately kypokalemic (K $=$ 3 to 3.4 mEq/L) patients, and 10 severely hypokalemic (K $<$ 2.9 mEq/L) patients.[475] The insensitivity of the eye or of even Holter recordings for short periods[476] (which seem not to have been obtained in this study) indicates that confirming studies are needed.

Other studies indicate that modest hypokalemia can have severe consequences.[477,478] Holland and co-workers[478] treated 21 patients with 50 mg hydrochlorothiazide twice a day for 4 weeks. These patients had a history of becoming hypokalemic during diuretic therapy; none of them had cardiac disease or was taking other medication. Before and after diuretic therapy, 24-hour ambulatory ECGs were recorded. This study is also subject to the limitations of Holter monitoring.[476] Seven of the 21 patients (33 percent) developed ventricular ectopy, including complex ventricular ectopy (multifocal PVCs, ventricular couplets, ventricular tachycardia). Potassium repletion decreased the number of ectopic ventricular beats per patient from 71.2 to 5.4 per hour. Apparently, some patients are sensitive to even minor potassium depletion. Therefore, although I recommend that hypokalemic patients be given potassium supplements, this issue is not clear.

My personal criteria for preoperative potassium therapy are as follows. As a rule, I believe all patients undergoing elective surgery should have normal serum potassium levels. However, I do not recommend delaying surgery if the serum potassium level is above 3.1 mEg/L or below 5.7 mEq/L, if the cause of potassium imbalance is known, and if the patient is in otherwise optimal condition. This range of safe potassium levels is arbitrary. I subject all patients with end-stage renal failure to dialysis (using the same arbitrary safe range) before all surgical procedures except truly emergency ones (as in the instance of imminent exsanguination). In 1978, Tanifuji and Eger[479] determined the relationships between electrolyte status and anesthetic requirement in dogs that may represent intraoperative considerations: hyponatremia and hypoosmolality decreased MAC, hypernatremia increased MAC, and hyperkalemia did not affect anesthetic requirement.

GASTROINTESTINAL AND LIVER DISEASE

The reader should also see the discussion of porphyrias in the section on neurologic disease; the discussion of nutritional deficiencies in the section on disorders of nutrition; and pediatric disorders, such as transesophageal fistula, in Chapters 49 & 67.

GASTROINTESTINAL DISEASE

THE PREOPERATIVE SEARCH FOR DIVERSE ASSOCIATED DISORDERS IN GASTROINTESTINAL DISEASE

Although preoperative preparation of the GI tract is usually the responsibility of the surgeon, and although the GI tract frequently does not need to be extensively evaluated by the anesthesiologist, GI disease can, and often does, cause derangements in many or all other systems. Such disturbances can affect the safety of anesthesia for the patient. Thus, the anesthesiologist may need not only to optimize the patient's condition through extensive preoperative preparation but also to have knowledge of disease processes and their effects in order to guide the patient smoothly through the perioperative period. The major advances of correcting fluid and electrolyte disorders and of optimizing nutritional status before surgery now allow surgery to be performed in patients with GI disease previously deemed to be at too great a risk and may have lessened the risk for others.[41,42,480-482] Still, in patients with GI disease, a thorough evaluation of intravascular fluid volume and electrolyte concentrations and nutrition is essential, including an evaluation of the supervening side effects of these therapies (e.g., hypophosphatemia from parenteral nutrition, hyperkalemia or cardiac dysrhythmias from too vigorous a treatment of hypokalemia, and congestive heart failure from too rapid or too vigorous treatment for hypovolemia).

In addition to vast alterations in fluids, electrolytes, and nutrition that can occur with such diverse GI diseases as neoplasms and pancreatitis, patients with GI disorders can have bowel obstruction, vomiting, or hypersecretion of acid. These effects may merit rapid induction of anesthesia with application of cricoid pressure or awake endotracheal intubation, preoperative nasogastric suctioning, or preoperative use of histamine-receptor blocking agents (also see Ch. 10).[481-483] Clotting abnormalities may need to be corrected, since the fat-soluble vitamin K (often malabsorbed) is necessary for synthesis of Factors V, VII, IX, and X in the liver (also see Ch. 34). Liver disease is often associated with GI disease and, if severe enough, can also result in deficiency of clotting factors synthesized by the liver.

Other factors should be remembered in any preoperative evaluation of the patient with GI disease. First, closed spaces containing gas expand by absorbing nitrous oxide. This expansion can lead to ischemic injury and/or GI viscus rupture.[484] Second, GI surgery predisposes the patient to sepsis; sepsis and decreased peripheral vascular resistance can lead to massive fluid requirements, cardiac failure, and renal insufficiency. Recently the wound infection rate has been declining; this decrease may be attributable to the use of better technique or to more appropriate prophylactic use of antibiotics.[485] Third, patients with GI disease may have many other associated disorders not directly related to the GI tract. For example, they may be anemic from deficiencies in iron, intrinsic factor, folate, or vitamin B_{12}. They may also manifest neurologic changes from combined-system disease. Respiration may be impaired because of heavy cigarette smoking, peritonitis, abscess, pulmonary obstruction, previous incisions, aspirations, or pulmonary embolism (as occurs with ulcerative colitis or with thrombophlebitis in the bedridden).[486] They may also have hepatitis, cholangitis, or side effects from antibiotic drugs or other medications, massive bleeding with anemia and shock, or psychological derangements. Since GI disease can be accompanied by so many diverse associated disorders, the clinician clearly must search for other system involvement and preoperatively assess and treat such disorders appropriately. Discussion of two specific diseases—ulcerative colitis and carcinoid tumors—will highlight the importance of other-system involvement in GI disease.

ULCERATIVE COLITIS AND CARCINOID TUMORS AS EXAMPLES OF GASTROINTESTINAL DISEASE AFFECTING OTHER SYSTEMS

Patients with ulcerative colitis often have psychological problems. They may also have phlebitis; deficiencies in iron, folate, or vitamin B_{12}; anemia; or clotting disorders caused by malabsorption. They may be malnourished, dehydrated, or have electrolyte abnormalities. In addition, ulcerative collitis can be accompanied by massive bleeding; bowel obstruction or perforation or toxic megacolon, causing respiratory compromise; hepatitis; arthritis; iritis; spondylitis; or diabetes secondary to pancreatitis.

Although carcinoid tumors usually arise from a primary tumor in the bowel, other sites (e.g., lung, liver, and stomach) have been considered as well. Carcinoid tumors frequently present as diarrhea with fluid and electrolyte abnormalities. Because these tumors secrete vasoactive substances such as serotonin, histamine, kinins, and prostaglandins,[487-489] patients can exhibit hypotension or hypertension with the flush of vasoactive substance release. Vasoactive substances can be released from the tumor by any number of substances including catecholamines. Thus, the anesthesiologist must tread a line between avoiding substances that release histamine (such as d-tubocurarine and morphine) and creating anesthesia so light that painful stimuli activate a sympathetic stress response.[491-496] The anesthesiologist must also be ready and able to treat hypotension, decreased peripheral vascular resistance, bronchospasm, and hypertension. α-Adrenergic receptor blockade with the phenothiazines, butyrophenones, or phenoxybenzamine and β-adrenergic receptor blockade with propranolol have been advocated to prevent catecholamine-mediated release of vasoactive substances; these practices, however, can lead to hypotension.

If severe hypotension occurs, the drug of choice is either angiotensin (now commercially unavailable in the United States) or vasopressin. However, the vasoactive substances released by carcinoid tumors cause fibrosis of heart valves, often resulting in pulmonic stenosis or tricuspid insufficiency. To increase cardiac output in the patient with tricuspid insufficiency, the anesthesiologist should avoid drugs or situations that increase pulmonary vascular resistance (e.g., angiotensin, vasopressin, acidosis, hypercarbia, hypothermia) (also see Chs. 28 & 32). In addition, if large amounts of serotonin are produced (equal to 200 mg/day of 5-hydroxyindoleacetic acid, a metabolic product of serotonin), then niacin deficiency with pellagra (as occurs with diarrhea, dermatitis, and dementia) can develop. These patients often are given serotonin antagonists (methysergide), anticholinergic drugs or histamine antagonists (cyproheptadine, ranitidine, or cimetidine), or prostaglandin-inhibiting drugs (aspirin, indomethacin, nonsteroidal antiinflammatory drugs). Many patients also develop bronchospasm with or without flushing when vasoactive substances are released. Thus, a patient with a carcinoid tumor may be well, or may be severely incapacitated by pulmonary, neurologic, nutritional, fluid, electrolyte, or cardiovascular disturbances.[487-490] Thus, the GI system by itself may not need extensive preoperative preparation, but GI disease can cause disturbances in any or all other systems that require both extensive preoperative preparation to optimize patient condition and preoperative knowledge of disease physiology and effects by anesthesiologists in order to guide patients through the perioperative period smoothly. In addition, the anesthesiologist's understanding of the nature of the surgery probably aids in determining the system involvement caused by GI disorder.[481,482,486]

LIVER DISEASE

What are the risks of giving anesthesia to patients with acute liver disease who require emergency surgery? What are the risks of giving anesthesia to patients with chronic impairment of liver function? What can be done to minimize these risks? Since hepatic function and physiology are discussed in Chapter 34, I will mention only that the liver performs many functions: it synthesizes (e.g., proteins, clotting factors), detoxifies the body of both drugs and the products of normal human metabolism, excretes waste products, and stores and supplies energy. Thus, tests of liver function assess synthesis (cholesterol levels, prothrombin time, albumin levels), cellular integrity (SGOT, alanine transaminase, LDH, alkaline phosphatase), the liver's ability to detoxify the body (e.g., ammonia, direct bilirubin, or lidocaine levels), and the liver's ability to excrete certain substances (BSP retention, total bilirubin levels).

In examining the effect of anesthesia (with or without surgery) on liver function, and in examining ways to reduce risk in patients with preexisting liver disease, investigators have often looked at one or more of these tests, or, more commonly, at major end points of morbidity (jaundice) or mortality. The evidence can be summarized as follows: without anesthesia or surgery, approximately 1 in 7 to 800 patients who are otherwise healthy and scheduled for surgery will have abnormal preoperative results for liver function tests; of these patients, one in three will develop jaundice (also see Ch. 8 for these studies).[497,498] All anesthetics tested (general, narcotic-nitrous oxide, and regional) have caused transient abnormalities in liver function tests. These abnormalities were magnified by upper intraabdominal surgery and occurred regardless of preexisting liver disease.[499-513] Patients with abnormal preoperative liver function tests obviously will have a higher incidence of abnormal results on postoperative liver function tests.[499,504-506,508,509] Lacking in the literature are investigations that studied patients with compromised hepatic function, to determine how to decrease the risk of surgery and anesthesia. In addition to preexisting hepatic disease and the operative site, hypokalemia, hypotension, sepsis, and the need for blood transfusion all contribute to postoperative hepatic dysfunction. Thus, anesthesia and surgery probably exacerbate hepatic disease and this obviously increases morbidity and mortality.[499,501,502,504-506,508,509]

The main goal of the anesthesiologist is to avoid making the hepatic disease (with perhaps its metabolic and CNS toxicity) worse and thereby increasing the chance of renal failure and death. Studies of portal hypertension have shown that mortality can be 50 percent when preoperative serum albumin concentrations are lower than 3 g/100 ml, preoperative serum bilirubin levels are greater than 3 mg/100 ml, and ascites and encephalopathy are present. By contrast, mortality decreases to 10 percent when preoperative serum albumin levels are 3 to 3.5 g/100 mg, preoperative serum bilirubin levels are 2 to 3 mg/100 ml, and encephalopathy is absent. The risks of anesthetizing a patient with chronic liver disease not requiring portacaval shunt are detailed only sporadically but appear to be greater than those associated with anesthetizing a healthy patient.[499-518]

Should halothane be given to patients with hepatitis or biliary tract disease? The National Halothane Study did not find that halothane caused massive hepatic necrosis, or any other hepatic abnormality, more frequently than did any other anesthetic agent,[509] and in fact demonstrated its safety in biliary tract surgery. Prospective studies have been contradictory at best as to whether repeat exposures to halothane within a short time elevate liver enzyme levels to a greater degree than do other anesthetic agents.[517-520] Because the incidence of hepatitis attributable only to halothane would be very low, very large groups would have to be studied. The incidence of postoperative jaundice and hepatitis not attributable to halothane is much greater than the incidence of hepatitis attributable only to halothane, and the absence of differentiating pathologic features makes halothane hepatitis difficult to exclude as a possibility. Thus, the strong bias of internists makes halothane hepatitis a popular diagnosis, despite the higher incidence of viral and drug hepatitides.[448,520-535] Another factor producing possible bias is the fact that animal models of halothane hepatitis incorporate liver hypoxia or pretreatment with polyvinylchlorides, conditions that can themselves adversely affect liver function. Thus, no irrefutable evidence exists implicating halothane as being better or worse than any other anesthetic for the patient with preexisting liver disease. However, should liver disease worsen postoperatively, the tendency is to blame halothane. Anesthesia is certainly less likely than hypoxia, trauma, viral hepatitis, drug-induced hepatitis, or sepsis to cause serious hepatic injury.[497-535] No one has yet determined whether a time limit exists within which repeat exposure to an anesthetic is more dangerous than exposure to various anesthetics, or after which repeat anesthesia is as safe as a first exposure to an anesthetic.

What should physicians do to avoid getting hepatitis from, or giving it to, patients? If the hepatitis B vaccine proves as safe as its initial trials suggest, and if the risk of anesthesia personnel acquiring the disease and perhaps its chronic sequelae is as great as studies suggest, it would be cost-effective for anesthesia personnel to be given the vaccine.[542] What should the physician with hepatitis B do to avoid infecting patients? That subject is discussed in detail elsewhere.[543]

Liver disease severe enough to affect hepatic synthesis adversely can impair the detoxification of many drugs,[432–434] including muscle relaxants[544] (also see Ch. 27) and can disturb coagulation (also see Ch. 39). Administration of fresh-frozen plasma may be needed to correct coagulation disorders.

HEMATOLOGIC DISORDERS AND ONCOLOGIC DISEASE

HEMATOLOGIC DISORDERS

ANEMIA AND POLYCYTHEMIA: GENERAL CONSIDERATIONS

Chapter 8 discussed the evidence that normovolemic anemia or polycythemia increases perioperative morbidity. Wasserman and Gilbert[545] evaluated two groups of patients undergoing major surgery. Of 28 patients with uncontrolled polycythemia (hemoglobin >16 g/dl), 22 (79 percent) had complications and 10 (36 percent) died. Of 53 patients having controlled polycythemia (hemoglobin <16 g/dl), 15 (28 percent) had complications and 3 (5 percent) died. In both groups, most of the complications were related to polycythemia (for example, hemorrhage or thrombosis). Although this study has deficiencies (e.g., the study was retrospective in design, no time frame of study was given, "minor" surgery was excluded, and no statement was provided as to why polycythemia was controlled preoperatively in some patients and not in others), its results indicate that knowledge and pretreatment of polycythemia might decrease perioperative morbidity and mortality.

No such evidence exists for normovolemic anemia. Rothstein[546] concluded that in children under 3 months of age, hemoglobin should be over 10 g/dl, whereas in older children, hemoglobin was adequate at the 9 g/dl level. For Slogoff,[547] hematocrit of 20 percent (hemoglobin of ~7 g/dl) was adequate for adults. However, no data confirm the hypothesis that treatment of moderate or mild normovolemic anemia prior to surgery decreases perioperative morbidity or mortality. Perhaps the duration of anemia is important also, because, with time, the cardiovascular system adjusts to anemia by increasing cardiac output.[547] Thus, there are no specific preoperative routines for anemia itself.

However, because anemia can be a hallmark of many other diseases possibly affecting perioperative anesthetic management, the presence of anemia preoperatively requires a search for, and treatment of, the underlying cause. For instance, anemia could indicate renal insufficiency or a drug reaction, both of which could alter anesthetic management. For this reason, the cause of anemia should be known preoperatively. Similarly, polycythemia can be a primary disease (such as polycythemia vera) or secondary to smoking, use of diuretic drugs, chronic use of androgens, hypoxia, or other forms of chronic lung/heart disease. Phlebotomies are quite effective for patients whose polycythemia is mild. Recently, cerebral blood flow was shown to improve when hematocrit was kept below 45 percent.[548–550] No prospective controlled study has been performed on humans regarding a possible decrease in perioperative morbidity or wound healing[550,551] from perioperative treatment of anemia or polycythemia. The time of most danger to the patient may be the early recovery room period, during which time oxygen delivery to the lungs is perhaps at its worst (also see Ch. 54). When religious convictions prohibit blood transfusion and the patient is anemic or may become anemic, therapeutic options include autotransfusion[552] and use of blood substitutes.[553] Although the latter have fallen into disrepute because of their effects on reticuloendothelial function, other substitutes probably will become available.[554] This subject is discussed in more detail in Chapter 39.

Several forms of anemia present special situations, such as sickle cell anemia, hereditary spherocytosis, and the autoimmune hemolytic anemias.

SICKLE CELL ANEMIA AND RELATED HEMOGLOBINOPATHIES

The sickle cell syndromes comprise a family of hemoglobinopathies caused by abnormal genetic transformation of amino acids in the heme portion or the hemoglobin molecule.[554-556] A major pathologic feature of sickle cell disease is the aggregation of irreversibly sickled cells in blood vessels. The molecular basis of sickling is aggregation of deoxygenated hemoglobin molecules along their longitudinal axis.[555,556] This abnormal aggregation distorts the cell membrane and produces a sickle shape. Irreversibly sickled cells become dehydrated and rigid and can cause tissue infarcts by impeding blood flow and oxygen to tissues.[557-559] Some other abnormal hemoglobins interact with hemoglobin S to various degrees, giving rise to symptomatic disease in patients heterozygous for hemoglobin S and one of the other hemoglobins such as the hemoglobin of thalassemia (hemoglobin C).

Two-tenths of 1 percent of the black population in America has sickle cell–thalassemia disease (hemoglobin SC); these patients also have end-organ disease and symptoms suggestive of organ infarction. For such patients, perioperative considerations should be similar to those for patients with sickle cell disease (hemoglobin SS), discussed below.

Whereas 8 to 10 percent of American blacks have the sickle cell trait (hemoglobin AS), 0.2 percent are homozygous for the sickle cell hemoglobin and have sickle cell anemia.

The sickle cell trait should not be considered a disease, because hemoglobin AS cells begin to sickle only when oxygen saturation of hemoglobin is below 20 percent. No difference has been found between normal persons (those with hemoglobin AA) and those with hemoglobin AS regarding survival rates or incidence of severe disease, with one exception: patients with hemoglobin AS have a 50 percent increase in pulmonary infarctions. However, single case reports of a perioperative death and a perioperative brain infarct in two patients with hemoglobin AS disease do exist.[560,561]

The pathologic end-organ damage that occurs in sickle cell states is attributable to three processes: the sickling of cells in blood vessels, an occurrence that causes infarcts and consequent tissue destruction secondary to tissue ischemia; hemolytic crisis secondary to hemolysis; and aplastic crises that occur with bone marrow exhaustion and can rapidly result in severe anemia. Logic dictates that patients currently in a crisis should not be operated upon except for extreme emergencies, and then only after exchange transfusion.[559-562]

Since sickling is increased with lowered oxygen tensions, acidosis, hypothermia, and the presence of more desaturated hemoglobin S, current therapy includes keeping the patient warm and well hydrated, giving supplemental oxygen, maintaining high cardiac output, and avoiding creating areas of stasis due to pressure. Meticulous attention to these practices in those periods when we usually do not pay most careful attention (i.e., waiting in the preinduction area) or when gas exchange may be most unmatched to cardiovascular-metabolic demands (early postoperative period) may be important in lessening morbidity. Even following these measures routinely with no special emphasis placed on the periods described reduced mortality to 1 percent in several series of patients with sickle cell syndromes.[559,561,562] Retrospective review of patient charts led the authors of those studies to conclude that, at most, a 0.5 percent mortality rate could be attributed to the interaction between sickle cell anemia and anesthetic agent.

Can this rate be decreased?[563-565] Several authors have advocated using partial exchange transfusions perioperatively. In children with sickle cell anemia and acute lung syndromes, partial exchange transfusion improved clinical symptoms and blood oxygenation. Also, serum bilirubin levels decreased in patients with acute liver injury. Clinical improvement of pneumococcal meningitis and cessation of hematuria in papillary necrosis also accompanied exchange transfusion.[566] The goal of exchange transfusion is to increase the concentration of hemoglobin A to 40 percent and the hematocrit to 35 percent. The 40 percent figure is an arbitrary one, as no controlled studies have established the threshold ratio of hemoglobin A to S that would render blood not able to sickle in vivo. To achieve the 40 percent ratio in a 70-kg adult, about 4 units of washed erythrocytes would have to be exchanged; the system is inexpensive but efficient. The possible decrease in perioperative morbidity after partial exchange transfusion has not been compared with the risks of exchange. Therefore, my recommendation is to pay meticulous attention to avoiding conditions that increase sickling and to limit exchange transfusion to crisis situations. Induction of hyponatremia has recently been shown to abort acute sickle cell crisis; however, this treatment is still experimental.[567]

In thalassemia, globin structures are normal but, because of gene deletion, the rate of synthesis of either the α or β chains of hemoglobin (α- and β-thalassemia, respectively) is reduced.[568] These syndromes are common in Southeast Asia, India, the Middle East, and in individuals of African descent. In thalassemia, facial deformity has been reported to make endotracheal intubation difficult.[568] This one case report has not been amplified upon, and there are no reports of this complication for patients with sickle cell anemia. However, the anemia associated with these syndromes often produces a compensatory hyperplasia of the erythroid marrow, which in turn is associated with severe skeletal abnormalities.[569]

Glucose 6-phosphate dehydrogenase (G6PD) deficiency (a sex-linked recessive trait) is also reported to occur in approximately 8 percent of black American men. A deficiency in this enzyme results in hemolysis of the erythrocyte and formation of Heinz bodies. Red cell hemolysis can also occur after administration of drugs that produce substances requiring G6PD for detoxification (e.g., methemoglobin,

glutathione, and hydrogen peroxide). Drugs to be avoided are sulfa drugs, quinidine, prilocaine, antimalarial drugs, antipyretic drugs, nonnarcotic analgesics, vitamin K analogues, and perhaps sodium nitroprusside.

HEREDITARY SPHEROCYTOSIS, ELLIPTOCYTOSIS, AND AUTOIMMUNE HEMOLYTIC ANEMIAS

Congenital abnormalities of the erythrocyte membrane are becoming better understood. In elliptocytosis and hereditary spherocytosis, the membrane is more permeable to cations and more susceptible to lipid loss when cell energy is depleted than is the membrane of the normal red blood cell. Both hereditary spherocytosis (present in 1 in 5,000 people) and hereditary elliptocytosis are inherited as autosomal dominant traits. In both, defects in the membrane are thought to result from mutation of spectrin, a structural protein of the membrane cytoskeleton.[570] Although the therapeutic role of splenectomy in these diseases is not fully defined, in severe disease, splenectomy is known to improve the shortened lifespan of the red blood cell 100 percent (from 20 to 30 days to 40 to 70 days). Because splenectomy does predispose the patient to gram-positive septicemia (particularly pneumococcal), perhaps patients should be given pneumococcal vaccine preoperatively prior to predictable bacteremic events. No specific problems relating to anesthesia have been reported for these disorders.

The autoimmune hemolytic anemias include cold antibody anemia, warm antibody anemia (idiopathic), and drug-induced anemias.[571,572] The cold antibody hemolytic anemias are mediated by immunoglobulin M or G antibodies, which, at room temperature and below cause red blood cells to clump. When these patients are given blood transfusions, the cells and all fluid infusions must be warm, and body temperature must be maintained meticulously at 37°C if hemolysis is to be avoided. Warm antibody (or "idiopathic" hemolytic anemia) is a difficult management problem characterized by chronic anemia, the presence of antibodies active against red blood cells, positive Coombs' test, and difficulty in cross-matching blood. For patients undergoing elective surgery, autologous transfusions and blood from rare Rh-negative red blood cell donors and/or the patient's first-degree relatives can be used. In emergency situations, the possibility of autotransfusions, splenectomy, or corticosteroid treatment should be discussed with a hematologist knowledgeable in this area. Drug-induced anemias have three mechanisms: receptor-type hemolysis, in which a drug (e.g., penicillin) binds to the membrane of the red blood cell, and the complex stimulates formation of an antibody against the complex; "innocent bystander" hemolysis, in which a drug (e.g., esquinidine, sulfuramide) binds to a plasma protein, thereby stimulating an antibody (IgM) that crossreacts with an erythrocyte; and autoimmune hemolysis, in which the drug stimulates production of an antibody (IgG) that crossreacts with the erythrocyte. Drug-induced hemolytic anemias generally cease when drug therapy ends. In emergency situations, the least incompatible cells available should be used for blood transfusion.

GRANULOCYTOPENIA

In patients who have fewer than 500 granulocytes/ml blood and established sepsis, granulocyte transfusion has been shown to prolong life.[573,574] One study has questioned this finding.[575] Although logic might appear to dictate giving granulocyte transfusions prophylactically to patients with fewer than 500 granulocytes/ml blood who will undergo bacteremic events, the effectiveness of this practice has not been studied extensively and is controversial.[576]

PLATELET DISORDERS

Although inherited platelet disorders are rare, acquired disorders are quite common. Both conditions cause skin and mucosal bleeding, whereas defects in plasma coagulation produce deep tissue bleeding or delayed bleeding. Perioperative treatment of inherited platelet

disorders (Glanzmann's thrombasthenia, Bernard-Souliep syndrome, Hermansky-Pudlak syndrome) consists of platelet transfusions. The much more common acquired disorders may respond to one of several therapies. Immune thrombocytopenias, such as those associated with lupus erythematosus, idiopathic thrombocytopenic purpura, uremia, hemolytic-uremic syndrome, and thrombocytosis may respond to steroids, splenectomy, platelet-pheresis, or alkylating agents, or may require platelet transfusions.[576–579] By far the largest number of platelet abnormalities consist of drug-related defects in the aggregation and release of platelets. Aspirin irreversibly acetylates platelet cyclooxygenase, the enzyme that converts arachidonic acid to prostaglandin endoperoxidases. Because cyclooxygenase is not regenerated in the circulation within the lifespan of the platelet, and because this enzyme is essential for the aggregation of platelets, one aspirin may affect platelet function for a week. All other drugs that inhibit platelet function (vitamin E, indomethacin, sulfinpyrazone, dipyrimadole, tricyclic antidepressant drugs, phenothiazines, furosemide, steroids) do not irreversibly inhibit cyclooxygenase function; thus, these drugs disturb platelet function for only 24 to 48 hours. If emergency surgery is needed before the customary 8-day period for platelet regeneration after aspirin, or if the 2-day period for other drugs has not elapsed, administration of 2 to 5 units of platelet concentrates will return platelet function in a 70-kg adult to an adequate level and platelet-induced clotting dysfunction to normal.[580–582] Only 30,000 to 50,000 normally functioning platelets/mm^3 are needed for normal clotting. One platelet transfusion will increase the platelet count from 4,000 to 20,000/ml blood; platelet half-life is about 8 hours.[580–582]

HEMOPHILIA AND RELATED CLOTTING DISORDERS

Abnormalities in blood coagulation owing to defects in plasma coagulation factor are either inherited or acquired. Inherited disorders include X-linked hemophilia A (a defect in Factor VIII activity), von Willebrand's disease (defect in von Willebrand's component of Factor VIII), hemophilia B (a sex-linked deficiency of Factor IX activity), and other less common disorders. The sex-linked origin of these disorders means that hemophilia occurs almost exclusively in male offspring of female carriers; men do not transmit the disease to their male offspring. In elective surgery, levels of the deficient coagulation factor should be assayed 48 hours before surgery and the level restored to 40 percent of normal before surgery. One unit of factor concentrate per kilogram of body weight normally increases factor concentration by 2 percent. Thus, in the individual essentially devoid of activity, administration of 20 units/kg body weight would be required as an initial dose. Since half-life is 6 to 10 hours for Factor VIII and 8 to 16 hours for Factor IX, one should give approximately 1.5 units/hr/kg of Factor VIII or 1.5 units/2 hr/kg of Factor IX. Additional administration of Factors VIII and IX should be guided by the activity of the clotting factors for about 6 to 10 days postoperatively.[583–587]

These factors are available in various preparations: cryoprecipitate, which contains 20 units/ml, is obtained from regular donors (the risk of hepatitis being 1:200 for 5-ml lots) or from fresh-frozen plasma (which contains 1 unit/ml). Some risk of transmitting hepatitis and AIDS accompanies these transfusions.[588,589] Factor IX, but not Factor VIII, is contained in prothrombin complex concentrates; however, these concentrates may contain activated clotting factors, leading to disseminated intravascular clotting and a high risk of hepatitis. In addition, although ϵ-aminocaproic acid or tranexamic acid (0.5 mg/kg) is sometimes administered as fibrinolytic inhibitors, these substances carry with them a significant risk of disseminated intravascular coagulation. Additional hazards of modern therapy include acute and chronic hepatitis, AIDS, hypersensitivity reactions; psychic trauma, chronic pain with narcotic addiction, and inhibition of factors, especially VIII.

Approximately 10 percent of patients with either hemophilia A or B develop an antibody that inactivates Factors VIII or IX (fresh-frozen plasma fails to increase clotting factor activity after incubation with the patient's plasma). These acquired anticoagulants are usually composed of immunoglobulin G, are poorly removed by plasmapheresis, and are variably responsive to immunosuppressive drugs. Use of prothrombin complex concentrates can be life-saving but carries the risk of disseminated intravascular coagulation and hepatitis.

Vitamin K deficiency is discussed in the section on liver disease. To review, vitamin K-dependent clotting factors (II, VII, IX, and X) require vitamin K for the postsynthetic addition of γ-carboxyl groups to glutamate residues; administration of vitamin K or fresh-frozen plasma can correct these deficiencies.

Patients who come to the operating room having received many units of blood (as in massive GI bleeding) may have deficient clotting. This impaired clotting is caused initially by depletion of platelets (which occurs after approximately 10 to 15 units of blood have been given and later, by depletion of coagulation factors (see Ch. 39).[590,591] Treatment of these deficiencies can be corrected with platelet concentrates (each concentrate is normally suspended in 50 ml of fresh plasma; thus, coagulation factors are also replaced).

Urokinase and streptokinase have been used to treat pulmonary embolism, deep-vein thrombosis, and arterial occlusive disease. Both enzymes accelerate the lysis of thrombi and emboli, in contrast to heparin, which may prevent but not dissolve a thrombus. Bleeding complications associated with these two fibrinolytic agents result from dissolution of hemostatic plugs and can be quickly reversed by discontinuing the medication and replenishing plasma fibrinogen with cryoprecipitate or plasma. However, cryoprecipitate and plasma are seldom needed preoperatively because the fibrinolytic activity or urokinase and streptokinase usually dissipates within an hour of discontinuing their administration.

The problem of patients on oral anticoagulants is discussed in the cardiovascular section of this chapter. Regional anesthetic techniques might be avoided in patients given anticoagulant drugs.[252–257] Whether these regional techniques should also be avoided in patients treated prophylactically with low-dose subcutaneous heparin has not been studied.[592] The effects of heparin sulfate can be reversed by titrating protamine, using activated clotting time as a guide. Our group usually gives approximately 1 mg of protamine per 3 to 4 mg of heparin administered within the last 8 hours. Pharmacologic research is searching for specific molecular subtypes of heparin that have different anticoagulant potency, binding affinities for antithrombin III, antithrombotic effects, and platelet aggregating effects. The search is for a "new" heparin preparation that will block thrombosis without causing clinical bleeding. Such a development might change our ways of monitoring clotting function. Determining bleeding time, platelet count, partial thromboplastin time (PTT) and prothrombin time will identify almost all problems in the patient with a suspected clotting or bleeding disorder (also see Ch. 39). As explained in Chapter 8, these screening tests probably should not be obtained in asymptomatic patients.

ONCOLOGIC DISEASE

Patients with malignant tumors may be otherwise healthy or desperately ill with nutritional, neurologic, metabolic, endocrinologic, electrolyte, cardiac, pulmonary, renal, hepatic, hematologic, or pharmacologic disabilities. Thus, determining the other disabilities accompanying malignant tumors requires evaluating all systems. Abnormalities frequently accompanying such tumors include hypercalcemia either by direct bone invasion or by ectopic elaboration of parathyroid hormone or other bone-dissolving substance, uric acid nephropathy, hyponatremia (especially with small cell, or oat cell, carcinoma of the lung), nausea, vomiting, anorexia and cachexia, fever, tumor-induced hypoglycemia, intracranial metastases (10 to 20 percent of all cancers), peripheral nerve or spinal cord disorders, meningeal carcinomatosis, toxic neuropathies secondary to anticancer therapy, and paraneoplastic neurologic syndromes (dermatomyositis, Eaton-Lambert syndrome, myopathies, and distal neuropathies). Many patients with malignant tumors are given large doses of analgesics and should be kept comfortable during the perioperative period; avoiding drug dependence is of no practical importance in terminally ill patients.[593-595] Marijuana (tetrahydro-

cannabinol) depresses the CNS vomiting center and may be more effective than the phenothiazines or butyrophenones in suppressing nausea associated with cancer and its therapy; it decreases anesthetic requirements 15 to 30 percent.[596]

The toxicity of cancer chemotherapy relates to the agents used and to the dose. For radiation therapy, damage occurs when the following doses are exceeded: lungs, 1,500 rad; kidneys, 2,400 rad; heart, 3,000 rad; spinal cord, 4,000 rad; intestine, 5,500 rad; brain, 6,000 rad; and bone, 7,500 rad. Alkylating agents cause bone marrow depression, including thrombocytopenia, alopecia, hemorrhagic cystitis, nausea, and vomiting. The antineoplastic alkaloids vincristine and vinblastine produce, respectively, peripheral neuropathies and SIADH and myelotoxicity. Nitrosoureas can cause severe hepatic and renal damage, as well as bone marrow toxicity, myalgias, and paresthesia. Folic acid analogues, such as methotrexate (MTX) produce bone marrow depression, ulcerative stomatitis, pulmonary interstitial infiltrates, GI toxicity, and occasionally severe liver dysfunction. Fluorouracil (5-FU) and floxuridine (FUDR), both pyrimidine analogues, cause bone marrow toxicity, megaloblastic anemia, nervous system dysfunction, and hepatic and GI alterations. Purine analogues (mercaptopurine, thioquanine) have bone marrow depression as their primary toxic effect. Anthracycline antibiotics (doxorubicin, daunorubicin, mithramycin, mitomycin C, bleomycin) can all cause pulmonary infiltrates, cardiomyopathies (especially doxorubicin and daunorubicin), myelotoxicity, and GI hepatic, and renal disturbances.

The wisdom of anesthetizing patients given bleomycin has been questioned. A retrospective study by Goldiner et al.[597] reported postoperative deaths in five consecutive patients given bleomycin. All five patients died of postoperative respiratory failure. Using the same anesthetic technique, Goldiner et al.[597] then anesthetized 12 patients, limited the inspired oxygen concentration to 22 to 25 percent perioperatively, and replaced much of the blood loss with colloids rather than crystalloids. None of the 12 patients died. These investigators postulated that bleomycin caused epithelial cell edema that progressed to necrosis of type I alveolar cells, fluid leakage into the alveolar space, and formation of "hyaline membranes" similar to that occurring in oxygen toxicity.[599] Goldiner et al. believe that this pathophysiologic similarity indicates a possible synergistic relationship between oxygen and bleomycin. However, LaMantia and co-workers[598] retrospectively analyzed charts of 16 patients undergoing surgery after bleomycin therapy. Thirteen patients were given oxygen at inspired concentrations of 37 to 45 percent. No instances of postoperative respiratory failure occurred. Thus, data are currently available to support all practices regarding oxygen administration to patients given bleomycin. My preference is to keep inspired oxygen concentrations at the lowest level providing adequate tissue oxygenation. When in doubt about side effects in patients undergoing cancer chemotherapy, my practice is to seek advice from two experts.

PATIENTS GIVEN DRUG THERAPY FOR CHRONIC AND ACUTE MEDICAL CONDITIONS

A steadily increasing number of potent drugs are being used to treat disease; the average hospitalized patient takes 10 drugs. Many drugs have side effects that might make anesthesia more risky or patient management more difficult. Knowing the pharmacologic properties and potential side effects of commonly used drugs helps the anesthesiologist avoid pitfalls during anesthesia and surgery. The first step in avoiding such pitfalls is to obtain a drug history from the patient. Then, for every drug, medicine, and over-the-counter preparation the patient is using, the anesthesiologist should know the name, classification of drug, diseases and conditions for which it is prescribed, and common side effects. Having such knowledge before surgery helps one to avoid making mistakes that can turn minor side effects into life-threatening situations. If necessary, the anes-

thesiologist should return to the patient's bedside to search for signs or symptoms of these effects. Unnecessary drugs should be discontinued for at least five half-lives of the drugs. This period should be longer if metabolites of the drug have activity and longer half-lives. For needed or beneficial drugs, the optimal dose should be determined in consultation with the treating physician; the optimal dose is that which maximizes the ratio of therapeutic value to risk of drug toxicity. Drug side effects should be sought and either corrected preoperatively or at least planned for in anesthetic management. For instance, if a patient is made hypokalemic with diuretic drugs, hypokalemia might be corrected before surgery or, at the very minimum, hyperventilation could be avoided during surgery (see earlier section on hypokalemia). This type of reasoning and planning is best done at least 1 week before surgery. Ideally, the surgeon, internist, and anesthesiologist should communicate regarding these topics well in advance of surgery. Understanding the side effects of chronic drug therapy that affect the sympathetic nervous system requires some knowledge of basic pharmacologic characteristics of the sympathetic nervous system.[600,601]

PHARMACOLOGIC PROCESSES IN THE SYMPATHETIC NERVOUS SYSTEM

The autonomic nervous system is discussed in detail in Chapter 28. A sympathetic neuron consists of a cell body and its nucleus, a long axon, and many nerve terminals. Enzymes responsible for synthesizing dopamine, norepinephrine, and epinephrine are made in the cell body, transported by a tube system (rapid axoplasmic transport) down the axon to the terminal where the neurotransmitters are made, and then stored in granules (Fig. 9-8). The sympathetic neuron makes neurotransmitters from either phenylalanine or tyrosine. Tyrosine hydroxylase, the rate-limiting enzyme, aids in converting tyrosine to dopa, which is decarboxylated by 1-aromatic acid decarboxylase to dopamine. Dopamine is taken up into granules, where it remains in that form

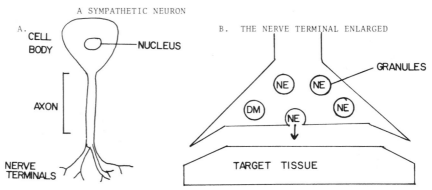

FIG. 9-8 A sympathetic neuron consists of (A) a cell body and its nucleus, a long axon, and (B) multiple nerve terminals. Enzymes responsible for the synthesis of dopamine (DM), norepinephrine (NE), and epinephrine are made in the cell body, transported by a tube system (rapid axoplasmic transport) down the axes to the terminal where the transmitters are made, and stored in granules. (Modified from Axelrod J: Neurotransmitters. Scientific American 230:58, 1974.)

or is converted by dopamine-α-hydroxylase to norepinephrine. The granules are little packets of neurotransmitters whose contents are released when an action potential reaches the nerve endings. In some nerve endings (and in the adrenal medulla), norepinephrine leaves the granules, is methylated in the cytoplasm to epinephrine, and then reenters a different group of intracellular granules.

Norepinephrine, dopamine, and epinephrine exert their physiologic effect by interacting with an appropriate receptor at the target tissue. The three major kinds of catecholamine receptors are α-adrenergic, β-adrenergic, and dopaminergic. These receptors are subdivided as follows:

α_1—stimulation constricts vascular smooth muscle and thus increases peripheral vascular resistance.

α_2—stimulation inhibits the release of norepinephrine itself (constituting negative feedback to the sympathetic neuron).

β_1—stimulation increases heart rate and the strength of cardiac contractions.

β_2—stimulation causes dilation of smooth muscles of the blood vessels and airway; relaxation of uterine smooth muscle; and a variety of endocrine effects, including secretion of renin.

β_3—stimulation results in a greater release of norepinephrine from the sympathetic neuron (constituting positive feedback to the sympathetic neuron).

Dopamine—stimulation causes dilation of renal blood vessels and may inhibit the release of acetylcholine.

These different effects may be caused by slight differences in receptor conformations.

The action of sympathomimetic substances is terminated through an unusual process: the nerve ending recaptures most norepinephrine from the target tissue using an active reuptake system (Fig. 9-9). Obviously, blockage of this system permits more norepinephrine to remain free to cause physiologic effects. In ad-

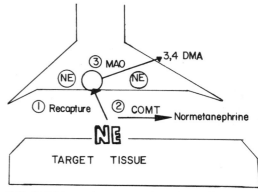

FIG. 9-9 The action of norepinephrine (NE) is terminated primarily through recapture of norepinephrine from the target tissue (i.e., recycling of NE back into the granules of the nerve terminal). The action of NE can also be terminated by metabolism of NE by catechol-O-methyltransferase (COMT) and/or monoamine oxidase (MAO).

dition to this reuptake system, two enzymes transform catecholamines metabolically: monamine oxidase (MAO) and catechol-O-methyltransferase (COMT) (Fig. 9-9).

ANTIHYPERTENSIVE DRUGS

Many antihypertensive agents and almost all mind-altering drugs affect sympathetic neuronal storage, uptake, metabolism, or release of neurotransmitters. For instance, the antihypertensive drug reserpine depletes the granules of norepinephrine, epinephrine, and dopamine in both the brainstem and periphery. The depletion of transmitters in sympathetic nerve endings renders drugs such as ephedrine and metaraminol ineffective, since such drugs act primarily by releasing catecholamines (Fig. 9-10). Guanethidine depletes granular norepinephrine and affects only the peripheral sympathetic system. In amounts used clinically, reserpine decreases MAC 20 to 30 percent, whereas guanethidine has no effect on anesthetic requirements.[168] In addition to causing a lack of response to indirectly acting vasopressors, reserpine may cause a denervation supersensitivity and hyperresponsiveness (with hypertension and/or tachycardia) to the usual doses of direct-acting sympathetic amines, such as phenylephrine (Neo-Synephrine™), isoproterenol, norepinephrine, epinephrine, and dopamine.[600–602] Thus, in patients who have been treated with drugs that alter sympathetic neurotransmitter release, uptake, metabolism, or receptor function, some problems

may occur: hypotension, hypertension, and/or bradycardia should be treated by titrating doses of direct-acting vasoconstrictors, such as phenylephrine (Neo-Synephrine™); vasodilators, such as nitroprusside; or chronotropic drugs, such as atropine, isoproterenol, or dopamine.

Another group of antihypertensive agents are the "false neurotransmitters." False neurotransmitters replace norepinephrine in the granules at the nerve ending. α-Methyldopa (Aldomet) becomes α-methyldopamine, which is further metabolized to α-methylnorepinephrine (Fig. 9-11). In some nerve endings and for some receptors, α-methyldopamine or α-methylnorepinephrine is more potent than dopamine or norepinephrine as dopaminergic or α-adrenergic receptor stimulants. However, at most nerve endings, the false neurotransmitters are less potent stimulants, and this lesser degree of stimulation is one means by which their antihypertensive action is produced. Alternately, α-methyldopa may act by stimulating the brainstem sympathetic nervous system. When this system antagonizes the peripheral sympathetic nervous system, the activity of the latter decreases and blood pressure is reduced. Through its central effect, α-methyldopa decreases anesthetic requirements 20 to 40 percent.[168]

In addition to altering the response to exogenously administered vasopressors, these neurotransmitter-depleting drugs can also produce side effects: psychic depression, nightmares, drowsiness, nasal stuffiness, diarrhea, bradycardia, and orthostatic hypotension with impotence (reserpine). Guanethidine can cause orthostatic hypotension, bradycardia, asthma,

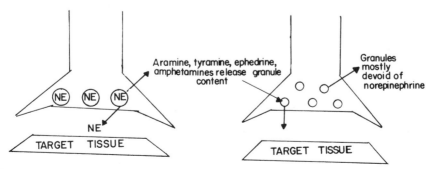

FIG. 9-10 Antihypertensive drugs such as metaraminol (Aramine), tyramine, and ephedrine release catecholamines from the granules of the nerve terminal. Therefore, if little norepinephrine (NE) is left within the granules (as after treatment with methyldopa, reserpine, or guanethidine), little norepinephrine is released.

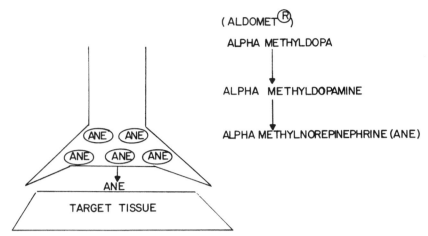

FIG. 9-11 In the granules of the nerve terminal, α-methyldopa (Aldomet) is converted enzymatically to α-methyldopamine by the same enzyme that converts dopa to dopamine. α-Methyldopamine is converted to α-methylnorepinephrine by the same enzyme that converts dopamine to norepinephrine.

diarrhea, and inhibition of ejaculation. α-Methyldopa is associated with drowsiness, orthostatic hypotension, bradycardia, diarrhea, acute or chronic hepatitis, cirrhosis, and autoimmune hemolytic anemia (i.e., positive Coombs' test).[603]

Catecholamine or sympathetic receptor blocking drugs affect the three major types of catecholamine receptors: α-adrenergic, β-adrenergic, and dopaminergic. The existence of subdivisions (e.g., β_1, β_2) suggested the possibility that some drugs would be found to affect only one set of receptors. For example, terbutaline is used more frequently than isoproterenol because terbutaline is said to exert a preferential effect on β_2-receptors (i.e., to dilate bronchial smooth muscle), thereby avoiding the cardiac stimulation produced by drugs that stimulate β_1-receptors. In fact, selectivity is dose related. At a certain dose, a direct β_2-receptor stimulating drug will affect only those receptors, but at a higher dose will stimulate both β_1- and β_2-receptors. The effect of a given dose varies with each patient. A certain dose may stimulate β_1- and β_2-receptors in one patient but neither receptor in another patient. More and more selective blocking drugs are being developed in hopes of widening the margin between β_1- and β_2- and α-adrenergic effects. However, ultimately, more selectivity is desired than even this. It would be advantageous to be able to decrease heart rate without changing myocardial contractility, or to increase contractility without changing heart rate. Such is the goal of much drug research and of the development of dobutamine (see Chs. 28 and 33). However, to date, all such selectivity appears to be dose related, even for dobutamine.[604]

Metoprolol (Lopressor) and atenolol (Tenormin) (both β_1-adrenergic receptor blocking drugs) and propranolol, timolol, and nadolol are the only widely available β-adrenergic receptor blocking drugs used for chronic therapy in the United States. Because nadolol has poor lipid solubility, it has a long elimination half-life (17 to 24 hours) and does not cross the blood-brain barrier readily. Although, nadolol should be associated with fewer CNS side effects such as fatigue, nightmares, and depression, we do not know that definitely yet. The ability to use it on a once daily basis should increase patient compliance. Although selective β-adrenergic receptor blocking drugs should be more appropriate in patients with increased airway resistance or diabetes, this advantage is apparent only when low doses are used. The use of β-adrenergic receptor blocking drugs has become widespread, as these drugs treat everything from angina and hypertension to priapism and stage fright. They appear to decrease morbidity and mortality in patients who have initially survived myocardial infarction.[605–607]

At present, propranolol is the standard for β-adrenergic receptor blocking drugs. Smulyan et al.[608] studied the problems of adult patients on long-term propranolol hydrochloride therapy who must undergo abdominal surgery. Because such patients cannot take oral medications postoperatively for many days, they must be protected against perioperative sympathetic stimulation and the propranolol withdrawal syndrome. A continuous intravenous infusion of propranolol (3 mg/hr, regardless of the patient's weight) given postoperatively accomplished these goals: postoperative serum propranolol levels and β-adrenergic receptor blockade returned to their "usual" preoperative levels. The hypotensive and bradycardic effects of propranolol and general anesthesia appear to be additive.[609] Propranolol does not affect anesthetic requirements.[610]

α-Adrenergic-receptor blocking drugs include phentolamine, prazosin, phenoxybenzamine, the phenothiazines, and the butyrophenones (such as droperidol). Dopaminergic receptor antagonists include the antischizophrenic medicines (phenothiazines and butyrophenones). The receptor-blocking drugs inhibit the action of sympathomimetic drugs at the receptor in a dose-related fashion. Thus, propranolol lowers blood pressure by blocking the tendency of norepinephrine and epinephrine to increase the rate and force of the contractions of the heart (and perhaps also their tendency to increase the secretion of renin). To overcome this blockade, one need only to provide more β-receptor stimulating drug. Thus, high doses of vasopressors may be needed to increase blood pressure in a patient given large doses of propranolol.

When administration of β-adrenergic receptor blocking drugs is terminated, sympathetic stimulation often increases, as if the body had responded to the presence of these drugs by increasing sympathetic neuron activity. Thus, propranolol withdrawal can be accompanied by a hyper-β-adrenergic condition that increases myocardial oxygen demands. Administering propranolol or metoprolol can cause bradycardia, CHF, fatigue, dizziness, depression, psychoses, bronchospasm, and Peyronie's disease.[603] Side effects of the dopaminergic receptor blocking drugs are discussed later in this chapter.

Prazosin (Minipress) is an α_1-adrenergic receptor blocking drug used to treat both hypertension and ischemic cardiomyopathy because it dilates both veins and arteries. It is associated with vertigo, palpitations, depression, dizziness, weakness, and anticholinergic effects.

Brainstem sympathomimetic drugs stimulate α-adrenergic receptors in the brainstem. Clonidine (Catapres), a drug with a half-life of 12 to 24 hours, is an α_2-adrenergic receptor stimulant. Presumably, clonidine lowers blood pressure through the central brainstem adrenergic stimulation referred to previously. It may also be used to treat opiate and tobacco withdrawal. Occasionally, withdrawal from clonidine can precipitate a sudden hypertensive crisis—analogous to that occurring on withdrawal from propranolol—causing a hyper-β-adrenergic condition. The degree of hypertensive crisis following clonidine withdrawal is now being debated. (Although intravenous clonidine is not available in the United States, a skin paste of clonidine is under FDA review.) Tricyclic antidepressant drugs, and presumably phenothiazines and the butyrophenones, interfere with the action of clonidine. Although administering a butyrophenone (e.g., droperidol) to a patient given clonidine chronically could theoretically precipitate a hypertensive crisis, none has been reported. Clonidine administration can be accompanied by drowsiness, dry mouth, orthostatic hypotension, bradycardia, and impotence. In dogs, acute clonidine administration decreases anesthetic requirements by 40 to 60 percent; chronic administration decreases requirements by 10 to 20 percent.[611,612]

Three other classes of antihypertensive drugs affect the sympathetic nervous system indirectly: diuretic drugs, arteriolar dilators, and slow (calcium) channel-blocking agents. Thiazide diuretic drugs are associated with hypochloremic alkalosis, hypokalemia, hyperglycemia, hyperuricemia, and hypercalcemia. The potassium-sparing diuretic drug spironolactone is associated with hyperkalemia, hyponatremia, gynecomastia, and impotence. All diuretic drugs can cause dehydration. The thiazide diuretics and furosemide appear to prolong neuromuscular blockade.[613] The arteriolar dilator hydralazine can cause a lupuslike condition (usually with renal involvement), nasal congestion, headache, dizziness, congestive heart failure, angina, and GI disturbances.

The slow-channel calcium ion antagonists (also called calcium channel blocking drugs) inhibit the transmembrane influx of calcium ions into cardiac and vascular smooth muscle. Such inhibition reduces heart rate (negative chronotropy), depresses contractility (negative inotropy), decreases conduction velocity (negative dromotropy), and dilates coronary, cerebral, and systemic arterioles (Fig. 9-12).[614] Verapamil, diltiazem, and nifedipine all produce such effects, but to varying degrees, and apparently by similar but different mechanisms.[615] Nifedipine is the most potent of the three as a smooth muscle dilator, while verapamil and diltiazem have negatively dromotropic and inotropic effects and vasodilating properties.

Diltiazem has weak vasodilating properties as compared with nifedipine and has less atrioventricular conduction effect than does verapamil. Thus, verapamil and diltiazem can increase the P-R interval and produce atrioventricular block. In fact, reflex activation of the sympathetic nervous system may be necessary during administration of diltiazem, and especially during verapamil therapy, to maintain normal conduction. Clearly, verapamil and diltiazem must be titrated very carefully when a patient is already taking a β-adrenergic receptor blocking drug,[616] or when adding β-blocking drugs to the patient already taking verapamil or diltiazem.

The use of calcium channel blocking drugs has several important implications for anesthetic management.[614,617-637] First, the effects of inhalational and narcotic anesthetic agents and

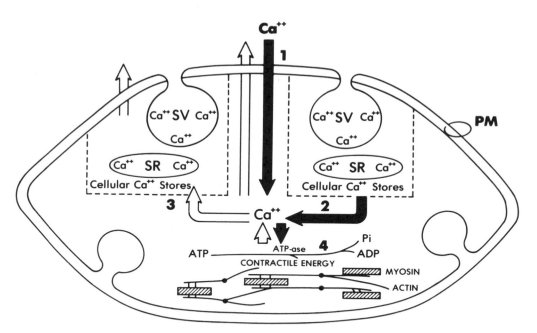

FIG. 9-12 Schematic drawing of smooth muscle cell showing calcium flux and possible sites of interference by halothane and nifedipine. The concentration of calcium (Ca^{++}) in the cytoplasm increases (black arrows) because of entry through the plasma membrane (PM) and release from surface vesicles (SV) or the sarcoplasmic reticulum (SR). When the concentration of cytoplasmic Ca^{++} is sufficiently high, ATP is activated. The splitting of ATP by ATPase provides the interaction and contraction of actin filaments and myosin particles constituting muscle fibers. The concentration of cytoplasmic Ca^{++} decreases (white arrows) with the return of Ca^{++} to cellular stores and the extracellular transport of Ca^{++}. Both halothane and nifedipine probably (1) inhibit the entry of Ca^{++} and (2) may also interfere with cytoplasmic Ca^{++} flux by reducing the release of Ca^{++} by the SR, by (3) reducing storage and reuptake, or by (4) blocking ATPase and/or the contractile mechanism. (Tosone SR, Reves JG, Kissin I, et al: Hemodynamic responses to nifedipine in dogs anesthetized with halothane. Anesth Analg 62:903, 1983.)

of nifedipine in decreasing systemic vascular resistance, blood pressure, and contractility may be additive.[614,619,621,623] Similarly, verapamil and anesthetics (inhalational anesthetics, nitrous oxide, and narcotics) increase atrioventricular conduction times and additively decrease blood pressure, systemic vascular resistance, and contractility.[617-619,623,625,627] Second, verapamil, and presumably the other calcium channel blocking drugs, have been found to decrease anesthetic requirements by 25 percent.[620] These agents can produce neuromuscular blockade; potentiate both depolarizing and nondepolarizing neuromuscular blocking drugs; and, in at least one type of myopathy (Duchenne's muscular dystrophy), can even precipitate respiratory failure.[630-634] Finally, since slow-channel activation of calcium is necessary to cause spasms of cerebral and coronary vessels, bronchoconstriction, and normal platelet aggregation, these drugs may have a role in treating ischemia of the nervous system, bronchoconstriction, and unwanted clotting disorders perioperatively.[628,633,635,636] All three drugs are highly protein bound and may displace or be displaced by other drugs that are also highly protein bound (e.g., lidocaine, bupivacaine, diazepam, disopyramide, and propranolol).[636] Adverse consequences can be minimized by titrating inhalational or narcotic agent to hemodynamic and anesthetic effects. By monitoring for side effects, the anesthetist can prevent side effects from becoming serious (S. Slogoff and co-workers, personal communication). Hemodynamic, but not electrophysio-ministering calcium.[637] Reversal of electrophysiologic effects may occur if industrial doses of beta adrenergic agonists are given.

MOOD-ALTERING DRUGS

Mood-altering drugs are the most frequently prescribed medications in the United States. They include MAO inhibitors (Fig. 9-9), phenothiazines, tricyclic antidepressant drugs, and drugs of abuse such as cocaine.

Monoamine oxidase inhibitors — isocarboxazide (Marplan), phenelzine (Nardil), pargyline (Eutonyl), and tranylcypromine (Parnate) — irreversibly bind to the enzyme MAO and thereby increase intraneuronal levels of amine neurotransmitters (serotonin, norepinephrine, dopamine, epinephrine, octopamine). This increase is associated with both an antidepressant and antihypertensive effect. Interactions between MAO inhibitors and a variety of foods and drugs containing indirectly acting sympathomimetic substances such as ephedrine or tyramine (found especially in the aged cheeses) can occur for as long as 2 weeks after the last dose of MAO inhibitor is given. The most serious effects of this interaction are convulsions, and hyperpyrexic coma (especially after narcotics). Anesthetic management for a patient given an MAO inhibitor can be chaotic: for this reason it is widely accepted practice to discontinue MAO inhibitors at least 2 to 3 weeks before any planned operation.[638-642] Emergency surgery on patients given MAO inhibitors can be punctuated by hemodynamic instability. Regional block can be attempted as treatment for postoperative pain to avoid having to give narcotics. Case reports of hyperpyrexic coma following administration of most narcotics exist in humans, and animal studies document a 10 to 50 percent incidence of hyperpyrexic coma in animals pretreated with MAO inhibitors that were then given a variety of narcotics.[375,638-641] These reactions appear to be treated best using therapy supporting vital functions.

Alternate drugs for the treatment of severe depression include the tricyclic antidepressant drugs: amitriptyline (Elavil, Endep), imipramine (Imavate, Tofranil, Presamine), desipramine (Norpramine), doxepin (Adapin, Sinequan), and nortriptyline (Aventyl). Tricyclic antidepressant drugs block the reuptake of neurotransmitters and cause their acute release. If given chronically, these drugs decrease noradrenergic catecholamine stores. Tricyclic antidepressant drugs also produce side effects similar to those produced by atropine (dry mouth, tachycardia, delirium, urinary retention) and can cause ECG changes (changes in T wave, prolongation of the QRS complex, bundle branch block or other conduction abnormalities, or premature ventricular contractions). Although dysrhythmias induced by tricyclic antidepressants have been treated successfully with physostigmine, bradycardia has sometimes occurred.[643] Drug interactions with tricyclic antidepressants include those related to the blockade of the reuptake of norepinephrine (such as interference with the action of guanethidine) and fatal dysrhythmias after halothane and pancuronium.[644,645] Such interactions, although predictable for a population of patients, may not alter an individual's threshold for dysrhythmias.

The effectiveness of phenothiazines and butyrophenones in schizophrenia suggests a dopamine-receptor blocking action. In addition, these drugs possess varying degrees of parasympathetic stimulation and ability to block α-adrenergic receptors. The phenothiazines include chlorpromazine (Thorazine, Chlor-PZ), promazine (Sparine), triflupromazine (Vesprin), fluphenazine (Prolixin), trifluoperazine, prochlorperazine (Compazine), and many others. The butyrophenones include droperidol and haloperidol (Haldol). Both phenothiazines and butyrophenones produce sedation, depression, and antihistaminic, antiemetic, and hypothermic responses. They are also associated with cholestatic jaundice, impotence, dystonia, and photosensitivity. Other side effects associated with phenothiazines include orthostatic hypotension (partly due to α-adrenergic blockade) and ECG abnormalities, such as prolongation of the Q-T or P-R intervals, blunting of T waves, depression of the S-T segment, and on rare occasion, premature ventricular contractions and Torsades du Pointes.[643,646-648]

Several important drug interactions are noteworthy for the phenothiazine derivatives. The effects of CNS depressants (especially narcotics and barbiturates) are enhanced by concomitant administration of phenothiazines. Also, CNS seizure threshold is lowered by administration of phenothiazines which should be avoided in patients who are epileptic or withdrawing from any drug that depresses the CNS. The antihypertensive effects of guanethidine are blocked by tricyclic antidepressant drugs and phenothiazines.[603] Lithium carbonate is used to treat manic depression; it is more effective in preventing mania than in relieving depression. In excitable cells, lithium mimics sodium, decreasing the release of neurotransmitters both centrally and peripherally. Lithium prolongs neuromuscular blockade,[649,650] and may decrease anesthetic requirements because it blocks brainstem release of norepinephrine, epinephrine, and dopamine.

Psychoactive drugs such as amphetamines and cocaine acutely release norepinephrine, epinephrine, and dopamine and block their reuptake. When taken chronically, they deplete the nerve endings of these neurotransmitters.

Drugs that appear to increase central α-adrenergic release increase anesthetic requirement, whereas drugs that appear to decrease central α-adrenergic release decrease anesthetic requirements. (This may not be the mechanism by which they alter anesthetic requirement, but it is a convenient way of remembering the alteration.) Drugs that affect only the β-adrenergic receptors do not alter anesthetic requirements.[168,610-612,651,652]

SYMPATHOMIMETIC DRUGS
(Also See Ch. 28)

Many antiasthmatic drugs (bronchodilators) such as terbutaline, aminophylline, and theophylline are sympathomimetic drugs that can interact with the volatile anesthetics to cause cardiac dysrhythmias. Halothane (and to some degree most other volatile anesthetics) sensitizes the myocardium to exogenous catecholamines.[653-656] Sensitization means that the minimum dose of exogenous epinephrine administered intravenously needed to produce premature ventricular contractions would be lower in individuals anesthetized with halothane than in awake individuals.

How much epinephrine is safe to give when halothane is the anesthetic? Katz and Bigger[653] reported that administering 0.15 ml/kg of a 1/100,000 epinephrine solution per 10-minute period (not to exceed 0.45 ml/kg of a 1/100,000 solution per hour) was safe. Several studies have shown that lidocaine given with epinephrine affords extra protection, and that enflurane and isoflurane are less sensitizing than halothane.[654-656] Since halothane is a potent bronchodilator,[657] it may be the best choice for anesthetizing patients with asthma.[658] However, this may not be the case; many asthmatic patients are already taking exogenous catecholamines such as xanthines as chronic bronchodilator therapy.

Xanthines are effective bronchodilators because they produce β-adrenergic stimulation in two ways: they cause release of norepinephrine[659,660] and also inhibit the breakdown of adenosine 3′,5′-cyclic monophosphate (cyclic AMP),[661] the mediator of many of the actions of β-adrenergic receptor agonists.[662] Phosphodiesterase catalyzes the breakdown of cyclic AMP. Thus, inhibition of phosphodiesterase by theophylline increases the concentration of cyclic AMP. Marcus et al.[659] and Westfall and Flemming[660] showed that at least 40 percent of the inotropic effects of aminophylline are due to its ability to release norepinephrine directly. Infusion of aminophylline also increases excretion of catecholamines in urine.[663] Experimentally, aminophylline decreases the threshold for ventricular fibrillation.[664]

Plasma theophylline levels of 5 mg/L are needed to reduce abnormally high airway resistance. No further beneficial effects are obtained when levels exceed 20 mg/L, and, instead, toxic effects appear.[665,666] Theophylline (aminophylline is a combination of 85 percent theophylline and 15 percent ethylenediamine) is metabolized largely by the liver, less than 10 percent being excreted unchanged in the urine. The average half-life is 4.4 ± 1.15 hours in adults, and clearance is 1.2 ml/min/kg.[665,666] Significant liver disease or pulmonary edema can decrease clearance of the drug by one-half and by one-third, respectively.[667] Cigarette smokers clear aminophylline more rapidly than nonsmokers.[668]

An interaction between aminophylline and halothane appears to be a predictable, frequent occurrence: of 16 dogs anesthetized with 1 percent halothane and given high-dose bolus injections of aminophylline, 12 had ventricular dysrhythmias and 8 had ventricular tachycardia or fibrillation.[669-671] Thus, it is advisable to wait three drug half-lives after the last dose of aminophylline is given (i.e., approximately 13 hours in normal individuals) before using halothane to anesthetize an asthmatic patient. Using another anesthetic that is a bronchodilator[657] but less likely to predispose the patient to catecholamine-induced dysrhythmias[654-656] (such as enflurane or isoflurane) might be an alternative in patients who must be given aminophylline or other exogenous sympathomimetic drugs before or during surgery.[672,673]

OTHER DRUGS

Drugs other than those discussed earlier in this chapter have implications for anesthetic management. These discussed therapies include anticoagulants (in hematologic section), endocrinologic preparations excluding birth control pills but including corticosteroids (in the section on endocrinologic disease), antihypertensives (earlier in this section and in cardiovascular diseases), anticonvulsants (in the section on neurologic disorders), and cancer chemotherapeutic agents (in the section on oncology).

ANTIDYSRHYTHMIC DRUGS

Antidysrhythmic drugs include local anesthetics (lidocaine, procaine), anticonvulsant (phenytoin) or antihypertensive (propranolol) drugs, calcium channel blocking agents, or primary antidysrhythmic drugs. These drugs are discussed elsewhere in this chapter or in Chapter 28. A useful reference with suggestions about drug therapy for cardiac dysrhythmias and monitoring of side effects was published by the *Medical Letter on Drugs and Therapeutics.*[674] Lack of adverse reports does not indicate that all these drugs should be continued through the time of surgery; pharmacokinetic studies have not yet determined whether anesthesia (or anesthesia with specific agents) alters the volume of distribution or clearance of these drugs to an extent sufficient to warrant changing the dosage or dosage schedule in the perioperative period. The dearth of reports on this subject may be due to a lack of significant drug interaction or to a lack of awareness that untoward events could be due to such an interaction.

The pharmacologic characteristics of the various antidysrhythmic drugs can affect anesthetic management. Disopyramide is similar to quinidine and procainamide in its antidysrhythmic effectiveness. Diisopyramide is mainly excreted by the kidneys, but hepatic disease increases its half-life. This drug often produces anticholinergic effects including tachycardia, urinary retention, and psychosis. Hepatitis has also been reported to have occurred after its use.[674] Little is known of the interaction of bretylium with anesthetic agents. Because bretylium blocks the release of catecholamines, chronic therapy with this drug has been associated with hypersensitivity to vasopressors.[674] Quinidine is dependent on the kidneys for excretion, can have vagolytic effects that can decrease atrioventricular block, and is associated with blood dyscrasias and GI disturbances.[674] Most of the antidysrhythmic agents enhance a nondepolarizing neuromuscular blockade. Reports confirm this enhancement for quinidine, phenytoin, lidocaine, procainamide, and propranolol.[675-684] No data document such an effect for depolarizing muscle relaxants.

ANTIBIOTICS

Many antibacterial agents are nephrotoxic and/or neurotoxic and many prolong neuromuscular blockade (also see Ch. 27).[678-684] The only antibiotics devoid of neuromuscular effects appear to be penicillin G and the cephalosporins.[683] Most enzyme-inducing drugs do not increase the metabolism of enflurane or isoflurane. However, isoniazid appears to induce the microsomal enzymes responsible for the metabolism of at least enflurane, increasing the possibility of fluorine-associated renal damage after enflurane.[685] Appropriate antibiotic prophylaxis for surgery requires knowledge of the probability of infection for that type of surgical procedure, and, if the incidence of infection warrants it, a drug regimen directed against the most likely infecting organisms.[686]

DIGITALIS

Digitalis preparations have a limited margin of safety, the risk of toxicity increasing with hypokalemia.[687] I avoid giving digitalis prophy-

lactically because potassium concentrations can fluctuate widely during anesthesia due to fluid shifts, ventilatory acid–base derangements, and adjuvant treatments;[688,689] and because intraoperative dysrhythmias caused by digitalis toxicity may be difficult to differentiate from those having other sources. Digitalis intoxication can present with such diverse cardiac dysrhythmias as junctional escape rhythm, premature ventricular contractions, ventricular bigeminy or trigeminy, junctional tachycardia, paroxysmal atrial tachycardia with or without block, sinus arrest, sinus exit block, Mobitz type I or II blocks, or ventricular tachycardia.[687] However, anesthetic agents appear to protect against digitalis toxicity, at least in animal studies.[689-692] A titrated cardioversion technique using at first 10, then 20, 30, 40, 50, 75, 100, 150, and 200 joule doses resulted in safe cardioversion in the presence of digitalis and diazepam analgesia.[693] For patients in atrial fibrillation, the ventricular response should guide the choice of dose of digitalis.

MEDICATIONS FOR GLAUCOMA
(Also See Ch. 52)

Medications for glaucoma include two organophosphates—echothiophate and isofluorophate. These drugs inhibit serum cholinesterase, which is responsible for hydrolysis and inactivation of succinylcholine and the ester-type local anesthetics such as procaine, chloroprocaine, and tetracaine.[694,695] These ester-type local anesthetics should be avoided in patients treated with eye drops containing organophosphate.

MAGNESIUM, CIMETIDINE, AND ORAL CONTRACEPTIVES

Magnesium is given to treat eclampsia; it can cause neuromuscular blockade by itself and potentiates neuromuscular blockade by both nondepolarizing and depolarizing muscle relaxants.[696,697] Cimetidine reduces hepatic blood flow and inhibits enzymatic degradation of drugs by the liver. Thus, higher blood levels and prolonged elimination half-lives may result when drugs that are metabolized by the liver (e.g., lidocaine, procaine, some narcotics, and propranolol) are given to patients chronically or acutely taking cimetidine.[698,699] The risk of postoperative venous thrombosis increases when oral contraceptives are used preoperatively.[700,701] Whereas some authorities recommend changing from oral contraceptives to topical methods of birth control 2 to 4 weeks before surgery,[702] no controlled study has established whether birth control pills should be stopped before surgery or what the resulting incidence of pregnancy would be. Other authorities recommend preventing venous thromboembolism by using low-dose heparin, guided by a determination of efficacy and cost-effectiveness.[703–705]

determine who is best able to care for the patient. Should one of these be best qualified, one should then watch that person care for the patient. Remember, few prospective controlled studies have been done to show that any preoperative technique, treatment, or management decreases perioperative risk. However, common sense and foreknowledge of potential pitfalls as well as diligence in avoiding those pitfalls should reduce avoidable perioperative complications.

INTERRUPTING A DRUG REGIMEN BEFORE SURGERY

As stated earlier, if a drug is needed for treatment preoperatively, it should be continued through surgery. The only exceptions to this general rule of not altering preoperative drug therapy would pertain to (1) MAO inhibitors; (2) anticoagulants, if surgical hemostasis is needed; (3) nicotinic acid; and (4) dosage adjustments for insulin and corticosteroids. These recommendations require that the anesthesiologist be aware of the pharmacologic characteristics, interactions, and anesthetic implications of drugs described earlier in this chapter.[375,702,706–709]

When in doubt about a disease or a drug, I consult the following textbooks: *Harrison's Principles of Internal Medicine; Anesthesia and Uncommon Diseases: Pathophysiologic and Clinical Correlations; Anesthesia and Co-Existing Disease; To Make the Patient Ready for Anesthesia: Medical Care of the Surgical Patient; Anesthetic Implications of Congenital Anomalies in Children; Medical Care of the Surgical Patient: A Problem-Oriented Approach to Management;* and *Goodman and Gilman's The Pharmacologic Basis of Therapeutics.* Following this, it is wise to consult two people who are experts about the drug or disease and then to

REFERENCES

1. Hamilton WK: Do let the blood pressure drop and do use myocardial depressants! Anesthesiology 45:273, 1976
2. Perioperative Evaluation in Medical Knowledge Self-Assessment Program VI. Philadelphia, American College of Physicians, 1982, pp 292–293
3. Cahill GF Jr: Diabetes mellitus: A brief overview. Johns Hopkins Med J 143:155, 1978
4. Cahill GF Jr, McDevitt HO: Insulin-dependent diabetes mellitus: the initial lesion. N Engl J Med 304:1454, 1981
5. Yoon J-W, Austin M, Onodera T, et al: Virus-induced diabetes mellitus. N Engl J Med 300:1173, 1979
6. The University Group Diabetes Program: A study of the effects of hypoglycemic agents on vascular complications in patients with adult-onset diabetes. Part I: Design, methods and baseline characteristics. Part II: Mortality results. Diabetes (suppl) 19:747, 1970
7. Camerini-Davalos RA, Velasco C, Glasser M, et al: Drug-induced reversal of early diabetic microangiopathy. N Engl J Med 309:1551, 1983
8. The University Group Diabetes Program: Effects of hypoglycemic agents on vascular complications in patients with adult-onset diabetes. VIII. Evaluation of insulin therapy: final report. Diabetes 31(suppl 5):1–81, 1982
9. Job D, Eschwege E, Guyot-Argenton C, et al: Effect of multiple daily insulin injections on the course of diabetic retinopathy. Diabetes 25:463, 1976

10. White NH, Waltman SR, Krupin T, et al: Reversal of neuropathic and gastrointestinal complications related to diabetes mellitus in adolescents with improved metabolic control. J Pediatr 99:41, 1981

11. Raskin P, Pietri AO, Unger R, et al: The effect of diabetic control on the width of skeletal-muscle capillary basement membrane in patient with Type I diabetes mellitus. N Engl J Med 309:1546, 1983

12. Engerman R, Bloodworth JMB, Helson S: Relationship of the microvascular disease in diabetes to metabolic control. Diabetes (suppl) 26:362, 1977

13. Pirart J: Diabetes mellitus and its degenerative complications: A prospective study of 4,000 patients observed between 1947 and 1973. Diabetes Care 1:168, 1978

14. Brenner BM: Hemodynamically mediated glomerular injury and the progressive nature of kidney disease. Kidney Int 23:647, 1983

15. Christlieb AR, Warram JH, Królewski AS, et al: Hypertension: The major risk factor in juvenile-onset insulin-dependent diabetics. Diabetes 30(suppl 2):90, 1981

16. Reported by Olson RL, Leichter S, Warram J, et al: Deaths among patients using continuous subcutaneous insulin infusion pumps — United States. MMWR 31:80, 1982

17. Goodson WH III, Hunt TK: Studies of wound healing in experimental diabetes mellitus. J Surg Res 22:221, 1977

18. Rosen RG, Enquist IF: The healing wound in experimental diabetes. Surgery 50:525, 1961

19. Walts LF, Miller J, Davidson MB, et al: Perioperative management of diabetes mellitus. Anesthesiology 55:104, 1981

20. Peterson L, Caldwell J, Hoffman J: Insulin adsorbance to polyvinyl chloride surfaces with implications for constant-infusion therapy. Diabetes 25:72, 1976

21. Meyer EJ, Lorenzi M, Bohannon NV, et al: Diabetic management by insulin infusion during major surgery. Am J Surg 137:323, 1979

22. Cruse PJ, Foord R: A 5-year prospective study of 23,649 surgical wounds. Arch Surg 107:206, 1973

23. Bagdade JD: Phagocytic and microbiological function in diabetes mellitus. Acta Endocrinol 83(suppl 205):27, 1976

24. Farrow SC, Fowkes FGR, Lunn JN, et al: Epidemiology in anaesthesia. II: Factors affecting mortality in hospital. Br J Anaesth 54:811, 1982

25. Galloway JA, Shuman CR: Diabetes and surgery. A study of 667 cases. Am J Med 34:177, 1963

26. Walsh DB, Eckhauser FE, Ramsburgh SR, et al: Risk associated with diabetes mellitus in patients undergoing gallbladder surgery. Surgery 91:254, 1982

27. Palumbo PJ: Blood glucose control during surgery (editorial). Anesthesiology 55:94, 1981

28. Garcia MJ, McNamara PM, Gordon T, et al: Morbidity and mortality in diabetics in the Framingham population. Sixteen year follow-up study. Diabetes 23:105, 1974

29. Muir JJ, Endres SM, Offord K, et al: Glucose management in patients undergoing operation for insulinoma removal. Anesthesiology 59:371, 1983

30. Havel RJ: Approach to the patient with hyperlipidemia. Med Clin North Am 66:319, 1982

31. Haskell WL, Camargo C Jr, Williams PT, et al: The effect of cessation and resumption of moderate alcohol intake on serum high-density-lipoprotein subfractions. N Engl J Med 310:805, 1984

32. Andres R: Effect of obesity on total mortality. Int J Obesity 4:381, 1980

33. Fox GS, Whalley DG, Bevan DR: Anaesthesia for the morbidly obese. Experience with 110 patients. Br J Anaesth 53:811, 1983

34. Vaughan RW, Bauer S, Wise L: Volume and pH of gastric juice in obese patients. Anesthesiology 43:686, 1975

35. Wilson SL, Mantena NR, Halverson JD: Effects of atropine, glycopyrrolate, and cimetidine on gastric secretions in morbidly obese patients. Anesth Analg 60:37, 1981

36. Bentley JB, Vaughan RW, Miller MS, et al: Serum inorganic fluoride levels in obese patients during and after enflurane anesthesia. Anesth Analg 58:409, 1979

37. Cork RC, Vaughan RW, Bentley JB: General anesthesia for morbidly obese patients — An examination of postoperative outcomes. Anesthesiology 54:310, 1981

38. Sours HE, Frattali VP, Brand CD, et al: Sudden death associated with very low calorie weight reduction regimens. Am J Clin Nutr 34:453, 1981

39. Harris RT: Bulimarexia and related serious eating disorders with medical complications. Ann Intern Med 99:800, 1983

40. Wharton BA, Howells GR, McCann RA: Cardiac failure in kwashiorkor. Lancet 2:384, 1967

41. Law DH: Current concepts in nutrition. Total parenteral nutrition. N Engl J Med 297:1104, 1977

42. Sheldon GF, Way L: Total parenteral nutrition: The state of the art. West J Med 127:398, 1977

43. Roizen MF, Lampe GH: Adrenal cortex mal-

function: Implications for the anesthetist. Semin Anesth III(3), 1984

44. Goldmann DR: The surgical patient on steroids, Medical Care of the Surgical Patient. Edited by Goldmann DR, Brown FH, Levy WK, et al. A Problem-Oriented Approach to Management. Philadelphia, JB Lippincott, 1982, p 113

45. Byyny RL: Preventing adrenal insufficiency during surgery. Postgrad Med 67:219, 228, 1980

46. Gold EM: The Cushing syndromes: Changing views of diagnosis and treatment. Ann Intern Med 90:829, 1979

47. Izenstein BZ, Dluhy RG, Williams GH: Endocrinology, To Make the Patient Ready for Anesthesia: Medical Care of the Surgical Patient. Edited by Vandam LD. Menlo Park, California, Addison-Wesley, 1980, p 112

48. White VA, Kumagai LF: Preoperative endocrine and metabolic considerations. Med Clin North Am 63:1321, 1979

49. Hanowell ST, Hittner KC, Kim YD, et al: Anesthetic management of primary aldosteronism. Anesthesiol Rev 9:36, 1982

50. Rabinowitz IN, Watson W, Farber EM: Topical steroid depression of the hypothalamic-pituitary-adrenal axis in psoriasis vulgaris. Dermatologica 154:321, 1977

51. Knudsen L, Christiansen LA, Lorentzen JE: Hypotension during and after operation in glucocorticoid-treated patients. Br J Anaesth 53:295, 1981

52. Oyama T: Hazards of steroids in association with anaesthesia. Can Anaesth Soc J 16:361, 1969

53. Plumpton FS, Besser GM, Cole PV: Corticosteroid treatment and surgery. 1. An investigation of the indications for steroid cover. Anaesthesia 24:3, 1969

54. Symreng T, Karlberg BE, Kågedal B, et al: Physiological cortisol substitution of long-term steroid-treated patients undergoing major surgery. Br J Anaesth 53:949, 1981

55. Axelrod L: Glucocorticoid therapy. Medicine (Baltimore) 55:39, 1976

56. Christy NP, Wallace EZ, Jailer JW: Comparative effects of prednisone and of cortisone in suppressing the response of the adrenal cortex to exogenous adrenocorticotropin. J Clin Endocrinol Metab 16:1059, 1956

57. Danowski TS, Bonessi JV, Sabeh G, et al: Probabilities of pituitary-adrenal responsiveness after steroid therapy. Ann Intern Med 61:11, 1964

58. Byyny RL: Withdrawal from glucocorticoid therapy. N Engl J Med 295:30, 1976

59. Graber AL, Ney RI, Nicholson WE, et al: Natural history of pituitary-adrenal recovery following long-term suppression with corticosteroids. J Clin Endocrinol Metab 25:11, 1965

60. Ackerman GL, Nolan GM: Adrenocortical responsiveness after alternate-day corticosteroid therapy. N Engl J Med 278:405, 1968

61. Jasani MK, Freeman PA, Boyle JA, et al: Studies of the rise in plasma 11-hydroxycorticosteroids (11-OHCS) in corticosteroid-treated patients with rheumatoid arthritis during surgery: Correlations with the functional integrity of the hypothalamo-pituitary-adrenal axis. Q J Med 37:407, 1968

62. Livanou T, Ferriman D, James VHT: Recovery of hypothalamo-pituitary-adrenal function after corticosteroid therapy. Lancet 2:856, 1967

63. Marx FW Jr, Barker WF: Surgical results in patients with ulcerative colitis treated with and without corticosteroids. Am J Surg 113:157, 1967

64. Nichols T, Nugent CA, Tyler FH: Diurnal variation in suppression of adrenal function by glucocorticoids. J Clin Endocrinol Metab 25:343, 1965

65. Prakash A, Tanga MC: Surgery and corticosteroids. An experimental study. Int Surg 49:143, 1968

66. Sampson PA, Brooke BN, Winstone NE: Biochemical confirmation of collapse due to adrenal failure. Lancet 1:1377, 1961

67. Sampson PA, Winstone NE, Brooke BN: Adrenal function in surgical patients after steroid therapy. Lancet 2:322, 1962

68. Streck WF, Lockwood DH: Pituitary adrenal recovery following short-term suppression with corticosteroids. Am J Med 66:910, 1979

69. Winstone NE, Brook BN: Effects of steroid treatment on patients undergoing operation. Lancet 1:973, 1961

70. Kaplan SA: Diseases of the adrenal cortex II. Congenital adrenal hyperplasia. Pediatr Clin North Am 26:77, 1979

71. Fauci AS, Dale DC, Balow JE: Glucocorticoid therapy: Mechanisms of action and clinical considerations. Ann Intern Med 84:304, 1976

72. Holaday JW, Law P-Y, Loh HH, et al: Adrenal steroids indirectly modulate morphine and β-endorphin effects. J Pharmacol Exp Ther 208:176, 1979

73. Krieger DT, Liotta AS, Brownstein MJ, et al: ACTH, β-lipoprotein, and related peptides in brain, pituitary, and blood. Recent Prog Horm Res 36:277, 1980

74. Hollenberg NK, Williams GH: Hypertension, the adrenal and the kidney: Lessons from pharmacologic interruption of the renin-angiotensin system. Adv Intern Med 25:327, 1980

75. Tyrrell JB, Brooks RM, Fitzgerald PA, et al: Cushing's disease. Selective trans-sphenoidal resection of pituitary microadenomas. N Engl J Med 298:753, 1978

76. Baker BL, Whitaker WL: Interference with wound healing by the local action of adrenocortical steroids. Endocrinology 46:544, 1950

77. Sandberg N: Time relationship between administration of cortisone and wound healing in rats. Acta Chir Scand 127:446, 1964

78. Ehrlich HP, Hunt TK: Effects of cortisone and vitamin A on wound healing. Ann Surg 167:324, 1968

79. Myerowitz RL, Medeiros AA, O'Brien TF: Bacterial infection in renal homotransplant recipients. A study of fifty-three bacteremic episodes. Am J Med 53:308, 1972

80. Dale DC, Fauci AS, Wolff SM: Alternate-day prednisone. Leukocyte kinetics and susceptibility to infections. N Engl J Med 291:1154, 1974

81. Ernest I, Ekman H: Adrenalectomy in Cushing's disease. A long-term follow-up. Acta Endocrinol (suppl) 160:3, 1972

82. Welbourn RB, Montgomery DAD, Kennedy TL: The natural history of treated Cushing's syndrome. Br J Surg 58:1, 1971

83. Weinberger MH, Grim CE, Hollifield JW, et al: Primary aldosteronism: diagnosis, localization, and treatment. Ann Intern Med 90:386, 1979

84. Herf SM, Teates DC, Tegtmeyer CJ, et al: Identification and differentiation of surgically correctable hypertension due to primary aldosteronism. Am J Med 67:397, 1979

85. Moore FD, Edelman IS, Olney JM, et al: Body sodium and potassium. III. Inter-related trends in alimentary, renal and cardiovascular disease; lack of correlation between body stores and plasma concentration. Metabolism 3:334, 1954

86. Jasani BM, Edmonds CJ: Kinetics of potassium distribution in man using isotope dilution and whole-body counting. Metabolism 20:1099, 1971

87. Johnson JE, Hartsuck JM, Zollinger RM Jr, et al: Radiopotassium equilibrium in total body potassium: studies using ^{43}K and ^{42}K. Metabolism 18:663, 1969

88. Surawicz B, Chlebus H, Mazzoleni A: Hemodynamic and electrocardiographic effects of hyperpotassemia: Differences in response to slow and rapid increases in concentration of plasma K. Am Heart J 73:647, 1967

89. Rao TLK, Jacobs KH, El-Etr AA: Reinfarction following anesthesia in patients with myocardial infarction. Anesthesiology 59:499, 1983

90. Oh SH, Patterson R: Surgery in corticosteroid-dependent asthmatics. J Allergy Clin Immunol 53:345, 1974

91. Schambelan M, Sebastian A: Hyporeninemic hypoaldosteronism. Adv Intern Med 24:385, 1979

92. Zusman RM: Prostaglandins and water excretion. Annu Rev Med 32:359, 1981

93. Oyama T, Taniguchi K, Jin T, et al: Effects of anaesthesia and surgery on plasma aldosterone concentration and renin activity in man. Br J Anaesth 51:747, 1979

94. Cooper GM, Paterson JL, Ward ID, et al: Fentanyl and the metabolic response to gastric surgery. Anaesthesia 36:667, 1981

95. Lehtinen A-M, Fyhrquist F, Kivalo I: The effects of fentanyl on arginine vasopressin and cortisol secretion during anesthesia. Anesth Analg 63:25, 1984

96. Stanley TH, Berman L, Green O, et al: Plasma catecholamine and cortisol responses to fentanyl-oxygen anesthesia for coronary-artery operations. Anesthesiology 53:250, 1980

97. Turton MB, Deegan T: Central and peripheral levels of plasma catecholamines, cortisol, insulin and non-esterified fatty acids. Clin Chim Acta 48:347, 1973

98. Namba Y, Smith JB, Fox GS, et al: Plasma cortisol concentrations during caesarean section. Br J Anaesth 52:1027, 1980

99. Wise L, Margraf H, Ballinger WF: The effect of surgical trauma on the excretion and conjugation pattern of 17-ketosteroids. Surgery 71:625, 1972

100. Knowlton AI: Addison's disease: A review of its clinical course and management, The Human Adrenal Cortex. Edited by Christy NR. New York, Harper & Row, New York, 1971, p 329

101. Liddle GW: Adrenal cortex, Cecil Textbook of Medicine. 15th Ed. Edited by Beeson PB, McDermott W, Wyngaarden JB. Philadelphia, WB Saunders, 1979, p 2144

102. Landon J, Greenwood FC, Stamp TCB, et al: The plasma sugar, free fatty acid, cortisol, and growth hormone response to insulin, and the comparison of this procedure with other tests of pituitary and adrenal function. II. In patients with hypothalamic or pituitary dysfunction or anorexia nervosa. J Clin Invest 45:437, 1966

103. Wood JB, Frankland AW, James VHT, et al: A rapid test of adrenocortical function. Lancet 1:243, 1965

104. Engquist A, Backer OG, Jarnum S: Incidence of postoperative complications in patients subjected to surgery under steroid cover. Acta Chir Scand 140:343, 1974

105. Winstone NE, Brooke BN: Effects of steroid treatment on patients undergoing operation. Lancet 1:973, 1961

106. Jensen JK, Elb S: Per- og postoperative kompli-

kationer hos tigligere kortikosteroidbehandlede patienter. Nord Med 76:975, 1966

107. St John Sutton MG, Sheps SG, Lie JT: Prevalence of clinically unsuspected pheochromocytoma. Review of a 50-year autopsy series. Mayo Clin Proc 56:354, 1981

108. Desmonts JM, le Houelleur J, Remond P, et al: Anaesthetic management of patients with pheochromocytoma: A review of 102 cases. Br J Anaesth 49:991, 1977

109. Roizen MF, Horrigan RW, Koike M, et al: A prospective randomized trial of four anesthetic techniques for resection of pheochromocytoma. Anesthesiology 57:A43, 1982

110. van Heerden JA, Sheps SG, Hamberger B, et al: Pheochromocytoma: current status and changing trends. Surgery 91:367, 1982

111. Roizen MF, Hunt TK, Beaupre PN, et al: The effect of alpha-adrenergic blockade on cardiac performance and tissue oxygen delivery during excision of pheochromocytoma. Surgery 94:941, 1983

112. Schaffer MS, Zuberbuhler P, Wilson G, et al: Catecholamine cardiomyopathy: An unusual presentation of pheochromocytoma in children. J Pediatr 99:276, 1981

113. Kopin IJ, Lake CR, Ziegler M: Plasma levels of norepinephrine. Ann Intern Med 88:671, 1978

114. Riley CM, Day RL, Greeley DM, et al: Central autonomic dysfunction with defective lacrimation. I. Report of five cases. Pediatrics 3:468, 1949

115. Shy GM, Drager GA: A neurologic syndrome associated with orthostatic hypotension: A clinico-pathologic study. Arch Neurol 2:511, 1960

116. Christensen NJ: Plasma noradrenaline and adrenaline measured by isotope-derivative assay, a review with special reference to diabetes mellitus. Dan Med Bull 26:17, 1979

117. Kontos HA, Richardson DW, Norvell JE: Mechanisms of circulatory dysfunction in orthostatic hypotension. Trans Am Clin Climatol Assoc 87:26, 1975

118. Ziegler MG, Lake CR, Kopin IJ: The sympathetic nervous system defect in primary orthostatic hypotension. N Engl J Med 296:293, 1977

119. Naftchi NE, Wooten GF, Lowman EW, et al: Relationship between serum dopamine-β-hydroxylase activity, catecholamine metabolism, and hemodynamic changes during paroxysmal hypertension in quadraplegia. Circ Res 35:850, 1974

120. Cohen CA: Anesthetic management of a patient with the Shy-Drager syndrome. Anesthesiology 35:95, 1971

121. Kirtchman MM, Schwartz H, Papper EM: Experiences with general anesthesia in patients with familial dysautonomia. JAMA 170:529, 1959

122. McCaughey TJ: Familial dysautonomia as an anaesthetic hazard. Can Anaesth Soc J 12:558, 1965

123. Meridy HW, Creighton RE: General anaesthesia in eight patients with familial dysautonomia. Can Anaesth Soc J 18:563, 1971

124. Ciliberti BJ, Goldfein J, Rovenstine EA: Hypertension during anesthesia in patients with spinal cord injuries. Anesthesiology 15:273, 1954

125. Desmond J: Paraplegia: Problems confronting the anaesthesiologist. Can Anaesth Soc J 17:435, 1970

126. Drinker AS, Helrich M: Halothane anesthesia in the paraplegic patient. Anesthesiology 24:399, 1963

127. Gronert GA, Theye RA: Pathophysiology of hyperkalemia induced by succinylcholine. Anesthesiology 43:89, 1975

128. Jousse AT, Wynne-Jones M, Breithaupt DJ: A follow-up study of life expectancy and mortality in traumatic transverse myelitis. Can Med Assoc J 98:770, 1968

129. Ewing DJ, Campbell IW, Clarke BF: Assessment of cardiovascular effects in diabetic autonomic neuropathy and prognostic implications. Ann Intern Med 92:308, 1980

130. Bevan DR: Shy-Drager syndrome. A review and a description of the anaesthetic management. Anaesthesia 34:866, 1979

131. Malan MD, Crago RR: Anaesthetic considerations in idiopathic orthostatic hypotension and the Shy-Drager syndrome. Can Anaesth Soc J 26:322, 1979

132. Wade JG, Larson CP, Hickey RF, et al: Carotid endarterectomy and carotid chemoreceptor and baroreceptor function in man. N Engl J Med 282:823, 1970

133. Hui KKP, Conolly ME: Increased numbers of beta receptors in orthostatic hypotension due to autonomic dysfunction. N Engl J Med 304:1473, 1981

134. Kendrick WW, Scott JW, Jousse AT, et al: Reflex sweating and hypertension in traumatic transverse myelitis. Treatm Serv Bull (Ottawa) 8:437, 1953

135. Amino N, Mori H, Iwatani Y, et al: High prevalence of transient postpartum thyrotoxicosis and hypothyroidism. N Engl J Med 306:849, 1982

136. Channick BJ, Adlin EV, Marks AD, et al: Hyperthyroidism and mitral-valve prolapse. N Engl J Med 305:497, 1981

137. Forfar JC, Miller HC, Toft AD: Occult thyrotoxicosis: A correctable cause of "idiopathic" atrial fibrillation. Am J Cardiol 44:9, 1979

138. Davis PJ, Davis FB: Hyperthyroidism in patients over the age of 60 years. Clinical features in 85 patients. Medicine (Baltimore) 53:161, 1974

139. Symons C: Thyroid heart disease. Br Heart J 41:257, 1979

140. Toft AD, Irvine WJ, Sinclair I, et al: Thyroid function after surgical treatment of thyrotoxicosis: a report of 100 cases treated with propranolol before operation. N Engl J Med 298:643, 1978

141. Feek CM, Sawers JSA, Irvine WJ, et al: Combination of potassium iodide and propranolol in preparation of patients with Graves' disease for thyroid surgery. N Engl J Med 302:883, 1980

142. Forfar JC, Muir AL, Sawers SA, Toft AD: Abnormal left ventricular function in hyperthyroidism. Evidence for a possible reversible cardiomyopathy. N Engl J Med 307:1165, 1982

143. Eriksson M, Rubenfeld S, Garber AJ, et al: Propranolol does not prevent thyroid storm. N Engl J Med 296:263, 1977

144. Roizen MF, Becker CE: Thyroid storm: A review of cases at University of California, San Francisco. Calif Med 115(4):5, 1971

145. Mackin JF, Canary JJ, Pittman CS: Thyroid storm and its management. N Engl J Med 291:1396, 1974

146. Murkin JM: Anesthesia and hypothyroidism: A review of thyroxine physiology, pharmacology, and anesthetic implications. Anesth Analg 61:371, 1982

147. Weinberg AD, Brennan MD, Gorman CA, et al: Outcome of anesthesia and surgery in hypothyroid patients. Arch Intern Med 143:893, 1983

148. Zwillich CW, Pierson DJ, Hofeldt FD, et al: Ventilatory control in myxedema and hypothyroidism. N Engl J Med 292:662, 1975

149. Bough EW, Crowley WF, Ridgway EC, et al: Myocardial function in hypothyroidism. Relation to disease severity and response to treatment. Arch Intern Med 138:1476, 1978

150. Babad AA, Eger EI II: The effects of hyperthyroidism and hypothyroidism on halothane and oxygen requirements in dogs. Anesthesiology 29:1087, 1968

151. Levine HD: Compromise therapy in the patient with angina pectoris and hypothyroidism: A clinical assessment. Am J Med 69:411, 1980

152. Paine TD, Rogers WJ, Baxley WA, Russell RO Jr: Coronary arterial surgery in patients with incapacitating angina pectoris and myxedema. Am J Cardiol 40:226, 1977

153. Bone HG III, Snyder WH III, Pak CYC: Diagnosis of hyperparathyroidism. Annu Rev Med 28:111, 1977

154. Weidmann P, Massry SG, Coburn WJ, et al: Blood pressure effects of acute hypercalcemia. Ann Intern Med 76:741, 1972

155. Rumancik WM, Denlinger JK, Nahrwold ML, et al: The QT interval and serum ionized calcium. JAMA 240:366, 1978

156. Frantz AG: Prolactin. N Engl J Med 298:201, 1978

157. Wilson CB, Dempsey LC: Transsphenoidal microsurgical removal of 250 pituitary adenomas. J Neurosurg 48:13, 1978

158. Thorner MO, Martin WH, Rogol AD, et al: Rapid regression of pituitary prolactinomas during bromocriptine treatment. J Clin Endocrinol Metab 51:438, 1980

159. March CM, Kletzky OA, Davajan V, et al: Longitudinal evaluation of patients with untreated prolactin-secreting pituitary adenomas. Am J Obstet Gynecol 139:835, 1981

160. McGuffin WL, Sherman BM, Roth J, et al: Acromegaly and cardiovascular disorders: A prospective study. Ann Intern Med 81:11, 1974

161. Southwick JP, Katz J: Unusual airway difficulty in the acromegalic patient — Indications for tracheostomy. Anesthesiology 51:72, 1979

162. Hassan SZ, Matz G, Lawrence AM, et al: Laryngeal stenosis in acromegaly: A possible cause of airway difficulties associated with anesthesia. Anesth Analg 55:57, 1976

163. Campkin TV: Radial artery cannulation. Potential hazard in patients with acromegaly. Anaesthesia 35:1008, 1980

164. Cobb WE, Spare S, Reichlin S: Neurogenic diabetes insipidus: Management with 1-dDAVP (1-desamino-8-D arginine vasopressin). Ann Intern Med 88:183, 1978

165. Smithwick RH, Thompson JE: Splanchnicectomy for essential hypertension. JAMA 152:1501, 1953

166. Brown BR: Anesthesia and essential hypertension, ASA Refresher Courses in Anesthesiology, Vol. 7. Edited by Hershey SG. Philadelphia, JB Lippincott, 1979, p 41

167. Sprague HB: The heart in surgery. An analysis of results of surgery on cardiac patients during the past ten years at the Massachusetts General Hospital. Surg Gynecol Obstet 49:54, 1929

168. Miller RD, Way WL, Eger EI II: The effects of alpha-methyldopa, reserpine, and guanethidine on minimum alveolar anesthetic requirement (MAC). Anesthesiology 29:1153, 1968

169. Veterans Administration Study on Antihypertensive Agents: Effects of treatment on morbidity in hypertension. JAMA 202:1028, 1967

170. Veterans Administration Cooperative Study Group on Antihypertensive Agents: Effects of treatment on morbidity in hypertension: Results in patients with diastolic blood pressure averaging 90 through 114 mm Hg. JAMA 213:1143, 1970

171. Berglund G, Wilhelmen L, Sannerstedt R, et al:

Coronary heart-disease after treatment of hypertension. Lancet 1:1, 1978

172. Hypertension Detection and Follow-up Program Cooperative Group: The effect of treatment on mortality in "mild" hypertension. N Engl J Med 307:976, 1982

173. Multiple Risk Factor Intervention Trial Research Group: Multiple risk factor intervention trial. Risk factor changes and mortality results. JAMA 248:1465, 1982

174. Ayobe MH, Tarazi RC: Reversal of changes in myocardial β-receptors and inotropic responsiveness with regression of cardiac hypertrophy in renal hypertensive rats (RHR). Circ Res 54:125, 1984

175. Prys-Roberts C, Meloche R, Foëx P: Studies of anesthesia in relation to hypertension. 1. Cardiovascular responses of treated and untreated patients. Br J Anaesth 43:122, 1971

176. Goldman L, Caldera DL: Risks of general anesthesia and elective operation in the hypertensive patient. Anesthesiology 50:285, 1979

177. Bedford RF, Feinstein B: Hospital admission blood pressure: A predictor for hypertension following endotracheal intubation. Anesth Analg 59:367, 1980

178. Asiddao CB, Donegan JH, Whitesell RC, et al: Factors associated with perioperative complications during carotid endarterectomy. Anesth Analg 61:631, 1982

179. Vacanti CJ, Van Houten RJ, Hill RC: A statistical analysis of the relationship of physical status to postoperative morbidity in 68,388 cases. Anesth Analg 49:564, 1970

180. Lewin I, Lerner AG, Green SH, et al: Physical class and physiologic status in the prediction of operative mortality in the aged sick. Ann Surg 174:217, 1971

181. Marx GF, Mateo CV, Orkin LR: Computer analysis of postanesthetic deaths. Anesthesiology 39:54, 1973

182. Urzua J, Dominguez P, Quiroga M, et al: Preoperative estimation of risk in cardiac surgery. Anesth Analg 69:625, 1981

183. Fleiss JL: Statistical Methods for Rates and Proportions. New York, Wiley, 1973, p 178

184. Schneider AJL, Knoke JD, Zollinger RM Jr, et al: Morbidity prediction using pre- and intraoperative data. Anesthesiology 51:4, 1979

185. Eerola M, Eerola R, Kaukinen S, et al: Risk factors in surgical patients with verified preoperative myocardial infarction. Acta Anaesthesiol Scand 24:219, 1980

186. Mauney FM, Ebert PA, Sabiston DC: Postoperative myocardial infarction: a study of predisposing factors, diagnosis and mortality in a high risk group of surgical patients. Ann Surg 172:497, 1970

187. Gordon T, Kannel WB: The Framingham, Massachusetts, study twenty years later, Community as an Epidemiologic Laboratory: A Casebook of Community Studies. Edited by Kessler II, Levin ML. Baltimore, Johns Hopkins Press, 1970, p 123

188. Benchimol A, Harris CL, Desser KB, et al: Resting electrocardiogram in major coronary artery disease. JAMA 224:1489, 1973

189. Tomatis LA, Fierens EE, Verbrugge GP: Evaluation of surgical risk in peripheral vascular disease by coronary angiography: A series of 100 cases. Surgery 71:429, 1972

190. Hertzer NR, Beven EG, Young JR, et al: Coronary artery disease in peripheral vascular patients. A classification of 1000 angiograms and results of surgical management. Ann Surg 199:223, 1984

191. Barnes RW, Liebman PR, Marszalek PB, et al: The natural history of asymptomatic carotid disease in patients undergoing cardiovascular surgery. Surgery 90:1075, 1981

192. Barnes RW, Marszalek PB: Asymptomatic carotid disease in the cardiovascular surgical patient: Is prophylactic endarterectomy necessary? Stroke 12:497, 1981

193. Ropper AH, Wechsler LR, Wilson LS: Carotid bruit and the risk of stroke in elective surgery. N Engl J Med 307:1388, 1982

194. Heyman A, Wilkinson WE, Heyden S, et al: Risk of stroke in asymptomatic persons with cervical arterial bruits. A population study in Evans County, Georgia. N Engl J Med 302:838, 1980

195. Borer JS, Brensike JF, Redwood DR, et al: Limitations of the electrocardiographic response to exercise in predicting coronary artery disease. N Engl J Med 293:367, 1975

196. Proudfit WL, Shirey EK, Sones FM: Selective CINE coronary angiography: Correlation with clinical finding in 1000 patients. Circulation 33:901, 1966

197. Goldschlager N: Use of the treadmill test in the diagnosis of coronary artery disease in patients with chest pain. Ann Intern Med 97:383, 1982

198. Weiner DA, Ryan TJ, McCabe CH, et al: Exercise stress testing. Correlations among history of angina, ST-segment response and prevalence of coronary-artery disease in the Coronary Artery Surgery Study (CASS). N Engl J Med 301:230, 1979

199. Arkins R, Smessaert AA, Hicks RG: Mortality and morbidity in surgical patients with coronary artery disease. JAMA 190:485, 1964

200. Topkins MJ, Artusio JF: Myocardial infarction and surgery: A five year study. Anesth Analg 43:715, 1964

201. Fraser JG, Ramachandran PR, Davis HS: Anes-

thesia and recent myocardial infarction. JAMA 199:318, 1972

202. Tarhan S, Moffitt EA, Taylor WF, et al: Myocardial infarction after general anesthesia. JAMA 199:318, 1972

203. Sapala JA, Ponka JL, Duvernow WFC: Operative and nonoperative risks in the cardiac patient. J Am Geriatr Soc 23:529, 1975

204. Steen PA, Tinker JH, Tarhan S: Myocardial reinfarction after anesthesia and surgery. JAMA 239:2566, 1976

205. Goldman L, Caldera DL, Southwick FS, et al: Cardiac risk factors and complications in noncardiac surgery. Medicine (Baltimore) 57:357, 1978

206. Schoeppel SL, Wilkinson C, Waters J, et al: Effects of myocardial infarction on perioperative cardiac complications. Anesth Analg 62:493, 1983

207. Knapp RB, Topkins MJ, Artusio JF Jr: The cerebrovascular accident and coronary occlusion in anesthesia. JAMA 182:332, 1962

208. Lowenstein E, Yusuf S, Teplick RS: Perioperative myocardial reinfarction: A glimmer of hope — A note of caution (editorial). Anesthesiology 59:493, 1983

209. Backer CL, Tinker JH, Robertson DM, et al: Myocardial reinfarction following local anesthesia for ophthalmic surgery. Anesth Analg 59:257, 1980

210. Wolf GL, Lynch S, Berlin I: Intra-ocular surgery with general anesthesia. Arch Ophthalmol 93:323, 1975

211. Bruschke AVG, Proudfit WL, Sones FM: Progress study of 590 consecutive nonsurgical cases of coronary disease followed 5–9 years. Circulation 47:1147, 1973

212. Mahar LJ, Steen PA, Tinker JH, et al: Perioperative myocardial infarction in patients with coronary artery disease with and without aorta-coronary bypass grafts. J Thorac Cardiovasc Surg 76:533, 1978

213. Kennedy JW, Kaiser GC, Fisher LD, et al: Clinical and angiographic predictors of operative mortality from the Collaborative Study in Coronary Artery Surgery (CASS). Circulation 63:793, 1981

214. Podrid PJ, Graboys TB, Lown B: Prognosis of medically treated patients with coronary-artery disease with profound ST-segment depression during exercise testing. N Engl J Med 305:1111, 1981

215. Rozanski A, Berman D, Gray R, et al: Preoperative prediction of reversible myocardial asynergy by postexercise radionuclide ventriculography. N Engl J Med 307:212, 1982

216. Mangano DT, Hedgcock MW, Wisneski JA: Noninvasive prediction of ventricular dysfunction:

coronary artery disease. Anesthesiology 57:A21, 1982

217. White CW, Wright CB, Doty DB, et al: Does visual interpretation of the coronary arteriogram predict the physiologic importance of a coronary stenosis? N Engl J Med 310:819, 1984

218. Benson H, McCallie DP: Angina pectoris and the placebo effect. N Engl J Med 300:1424, 1979

219. Oberman A, Kouchoukos NT, Harrell RR, et al: Surgical versus medical treatment in disease of the left main coronary artery. Lancet 2:591, 1976

220. Takaro T, Hultgren HN, Lipton MJ, et al: The VA cooperative randomized study of surgery for coronary arterial occlusive disease. II. Subgroup with significant left main lesions. Circulation 54:6(suppl 3),III107, 1976

221. Vliestra RE, Assad-Morell JL, Frye RL, et al: Survival predictors in coronary artery disease. Medical and surgical comparisons. Mayo Clin Proc 42:85, 1977

222. Reed RC, Murphy ML, Hultgren HN, et al: Survival of men treated for chronic stable angina pectoris. A cooperative randomized study. J Thorac Cardiovasc Surg 75:1, 1978

223. Scher KS, Tice DA: Operative risk in patients with previous coronary artery bypass. Arch Surg 111:807, 1976

224. McCollum CH, Giarcia-Rinaldi R, Graham JM, et al: Myocardial revascularization prior to subsequent major surgery in patients with coronary artery disease. Surgery 81:302, 1977

225. Crawford ES, Morris GC, Howell JF, et al: Operative risk in patients with previous coronary artery bypass. Ann Thorac Surg 26:215, 1978

226. Hultgren HN, Pfeifer JF, Angell WW, et al: Unstable angina: Comparison of medical and surgical management. Am J Cardiol 39:734, 1977

227. Roizen MF, Beaupre PN, Alpert RA, et al: Monitoring with two-dimensional transesophageal echocardiography. J Vasc Surg 1:300, 1984

228. The Criteria Committee of the New York Heart Association, Kossman CE (chairman): Diseases of the heart and blood vessels, Nomenclature and Criteria for Diagnosis. 6th Ed. Boston, Little, Brown, 1964

229. Nachlas MM, Abrams SJ, Goldberg MM: The influence of arteriosclerotic heart disease on surgical risk. Am J Surg 101:447, 1961

230. Santos AL, Gelperin A: Surgical mortality in the elderly. J Am Geriatr Soc 23:42, 1975

231. Ziffren SE, Hartford CE: Comparative mortality for various surgical operations in older versus younger age groups. J Am Geriatr Soc 20:485, 1972

232. Cogbill CL: Operation in the aged. Arch Surg 94:202, 1967

233. Driscoll AC, Hobika JH, Etsen BE, et al: Clini-

cally unrecognized myocardial infarction following surgery. N Engl J Med 264:633, 1961

234. Cohn PF, Gorlin R, Cohn LH, et al: Left ventricular ejection fraction as a prognostic guide in surgical treatment of coronary and valvular heart disease. Am J Cardiol 34:136, 1974

235. Riles TS, Kopelman I, Imparato AM: Myocardial infarction following carotid endarterectomy: A review of 683 operations. Surgery 85:249, 1979

236. Sanz G, Castañer A, Bertriu A, et al: Determinants of prognosis in survivors of myocardial infarction. A prospective clinical angiographic study. N Engl J Med 306:1065, 1982

237. Epstein SE, Palmeri ST, Patterson RE: Evaluation of patients after acute myocardial infarction. Indications for cardiac catheterization and surgical intervention. N Engl J Med 307:1487, 1982

238. Roy WL, Edelist G, Gilbert B: Myocardial ischemia during non-cardiac surgical procedures in patients with coronary-artery disease. Anesthesiology 51:393, 1979

239. Kaplan JA, King SB: The precordial electrocardiographic lead (V_5) in patients who have coronary-artery disease. Anesthesiology 45:570, 1976

240. Braunwald E: Thirteenth Bowditch Lecture. The determinants of myocardial oxygen consumption. Physiologist 12:65, 1969

241. Robinson BF: Relation of heart rate and systolic blood pressure to the onset of pain and angina pectoris. Circulation 25:1073, 1967

242. Gobel FL, Nordstrom LA, Nelson RR, et al: The rate pressure product as an index of myocardial oxygen consumption during exercise in patients with angina pectoris. Circulation 57:549, 1978

243. Cannon DS, Levy W, Cohen LS: The short- and long-term prognosis of patients with transmural and nontransmural myocardial infarction. Am J Med 61:452, 1976

244. Mills P, Rose J, Hillingsworth J, et al: Long-term prognosis of mitral-valve prolapse. N Engl J Med 297:13, 1977

245. Schlant RC, Felner JM, Miklozek C, et al: Mitral valve prolapse. DM 26(10):1, 1980

246. Bor DH, Himmelstein DU: Endocarditis prophylaxis for patients with mitral valve prolapse. A quantitative analysis. Am J Med 76:711, 1984

247. Swartz MH, Teicholz LE, Donoso F: Mitral valve prolapse: A review of associated arrhythmias. Am J Med 62:377, 1977

248. Clemens JD, Horwitz RI, Jaffe CC, et al: A controlled evaluation of the risk of bacterial endocarditis in persons with mitral-valve prolapse. N Engl J Med 307:776, 1982

249. Berry FA, Blankenbaker WL, Ball CG: A comparison of bacteremia occurring with nasotracheal and orotracheal intubation. Anesth Analg 52:873, 1973

250. Shull HJ, Greene BM, Allen SD, et al: Bacteremia with upper gastrointestinal endoscopy. Ann Intern Med 83:212, 1975

251. Committee on Prevention of Rheumatic Fever and Bacterial Endocarditis of the American Heart Association: Prevention of bacterial endocarditis. Circulation 56:139A, 1977

252. Tinker JH, Tarhan S: Discontinuing anticoagulant therapy in surgical patients with cardiac valve prostheses. Observations in 180 operations. JAMA 239:738, 1978

253. Cade JF, Hunt D, Stubbs KP, et al: Guidelines for the management of oral anticoagulant therapy in patients undergoing surgery. Med J Aust 2:292, 197

254. Katholi RE, Nolan SP, McGuire LB: The management of anticoagulation during noncardiac operations in patients with prosthetic heart valves. A prospective study. Am Heart J 96:163, 1978

255. De Angelis J: Hazards of subdural and epidural anesthesia during anticoagulant therapy: A case report and review. Anesth Analg 51:676, 1972

256. Edelson RN, Chernik NL, Posner JB: Spinal subdural hematomas complicating lumbar puncture. Arch Neurol 31:134, 1974

257. Brem SS, Hafler DA, Van Uitert RL, et al: Spinal subarachnoid hematoma. A hazard of lumbar puncture resulting in reversible paraplegia. N Engl J Med 303:1020, 1981

258. Lutz DJ, Noller KL, Spittell JA Jr, et al: Pregnancy and its complications following cardiac valve prostheses. Am J Obstet Gynecol 131:460, 1978

259. Smith ND, Raizada V, Abrams J: Auscultation of the normally functioning prosthetic valve. Ann Intern Med 95:594, 1981

260. Pastore JO, Yurchak PM, Janis KM, et al: The risk of advanced heart block in surgical patients with right bundle branch block and left axis deviation. Circulation 57:677, 1978

261. Berg GR, Kotler MN: The significance of bilateral bundle branch block in the preoperative patient. A retrospective electrocardiographic and clinical study in 30 patients. Chest 59:62, 1971

262. Rooney S-M, Goldiner PL, Muss E: Relationship of right bundle-branch block and marked left axis deviation to complete heart block during general anesthesia. Anesthesiology 44:64, 1976

263. Kunstadt D, Punja M, Cagin N, et al: Bifascicular block: A clinical and electrophysiologic study. Am Heart J 86:173, 1973

264. Venkataraman K, Madias JE, Hood WB Jr: Indications for prophylactic preoperative insertion of pacemakers in patients with right bundle

branch block and left anterior hemiblock. Chest 68:501, 1975

265. McAnulty JH, Rahimtoola SH, Murphy E, et al: Natural history of "high-risk" bundle-branch block. Final report of a prospective study. N Engl J Med 307:137, 1982

266. Ruskin JN, DiMarco JP, Garan H: Out-of-hospital cardiac arrest. Electrophysiologic observations and selection of long-term antiarrhythmic therapy. N Engl J Med 303:607, 1980

267. Ruberman W, Weinblatt E, Frank CW, et al: Repeated 1 hour electrocardiographic monitoring of survivors of myocardial infarction at 6 month intervals: Arrhythmia detection and relation to prognosis. Am J Cardiol 47:1197, 1981

268. Bigger JT Jr, Weld FM, Rolnitzky LM: Prevalence, characteristics and significance of ventricular tachycardia (three or more complexes) detected with ambulatory electrocardiographic recording in the late hospital phase of acute myocardial infarction. Am J Cardiol 48:815, 1981

269. Josephson ME, Horowitz LN, Spielman SR, et al: Electrophysiologic and hemodynamic studies in patients resuscitated from cardiac arrest. Am J Cardiol 46:948, 1980

270. Gallagher JJ, Pritchett ELC, Sealy WC, et al: The pre-excitation syndromes. Prog Cardiovasc Dis 20:285, 1978

271. Sadowski AR, Moyers JR: Anesthetic management of the Wolff-Parkinson-White syndrome. Anesthesiology 51:553, 1979

272. Kruse I, Arnman K, Conradson T-B, et al: A comparison of the acute and long-term hemodynamic effects of ventricular inhibited and atrial synchronous ventricular inhibited pacing. Circulation 65:846, 1982

273. Josephson ME, Kastor JA: Supraventricular tachycardia: Mechanisms and management. Ann Intern Med 87:346, 1977

274. Simon AB: Perioperative management of the pacemaker patient. Anesthesiology 46:127, 1977

275. Shapiro WA, Roizen MF, Singleton MA, et al: Intraoperative pacemaker complications. Anesthesiology (in press)

276. Thiagarajah S, Azar I, Agres M, et al: Pacemaker malfunction associated with positive-pressure ventilation. Anesthesiology 58:565, 1983

277. Stein M, Cassara EL: Preoperative pulmonary evaluation and therapy for surgery patients. JAMA 211:787, 1970

278. Collins CD, Darke CS, Knowelden J: Chest complications after upper abdominal surgery: Their anticipation and prevention. Br Med J 1:401, 1968

279. Bartlett RH, Brennan ML, Gazzaniga AB, et al: Studies on the pathogenesis and prevention of postoperative pulmonary complications. Surg Gynecol Obstet 137:925, 1973

280. Lyager S, Wernberg M, Rajani N, et al: Can postoperative pulmonary conditions be improved by treatment with the Bartlett-Edwards incentive spirometer after upper abdominal surgery? Acta Anaesthesiol Scand 23:312, 1979

281. Tisi GM: Preoperative evaluation of pulmonary function: Validity, indications, benefits. Am Rev Respir Dis 119:293, 1979

282. Hedley-Whyte J, Burgess GE, Feeley TW, et al: Critical analysis of preventive measures, p. 119. In Applied Physiology of Respiratory Care. Boston, Little, Brown, 1976

283. Pontoppidan H: Mechanical aids to lung expansion in non-intubated surgical patients. Am Rev Respir Dis 122:109, 1980

284. Graham WGB, Bradley DA: Efficacy of chest physiotherapy in the resolution of pneumonia. N Engl J Med 299:624, 1978

285. Connors AF Jr, Hammon WE, Martin RJ, et al: Chest physical therapy. The immediate effect on oxygenation in acutely ill patients. Chest 78:559, 1980

286. Cottrell JE, Siker ES: Preoperative intermittent positive pressure breathing therapy in patients with chronic obstructive lung disease: Effect on postoperative pulmonary complications. Anesth Analg 52:258, 1973

287. Forthman HJ, Shepard A: Postoperative pulmonary complications. South Med J 62:1198, 1969

288. Boushy SF, Billing DM, North LB, et al: Clinical course related to preoperative pulmonary function in patients with bronchogenic carcinoma. Chest 59:383, 1971

289. Mittman C: Assessment of operative risk in thoracic surgery. Am Rev Respir Dis 84:197, 1961

290. Reichel J: Assessment of operative risk of pneumonectomy. Chest 62:570, 1972

291. Fischl MA, Pitchenik A, Gardner LB: An index predicting relapse and need for hospitalization in patients with acute bronchial asthma. N Engl J Med 305:783, 1981

292. Hall WJ, Douglas RG, Hyde RW, et al: Pulmonary mechanics after uncomplicated influenza A infection. Am Rev Respir Dis 113:141, 1976

293. Green GM, Jakab GJ, Low RB, et al: Defense mechanisms of the respiratory membrane. Am Rev Respir Dis 115:479, 1977

294. Tait AR, Ketcham TR, Klein MJ, et al: Perioperative respiratory complications in patients with upper respiratory tract infections. Anesthesiology 59:A433, 1983

295. Latimer RG, Dickman M, Day WC, et al: Ventilatory patterns and pulmonary complications after upper abdominal surgery determined by

preoperative and postoperative computerized spirometry and blood gas analysis. Am J Surg 122:622, 1971

296. Tarhan S, Moffitt EA, Sessler AD, et al: Risk of anesthesia and surgery in patients with chronic bronchitis and chronic obstructive pulmonary disease. Surgery 74:720, 1973

297. Gould AB: Effect of obesity on respiratory complications following general anesthesia. Anesth Analg 41:448, 1962

298. Buist AS, Sexton GJ, Nagy JM, et al: The effect of smoking cessation and modification on lung function. Am Rev Respir Dis 114:115, 1976

299. McCarthy DS, Craig DB, Cherniack RM: Effect of modification of the smoking habit on lung function. Am Rev Respir Dis 114:103, 1976

300. Kark JD, Lebiush M, Rannon L: Cigarette smoking as a risk factor for epidemic $A(H_1N_1)$ influenza in young men. N Engl J Med 307:1042, 1982

301. Neiwoehner DE, Kleinerman J, Rice DB: Pathologic changes in the peripheral airways of young cigarette smokers. N Engl J Med 291:755, 1974

302. Enson Y: Pulmonary heart disease: Relation of pulmonary hypertension to abnormal lung structure and function. Bull NY Acad Med 53:551, 1977

303. Edwards WD, Edwards JE: Clinical primary pulmonary hypertension: Three pathologic types. Circulation 56:884, 1977

304. UCLA Conference, Crandall ED (moderator): Recent developments in pulmonary edema. Ann Intern Med 99:808, 1983

305. Stein PD, Willis PW III, DeMets DL: History and physical examination in acute pulmonary embolism in patients without preexisting cardiac or pulmonary disease. Am J Cardiol 47:218, 1981

306. Alpert JS, Irwin RS, Dalen JE: Pulmonary hypertension. Curr Probl Cardiol 5(10):1, 1981

307. Cohen ML, Kronzon I: Adverse hemodynamic effects of phentolamine in primary pulmonary hypertension. Ann Intern Med 95:591, 1981

308. Packer M, Greenberg B, Massie B, et al: Deleterious effects of hydralazine in patients with pulmonary hypertension. N Engl J Med 306:1326, 1982

309. Domino KB, Wetstein L, Glasser SA, et al: Influence of mixed venous oxygen tension ($P\overline{v}O_2$) on blood flow to atelectatic lung. Anesthesiology 59:428, 1983

310. Mendella LA, Manfreda J, Warren CPW, et al: Steroid response in stable chronic obstructive pulmonary disease. Ann Intern Med 96:17, 1982

311. Settipane GA, Dudupakkam RK: Aspirin intolerance. III. Subtypes, familial occurrence and cross reactivity with tartrazine. J Allergy Clin Immunol 56:215, 1975

312. Aubier M, De Troyer A, Sampson M, et al: Aminophylline improves diaphragmatic contractility. N Engl J Med 305:249, 1981

313. Keogh BA, Hunninghake GW, Line BR, et al: The alveolitis of pulmonary sarcoidosis. Evaluation of natural history and alveolitis-dependent changes in lung function. Am Rev Respir Dis 128:256, 1983

314. Fabbri LM, Aizawa H, Alpert SE, et al: Airway hyperresponsiveness and changes in cell counts in bronchoalveolar lavage after ozone exposure in dogs. Am Rev Respir Dis 129:288, 1984

315. Baughman RP, Fernandez M, Bosken CH, et al: Comparison of gallium-67 scanning, bronchoalveolar lavage, and serum angiotensin-converting enzyme levels in pulmonary sarcoidosis. Predicting response to therapy. Am Rev Respir Dis 129:676, 1984

316. Williams DE, Pairolero PC, Davis CS, et al: Survival of patients surgically treated for stage I lung cancer. J Thorac Cardiovasc Surg 82:70, 1981

317. Pitlik SD, Fainstein V, Bodey GP: Tuberculosis mimicking cancer—A reminder. Am J Med 76:822, 1984

318. Levy JH, Roizen MF, Morris JM: Anaphylactic and anaphylactoid reactions: A review. Spine (in press)

319. Watkins J: Anaphylactoid reactions to I.V. substances. Br J Anaesth 51:51, 1979

320. Bristow MR, Ginsburg R, Harrison DC: Histamine and the human heart: The other receptor system. Am J Cardiol 49:249, 1982

321. Austen KF: Systemic anaphylaxis in the human being. N Engl J Med 291:661, 1974

322. Goetzl EJ: Mediators of immediate hypersensitivity derived from arachidonic acid. N Engl J Med 303:822, 1980

323. Michelassi F, Landa L, Hill RD, et al: Leukotriene D_4: A potent coronary artery vasoconstrictor associated with impaired ventricular contraction. Science 217:841, 1982

324. Smith PL, Kagey-Sobotka A, Bleecker ER, et al: Physiologic manifestations of human anaphylaxis. J Clin Invest 66:1072, 1980

325. Delage C, Irey NS: Anaphylactic deaths: A clinicopathologic study of 43 cases. J Forensic Sci 17:525, 1972

326. Murano G: The "Hageman" connection: Interrelationships of blood coagulation, fibrino(geno)lysis, kinin generation, and complement activation. Am J Hematol 4:409, 1978

327. Radford SG, Lockyer JA, Simpson PJ: Immunological aspects of adverse reactions to Althesin. Br J Anaesth 54:859, 1982

328. Lasser EC, Lang JH, Hamblin AE, et al: Activation systems in contrast idiosyncrasy. Invest Radiol 15(suppl 6):S2, 1980

329. Lasser EC, Lang JH, Lyon SG, et al: Complement and contrast material reactors. J Allergy Clin Immunol 64:105, 1979

330. Chenoweth DE, Cooper SW, Hugli TE, et al: Complement activation during cardiopulmonary bypass. N Engl J Med 304:497, 1981

331. Craddock PR, Fehr J, Brigham KL, et al: Complement and leukocyte-mediated pulmonary dysfunction in hemodialysis. N Engl J Med 296:769, 1977

332. Vercellotti GM, Hammerschmidt DE, Craddock PR, et al: Activation of plasma complement by perfluorocarbon artificial blood: Probable mechanism of adverse pulmonary reactions in treated patients and rationale for corticosteroid prophylaxis. Blood 59:1299, 1982

333. Lorenz W, Doenicke A, Schöning B, et al: The role of histamine in adverse reactions to intravenous agents, Adverse Reactions of Anaesthetic Drugs. Edited by Thornton JA. Amsterdam, Elsevier/North Holland Biomedical Press, 1981, p 169

334. Rosow CE, Moss J, Philbin DM, et al: Histamine release during morphine and fentanyl anesthesia. Anesthesiology 56:93, 1982

335. Moss J, Rosow CE, Savarese JJ, et al: Role of histamine in the hypotensive action of d-tubocurarine in humans. Anesthesiology 55:19, 1981

336. Hirshman CA, Peters J, Cartwright-Lee I: Leukocyte histamine release to thiopental. Anesthesiology 56:64, 1982

337. Moss J, McDermott DJ, Thisted RA, et al: Anaphylactic/anaphylactoid reactions in response to Chymodiactin (chymopapain). Anesth Analg 63:253, 1984

338. Hall BB, McCulloch JA: Anaphylactic reactions following the intradiscal injection of chymopapain under local anesthesia. J Bone Joint Surg 65A:1215, 1983

339. Javid MJ: Treatment of herniated lumbar disk syndrome with chymopapain. JAMA 243:2043, 1980

340. Watts C: Complications of chemonucleolysis for lumbar disc disease. Neurosurgery 1:2, 1977

341. Brown MD: Intradiscal Therapy. Chymopapain or Collagenase. Chicago, Year Book, 1983, pp 91–92, 101–109

342. McCulloch JA: Chemonucleolysis: Experience with 2000 cases. Clin Orthop 146:128, 1980

343. Millbern SM, Bell SD: Prevention of anaphylaxis to contrast media. Anesthesiology 50:56, 1979

344. Zweiman B, Mishkin MM, Hildreth EA: An approach to the performance of contrast studies in contrast material-reactive persons. Ann Intern Med 83:159, 1975

345. Miller WL, Doppman JL, Kalan AP: Renal arteriography following systemic reaction to contrast material. J Allergy Clin Immunol 56:291, 1975

346. Kaliner M, Sigler R, Summers R, et al: Effects of infused histamine: Analysis of the effects of H-1 and H-2 histamine receptor antagonists on cardiovascular and pulmonary responses. J Allergy Clin Immunol 68:365, 1981

347. Philbin DM, Moss J, Akins CW, et al: The use of H_1 and H_2 histamine antagonists with morphine anesthesia: A double-blind study. Anesthesiology 55:292, 1981

348. Hammerschmidt DE, White JG, Craddock PR, et al: Corticosteroids inhibit complement-induced granulocyte aggregation. A possible mechanism for their efficacy in shock states. J Clin Invest 63:798, 1979

349. Halevy S, Altura BT, Altura BM: Pathophysiological basis for the use of steroids in the treatment of shock and trauma. Klin Wochenschr 60:1021, 1982

350. Ring J, Messmer K: Incidence and severity of anaphylactoid reactions to colloid volume substitutes. Lancet 1:466, 1977

351. Ring J, Stephan W, Brendel W: Anaphylactoid reactions to infusions of plasma protein and human serum albumin. Clin Allergy 9:89, 1979

352. Ellison N, Behar M, MacVaugh H, et al: Bradykinin, plasma protein fraction, and hypotension. Ann Thorac Surg 29:15, 1978

353. Milner LV, Butcher K: Transfusion reactions reported after transfusion of red blood cells and of whole blood. Transfusion 18:493, 1978

354. Owen DAA, Harvey CA, Boyce MJ: Effects of histamine on the circulatory system. Klin Wochenschr 60:972, 1982

355. Barach EM, Nowak RM, Lee TG, et al: Epinephrine for treatment of anaphylactic shock. JAMA 251:2118, 1984

356. Schleimer RP, MacGlashan DW, Gillespie E, et al: Inhibition of basophil release by anti-inflammatory steroids. J Immunol 129:1632, 1982

357. Del Pizzo A: Hereditary angioneurotic edema. Anesthesiol Rev 5:41, 1978

358. Hosea SW, Santaella ML, Brown EJ, et al: Long-term therapy of hereditary angioedema with danazol. Ann Intern Med 93:809, 1982

359. Oxelius V-A, Laurell A-B, Lindquist B, et al: IgG subclasses in selective IgA deficiency. Importance of IgG2-IgA deficiency. N Engl J Med 304:1476, 1981

360. Levy DE, Bates D, Caronna JJ, et al: Prognosis in nontraumatic coma. Ann Intern Med 94:293, 1981

361. Plum F, Posner JB: The Diagnosis of Stupor and Coma. 2nd Ed. Philadelphia, FA Davis, 1972

362. Caplan LR, Thomas C, Banks G: Central nervous system complications of addition to "T's and Blues." Neurology (NY) 32:623, 1982

363. Drugs for epilepsy. Med Lett Drugs Ther 21:25, 1979

364. Montouris GD, Fenichel GM, McLain LW Jr: The pregnant epileptic. A review and recommendations. Arch Neurol 36:601, 1979

365. Delgado-Escueta AV, Wasterlain C, Treiman DM, et al: Management of status epilepticus. N Engl J Med 306:1337, 1982

366. Penry JK, Newmark ME: The use of antiepileptic drugs. Ann Intern Med 90:207, 1979

367. Joas TA, Stevens WC, Eger EI II: Electroencephalographic seizure activity in dogs during anesthesia. Br J Anaesth 43:739, 1971

368. Lebowitz MH, Blitt CD, Dillon JB: Enflurane-induced central nervous system excitation and its relation to carbon dioxide tension. Anesth Analg 51:355, 1972

369. Buzello W, Jantzen K, Scholler KL: The influence of Ethrane on the electro- and pentylenetetrazol-convulsions in mice. Anaesthesist 24:118, 1975

370. Kitagawa J, Iwatsubo K, Shigenaga Y, et al: Pharmacologic comparison between enflurane and halothane. Folia Pharmacol Jpn 72:211, 1976

371. Wollman H, Smith AL, Neigh JL, et al: Cerebral blood flow and oxygen consumption in man during electroencephalographic seizure patterns associated with Ethrane anesthesia, Cerebral Blood Flow. Edited by Brock M, Fieschi C, et al. Berlin, Springer-Verlag, 1969, p 246

372. Opitz A, Brechts B, Stenzel E: Enflurane anaesthesia for epileptic patients. Anaesthesist 26:329, 1977

373. Preventing spread of meningococcal disease. Med Lett Drugs Ther 23:37, 1981

374. Weiner WJ, Koller WC, Perlik S, et al: Drug holiday and management of Parkinson disease. Neurology (NY) 30:1257, 1980

375. Schwartz AJ, Wollman H: Anesthetic considerations for patients on chronic drug therapy: L-dopa, monamine oxidase inhibitors, tricyclic antidepressants and propranolol, ASA Refresher Courses in Anesthesiology. Vol. 4. Edited by Hershey SG. Philadelphia, JB Lippincott, 1976, p 99

376. Ngai SH: Parkinsonism, levodopa, and anesthesia. Anesthesiology 37:344, 1972

377. Wiklund RA, Ngai SH: Rigidity, and pulmonary edema after Innovar in a patient on levodopa therapy: Report of a case. Anesthesiology 35:545, 1971

378. Terry RD, Katzman R: Senile dementia of the Alzheimer type. Ann Neurol 14:497, 1983

379. Raskin NH, Appenzeller O: Major Problems in Internal Medicine. Vol. 19: Headache. Philadelphia, WB Saunders, 1980

380. Kudrow L: Comparative results of prednisone, methylsergide, and lithium therapy in cluster headache, Current Concepts in Migraine Research. Edited by Greene R. New York, Raven Press, 1978, p 159

381. Ovassapian A, Land P, Schafer MF, et al: Anesthetic management for surgical corrections of severe flexion deformity of the cervical spine. Anesthesiology 58:370, 1983

382. Dahm LS, Dickson JH, Harrison, GH: Perioperative and anesthetic management in the patient with scoliosis. Anesthesiol Rev 9:13, 1982

383. Baskett PJF, Armstrong R: Anaesthetic problems in multiple sclerosis. Are certain agents contraindicated? Anaesthesia 25:397, 1970

384. Tschudy DP, Valsamis M, Magnussen CR: Acute intermittent porphyria: Clinical and selected research aspects. Ann Intern Med 83:851, 1975

385. Ellefson RD: Porphyrinogens, porphyrins, and the porphyrias. Mayo Clin Proc 57:454, 1982

386. Mees DE Jr, Frederickson EL: Anesthesia and the porphyrias. South Med J 68:29, 1975

387. Risk SF, Jacobson JH, Silvay G: Ketamine as an induction agent for acute intermittent porphyria. Anesthesiology 46:305, 1977

388. Blekkenhorst GH, Harrison GG, Cook ES, et al: Screening of certain anaesthetic agents for their ability to elicit acute porphyric phases in susceptible patients. Br J Anaesth 52:759, 1980

389. Drachman DB: Myasthenia gravis (second of two parts). N Engl J Med 298:186, 1978

390. Rowland LP: Controversies about the treatment of myasthenia gravis. J Neurol Neurosurg Psychiatry 43:644, 1980

391. Drachman DB, Adams RN, Josifek LF, et al: Functional activities of autoantibodies to acetylcholine receptors and the clinical severity of myasthenia gravis. N Engl J Med 307:769, 1982

392. Miller RD: Myasthenia gravis, Clinical Anesthesia. Case Selections from the University of California, San Francisco. Edited by Wilkinson PL, Ham J, Miller RD. St Louis, CV Mosby, 1980, p 148

393. Hedley-Whyte J, Borgess GE, Feeley TW, et al: Respiratory management of peripheral neurologic disease, p. 245. In Applied Physiology of Respiratory Care. Boston, Little, Brown, 1976

394. Schmidt GB, Patel KP, Grundy EM, et al: The perioperative management of patients with myasthenia gravis: A review. Anesthesiol Rev 4:29, 1977

395. Rolbin SH, Levinson G, Shnider SM, et al: Anes-

thetic considerations for myasthenia gravis and pregnancy. Anesth Analg 57:441, 1978

396. Leventhal SR, Orkin FK, Hirsh RA: Prediction of the need for postoperative mechanical ventilation in myasthenia gravis. Anesthesiology 53:26, 1980

397. Miller J, Lee C: Muscle diseases, Anesthesia and Uncommon Diseases. Pathophysiologic and Clinical Correlations. Edited by Katz J, Benumof J, Kadis LB. 2nd Ed. Philadelphia, WB Saunders, 1981, p 530

398. Rosenberg H, Durbin CG: Anesthesia in the presence of neuromuscular disease. Anesthesiol Update 1:20, 1978

399. Britt BA (editor): Malignant hyperthermia. Int Anesthesiol Clin 17:1, 1979

400. Kobel M, Creighton RE, Steward DJ: Anaesthetic considerations in Down's syndrome: Experience with 100 patients and a review of the literature. Can Anaesth Soc J 29:593, 1982

401. Bedford RF, Morris L, Jane JA: Intracranial hypertension during surgery for supratentorial tumor: Correlation with preoperative computed tomography scans. Anesth Analg 61:430, 1982

402. Ramirez-Lassepas M, Quinones MR: Heparin therapy for stroke: hemorrhagic complications and risk factors for intracerebra hemorrhage. Neurology (NY) 34:114, 1984

403. Walshaw MJ, Pearson MG: Hypoxia in patients with acute hemiplegia. Br Med J 288:15, 1984

404. Allen GS, Ahn HS, Preziosi TJ, et al: Cerebral arterial spasm — A controlled trial of nimodipine in patients with subarachnoid hemorrhage. N Engl J Med 308:619, 1983

405. Drugs for psychiatric disorders. Med Lett Drugs Ther 25:45, 1983

406. Appel GB, Neu HC: The nephrotoxicity of antimicrobial agents. N Engl J Med 296:663, 722, 784, 1977

407. Fischer RP, Polk HC Jr: Changing etiologic patterns of renal insufficiency in surgical patients (editorial). Surg Gynecol Obstet 140:85, 1975

408. Yamauchi H, Hopper J Jr: Hypovolemic shock and hypotension as a complication in the nephrotic syndrome. Report of ten cases. Ann Intern Med 60:242, 1964

409. Venkatachalam MA, Rennke HG, Sandstrom DJ: The vascular basis for acute renal failure in the rat. Circ Res 38:267, 1976

410. Tasker PRW, MacGregor GA, De Wardener HE: Prophylactic use of intravenous saline in patients with chronic renal failure undergoing major surgery. Lancet 2:911, 1974

411. Brenowitz JB, Williams CD, Edwards WS: Major surgery in patients with chronic renal failure. Am J Surg 134:765, 1977

412. Bennett WM, Luft F, Porter GA: Pathogenesis of renal failure due to aminoglycosides and contrast media used in roentgenography. Am J Med 69:767, 1980

413. Warren SE, Blantz RC: Mannitol. Arch Intern Med 141:493, 1981

414. Feldman HA, Singer I: Endocrinology and metabolism in uremia and dialysis: A clinical review. Medicine (Baltimore) 54:345, 1975

415. Walser M: Nutritional management of chronic renal failure. Am J Kidney Dis 1:261, 1982

416. Raskin NH, Fishman RA: Neurologic disorders in renal failure. N Engl J Med 294:143, 204, 1976

417. Vincenti F, Duca RM, Amend W, et al: Immunologic factors determining survival of cadaver-kidney transplants: The effect of HLA serotyping, cytotoxic antibodies and blood transfusions on graft survival. N Engl J Med 299:793, 1978

418. Rao KV, Anderson RC, O'Brien TJ: Factors contributing for improved graft survival in recipients of kidney transplants. Kidney Int 24:210, 1983

419. Burke GR, Gulyassy PF: Surgery in the patient with renal disease and related electrolyte disorders. Med Clin North Am 63:1191, 1979

420. Oh MS, Carroll HS: The anion gap. N Engl J Med 297:814, 1977

421. Rowe JW, Andres R, Tobin JD, et al: The effect of age on creatinine clearance in men: A cross-sectional and longitudinal study. J Gerontol 31:155, 1976

422. Ansari Z, Baldwin DS: Acute renal failure due to radio-contrast agents. Nephron 17:28, 1976

423. Byrd L, Sherman RL: Radiocontrast induced acute renal failure: A clinical and pathophysiological review. Medicine (Baltimore) 58:270, 1979

424. Eisenberg RL, Bank WO, Hedgecock MW: Renal failure after major angiography. Am J Med 68:43, 1980

425. Abel RM, Buckley MJ, Austen WL: Etiology, incidence and prognosis of renal failure following cardiac operations. J Thorac Cardiovasc Surg 71:323, 1976

426. Smolens P, Stein JH: Pathophysiology of acute renal failure. Am J Med 70:479, 1981

427. Kleinknecht D, Ganeval D, Gonzalez-Duque LA, et al: Furosemide in acute oliguric renal failure: A controlled trial. Nephron 17:51, 1976

428. Anderson RJ, Linas SL, Berns AS, et al: Nonoliguric acute renal failure. N Engl J Med 296:1134, 1977

429. Alpert RA, Roizen MF, Hamilton WK, et al: Intraoperative urinary output does not predict postoperative renal function in patients undergoing abdominal aortic revascularization. Surgery 95:707, 1984

430. Dolan MJ, Whipp BJ, Davidson WD, et al: Hypopnea associated with acetate hemodialysis: Carbon dioxide-flow-dependent ventilation. N Engl J Med 305:72, 1981

431. Advisory Committee to the Renal Transplant Registry: The 13th report of the human renal transplant registry. Transplant Proc 9:9, 1977

432. Bennett WM, Aronoff GR, Morrison G, et al: Drug prescribing in renal failure: Dosing guidelines for adults. Am J Kidney Dis 3:155, 1983

433. Rubin AL, Stenzel KH, Reidenberg MM: Symposium on drug action and metabolism in renal failure. Am J Med 62:459, 1977

434. Benet L (editor): The Effect of Disease States on Drug Pharmacokinetics. Washington, D.C., Am Pharmaceutical Assoc/Am Pharmaceutical Sci, 1976

435. Keighley MRB: Antibiotics in biliary disease: The relative importance of antibiotic concentrations in the bile and serum. Gut 17:495, 1976

436. Root RK, Hierholzer WJ Jr: Infectious disease, Clinical Pharmacology: Basic Principles in Therapeutics. 2nd Ed. Edited by Melmon KL, Morelli HF. New York, Macmillan, 1978, p 709

437. Antimicrobial prophylaxis for surgery. Med Lett Drugs Ther 25:113, 1983

438. Everett EO, Hirschmann JV: Transient bacteremia and endocarditis prophylaxis: A review. Medicine (Baltimore) 56:61, 1977

439. Robinson JA, Klodnycky ML, Loeb HS, et al: Endotoxin, prekallikrein, complement and systemic vascular resistance. Sequential measurements in man. Am J Med 59:61, 1975

440. The Medical Letter on Drugs and Therapeutics Handbook of Antimicrobial Therapy. New Rochelle, NY, The Medical Letter, 1982

441. Platt R, Polk BF, Murdock B, et al: Mortality associated with nosocomial urinary-tract infection. N Engl J Med 307:637, 1982

442. Albert RK, Condie F: Hand-washing patterns in medical intensive-care units. N Engl J Med 304:1465, 1981

443. Farber BF, Kaiser DL, Wenzel RP: Relation between surgical volume and incidence of postoperative wound infection. N Engl J Med 305:200, 1981

444. Band JD, Maki DG: Steel needles used for intravenous therapy. Morbidity in patients with hematologic malignancy. Arch Intern Med 140:31, 1980

445. Gross PA, Neu HC, Aswapokee P, et al: Deaths from nosocomial infections: Experience in a university hospital and a community hospital. Am J Med 68:219, 1980

446. Young LS: Nosocomial infections in the immunocompromised adult. Am J Med 70:398, 1981

447. Popovic M, Sarngadharan MG, Read E, et al: Detection, isolation, and continuous production of cytopathic retroviruses (HTLV-III) from patients with AIDS and pre-AIDS. Science 224:497, 1984

448. Aach RD, Szmuness W, Mosley JW, et al: Serum alanine aminotransferase of donors in relation to the risk of non-A, non-B hepatitis in recipients. The transfusion-transmitted viruses study. N Engl J Med 304:989, 1981

449. Dworsky ME, Welch K, Cassady G, et al: Occupational risk for primary cytomegalovirus infection among pediatric health-care workers. N Engl J Med 309:950, 1983

450. Committee on Infections Within Hospitals, American Hospital Association: Infection Control in the Hospital. Chicago, American Hospital Association, 1979

451. Committee on Control of Surgical Infections, Altemeier WA (editor): Manual of Control of Infection in Surgical Patients. Philadelphia, JB Lippincott, 1976

452. Arieff AI, Llacki F, Massry SG: Neurologic manifestations and morbidity of hyponatremia: Correlation with brain water and electrolytes. Medicine (Baltimore) 55:121, 1976

453. Seeley JF, Dirks JH: Site of action of diuretic drugs. Kidney Int 11:1, 1977

454. Hantman O, Rossier B, Zohlman R, et al: Rapid correction of hyponatremia in the syndrome of inappropriate antidiuretic hormone. Ann Intern Med 78:870, 1973

455. Forrest JN Jr, Cox M, Hong C, et al: Superiority of demeclocycline over lithium in the treatment of chronic inappropriate secretion of antidiuretic hormone. N Engl J Med 298:173, 1978

456. Muldowney FP, Williams RT: Clinical disturbances in serum sodium and potassium in relation to alteration in total exchangeable sodium, exchangeable potassium and total body water. Am J Med 35:768, 1963

457. Surawicz B: Relationship between electrocardiogram and electrolytes. Am Heart J 73:814, 1967

458. Sack D, Kim ND, Harrison CE Jr: Contractility and subcellular calcium metabolism in chronic potassium deficiency. Am J Physiol 226:756, 1974

459. Wong KC, Vitez TS: Electrolyte imbalance. Semin Anesth 2:161, 1983

460. Goggin MJ, Joekes AM: Gas exchange in renal failure. I. Dangers of hyperkalaemia during anaesthesia. Br Med J 2:244, 1971

461. Wright BD, Di Giovanni AJ: Respiratory alkalosis, hypokalemia and repeated ventricular fibrillation associated with mechanical ventilation. Anesth Analg 48:467, 1969

462. Sack D, Kim ND, Harrison CE Jr: Contractility

and subcellular calcium metabolism in chronic potassium deficiency. Am J Physiol 226:756, 1974

463. Edwards R, Winnie AP, Ramamurthy S: Acute hypocapneic hypokalemia: An iatrogenic anesthetic complication. Anesth Analg 56:786, 1977

464. Lawson NW, Butler GH, Rat CT: Alkalosis and cardiac arrhythmias. Anesth Analg 52:951, 1973

465. Aldinger KA, Samaan NA: Hypokalemia with hypercalcemia. Prevalence and significance in treatment. Ann Intern Med 87:571, 1977

466. Wong KC, Kawamura R, Hodges MR, et al: Acute intravenous administration of potassium chloride to furosemide pretreated dogs. Can Anaesth Soc J 24:203, 1977

467. Kawamura R, Wong KC, Hodges MR: Intravenous potassium chloride in hypokalemic dogs pretreated with digoxin. Anesth Analg 57:108, 1978

468. Kunin AS, Surawicz B, Sims EAH: Decrease in serum potassium concentrations and appearance of cardiac arrhythmias during infusion of potassium with glucose in potassium-depleted patients. N Engl J Med 266:228, 1962

469. Wilkinson PL, Ham J, Miller RD: Preoperative hyperkalemia and elective surgery, Clinical Anesthesia. Case Selections from the University of California, San Francisco. Edited by Wilkinson PL, Ham J, Miller RD. St Louis, CV Mosby, 1980, p 54

470. Lawson DH: Adverse reactions to potassium chloride. Q J Med 43:433, 1974

471. Kassirer JP, Harrington JT: Diuretics and potassium metabolism: A reassessment of the need, effectiveness and safety of potassium therapy. Kidney Int 11:505, 1977

472. Sullivan JM, Dluhy RG, Wacker WEC, et al: Interrelationships among thiazide diuretics and calcium, magnesium, sodium, and potassium balance in normal and hypertensive man. J Clin Pharmacol 18:530, 1978

473. Dyckner T, Wester PO: Ventricular extrasystoles and intracellular electrolytes before and after potassium and magnesium infusions in patients on diuretic treatment. Am Heart J 97:12, 1979

474. McMahon FG: Thiazides. Management of Essential Hypertension. Mt Kisco, NY, Futura, 1978, p 21

475. Vitez TS, Soper LE, Soper PG: Chronic hypokalemia does not increase anesthetic dysrhythmias. Anesth Analg 61:221, 1982

476. Morganroth J, Michelson EL, Horowitz LN, et al: Limitations of routine long-term electrocardiographic monitoring to assess ventricular ectopic frequency. Circulation 58:408, 1978

477. Duke M: Thiazide-induced hypokalemia. Association with acute myocardial infarction and ventricular fibrillation. JAMA 239:43, 1978

478. Holland OB, Nixon JV, Kuhnert L: Diuretic-induced ventricular ectopic activity. Am J Med 70:762, 1981

479. Tanifuji Y, Eger EI II: Brain sodium, potassium and osmolality: Effect on anesthetic requirement. Anesth Analg 57:404, 1978

480. Heymsfield SB, Bethel RA, Ansley JD: Enteral hyperalimentation: An alternative to central venous hyperalimentation. Ann Intern Med 90:63, 1979

481. Bull DM (moderator): Crohn's disease of the colon. Gastroenterology 76:607, 1979

482. Weser E: Nutritional aspects of malabsorption. Short gut adaptation. Am J Med 67:1014, 1979

483. May RJ, Long BW, Gardner JD: H_2-histamine receptor blocking agents in the Zollinger-Ellison syndrome. Ann Intern Med 87:668, 1977

484. Eger EI II, Saidman LJ: Hazards of nitrous oxide anesthesia in bowel obstruction and pneumothorax. Anesthesiology 26:61, 1965

485. [Reported by Hospital Infections Branch, Bacterial Diseases Bureau of Epidemiology, CDC]: Trends in surgical wound infection rates. MMWR 29:27, 33, 1980

486. Ross AHM, Smith MA, Anderson JR, et al: Late mortality after surgery for peptic ulcer. N Engl J Med 307:519, 1982

487. Tilson MD: Carcinoid syndrome. Surg Clin North Am 54:409, 1974

488. Dory A: Theoretical and clinical considerations in anaesthesia for secreting carcinoid tumors. Can Anaesth Soc J 18:245, 1971

489. Mason RA, Steane PA: Carcinoid syndrome: Its relevance to the anaesthetist. Anaesthesist 31:228, 1976

490. Koppolu SRD, Miller R: Atypical carcinoid syndrome during anesthesia. Anesthesiol Rev 4:27, 1977

491. Roizen MF, Moss J, Henry DP, et al: Effect of general anesthetics on handling- and decapitation-induced increases in sympathoadrenal discharge. J Pharmacol Exp Ther 204:11, 1978

492. Roizen MF, Wilkinson PL, Chatterjee K, et al: Does anesthesia alter myocardial stress during coronary artery surgery . . . A-V myocardial norepinephrine differences, a new index of myocardial stress, Catecholamines and Stress: Recent Advances. Edited by Usdin E, Kvetňanský R, Kopin IJ. New York, Elsevier, 1980, p 211

493. Shnider SM, Wright RG, Levinson G, et al: Uterine blood flow and plasma norepinephrine changes during maternal stress in the pregnant ewe. Anesthesiology 50:524, 1979

494. Philbin DM, Coggins CH: Plasma antidiuretic hormone levels in cardiac surgical patients dur-

ing morphine and halothane anesthesia. Anesthesiology 49:95, 1978

495. Madsen SN, Brandt MR, Engquist A, et al: Inhibition of plasma cyclic AMP, glucose and cortical response to surgery by epidural analgesia. Br J Surg 64:669, 1977

496. Muldoon SM, Moss J, Freas W, et al: The effects of anaesthetics on the sympathoadrenal system. Clin Anaesthesiol 2:289, 1984

497. Wataneeyawech M, Kelly KA Jr: Hepatic diseases, unsuspected before surgery. NY State J Med 75:1278, 1975

498. Schemel WH: Unexpected hepatic dysfunction found by multiple laboratory screening. Anesth Analg 55:810, 1976

499. Clark R, Doggart J, Tavery T: Changes in liver function after different types of surgery. Br J Anaesth 48:119, 1976

500. Stevens WC, Eger EI II, Joas TA, et al: Comparative toxicity of isoflurane, halothane, fluroxene, and diethyl ether in human volunteers. Can Anaesth Soc J 20:357, 1973

501. Gelman SI, Fowler KC, Smith LR: Liver circulation and function during isoflurane and halothane anesthesia. Anesthesiology 61:726–730, 1984

502. Akdikem S, Flanagan TV, Landmesser CM: A comparative study of serum glutamic pyruvic transaminase changes following anesthesia with halothane, methoxyflurane, and other inhalation agents. Anesth Analg 45:819, 1966

503. Strunin L: Preoperative assessment of the patient with liver dysfunction. Br J Anaesth 50:25, 1978

504. Harville DD, Summerskill WH: Surgery in acute hepatitis—Cause and effects. JAMA 184:257, 1963

505. Farman JV: Anaesthesia in the presence of liver disease and for hepatic transplantation. Br J Anaesth 44:946, 1972

506. Viegas O, Stoelting RK: LDH$_5$ changes after cholecystectomy and hysterectomy in patients receiving halothane, enflurane or fentanyl. Anesthesiology 51:556, 1979

507. Smith AA, Volpitto PP, Gramling ZW, et al: Chloroform, halothane and regional anesthesia: A comparative study. Anesth Analg 52:1, 1973

508. Ronk W: Liver function chemistries after enflurane and narcotic-N$_2$O anesthesia. AANA J 46:507, 1978

509. The National Halothane Study, Bunker JP, Forrest WH, Mosteller F, et al (editors): A Study of the Possible Association Between Halothane Anesthesia and Postoperative Hepatic Necrosis. Washington, DC, US Government Printing Office, 1969

510. McEvan J: Liver function tests following anesthesia. Br J Anaesth 48:1065, 1976

511. Evans C, Evans M, Pollock AV: The incidence and causes of postoperative jaundice. Br J Anaesth 46:520, 1974

512. Shingu K, Eger EI II, Johnson BH, et al: Effect of oxygen concentration, hyperthermia, and choice of vendor on anesthetic-induced hepatic injury in rats. Anesth Analg 62:146, 1983

513. La Mont JT: Postoperative jaundice. Surg Clin North Am 54:637, 1974

514. Dawson JL: The incidence of postoperative renal failure in obstructive jaundice. Br J Surg 52:663, 1965

515. Child CG, Turcolte JG: The Liver and Portal Hypertension. Philadelphia, WB Saunders, 1964

516. Resnick RH, Iber FL, Ishihara AM, et al: A controlled study of the therapeutic portacaval shunt. Gastroenterology 67:843, 1974

517. Wright R, Eade OE, Chisholm M, et al: Controlled prospective study of the effect on liver function of multiple exposures to halothane. Lancet 6:817, 1975

518. Trowell J, Peto R, Smith AC: Controlled trial of repeated halothane anaesthetics in patients with carcinoma of the uterine cervix treated with radium. Lancet 1:821, 1975

519. Allen PJ, Downing JW: A prospective study of hepatocellular function after repeated exposures to halothane or enflurane in women undergoing radium therapy for cervical cancer. Br J Anaesth 49:1035, 1977

520. Fee JPH, Black GW, Dundee JW, et al: A prospective study of liver enzyme and other changes following repeat administration of halothane and enflurane. Br J Anaesth 51:1133, 1979

521. Carney FMT, Van Dyke RA: Halothane hepatitis: A critical review. Anesth Analg 51:135, 1972

522. Vergani D, Tsantoulas D, Eddleston ALWF, et al: Sensitization to halothane—Altered liver components in severe hepatic necrosis after halothane anesthesia. Lancet 2:801, 1978

523. Dykes MHM: Is halothane hepatitis chronic active hepatitis? (editorial). Anesthesiology 46:233, 1977

524. Bréchot C, Nalpas B, Courouce A-M, et al: Evidence that hepatitis B virus has a role in liver-cell carcinoma in alcoholic liver disease. N Engl J Med 306:1384, 1982

525. Thomas FB: Chronic aggressive hepatitis induced by halothane. Ann Intern Med 81:487, 1974

526. Rakela J, Redeker AG: Chronic liver disease after acute non-A, non-B viral hepatitis. Gastroenterology 77:1200, 1979

527. Berman M, Alter JH, Ishak KG, et al: The chronic sequelae of non-A, non-B hepatitis. Ann Intern Med 91:1, 1979

528. Dykes MHM: Unexplained postoperative fever. JAMA 216:641, 1971

529. Sipes I, Brown B: An animal model of hepatotoxicity associated with halothane anesthesia. Anesthesiology 45:622, 1976

530. Klatskin G, Kimberg DV: Recurrent hepatitis attributable to halothane sensitization in an anesthetist. N Engl J Med 280:515, 1969

531. Douglas HJ, Eger EI II, Biava CG, et al: Hepatic necrosis associated with viral infection after enflurane anesthesia. N Engl J Med 296:553, 1977

532. Gall EA: Report of the pathology panel: National Halothane Study. Anesthesiology 29:233, 1968

533. Dykes MHM, Gilbert JP, Schur PH, et al: Halothane and the liver: A review of the epidemiologic, immunologic and metabolic aspects of the relationship. Can J Surg 15:1, 1972

534. Wright EC, Seeff LB, Berk PD, et al: Treatment of chronic active hepatitis. An analysis of three controlled trials. Gastroenterology 73:1422, 1977

535. Reynolds TB: Chronic hepatitis: Current dilemmas. Am J Med 69:485, 1980

536. Hepatitis B virus vaccine safety: Report of an inter-agency group. MMWR 31:465, 1982

537. Centers for Disease Control, Department of Health and Human Services: Inactivated hepatitis B virus vaccine. Recommendation of the Immunization Practice Advisory Committee. Ann Intern Med 97:379, 1982

538. Gerety RJ, Tabor E: Newly licensed hepatitis B vaccine. Known safety and unknown risks. JAMA 249:745, 1983

539. Richter JM, Silverstein MD, Schapiro R: Suspected obstructive jaundice: A decision analysis of diagnostic strategies. Ann Intern Med 99:46, 1983

540. Berry AJ, Isaacson IJ, Hunt D, et al: The prevalence of hepatitis B viral markers in anesthesia personnel. Anesthesiology 60:6, 1984

541. Van Thiel DH, Schade RR, Starzl TE: After 20 years, liver transplantation comes of age. Ann Intern Med 99:854, 1983

542. Mulley AG, Silverstein MD, Dienstag JL: Indications for use of hepatitis B vaccine, based on cost-effectiveness analysis. N Engl J Med 307:644, 1982

543. Naulty JS, Reves JG, Tobey RR, et al: Hepatitis and operating room personnel: An approach to diagnosis and management. Anesth Analg 56:360, 1977

544. Duvaldestin P, Agoston S, Henzel D, et al: Pancuronium pharmacokinetics in patients with liver cirrhosis. Br J Anaesth 50:1131, 1978

545. Wasserman LR, Gilbert HS: Surgical bleeding in polycythemia vera. Ann NY Acad Sci 115:122, 1964

546. Rothstein P: What hemoglobin level is adequate in pediatric anesthesia? Anesthesiol Update 1(24):2, 1978

547. Slogoff S: Anesthesia considerations in the anemic patient. Anesthesiol Update 2(7):1, 1979

548. Thomas DJ, Du Boulay GH, Marshall J, et al: Effect of hematocrit on cerebral blood flow in man. Lancet 2:941, 1977

549. York EL, Jones RL, Menon D, et al: Effects of secondary polycythemia on cerebral blood flow in chronic obstructive pulmonary disease. Am Rev Respir Dis 121:813, 1980

550. Thomas DJ: Whole blood viscosity and cerebral blood flow (editorial). Stroke 13:285, 1982

551. Heughan C, Grislis G, Hunt TK: The effect of anemia on wound healing. Ann Surg 179:163, 1974

552. Lichtiger B, Dupuis JF, Seski J: Hemotherapy during surgery for Jehovah's Witnesses: A new method. Anesth Analg 61:618, 1982

553. Tremper KK, Friedman AE, Levine EM, et al: The preoperative treatment of severely anemic patients with a perfluorochemical oxygen-transport fluid, Fluosol-DA. N Engl J Med 307:277, 1982

554. Greenburg AG: Blood substitutes: Where are we? Surg Annu 15:13, 1983

555. Vichinsky EP, Lubin BH: Sickle cell anemia and related hemoglobinopathies. Pediatr Clin North Am 27:429, 1980

556. Sheehy TW, Plumb VJ: Treatment of sickle cell disease. Arch Intern Med 137:779, 1977

557. Sears DA: The morbidity of sickle cell trait: A review of the literature. Am J Med 64:1021, 1978

558. Heller P, Best WR, Nelson RB, et al: Clinical implication of sickle cell trait and glucose-6-phosphate dehydrogenase deficiency in hospitalized black male patients. N Engl J Med 300:1001, 1979

559. Price HL: Anesthesia in sickle-cell states. Anesthesiol Update 2(17):1, 1979

560. Dalal FY, Schmidt GB, Bennett EJ, et al: Sickle-cell trait, a report of a postoperative neurological complication. Br J Anaesth 46:387, 1974

561. Oduro KA, Searle JF: Anaesthesia in sickle-cell states: A plea for simplicity. Br Med J 4:596, 1972

562. Homi J, Reynolds J, Skinner A, et al: General anesthesia in sickle-cell disease. Br Med J 1:1599, 1979

563. Trubowitz S: The management of sickle cell anemia. Med Clin North Am 60:933, 1976

564. Morrison JC, Wiser WL: The use of prophylactic partial exchange transfusion in pregnancies associated with sickle cell hemoglobinopathy. Obstet Gynecol 48:516, 1976

565. Morrison JC, Whybrew WD, Bucovaz ET: Use of partial exchange transfusion preoperatively in patients with sickle cell hemoglobinopathies. Am J Obstet Gynecol 132:59, 1978

566. Lanzkowsky P, Shende A, Karayalcin G, et al:

Partial exchange transfusion in sickle cell anemia: Use in children with serious complications. Am J Dis Child 132:1206, 1978

567. Rosa RM, Bierer BE, Thomas R, et al: A study of induced hyponatremia in the prevention and treatment of sickle-cell crisis. N Engl J Med 303:1138, 1980

568. Orr D: Difficult intubation: A hazard in thalassemia. A case report. Br J Anaesth 39:585, 1967

569. Pootrakul P, Hungsprenges S, Fucharoen S, et al: Relation between erythropoiesis and bone metabolism in thalassemia. N Engl J Med 304:1470, 1981

570. Lux SE, Wolfe LC: Inherited disorders of the red cell membrane skeleton. Pediatr Clin North Am 27:463, 1980

571. Frank MM, Schreiber AD, Atkinson JP, et al: Pathophysiology of immune hemolytic anemia. Ann Intern Med 87:210, 1979

572. Loque G, Rosse W: Immunologic mechanisms in autoimmune hemolytic disease. Semin Hematol 13:277, 1976

573. Herzig RH, Herzig GP, Graw RG Jr, et al: Successful granulocyte transfusion therapy for gram negative septicemia. N Engl J Med 296:701, 1977

574. Alavi JB, Root RK, Djerassi I, et al: A randomized clinical trial of granulocyte transfusion for infection in acute leukemia. N Engl J Med 296:706, 1977

575. Winston DJ, Ho WG, Gale RP: Therapeutic granulocyte transfusions for documented infections. A controlled trial in ninety-five infectious granulocytopenic episodes. Ann Intern Med 97:509, 1982

576. Strauss RG, Connett JE, Gale RP, et al: A controlled trial of prophylactic granulocyte transfusions during initial induction chemotherapy for acute myelogenous leukemia. N Engl J Med 305:597, 1981

577. Lacey JV, Penner JA: Management of idiopathic thrombocytopenic purpura in the adult. Semin Thromb Hemost 3:160, 1977

578. Kelton JG: Management of the pregnant patient with idiopathic thrombocytopenic purpura. Ann Intern Med 99:796, 1983

579. Tyler DC: Anesthetic management of hemolytic-uremic syndrome. Anesthesiol Rev 9:23, 1982

580. Simpson MB: Platelet function and transfusion therapy in the surgical patient, Platelet Physiology and Transfusion. Edited by Schiffer CJ. Washington, DC, American Association of Blood Banks, 1978, p 51

581. Davis DW, Steward DT: Unexplained excessive bleeding during operation: Role of acetylsalicylic acid. Can Anaesth Soc J 24:452, 1977

582. Majerus PW, Miletich JP: Relationships between platelets and coagulation factors in hemostasis. Annu Rev Med 29:41, 1978

583. Evans BE: Dental treatment for hemophiliacs: Evaluation of dental program (1975–1976) at the Mount Sinai Hospital International Hemophilia Training Center. Mt Sinai J Med 44:409, 1977

584. Zauber NP, Levin J: Factor IX levels in patients with hemophilia B (Christmas Disease) following transfusion with concentrates of factor IX or fresh frozen plasma (FFP). Medicine (Baltimore) 56:213, 1977

585. Gralnick HR, Coller BS, Schulman NR, et al: Factor VIII. Ann Intern Med 86:598, 1977

586. Aledort LM: Recent advances in hemophilia. Ann NY Acad Sci 240:1, 1975

587. Blatt PM, Brinkhous KM, Culp HR, et al: Antihemophilic factor concentrate therapy in von Willebrand's disease. JAMA 236:2770, 1976

588. Curran JW, Lawrence DN, Jaffe H, et al: Acquired immunodeficiency syndrome (AIDS) associated with transfusions. N Engl J Med 310:69, 1984

589. Bove JR: Transfusion-associated AIDS—A cause for concern (editorial). N Engl J Med 310:115, 1984

590. Miller RD: Complications of massive blood transfusions. Anesthesiology 39:82, 1973

591. Sherman LA: Alterations in hemostasis during massive transfusion, Massive Transfusion. Edited by Nusbacher J. Washington, DC, American Association of Blood Banks, 1978, p 51

592. Halkin H, Goldberg J, Modan M, et al: Reduction of mortality in general medical in-patients by low-dose heparin prophylaxis. Ann Intern Med 96:561, 1982

593. Marks RM, Sachar EJ: Undertreatment of medical inpatients with narcotic analgesics. Ann Intern Med 78:173, 1973

594. Catalano RB: The medical approach to management of pain caused by cancer. Semin Oncol 2:379, 1975

595. Twycross RBG: Choice of strong analgesics in terminal cancer: Diamorphine or morphine. Pain 3:93, 1977

596. Vitez TS, Way WL, Miller RD, et al: Effect of delta-9-tetrahydrocannabinol on cyclopropane MAC in the rat. Anesthesiology 38:525, 1973

597. Goldiner P, Carlon GC, Cvitkovic E, et al: Factors influencing postoperative morbidity and mortality in patients treated with bleomycin. Br Med J 1:1664, 1978

598. LaMantia KR, Glick JH, Marshall BE: Supplemental oxygen does not cause respiratory failure in bleomycin-treated surgical patients. Anesthesiology 60:65, 1984

599. Singer MM, Wright F, Stanley LK, et al: Oxygen toxicity in man. A prospective study in patients after open-heart surgery. N Engl J Med 283:1473, 1970

600. Mayer SE: Neurohumoral transmission and the autonomic nervous system, Goodman and Gilman's The Pharmacological Basis of Therapeutics. 6th Ed. Edited by Gilman AG, Goodman LS, Gilman A. New York, Macmillan, 1980, p 56

601. Lake CR, Chernow B, Feuerstein G, et al: The sympathetic nervous system in man: Its evaluation and the measurement of plasma NE, Norepinephrine. Edited by Ziegler MG, Lake CR. Baltimore, Williams & Wilkins, 1984, p 1

602. Burn JH, Rand MJ: Actions of sympathomimetic amines on animals treated with reserpine. J Physiol (Lond) 144:314, 1958

603. Drugs for hypertension. Med Lett Drugs Ther 23:45, 1981

604. Sethna DH, Gray RJ, Moffitt EA, et al: Dobutamine and cardiac oxygen balance in patients following myocardial revascularization. Anesth Analg 61:917, 1982

605. The Norwegian Multicenter Study Group: Timolol-induced reduction in mortality and reinfarction in patients surviving acute myocardial infarction. N Engl J Med 304:801, 1981

606. Sleight P: Beta-adrenergic blockade after myocardial infarction (editorial). N Engl J Med 304:837, 1981

607. Frishman WH, Furberg CD, Friedewald WT: β-Adrenergic blockade for survivors of acute myocardial infarction. N Engl J Med 310:830, 1984

608. Smulyan H, Weinberg SE, Howanitz PJ: Continuous propranolol infusion following abdominal surgery. JAMA 247:2539, 1982

609. Slogoff S, Keats AS, Hibbs CW, et al: Failure of general anesthesia to potentiate propranolol activity. Anesthesiology 47:504, 1977

610. Tanifuji Y, Eger EI II: Effect of isoproterenol and propranolol on halothane MAC in dogs. Anesth Analg 55:383, 1976

611. Kaukinen S, Pyykkö K: The potentiation of halothane anaesthesia by clonidine. Acta Anaesthesiol Scand 23:107, 1979

612. Bloor BC, Flacke WE: Reduction in halothane anesthetic requirement by clonidine, an alpha-adrenergic agonist. Anesth Analg 61:741, 1982

613. Miller RD, Sohn YJ, Matteo RS: Enhancement of d-tubocurarine neuromuscular blockade by diuretics in man. Anesthesiology 45:442, 1976

614. Tosone SR, Reves JG, Kissin I, et al: Hemodynamic responses to nifedipine in dogs anesthetized with halothane. Anesth Analg 62:903, 1983

615. Millard RW, Grupp G, Grupp IL, et al: Chronotropic, inotropic, and vasodilator actions of diltiazem, nifedipine, and verapamil. Circ Res 52(suppl I):I29, 1983

616. Braunwald E: Mechanism of action of calcium-channel-blocking agents. N Engl J Med 307:1618, 1982

617. Zimpfer M, Fitzal S, Tonzcar L: Verapamil as a hypotensive agent during neuroleptanaesthesia. Br J Anaesth 53:885, 1981

618. Kapur PA, Flacke WE: Epinephrine-induced arrhythmias and cardiovascular function after verapamil during halothane anesthesia in the dog. Anesthesiology 55:218, 1981

619. Reves JG, Kissin I, Lell WA, et al: Calcium entry blockers: Uses and implications for anesthesiologists. Anesthesiology 57:504, 1982

620. Maze M, Mason DM: Verapamil decreases the MAC for halothane in dogs. Anesth Analg 62:274, 1983

621. Springman SR, Redon D, Rusy BF: The effect of nifedipine on the circulation during morphine-N_2O and halothane anesthesia in dogs. Anesth Analg 62:284, 1983

622. Marshall AG, Kissin I, Reves JG, et al: Interaction between negative inotropic effects of halothane and nifedipine in the isolated rat heart. J Cardiovasc Pharmacol 5:592, 1983

623. Zaggy AP, Kates RA, Norfleet EA, et al: The comparative cardiovascular effects of verapamil, nifedipine, and diltiazem during halothane anesthesia. Anesthesiology 59:A44, 1983

624. Casthely PA, Villanueva R, Schneider A: Shunting during hypotension with nifedipine. Anesthesiology 59:A510, 1983

625. Norfleet EA, Heath KR, Kopp VJ, et al: Verapamil—Different cardiovascular responses during N_2O analgesia and halothane anesthesia. Anesthesiology 57:A75, 1982

626. Hantler CB, Felbeck PG, Kroll DA, et al: Effects of verapamil on sinus and AV nodal function in the presence of volatile anesthetics. Anesthesiology 59:A38, 1983

627. Kates RA, Kaplan JA: Cardiovascular responses to verapamil during coronary artery bypass graft surgery. Anesth Analg 62:821, 1983

628. Fanta CH, Drazen JM: Calcium blockers and bronchoconstriction (editorial). Am Rev Respir Dis 127:673, 1983

629. Epstein SE, Rosing DR: Verapamil: Its potential for causing serious complications in patients with hypertrophic cardiomyopathy. Circulation 64:437, 1981

630. Kraynack BJ, Lawson NW, Gintautas J: Verapamil reduces indirect muscle twitch amplitude and potentiates pancuronium in vitro. Anesthesiology 57:A265, 1982

631. Durant NN, Nguyen N, Briscoe JR, et al: Potentiation of pancuronium and succinylcholine by verapamil. Anesthesiology 57:A267, 1982

632. Williams JP, Broadbent MP, Pearce AC, et al: Verapamil potentiates the neuromuscular blocking effects of enflurane in vitro. Anesthesiology 59:A276, 1983

633. Dale J, Landmark KH, Myhre E: The effects of nifedipine, a calcium antagonist, on platelet function. Am Heart J 105:103, 1983

634. Zalman F, Perloff JK, Durant NN, et al: Acute respiratory failure following intravenous verapamil in Duchenne's muscular dystrophy. Am Heart J 105:510, 1983

635. White BC, Gadzinski DS, Hoehner PJ, et al: Effect of flunarizine on canine cerebral cortical blood flow and vascular resistance post cardiac arrest. Ann Emerg Med 11:119, 1982

636. McAllister RG Jr: Clinical pharmacokinetics of calcium channel antagonists. J Cardiovasc Pharmacol 4(suppl 3):S340, 1982

637. Merin RG: Calcium (slow) channel blocking drugs, ASA Refresher Courses in Anesthesiology. Vol. 10. Edited by Hershey S. Philadelphia, JB Lippincott, 1982, p 143

638. Evans-Prosser CDG: The use of pethidine and morphine in the presence of monamine oxidase inhibitors. Br J Anaesth 40:279, 1968

639. Campbell GD: Dangers of monamine oxidase inhibitors. Br Med J 1:750, 1963

640. Rogers KJ, Thornton JA: The interaction between monamine oxidase inhibitors and narcotic analgesics in mice. Br J Pharmacol 36:470, 1969

641. Sjoqvist F: Psychotropic drugs. 2: Interaction between monamine oxidase (MAO) inhibitors and other substances. Proc R Soc Med 58:967, 1965

642. Monamine oxidase inhibitors for depression. Med Lett Drugs Ther 22:58, 1980

643. Drugs for psychiatric disorders. Med Lett Drugs Ther 25:45, 1983

644. Edwards RE, Miller RD, Roizen MF, et al: Cardiac effects of imipramine and pancuronium during halothane and enflurane anesthesia. Anesthesiology 50:421, 1979

645. Kosanin R: Anesthetic considerations in patients on chronic tricyclic antidepressant therapy. Anesthesiol Rev 8:38, 1981

646. Veith RC, Raskind MA, Caldwell JH, et al: Cardiovascular effects of tricyclic antidepressants in depressed patients with chronic heart disease. N Engl J Med 306:954, 1982

647. Richelson E, El-Fakahany E: Changes in the sensitivity of receptors for neurotransmitters and the actions of some psychotherapeutic drugs. Mayo Clin Proc 57:576, 1982

648. Adverse interactions of drugs: Med Lett Drugs Ther 23:17, 1981

649. Hill GE, Wong KC: Lithium carbonate and neuromuscular blocking agents. Anesthesiology 46:122, 1977

650. Martin BA, Kramer PM: Clinical significance of the interaction between lithium and a neuromuscular blocker. Am J Psychiatry 139:1326, 1982

651. Johnston RR, Way WL, Miller RD: Alteration of anesthetic requirements by amphetamine. Anesthesiology 36:357, 1972

652. Stoelting RK, Creasser CW, Martz RC: Effect of cocaine administration on halothane MAC in dogs. Anesth Analg 54:422, 1975

653. Katz RL, Bigger JT: Cardiac arrhythmias during anesthesia and operation. Anesthesiology 33:193, 1970

654. Joas TA, Stevens WC: Comparison of the arrhythmic doses of epinephrine during Forane, halothane and enflurane anesthesia in dogs. Anesthesiology 35:48, 1971

655. Johnston RR, Eger EI II, Wilson C: A comparative interaction of epinephrine with enflurane, isoflurane and halothane in man. Anesth Analg 55:709, 1976

656. Horrigan RW, Eger EI II, Wilson CB: Epinephrine-induced arrhythmias during enflurane anesthesia in man: A nonlinear dose–response relationship and dose-dependent protection from lidocaine. Anesth Analg 57:547, 1978

657. Hirshman CA, Bergman NA: Halothane and enflurane protect against bronchospasm in an asthma dog model. Anesth Analg 57:629, 1978

658. Shnider SM, Papper EM: Anesthesia for the asthmatic patient. Anesthesiology 22:886, 1961

659. Marcus ML, Skelton CL, Graver LE, et al: Effects of theophylline on myocardial mechanics. Am J Physiol 222:1361, 1972

660. Westfall DP, Flemming WW: Sensitivity changes in the dog heart to norepinephrine, calcium and aminophylline resulting from pretreatment with reserpine. J Pharmacol Exp Ther 159:98, 1968

661. Rall TW, West TC: The potentiation of cardiac inotropic responses to norepinephrine by theophylline. J Pharmacol Exp Ther 139:269, 1963

662. Webb-Johnson DC, Andrews JL: Bronchodilator therapy I. N Engl J Med 297:476, 1977

663. Atuk NO, Blaydes C, Westervelt FB, et al: Effect of aminophylline on urinary excretion of epinephrine and norepinephrine in man. Circulation 35:745, 1967

664. Horwitz LN, Spear JF, Moore EN, et al: Effect of aminophylline on the threshold for initiating ventricular fibrillation during respiratory failure. Am J Cardiol 35:376, 1975

665. Mitenko PA, Ogilvie RI: Pharmacokinetics of intravenous theophylline. Clin Pharmacol Ther 14:509, 1973

666. Patterson JW, Shenfield GM: Bronchodilators. Parts I and II. Br Thorac Tuberc Assoc Rev 4:25, 61, 1974

667. Piafsky KM, Ogilvie RI: Dosage of theophylline in bronchial asthma. N Engl J Med 292:1218, 1975

668. Hunt SN, Jusko WJ, Yurchak AM: Effect of smoking on theophylline disposition. Clin Pharmacol Ther 19:546, 1975

669. Takaori M, Loehning RW: Ventricular arrhythmias induced by aminophylline during halothane anaesthesia in dogs. Can Anaesth Soc J 14:79, 1967

670. Takaori M, Loehning RW: Ventricular arrhythmias during halothane anaesthesia: Effect of isoproterenol, aminophylline, and ephedrine. Can Anaesth Soc J 12:275, 1965

671. Roizen MF, Stevens WC: Multiform ventricular tachycardia due to the interaction of aminophylline and halothane. Anesth Analg 57:738, 1978

672. Berger JM, Stirt JA, Sullivan SF: Enflurane, halothane, and aminophylline — Uptake and pharmacokinetics. Anesth Analg 62:733, 1983

673. Stirt JA, Berger JM, Sullivan SF: Lack of arrhythmogenicity of isoflurane following administration of aminophylline in dogs. Anesth Analg 62:568, 1983

674. Treatment of cardiac arrhythmias. Med Lett Drugs Ther 25:21, 1983

675. Harrah MD, Way WL, Katzung BG: The interaction of d-tubocurarine with antiarrhythmic drugs. Anesthesiology 33:406, 1970

676. Telivuo L, Katz RL: The effects of modern intravenous local anesthetics on respiration during partial neuromuscular block in man. Anaesthesia 25:30, 1970

677. Miller RD, Way WL, Katzung BG: The potentiation of neuromuscular blocking agents by quinidine. Anesthesiology 28:1036, 1967

678. Pittinger CB, Eryasa Y, Adamson R: Antibiotic-induced paralysis. Anesth Analg 49:487, 1970

679. Singh YN, Harvey AL, Marshall IG: Antibiotic induced-paralysis of the mouse phrenic nerve-hemidiaphragm preparation, and reversibility by calcium and by neostigmine. Anesthesiology 48:418, 1978

680. Pittinger CB, Adamson R: Antibiotic blockade of neuromuscular function. Annu Rev Pharmacol 12:169, 1972

681. Becker LD, Miller RD: Clindamycin enhances a non-depolarizing neuromuscular blockade. Anesthesiology 45:84, 1976

682. Sampson IH, Miller R: Antibiotics: Their relevance to the anesthesiologist, a review. Anesthesiol Rev 5:43, 1978

683. Snavely SR, Hodges GR: The neurotoxicity of antibacterial agents. Ann Intern Med 101:92, 1984

684. McIndewar IC, Marshall RJ: Interactions between the neuromuscular blocking drug Org NC45 and some anaesthetic, analgesic and antimicrobial agents. Br J Anaesth 53:785, 1981

685. Rice SA, Sbordone L, Mazze RI: Metabolism by rat hepatic microsomes of fluorinated ether anesthetics following isoniazid administration. Anesthesiology 53:489, 1980

686. Antimicrobial prophylaxis for surgery. Med Lett Drugs Ther 23:77, 1981

687. Beller GA, Smith TW, Abelmann WH, et al: Digitalis intoxication. N Engl J Med 284:989, 1971

688. Hurlbert BJ, Edelman JD, David K: Serum potassium levels during and after terbutaline. Anesth Analg 60:723, 1981

689. Morrow DH: Anesthesia and digitalis toxicity. VI. Effect of barbiturates and halothane on digoxin toxicity. Anesth Analg 49:305, 1970

690. Pratila MG, Pratilas V: Anesthetic agents and cardiac electromechanical activity. Anesthesiology 49:338, 1978

691. Logic JR, Morrow DH: The effect of halothane on ventricular automaticity. Anesthesiology 36:107, 1972

692. Ivankovich AD, Miletich DJ, Grossman RK, et al: The effect of enflurane, isoflurane, fluroxene, methoxyflurane and diethyl ether on ouabain tolerance in the dog. Anesth Analg 55:360, 1976

693. Ali N, Dais K, Banks T, Sheikh M: Titrated electrical cardioversion in patients on digoxin. Clin Cardiol 5:417, 1982

694. Adverse systemic effects from ophthalmic drugs. Med Lett Drugs Ther 24:53, 1982

695. Pantuck EJ, Pantuck CB: Cholinesterases and anticholinesterases, Muscle Relaxants. Edited by Katz RL. Amsterdam, Excerpta Medica, 1975, p 143

696. Ghoneim MM, Long JP: The interaction between magnesium and other neuromuscular blocking agents. Anesthesiology 32:23, 1970

697. Del Castillo J, Engback L: The nature of neuromuscular block produced by magnesium. J Physiol (Lond) 124:370, 1954

698. Feely J, Wilkinson GR, McAllister CB, et al: Increased toxicity and reduced clearance of lidocaine by cimetidine. Ann Intern Med 96:592, 1982

699. Lam AM, Parkin JA: Cimetidine and prolonged post-operative somnolence. Can Anaesth Soc J 28:450, 1981

700. Vessey MD, Doll R, Fairbairn AS, et al: Postoperative thromboembolism and the use of oral contraceptives. Br Med J 3:123, 1970

701. Greene GR, Sartwell PE: Oral contraceptive use in patients with thromboembolism following surgery, trauma, or infection. Am J Public Health 62:680, 1972

702. Interruption of a drug regimen before anesthesia. Med Lett Drugs Ther 16:19, 1974

703. Salzman EW, Davies GC: Prophylaxis of venous thromboembolism. Analysis of cost effectiveness. Ann Surg 191:207, 1980

704. Leyvraz PF, Richard J, Bachmann F, et al: Adjusted versus fixed-dose subcutaneous heparin in the prevention of deep-vein thrombosis after total hip replacement. N Engl J Med 309:954, 1983

705. Salzman EW: Progress in preventing venous thromboembolism (editorial). N Engl J Med 309:980, 1983

706. Cascorbi HF: Perianesthetic problems with nonanesthetic drugs, ASA Refresher Courses in Anesthesiology. Vol. 6. Edited by Hershey SG. Philadelphia, JB Lippincott, 1978, p 15

707. Cullen BF, Miller MG: Drug interactions and anesthesia: A review. Anesth Analg 58:413, 1979

708. Smith NT, Miller RD, Corbascio AN: Drug Interactions in Anesthesia. Philadelphia, Lea & Febiger, 1981

709. Update: Drugs in breast milk. Med Lett Drugs Ther 21:21, 1979

10

Anesthesia Risk

John H. Tinker, M.D.
Sandra L. Roberts, M.D.

Perhaps the most insidious hazard of anesthesia is its relative safety.

Jeffrey B. Cooper

The first so-called anesthetic deaths were described in a remarkable 1858 treatise by John Snow, entitled *On Chloroform and Other Anaesthetics*.[1] As A.S. Keats has pointed out,[2] few if any subsequent investigators have gone into such detail or performed specific experiments in an effort to ascertain whether particular deaths were actually due to anesthesia. Again, using the words of Keats[2]:

No control study of the hazards of operation without anesthesia or conversely anesthesia without operation will ever be performed. The hazards of anesthesia can never be considered independent of a second procedure.

Nonetheless, mortality and morbidity obviously can be directly attributed to anesthesia. To some extent, we have become victims of the admonishments of prominent anesthetists such as Sir Robert Macintosh,[3] who in a 1948 treatise entitled *Deaths under Anaesthetics* convinced many that anesthetic drugs and practices were (are, should be) safe, and that there could seldom, if ever, be a death in the operating room without error on the part of someone. The idea that anesthesia risk per se would approach zero if errors and mistakes could be eliminated resulted in suggestions by Ruth[4] in 1945 that "anesthesia study commissions" be set up to adjudicate blame, ferret out exact causes for each anesthetic misadventure, and by so doing permit anesthetists to develop methods to assure that such failings would not recur. No reasonable anesthetist can argue that deaths and morbidity are occasionally due to errors, lapses, and preventable failures. However, the possible benefit of such study commissions in preventing future recurrences is open to question. Many currently accepted techniques might have been judged to constitute malpractice just 20 years ago. To use Keats's[2] example, if a critically ill cardiac pa-

359

tient who had received 2 mg/kg morphine was then given a vasodilator such as nitroprusside and later died in the operating room, the Beecher and Todd study commission[5] would most likely have considered it an anesthetic death. Adoption of innovations in the management of critically ill, inherently high-risk patients could be hindered if death should be judged due to technical error or flaw associated with the innovation rather than to severe patient instability. In today's legal climate, the judgment of "anesthetic death" by such a commission—legal or quasilegal—could probably not be kept confidential.

Another problem in assuming every anesthetic death to be due to error is the fact that each year countless deaths suddenly occur with no discernible cause, even after autopsy. There is no reason to believe that anesthesia magically protects a patient from this risk of unexplainable sudden death. Everyone accepts that some people die during natural sleep; indeed this is often regarded as "the best way to go." The lay public would like to believe that being "put to sleep" carries no risk at all—not even that of an afternoon nap. The idea that if a patient dies or sustains injury, error must have played a causal role has spawned much legal profit. Juries are led to believe, and indeed often want to believe, that any untoward outcome must be rooted in physician fault. Although this misbelief is exploited by lawyers, it is rooted in long-standing self-deprecatory thinking within anesthesiology in particular, but also by medicine in general.

Present-day buzzwords such as "risk/cost–benefit ratio" and "outcome studies" have useful roles in assessing anesthetic techniques as long as extrapolation is not overdone. To deduce that anesthetic risk can and must be zero because there is little or no therapeutic benefit of anesthesia per se is fallacious. No one educated in the myriad complexities and possible disasters inherent in such separate categories as muscle relaxants, inhaled anesthetics, local anesthetics, hypnotics, all the above plus preexistent patient disease, all the above plus surgical stress and trespass, plus electromechanical quasicomputerized monitors and drug delivery systems could rationally conclude that the sum total risk of an "anesthetic" could or should be zero. Anesthesia performed com-

pletely in accordance with current accepted standards can still be associated with major morbidity or mortality.

Some educators hold that browbeating anesthetists-in-training with the concept that all untoward outcomes are due to preventable errors will result in optimal vigilance. But we believe that truth, including the admission of ignorance where such exists, is a better educational tool. For example, the self-deprecatory approach to instances in which intraoperative death was not due to anesthetic error produces a self-doubt and guilt in trainees that may adversely affect their future ability and judgment rather than result in "optimal vigilance." For the beginning anesthetist reading this chapter, our message is that while lack of vigilance and poor judgment certainly do result in "anesthetic death," nonetheless patients can and do die despite state-of-the-art anesthetic and perioperative care.

IS THERE AN AGREED-UPON DEFINITION OF "ANESTHETIC RISK"?

Previously, perioperative death and, by extension, perioperative morbidity, were categorized as primarily anesthesia, anesthesia contributory, primarily surgery, surgery contributory, or primarily patient disease.[4-14] Obviously, the causes of mortality and morbidity are of prime importance. Yet, among 15 institutions performing coronary artery bypass surgery (CABG), Kennedy et al.[15] reported that perioperative mortality ranged from 0.3 to more than 6 percent for the same operation in groups of patients that could not be told apart by standard disease-severity criteria. In this report, the mortality rates were nearly linearly distributed between these extremes. The idea here is that such disparate overall outcomes need explanations. Perhaps detailed explanations can yield specific improvements in care. Another example of such disparate outcomes can be seen by comparing the outcome results published for carotid endarterectomy. Sundt et al.[16] reported an overall stroke/mortality outcome of 3.6 percent (when minor new deficits were included) and 2.5 percent for major deficits plus mortalities, following 1,145 operations. By sharp contrast, Easton and Sherman,[17] examining 228 of the same operations, reported a stroke-plus-death rate nearly 10 times greater, namely 21.1 percent. Modern outcome studies, when carefully compared and subjected to further detailed analysis, may yield more useful information than the "anesthetic risk" studies of the past.

There are problems with outcome-type studies when the overall result is nearly all that is known.[18] For example, if perioperative mortality (from whatever cause) is assumed to be 3 percent in hospital A and 6 percent in hospital B for the same operation, are both hospitals really doing the same operation? Were the patients equally sick? Have things changed so much since the (presumably retrospective) studies mentioned above that neither number has any current likely validity?[18] Consider the most recent studies of anesthetic morbidity and mortality[19-25] done retrospectively in Great Britain. Despite their recent publication (1982– 1983), still 8.1 percent of cases were reported wherein ether, trichloroethylene, or cyclopropane was used, probably indicating a considerable time lag with current practice.

These studies, by Lunn and associates [19-25] in Cardiff, Wales, are nonetheless examples of thoughtful and rigorous modern attempts to attack the problem of identification of "anesthetic risk." A total of 108,878 anesthetics were reported, having been administered between 1972 and 1977 (illustrative in itself of the time lag necessary in bringing retrospective studies to publication — 1982).[19,24] In the initial evaluation, no attempt was made to assign specific causes to the deaths, 102 of which occurred in the operating room (0.09 percent), 27 in the recovery room (0.02 percent), and 2,262 (2.08 percent) within 6 days elsewhere in hospital. The overall in-hospital mortality was therefore 2.19 percent, taking into account all those patients who received anesthetics.

Next, Lunn and colleagues constructed five "overall risk" categories based on subjective assessment of degree of overall illness —

nearly identical to the familiar ASA classifications. As expected, the in-hospital mortality ranged from 0.3 percent for those judged to be "good risks," to 57.8 percent for those judged "moribund."[19,24] These workers also analyzed the overall mortality by anatomic location of surgery. More or less as expected, intracranial (9.7 percent), intrathoracic (8.6 percent), and upper abdomen (6.6 percent) were the highest risk groups by region. The most common associated risk factors predictive of mortality were, again as expected, concomitant coronary artery disease and/or chronic pulmonary disease.

As pointed out in Schneider's analysis[18] of the Cardiff data,[19-25] there seems to be a set of "simple fractions" to which this reasonably modern overall risk data can be reduced. If the patient was healthy, with no added risk factors, total perioperative mortality was about 1 in 500. Add a single risk factor, but assume a patient in otherwise good condition, and the patient's overall in-hospital mortality was about 1 in 100. If, in addition to a systemic disease, there was some preoperative impairment of ability to function normally, the risk jumped to roughly 1 in 50. If that impairment was cardiac failure, the overall risk was 1 in 25. Next, severe global preoperative impairment yielded an overall perioperative mortality of 1 in 5. Finally, for patients judged to be moribund or nearly so, the mortality was at least 1 in 2.

How useful is all this to the anesthesiologist? How much of this risk is due to anesthesia? How much of that which is even remotely related to anesthesia can in fact be classified as preventable? Once again, the notable efforts of Lunn and colleagues in Cardiff[20] provide some answers. After establishing an elaborate data collection system as well as credibility for confidentiality, these investigators received many in-depth reports of deaths occurring within 6 days of anesthesia. They were careful to establish the fact that their detailed analyses of these deaths would remain out of the legal system and anonymous. This is, perhaps, possible in Great Britain — just as it is probably impossible in the United States. Nonetheless, the "response rate was considerably less than in the previous study and this itself is a source of considerable disappointment."[20] Lunn et al. were doubtful, however, that overall death rates had changed much in the interval between their studies.

In the later study,[20] reports of 197 deaths that occurred within 6 days of anesthesia and surgery were analyzed by a "blinded assessor" from the same geographic region as the hospital in question. Forty-three percent of the 197 deaths were believed by the assessors to have had nothing to do with anesthesia, 41 percent to be partly due to anesthesia, and 16 percent to be "totally" due to anesthesia. At the same time, opinions as to responsibility for the death were asked of both attending anesthetist and surgeon. The independent assessor agreed with the anesthetist alone in 33 percent of cases, with the surgeon alone in 29 percent of cases, with neither in 19, and with both in only 18 percent of cases. It is important to point out that the anesthetist, the surgeon, and the assessor were guaranteed immunity from each other and the legal system in this study.

An example taken from the Cardiff study might serve to point out the difficulties inherent in any study of anesthetic risk[20]:

> **A six month old infant was to have a pyloromyotomy. No vagolytic drug was given but 2 percent halothane was administered after 12.5 mg suxamethonium [succinylcholine], with manual intermittent positive pressure ventilation of the lungs.**

Although both the anesthetist and surgeon believed that anesthesia played some part in the death that occurred during the anesthetic, the assessors considered anesthesia to be totally responsible.[20] Add the United States opportunistic adversarial legal system, plus the curious but well-rooted idea that pain, suffering, loss of companionship, and loss of "consortium," all can and should somehow be financially compensated, and it is easy to see why the climate is indeed difficult for valid assessment of "anesthetic risk."

Of the deaths adjudicated by the Cardiff group to be due to anesthesia, how many were classed as "preventable"? Of 32 deaths judged totally due to anesthesia, five were described as unavoidable, that is, not due to detectable errors in judgment, to wrong drug, to lapses in vigilance, or to departures from "standard of care." This supports Keats's claim[2] that not all "anesthesia deaths" are necessarily (avoid-

ably) due to errors and lapses. Some examples seem indicated here too, again taken from the Cardiff study[20]:

> **The induction of anaesthesia in one patient with ischemic heart disease had only just commenced, prior to coronary artery bypass grafting, but the patient immediately died despite resuscitative efforts. [Another] patient apparently developed malignant hyperpyrexia in the ward following an ophthalmic operation and after the anaesthetist had left the hospital. [Another patient developed] an immediately fatal, possibly anaphylactoid, reaction to either thiopentone or suxamethonium.**

In the remaining 27 deaths, there were "avoidable features," but even in these cases, the investigators could not always find convincing evidence that if the discovered errors and/or lapses had not occurred, the results might have been improved. This 1983 paper[20] is cited to students of anesthesiology as a serious and dedicated attempt to ascertain whether "anesthetic risk" is possible to assess. Lunn et al. concluded (1) that some form of independent adjudication of "blame" is essential, and (2) that some form of mandatory reporting system, rather than reliance on volunteers, is required before the magnitude of the problem can be elucidated, but that the reporting system must somehow be protected from the legal vicissitudes of discovery tactics and procedures.

Our experience[26-29] with retrospective studies has convinced us that although such studies miss much that may have occurred due to lack of documentation, they nonetheless "tell it like it was" often disconcertingly so. Findings that the profession might rather not admit may emerge. For example, we reported that a significantly greater number of "emergency" coronary artery bypass graft operations occurred on Friday afternoons than would have been expected on the basis of chance alone.[29] Since that report, fewer of these operations have been performed as emergencies at that institution, leading to more uniform distribution through the week. Lunn[25] was able to make some rather startling projections from the data gathered by the Cardiff group in England:

TABLE 10-1. Overall Summary of Cardiff Data*

Risk Factor	Incidence
1. Overall 6-day mortality after surgery	0.6% (60 per 10,000)
2. Overall deaths related at all to anesthesia	0.05% (5 per 10,000)
3. Anesthesia believed causative of death	0.8–0.9 per 10,000
4. Anesthesia partly or totally causative of death (includes No. 3 above)	1–2 per 10,000

* Most recent major studies of overall risk of anesthesia, performed by Lunn and associates (refs. 19–25).

If, and the extrapolation may not be valid, the study population represents the practice of anaesthesia in the whole country [Great Britain], 300,000 patients per year are not seen by their anaesthetist preoperatively, 468,000 do not have their blood pressure recorded during their operations, 534,000 have operations prior to which their anaethetists have not tested the anaesthetic machine and during which, in 1,290,000 cases their ECG is not monitored.

The approximations noted in Table 10-1, seem a reasonable summary of the Cardiff studies of Lunn and colleagues[19-25].

Other relatively recent studies[26,30-32] from Australia, Finland, South Africa, Canada, and the United States seem to be in reasonable agreement with the Cardiff data. Approximately one death per 10,000 anesthetics was totally attributable to anesthesia, and approximately 2 deaths per 10,000 anesthetics were either totally or in major part due to anesthesia management. If these relatively recent studies are indicative, then there has been improvement in anesthesia-related mortality risk, as will be apparent from the following discussion of past studies.

CAN PAST STUDIES BE USED TO BETTER UNDERSTAND MODERN "ANESTHETIC RISK"?

In 1970, Goldstein and Keats[33] published a definitive summary of the various attempts to define "anesthetic risk" up to that time. This review is significant for its completeness and because the onrush of medical malpractice lawsuits in the United States seems to have effectively discouraged most American investigators from making subsequent detailed attempts to discover "anesthetic risk"—especially those in which "error" might have to be admitted. The idea that all anesthetic deaths must have been due to "errors" assumed that anesthetic drugs and adjuvants are unique, that is, have no inherent toxicity.[7,34] Although this bias permeates many past as well as recent studies, biases in other curious directions have occurred. Beecher and Todd[5] decided that the leading culprit in anesthetic risk was curare. Eight other drugs did not receive any such label, one way or the other. Their bias, nearly opposite the bias that all anesthetic deaths are due to error, was such that they attributed only 10 of 384 "anesthetic deaths" (7.5 percent) to error. The National Halothane Study,[35] although it did not discount error, assumed that if a particular drug or technique had a higher risk, some part of said risk was due to the potential of the technique itself to produce error. Dripps et al.[8] found error in 87 percent of 80 deaths, Clifton and Hotten[36] reported error in 65 percent of 52 deaths, Dornette and Orth[10] found error in 87 percent of 47 deaths, Memery[37] noted error in 73 percent of 64 deaths, and Edwards, et al.[38] found error in 89 percent of 1,000 deaths. It is important to recall Goldstein and Keats's analysis[33] of the above data that "one should not resort to self-flagellation." Thus, the role of "error" in the production of "anesthetic death" appears to be between 8 and 100 percent, with the remainder if any, due to "inherent toxicity." The recent Cardiff studies of Lunn and colleagues[19-25] carefully skirt this issue. Their analysis of 197 reports of deaths within 6 days revealed 32 probable anesthetic deaths of which 27 were classed as avoidable, for a 77 percent error rate, not different from numerous past studies. What about overall "anesthesia death" rates prior to 1970? Table 10-2 is redrawn from the data of Goldstein and Keats.[33]

These retrospective studies obviously varied widely in methodology and rates of "anesthesia risk." Although a trend toward improvement did not occur during those years, a major improvement has recently appeared, as shown by the Cardiff data. What can be learned from these older studies? First, definitive large-scale studies of anesthesia risk from American institutions that attempt to label individual cases as "anesthesia causative" and/or "anesthesia contributory" have not been performed for the past 15 years. Although it would be sensible to permit such data to be collected in a fashion that is not "discoverable," that is, available for individual legal cases, no such definitive legal protection exists in the United States. We doubt that a modern Beecher and Todd[5]-type study, valuable though it would be, could be performed in the United States today. Second, studies that attributed death to anesthesia as opposed to other causes have been replaced by studies of incidence of untoward occurrences, lapses, misadventures, and errors in judgment, in which investigators are careful to avoid connecting such events with specific cases wherein poor outcome occurred. Even so, possible legal disclosures of in-house questionnaires, such as "anesthetic mishap report" forms, impede frank discussion and reportage.

THE FRENCH SURVEY OF ANESTHESIA ACCIDENTS AND MORTALITY[40]

Beginning in 1977, the French Health Ministry carried out a nationwide survey of accidents that occurred during anesthesia. The results were reported in 1983,[40] reflecting 190,389 anesthetics surveyed in 2,000 institutions between May 1978 and March 1982. During administration of these anesthetics, 265 accidents occurred that were associated with 66 deaths plus 13 comas lasting longer than 24 hours, for an overall frequency of one accident per 718 and 1 death in 2,885 anesthetics. These investigators reported a rate of 1 death per 13,599 anesthetics attributed totally to improper anesthesia practice. This is numerically better than the 1 per 10,000 figure reported from just a few years previously by the Cardiff group,[19-25] but it is not possible to say with certainty that it represents a favorable trend. It is not unreasonable that an anesthesiologist will perform or be responsible for 1,000 anesthetics per year. Therefore, it is not unlikely that each of us will be responsible if these statistics hold, irrespective of skill or experience level, for 1 death every 10 to 15 years; that is, two to three deaths totally attributable to improper anesthesia practice for each anesthesiologist during his or her career in the specialty. In the French study,[40] accidents were most common at extremes of age, although there seemed to be fewer accidents when extremely elderly patients were anesthetized (possibly this is real, representing more careful anesthesia, better monitoring, distribution of those cases to more experienced anesthetists, and so on). Emergency operations had almost three times the accident rate of elective ones, confirming other observations.[29]

In the French study,[40] "accidents" were classified into four groups: technical difficulty, respiratory failure, cardiovascular failure, and neurologic catastrophe. Circulatory failure accounted for the greatest numbers of deaths. This finding is in contrast to the widely held belief that most anesthesia "accidents" are due to respiratory misadventures such as endotracheal tube dislodgements, obstructions, and disconnections. During induction, if an accident were going to occur, it would most likely be due to circulatory collapse and/or anaphylaxis. Although there were 11 accidents due to technical difficulties during induction, none resulted in death.

During maintenance of anesthesia, circulatory collapse again led the list of "accidents," accounting for the greatest number of complications and deaths. It was not until the recovery period that respiratory difficulties replaced cardiac problems as the most likely untoward events. Twenty-two deaths and comas were considered totally related to anesthesia. Of these, 20 were considered "probably avoidable," including 11 cases wherein respiratory depression occurred postoperatively in unsupervised patients, five cases of aspiration, three

TABLE 10-2. Estimates of Anesthetic Risk Prior to 1970

Investigators	Year	Number of Anesthetics	Overall Incidence of Death	
			Anesthesia Primary	Anesthesia Primary plus Contributory
Beecher and Todd[5]	1954	599,584	1 : 2,680	1 : 1,560
Dornette and Orth[10]	1956	63,150	1 : 2,429	1 : 1,344
Dripps et al.[8]*	1961	33,224	1 : 852	1 : 415
Clifton and Hotten[36]†	1963	205,640	1 : 6,048	1 : 3,955
Memery[37]	1965	69,291	1 : 3,145	1 : 1,082
Harrison[39]‡	1968	177,928	—	1 : 3,007

* Considered only spinal anesthesia plus general anesthesia with muscle relaxants.
† Considered only deaths during anesthesia or failure to return to consciousness.
‡ Considered only deaths within 24 hours of anesthesia or failure to return to consciousness.

cases of equipment failure, and one overdosage. The two situations wherein anesthesia management was considered causative but unavoidable were both anaphylactic responses despite negative histories.[40]

HOW ACCURATE IS THE ASA PHYSICAL STATUS RATING AS A PREDICTOR OF RISK?

The ASA physical status rating is applied to patients before anesthesia and surgery. It has evolved somewhat since its original description.[8] Currently,[18] five categories are recognized, as noted in Table 10-3.

In the 1970 review by Goldstein and Keats[33] of deaths attributable in whole or in part to anesthesia, a total of 41 percent of all such deaths occurred in ASA class I or II patients. Their conclusion was that ASA physical status was "not a sensitive predictor of anesthetic mortality." If most "anesthetic deaths" are due to errors, lapses, or technical difficulties, then ASA physical status might not be expected to be very predictable of risk. Nonetheless, most practitioners strongly believe ASA

physical status to be capable of prediction of overall outcome. Vacanti et al.,[41] in 1970, collected 68,388 cases from 11 U.S. Naval hospitals and reported that ASA physical status was somewhat predictive, at least of overall outcome (Table 10-4).

None of the ASA I patients in the Naval Hospital Study[41] should have died; that is, death was due to anesthesia error (a speculation probably in error for the reasons mentioned earlier). Therefore, assuming a basal "error" percentage of 0.08 percent, the much lower overall percentages of "error" in the numerous studies of anesthetic death, including the recent Cardiff studies,[19-25] cannot be easily explained. To conclude that the likelihood of "error" must increase with the degree of illness of the patient is a dangerous and unfounded assumption, although poor patient reserves may lower patient tolerance for error. The above statistics cover overall death risks, not simply those judged attributable to anesthesia.

Table 10-5, taken from the work of Marx et al.[12] from a 1973 study of 34,145 patients, also shows ASA physical status to be a reasonable predictor of overall outcome, although again not necessarily of anesthesia involvement.

Comparing these two studies,[12,41] definitions of ASA physical status IV and V, that is,

TABLE 10-3. ASA Physical Status*

Category	Description
I	Healthy patient
II	Mild systemic disease — no functional limitation
III	Severe systemic disease — definite functional limitation
IV	Severe systemic disease that is a constant threat to life
V	Moribund patient unlikely to survive 24 hours with or without operation

* American Society of Anesthesiologists classifications as described by Schneider.[18]

TABLE 10-4. ASA Physical Status versus Overall Death Rates

Physical Status	Number of Cases	Deaths	Mortality Rate* (%)
I	50,703	43	0.08
II	12,601	34	0.27
III	3,626	66	1.82
IV	850	66	7.76
V	608	57	9.38
Total	68,388	266	0.39

* Note that this is overall mortality, not specifically attributable to anesthesia. (Modified from Vacanti CJ, Van Houten RJ, Hill RC: A statistical analysis of the relationship of physical status to postoperative mortality in 68,388 cases. Anesth Analg 49:564, 1970.)

TABLE 10-5. ASA Physical Status versus Overall Death Rates

Physical Status	Mortality	
	N	%
I	(11/18,320)	0.06
II	(50/10,609)	0.4
III	(168/3,820)	4.3
IV	(252/1,073)	23.4
V	(164/323)	50.7

(Modified from Marx GF, Mateo CV, Orkin LR: Computer analysis of post-anesthetic deaths. Anesthesiology 39:54, 1973.)

assessment of risk categories obviously were not applied similarly. In the Vacanti et al.[41] study, only 9.4 percent of the ASA V patients died, whereas fully one-half succumbed in the Marx et al.[12] report. The ASA category V definition is that of a patient who is not expected to survive 24 hours with or without surgery. So although ASA physical status is widely accepted, it is only a gross predictor of overall outcome and is most certainly not a predictor of "anesthetic risk." It is worth mentioning here that ASA physical status was shown by Waters et al.[42] to be just as or more predictive of cardiovascular risk-related outcome in patients who underwent anesthesia and surgery than the oft-quoted "cardiac risk index" of Goldman et al.[43] (see the following discussion and Ch. 9).

tions. Circulatory (47.4 percent) and respiratory (36.2 percent) problems accounted for the bulk of the difficulties. Regional anesthesia was not associated with a significantly different percentage of complications. Cardiac arrest constituted 23 percent of all these complications and seemed to occur at about the same frequency whether the preoperative assessment of cardiac risk was high or low. Although the percentage of ICU admissions caused by anesthetic complications was low (2.2 percent), these patients had a high mortality, namely 32 percent. When intraoperative circulatory complications occurred, 21 percent of the patients died, and if there was an intraoperative arrest with immediately successful resuscitation, only 48 percent survived the ICU admission. Of all the anesthetic complications prompting ICU admission, 76 percent required prolonged ventilator support. The authors concluded that "the intensive therapy of these complications is still not successful compared to that of the other cases treated in the ICU."[44]

WHAT IS THE MORBIDITY/ MORTALITY OF "ANESTHETIC MISADVENTURES"?

A Polish institution reported on 81,559 anesthetics performed between 1977 and 1981, all in adults, wherein "anesthetic complications" occurred in 2.05 percent, with death in the operating room in 0.04 percent (4 per 10,000) of cases.[44] Of the 4,955 adults given postoperative intensive care unit (ICU) care, 100 (2.2 percent) were admitted due to anesthetic complica-

ACCIDENTS, LAPSES, FAILURES, AND "CRITICAL INCIDENTS": THE STUDIES OF COOPER AND COLLEAGUES
(Also See Ch. 12)

Cooper et al. developed and used a "critical incident" reporting and analysis method first described by Flanagan[45] in 1954. A "critical incident" was defined by Cooper et al.[46] as follows:

A critical incident is a human error or equipment failure that could have led (if not dis-

covered or corrected in time) or did lead to an undesirable outcome, ranging from increased length of hospital [or recovery room/ICU] stay to death.

Reports of these "critical incidents" were obtained from volunteer anesthesiologists in the Boston community. These incidents were reported voluntarily at first. The 1984 report[46] involved a total of 616 such events collected in that manner. Next, trained nonphysician interviewers contacted the volunteer anesthesiologists and were able to elicit reports of 234 additional "critical incidents" from the same anesthetists. In a third round of reporting, another 239 incidents came to light. In addition to the 1089 incidents that met the above criteria, they collected 798 more "occurrences" that fell short of being "critical incidents" in one way or another.

These critical incidents were then classified as being due primarily to human error (70 percent); airway, IV, or arterial line disconnections (13 percent); equipment failure (11 percent) and other causes (6 percent). Human error, by far the largest causative category, was subdivided into errors involving drug administration (24 percent); improper use of anesthesia machine (22 percent); airway management errors (16 percent); and several other categories. Most "disconnections" involved the breathing circuit (71 percent), but there were substantial numbers of disconnections involving IVs and/or invasive monitoring equipment that constituted "critical incidents."[46]

Cooper et al.[46–49] made no attempt to ascertain the absolute ocurrence rate (per operation or per hour of anesthesia) of any type of critical incident. Their purpose is to elucidate patterns by which errors and lapses develop and thereby to attempt to understand mechanisms and provide preventive measures. They have been able to group human errors into three categories as they relate to anesthesia. Technical errors, wherein the action actually taken was not the one intended,* arose, in their opinion, from both skill deficiencies and poor "human factors" engineering. *Judgmental errors*,

wherein the action taken was a "bad" decision, were considered by Cooper et al.[46] to have arisen from "lapses in training or poorly developed decision making skills." The third category of human error was termed monitoring and vigilance failures, defined as "failure to recognize or act upon visible data requiring a response."[46]

Not all the "critical incidents" discovered by Cooper and colleagues led to "substantial negative outcomes." No clear case could be made as to why some were discovered and corrected in time to prevent damage while others were not. Probably, the sicker the patient, the more likely a critical incident was to have a negative outcome.

Another area Cooper et al.[49] have studied is the question of whether the common practice of exchanges between anesthesia personnel during long procedures (for short "breaks") is beneficial or harmful. Of 1089 reports of critical incidents, 96 involved a relief anesthetist. Of the latter, in 28 cases the relief anesthetist discovered an error (and presumably corrected it if possible). In only 10 incidents, the process of exchange was thought to have contributed to or to have caused the error. None of the incidents associated with substantial negative outcome involved a relief anesthetist. This unique report strongly implies that reasonable relief (by competent personnel) during long procedures improves vigilance and thereby quality of care.[49] Airline pilots know and take advantage of this, but some hospitals have rigid prohibitions against such practices.

What about strategies to improve (lower) the incidence and severity of these critical incidents? Clearly, improved training and supervision, with more and improved experience for trainees is often cited as important.[46] About one-third of the incidents that led to negative outcomes could have been ameliorated by better preoperative assessment and/or better equipment and apparatus inspection. Also cited are needs for better-designed monitors and equipment, that is, human factors engineering.[46] Organizational improvements, including better matching of cases to experience levels of trainees are also important.[46]

Cooper et al.[46] estimate that roughly one-half the anesthesia-related mortality would likely fall within one or another "preventable" category. This finding is in agreement with the

---

* The term "inadvertent" was applied here in an earlier publication.[47] Unfortunately, the use of this word may be sufficient to bind legal defenses unnecessarily. Cooper and co-workers avoided the term in their 1984 report.[46]

studies of Lunn and colleagues.[19-25] If there are 2,000 "anesthetic deaths" in the United States per year, according to the 1978 estimate of Epstein,[50] and if 20 million anesthetics are given in the United States annually, the anesthesia-related death risk of 1 per 10,000 cases is relatively low compared with most other causes of death but relatively high if compared with the 125 deaths per year attributed to scheduled commercial aviation.[46] Cooper et al.[46] wonder whether a "point of diminishing returns" has not been reached whereby the improvements in vigilance, safety of drugs, reliability of equipment, greater awareness in training, and so forth may now be offset by our increasingly complex and invasive monitoring methods, more elderly and probably sicker patients, and increasingly major surgical trespass.

The efforts of Cooper et al. are important because they represent a way to study these critical incidents anonymously, without fear of legal implications. Unfortunately, they may represent "preaching to the already convinced." We still do not know whether these critical incidents are random or whether they occur with significantly greater frequencies to relatively few patients. They are not able to identify anesthetists who are chronically "incident prone," let alone improve their practices or weed them out if they are incorrigible. By contrast, airline pilots are required to take frequent recertification examinations and unannounced check rides. Their safety record is enviable.

ANESTHETIC RISKS IN CERTAIN CLINICAL SITUATIONS

OBSTETRICS
(Also See Ch. 47)

In England, a comprehensive system of maternal death reporting and inquiry was begun in 1952.[51] The overall trend has been steadily toward safer pregnancies. Despite this progress in other areas, Rosen[51] comments: "The progress in making anaesthesia safer for pregnant patients is unimpressive." In 1964–1965, there were 50 anesthesia-related deaths in England in these patients. Most recent data, for 1978, show a nearly equal 17.2 such deaths per million maternities, a rate of 0.17 per 10,000, much lower than the overall anesthesia risk reported above. Most of these deaths were associated with emergency cesarean sections. The most common proximate causes were aspiration and/or difficult intubation. In France,[52] although less comprehensive data are available, similar statistics seem to apply. Again, emergency cesarean operation was associated with greatest risk of anesthetic-related maternal death.

PEDIATRICS
(Also See Ch. 49)

Delegue et al.[53] recently reported on 54,100 children anesthetized between 1974 and 1982 in France. There were 32 deaths, of which 40 percent (13) were considered to be due exclusively to anesthesia, and another 28 percent were due in part to anesthesia. Their figure of approximately 6 per 10,000 is higher than the 1.4 per 10,000 reported by Smith up to 1968 at the Boston Children's Hospital.[54] It is logical that anesthesia risk in a pediatric patient population might depend on the percentages of patients operated on who were less than 1 year of age, rather than simply using the designation "pediatric." It is logical, although not demonstrated, that anesthesia-related mortality and morbidity should decrease rapidly in pediatric patients older than 1 year.

GERIATRICS
(Also See Ch. 50)

In a prospective study of 500 consecutive patients over 70 years of age, Filzweiser and List[55] reported in 1983 that 90 percent of these patients were classed as ASA III or worse. There were 164 (32.8 percent) intraoperative, plus 211 (42.2 percent) postoperative complications. Despite this, there were no intraoperative deaths. Hospital mortality was 3.4 percent, none of which was attributed to anesthesia. Gersh et al.[56] reported excellent results for coronary artery surgery in elderly patients. In another study of the elderly patient, in women at least, accidents due to anesthesia (and mortality therefrom) actually were reduced in incidence in extremely elderly patients (over age 85).[40] Thus, it is not necessarily valid to assume that greater anesthetic risk attends these patients, although any experienced anesthetist will agree that there is often little margin for error. The latter impression may be selective; the most experienced and/or competent anesthetist may often get selected to anesthetize these patients.

CORONARY ARTERY DISEASE
(Also See Chs. 9 & 41)

Patients who undergo anesthesia and noncardiac surgery who have concomitant coronary artery disease (CAD) have well-documented higher risks of perioperative (within 7 days of anesthesia) myocardial infarction (MI) and death. Several large retrospective studies of patients with documented prior myocardial infarctions who underwent anesthesia and (noncardiac) surgery[26,57-62] show remarkable agreement: (1) adult patients without prior MI have a 0.15 to 0.65 percent risk of a perioperative MI; (2) patients with prior MI have an overall reinfarction risk of about 6 percent; (3) patients with recent MI (within 3 months) have an approximate 30 percent reinfarction risk; (4) patients with a relatively recent MI (3 to 6 months old) have an approximate 15 percent reinfarction risk; and (5) the risk of death from such a perioperative reinfarction is very high, namely 50 to 70 percent, much higher than the risk of death from an MI not temporally related to anesthesia and surgery. Also important is the fact that if a patient with CAD does succumb within the first week after any surgery, it is almost always of cardiac etiol-

ogy, no matter what the surgery or the patient's primary disease. This is why the subject has excited such wide interest among anesthesiologists.

Attempts to study this important problem prospectively have been controversial. Goldman et al.[43] in 1977 carefully examined 1,001 patients before surgery, documented the outcomes, and attempted to find those risk factors predictive of statistically significant morbidity and mortality. These workers concluded that S3 gallop or jugular venous distention; MI in the preceding 6 months; rhythm other than sinus; more than five premature ventricular contractions per minute any time before operation; intraperitoneal, intrathoracic, or aortic operation; age >70 years; significant valvular aortic stenosis; emergency operations; and "poor general medical condition" were all predictors of poor outcome. Furthermore, they constructed a point scale that enabled the establishment of four cardiac risk categories.[43]

While this study[43] was a landmark attempt to quantify perioperative cardiac risk, it has not proved a complete success. One subsequent independent attempt[42] at validation of the Goldman cardiac risk index has shown that index to be no more predictive of perioperative cardiac risk than the long-used subjective ASA physical status rating. A second validation attempt showed the Goldman cardiac risk index to grossly underestimate risk for those patients who underwent abdominal aortic aneurysm resections and did not have histories of coronary artery disease.[63]

Although the numerical perioperative MI risks quoted above from retrospective studies probably still apply in many, if not most, hospitals, recently Rao et al.[64] reported a series of patients who underwent anesthesia and surgery in the presence of recent MI who had much improved outcomes. They retrospectively examined 364 prior MI patients who had surgery during 1973–1976 to obtain a baseline, then prospectively examined 733 prior MI patients operated on from 1977–1982 using aggressive "contemporary" management. Patients with MI's less than 3 months old had a reinfarction rate of 5.8 percent, compared with the 36 percent found in their own previous retrospective series. Patients with MI between 3 and 6 months of age had a 2.3 percent reinfarction rate, compared with a 26 percent rate in the previous retrospective population. Rao et al.[64] attributed the much lower rates than those they had obtained in prior years to extensive use of invasive hemodynamic monitoring (PA catheters) as well as the data derived from such evaluations, which led to aggressive use of β-blockers and vasodilators. Serious questions are raised whenever any outcome study, whether prospective or retrospective, attempts to state or imply that the reasons for improved outcome are due to specifically selected changes in therapy. The reader interested in this controversy is referred to the editorial accompanying this study.[65] Nonetheless, the Rao et al.[64] report represents a significant improvement in outcome. If it can be confirmed elsewhere, and the reasons for it conclusively demonstrated, a significant advance in the care of these high-risk patients may indeed have occurred.

Patients who have previously undergone coronary artery bypass grafting operations (CABG) often present for subsequent surgery. Mahar et al.[28] reported 99 patients who underwent 168 noncardiac operations after CABG. Not a single perioperative MI occurred. This finding was confirmed in several other studies.[66-68] This may indicate that prior CABG somehow "protected" these CAD patients against the risks noted above, or it may indicate that the "event," namely a perioperative MI, had already occurred surrounding the CABG and was therefore no longer "available" to happen. This is less important to anesthesiologists assessing individual patients than the fact that post-CABG patients, presenting for subsequent surgery, apparently pose much less cardiac risk than do patients with CAD or prior MI who have not undergone CABG.[28,66-68] Such "event" analysis, that is, the concept that once an event has occurred, it may not be as likely to happen again soon, might be applicable in cases wherein "error" has occurred.

Ophthalmologic surgery is often undertaken in elderly patients with CAD. In an attempt to discover whether the magnitude of the surgery or the performance of anesthesia influenced the occurrence of perioperative MI, Backer et al.[69] studied more than 10,000 such procedures. Of 288 separate operations in pa-

tients who had suffered a well-documented prior MI, not a single perioperative MI occurred. Numerous others with probably extensive preoperative CAD had similarly good outcomes. These operations were done with retrobulbar block plus local anesthesia, but there is evidence that the same results apply to patients given general anesthesia for ophthalmic operations.[70] This indicates that magnitude of surgery probably plays a more major role than general versus regional or local anesthesia, at least with respect to risks of perioperative cardiac complications.

Many of the retrospective studies mentioned have attempted to elucidate risk factors that increase risk of perioperative MI in CAD patients. Intrathoracic, great vessel, and upper abdominal operations are clearly associated with increased risk. Especially high risks are operations on the aorta in patients with known or suspected CAD.[26,63] Location of the prior MI has not been statistically shown to affect incidence or severity of reinfarctions, although it seems logical that patients with prior subendocardial infarction might be candidates for "completion" into transmural MI.[26] Increasing age probably poses increased perioperative MI risk.[26,71,72] Steen et al.[26] reported that thoracic, great vessel, and upper abdominal operations lasting more than 4 hours were associated with the greatest cardiac risk. For other operations, time under anesthesia could not be definitely associated with increased risk. Several groups have reported that intraoperative hypotension either was associated with or heralded (or was caused by) a perioperative MI.[26,64] Peak incidence of perioperative MI is not, however, in the operating room, but rather on the first to third postoperative day.[26,58] Although avoidance of hypertension and tachycardia is widely believed to be protective, no retrospective study has shown that absence of either was associated with better outcome. The prospective study of Rao et al.[64] can be cited as evidence that such hemodynamic control may be beneficial. Severity of preexisting coronary artery disease is assessable only if the patient has had a prior coronary angiogram. The prospective multiinstitutional Coronary Artery Surgery Study (CASS)[15,49] clearly showed that severity of CAD is associated with increased risk of performance of CABG, as expected. Also associated with high perioperative risk is evidence of decreased ventricular performance (decreased left ventricular ejection fraction, increased left ventricular end-diastolic pressure). A recent CASS report[49] showed that elderly individuals with severe CAD can undergo CABG with reasonably low risk, although higher than that of younger patients.

Coronary artery disease is often associated with chronic obstructive pulmonary disease (COPD). Patients with documented severe impairment of pulmonary function can still undergo CABG without added mortality risk, according to a recent study by Warner et al.[73] These patients had a high incidence of pulmonary morbidity as expected but also had an approximate doubling of the perioperative MI rate.

Another way to examine the "benefit" side of the risk – benefit equation is to attempt to ascertain whether a particular operation actually resulted in claimed benefits. Clearly, CABG itself is associated with a significant percentage of perioperative MI.[15,56,72,74-76] Literature reports range from <5 to >10 percent, although reported rates may be in part dependent on extent of postoperative examination of these patients. These postoperative MIs do result in impaired long-term survival.[77] Coronary artery bypass surgery has been controversial in this regard, and numerous attempts have been made to study its efficacy. One of these, namely the Veterans Administration Cooperative Study[72,74-75] concluded that few patients except those with significant left mainstem coronary disease were actually benefited. Another study[78] concluded that expert medical therapy could produce mortality results equal to or better than surgery in patients with severe CAD despite the fact that the diagnosis of CAD in their patients was poorly documented at best, namely by ST depression on exercise electrocardiogram (ECG), without coronary angiography. Two recent studies of outcome after CABG have appeared, both with randomized allocation of CAD patients with equivalent degrees of disease to either medical or surgical groups, both with long-term (5 year) follow-up with exercise testing and repeat angiography. One study reported significant benefit from

CABG,[79] the other reported no difference between CABG and medical therapy.[80] The reason for presenting these studies in a chapter on anesthetic risk is to provide a graphic illustration of the difficulties in trying to use an outcome (risk) study to advocate a particular treatment. Nowhere is this better illustrated than in the controversies over efficacy of invasive monitoring in CAD patients[64,65] and over timing[29] and efficacy[78-80] of CABG itself.

Percutaneous transluminal coronary angioplasty (PTCA) has recently come into widespread usage. A report from the Registry established among several institutions illustrates another problem with interpreting outcome (risk) studies.[81] The interested reader is referred to this report for details, but suffice it to state here that after perusing the list and incidence of various major complications in this report, many readers may come to the opposite conclusion from that of the report's authors. The latter concluded that PTCA is generally safe and effective. Despite 121 episodes of prolonged angina, 72 myocardial infarctions, 70 coronary occlusions, 63 instances of coronary spasm, 43 dissections and/or tears of coronary arteries, plus numerous other less frequent difficulties (a total of 543 complications in only 1,500 patients), the authors concluded that the PTCA procedure is both safe and effective.[81] Their conclusions are at least open to reinterpretation by other physicians. Although "outcome" studies of overall risk are currently in vogue, interpretation of their results may be difficult and controversial.

What was the role of anesthesia per se? If an apparently healthy patient dies during or just after an anesthetic, suspicion descends upon the anesthetic and/or its administration. When a significant risk factor is present, such as a preoperative myocardial infarction, the difficulty of assigning blame is not confounded only by the presence of the major risk factor but also by the fact that the causes, proper treatment, and subtle nuances of the other disease (in this case, coronary atherosclerosis) are themselves not well understood, not to mention the possible interactions of anesthetic-related hemodynamic – metabolic – neuromuscular (and other) effects with the underlying disease processes.

CARDIAC RISK FACTORS OTHER THAN CORONARY ARTERY DISEASE

A patient who has a bed-chair existence due to congestive heart failure would be expected to be at increased anesthetic risk. Surprisingly, there have been no classifications of anesthetic risk compared with New York Heart Association's classifications of cardiac patients. The problem is that unlike atherosclerotic heart disease, most other types of heart disease are associated with few discrete events. The degree of heart failure, which is difficult to assess, has an uneven continuum. Assessment of anesthetic or perioperative risk is more possible if groups of patients who have suffered a discrete prior event are studied. Patients who have had cardiac valve prostheses have been studied after they returned for needed subsequent noncardiac surgery.[27,82] Cessation of anticoagulants for a few days did not result in major thromboembolic complications. Other complications attributable to residual anticoagulation were present in relatively high incidences. The CASS,[15,49] the VA Cooperative Studies[74-75,83] and the Goldman et al. studies[43] do provide clear evidence that myocardial dysfunction, whether documented by history of exercise intolerance, left ventricular end-diastolic pressure elevations, decreased ejection fractions, or abnormal ventricular wall motion, does result in greatly increased risk, not only for performance of coronary artery bypass but for other noncardiac operations as well. The studies conducted by Jeffrey et al.[63] indicate that extent of accompanying myocardial dysfunction clearly affects outcome for abdominal aortic operations. Carotid endarterectomy results have been similarly shown by Sundt et al.[16] to be affected by accompanying cardiac disease.

HYPERTENSION
(Also See Ch. 9)

Although a 1979 report by Goldman et al.[84] suggested that hypertensives present little if any added risk for anesthesia and surgery, the accompanying editorial[85] points out that too small a number of patients with genuinely severe hypertension was studied to permit the null hypothesis (i.e., that there was no added risk) to be verified. Clearly, the VA Cooperative Studies of hypertension[86,87] indicate that antihypertensive therapy is beneficial in numerous ways, although these investigations do not specifically address anesthetic risk. The studies conducted by Prys-Roberts et al.[88] are usually cited as evidence for postponement of surgery in patients if control of hypertension is less than optimal. Steen et al.[26] found approximately double the reinfarction rate perioperatively in patients who carried a diagnosis of hypertension (with treatment) preoperatively. The latter study made no attempt to classify said treatment into "adequate" versus "inadequate." The reader is referred to Chapter 9 for details of this troublesome preoperative evaluation controversy.

PULMONARY DISEASE
(Also See Chs. 59, 63, & 64)

A 1973 paper by Tarhan et al.[89] is sometimes cited as evidence that patients with severe chronic obstructive pulmonary disease (COPD) have less risk of postoperative morbidity or mortality if they are operated on under regional as opposed to general anesthesia. In fact, the differences cited are not statistically significant, nor was there any attempt to adjust the study group data with respect to age, type or location of operation, length of surgery, and other factors. This study showed that severe COPD is a definite additional risk factor in most types of surgery. Warner et al.[73] studied patients with severely limited pulmonary function, as measured by extensive preoperative pulmonary function testing, prior to undergoing cardiac surgery. Surprisingly, there was not one hospital death among 62 patients with severe COPD who underwent CABG. By contrast, patients with severe COPD who underwent cardiac valve replacement had approximately double the expected mortality. This is mentioned to point out the possibility that the presence of a significant potential risk factor might actually serve to alert the medical care team sufficiently, so that more competent, vigilant care actually may result in less mortality.

Norlander and Hallen[90] reported that following abdominal surgery, postoperative pulmonary complications occur with "relatively stable" frequencies. When the studies were done retrospectively, complication rates of 2 to 20 percent were reported, compared with 20 to 50 percent when prospective studies were performed.[90] Although it is well accepted that preexisting COPD leads to much higher rates of postoperative pulmonary morbidity, there is no agreement as to which (if any) preoperative lung function criteria are in fact predictive of outcome.[90] Actually, in a 1980 study, a history of degree of smoking (number of pack-years) was just as good a predictor of outcome as any pulmonary function test (with a specificity of 72 percent!).[91] At the Karolinska Institute in Stockholm, Sweden, in an experience of more than 40,000 cases, there were perioperative respiratory complications in more than 7 percent of patients not known to have abnormal preoperative respiratory function.[90] If COPD was present, major pulmonary complications could be expected after approximately every tenth anesthetic.[90] Norlander and colleagues[90] also commented on the lack of predictive value of routine preoperative chest roentgenograms stating that:

> **Our figures from 1981 indicate that there are no major differences between the intra-anesthetic frequency of respiratory complication if the chest x-ray is normal or if it is pathological.**

ARE THERE OTHER WELL-DOCUMENTED RISK FACTORS?
(Also See Ch. 9)

The assumption behind the concept that extensive appreciation of the patient's medical and surgical problems, and the idea that these problems should be in the best possible state of repair preoperatively, is that such knowledge and optimization will make anesthesia inherently safer. Yet anesthetic errors, accidents, lapses, and misadventures do not necessarily happen only during anesthesia for the sickest patients. There is also a natural bias in any group of anesthetists toward assigning the most experienced, presumably competent, persons to handle the most complex cases. Boredom during a "routine" case is a risk factor but is probably not quantifiable. Clearly all anesthesia risk is not related to extent of preoperative disease or degree to which its therapy has been optimized. Another trap that has claimed some investigators is the study of a small number of patients who have a probable risk factor. If the group does well, the authors conclude that the condition does not, in fact, add risk. Goldman et al.[84] concluded in 1979 that hypertension was not a significant perioperative risk factor. In an accompanying editorial, Prys-Roberts[85] pointed out that too few patients studied actually had significant hypertension. The reader must bear in mind that as the number of subjects studied approaches zero, the probability of acceptance of the null hypothesis (that there is no difference between groups) approaches 100 percent.[92] Does one disease carry a worse risk factor than another? Should we give one drug over another to treat a given disease? What about all the possible drug–drug interactions that could occur preoperatively? Ponder these permutations and combinations and it will become obvious why investigators have limited themselves to such events as preoperative MI, intraoperative cardiac arrest, and the like as subjects for analysis of perioperative risk. The potential anesthesia interactions with vital organ diseases, drugs, treatments, and injuries, all discussed in the chapters on preoperative evaluation (Chs. 8 and 9), are logical, but are likely to remain difficult to quantitate.

THE RISK OF ANESTHESIA TO ANESTHESIOLOGISTS

In addition to examining "anesthetic risk" to the patient, does the administration of anesthesia pose a hazard to anesthesiologists? Male physician anesthetists have been reported to have an increased rate of suicide,[93] although there is disagreement as to whether this significantly differs from the overall increased occurrence of suicide among male physicians in general.[94] The Georgia Impaired Physician's Program estimates overall physician incidence of alcoholism and other drug addiction to be roughly 14 percent, with the highest incidences among physician anesthetists, obstetrician-gynecologists, and psychiatrists.[95] A survey of southeastern academic anesthesia department chairmen reported that 1 to 2 percent of personnel came to their attention because of drug or alcohol abuse.[96] Type B hepatitis, non-A non-B hepatitis, and herpes simplex infections, particularly herpetic whitlow, have been documented to be occupational hazards of anesthesia.[97] With respect to chronic major toxicity, there has been intense interest in studies of anesthetic agent mutagenicity, carcinogenicity, and teratogenicity. In addition to laboratory studies of these questions, numerous epidemiologic studies have been performed—some controlled enough to permit sober conclusion—others sensational enough to stir emotions and spark governmental regulatory activity.

MUTAGENICITY
(Also See Ch. 22)

Mutagenicity can be studied a number of ways, but a common method involves a bacterial screening analysis, using a specialized strain of *Salmonella* (the Ames test). Various mutagenic studies have shown that fluroxene, divinyl ether, and trichloroethylene are mutagenic, again at least in these bacterial in vitro systems. There is no way to document human mutagenicity in just one or two generations.[98] By sharp contrast, these same bacterial mutagenicity studies have been entirely negative for halothane, enflurane, isoflurane, and nitrous oxide.[98] The famous fruit fly, *Drosophila melanogaster*, given huge doses of halothane, was shown to produce chromosomal nondisjunctions, indicative of weak mutagenicity in that

easily mutated species.[99] Extensive studies in mammals have shown no mutagenicity attributable to halothane, enflurane, or isoflurane.[100]

CARCINOGENICITY
(Also See Ch. 22)

These studies are almost always performed using rodents. Chloroform clearly is a carcinogen, at least in large doses. Trichloroethylene has also been shown productive of hepatic malignancy.[98] In 1976, an unfortunate suboptimally controlled study by Corbett[101] implicated isoflurane as responsible for producing hepatic tumors in mice. Subsequently, controlled studies by Eger et al.[102] showed that chronic exposure to isoflurane, enflurane, halothane, methoxyflurane, or nitrous oxide did not increase the incidence of mouse liver tumors as compared with control groups given either oxygen or air. Baden et al.[103] in 1982 gave lifetime exposures of maximally tolerated amounts of halothane and enflurane to mice and found no carcinogenicity. Similarly, Coate et al.[104] exposed mice to nitrous oxide 50 parts per million (ppm), or halothane 10 ppm plus nitrous oxide 500 ppm, for 104 weeks, 7 hours per day, 5 days per week. They found no tumor incidence greater than that seen in appropriate controls. Thus, there is no credible evidence that the currently used volatile agents, plus nitrous oxide, are either mutagenic or carcinogenic. The various metabolites of these agents have also been evaluated and found not to be toxic in these ways.

TERATOGENICITY
(Also See Ch. 22)

The subject of teratogenicity does not involve the same question as the epidemiologic question, that anesthetics might interfere with human reproduction. It is known that nitrous oxide is a weak teratogen in rodents.[98] Pregnant rodents given lengthy exposures to halothane also have significantly increased numbers of malformed fetuses.[98] Baden[98] has questioned whether the effects might not be due merely to the length of the required anesthetic exposure, with possible interference in oxygen delivery and nutrition. With respect to enflurane and isoflurane, all teratogenic studies through 1984 are negative, with the single exception of increased cleft palate incidence in mice given isoflurane found by Mazze et al.[105] Human teratogenicity of anesthetics has been studied by Wyrobek et al.,[106] who examined the semen of 46 experienced anesthesiologists, all of whom had been working regularly in operating rooms for at least the previous year. The "controls" were semen samples obtained from 26 beginning anesthesia residents who had spent virtually no time in the operating room. No morphologic sperm differences were noted between the groups. This is, to our knowledge, the only human teratologic study that is not of an epidemiologic nature. Mazze et al.[105] believe their rodent evidence is strong enough to recommend that isoflurane not be given in the first trimester of human pregnancy.

CHRONIC ANESTHETIC TOXICITY: EPIDEMIOLOGIC STUDIES (Also See Ch. 22)

In 1929, in a paper from the Institute of Hygiene in Berlin, it was noted that mechanical means of removing anesthetic vapors from that institution's operating rooms had been in place for the preceding 10 years![107] The workers considered it likely that the vapors were potentially harmful. They also contended that environmental factors such as standing, humidity, and poor illumination all would be likely to contribute to the health of operating room workers. Although they had no animal or human scientific evidence, these investigators recommended that immediate action be taken throughout Germany to remove these vapors from the operating room arena and that it would be unwise to await conclusive evidence[107] (a sad theme we still contend with).

The "modern" era probably starts in 1970; since that time, various authors have attempted to build an epidemiologic case that

groups of workers exposed to trace amounts (or more) of waste anesthetic gases had reproductive or other health problems of various types.[108] These early epidemiologic studies suffered from numerous design problems, not the least of which is called "response bias." It is important to understand this bias, which is perhaps best explained by examining the findings reported by Axelson and Reilander in 1982.[109] These workers studied 655 pregnancies in Swedish hospital workers, some of whom had been exposed to waste anesthetics in operating rooms, while others had not. Of the workers not exposed (and undoubtedly not concerned), fully one-third of the independently obtained incidence of spontaneous abortions (as proved by medical records) were not reported on the questionnaires that had been filled out by workers. In sharp contrast, every single spontaneous abortion that did occur (by medical record check) in the exposed (and undoubtedly concerned) workers was actually reported by them on the questionnaire. This is dramatic evidence for what biostatisticians call response bias.[109] It is nothing new to epidemiologists that questionnaires and/or surveys do not correspond very well with actual medical records. In a recent review, Mazze[108] cites a study showing that the "match" between surveys and actual medical records can be as poor as 24 percent!

By far the best way to perform such a study is therefore prospectively and with actual medical records rather than surveys. Such a study was reported by Ericson and Kallen in 1979.[110] These workers studied 494 women who had worked in operating rooms throughout their pregnancies. This group's medical record-proven spontaneous abortion rate was 4.5 percent. The control group, namely female medical workers employed outside anesthetizing locations, had a similarly proven spontaneous abortion rate of 5.2 percent.[110]

A massive study of dentists (nearly all male) and their chairside assistants (nearly all female) was completed by Cohen et al. in 1980.[111] Dental operatories wherein nitrous oxide was in use were compared with those in which local anesthesia alone was used. This is the only epidemiologic study in which halothane and the other volatile agents were completely eliminated. A two- to threefold increase in neurologic disorders of various sorts occurred in the workers, both male and female, who had been exposed to nitrous oxide. On the other hand, few dental operatories were scavenged in those days, with estimated nitrous oxide concentrations sometimes exceeding 1,500 ppm. Whether working in a dental operatory in which general anesthesia was in use was more generally stressful, especially given the recent publicity about the dangers of anesthesia, cannot be ascertained. Nonetheless, the study convinced most dentists to employ scavenging devices. Reproductive abnormalities in the female chairside assistants attributable to nitrous oxide were not conclusively demonstrated.[111]

The American Society of Anesthesiologists, properly concerned with this question, contracted with an independent group of biostatisticians (Epistat) to evaluate the entire literature and all data on this important subject. As reported to the 1981 ASA meeting, this group reached four conclusions: (1) adverse reproductive outcomes for females directly exposed to anesthetics are "the only health effect for which there is reasonable consistent evidence"; (2) many existing data are not worth reanalysis; (3) epidemiologic data thus far obtained, or likely to be obtained, are inadequate for setting exposure limits for anesthetic gases in operating rooms; and (4) future studies should be cohort types, should be prospective, and should employ near-total participation of exposed groups plus near-total follow-up.[112]

Should we scavenge trace (waste) anesthetic gases from operating rooms? In a complete, recent, and carefully written review of this controversial subject, Mazze[108] clearly answers "yes" to that question. In 1977, the U.S. National Institute of Occupational Safety and Health (NIOSH) suggested a proposed standard for average operating room concentrations of halothane at 0.5 ppm and of nitrous oxide at 25 ppm. Exactly what "average" concentrations mean, where they should be measured, and when is unclear. Worse, these concentrations were quite arbitrary, because there is no evidence to show that degree of toxicity is necessarily even related to degree of exposure (and whether length of exposure is more or less important than concentrations to which workers are exposed). Clearly, these proposed standards, if enacted, would have been costly and may not have even been possible to maintain. There is no safe limit known for trace anesthetics in operating rooms. The NIOSH-proposed regulation is postponed as of 1984. Still, scavenging makes sense, as does routine monitoring to check for hose connection leaks and other failures. Records of the monitoring results should be kept. What is needed is an anesthetic gas personal dosimeter that can be worn before actual exposure to these agents can be quantitated.

SUMMARY: WHAT IS "ANESTHETIC RISK"?

Because of the legal implications of publication of frank and honest assessments of blame, coupled with a well-founded doubt that anonymity can nowadays be maintained, it is doubtful that we will be able, in the 1980s, in the United States at least, to update the old studies of anesthetic risk. The Cardiff studies[19-25] are probably our modern standards. Cooper and colleagues[46-49] have provided us with renewed awareness of the need for studies of vigilance and of improved design of equipment in an effort to decrease the incidence of human errors. Our ability to regulate and/or analyze our performance is primitive indeed as compared with that, for example, required for the airline industry. To be sure, we deal with many more unknowns, but in the face of the legal liabilities of the 1980s, we may have become more secretive, that is, more willing to hide and cover our errors than ever before. Clearly there is risk to anesthesia. Errors and lapses do account for some, perhaps a majority, of "anesthetic deaths." Nonetheless, there is inherent toxicity in the drugs and techniques we use, which will likely always be so; that is, not every "anesthetic death" need necessarily be due to an error or lapse. It is appropriate to conclude that for every 10,000 anesthetics given, between one and three patients will die primarily as a result of the administration of anesthesia, and that a high percentage (more than 50) of those deaths probably would be judged preventable in light of knowledge available concurrently. To those who say that because anesthesia is not therapeutic, nothing less than zero risk should be tolerated, we retort that although anesthesia may not be therapeutic, it most certainly is beneficial. The concept of risk versus benefit is applicable to anesthesia. We are not saying that anesthesia risks of between 1 and 3 per 10,000 anesthetics are an irreducible minimum. We are implying that such a risk–benefit ratio is, in fact, quite excellent as compared with medicine in general. We reiterate that anesthesia risk is not linearly dependent on severity of patient disease or complexity of surgical procedure. Although the legal concept that no patient should ever die or be injured from anesthesia must be stopped, we must be prepared to critically assess our individual performances. We close with a quote from Dr. Arthur Keats[2]:

To every benefit, there is a risk. The only way to guarantee immunity from risk is to do nothing at all.

REFERENCES

1. Snow J: On Chloroform and Other Anaesthetics. London, John Churchill, 1858, pp 107–251
2. Keats AS: What do we know about anesthetic mortality. Anesthesiology 50:387, 1979
3. Macintosh RR: Deaths under anaesthetics. Br J Anaesth 21:107, 1948
4. Ruth HS: Anesthesia study commissions. JAMA 127:514, 1945
5. Beecher HK, Todd DP: A study of the deaths associated with anesthesia and surgery. Ann Surg 140:2, 1954
6. Trent JC, Gaster E: Anesthetic deaths in 54,128 consecutive cases. Ann Surg 119:954, 1944
7. Phillips OC, Frazier TM, Graff TD, et al: The Baltimore Anesthesia Study Committee: Review of 1024 postoperative deaths. JAMA 174:2015, 1960
8. Dripps RD, Lamont A, Eckenhoff JE: The role of anesthesia in surgical mortality. JAMA 178:261, 1961
9. Special Committee Investigating Deaths Under Anaesthesia: Report On 745 Classified Cases, 1960–1968. Med J Aust 1:573, 1970
10. Dornette WHL, Orth OS: Death in the operating room. Anesth Analg 35:545, 1956
11. Gebbie D: Anesthesia and death. Can Anaesth Soc J 13:390, 1966
12. Marx GF, Mateo CV, Orkin LR: Computer analysis of post-anesthetic deaths. Anesthesiology 39:54, 1973
13. Bodlander FM: Deaths associated with anesthesia. Br J Anaesth 47:36, 1975
14. Gordon T, Larson CP, Prestwick R: Unexpected cardiac arrest during anesthesia in surgery: An environmental study. JAMA 236:2758, 1976
15. Kennedy JW, Kaiser GC, Fisher LD, et al: Clinical and angiographic predictors of operative mortality from the collaborative study in coronary artery surgery (CASS). Circulation 63:793, 1981
16. Sundt TM, Sharbrough FW, Piepgras DG, et al: Correlation of cerebral blood flow and electroencephalographic changes during carotid endarterectomy. Mayo Clin Proc 56:533, 1981
17. Easton JD, Sherman DG: Stroke and mortality rate in carotid endarterectomy: 228 consecutive operations. Stroke 8:565, 1977
18. Schneider AJL: Assessment of risk factors and surgical outcome. Surg Clin North Am 63:1113, 1983
19. Lunn JN, Mushin WW: Mortality Associated With Anaesthesia. London, Nuffield Provincial Hospitals Trust, 1982
20. Lunn JN, Hunter AR, Scott DB: Anaesthesia related surgical mortality. Anaesthesia 38:1090, 1983
21. Farrow SC, Fowkes FGR, Lunn JN, et al: Epidemiology in anaesthesia. II. Factors affecting mortality in hospital. Br J Anaesth 54:811, 1982
22. Fowkes, FGR, Lunn JN, Farrow SC, et al: Epidemiology in anaesthesia. III. Mortality risk in patients with coexisting physical disease. Br J Anaesth 54:819, 1982
23. Lunn JN, Farrow SC, Fowkes FGR, et al: Epidemiology in anaesthesia. I. anaesthetic practice over twenty years. Br J Anaesth 54:803, 1982
24. Lunn JN: The role of mortality studies, Quality of Care in Anesthetic Practice. Edited by Lunn JN. Basingstoke, Macmillan, 1983, pp 163–168
25. Vickers MD, Lunn JN: Mortality in Anaesthesia. Berlin, Springer-Verlag, 1983 pp 19–24
26. Steen PA, Tinker JH, Tarhan S: Myocardial reinfarction after anesthesia in surgery. JAMA 239:2566, 1978

27. Tinker JH, Tarhan S: Discontinuing anticoagulant therapy in surgical patients with cardiac valve prostheses. JAMA 239:738, 1978

28. Mahar LJ, Steen PA, Tinker JH, et al: Perioperative myocardial infarction in patients with coronary artery disease with and without aorto-coronary artery bypass grafts. J Thorac Cardiovasc Surg 76:533, 1978

29. Mears JH, Plitt K, Tinker JH: Coronary bypass: Are there legitimate emergencies? Anesthesiology 55:A22, 1981

30. Hovi-Viander M: Death associated with anaesthesia. Br J Anaesth 52:483, 1980

31. Harrison GG: Anaesthetic-associated mortality. South Afr Med J 48:550, 1974

32. Turnbull KW, Fancourt-Smith PF, Banting GC: Death within 48 hours of anaesthesia at the Vancouver General Hospital. Can Anaesth Soc J 27:159, 1980

33. Goldstein A, Keats AS: The risk of anesthesia. Anesthesiology 33:130, 1970

34. Boba A, Landmesser CM: Total cardiorespiratory collapse (cardiac arrest). NY J Med 61:2928, 1961

35. Bunker JP, Forrest WH, Mosteller F, et al: The National Halothane Study: A study of the possible association between halothane anesthesia and postoperative hepatic necrosis. Bethesda, National Institute of Health, National Institute of General Medical Sciences, 1969

36. Clifton BS, Hotten WIT: Deaths associated with anaesthesia. Br J Anaesth 35:250, 1963

37. Memery HN: Anesthesia mortality in private practice: A ten year study. JAMA 194:1185, 1965

38. Edwards G, Morton HJV, Pask EA, et al: Deaths associated with anaesthesia: Report on 1000 cases. Anaesthesia 11:194, 1956

39. Harrison GG: Anaesthetic contributory death — Its incidence and causes. Part I: Incidence; Part II: Causes. South Afr Med J 42:514, 1968

40. Hatton F, Tiret L, Vourc'h G, et al: Morbidity and mortality associated with anaesthesia — French survey: Preliminary results, Mortality in Anaesthesia. Edited by Vickers MD, Lunn JN. Berlin, Springer-Verlag, 1983, pp 25–38

41. Vacanti CJ, Van Houten RJ, Hill RC: A statistical analysis of the relationship of physical status to postoperative mortality in 68,388 cases. Anesth Analg 49:564, 1970

42. Waters J, Wilkinson C, Golmon M: Evaluation of cardiac risk in noncardiac surgical patients. Anesthesiology 55:A343, 1981

43. Goldman L, Caldera DL, Nussbaum SR, et al: Multifactorial index of cardiac risk in noncardiac surgical procedures. N Engl J Med 297:845, 1977

44. Jurczyk W, Wolowicka L, Szulc R, et al: Complication of anaesthesia as subjects for intensive therapy, Mortality in Anaesthesia. Edited by Vickers MD, Lunn JN. Berlin, Springer-Verlag, 1983, pp 83–87

45. Flanagan JC: The critical incident technique. Psychol Bull 51:327, 1954

46. Cooper JB, Newbower RS, Kitz RJ: An analysis of major errors and equipment failures in anesthesia management: Considerations for prevention and detection. Anesthesiology 60:34, 1984

47. Cooper JB, Newbower RS, Long CD, et al: Preventable anesthesia mishaps — A study of human factors. Anesthesiology 49:399, 1978

48. Cooper JB, Long CD, Newbower RS: Human error in anesthesia management, Quality of Care in Anesthesia. Edited by Grundy BL, Gravenstein JS. Springfield, Ill, Charles C Thomas, 1982, pp 114–130

49. Cooper JB, Newbower RS, Long CD, et al: Critical incidents associated with intraoperative changes of anesthesia personnel. Anesthesiology 56:456, 1982

50. Epstein RM: Morbidity and mortality from anesthesia: A continuing problem. Anesthesiology 49:388, 1978

51. Rosen M: Maternal mortality associated with anaesthesia in England and Wales, Mortality in Anaesthesia. Edited by Vickers MD, Lunn JN. Berlin, Springer-Verlag, 1983, pp 39–44

52. Barrier G: Anaesthesia and maternal mortality in France, Mortality in Anaesthesia. Edited by Vickers MD, Lunn JN. Berlin, Springer-Verlag, 1983, pp 45–48

53. Delegue L, Ghnassia MD, Reiner SR, et al: An analysis of anaesthetic mortality among children, Mortality in Anaesthesia. Edited by Vickers MD, Lunn JN. Berlin, Springer-Verlag, 1983, pp 69–74

54. Smith RM: Anesthesia for infants and children. 3rd ed. St Louis, Mosby Co, 1968, p 504

55. Filzweiser G, List WF: Morbidity and mortality in elective geriatric surgery, Mortality in Anaesthesia. Edited by Vickers MD, Lunn JN. Berlin, Springer-Verlag, pp 75–82, 1983

56. Gersh BJ, Kronmal RA, Frye RL, et al: Coronary arteriography and coronary artery bypass surgery: Morbidity and mortality in patients ages 65 years or older. Circulation 67:483, 1983

57. Topkins MJ, Artusio JF: Myocardial infarction in surgery, a five year study. Anesth Analg 23:716, 1964

58. Tarhan S, Moffitt EA, Taylor WF, et al: Myocardial infarction after general anesthesia. JAMA 220:1451, 1972

59. Eerola M, Eerola R, Kaukinen S, et al: Risk fac-

tors in surgical patients with verified preoperative myocardial infarction. Acta Anaesthesiol Scand 24:219, 1980

60. Fraser JG, Ramachandran PR, Davis HS: Anesthesia and recent myocardial infarction. JAMA 199:318, 1967

61. Arkins R, Smessaert AA, Hicks RG: Mortality and morbidity in surgical patients with coronary artery disease. JAMA 190:485, 1964

62. Sapala JA, Ponka JL, Duvernow WSC: Operative and nonoperative risks in the cardiac patient. J Am Geriatr Soc 23:529, 1975

63. Jeffrey CC, Kunsman J, Cullen D, et al: A prospective evaluation of cardiac risk. Anesthesiology 58:462, 1983

64. Rao TL, Jacobs KH, El-Etr AA: Reinfarction following anesthesia in patients with myocardial infarction. Anesthesiology 59:499, 1983

65. Lowenstein E, Yusuf S, Teplick R: Perioperative myocardial reinfarction: A glimmer of hope — A note of caution. Anesthesiology 59:493, 1983

66. Scher KS, Tice DA: Operative risk in patients with previous coronary artery bypass. Arch Surg 111:807, 1976

67. McCollum CH, Garcia-Rinoldi R, Graham JM, et al: Myocardial revascularization prior to subsequent major surgery in patients with coronary artery disease. Surgery 81:302, 1977

68. Crawford SE, Morris GC, Howel JF, et al: Operative risk in patients with previous coronary artery bypass. Ann Thorac Surg 26:215, 1978

69. Backer CL, Tinker JH, Robertson DM, et al: Myocardial reinfarction following local anesthesia for ophthalmic surgery. Anesth Analg 59:257, 1980

70. Lang D: Massachusetts Eye and Ear Infirmary, personal communication.

71. Ziffren SE, Hartford CE: Comparative mortality for various surgical operations in older versus younger age groups. J Am Geriatr Soc 20:485, 1972

72. Santos AL, Gelperin A: Surgical mortality in the elderly. J Am Geriatr Soc 23:42, 1975

73. Warner MA, Tinker JH, Frye RL, et al: Risk of cardiac operations in patients with concomitant pulmonary dysfunction. Anesthesiology 57:A57, 1982

74. Takaro T, Hultgren HN, Lipton MJ, et al: The VA cooperative randomized study of surgery for coronary occlusive disease. II Subgroup with significant left main lesion. Circulation 54 (suppl 3):III–107, 1976

75. Hultgren HN, Pfeifer JF, Angell WW, et al: Unstable angina: Comparison of medical and surgical management. Am J Cardiol 39:734, 1977

76. Vlietstra RE, Assad-Morell JL, Frye RL, et al: Survival predictors in coronary artery disease. Medical and surgical comparisons. Mayo Clin Proc 42:85, 1977

77. Namay DL, Hammermeister KE, Zia MS, et al: Effect of perioperative myocardial infarction on late survival in patients undergoing coronary artery bypass surgery. Circulation 65:1066, 1982

78. Podrid PJ, Grayboys TB, Lown B: Prognosis of medically treated patients with coronary artery disease with profound ST segment depression during exercise testing. N Engl J Med 305:111, 1981

79. Frick MH, Harjola PT, Valle M: Persistant impairment after coronary bypass surgery: ergometric and angiographic correlations in five years. Circulation 67:491, 1983

80. Pantely GA, Kloster FE, Morris CD: Late exercise test results from a prospective randomized study of bypass surgery for stable angina. Circulation 68:413, 1983

81. Dorros G, Cowley MJ, Simpson J, et al: Percutaneous transluminal coronary angioplasty: Report of complications from the National Heart and Lung and Blood Institute PTCA registry. Circulation 67:723, 1983

82. Katholi RE, Nolan FP, McGuire LB: The management of anticoagulation during noncardiac operations in patients with prosthetic heart valves. Am Heart J 96:163, 1978

83. Reed RC, Murphy ML, Hultgren HN, et al: Survival of men treated for chronic stable angina pectoris. A cooperative randomized study. J Thorac Cardiovasc Surg 75:1, 1978

84. Goldman L, Caldera DL: Risks of general anesthesia in elective operation in the hypertensive patient. Anesthesiology 50:285, 1979

85. Prys-Robert C: Hypertension and anesthesia — Fifty years on. Anesthesiology 50:281, 1979

86. Veterans Administration study on antihypertensive agents: Effects of treatment on morbidity in hypertension. JAMA 202:1028, 1967

87. Veterans Administration Cooperative Study Group on Antihypertensive Agents: Effects of treatment on morbidity in hypertension: Results in patients with diastolic blood pressure averaging 90 through 114 millimeters of mercury. JAMA 213:1143, 1970

88. Prys-Roberts C, Meloche R, Foex P: Studies of the anaesthesia in relation to hypertension. I. Cardiovascular responses of treated and untreated patients. Br J Anaesth 43:122, 1971

89. Tarhan S, Moffitt EA, Sessler AD, et al: Risk of anesthesia in surgery in patients with chronic bronchitis and chronic obstructive pulmonary disease. Surgery 74:720, 1973

90. Norlander O, Hallen B: Anaesthetics mortality

and pulmonary function, Mortality in Anaesthesia. Edited by Vickers MD, Lunn JN. Berlin, Springer-Verlag, 1983 pp 59–68

91. Hedenstierna G, Wiklund L: Postoperative lunkomplikationer. Preoperative assessment. Lakartidningen 77:2897, 1980

92. Brown B: Statistical problems in comparing outcomes of low incidence, Health Care Delivery in Anesthesia. Edited by Hirsh RA, Forrest WH, Orkin FK, Wallman H. Philadelphia, Stickley, 1980, pp 157–162

93. Lew EA: Mortality experience among anesthesiologists, 1954–1976. Anesthesiology 51:195, 1979

94. Bruce DL, Eide KA, Smith NJ, et al: A prospective survey of anesthesiologist mortality, 1967–1971. Anesthesiology 41:71, 1974

95. Farley WJ, Talbott GD: Anesthesiology and addiction. Anesth Analg 62:465, 1983

96. Gravenstein JS, Kory WP, Marks RG: Drug abuse by anesthesia personnel. Anesth Analg 62:467, 1983

97. du Moulin GC, Hedley-Whyte J: Hospital-associated viral infection and the anesthesiologist. Anesthesiology 59:51, 1983

98. Baden JM: Chronic toxicity of inhalation anaesthetics. Clin Anaesthesiol 1:441, 1983

99. Clements J, Todd NK: Halothane in nondysjunctions in *Drosophila*. Mutat Res 91:225, 1981

100. Basler A, Rohrborn G: Lack of mutagenic effects of halothane in mammals in vivo. Anesthesiology 55:143, 1981

101. Corbett TH: Cancer and congenital anomaly associated with anesthesia. Ann NY Acad Sci 271:58, 1976

102. Eger EI, White AE, Brown CL, et al: A test of the carcinogenicity of enflurane, isoflurane, halothane, methoxyflurane and nitrous oxide in mice. Anesth Analg 57:678, 1978

103. Baden JN, Egbert B, Mazze RI: Carcinogen bioassay of enflurane in mice. Anesthesiology 56:9, 1982

104. Coate WB, Ulland BN, Lewis TR: Chronic exposure to low concentrations of halothane–nitrous oxide: Lack of carcinogenic effect in the rat. Anesthesiology 50:306, 1979

105. Mazze RI, Wilson AI, Rice SA, et al: Effects of isoflurane on reproduction and fetal development in mice. Abstracts, 1984, International Anesthesiology Research Society Meeting, Reno, Nevada, p 27

106. Wyrobek AJ, Brodsky J, Gordon L, et al: Sperm studies in anesthesiologists. Anesthesiology 55:527, 1981

107. Buxton-Hopkin DA: Hazards and Errors in Anaesthesia. Berlin, Springer-Verlag, 1980, p 34

108. Mazze RI: Waste anaesthetic gases: A health hazard? Clin Anaesthesiol 1:431, 1983

109. Axelsson G, Rylander R: Exposure to anaesthetic gases in spontaneous abortion: Response bias in a postal questionnaire study. Int J Epidemiol 11:250, 1982

110. Ericson A, Kallen B: Survey of infants born in 1973 to 1975 to Swedish women working in operating rooms during their pregnancy. Anesth Analg 58:302, 1979

111. Cohen EN, Brown BW, Wu ML, et al: Occupational disease in dentistry and chronic exposure to anesthetic gases. J Am Dent Assoc 101:21, 1980

112. Colton SC: Evaluation of the epidemiologic evidence for occupational hazards of anesthetic gases. Proceedings of the 1982 ASA Meeting.

11

Psychological Preparation and Preoperative Medication

Robert K. Stoelting, M.D.

INTRODUCTION

Anesthetic management begins with the preoperative psychological preparation of the patient and administration of a drug or drugs selected to produce specific pharmacologic responses prior to the induction of anesthesia. Traditionally, this initial psychological and pharmacologic component of anesthetic management is referred to as preoperative medication. Ideally, preoperative medication should increase the likelihood that patients will enter the preoperative period free from apprehension, sedated but easily arousable and fully cooperative.

PREOPERATIVE PSYCHOLOGICAL PREPARATION

The psychological component of preoperative preparation is provided by the anesthesiologist's preoperative visit and interview with the patient and family members. A thorough description of anesthetic management and events to anticipate during the perioperative period serves as a nonpharmacologic antidote to anxiety by reducing the unknown and establishing a personal relationship. The value of this interview is evidenced by its demonstrable calming effect.[1,2] For example, fewer adult patients are nervous before the induction of anes-

TABLE 11-1.   Value of Preoperative Interview Compared with Pentobarbital

	Percentage of Patients			
	Interview	Pentobarbital*	Interview and Pentobarbital*	No Interview and No Pentobarbital
Feel nervous	40	61	38	58
Feel drowsy	26	30	38	18
Judged adequately sedated	65	48	71	35

* 2 mg/kg intramuscularly 1 hour before surgery. (Data from Egbert LD, Battit GE, Turndorf, et al: The value of the preoperative visit by an anesthetist. JAMA 185:553, 1963.)

thesia when a preoperative interview has been conducted as compared with patients receiving pentobarbital but not an interview (Table 11-1).[1] In addition, more patients are judged to be adequately sedated before surgery when an interview has been conducted. A booklet containing information about anesthesia was less effective than a preoperative interview in reducing anxiety.[2] In children, careful psychological preparation and well-informed parents to support the child are extremely valuable. Nevertheless, a shortage of time and the fact that some patients' problems do not lend themselves to reassurance may limit the value of the preoperative interview. Therefore, preoperative pharmacologic preparation is often indicated.

PREOPERATIVE PHARMACOLOGIC PREPARATION

Pharmacologic premedication is typically administered in the patient's hospital room 1 to 2 hours before the anticipated induction of anesthesia. The goals for pharmacologic premedication are multiple and must be individualized to meet each patient's unique requirements (Table 11-2). Some previously accepted goals of pharmacologic premedication are either no longer valid or are better achieved by intravenous administration of the drug at a time more likely to correspond to the time when a pharmacologic effect is necessary (e.g., induction of anesthesia or near the conclusion of anesthe-

TABLE 11-2.   Goals for Preoperative Medication

Anxiety relief
Sedation
Analgesia
Amnesia
Antisialagogue effect
Elevation of gastric fluid pH
Reduction of gastric fluid volume
Prophylaxis against allergic reactions

(Modified from Stoelting RK, Miller RD: Basics of Anesthesia. New York, Churchill Livingstone, 1984.)

sia) (Table 11-3). The best drug or drug combination to achieve the desired goals of pharmacologic premedication is often influenced by the individual physician's previous experience. Indeed, the number of published articles devoted to preoperative medication emphasizes that the ideal drug or drug combination, if such exists, has yet to be discovered.

Pharmacologic preparation should never be routine. The appropriate drug(s) and doses can be selected only after the psychological and physiologic condition of the patient have been

TABLE 11-3.   Low-Priority Goals for Preoperative Premedication

Reduction of cardiac vagal activity—better achieved with an intravenous injection just before the time of anticipated need
Facilitation of induction of anesthesia—not necessary in view of availability of potent intravenous induction drugs
Decreased anesthetic requirements—not of sufficient magnitude to be clinically significant
Postoperative analgesia—better achieved with an intravenous injection just before the time of anticipated need
Prevention of postoperative nausea and emesis—better achieved with an intravenous injection just before the time of anticipated need

(Modified from Stoelting RK, Miller RD: Basics of Anesthesia. New York, Churchill Livingstone, 1984.)

TABLE 11-4. Is Depressant Preoperative Medication Indicated?

No	Yes
Less than 1 year of age	Cardiac surgery
Elderly	Cancer surgery
Most outpatients	Most inpatients
Decreased level of consciousness	Regional anesthesia
Intracranial pathology	
Severe chronic lung disease	
Hypovolemia	

(Modified from Stoelting RK, Miller RD: Basics of Anesthesia. New York, Churchill Livingstone; 1984.)

evaluated. Drug choice and dose must take into account patient age, weight, physical status, degree of anxiety, tolerance for depressant drugs, prior hospitalizations (especially in children), previous adverse experiences with drugs used for preoperative medication (dizziness, nausea, vomiting, "allergy"), duration, and type of surgery (emergency or elective, inpatient or outpatient). After a thorough evaluation of the patient, it may be appropriate not to include drugs in the preoperative preparation (Table 11-4). In contrast, other patients undergoing life-threatening surgery may deserve aggressive pharmacologic attempts to decrease preoperative anxiety and produce sedation (Table 11-4). Finally, the patient who requests to be "asleep" before being transported to the operating room must be reassured this is neither a desired nor safe goal of pharmacologic premedication.

DRUGS FOR PREOPERATIVE MEDICATION

Several classes of drugs are available to facilitate achievement of the desired goals for preoperative medication in each individual patient (Table 11-5). These drugs are often administered intramuscularly but, when possible, the oral route of administration should be considered to improve patient comfort. The small amount of water (30 to 60 ml) used to facilitate oral administration of drugs introduces no hazards related to gastric fluid volume. Ultimately, the specific drug choices are based on a consideration of the goals one wishes to achieve with preoperative pharmacologic preparation balanced against the potential undesirable effects these drugs may produce.

BARBITURATES

Secobarbital and pentobarbital are examples of barbiturates used for preoperative medication. Advantages cited for these drugs include sedation, minimal respiratory depressant effects as evidenced by an unchanged ventilatory response to carbon dioxide, minimal circulatory depression, rarity of nausea and vomiting, and effectiveness when administered orally.[3] Disadvantages include lack of analgesia, disorientation, especially if administered to patients in pain, and absence of a specific pharmacologic antagonist. Enzyme induction is not a consideration with the doses used for preoperative medication. The rare patient with acute intermittent porphyria should not receive barbiturates, as these drugs may precipitate an acute exacerbation of this disease.

NARCOTICS

Morphine and meperidine are the narcotics most frequently used for preoperative medication. Fentanyl does not have an appro-

TABLE 11-5. Drugs and Doses Used for Preoperative Premedication

Classification	Drug	Typical Adult Dose (mg)	Route of Administration
Barbiturates	Secobarbital	50–150	Oral, IM
	Pentobarbital	50–150	Oral, IM
Narcotics	Morphine	5–15	IM
	Meperidine	50–100	IM
Benzodiazepines	Diazepam	5–10	Oral
	Lorazepam	2–4	Oral, IM
Butyrophenones*	Droperidol	1.25	IV
Antihistamines	Diphenhydramine	25–75	Oral, IM
	Promethazine	25–50	IM
	Hydroxyzine	50–100	IM
Anticholinergics	Atropine	0.3–0.6	IM
	Scopolamine	0.3–0.6	IM
	Glycopyrrolate	0.1–0.3	IM
H_2-Antagonists	Cimetidine	300	Oral, IM, IV
	Ranitidine	150	Oral
Antacids	Particulate	15–30 ml	Oral
	Nonparticulate	15–30 ml	Oral
Stimulants of gastric motility	Metoclopramide	5–10	Oral, IM, IV

* Recommended for use as an antiemetic to be administered near the conclusion of surgery.
Abbreviations used: IM, intramuscular; IV, intravenous.
(Modified from Stoelting RK, Miller RD: Basics of Anesthesia. New York, Churchill Livingstone, 1984.)

priate onset and duration of action to justify recommending its use as preoperative medication. Advantages sited for narcotics include facilitation of anesthetic induction, reduction in anesthetic requirements, production of preoperative and postoperative analgesia, ease of controlled ventilation of the lungs intraoperatively, and reversibility with naloxone. Many of these advantages are no longer valid. For example, potent and rapidly acting intravenous drugs ensure a rapid and pleasant induction of anesthesia regardless of preoperative medication. The decrease in inhalation anesthetic requirements produced by morphine is probably clinically insignificant.[4] Pain is rare preoperatively, while postoperative analgesia is best achieved with intravenous drugs administered near the end of surgery. When a nitrous oxide–narcotic anesthetic technique is planned, initial narcotic administration is more logically given intravenously before induction of anesthesia rather than intramuscularly as part of the preoperative medication.

Adverse side effects of narcotics when used for preoperative medication are several. Although narcotics exert no significant depres-sant effects on the myocardium, they do produce relaxation of peripheral vascular smooth muscle manifested as orthostatic hypotension. Orthostatic hypotension will be further exaggerated if a narcotic is administered to a patient with decreased intravascular fluid volume. In contrast to barbiturates, narcotics used for preoperative medication depress the medullary respiratory center as evidenced by decreased responsiveness to carbon dioxide.[3] The euphoric effect of narcotics in patients with pain may be dysphoria in the absence of pain. Nausea and vomiting most likely reflect narcotic stimulation of the chemoreceptor trigger zone in the medulla. Recumbency seems to minimize nausea and vomiting after administration of a narcotic suggesting stimulation of the vestibular apparatus may also be important in production of this undesirable effect. Narcotic-induced smooth muscle constriction may be manifest as choledochoduodenal sphincter spasm, causing some to question the use of narcotics in patients with biliary tract disease.[5] Complaints of right upper quadrant pain following preoperative medication with a narcotic should arouse suspicion of this adverse response. Confirmation of the diagnosis is disappearance of the pain following administration of intravenous naloxone 1 μg/kg. Antidiuretic hormone release, although attributed to morphine, has not been documented to occur in humans.[6]

BENZODIAZEPINES

Benzodiazepines are considered to be specific for anxiety relief. For example, diazepam and lorazepam act on specific brain receptors to produce selective antianxiety effects at doses that do not produce excessive sedation, cardiopulmonary depression, nausea, or vomiting. It is speculated that benzodiazepines increase the responsiveness of brain receptors to the inhibitory neurotransmitter, gamma aminobutyric acid (GABA).[7] In addition, these drugs, particularly lorazepam, produce a suppression of recall of events that occur during the period following their administration (anterograde amnesia).[8] Suppression of recall of preceding events (retrograde amnesia) is less predictable. In animals, diazepam 0.25 mg/kg intramuscularly increases the seizure threshold for lidocaine, but there is no evidence in humans that doses of benzodiazepines as used for pharmacologic premedication reduce the likelihood of local anesthetic toxicity.[9]

A disadvantage of benzodiazepines as used for pharmacologic premedication is excessive and prolonged sedation in occasional patients. This is particularly likely in patients who receive lorazepam in a dose exceeding 50 μg/kg (total dose should not exceed 4 mg). Physostigmine may be effective in reversing sedation produced by benzodiazepines.[10] In the future, specific pharmacologic antagonists of benzodiazepines may become available.[11] Elderly patients or those with severe liver dysfunction may be unusually sensitive to the depressant effects of diazepam.[12]

Cimetidine has been shown to delay the clearance of diazepam from the plasma, introducing the theoretical possibility of an adverse drug interaction when these drugs are administered together for pharmacologic premedication.[13] The clinical significance of the delayed

clearance of diazepam when this drug is administered with cimetidine as pharmacologic premedication is unknown. Nevertheless, the same concern is not relevant for lorazepam, as this drug depends on glucuronidation in the liver, which is not influenced by cimetidine.

Pain at the intramuscular injection site of diazepam plus poor systemic absorption account for the popularity of the oral route of administration of diazepam when used for pharmacologic premedication.[14] In contrast, lorazepam is equally well absorbed after intramuscular or oral administration. Furthermore, lorazepam metabolites are inactive in contrast to the significant pharmacologic activity of the major metabolite of diazepam. Finally, midazolam is rapidly absorbed after intramuscular administration, producing desirable effects that peak within 30 minutes and begin to wane by 60 minutes.[15] As such, midazolam may be an ideal selection for preoperative medication when a short interval between drug administration and induction of anesthesia is anticipated.

BUTYROPHENONES

The use of droperidol as preoperative medication is limited because of the occasional production of dysphoria following its administration.[16] Dysphoric patients express a fear of death and may refuse a previously agreed-upon elective operative procedure. Another disadvantage of droperidol is production of dopaminergic receptor blockade, which may produce extrapyramidal symptoms in normal patients as well as in those with coexisting paralysis agitans.[17] Finally, droperidol is a mild α-adrenergic antagonist, which may detract from its use in patients with a decreased intravascular fluid volume.

As a dopaminergic receptor blocker, droperidol counters the inhibitory effect of dopamine on the carotid body and the ventilatory response to hypoxia. By virtue of this ability to preserve carotid body responsiveness, droperidol may be a relatively safe drug in patients dependent on hypoxic ventilatory drive.[18]

The most important use for droperidol is as

an antiemetic. Ideally, the drug is administered intravenously to high-risk patients (e.g., those who have had eye surgery, who are obese, or who have a history of prior vomiting, or females in the late part of the menstrual cycle) toward the conclusion of surgery to provide protection in the early postoperative period. For example, droperidol 1.25 mg administered intravenously 5 minutes before the conclusion of general anesthesia for orthopedic surgery significantly decreased the incidence of nausea and vomiting.[19] Likewise, droperidol 2.5 mg administered intravenously following clamping of the umbilical cord significantly decreased the incidence of nausea and vomiting in patients receiving spinal anesthesia for elective cesarean section (Fig. 11-1).[20] Nevertheless, routine prophylactic use of antiemetics is not indicated, as not all patients experience this adverse effect. Furthermore, droperidol is not always an effective antiemetic and may be as-

sociated with delayed awakening from anesthesia as well as an increased incidence of postoperative dizziness.[21]

ANTIHISTAMINES

Drugs such as promethazine and hydroxyzine may be classified as antihistamines or tranquilizers. These drugs are used for preoperative medication because of their sedative and antiemetic properties. For example, promethazine combined with meperidine does not increase depression of ventilation produced by meperidine but does produce an additive sedative effect.[22]

Diphenhydramine (0.5 to 1 mg orally or intramuscularly) in combination with cimetidine (4 to 6 mg/kg orally) has been recommended as pharmacologic premedication to provide prophylaxis against intraoperative allergic reactions in patients with chronic atopy or who are undergoing procedures (dye studies, chemonucleolysis) known to be associated with allergic reactions.[23] The combination of an H_1-receptor antagonist (diphenhydramine) and H_2-receptor antagonist (cimetidine) acts to occupy peripheral receptor sites normally responsive to histamine, thereby reducing manifestations of any subsequent drug-induced release of histamine. Prednisone (50 mg every 6 hours for four doses) may also be added to this regimen.

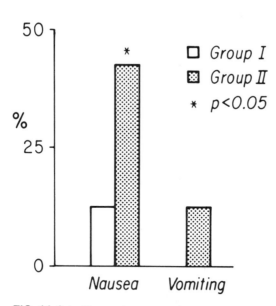

FIG. 11-1 Incidence of nausea and vomiting following elective cesarean section with spinal anesthesia was determined in 50 patients receiving alternately droperidol 2.5 mg (group 1) or saline 1 ml (group II) immediately after clamping the umbilical cord. Droperidol significantly reduced the incidence of postoperative nausea, and none of the drug-treated patients vomited. (Santos A, Datta S: Prophylactic use of droperidol for control of nausea and vomiting during spinal anesthesia for cesarean section. Anesth Analg 63:85, 1984.)

ANTICHOLINERGICS

Atropine, scopolamine, and glycopyrrolate are examples of anticholinergics used in preoperative medication. These drugs are competitive inhibitors of the muscarinic actions of acetylcholine. Atropine and scopolamine are tertiary amines and can cross lipid barriers such as the blood-brain barrier, placenta, and gastrointestinal tract. By contrast, glycopyrrolate acts only on peripheral cholinergic receptors, as its quaternary ammonium structure prevents it from crossing lipid barriers in significant amounts.[24]

The sensitivity of peripheral cholinergic receptors differs such that low doses of an anticholinergic may be sufficient to inhibit salivation but large doses are necessary for cardiac or gastrointestinal effects.[24] Furthermore, responses to the various anticholinergics differ with the doses used for preoperative medication. For example, scopolamine has significant effects on the CNS and is a potent antisialagogue. By contrast, atropine has minimal effects on the CNS and is a more effective cardiac vagolytic than scopolamine. Glycopyrrolate has no CNS effects and produces minimal cardiovascular and visual effects. As an antisialagogue, glycopyrrolate is more potent and longer lasting than atropine.

Routine inclusion of an anticholinergic in the preoperative medication is not necessary. The most frequent reasons for administering an anticholinergic are for the purpose of (1) producing an antisialagogue effect, (2) providing sedative and amnesic effects, (3) decreasing gastric hydrogen ion secretion, and (4) preventing reflex bradycardia. In addition, intramuscular atropine or glycopyrrolate may serve as a placebo in patients who expect a preoperative injection.

ANTISIALAGOGUE EFFECT

The need for including an anticholinergic in the preoperative medication to produce an antisialagogue effect has been questioned, since currently used inhalation anesthetics do not stimulate excessive upper airway secretions. Nevertheless, more satisfactory conditions during general anesthesia due to decreased secretions are likely when an anticholinergic is administered preoperatively, particularly when a tracheal tube is in place.[25] An antisialagogue effect is especially important for intraoral operations or when topical anesthesia is necessary, as excessive secretions may interfere with the surgery or impair production of topical anesthesia by diluting the local anesthetic. Administration of an anticholinergic for an antisialagogue effect is not necessary when regional anesthesia is planned.

Glycopyrrolate and scopolamine are more potent antisialagogues than atropine. Since the discomfort of a dry mouth and throat in an awake patient is an important consideration, it is reasonable to administer the anticholinergic just before the patient leaves the hospital room for transportation to the operating room. Nevertheless, anxiety, fluid deprivation, and other drugs used in the preoperative medication may produce a dry mouth even in the absence of an anticholinergic.[26]

PRODUCTION OF SEDATIVE AND AMNESIC EFFECTS

Atropine and scopolamine are tertiary amines that can cross lipid barriers including the blood–brain barrier. Resulting sedative and amnesic effects reflect penetrance of these drugs into the CNS. Scopolamine is eight to nine times more potent than atropine as an amnesic.[24] Patient acceptance of morphine as preoperative medication is better when this drug is combined with scopolamine rather than with atropine.[27] Sedative or amnesic effects following glycopyrrolate administration would be unlikely, since the quaternary ammonium structure of this drug prevents easy passage into the CNS.

Despite the clinical impression that scopolamine is a potent amnesic, at least one study does not support this view when the drug is used alone.[28] In this report, all patients receiving scopolamine 0.5 mg intravenously remembered their arrival in the operating room when questioned 24 hours later. In contrast, the incidence of amnesia for entering the operating room was 32 percent with 5 to 10 mg of intravenous diazepam and 50 percent with diazepam plus scopolamine, confirming that scopolamine contributed significantly to the amnesic effects of diazepam.

DECREASED GASTRIC HYDROGEN ION SECRETION

The value of an anticholinergic in elevating gastric fluid pH is questionable. Atropine or glycopyrrolate administered intramuscularly 1 to 1.5 hours before induction of anesthesia in

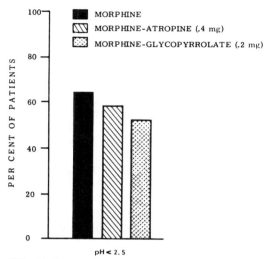

FIG. 11-2 The percentage of patients with a gastric fluid pH below 2.5 at the time of induction of anesthesia was not different (*P* <0.05) with or without the inclusion of an anticholinergic in the preoperative medication. All drugs were administered intramuscularly 1 to 1.5 hours before the induction of anesthesia. (Data from Stoelting RK: Response to atropine, glycopyrrolate, and Riopan of gastric fluid pH and volume in adult patients. Anesthesiology 48:367, 1978.)

adult patients is not effective in significantly raising gastric fluid pH or reducing gastric fluid volume as compared with patients not receiving an anticholinergic.[29,30] For example, about 60 percent of patients have a gastric fluid pH below 2.5 immediately following induction of anesthesia with or without inclusion of atropine (0.4 mg) or glycopyrrolate (0.2 mg) in the preoperative medication (Fig. 11-2).[29] Increasing the glycopyrrolate dose to 0.3 mg does not prove more effective in increasing gastric fluid pH above 2.5.[31] Furthermore, adding glycopyrrolate to cimetidine does not produce an effect different from cimetidine alone.[32]

PREVENTION OF REFLEX BRADYCARDIA

Prevention of reflex bradycardia seems unlikely with the timing and dose of intramuscular anticholinergic typically administered for preoperative medication. If an anticholinergic is selected to prevent reflex bradycardia, the most logical approach is to administer atropine or glycopyrrolate intravenously shortly before the anticipated need.[33] Indeed, intravenous administration of glycopyrrolate or atropine 3 minutes before induction of anesthesia with thiopental prevented heart rate slowing in response to repeated doses of succinylcholine.[34] Vagal responses may be more active in children; therefore, intravenous atropine is often administered immediately before induction of anesthesia.

SIDE EFFECTS

Undesirable side effects of anticholinergics may include (1) CNS toxicity, (2) relaxation of the lower esophageal sphincter, (3) heart rate changes, (4) mydriasis and cycloplegia, (5) elevation of body temperature, (6) drying of airway secretions, and (7) increased physiologic dead space.

CENTRAL NERVOUS SYSTEM TOXICITY

The central anticholinergic syndrome represents toxic CNS effects of anticholinergics. Symptoms include restlessness, agitation, prolonged somnolence after anesthesia, and, in extreme cases, convulsions and coma. Toxicity is most likely to follow scopolamine, but the incidence should be low with the doses used for preoperative medication. CNS toxicity is even less likely with atropine. Nevertheless, elderly patients may be particularly susceptible to CNS toxic effects from both scopolamine and atropine.[35] A central anticholinergic syndrome after glycopyrrolate is unlikely, since this drug is unable to easily cross the blood–brain barrier.

Physostigmine 1 to 2 mg intravenously is effective in reversing the central anticholinergic syndrome produced by atropine or scopolamine.[36] Simultaneous administration of glycopyrrolate intravenously should be an effective method for preventing undesirable peripheral muscarinic effects (bradycardia, salivation) produced by physostigmine. Toxicity attributed to scopolamine or atropine may also represent an uninhibited response to pain as the depressant effects of the anesthetic dissipate.

RELAXATION OF THE LOWER ESOPHAGEAL SPHINCTER

The lower esophageal sphincter is a 2- to 5-cm zone of increased intraluminal pressure at the gastroesophageal junction and is assumed to be an important determinant in the prevention of gastric reflux. When barrier pressure (lower esophageal sphincter pressure minus gastric pressure) is less than 13 cm H_2O, the patient becomes vulnerable to gastroesophageal reflux and the hazards of aspiration pneumonitis should inhalation of gastric fluid occur.[37] Intravenous administration of an anticholinergic results in relaxation of the lower esophageal sphincter.[38] It is assumed, but not documented, that intramuscular administration of these drugs as used for preoperative medication would also lower esophageal sphincter pressure.

Conceivably, inclusion of an anticholinergic in the preoperative medication could increase the risk of gastroesophageal reflux. This remains a theoretical hazard of anticholinergics, as there is no evidence that the incidence of aspiration pneumonitis is increased in patients receiving these drugs as preoperative medication.

HEART RATE CHANGES

Theoretically, heart rate may increase after intramuscular anticholinergic administration. When a tachycardia would be undesirable, scopolamine or glycopyrrolate are better choices than atropine because these drugs manifest fewer cardioaccelerator effects.[24] Nevertheless, the most likely cardiac response after intramuscular atropine as used in preoperative medication is heart rate slowing. This is believed to be secondary to central vagal stimulation before a sufficient atropine blood concentration is established in the periphery to offset this central effect.[24]

Atropine administered to a pregnant patient may result in loss of fetal beat-to-beat heart rate variability, removing an early sign of fetal hypoxemia. Glycopyrrolate would seem less likely to produce this effect, since it is unable to cross the placenta easily.

MYDRIASIS AND CYCLOPLEGIA

Atropine and scopolamine may produce mydriasis and cycloplegia such that patients may experience visual impairment postoperatively. Scopolamine has a greater mydriatic effect than atropine.[39] Conceivably, mydriasis could interfere with drainage of aqueous humor from the anterior chamber of the eye. Despite this response, an anticholinergic may be safely included in the preoperative medication of a patient with glaucoma. However, miotic eye drops should be continued, and atropine or glycopyrrolate would seem a more prudent choice than scopolamine.

ELEVATION OF BODY TEMPERATURE

An anticholinergic may result in elevation of body temperature by suppressing sweat glands, which are innervated by cholinergic nerves via the sympathetic nervous system.[24] Prevention of sweating by this mechanism in children may further increase body temperature, especially if there is preexisting fever.

DRYING OF AIRWAY SECRETIONS

In addition to the discomfort of a dry mouth, the drying and thickening of mucus makes it difficult for cilia to clear secretions. Therefore, it may be best to avoid anticholinergics in patients who benefit from thin secretions.

INCREASED PHYSIOLOGIC DEAD SPACE

Atropine or scopolamine increase physiologic dead space 20 to 25 percent.[3] This is compensated for by increased minute ventilation such that arterial PCO_2 does not increase. This increased minute ventilation should not be interpreted as antagonism of ventilatory depression produced by concomitantly administered drugs such as narcotics. Alone, anticholinergics do not alter the ventilatory responses to carbon dioxide.[3]

HISTAMINE H₂-RECEPTOR ANTAGONISTS

Histamine H_2-receptor antagonists (cimetidine, ranitidine) counter the ability of histamine to induce secretion of gastric fluid with a high hydrogen ion concentration. Therefore, these drugs offer a pharmacologic approach for increasing gastric fluid pH preoperatively. Elevation of gastric fluid pH above 2.5 is desirable, since the severity of aspiration pneumonitis is accentuated by inhalation of fluid with a pH below 2.5.

Administration of cimetidine (300 mg orally) 1 to 1.5 hours before induction of anesthesia increases the gastric fluid pH above 2.5 in more then 80 percent of patients (Fig. 11-3).[40] In this study, gastric fluid volume was not detectably altered by cimetidine. In another report, administration of cimetidine (300 mg intravenously) 2 hours before induction of anesthesia, reduced gastric fluid volume and increased gastric fluid pH above 2.5 in 11 of 11 patients.[41]

Routine inclusion of a histamine H_2-receptor antagonist in the preoperative medication has been suggested.[42] This recommendation is based on the presumed low risk : benefit ratio of these drugs and on the observation that most patients have a gastric fluid pH below 2.5 prior to elective surgery. These drugs would be particularly appropriate before emergency surgery in unprepared patients, in patients with symptoms of gastroesophageal reflux or hiatal hernia, and when anesthesia administered via a face mask is planned or when prolonged induction of anesthesia is anticipated. Obese patients may have a lower gastric fluid pH and higher gastric fluid volume than their nonobese counterparts, and therefore cimetidine or ranitidine administration would seem logical.[43] Likewise, outpatients may have large acidic gastric fluid volumes that may reflect the lack of a preoperative interview and medication to decrease anxiety.[44] Use of an H_2-receptor antagonist in pregnant patients is attractive and has not been shown to produce adverse fetal effects despite placental passage of the drugs.[45] Intravenous administration of an H_2-receptor antagonist is a consideration for patients requiring emergency surgery or for those who cannot receive oral medications. Small

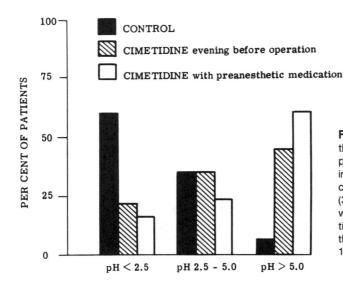

FIG. 11-3 Compared with control patients, the percentage of patients with a gastric fluid pH above 2.5 and 5.0 immediately following induction of anesthesia was significantly increased in those patients receiving cimetidine (300 mg orally) the evening before surgery or with the preoperative (preanesthetic) medication. (Stoelting RK, Miller RD: Basics of Anesthesia. New York, Churchill Livingstone, 1984, and based on data in ref. 40.)

bowel obstruction represents an increased risk for aspiration but H_2-receptor antagonists are probably not indicated as gastric fluid is already alkaline.[42]

Despite convincing evidence that H_2-receptor antagonists increase gastric fluid pH, there are no data to demonstrate that increased patient safety is present should inhalation of gastric contents occur in those pretreated with these drugs.[42] Indeed, in animals, respiratory epithelial damage occurred following aspiration of fluid with a pH 5.9 and devoid of particulate matter, suggesting that control of gastric fluid pH is not the final solution.[46] Furthermore, it must be appreciated that an inherent failure rate is associated with these drugs that is unpredictable despite what is considered the administration of an optimal dose and use of an appropriate timing interval. Although unlikely with the doses used for preoperative medication, it is important to recognize that cimetidine has been associated during chronic use with CNS depression and inhibition of cytochrome P-448 and P-450 enzymes with impaired elimination of several drugs.[42] Ranitidine may be less likely than cimetidine to produce CNS effects or to alter metabolism of drugs by inhibition of hepatic microsomal enzyme systems.[47] Administration of an H_2-receptor antagonist to a patient with bronchial asthma is questionable, as blockade of bronchodilating effects mediated by H_2-receptors would leave unopposed H_1-receptor mediated bronchoconstriction. It must be appreciated that these drugs will not alter the pH of gastric fluid present before administration of the drug nor will cimetidine facilitate gastric emptying. Finally, an H_2-antagonist will not influence the incidence of vomiting or regurgitation.

Under no circumstances can preoperative medication with an H_2-antagonist be substituted for anesthetic techniques (e.g., intubation of the trachea with a cuffed tube or maintenance of consciousness) known to protect the lungs from inhalation of gastric fluid. Aspiration is also a hazard at the conclusion of surgery when the tracheal tube is removed. In this regard, cimetidine administered as pharmacologic premedication is unlikely to offer protection at the conclusion of operations lasting more than 3 hours.[48] Conversely, ranitidine may provide protection for up to 9 hours.[48]

ANTACIDS

Antacids administered 15 to 30 minutes before the induction of anesthesia are nearly 100 percent effective in elevating the gastric fluid pH above 2.5 (Fig. 11-4).[29,49,50] Inhalation of gastric fluid containing particulate antacids, however, may be associated with severe and persistent pulmonary dysfunction despite a high pH of the aspirated material.[51,52] In contrast, the nonparticulate antacid, 0.3 M sodium citrate does not produce significant pulmonary dysfunction should inhalation of fluid containing this antacid occur.[53] Bicitra is a commercially available antacid containing sodium citrate and citric acid.[54]

Compared with H_2-receptor antagonists, the administration of an antacid is effective in raising the pH of gastric fluid present in the stomach at the time of administration. For this reason, administration of an antacid is more logical than an H_2-receptor antagonist when

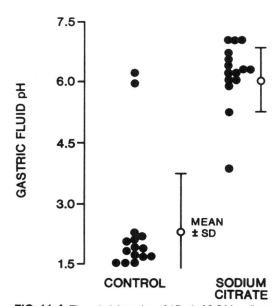

FIG. 11-4 The administration of 15 ml of 0.3 M sodium citrate 15 to 20 minutes before the induction of anesthesia raised the gastric fluid pH above 2.5 in every patient. The mean gastric fluid pH was 6.0 in patients treated with sodium citrate compared with 2.4 in the control patients. (Stoelting RK, Miller RD: Basics of Anesthesia. New York, Churchill Livingstone, 1984, and based on data in ref. 49.)

emergency surgery (e.g., cesarean section) is necessary. The use of an antacid to elevate gastric fluid pH is associated with a modest increase in gastric fluid volume that does not occur with H_2-receptor antagonists.[40,55] Furthermore, antacids may slow the speed of gastric emptying. Since the severity of aspiration pneumonitis depends on both the volume (greater than 0.4 ml/kg) and pH (below 2.5) of the inhaled fluid, this increased gastric fluid volume effect of antacids must be considered. In addition, mixing of antacids with gastric fluid may not occur in patients who remain immobile. Finally, the efficacy of antacids or H_2-receptor antagonists in raising the pH of undigested food particles is not proven.

METOCLOPRAMIDE

Metoclopramide speeds gastric emptying by selectively stimulating motility of the upper gastrointestinal tract and relaxing the pyloric sphincter.[56,57] The onset of this metoclopramide effect is 30 to 60 minutes after oral administration and 1 to 3 minutes following a similar dose administered intravenously or intramus-cularly (Fig. 11-5).[56] Conceivably, this drug may find a place in pharmacologic premedication for use in reducing gastric fluid volume, particularly in the patient with diabetes mellitus and associated gastroparesis, in the parturient, and in the patient who has recently ingested food and subsequently requires emergency surgery for disease unrelated to the gastrointestinal tract. Nevertheless, substantial gastric fluid volumes can still be present despite administration of metoclopramide.[42] Furthermore, the administration of a narcotic or anticholinergic with metoclopramide is questionable, since the impact of metoclopramide on gastric motility may be offset by these drugs.

Metoclopramide alone increases lower esophageal sphincter tone and, when combined with an anticholinergic, offsets the reduction in sphincter tone normally produced by these drugs (Table 11-6).[58] Nevertheless, the clinical significance of this effect on lower esophageal sphincter tone has not been documented.

Metoclopramide is alleged to reduce the incidence of postoperative nausea and vomiting.[59] Despite these alleged effects, the incidence of vomiting in the first 24 hours postoperatively was not reduced by metoclopramide administered intravenously 5 minutes before

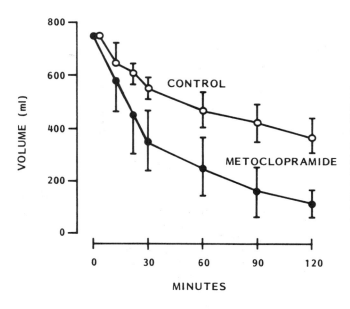

FIG. 11-5 Gastric emptying time was measured in parturients during labor. Following administration of 750 ml of water via a nasogastric tube, the gastric fluid volume decreased at a faster rate in those patients treated with metoclopramide (10 mg intramuscularly) as compared with patients not receiving this drug (control). (Stoelting RK, Miller RD: Basics of Anesthesia. New York, Churchill Livingstone, 1984, and based on data in ref. 56.)

TABLE 11-6. Effect of Metoclopramide and/or Atropine on Barrier Pressure*

	Barrier Pressure (cm H_2O)
Metoclopramide	Increase 12.4
Atropine	Decrease 8.4
Metoclopramide followed by atropine	Increase 11.1
Atropine followed by metoclopramide	Increase 3.0

* Barrier pressure = lower esophageal spincter pressure minus gastric pressure.
(Modified from Brock-Utne JG, Dimopoulos GE, Downing JW, et al: Effect of metoclopramide given before atropine sulphate on lower oesophageal sphincter tone. South A Med J 61:465, 1982.)

the conclusion of surgery.[19] Failure of metoclopramide to prevent postoperative emesis suggests that a drug that increases gastrointestinal motility is not useful as an antiemetic when the gastrointestinal tract is hyporeactive following surgery.

Side effects of metoclopramide are related to its passage into the CNS and production of dopaminergic receptor blockade manifesting as extrapyramidal symptoms. Finally, metoclopramide has no effect on the pH of gastric fluid.

EVALUATION OF DRUGS USED FOR PREOPERATIVE MEDICATION

Precise methods to quantify the value of drugs used for preoperative medication are not available.[60] Although anxiety relief is an important goal of preoperative medication, there is no reliable method to measure this subjective response. Sedation is a more objective measurement, but it must be remembered that drowsiness does not ensure anxiety relief.[26] Comparison of studies on preoperative medication is hampered by different drug doses, sites, and methods of injection, as well as by varying times for measuring responses. Differences in emotional states of patients and what the patient expects from the preoperative medication may also play a role in the evaluation of a drug or drug combination.

Despite these complexities, Forrest et al.[26] provided useful information on preoperative medication administered to adult patients prior to elective operations (Table 11-7). These investigators evaluated responses following intramuscular pentobarbital, secobarbital, diazepam, hydroxyzine, morphine, and meperidine. With the exception of diazepam, all drugs produced dose-related sedation 0.5 to 1 hour after injection. According to patient evaluation, no drug at any dose had a significant effect on apprehension relative to the placebo, emphasizing that sedation does not equal anxiety relief. Those who received a placebo, however, were more apprehensive in the operating room than when interviewed earlier in their rooms. Interestingly, anesthesiologists, who did not know which drug had been given, rated preoperative medication satisfactory in 37 to 63 percent of patients receiving placebo and in 43 to 67 percent of drug-treated patients. The two most frequent side effects described by patients were dry mouth and slurred speech. Nausea was an infrequent complaint, and vomiting did not occur in any patient. Severe pain at the intramuscular injection site was infrequent, and the incidence was not increased for any specific drug. These data cast doubt on the ability to measure predictably and confirm the value of drugs used for preoperative medication but should not be accepted as evidence that drugs never produce a more comfortable patient during the preoperative period.

TABLE 11-7. Percentage of Patients Reporting Side Effects After Intramuscular Preoperative Medication

Medication	Dry Mouth	Slurred Speech	Dizzy	Nauseated	Vomiting
Pentobarbital, 50 mg	30	20	10	7	0
Pentobarbital, 150 mg	28	38	10	7	0
Secobarbital, 50 mg	34	21	3	7	0
Secobarbital, 150 mg	47	43	13	10	0
Placebo	26	23	6	10	0
Diazepam, 5 mg	30	10	3	3	0
Diazepam, 10 mg	37	30	13	0	0
Hydroxyzine, 50 mg	50	27	3	3	0
Hydroxyzine, 100 mg	37	30	3	0	0
Placebo	27	23	3	10	0
Morphine, 5 mg	77	33	13	3	0
Morphine, 10 mg	88*	33	17	10	0
Meperidine, 50 mg	83*	33	17	20	0
Meperidine, 100 mg	87*	57*	23	3	0
Placebo	50	17	13	17	0

* Significantly different from placebo control ($P < 0.05$).
(Modified from Forrest WH, Brown CR, Brown BW: Subjective responses to six common preoperative medications. Anesthesiology 47:241, 1977.)

RECOMMENDED APPROACH TO PREOPERATIVE MEDICATION

An outline of the recommended approach to preoperative medication is presented in Table 11-8. Preoperative medication begins with the anesthesiologist's interview, explanation of the planned anesthetic management, and discussion of any questions or concerns the patient or other interested parties may pose. The importance of this personal contact, ideally the day before elective surgery, is well documented.[1] After the interview is concluded, the decision as to the need for pharmacologic preparation is made and the specific drug(s) and doses to be administered are determined.

Timing of drug administration is as important as the drug or drugs selected for preoperative medication. Preoperative medication designed to decrease anxiety and produce sedation is most appropriately administered 1 to 2 hours before induction of anesthesia. Oral administration of a benzodiazepine is ideal. Oral cimetidine is also conveniently administered at this time. Metoclopramide administered orally is a logical consideration for inclusion in the preoperative medication when a predictable reduction in gastric fluid volume is important. The small amount of water (30 to 60 ml) needed for oral administration of drugs is negligible with respect to gastric fluid volume. Intramuscular administration of morphine is an alternative to a benzodiazepine if analgesia is an important objective. For example, analgesia

TABLE 11-8. Recommended Preoperative Medication for Adult Patients Prior to Elective Surgery

1. Patient interview by anesthesiologist the day before surgery
2. Flurazepam (oral) to treat insomnia the night before surgery
3. Diazepam or lorazepam orally 1 to 2 hours before induction of anesthesia
4. Substitute morphine intramuscularly for number 3 if analgesia is desired
5. Scopolamine intramuscularly 1 to 2 hours before induction of anesthesia if reliable sedation and amnesia are desired—otherwise do not administer an anticholinergic, or follow recommendation number 8
6. Cimetidine orally 1 to 2 hours before induction of anesthesia
7. Metoclopramide orally 1 to 2 hours before induction of anesthesia—not routine at present
8. Glycopyrrolate (intramuscular) when patient is ready to be transported to the operating room if an antisialagogue effect is desired

provided by the preoperative medication is important when pain is present preoperatively or preparation for anesthesia is likely to be uncomfortable due to placement of invasive monitors or performance of nerve blocks. Emergency surgery requiring general anesthesia in a patient who has recently eaten would seem a logical situation for intravenous administration of cimetidine and metoclopramide. An alternative to cimetidine administered intravenously is a nonparticulate antacid.

Intramuscular administration of scopolamine at the same time as an oral drug or intramuscular narcotic is indicated when it is desirable to exploit the amnesic and sedative effects of this anticholinergic. It seems to be a valid clinical impression that scopolamine contributes significantly to the sedative and amnesic effects of concomitantly administered drugs. Indeed, the combination of intramuscular morphine and scopolamine is ideal for producing tranquility and sedation in patients most deserving of aggressive pharmacologic premedication.

An anticholinergic drug selected solely to produce an antisialagogue effect is most appropriately administered intramuscularly immediately before the patient is transported to the operating room. An anticholinergic drug given 1 to 2 hours before the induction of anesthesia serves only to prolong the uncomfortable sensation of a dry mouth and throat experienced by the patient. Glycopyrrolate is the most logical drug if an antisialagogue response without CNS effects is desired.

Drugs to decrease vagal activity (atropine, glycopyrrolate), protect against postoperative emesis (droperidol) or provide postoperative analgesia are most logically administered intravenously at a time just preceding the desired effect. Certainly, routine antiemetic therapy is not necessary, since most patients do not need this type of prophylaxis. It is better to identify those at risk and administer an intravenous antiemetic 15 to 20 minutes before the end of the operation.

Finally, it must be remembered that insomnia is predictable the night before elective surgery. Flurazepam or temazepam administered orally are an effective treatment of insomnia.

REFERENCES

1. Egbert LD, Battit GE, Turndorf H, et al: The value of the preoperative visit by an anesthetist. JAMA 185:553, 1963
2. Leigh JM, Walker J, Janaganathan P: Effect of preoperative anaesthetic visit on anxiety. Br Med J 2:987, 1977
3. Smith TC, Stephen GW, Zeiger L, et al: Effects of premedicant drugs on respiration and gas exchange in man. Anesthesiology 28:883, 1967
4. Saidman LJ, Eger EI II: Effect of nitrous oxide and of narcotic premedication on the alveolar concentration of halothane required for anesthesia. Anesthesiology 25:302, 1964
5. Greenstein AJ, Kayman A, Singer A, et al: A comparative study of pentazocine and meperidine on the biliary passage pressure. Am J Gastroenterol 58:417, 1972
6. Philbin DM, Coggins CH: Plasma antidiuretic hormone levels in cardiac surgical patients during morphine and halothane anesthesia. Anesthesiology 49:95, 1978
7. Study RE, Barker JL: Cellular mechanisms of benzodiazepine action. JAMA 247:2147, 1982
8. Bradshaw EG, Ali AA, Mulley BA, et al: Plasma concentrations and clinical effects of lorazepam after oral administration. Br J Anaesth 53:517, 1981
9. Moore DC, Balfour RI, Fitzgibbons D: Convulsive arterial plasma levels of bupivacaine and the response to diazepam therapy. Anesthesiology 50:454, 1979
10. Caldwell CB, Gross JB: Physostigmine reversal of midazolam-induced sedation. Anesthesiology 57:123, 1982
11. O'Boyle C, Lambe R, Darragh A, et al: RO 15-1788 antagonizes the effects of diazepam in man without affecting its bioavailability. Br J Anaesth 55:349, 1983
12. Koltz U, Avant GR, Hoyumpa A, et al: The effects of age and liver disease on the disposition and elimination of diazepam in adult man. J Clin Invest 55:347, 1975
13. Feely J, Wilkinson GR, Wood AJJ: Reduction of liver blood flow and propranolol metabolism by cimetidine. N Engl J Med 304:693, 1981
14. Hillestad L, Hansen T, Melsom H, et al: Diazepam metabolism in normal man 1. Serum concentrations and clinical effects after intravenous, intramuscular and oral administration. Clin Pharmacol Ther 16:479, 1974

15. Fragen RJ, Dunk DI, Avram MJ, et al: Midazolam versus hydroxyzine as intramuscular premedicant. Can Anaesth Soc J 30:136, 1983

16. Lee CM, Yeakel AE: Patient refusal of surgery following Innovar premedication. Anesth Analg 54:225, 1975

17. Patton CM: Rapid induction of acute dyskinesia by droperidol. Anesthesiology 43:126, 1975

18. Ward DS: Stimulation of hypoxic ventilatory drive by droperidol. Anesth Analg 63:106, 1984

19. Korttila K, Kauste A, Auvinen J: Comparison of domperidone, droperidol, and metoclopramide in the prevention and treatment of nausea and vomiting after balanced general anesthesia. Anesth Analg 58:396, 1979

20. Santos A, Datta S: Prophylactic use of droperidol for control of nausea and vomiting during spinal anesthesia for cesarean section. Anesth Analg 63:85, 1984

21. Cohen SE, Woods WA, Wyner J: Antiemetic efficacy of droperidol and metoclopramide. Anesthesiology 60:67, 1984

22. Keats AS, Telford J, Jurosu Y: "Potentiation" of meperidine by promethazine. Anesthesiology 22:34, 1961

23. Beaven MA: Anaphylactoid reactions to anesthetic drugs. Anesthesiology 55:3, 1981

24. Mirakhur RK: Anticholinergic drugs. Br J Anaesth 51:671, 1979

25. Falick YS, Smiler BG: Is anticholinergic premedication necessary? Anesthesiology 43:472, 1975

26. Forrest WH, Brown CR, Brown BW: Subjective responses to six common preoperative medications. Anesthesiology 47:241, 1977

27. Conner JT, Bellville JW, Wender R, et al: Morphine, scopolamine, and atropine as intravenous surgical premedicants. Anesth Analg 56:606, 1977

28. Frumin MJ, Hereker VR, Jarvik ME: Amnesic actions of diazepam and scopolamine in man. Anesthesiology 45:406, 1976

29. Stoelting RK: Responses to atropine, glycopyrrolate, and Riopan of gastric fluid pH and volume in adult patients. Anesthesiology 48:367, 1978

30. Manchikanti L, Roush JR: Effect of preanesthetic glycopyrrolate and cimetidine on gastric fluid pH and volume in outpatients. Anesth Analg 63:40, 1984

31. Baraka A, Saab M, Salem MR, et al: Control of gastric acidity by glycopyrrolate premedication in the parturient. Anesth Analg 56:642, 1977

32. Manchikanti L, Kraus JW, Edds SP: Cimetidine and related drugs in anesthesia. Anesth Analg 61:595, 1982

33. Meyers EF, Tomeldan SA: Glycopyrrolate compared with atropine in prevention of the oculocardiac reflex during eye-muscle surgery. Anesthesiology 51:350, 1979

34. Sorensen O, Eriksen S, Hommelgaard P, et al: Thiopental nitrous-halothane anesthesia and repeated succinylcholine: Comparison of preoperative glycopyrrolate and atropine administration. Anesth Analg 59:686, 1980

35. Smith DS, Orkin FK, Gardner SM, et al: Prolonged sedation in the elderly after intraoperative atropine administration. Anesthesiology 51:348, 1979

36. Holzgrafe RE, Vondrell JJ, Mintz SM: Reversal of postoperative reactions to scopolamine with physostigmine. Anesth Analg 52:921, 1973

37. Haddad JK: Relation of gastroesophageal reflux to yield sphincter pressures. Gastroenterology 58:175, 1970

38. Brock-Utne JG, Rubin J, Welman S, et al: The effect of glycopyrrolate (Robinul) on the lower oesophageal sphincter. Can Anaesth Soc J 25:144, 1978

39. Garde JF, Aston R, Endler GC, et al: Racial mydriatic responses to belladonna premedication. Anesth Analg 57:572, 1978

40. Stoelting RK: Gastric fluid pH in patients receiving cimetidine. Anesth Analg 57:675, 1978

41. Maliniak K, Vakil AH: Pre-anesthetic cimetidine and gastric pH. Anesth Analg 58:309, 1979

42. Coombs DW: Aspiration pneumonia prophylaxis (Editorial). Anesth Analg 62:1055, 1983

43. Vaughn RW, Bauer S, Wise L: Volume and pH of gastric juice in obese patients. Anesthesiology 43:686, 1975

44. Ong BY, Palahniuk RJ, Cumming M: Gastric volume and pH in out-patients. Can Anesth Soc J 25:36, 1978

45. Hodgkinson R, Glassenberg R, Joyce TH, et al: Comparison of cimetidine (Tagamet) with antacid for safety and effectiveness in reducing gastric acidity before elective cesarean section. Anesthesiology 59:86, 1983

46. Wynne JW, Ramphal R, Hood CI: Tracheal mucosal damage after aspiration: a scanning electron microscope study. Am Rev Respir Dis 124:728, 1981

47. Zeldis JE, Freidman LS, Isselbacher KJ: Ranitidine: A new H_2-receptor antagonist. N Engl J Med 309:1368, 1983

48. Coombs DW, Hooper DW: Cimetidine as a prophylactic against acid aspiration at tracheal extubation. Can Anaesth Soc J 28:33, 1981

49. Viegas OJ, Ravindran RS, Shumacker CA: Gastric fluid pH in patients receiving sodium citrate. Anesth Analg 60:521, 1981

50. Gibbs CP, Spohr L, Schmidt D: The effectiveness of sodium citrate as an antacid. Anesthesiology 57:44, 1982

51. Gibbs CP, Schwartz DJ, Wynne JW, et al: Antacid pulmonary aspiration in the dog. Anesthesiology 51:380, 1979

52. Bond VK, Stoelting RK, Gupta CD: Pulmonary aspiration syndrome after inhalation of gastric fluid containing antacids. Anesthesiology 51:452, 1979

53. Gibbs CP, Hempling RE, Wynne JW, et al: Antacid pulmonary aspiration. Anesthesiology 51:S290, 1979

54. Reisner LS: Bicitra is 0.3 molar sodium citrate (letter). Anesth Analg 61:801, 1982

55. Foulkes E, Jenkins LC: A comparative evaluation of cimetidine and sodium citrate to decrease gastric acidity: Effectiveness at the time of induction of anaesthesia. Can Anaesth Soc J 23:29, 1981

56. Howard FA, Sharp DS: Effect of metoclopramide on gastric emptying during labour. Br Med J 1:446, 1973

57. Wyner J, Cohen SE: Gastric volume in early pregnancy: Effect of metoclopramide. Anesthesiology 57:209, 1982

58. Brock-Utne JG, Dimopoulos GE, Downing JW, et al: Effect of metoclopramide given before atropine sulphate on lower oesophageal sphincter tone. South Afr Med J 61:465, 1982

59. Winning TJ, Brocke-Utne JG, Downing JW: Nausea and vomiting after anesthesia and minor surgery. Anesth Analg 56:674, 1977

60. Norris W: The quantitative assessment of premedication. Br J Anaesth 41:778, 1969

12

The Immediate Preinduction Period

Ronald D. Miller, M.D.

INTRODUCTION

One of the main obligations of the anesthesiologist is to prepare the patient and operating room for a safe anesthetic. In this chapter, the tasks that should be completed from the time the patient enters the operating room until induction of anesthesia are described. The considerations presented in this chapter apply to all patients undergoing all types of anesthesia and surgery, even the most simple and routine types. More specific preparation and monitoring for specialized types of anesthesia and surgery will be covered in the appropriate chapters (e.g., Swan-Ganz catheters in Ch. 13).

The anesthesiologist should develop a routine which assures that the operating room, its equipment, and the patient are prepared for safe anesthesia. Apparently, some anesthesiologists are not using an adequate routine. Cooper et al.,[1] using a modified critical-incident analysis technique, evaluated preventable mishaps resulting from human error that could have or actually did contribute to anesthetic risk. Of 277 incidents, 47 percent of them occurred during the time from entry of the patient into the operating room until the surgical incision; 82 percent of these incidents were secondary to human error and 14 percent were due to overt equipment error. The most common errors, in order of frequency, are breathing circuit disconnection, accidental gas flow change, syringe swap, gas supply problem, intravenous apparatus disconnection, and laryngoscope malfunction.

Cooper et al.[1] concluded that associated factors also contributed to errors, some of which, listed in order of occurrence, are inadequate total experience, inadequate familiarity with equipment, poor communication with other members of the surgical team, haste, inattention or carelessness, fatigue, excessive dependence on other personnel, and failure to perform a normal check.

Although several factors obviously contribute to these preventable mishaps in the preinduction of anesthesia period, knowing how the anesthetic equipment works and ensuring that this equipment is functioning properly will eliminate many of the errors. Obviously, the anesthesiologist must develop a checklist and acquire the discipline to utilize it every time an anesthetic is administered. Airline pilots run through a mandatory checklist before starting a flight; this same principle applies to starting an anesthetic. The following questions are the most important ones for the anesthesiologist to ask.

QUESTIONS THE ANESTHESIOLOGIST SHOULD ASK

IS THE CENTRAL AND CYLINDER SOURCE OF OXYGEN AND NITROUS OXIDE FUNCTIONING?

Most hospitals pipe oxygen and often nitrous oxide from large cylinders in central locations in the hospital. Coupling systems at wall outlets and machines are designed to prevent accidental interchange of nitrous oxide and oxygen. Despite this system, nitrous oxide and oxygen lines have been accidentally switched on occasion, resulting in severe morbidity and even death.

Feeley and Hedley-Whyte[2] surveyed hospitals with anesthesia residency training programs to ascertain the frequency and types of complications encountered with the use of bulk supplies of oxygen and nitrous oxide. A total of 76 incidents were reported, 3 of which led to death. In one hospital, tanks used for central oxygen were marked to contain oxygen but in fact contained nitrogen. Use of these tanks was felt to contribute to the deaths of two in-

fants. Another patient died while being anesthetized in a new operating room where the oxygen and nitrous oxide pipes were crossed. I am aware of three deaths caused by this same mistake; fortunately these problems are usually, but not always, detected before serious damage to a patient occurs. The most frequent malfunction was insufficient oxygen pressure (Table 12-1). Feeley and Hedley-Whyte[2] concluded that the major problem was that most hospitals have no formal system of inspection to ensure that hospitals and gas suppliers comply with the National Fire Protection Association regulations. Although compliance is required by the Joint Commission on Accreditation of Hospitals, their inspection apparently is often inadequate. Obviously, all physicians should be aware of the designs and hazards of medical gas delivery systems and whether their own hospital complies with regulations. On a day-by-day basis, routine use of an oxygen analyzer in the anesthetic system should allow the anesthesiologist to immediately detect when defects in central gas delivery systems have occurred.

Small cylinders attached to the anesthetic machine should be available as a backup in case the central source of gases fails. These smaller cylinders should be checked before each administration of anesthetic. The anesthetic machines have pressure gauges to determine the gas pressure in these smaller cylin-

TABLE 12-1. Reported Malfunctions of Gas Delivery Systems

Malfunction	Number of Reports
Insufficient oxygen pressure	37
Excessive oxygen and nitrous oxide pressure	7
Crossed pipelines	6
Depletion of nitrous oxide	5
Failure of low-pressure alarm	4
Leaks in nitrous oxide pipeline	3
Leaks in wall connectors	2
Freezing of nitrous oxide regulators	2
Low oxygen flow	2
Others	8
Total	76

(Modified from Feeley TW, Hedley-Whyte J: Bulk oxygen and nitrous oxide delivery systems. Anesthesiology 44:301, 1976.)

ders. In the case of oxygen, the pressure on the gauge is proportional to the volume of gas in the cylinder. This is because the temperature in the operating room is above the critical temperature of oxygen (the critical temperature is that at which a gas cannot be liquefied by pressure). Therefore, when the pressure gauge reads 1200 psi, the tank is 66 percent full of oxygen, as compared to a pressure of 1800 psi.

In the case of nitrous oxide, the cylinder pressure does not reflect the volume of gas available. This is because nitrous oxide is stored as a liquid. As gas is withdrawn from the cylinder, it is replaced by an equal volume vaporized from the liquid without change in pressure until all the liquid is exhausted. In this manner, greater volumes can be stored in cylinders if they liquefy at room temperature. For example, 420 gallons of nitrous oxide can be stored in an E cylinder at 750 psi, while only 165 gallons of oxygen can be stored in an E cylinder at 1800 psi.

HAS THE ANESTHETIC MACHINE BEEN CHECKED THOROUGHLY?

As outlined by Cooper et al.,[1] the failure to perform a proper check is associated with a large fraction of errors designated as preventable mishaps. Although the check will vary somewhat, depending on the anesthetic system being used (see Ch. 5 for a detailed description of various anesthetic systems), several checks apply to all anesthetic systems (see Table 12-2). In essence, the anesthesiologist should confirm that the gas sources from the central source and cylinders are adequate. Is the vaporizer full of anesthetic? Does the circuit have any leaks or unexpected resistance? Is the absorbent satisfactory? I strongly recommend that the anesthesiologist apply the mask to his own face and breathe through the circuit; this will confirm that the circuit does not offer a high resistance to breathing such as from a malfunctioning valve. Also, an excessive concentration of anesthetic that could occur from an undetected open flowmeter may be perceived. Lastly, by smelling the outflow from the anesthetic machine, the anesthesiologist can even check to

TABLE 12-2. Checklist for Evaluation of an Anesthetic Machine *Prior* to Its Use

1. Date of last inspection and servicing. (Ideally, maintenance should be performed every 3 to 6 months.)
2. Oxygen tank pressure (with flowmeters off) indicates an oxygen supply sufficient for the expected duration of the case.
3. Oxygen flowmeter ball or float rotates freely without sticking to side or top of flowmeter tube.
4. Nitrous oxide flowmeter ball or float rotates freely and is not jammed at top of flowmeter tube; nitrous oxide is turned off before starting anesthesia.
5. Oxygen flush valve fills reservoir bag rapidly when it is opened and the breathing circuit is closed (i.e., by the anesthesiologist placing a thumb over the mask of endotracheal tube connector and with the pop-off valve closed).
6. Breathing circuit holds a steady positive pressure when circuit is closed and flow of fresh oxygen is turned off to ascertain the absence of leaks.
7. Pop-off valve releases positive pressure when it is opened.
8. The anesthesiologist breathes through the anesthetic system to detect any unexpected resistance in the circuit (e.g., malfunctioning valve).
9. Carbon dioxide absorbent is not depleted (i.e., see color indicator).
10. Volatile anesthetic vaporizers are filled adequately.
11. Sniff test — no smell of anesthetic when vaporizer is off: intensity of odor is appropriate when vaporizer is turned on to a low or medium concentration.
12. Suction bottle is empty and suction apparatus develops greater than 25 mm Hg of negative pressure.
13. Oxygen analyzer is turned on and is calibrated appropriately.

see whether the vaporizer is functioning. The "calibrated nose" is a very useful clinical tool. As stated by Cullen and Larson,[3] the advantages of preventing inadvertent exposure to the patient of dangerously high concentrations of anesthetic outweigh the highly unlikely toxic effects to the anesthesiologist from an occasional sniff of the machine outflow.

IS THE ANESTHETIC WORK AREA ORGANIZED PROPERLY?

A carefully organized work space should lessen the chance of overt error and increase the chance of being effective in a crisis situation. As indicated earlier, an accidental syringe swap is a common cause of preventable anesthetic mishaps. These errors probably could be prevented by simply labeling the syringes. The anesthesiologist must develop a checklist that is meticulously followed. Although several such checklists have been recommended,[4] the anesthesiologist probably should develop one that best suits his or her needs. Obviously, surgery can be delayed by the anesthesiologist who has an unrealistic checklist that takes too much time to follow. However, if the operating room and, specifically, anesthetic work area are adequately prepared before the first case, an adequate check between cases should take less than 5 minutes.

IS THE INTRAVENOUS LINE FUNCTIONING PROPERLY?

A well-functioning intravenous line is an obvious necessity for most anesthetics and surgery. Although the techniques of establishing an intravenous line have been adequately described in most introductory texts of anesthesia,[3] I have a few preferences.

Often, patients are subjected to unnecessary discomfort in an effort to establish a large-bore intravenous line prior to induction of anesthesia. Patients enter the operating room with veins that are often collapsed due to fear or cold. In this situation, I prefer to use an inhalational induction of anesthesia or to find a small vein with a fine needle through which drugs such as thiopental can be infused. After anesthesia has been induced, these veins probably will be dilated and a larger, more suitable line can then be established.

Basically, three kinds of needles are used: "butterfly needle," intracath, and extracath. The butterfly is very good for small veins, such as the scalp vein of an infant; however, movement will cause the solid needle to puncture the vein and "infiltrate." The intracath has a plastic catheter introduced through the needle, while an extracath has the plastic catheter introduced over the needle. The latter is preferred because it causes less bleeding at the puncture site of the vein.

A vein that is easily seen and reasonably straight should be selected. The dorsum of the hand frequently has such veins. If the vein is collapsed because of cold or the patient's fear, measures can be taken to dilate the vein. These measures are dependent on drainage, application of moist heat, or gentle rubbing or tapping of the puncture site. Too often the novice will firmly pound the patient's hand or arm instead of gently rubbing it. The former is unproductive and uncomfortable for the patient.

Details of venipuncture have been described in various introductory texts of anesthesia.[3,5] Whether the bevel of the needle should be up or down when puncturing the vein is one aspect of the technique on which there is disagreement. Cullen and Larson[3] advocate having the bevel down. They argue that there is less possibility of puncturing the vein wall furthermost from the skin and less likelihood of leakage from part of the bevel being out of the vein. Also, the bevel-down technique allows one to see the dimple produced in the vein ahead of the needle just before the needle enters the vein. Lastly, the bevel-down technique facilitates securing the needle flat against the skin, a procedure that Cullen and Larson[3] feel is advantageous. Despite these convincing reasons, many clinicians recommend keeping the bevel up until the vein has been punctured; this is my preference, because it facilitates entry into the vein. If the bevel-up technique is selected, the needle should be rotated 180° after the vein has been entered to lessen the chance of puncturing the vein wall that is furthermost from the skin. A common error of the novice is attempting to slide the catheter off the introducing needle prematurely. Too often, although the needle has penetrated the vein, the plastic catheter is still outside the vein. Therefore, if an extracath is used, the entire unit should be advanced into the vein a few millimeters before sliding the catheter off the introducing needle.

Probably the most common complication in using a plastic catheter is thrombophlebitis. My practice is to use 1 percent iodine or Betadine as an antiseptic. I then apply an antibiotic ointment to the insertion site and cover it with a small sterile dressing. Admittedly, the efficacy of each one of these maneuvers has not been established.

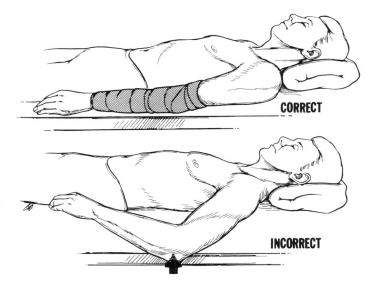

FIG. 12-1 If the arm is allowed to hang over the edge of the operating table in the supine position, an ulnar nerve neuropathy may result. (Stoelting RK, Miller RD: Basics of Anesthesia, New York, Churchill Livingstone, 1984.)

IS THE PATIENT IN A POSITION THAT WILL NOT CAUSE COMPLICATIONS?

Under anesthesia, the patient obviously does not know whether he is in a position that may lead to a peripheral neuropathy or pressure necrosis. Placing the patient in the position of surgery before anesthesia is induced will help identify areas of undue pressure. Frequently, however, the patient can be positioned only after anesthesia has been induced. Thus the anesthesiologist must be aware of

areas of the body that are especially vulnerable to injury. This usually occurs where nerves are in their long anatomic course and often superficially distributed.

SUPINE POSITION

Of 72 postoperative peripheral nerve complications, 33 occurred in the supine position. Of these, 14 involved the brachial plexus,[5] with

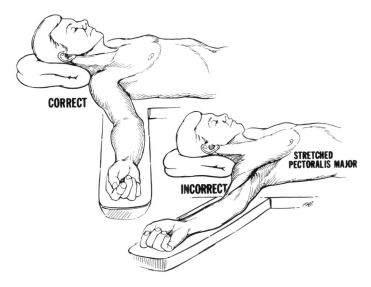

FIG. 12-2 When the arm is extended more than 90°, the brachial plexus may be injured. This possibility can be detected by palpation of the pectoralis major muscle. If the muscle is tense, it is likely that the brachial plexus is being unduly stretched. (Stoelting RK, Miller RD: Basics of Anesthesia. New York, Churchill Livingstone, 1984.)

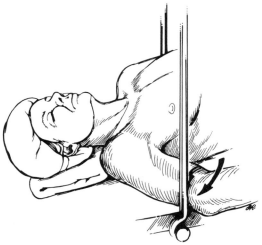

the ulnar nerve being the most common,[6] probably because of its superficial path along the median elbow. This injury can be prevented by proper padding and positioning (Fig. 12-1). If the arm is extended, then risk of brachial plexus injury develops; stretch to the brachial plexus should be avoided. A guide to follow is to palpate the tension of the pectoralis major muscle (Fig. 12-2). If it is relaxed, then tension on the brachial plexus is unlikely. Also, compression against a frame for surgical drapes can cause a radial neuropathy (Fig. 12-3).

PRONE POSITION

This position can result in several complications from pressure. The eye may be contused or penetrated from pressure with the face down. To ensure that pressure is not being applied to the eye, the bony orbit should be palpated. If the entire orbit can be easily palpated

FIG. 12-3 Compression of the arm against a frame for surgical drapes (ether screen) either in the supine or head-down position can cause compression and resultant neuropathy of the radial nerve. (Stoelting RK, Miller RD: Basics of Anesthesia. New York, Churchill Livingstone, 1984.)

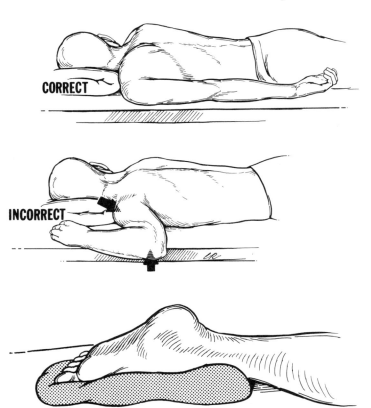

FIG. 12-4 Proper padding in the prone position can minimize damage to the brachial plexus, especially the ulnar nerve. (Stoelting RK, Miller RD: Basics of Anesthesia. New York, Churchill Livingstone, 1984.)

FIG. 12-5 Injury to the foot can be minimized by proper padding in the prone position. (Stoelting RK, Miller RD: Basics of Anesthesia. New York, Churchill Livingstone, 1984.)

FIG. 12-6 This position indicates the multiple problems that can occur with an improperly positioned patient in the flexed prone position. If excessively stretched, the brachial plexus can be damaged. The ulnar nerve can be damaged by inadequate padding of the elbow. Inadequate padding under the head can cause eye damage or undue pressure to the face or lower eyelid. Excessive compression to the inferior vena cava can be minimized by padding under the inferior iliac spine. (Stoelting RK, Miller RD: Basics of Anesthesia. New York, Churchill Livingstone, 1984.)

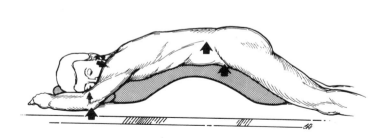

with no obstruction, then probably no undue pressure is being applied to the eye. The brachial plexus can be injured if it is stretched or by pressure from improperly placed support. The ulnar nerve is especially vulnerable when the elbow is placed against sharp edges of the table; flexion of the table makes the danger more likely (Fig. 12-4). Injury to the nerves and tendons of the dorsum of the foot may occur if the foot rests against the metal edge of the table; proper padding can prevent this complication (Fig. 12-5). The femoral cutaneous nerve of the thigh can be compressed against the supporting devices under the plexus, causing a syndrome called meralgia paresthetica. These are only a few of the many problems that can result from the prone position (Fig. 12-6). The reader is referred to an excellent chapter by Smith that deals with the problems associated with the prone position.[7]

LATERAL DECUBITUS POSITION

In this position, padding or pillows should be placed under the head (Fig. 12-7) and between the knees and elbows (Fig. 12-8). If the head is improperly supported (Fig. 12-7), compression to the dependent arm may occur and may impair neurovascular function to that extremity. The pillow between the knees and elbows will help distribute the weight of the upper extremity to the dependent extremity

more evenly. Lastly, the brachial plexus can be compressed if the body is pressing on the dependent axilla. A small roll under the upper chest and not the axilla will take the weight off the arm (Fig. 12-8).[8]

LITHOTOMY POSITION

Four nerves are most likely to be damaged in the lithotomy position.[9] The obturator nerve can be compressed by undue flexion of the

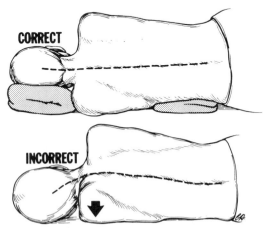

FIG. 12-7 Injury to the nondependent brachial plexus can be minimized by proper padding underneath the head. (Stoelting RK, Miller RD: Basics of Anesthesia. New York, Churchill Livingstone, 1984.)

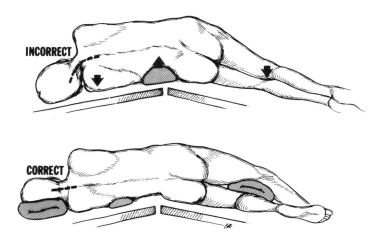

FIG. 12-8 In the lateral decubitus position, pillows between the legs and elbows help distribute the weight of the upper extremity to that of the lower extremity. (Stoelting RK, Miller RD: Basics of Anesthesia. New York, Churchill Livingstone, 1984.)

thigh to the groin. The saphenous nerve may be compressed against the medial aspect of the knee brace. The femoral nerve can be damaged by excessive angulation of the thigh with consequent compression to the nerve trunk. Lastly, the common peroneal nerve courses around the head of the fibula at the tibial condyles after penetrating various fascial planes; prolonged pressure at this point, by compression on the lateral aspect of the knee, can dam-

age this nerve. These neuropathies can be prevented by cushioning the ankle and the knee against pressure from the metal stirrup. Wrapping a towel around the knee and ankle is effective in attenuating pressure (Fig. 12-9). When the patient is being positioned, the legs should be elevated and flexed together. The thighs should be flexed no more than 90° before rotating the stirrups laterally.[9]

In summary, there obviously are many other less commonly used positions. The reader is referred to an excellent book edited by Martin[7-9] in which the various positions are discussed in detail. Most complications can be prevented by using good sense by which excessive pressure or angulation of the body is avoided.

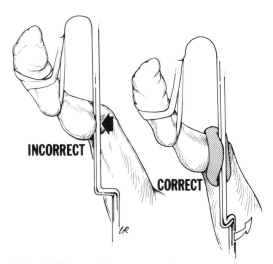

FIG. 12-9 In the lithotomy position, the saphenous nerve can be compressed by the stirrups used to elevate the legs when padding is inadequate (Stoelting RK, Miller RD: Basics of Anesthesia. New York, Churchill Livingstone, 1984, and adapted from Britt BA, Gordon RA: Peripheral nerve injuries associated with anaesthesia. Can Anaesth Soc J 11:514, 1964.)

PROBLEMS FROM AN ANESTHETIC MASK

Several problems can occur from improper application of an anesthetic mask, strap, or tracheal tube connector (Figs. 12-10 and 12-11). Necrosis to the bridge of the nose can be prevented by massage of the nose every 5 minutes or so. Compression to various nerves or the outer third of the eyebrow can be prevented by putting a soft pad underneath the mask strap.

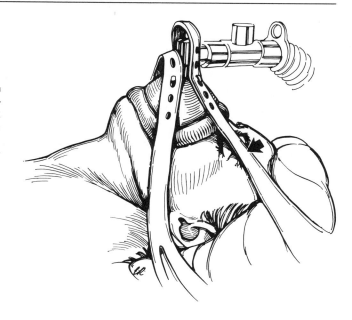

FIG. 12-10 Several complications can occur from excessive pressure with application of an anesthetic mask and mask strap. The outer third of the eyebrow can disappear with excessive compression from the strap. The buccal branch of the facial nerve can be injured from the mask strap, and also necrosis of the bridge of the nose can occur from excessive pressure by the anesthetic mask. (Stoelting RK, Miller RD: Basics of Anesthesia. New York, Churchill Livingstone, 1984.)

SUMMARY

To prepare the patient and operating room for a safe anesthetic, the following preanesthetic checklist is recommended (E. I. Eger II, personal communication).

Recommended Preanesthetic Checklist

A. Before first case of day
  1. Machine checkout (Table 12-2)
  2. Check and calibrate monitors
    a. Electrocardiogram
    b. Strain gauge
    c. Thermometers
    d. Other transducers
  3. Check emergency drug supply
    a. Lidocaine
    b. Bicarbonate

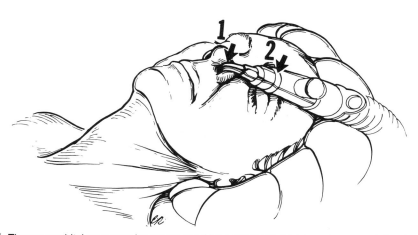

FIG. 12-11 The supraorbital nerve can be compressed by a tracheal tube connector, especially when padding is insufficient. Pressure on the nasal opening by the connector can result in tissue ischemia and damage. (Stoelting RK, Miller RD: Basics of Anesthesia. New York, Churchill Livingstone, 1984.)

c. Cardiotonics (isoproterenal, epinephrine, ephedrine, and other pressors)
d. Propranolol
e. Atropine

B. Before each case of day
1. Recheck machine for leaks
2. Set up intravenous and infusion devices
3. Check airways (oropharyngeal, nasopharyngeal, endotracheal, bite blocks)
4. Check laryngoscope (extra blade available)
5. Minimum drugs drawn up and labeled — thiopental, succinylcholine (vasopressor if regional technique)
6. Patient arrives: check
   a. Identification, consent
   b. NPO
   c. Permits
   d. Premedications and effect
   e. Special orders (steroids, diabetes, etc)
   f. Laboratory work not available previous evening
   g. Status of ordered blood
   h. Dentures
   i. Intravenous (contains additives?)
7. Attach to the patient:
   a. Blood pressure cuff and stethoscope
   b. Precordial stethoscope
   c. Other monitors
   d. Intravenous line
   e. Electrocardiogram
8. Check all monitors — record initial values
9. Position patient for induction of anesthesia
   a. Prevent nerve injury
   b. Use comfortable restraints as indicated

REFERENCES

1. Cooper JB, Newbower RS, Long CD, et al: Preventable anesthesia mishaps: A study of human factors. Anesthesiology 49:339, 1978
2. Feeley TW, Hedley-Whyte J: Bulk oxygen and nitrous oxide delivery systems: design and dangers. Anesthesiology 44:301, 1976
3. Cullen SC, Larson CP Jr: Essentials of Anesthetic Practice. Chicago, Yearbook Medical Publishers, 1974, pp 112–118
4. Friedman G, Cunningham MA: Preanesthetic checklists of equipment and drugs. Anesth Rev 10:44, 1979
5. Parks BJ: Postoperative peripheral neuropathies. Surgery 74:348, 1973
6. Miller RG, Camp PE: Postoperative ulnar neuropathy. JAMA 242:1636, 1979
7. Smith RH: The prone position, Positioning in Anesthesia and Surgery, Edited by Martin JT. Philadelphia, WB Saunders, 1978, pp 32–43
8. Thomas AN: The lateral decubitus position, Positioning in Anesthesia and Surgery. Edited by Martin JT. Philadelphia, WB Saunders, 1978, pp 116–124
9. Goldstein PJ: The lithotomy position, Positioning in Anesthesia and Surgery. Edited by Martin JT. Philadelphia, WB Saunders, 1978, pp 142–151

SECTION IV

PREPARATION OF THE PATIENT/USE OF ANESTHETIC AGENTS: INTRAOPERATIVE

13

Monitoring

Carl C. Hug, Jr., M.D., Ph.D.

INTRODUCTION

A definition of the verb *to monitor* is, "to watch, observe, or check, especially for a special purpose," and a definition of the noun *monitor* is, "that which warns or instructs." There are several important implications of both definitions: (1) a person is involved in establishing the process and in responding to its results; (2) mere data collection alone is insufficient, since rules and logic must accompany any data in order for it to warn; (3) a special purpose exists, that is, monitoring is focused on a specific objective and goes beyond the generalized, noncritical collection of data. It fits with the adage, "you see what you look for."

In the practice of anesthesiology, we have a special concern about monitoring. Ideally anesthesia is a totally reversible process. The patient's primary objective is to have an examination or surgical operation, not to have anes-

thesia for its own sake. This by no means diminishes the importance of the anesthesiologist; rather, his importance is all the greater because of the nature of the anesthetics. Not only are they potent drugs with potential for producing toxicity, but the anesthesiologist is more and more frequently called upon to administer them to critically ill patients with little capacity to tolerate any kind of stress. Beyond providing anesthesia, the anesthesiologist is responsible for the support of life itself during the procedure. It is no wonder, then, that the anesthesiologist is the monitor of drug effects and of vital functions intraoperatively and beyond, at least until the effects of anesthetic drugs and procedures are fully reversed. Although he uses monitoring devices to accomplish his objectives, the anesthesiologist is the monitor.

Because the modern anesthesiologist is faced with the challenges of potent drugs and of severe disease, a more sophisticated and precise evaluation of the status of the patient and responses to anesthetic drugs and surgery is required now than in the past. Monitoring devices have become correspondingly more complex and expensive in terms of money and, in some cases, in terms of risk to the patient. The anesthesiologist must therefore use carefully considered judgment in deciding which monitoring techniques are to be used in each patient.

Monitoring of patients during anesthesia and surgery has three important objectives: diagnosis of a problem or early recognition of a deleterious trend; estimation of the severity of the situation; and evaluation of the response to therapy, including both its effectiveness and side effects or toxicity. Monitoring can be performed at several levels:

Routine monitoring, applicable to all patients regardless of their pathophysiologic status;

Specialized monitoring for a particular pathologic problem (e.g., serum glucose determinations in the diabetic patient) or for the use of a specialized technique (e.g., controlled hypotension);

Extensive monitoring of all major systems in the critically ill patient and in those undergoing extensive operations potentially affecting all organ and tissue functions (e.g., cardiac surgery with cardiopulmonary bypass).

SCOPE OF THE CHAPTER

This chapter surveys monitoring techniques that are or potentially will become useful in the anesthetic management of adult patients undergoing surgery. Emphasis is placed on monitoring of the CNS, ventilation, hemodynamics, and body temperature, which are important in every case. The reader is referred to other chapters for discussions of the monitoring of blood volume (Chs. 38 & 39), coagulation (Ch. 39), hepatic and renal function (Chs. 34 & 35), and neuromuscular transmission (Ch. 26); and since monitoring techniques have become specialized just as the practice of anesthesiology has, the reader should consult the chapters dealing with pediatric (Ch. 49) and ob-

stetric (Ch. 47) patients and with anesthesia for neurologic (Ch. 43) and cardiac (Ch. 41) surgery.

A number of reviews on the subject of monitoring surgical patients in the operating room and intensive care unit (ICU) have been published in recent years.[1-5] They clearly indicate the evolution of and potential for new developments in the monitoring of patients by anesthesiologists.

ROUTINE MONITORING

Basic monitoring of the patient under anesthesia is an extension of the basic elements of physical diagnosis, including inspection, palpation, percussion, and auscultation (Table 13-1). Some of the individual items provide information about the function of several organ systems. For example, normal skin color is indicative of normal circulation, ventilation, and body temperature. If the skin color is abnormal, problems may exist in one or more organ systems, and further investigation is necessary to diagnose the cause or causes.

This level of monitoring may seem simple and obvious, and its value may be overlooked in this highly technical age to the detriment of the patient. The value of physical diagnosis lies in its use to corroborate data, especially that which is unexpected, from monitoring devices; as a backup measure when the devices fail; and to extend the usefulness of some monitoring devices. For example (1) a sphygmomanometer can be used in conjunction with direct arterial blood pressure monitoring to verify the accuracy of systolic pressure measurements by the transducer system; (2) palpation of a full and regular pulse indicates that the fibrillation-like pattern in the electrocardiogram (ECG) is an artifact; and (3) the use of an esophageal stethoscope in combination with central venous pressure (CVP) monitoring can detect signs of fluid overload and heart failure; auscultation of

TABLE 13-1. **Physical Diagnosis in Monitoring of Anesthetized Patients**

Inspection
  Skin — color, capillary refill, rash, edema, hematoma
  Nail beds — color, capillary refill
  Mucous membrane — color, moisture, edema
  Surgical field — color of tissues and blood, rate of blood loss, muscular relaxation
  Blood loss — surgical drapes, gowns, sponges, suction bottles
  Position — potential for trauma (joints, nerves, circulation)
  Movement — purposeful or reflex (nonparalyzed patient), ventilation
  Eyes — conjunctiva (color, edema), pupils (size, direct and consensual reactivity, change with noxious stimulation)

Palpation
  Skin — temperature, texture (e.g., papular rash), edema, hematoma, subcutaneous emphysema (crepitation)
  Pulses — fullness, rate, and rhythm
  Muscle tone

Percussion
  Urinary bladder distention — urine
  Gastric distention — air
  Pneumothorax

Auscultation
  Ventilation — breath sounds (normal, pathologic, absent; distribution over lung fields); proper placement of endotracheal tube.
  Heart sounds — rate, rhythm, extrasounds, murmurs
  Blood pressure — sphygmomanometry
  Location of nasogastric tube — injection or aspiration of gastric air

abnormal breath (rales) and heart sounds (S_3) will herald the development of left heart failure even if the CVP remains within normal limits.

Routine monitoring of the anesthetized patient involves the physical diagnostic items listed in Table 13-1, including the use of a precordial or esophageal stethoscope to listen to breath and heart sounds continuously and a sphygmomanometer to measure blood pressure regularly. In addition, many anesthesiologists routinely monitor the ECG and body temperature because the risks and costs of doing so are minimal and the potential benefits are substantial. The frequency of dysrhythmias under anesthesia is considerable, and it is necessary to distinguish innocuous premature beats and dysrhythmias from those that are, or that may progress to, a life-threatening type. Also, the high incidence of coronary artery disease in the adult patient population makes it worthwhile to be on the lookout for ECG signs of myocardial ischemia in the anesthetized patient, who is unable to complain of angina pectoris. Changes in body temperature are common during anesthesia and surgery and can affect organ function as well as the interpretation of certain monitoring data (e.g., blood-gas values). Malignant hyperpyrexia is a life-threatening consequence of anesthesia. Consequently, the routine monitoring of body temperature is not only justified but is considered mandatory by many anesthesiologists.

A peripheral nerve stimulator to determine the degree of neuromuscular junction blockade is used routinely by many anesthesiologists in any patient who receives a muscle relaxant. Some anesthesiologists consider the routine use of a ventilator–anesthetic circuit–patient disconnect alarm system essential in patients whose ventilation is supported mechanically in the operating room. Monitoring of the oxygen concentration in the inspired gas mixture and of anesthetic contamination of the operating room is routinely done under the direction of the anesthesiologists in some hospitals.

There are reasons to go beyond the routine monitoring described above, even in fairly healthy patients undergoing common types of anesthesia and surgery. It may be worthwhile to verify the adequacy of ventilation by analysis of arterial blood gases. If a particular item is needed for one purpose, why not take advantage of it for monitoring purposes? For example, one can measure urine flow if an indwelling urinary catheter is used, measure CVP if an external jugular vein is to be cannulated, and measure arterial blood pressure directly if an arterial cannula is inserted for blood-gas analysis.

Specialized monitoring techniques may be indicated for rapid detection of trends, precision of measurement, specific diagnosis of abnormalities that exist or are likely to develop, and to free the hands of the anesthesiologist for other tasks. The methods most frequently used by the anesthesiologist are discussed below and in other chapters of this book.

MONITORING PATIENT SAFETY

Ensuring patient safety and comfort should be considered as part of the routine monitoring of all patients undergoing anesthesia. Mechanisms of self-protection, including warning signs (e.g., pain) and escape or withdrawal movements, are lost with the induction of anesthesia. The anesthesiologist and others caring for the patient in this vulnerable state must act on the patient's behalf to prevent in-

jury. The first step is to remain keenly aware of the potential for harm, the second is to recognize the body areas most susceptible to injury, and the third is to monitor these sites for breakdown of protection and early signs of injury.

The areas of particular concern are listed in Table 13-2. Some suggestions for protection follow.

POSITIONING

It is important to have the patient assume a position as close as possible to that required for surgery (also see Ch. 12). Protective padding should be applied to vulnerable sites at risk of injury due to pressure and other factors. When moving the head and extremities of an anesthetized patient, the usual direction and range of motion for that particular patient should be followed, without forcing any movement (e.g., arthritic joints).

Monitoring devices and connecting lines should be arranged in anticipation of positional changes that will be made later in the procedure; this is done to minimize the difficulties of moving the patient, to avoid accidental disruption or distortion of monitoring, and to prevent complications related to dislodgment of cannulae and other devices from the patient.

TABLE 13-2.   Body Sites Especially Vulnerable to Injury in the Anesthetized Patient

Region	Part	Consequences
Head	Eyes	Corneal abrasion; retinal damage by pressure on globe (especially with glaucoma)
	Ears	Tympanic membrane perforation by foreign objects; cauliflower ear from folding the pinna
Airway	Lips and tongue	Lacerations and bruising from teeth, airway devices, and instruments
	Teeth	Cracking, chipping, dislodgment by airway devices
	Pharynx	Silent aspiration of stomach contents, teeth, and other objects loose in the pharynx; causes of airway obstruction
Neck	Vasculature	Impairment of cerebral blood flow by rotation of the neck
	Brachial plexus	Neuropathy from stretching of plexus by neck rotation and arm abduction
Extremities	Nerves	Pressure on ulnar nerve at elbow (olecranon fossa), peroneal nerve lateral to the fibula
	Joints	Overextension, especially of arthritic joints
	Vasculature	Distal ischemia and edema from circulatory occlusion
Skin		Burns from antiseptic solutions, warming blankets, electrocautery, improper grounding of electrical equipment

EYES

The eyes must be protected from corneal abrasion, pressure, and other injuries. Eyelids should be taped securely in the closed position without the tape exerting pressure on the cornea. The method of taping should permit its periodic removal and examination of the pupils and conjunctiva. If the head is covered under surgical drapes, the anesthesiologist should monitor the actions of others to avoid any pressure being exerted on the eyes or any part of the face (e.g., by the surgeon's elbow, instruments).

INFECTION

The anesthesiologist and others should be alert to any breakdown in sterile technique that may lead to the introduction of infectious organisms through percutaneous vascular cannulation sites, urinary bladder catheter, airway, or surgical wound.

MEDICATION AND BLOOD ADMINISTRATION ERRORS

Obviously, labels should be read carefully. When practical, drugs packaged in containers that are distinctively shaped and labeled should be chosen over those that closely resemble one another.

ELECTRICAL BURNS

An alarm mechanism, preferably both audible and visible, should be incorporated into the electrical cautery unit to indicate the lack of appropriate grounding of the patient. The cause triggering any electrical malfunction alarm in the operating room or piece of equipment should be identified.

OTHER SOURCES OF INJURY

Any small or dangerous objects should not be left lying loosely around the patient (e.g., needles, bottle caps). Proper procedures including the use of restraints should be employed to prevent self-inflicted injuries by the deleterious, semicomatose patient. Bed rails and safety straps should be used even for the fully conscious patient, who should never be left unattended or unobserved in the operating or recovery rooms.

DEPTH OF ANESTHESIA
(Also See Ch. 17)

The anesthesiologist's goals are the patient's comfort and facilitation of the surgeon's work. In terms of the patient's comfort, the most important goals are prevention of pain and reduction of anxiety. The surgeon's work is facilitated by proper positioning of the patient and, in the case of abdominal and certain orthopedic operations, relaxation of skeletal muscle may be needed to permit good exposure of the surgical field. Of course, sudden and unexpected movement of the patient in response to noxious stimuli is undesirable from all points of view: the patient may be injured, the surgeon's work may be impeded, and the anesthesiologist may be embarrassed by the apparent failure to have the patient anesthetized and under control. Satisfying all concerned presents the anesthesiologist with a considerable challenge, which is made all the more difficult in the sick patient with limited physiologic reserves and for whom the maintenance of vital functions in a stable state close to normal is considered to be desirable. For the ensuing discussion, it is useful to bear in mind the discrete objectives of anesthesia: analgesia, relief of anxiety, amnesia or unconsciousness; muscular relaxation; suppression of somatic, autonomic, and endocrine reflex responses to noxious stimuli; and hemodynamic stability.

Regional anesthesia can be used to provide analgesia, muscular relaxation, and reflex suppression. Cardiovascular changes may contraindicate its use in some situations, but measures can be taken to prevent deleterious effects in many patients. Anxiety can be prevented or controlled by (1) discussing the circumstances with the patient preoperatively, (2) comforting and reassuring the patient intraoperatively, and, if necessary, (3) administering sedative (anxiolytic) and hypnotic drugs before or during the operation. Even though patients are awake during operations under regional anesthesia and can recall intraoperative events, they are usually satisfied as long as they do not experience pain or other discomforts (e.g., lengthy maintenance of the same position, urinary bladder distention, unpleasant environmental conditions). The awake or easily arousable patient can tell the anesthesiologist about his discomforts and can also provide useful information about the general well being of his vital organ systems.

The goal of general anesthesia is to render the patient unconscious thereby preventing pain, anxiety, and recall of intraoperative events. Potent inhaled anesthetics (e.g., halothane) readily produce unconsciousness and high concentrations can be used to produce muscular relaxation and reflex suppression, providing depression of the cardiovascular system and other side effects of the agent are not detrimental to the patient. Narcotic analgesics alone (in very high doses) or in combination with intravenous hypnotics or low concentrations of inhaled anesthetics can produce unconsciousness and reflex suppression, but they do not produce skeletal muscle relaxation (and may produce muscular rigidity). Thus, it is a common practice, although not always necessary, to administer skeletal muscle relaxants during general anesthesia. Relaxants eliminate the need for high concentrations of potent inhaled anesthetics, eliminate rigidity and facilitate artificial ventilation in the apneic, narcotized patient, and make the anesthetic appear to be successful to observers. It is difficult to differentiate between general anesthesia and paralysis. Herein lies a problem. How will the anesthesiologist know whether the patient becomes aroused by noxious surgical stimuli and is aware of intraoperative events? Before attempting to suggest a solution to this dilemma, several important points should be noted.

1. Complete muscular paralysis is seldom necessary, and the peripheral nerve stimulator can be used to titrate relaxant drug dosage to the desired degree of incomplete paralysis. Moreover, the desirable intensity of relaxation does not remain constant throughout the operation. Advantage can be taken of periods when paralysis is unnecessary to evaluate the depth (adequacy) of general anesthesia by allowing muscle relaxant effects to wear off and by observing the patient for responses to commands and to noxious stimulation. The anesthesiologist has to educate the surgeon and other members of the team about the reasons for doing this. Patient movements can be a disconcerting experience for the uninformed.

2. General anesthesia represents a balance between CNS depression by drugs and CNS arousal by noxious stimuli. The intensity of stimulation varies during the operation. Tracheal intubation, airway manipulation, skin incision and suturing, electrocauterization, periostial scraping, and bone sawing are examples of relatively intense stimuli, and in some cases are very transient.

3. The dose–response relationships are quantitatively different for different effects of the same drug in the same patient. Thus, a given dose or concentration of the drug may produce relatively more depression of the heart than of the nervous system, or vice versa. Under general anesthesia some patients react to surgical stimulation primarily by moving or grimacing (when not paralyzed). Others do not show these somatic responses, but their heart rate and blood pressure increase, and still others show only a few sympathetic signs (e.g., tearing, sweating). Many patients exhibit all these signs, including somatic, hemodynamic, and sympathetic; but others do not.[7,8] It is not uncommon to observe a patient open his/her eyes in response to command or to a noxious stimulus and maintain an absolutely stable blood pressure and heart rate within his/her usual and normal range.[9]

4. Patients differ in their sensitivities to anesthetic drugs and to noxious stimuli. The range of anesthetic doses and concentrations

required for adequate levels of anesthesia are relatively broad. Therefore, a dose or concentration that provides just an adequate depth of anesthesia for one patient under one set of circumstances is inadequate in other circumstances or in other patients, and it may represent an unnecessarily excessive dose in still other patients and under other conditions.[10-14]

5. The narcotic analgesics are capable of producing profound analgesia without inducing unconsciousness. When very large doses induce unconsciousness, it is not uncommon for the patient to exhibit a startle response and to arouse suddenly in response to stimulation during the recovery period. No one has described a means of recognizing the patient's susceptibility to arousal in advance. It is difficult to control the patient's thrashing about, often with elevations of heart rate and blood pressure, especially if the stimulation continues. If the stimulation is stopped, the patient often dozes off and remains quiet until stimulated again, and the arousal response is repeated. Obviously, the paralyzed patient does not exhibit somatic arousal responses.

6. The intensity of anesthetic drug effect is proportional to its concentration or partial pressure (inhaled anesthetics) at its sites of action in the CNS.[10-15] The pharmacokinetics of inhaled and intravenous anesthetics are such that their levels in the CNS (and blood) vary widely and continuously unless they are administered continuously at a rate equaling their distribution in and elimination from the body. The actual measurement of anesthetic concentrations or partial pressures in the operating room is becoming practical (i.e., infrared and mass spectroscopy). Such measurements are certainly useful in verifying correct function of the anesthesia delivery system (vaporizer, infusion pump) and in identifying the patient with pharmacokinetic abnormalities. However, there is a considerable range of variation in response to a given drug concentration among patients and in any one patient under different conditions (e.g., variable stimulus intensity). Therefore, the achievement of a concentration effect in 95 percent of patients (EC95) does not guarantee that some patients (5 percent) will be adequately anesthetized, and the EC95 represents an overdose (an excessive concentration) for most patients.

7. The consequences of inadequate analgesia are obvious.[16-18] The implications of the patient's awareness of intraoperative events in the absence of pain are not so clear.[18,19] First, the patient given a regional anesthetic is aware of events; some become quite anxious unless drugs or reassurance are provided. In addition, the patient under regional anesthesia remains able to express himself. By contrast, the patient under general anesthesia expects to be unconscious and, if he finds himself awake during the operation, it is likely that (1) he will assume something is going wrong and become anxious, (2) he will expect to experience pain and other frightening consequences, and (3) he will feel trapped and unable to escape or to express his fear, especially if paralyzed and intubated. The recall of such unexpected and frightening circumstances has longer-term psychological implications for the patient and some practical consequences for the physicians (e.g., professional embarrassment, charges of malpractice). The prior administration of an amnesic drug may prevent the patient's recall, but it may not alleviate, and may actually exacerbate, the psychological consequences.[19]

Given these observations, the anesthesiologist can choose between two basic approaches to minimizing the risk of arousal or awakening intraoperatively. First, the dose or concentration of the anesthetic drug can be maintained at a level sufficiently high to render virtually all patients unconscious (MAC × 1.3 = ED99). This has the disadvantage of overdosing almost every patient, of producing adverse anesthetic side effects, and of greatly extending the time to recovery. Alternatively, the anesthesiologist can hone his clinical skills to provide satisfactory anesthesia with minimal doses of muscle relaxants used only when they are necessary. Preserving as much neuromuscular function as possible will allow him to detect somatic as well as other signs of inadequate general anesthesia and to titrate anesthetic drug dosages against the patient's responses to graded degrees of noxious stimulation.

If the anesthesiologist cannot be certain that the patient is unconscious, he should assume that the patient is arousable or awake and should treat the patient accordingly, much as he would during regional anesthesia. That is, minimize extraneous noise and unpleasant environmental conditions and offer reassuring words of comfort to the patient. The use of amnesic drugs is questionable.[19]

One or more methods of detecting arousal and awareness in the paralyzed patient should be developed. One prospect currently receiving renewed attention is the electroencephalogram, especially in a computer-processed form that is both convenient and practical.

ELECTROENCEPHALOGRAPHY[20-23]

The most direct monitor of CNS function in the anesthetized or comatose patient is the electroencephalogram (EEG). Depending on the number and location of the electrodes, it can provide an overview of CNS electrical activity and it can be used to detect relatively localized changes in CNS function. The anesthesiologist is interested in the EEG for two purposes: to measure anesthetic depth and to detect CNS hypoxia.

Measurements of anesthetic depth would be most useful in paralyzed patients (see above) and in patients receiving anesthetic drugs to suppress electrical (cerebral metabolic) activity for CNS protection or resuscitation (also see Ch. 61). In the latter circumstances, EEG monitoring is essential to assure attainment of the desired isoelectric end point without using excessive doses of the anesthetic drug with its attendant cardiovascular depression and other toxicities.

In the usual circumstances of general anesthesia for surgical operations and other procedures, the usefulness of the EEG as a monitor of anesthetic depth has been limited for several reasons. Each anesthetic drug and each combination of CNS drugs (i.e., sedatives, hypnotics, analgesics, anesthetics, and some autonomic drugs) produce somewhat different EEG patterns as the doses are changed.[22,24,25] This certainly makes EEG interpretation difficult under most anesthetic conditions. When anesthesia is produced by a single drug, the change

in EEG patterns may be a useful guide to anesthetic depth providing other factors affecting the EEG are kept constant (Table 13-3). The standard EEG recording techniques used by neurologists are not practical for monitoring anesthetic depth in the operating room. Investigators and manufacturers are seeking to make EEG monitoring practical for the anesthesiologist by computer processing of the signal in order to provide a simplified presentation of data that can be interpreted rapidly, is easily quantitated, allows trend analysis, and can be permanently recorded on paper. Although several devices incorporating these characteristics are commercially available or in clinical trials, their usefulness as monitors of anesthetic depth has yet to be established.

Global or diffuse cerebral ischemia as a consequence of severe systemic hypotension or hypoxemia is manifest on any and all scalp leads by slowing of the EEG (i.e., diminished high frequency and increased low-frequency activity). As the ischemia continues, the low-frequency activity progressively decreases to burst suppression (transient, intermittent isoelectric pattern) and then to a continuous isoelectric state. The magnitude of change in EEG amplitude or frequency does not necessarily indicate the severity of the ischemia nor correlate with the degree of irreversibility of neuronal dysfunction. The duration of the ischemic episode does have a bearing on the outcome.[26] For example, incomplete focal ischemia during carotid endarterectomy that persists for more than 10 minutes is associated with the accumulation of serious neurologic deficiencies. Ischemic episodes of less than 10 minutes are usually followed by rapid normalization of the EEG as the hypoxemia and hypotension are corrected and there are no serious (obvious) neurologic sequelae.[27] There is uncertainty about the possibility of subtle neurologic deficits (e.g., memory loss, mood alteration) following brief ischemic episodes. Monitoring the EEG for signs of global ischemia is appropriate in patients undergoing cardiac surgery and extracorporeal circulation (also see Ch. 41), who are subjected to deliberate hypotension (also see Ch. 55), or who are otherwise at risk of sudden reductions of cerebral blood flow (CBF) or hypoxemia.[28-30]

It is more difficult to detect localized cere-

TABLE 13-3. Factors Altering the Electroencephalogram

Anesthetic and premedicant drugs
Different EEG patterns for different drugs, even within the same pharmacologic class; activation and suppression of EEG activity can occur at different doses of the same drug.

Sensory stimulation
Stimulates the ascending reticular activating system and increases EEG activity; the EEG pattern reflects the net effect of sensory stimulation and anesthesia.

Oxygenation of CNS tissue
Determined by both oxygen content of blood and cerebral perfusion rate; hypoxia may initially produce EEG activation through peripheral chemoreceptor activation of the ascending reticular activating system; persistent hypoxia will lead first to EEG slowing and then to an isoelectric EEG.

Carbon dioxide
Mild hypercarbia activates the EEG through stimulation of the ascending reticular activating system; marked hypercarbia causes narcosis and EEG slowing.

Body temperature
Progressively greater degrees of hypothermia produce progressive EEG slowing.

Serum glucose
Hypoglycemia produces coma and EEG slowing due to inadequate substrate availability for metabolic energy production; hyperglycemia (>600 mg/dl) produces hyperosmolar coma and EEG slowing due to brain dehydration.

Electrolytes
Hyponatremia (<120 mEq/L) results in progressive obtundation and EEG slowing; hypernatremia (>150 mEq/L) produces hyperosmolar coma.

Convulsions
Variable EEG patterns depending on the factor precipitating convulsions; seizures are followed by postictal depression characterized by reduced EEG activity.

bral ischemia, which is to be expected in patients with cerebrovascular disease, arterial embolic obstructions, or discrete intracranial pathology. In such cases, the EEG changes indicative of ischemia will be evident only if the scalp leads are in a position, to "see" the electrical changes and the recording technique is appropriate to detect the change. Obviously the changes will be more evident the nearer the electrode is to the site of ischemia. If the recording technique amplifies the difference between two leads, only one of which is over an ischemic area, EEG slowing may not be evident in the tracing, which represents the difference in electrical activity detected by the two leads.[21] One means of increasing the chance of detecting signs of ischemia is to monitor the EEG bilaterally and to look for hemispheric differences in the EEG patterns. This is particularly appropriate for the patient with evidence of a unilateral carotid arterial obstruction. During carotid endarterectomy, ipsilateral slowing of the EEG at the time of arterial clamping is indicative of the need for a shunt; the contralateral EEG should remain unchanged and reflect the anesthetized ("control") state.[31]

The technical details of EEG monitoring are crucial to the recording of reliable data.[21] The EEG signal is of very low energy (10 to 100 μV) compared with other electrical potentials (e.g., ECG 500 to 1,000 mV, electrical equipment 120 V). From a practical viewpoint, it is necessary (1) to establish good electrode contact (i.e., minimum impedance) with the patient's scalp, and (2) to minimize extraneous electrical interference or to compensate for its presence.

To keep impedance at a minimum, the following steps are recommended: (1) Degrease and abrade the scalp in a relatively hairless area (forehead and behind the ear over the mastoid process); (2) apply silver disc electrodes filled with conductive paste to the prepared scalp areas and use collodion to fix them in place; (3) measure the impedance (should be a built-in feature of the EEG recording device) to determine that it is less than 5,000 to 10,000 Ω (varies depending on the amplifier) and that it is equivalent for the individual electrodes; and (4) make sure that the EEG amplifying and recording device have a signal to warn of increased impedance—the operator should intermittently verify that it is satisfactory during the period of monitoring.

Platinum or gold needles have been used as electrodes, especially if it is necessary to sterilize them and include the EEG lead site within the surgical field. Except for this situation, they are inferior to the silver discs because needles may produce discomfort in the awake patient, are less easily stabilized to avoid motion artifacts, have a small surface area (higher impedance), and can produce hematoma, edema, and infection, all of which result in variable increases in impedance.

In order to record the EEG with the highest fidelity, it is necessary to screen out all other electrical activity in the environment. This is possible in a research laboratory but impractical in a modern operating room. Consequently, equipment manufacturers build in filters to reduce or eliminate electrical frequencies below 0.5 Hz and above 35 Hz. The loss of fidelity that results is not significant for routine EEG monitoring. The usual EEG frequency ranges ($\delta < 4$ Hz, θ 4 to 7 Hz, α 8 to 13 Hz, $\beta > 13$ Hz) are seldom meaningful in the anesthetized patient in whom there is a continuum of rapidly shifting frequencies. Rather, the patterns may be defined as "activated," characterized by low voltage and high frequencies; "depressed," high voltage and low frequency; or "isoelectric," which occurs with ischemia, hypothermia, barbiturate coma, 2+ MAC isoflurane anesthesia, or death. Thus, even dramatic changes in the EEG do not necessarily indicate CNS ischemia. Very often it is the change in amplitude and frequency over time or in association with some event that signals a significant change in cerebral function and well-being.

The differential amplifier is another device that is included in EEG machines. Since much electrical artifact (especially 60-Hz current) is detected by all scalp leads, it can be removed by measuring the difference in potential between two "active" scalp electrodes that are each referenced to a neutral third electrode. The differential amplifier subtracts the electrical frequencies that are common between the active and neutral electrodes leaving the difference in electrical potential between the two "active" electrodes to be amplified. Typically, the neutral electrode is placed in the midline on the forehead, one of the active elec-

trodes is placed on the forehead over the eye, and the other active electrode is placed behind the ipsilateral ear over the mastoid process. This arrangement records a unilateral (single-hemisphere) EEG. Another pair of active electrodes can be placed in the corresponding contralateral positions and referenced to the same neutral electrode to monitor the other hemisphere (i.e., for bilateral EEG monitoring). Bilateral EEG monitoring is most useful in detecting the subtle changes in cerebral electrical activity associated with modest reduction in cerebral blood flow to one hemisphere (e.g., crimping of a carotid artery shunt during endarterectomy).[31] Alternatively, as a monitor of global function, one pair of active electrodes can be placed contralaterally opposite each other to record potential differences between the two cerebral hemispheres.

Various types of computer processing and displays of the EEG are being investigated for their applicability to the operating room setting.[20,21] Such processing is designed to reject artifacts, provide quantitative data, permit continuous monitoring with easy recognition of trends, provide a permanent compact record, and eliminate the bulkiness and complexity of the standard EEG machine that spews out 300 pages of recording paper hourly. The reader is referred to the manufacturers' representatives and to other sources for descriptions of specific devices, all of which present over time some representation of the frequency and amplitude of cerebral electrical activity.

In *period analysis* of the EEG, the frequency of some change in amplitude (e.g., change in polarity) is presented as a function of time. As the EEG slows, this frequency of change decreases.

In *aperiodic analysis*, each waveform is analyzed; it is not an averaging technique. The power (amplitude) present at each frequency is displayed over time. The information is presented as a three-dimensional display showing all three axes of power (amplitude) vs frequency vs time (Fig. 13-1A). This technique was developed by Demetrescu and is commercially available (Lifescan EEG, Neurometrics, Inc.).

In *power spectrum analysis*, the computer performs a Fourier analysis, actually a fast-

Fourier transformation, to convert the complex and irregular EEG signal to equivalent sine waves of known frequencies and amplitudes. This information can be presented in one of two ways. One method involves a three-dimensional display of the power spectrum in which time and amplitude are compressed on the same vertical axis—compressed spectral array (CSA, Fig. 13-1B)—with the disadvantages of the loss of some amplitude data and difficulties in evaluating temporal relationships of the data to events. The CSA format is available commercially as the Neurotrac (by Interspec). Alternatively, a two-dimensional display with frequency vs time is displayed in the form of a dot matrix, in which amplitude is represented as the intensity of shading or dot size—density-modulated spectral array (DSA, Fig. 13-1C). Because the display is two-dimensional, the DSA can be printed on a recorder along with blood pressure, ECG, and other information, thereby facilitating correlations of physiologic data and permitting trend analysis.

The anesthesiologist is most interested in rather large shifts in EEG frequency and amplitude (power). As anesthesia deepens or ischemia occurs, there is a loss of amplitude or power at the higher frequencies, and most of the total power remaining in the EEG is concentrated at lower frequencies. A convenient way to express power shifts of this type is to identify the highest frequency containing any power. Some have attempted to eliminate very small high-frequency activity (which often represents random noise) by identifying the frequency below which a certain percentage of the total power is present. For example, the spectral edge frequency (SEF) is the frequency below which 95 percent of the EEG power is located.[32] One commercially available device, the Neurotrac, shows the SEF on the CSA display (Fig. 13-1B). Decreases in cerebral blood flow or increases in anesthetic depth with certain drugs (e.g., narcotic anesthetics) are represented by a shift of the SEF to the left (i.e., to a slower frequency). There are clearly limitations in attempting to describe the EEG and all the variables it represents by a single number.[33]

Another commercial device, the cerebral function monitor (CFM), filters out low (< 2 Hz) and high (> 15 Hz) frequency activity and plots a product of rectified power and frequency against time. Severe cerebral ischemia is evident as a marked reduction in the frequency-power product. The device has not been demonstrated to be useful as a monitor of anesthetic depth for any single drug, or combination of drugs, and the data it presents cannot be correlated with a standard EEG. The power spectrum analyzer (PSA) is another device similar to the CFM and should not be confused with either CSA or DSA. The utility of the CFM and PSA for the anesthesiologist's purposes remains to be demonstrated.

Another attempt to monitor CNS functional integrity in the unconscious or anesthetized patient is the use of evoked potentials.[21,34] Various types of stimuli (e.g., visual, auditory, discrete somatosensory) produce an electrical response in the corresponding areas of the cerebral cortex. The primary response reflecting activity evoked by transmission of the sensory impulse to the specific sensory area occurs with a specific latency (approximately 15 msec) followed by nonspecific secondary waves lasting up to 100 msec and representing electrical activity in sensory association sites and in other areas of the CNS. The prolongation of latency or the disappearance of the early specific wave correlates well with focal neuropathology along the neural transmission route. This technique has been applied to detect functional impairment in the sensory system related to surgical maneuvers (e.g., compression of the spinal cord during operations on the spine). The primary wave is minimally affected by general anesthetic drugs, which do modify the later nonspecific waves. The applications and limitations of evoked potential techniques for the monitoring of anesthetic depth or for the detection of CNS hypoxia have not been explored fully[35] (also see Chs. 36, 43, & 44).

Methods for measuring CBF and intracranial pressure are presented in Chapters 36 and 43. Their monitoring applications are primarily in the anesthetic management and critical care of patients with intracranial neuropathology. The measurement of CBF during carotid endarterectomy (also see Ch. 44) is done in relatively few university medical centers. The direct measurement of blood flow through an exposed carotid artery shunt is possible but its

10:44:07   100uVOLTS

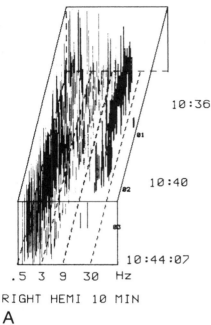

10:36

10:40

10:44:07

.5 3 9 30 Hz

RIGHT HEMI 10 MIN

A

FIG. 13-1 Examples of EEG data presentation by three methods. (A) Aperiodic analysis (Neurometrics, Lifescan). The height of each vertical line represents amplitude, and the maximum amplitude is set at 100 microvolts (vertical axis or vertical height of the box image). The location of each vertical line on the floor of the box corresponds to frequency (Hz on horizontal axis) and to time (shown along right hand side of box as 10:36, 10:40, 10:40:07). The recording is from a 66-year-old female patient (60 kg) who had been premedicated with diazepam and morphine approximately 30 minutes earlier. At 10:38 (even marker "01" on the recording) she received 40 μg sufentanil (0.7 μg/kg). Just after 10:40 ("02"), she became unresponsive and apneic, ventilation by mask was begun, and the blood pressure declined from 170/90 to 80/60 mm Hg. The trachea was intubated at approximately 10:42 ("03") and the blood pressure returned to 170/85 mm Hg. Notice that there was a sudden loss of high frequency activity and an increase in low frequency activity with the onset of unconsciousness (and hypotension). These EEG changes persisted beyond the restoration of blood pressure and are typical of the EEG changes seen with the induction of narcotic anesthesia. (B) Compressed spectral array (CSA) and spectral edge frequency (SEF) recording from the Neurotrak EEG analyser. A left carotid endarterectomy was being performed with a shunt in place during isoflurane-fentanyl anesthesia. At "08" the left carotid artery was clamped and the shunt removed while the systemic blood pressure remained unchanged at 150/70 mm Hg. AT the "X" the external carotid artery was unclamped, and at "y" the internal carotid artery was unclamped with almost immediate restoration of EEG activity and return of the SEF to the previous level.

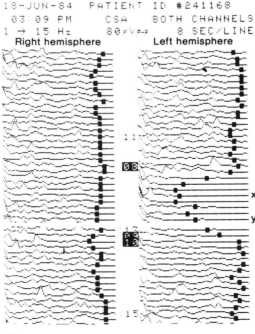

18-JUN-84   PATIENT ID #241168
03:09 PM   CSA   BOTH CHANNELS
1 → 15 Hz   80uVp-p   8 SEC/LINE
Right hemisphere   **Left hemisphere**

B

Power Spectrum vs. Spectral Edge

FIG. 13-1 (continued) (C) Density-modulated spectral array (DSA) and spectral edge frequency (SEF) recorded during the induction of enflurane anesthesia in an unpremedicated patient. The amplitude of a low frequency band gradually decreased from A to B at which point tracheal intubation occurred and the low frequency activity terminated abruptly. A higher frequency band decreased in frequency and increased in amplitude from A to B. The SEF remained almost constant. (Levy WJ: Intraoperative EEG patterns: implications for EEG monitoring. Anesthesiology 60:430, 1984).

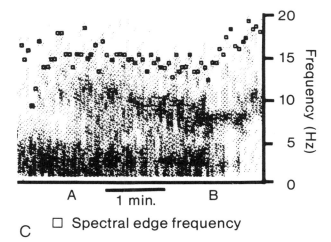

C □ Spectral edge frequency

importance as a routine monitoring technique in carotid artery surgery remains to be determined.[36]

VENTILATION

Ventilation is a vital function that is altered to some degree by all anesthetic techniques and by many surgical procedures (also see Chs. 21 & 32). Patients requiring surgery may have pulmonary disease, and this may increase the difficulty of achieving satisfactory ventilation during and after anesthesia and surgery. The anesthesiologist assumes responsibility for the adequacy of the patient's ventilation intraoperatively and in many cases finds it necessary to assist or to support ventilation completely. Monitoring the effectiveness of ventilation is essential under these conditions, especially since most causes of ventilatory insufficiency during the perioperative period are both avoidable and correctable.

Ventilation has as its primary purpose the provision of O_2 to and the removal of CO_2 from blood. The single, definite monitor of the adequacy of ventilation is the analysis of O_2 and CO_2 partial pressures in arterial blood, and these laboratory tests are commonly used for patients in the operating room. Other measures of ventilatory function can be especially useful in diagnosing the cause of ventilatory insufficiency; early warning signs and devices can alert the anesthesiologist to problems before they result in ventilatory insufficiency and its consequences.

There are a number of signs of hypoxemia and hypercarbia in the normal, awake subject (Table 13-4). These signs may prove unreliable in the anesthetized surgical patient under some circumstances. For example, the presence of anemia or cutaneous vasoconstriction may mask cyanosis. Certain anesthetic drugs (e.g., spinal anesthesia) may obtund the hemodynamic manifestations of sympathetic stimulation produced by hypercarbia and/or hypoxemia. Also, these signs and symptoms are not useful in quantifying the severity of ventilatory insufficiency and often cannot be used to distinguish between ventilatory and circulatory problems, hence the need for accurate and reliable monitoring of ventilation during anesthesia and surgery, especially in patients who have a high risk of ventilatory insufficiency as a re-

---

TABLE 13-4.   Signs of Hypoxemia and Hypercarbia in the Normal, Awake Patient

Ventilation
  Increased ventilatory effort, frequency, and tidal volume in response to chemoreceptor stimulation by hypoxia (carotid body) and by hypercarbia (medullary respiratory centers).

Circulation
  Sympathetic nervous system stimulation by hypoxia and/or hypercarbia leads to increased heart rate and blood pressure.
  Direct effects of hypoxia on the heart lead to slowing of the rate, dysrhythmias, ECG signs of ischemia, and progressive impairment of myocardial contractility.
  Carbon dioxide acts directly on vascular smooth muscle to produce vasodilation; respiratory acidosis leads to cardiac dysrhythmias.

Skin, mucous membranes, conjunctiva
  Hypoxemia produces cyanosis in the absence of cutaneous vasoconstriction and anemia.

Surgical site
  Hypoxemia darkens the color of blood.
  Hypercarbia increases bleeding.

Central nervous system
  Hypercarbia may produce muscular twitching and convulsions before the onset of coma ($PaCO_2 > 250$ mm Hg); halothane MAC is reduced progressively at $PaCO_2 > 90$ mmHg.
  Hypoxia produces coma.

---

sult of their disease state, type of surgery, or both.

The most important aspect of ventilation is providing sufficient oxygen to the CNS and heart. Of course, the elimination of CO_2 is also important, but the effects of hypercarbia are reversible, whereas a relatively brief period of brain hypoxia results in severe and irreversible damage.[26,27] Almost all causes of brain damage due to ventilatory insufficiency during anesthesia are preventable and, when not recognized and corrected promptly, the anesthesiologist bears primary responsibility. Continuous monitoring of oxygenation is absolutely mandatory, and the anesthesiologist must be aware of all possible clues to the existence of inadequate ventilation and oxygen delivery to the patient (Tables 13-4 and 13-8). The causes of hypoxemia are discussed in Chapter 32.

Problems with ventilation during anesthesia can be classified in terms of the following: inspired gas mixture, ventilation of the lungs, pulmonary blood flow, and gas exchange. Monitoring techniques and devices can also be considered in relation to these aspects of ventilation. Techniques and devices limited to one aspect of ventilation are particularly useful in identifying the cause of ventilatory insufficiency, but accurate assessment of the degree of ventilatory failure can be accomplished only with analysis of arterial blood gases.

ANALYSIS OF BLOOD GASES (Also See Ch. 37)

Routine analysis of blood gases in the clinical laboratory involves measurement of pH and of the partial pressures of O_2 and CO_2. The hematocrit (or hemoglobin concentration*) is usually determined simultaneously to calculate the oxygen content of the blood and to estimate the base deficit or excess. The reader is referred elsewhere for a discussion of the methods of these analyses.[37,38] Physiologic and pathologic changes in arterial blood gases are summarized in Chapter 37. The following discussion focuses on the pitfalls in interpretation of the results of blood-gas analysis.

SAMPLE COLLECTION

Blood-gas analysis is usually performed on arterial blood in order to evaluate the adequacy of ventilation. When it is impractical to obtain an arterial sample (e.g., newborn infant), capillary blood from a finger or toe on a warmed and well-perfused extremity may provide a close

---

* The hemoglobin concentration (in g/dl) of blood is approximately one-third of the hematocrit in percent.

approximation of arterial blood. Venous blood-gas analysis does not provide an estimate of pulmonary function in terms of oxygenation of blood, but it can give indications of the degree of oxygen extraction by peripheral tissues, of hypercarbia or hypocarbia (assuming the usual arteriovenous differences of 4 to 6 mm Hg in PCO_2), and of acid–base balance. Obviously, it is important to recognize the differences between arterial and venous blood (Table 13-5) in interpreting the results of blood-gas analysis.

Certain precautions are necessary in withdrawing and preserving the blood sample in order to ensure that it accurately represents the circulating blood:

1. The syringe should be airtight and rinsed with heparin (1,000 units/ml), and the plunger should be depressed completely to expel the excess heparin from the syringe. Fifteen μl of a 1,000-unit/ml solution contains 15 units of heparin, which is sufficient to anticoagulate 3 ml of whole blood.

2. If the blood sample is to be taken from an indwelling cannula, old blood and flush solution contained in the cannula should be withdrawn and discarded before the sample is collected in order to ensure that it will be representative of the blood circulating at the time of sampling.

3. Air bubbles should be eliminated from the sample, and the syringe should be immediately sealed and placed in ice to prevent uptake or loss of gases (i.e., from the ambient air, by metabolism in the blood cells).

4. The temperature of the patient should be noted so that appropriate corrections can be made; typically, blood-gas analysis is performed in vitro at 37°C. Temperature devia-

tions alter the solubility of gases in blood and hence their partial pressures. Nomograms and slide rules are available to correct blood PO_2, PCO_2, and pH for temperature differences between the patient and electrode system.[39,40] There is considerable controversy about the appropriateness of correcting CO_2 tensions and pH for temperature deviations from 37°C, especially in the case of deliberate hypothermia.[41-43]

INTERPRETATION

Oxygen has a very limited solubility in blood; most of the oxygen is carried in combination with hemoglobin (Hb), which is essentially saturated at an oxygen partial pressure of 100 mm Hg. The total oxygen content of blood can be calculated as follows:

1. Determine the Hb saturation by actual measurement or by reference to the appropriate oxyhemoglobin dissociation curve.*

2. Multiply the oxygen content of saturated Hb (1.3 cc O_2/g Hb) by the percentage saturation to determine the amount of oxygen carried by Hb in blood. Hemoglobin concentrations in whole blood are usually expressed as g/dl. (One dl is 100 ml. Volume percent is the volume of gas (cc) in 100 ml or 1 dl.)

3. Multiply the oxygen solubility factor (0.003 ml O_2/dl blood/mm Hg) by the PaO_2 to determine the amount of oxygen carried in physical solution in blood.

4. Sum the values of steps 2 and 3 to determine the total oxygen content of blood. For example, Hb 15 g/dl blood, PaO_2 = 100 mm Hg
   1. Hb 100% saturated at PaO_2 of 100 mm Hg
   2. 15 g/dl × 100% × 1.3 cc O_2/g Hb = 19.5 cc O_2/dl blood
   3. 100 mm Hg × 0.003 ml/dl/mm Hg = 0.3 cc O_2/dl blood
   4. 19.5 + 0.3 = 19.8 cc O_2/dl blood

TABLE 13-5. Normal Blood-Gas Values

		Arterial	Mixed Venous
pH		7.40	7.36
$PaCO_2$ (mm Hg)		40.0	46.0
PaO_2 (mm Hg)	*years of age**		40.0
	20–29	84–104	
	30–39	81–101	
	40–49	78–98	
	50–59	74–94	
	60–69	71–91	

* Mean $PaO_2 = 100 - \dfrac{\text{years of age}}{3}$

---

* The relationship between Hb saturation and PaO_2 is affected by temperature, pH, base excess, ionic strength, type of hemoglobin, and the concentration of 2,3-diphosphoglycerate in the erythrocyte.[44]

Carbon dioxide is hydrated to carbonic acid, which dissociates to bicarbonate and hydrogen ions. Thus, there is a relationship between PCO_2 and pH, which can be summarized on a nomogram[39] or Severinghaus slide rule.[40] Deviations from this relationship are due to the presence of other (metabolic or fixed) acids and bases and are expressed in terms of a base deficit or excess. Dripps et al.[45] summarized the relationships in two tables designed for memorization (Table 13-6).

INDWELLING AND CUTANEOUS PROBES

Oxygen, CO_2, and pH-sensitive probes have been developed for insertion in peripheral arteries for continuous monitoring of these variables in blood.[37,46] Their place in intraoperative monitoring has not yet been determined in relationship to their cost and to their relative advantages and disadvantages over current practices of intermittent sampling of blood for in vitro analysis of gases.

Transcutaneous oximetry and CO_2 measurement are indirect methods of estimating gas tensions in blood passing through capillaries or veins of the skin. Accuracy of the devices depends on their proper calibration and on the maintenance of a brisk blood flow through the skin. Although the devices may be less accurate than direct measurement of arterial blood gases in the hemodynamically unstable patient, they offer the advantages of continuous monitoring and can indicate adverse trends due to either respiratory or circulatory impairment.[46,47] Unfortunately, they cannot replace periodic direct arterial blood-gas analysis in critically ill and unstable patients.

INSPIRED GAS MIXTURE

The formulation of the inspired mixture of gases in the operating room is usually accomplished by the anesthesia machine, the function of which should be evaluated before the induction of anesthesia, and preferably before the patient arrives at the anesthetizing location (also see Chs. 5 & 12).* Despite the best preparations, malfunction of the anesthesia machine can occur, and there are four potential problems related to the inspired gas mixture: inadequate oxygen content, presence of CO_2 (rebreathing), inappropriately high or low anesthetic concentrations, and contamination of the mixture with infectious irritating or toxic volatile substances. Precise analysis of the components of the inspired gaseous mixture is becoming a reality with the use of mass spectrometers and other sophisticated and expensive devices (e.g., infrared analyzers for carbon dioxide, halothane, and enflurane). However, most anesthesiologists do not have access to such equipment and are required to use other means of evaluating the gas mixture they administer to their patients.

The single most important constituent of any anesthetic mixture is oxygen. Oxygen analyzers (e.g., paramagnetic, fuel cell, and polarographic) are relatively inexpensive (less than $500) and provide the only reliable means of quantifying the oxygen content in the inspired mixture.[48] An oxygen analyzer is absolutely required for low-flow or closed-circuit administration of anesthetic mixtures containing nitrous oxide. Oxygen analyzers measure the percentage oxygen in the gas mixture; nitrous oxygen concentrations can be estimated as the difference between oxygen percentage and 100 percent.

The presence of CO_2 in the inspired gas (rebreathing) cannot be detected without relatively expensive equipment, the cost of which may be justified by the other functions it performs.[46,49] In the absence of sophisticated equipment, the risk of rebreathing can be reduced by maintaining high flows of fresh gas mixture (with the disadvantages of wasting anesthetic gases and pollution of the operating room atmosphere) or by using a carbon dioxide absorber in a low-flow system. Function of the absorber can be checked by feeling its surface (CO_2 absorption produces heat) and by incorpo-

---

* The patient's anxiety can only increase when he hears comments such as "That doesn't work!" or "What's gone wrong with this?" and observes last-minute repairs that suggest the imperfect functioning of equipment upon which his life will depend.

TABLE 13-6. Relationships Among PaCO$_2$, pH, and Base Excess or Deficit

A. Predicted pH at different PaCO$_2$ levels (No metabolic acid–base abnormality)

PaCO$_2$ (mm Hg)	pH	
70	7.25	
60	7.30	$\pm$ 0.05 pH units/10 mm Hg PCO$_2$
50	7.35	
40	7.40	
30	7.5	
20	7.6	$\pm$ 0.1 pH units/10 mm Hg PCO$_2$
10	7.7	

B. Predicted pH at different levels of metabolic acidosis or alkalosis (PaCO$_2$ = 40 mm Hg)

pH	Base (mEq/L)
7.1	−21
7.2	−14
7.3	− 7
7.4	0 $\pm$ 7 mEq/0.1 pH unit
7.5	+ 7
7.6	+14
7.7	+21

C. To estimate a base deficit or excess at a given pH and PCO$_2$
   1. Adjust the pH for the contribution of respiratory acidosis or alkalosis by the amount corresponding to the difference between the given PCO$_2$ and 40 mm Hg (part A)
   2. Estimate the base deficit or excess from part B
   e.g., Given a pH = 7.25 and a PCO$_2$ = 50
     (1) PCO$_2$ 50 → 40
        pH 7.25 → 7.30
     (2) 7.30 corresponds to a base of −7 mEq/L (i.e., a base deficit of 7 mEq/L)

(Modified from Dripps RD, Eckenhoff JE, Vandam LD: Introduction to Anesthesia. The Principles of Safe Practice. 6th Ed. Philadelphia, WB Saunders, 1982.)

rating an indicator that turns a different color when the absorbent is exhausted. Of course, the anesthesiologist should be alert to physiologic changes suggestive of hypercarbia.

The presence of inappropriate concentrations of volatile anesthetics or of irritating contaminants can often be detected by the anesthesiologist himself inhaling the anesthetic mixture for one or two breaths ("sniff test"). This practice is condemned by some because it is not a very sensitive test and because it repeatedly exposes the anesthesiologist to anesthetics with the risk of their accumulation and toxicity. An ultraviolet analyzer for halothane (Cavitron) is available at a moderate cost and is adequate for clinical use. The Narkotest meter (Drager) is inexpensive and sensitive to all volatile anesthetics. However, it is not particularly accurate and has the disadvantages of a very slow response time and of being affected by water vapor. All the other commercially available devices (i.e., infrared analyzer, gas chromatograph, mass spectrograph) offer specificity and precision of gas analysis, but currently they are very expensive. Systems have been, and continue to be, developed for the timesharing use of a single analyzer by multiple rooms within an operating suite. Such systems spread the costs among patients and, given the multiple functions the systems serve and the potential benefits in reductions of risk, their installation in hospitals outside academic medical centers will probably increase. The anesthesiologist and patient are probably best served by regular inspection and maintenance of the anesthesia machine, including the anesthetic vaporizers.

LUNG VENTILATION
(Also See Chs. 32 & 59)

Ventilation of the lungs is measured in terms of the volume of gas inspired (I) or exhaled (E) in a single breath (tidal volume, V$_T$) or

TABLE 13-7. Normal Values of Ventilatory Variables for Adult Males at Rest

Variables	Abbreviation	Normal, Average Values
Frequency	f	12 breaths/min
Tidal volume	$\dot{V}T$	500 cc (3 to 4 cc/lb body wt)
Expired minute ventilation (total)	$\dot{V}E$	6,000 cc/min
Anatomic dead space	$\dot{V}D$	150 cc (1 cc/lb body wt)
Alveolar minute ventilation	$\dot{V}A$	4,200 cc/min
Vital capacity	VC	4,800 cc
Compliance of lung and thorax	C	0.1 L/cm H_2O

over a minute's time (minute ventilation, $\dot{V}$). Minute ventilation is the product of tidal volume and frequency (f) of breaths per minute:

$$\dot{V} = \dot{V}T \times f$$

Normal values for these ventilatory variables are shown in Table 13-7. The focus of this discussion is on monitoring the effectiveness of ventilation regardless of the particular mode of ventilation that is being used. Again, the definitive test of ventilation is the analysis of arterial blood gases. But there are other means of monitoring ventilatory variables that may be especially useful in diagnosing the causes of hypoxemia, hypercarbia, and acidosis (Table 13-8); and there are useful alarms for early warnings of impending or existing problems (e.g., apnea alarms).

Apnea alarms respond to the failure of airway or anesthetic circuit pressure to rise within a set period of time. Such alarms are probably indicated any time the anesthesiologist is not directly in touch with the patient and especially when a mechanical ventilator is

being used. Early detection of a disconnection between the patient and the breathing circuit is obviously necessary if the development of hypoxemia and hypercarbia are to be avoided.

The measurement of inspired or exhaled gas volumes is most accurately done with a watersealed bell spirometer. However, this instrument is too bulky and cumbersome for routine clinical use. There are a number of more portable though less accurate devices (e.g., gas meter, anemometer, and pneumotachograph) that can adequately fill clinical needs, provided they are calibrated regularly and handled carefully to avoid damage to their relatively delicate mechanisms. Probably the most widely used instrument is the Wright respirometer. Its performance is affected by the composition of the gas, humidity, and instantaneous rates of gas flow. Nevertheless, its use is justified for clinical purposes.[44]

Another aspect of lung ventilation that changes with anesthesia, surgery, and disease states is the compliance of the lungs and chest wall. Compliance is the volume change per

TABLE 13-8. Monitoring of Lung Ventilation

Visual
  Regular, normal movement of the diaphragm, chest and anesthesia reservoir bag or ventilator bellows; alternate condensation and vaporization of water in the endotracheal tube; rise and fall of anesthesia circuit pressure gauge. The ventilator bellows should be filled from below so that they will collapse to signal loss of pressure in the ventilator-anesthesia circuit.

Auditory
  Breath sounds through an esophageal or precordial stethoscope, at the lips, or in the anesthesia circuit.
  Regular cycling of ventilator which should be equipped with auditory alarms to signal malfunction. Auditory alarm on oxygen analyzer to signal inadequate oxygen in the inspired gas mixture.

Volume measurement
  Bellows of the ventilator (e.g., Ventimeter), spirometers, pneumotachograph

Carbon dioxide measurement (e.g., capnograph, mass spectrometer)
  Rise and fall of carbon dioxide concentration in airway gases with ventilation by fresh gas (i.e., nonrebreathing or CO_2 absorber systems).

Apnea monitor
  Sounds an alarm when pressures within the anesthesia system do not change over a 15- to 20-second interval.

$$\text{Total compliance} = \frac{\text{change in lung volume}}{\text{change in alveolar-ambient pressure gradient}} \tag{1}$$

$$\text{Lung compliance} = \frac{\text{change in lung volume}}{\text{change in alveolar-intrathoracic pressure gradient}} \tag{2}$$

$$\text{Chest wall compliance} = \frac{\text{change in lung volume}}{\text{change in intrathoracic-ambient pressure gradient}} \tag{3}$$

$$\frac{1}{\text{total compliance}} = \frac{1}{\text{lung compliance}} + \frac{1}{\text{chest wall compliance}} \tag{4}$$

unit change of the transmural pressure gradient and can be defined as above (Eqs. 1-3).[44] The total compliance of the lungs plus the chest wall is related to their individual compliances (Eq.4).

In the usual clinical setting of the anesthetized patient, the anesthesiologist may utilize the pressure gauge in the anesthesia breathing system to monitor the lung inflation pressure produced by a given volume of ventilation. (Alternatively, the volume of inspired or exhaled gas can be measured for a given inflation pressure.) High inflation pressures indicate low compliance and may signify changes in skeletal muscle tone (intercostal, diaphragmatic, abdominal) as a result of a lessening of anesthetic depth or muscular paralysis, development of tension pneumothorax or increased intraabdominal pressure, changes in lung compliance (e.g., interstitial edema), or the presence of airway obstruction from any of a large number of potential causes. Besides signifying alterations in the above, reduced compliance affects the volume of ventilation delivered by a pressure-driven ventilator.

More precise determinations of compliance, both static and dynamic, are required for research purposes but add little to the clinical management of patients. Similarly, measurements of airway resistance are largely a research tool.

The prompt diagnosis of airway obstruction is of vital importance. Causes of airway obstruction are listed in Table 13-9. Airway obstruction can be partial or complete. Complete airway obstruction is more obvious, because there is no exchange of gas between the lungs and the anesthesia system or ambient air. It can be recognized most directly by the absence of breath sounds. Other signs of airway obstruction are listed in Table 13-10. If the location of the obstruction is in the trachea or upper airway, the cause obviously must be identified and remedied promptly. In the setting of anesthesia and surgery four possibilities should be considered:

1. Upper airway obstruction due to the tongue; usually corrected by proper positioning

TABLE 13-9. Causes of Airway Obstruction

Lips
Tongue
Epiglottis
Edematous tissue
Secretions
Laryngospasm
Bronchospasm
Clamping of trachea or bronchus by surgeon
Low lung compliance
    Pulmonary edema
    Emphysema
Low thoracic compliance
    Muscular rigidity
    Circumferential bandaging of trunk
    Surgeon leaning on patient's chest and/or abdomen
Hemothorax, pleural effusion
Tension pneumothorax
Herniation of abdominal structures into thorax
Ascites, obesity
Foreign objects in airway
Endotracheal tube
    Kinking
    Balloon cuff overlying tip
    Overinflation of balloon cuff with invagination of endotracheal tube
    Single lumen occluded against mucosa
    Plugged with secretions or blood
    Endobronchial position

TABLE 13-10. Signs of Airway Obstruction

Spontaneous ventilation
  Increasing ventilatory effort (reflex due to hypercarbia, hypoxia)
  Retraction of intercostal, supraclavicular, and abdominal tissues
  Reduced or absent breath sounds over lung fields
  Abnormal breath sounds due to turbulence especially in upper airway
  Reduced or absent exchange of gas (i.e., absence of sound, temperature change, moisture condensation at lips or in endotracheal tube; reduced or absent movement of reservoir bag; spirometer records low or no tidal volume)
  Signs of hypoxemia and hypercarbia

Positive-pressure ventilation
  High lung inflation pressure
  Reservoir bag does not empty (i.e., inspiratory obstruction) or does not refill normally (i.e., expiratory obstruction)
  Absence of condensation in endotracheal tube
  Reduced or absent breath sounds over lung fields and in breathing circuit
  Little or no movement of thorax or abdominal wall with application and release of positive pressure
  Signs of hypoxemia and hypercarbia

---

of the head and mandible and by insertion of an oral airway or endotracheal tube.

2. Foreign object in the airway from the patient (e.g., dental work, tobacco), the anesthesiologist (e.g., improperly positioned airway device), or the surgeon (e.g., pharyngeal packing). Examination of the airway and possibly laryngoscopy or bronchoscopy assists in making the diagnosis and offers the means of removal of the obstructing object. An emergency tracheotomy may be necessary.

3. Laryngospasm is almost always associated with airway manipulation or with the presence of foreign material in the larynx of a lightly anesthetized patient. The diagnosis is often obvious; laryngoscopy makes it definite but is not often indicated or appropriate (wastes time and further stimulates the airway). Therapy involves maximal cephalad displacement of the mandible,[50] maintenance of positive airway pressure with pure oxygen and, if necessary, administration of a muscle relaxant (e.g., 10 to 20 mg of succinylcholine IV).

4. Obstruction of the endotracheal tube is most easily ruled out by the passage of a lubricated suction catheter completely through the length of the tube. If the catheter cannot be passed, the endotracheal tube must be manipulated (e.g., deflation of the balloon or elimination of kinking) or removed for inspection (e.g., occlusion by clotted blood). When the operation involves the neck or upper mediastinum, the possibility of the surgeon obstructing the trachea should be considered.

Partial airway obstruction presents more subtle signs than does complete obstruction (Table 13-10). The exchange of gases continues through a partial obstruction and results in sounds that are useful in identifying the cause and location of the obstruction. Partial obstruction by the tongue creates rough, irregular stertorous (snoring) sounds that are loudest over the neck. Fluid in the pharynx is associated with a gurgling type of noise. Laryngospasm produces a high-pitched whistle or squeak. Foreign objects produce a variety of noises, depending on the degree of the obstruction (pitch) and on their mobility in the airway (e.g., rattling or fluttering sounds). Bronchiolar constriction among other factors produces wheezing, bronchiolar secretions result in rhonchi, and alveolar fluid (edema) causes rales. Absent or distant breath sounds over a portion of the lung may signify bronchial obstruction, atelectasis, or pneumothorax.

In addition to sounds, partial airway obstruction can be evaluated in the more quantitative terms of tidal volume, duration of inspiration or expiration, compliance, and arterial blood gases.

The measurement of lung volumes is not done by the anesthesiologist in the usual clinical setting except for the occasional estimation of functional residual capacity (FRC) during mechanical ventilation of patients under intensive care for acute respiratory failure. The closed-circuit helium-dilution technique is the simplest, most accurate method.[51]

Estimates of wasted ventilation, that is dead space ventilation as a fraction of total ventilation (V_D/V_T), involves the measurements of the partial pressure of CO_2 in arterial ($PaCO_2$) blood and in mixed expired gas ($PECO_2$) collected for several minutes in a large gas-tight bag (30 L). The ratio can then be calculated:

$$\frac{V_D}{V_T} = \frac{PaCO_2 - PECO_2}{PaCO_2}$$

Again, these measurements by the anesthesiologist are usually confined to the clinical setting of the ICU and are made in an attempt to explain discrepancies between $PaCO_2$ and minute ventilation.

PULMONARY BLOOD FLOW AND GAS EXCHANGE (Also See Ch. 32)

The uptake of oxygen by and elimination of CO_2 from venous blood occurs at the alveolar-capillary membrane. This exchange obviously depends on ventilation and perfusion of the alveoli and on the condition of the membrane. Even under normal conditions in healthy persons, some of the pulmonary blood flow is not exposed to ventilated alveoli, and the mismatch of ventilation and perfusion tends to increase under conditions of anesthesia, surgery, and disease (also see Ch. 32). Disease can also affect the condition of the alveolar-capillary membrane.

The effectiveness of the lungs in converting venous blood to arterial is most conveniently measured in terms of oxygenation.* Pulmonary blood flow through unventilated alveoli and right-to-left shunts represents wasted blood flow ($\dot{Q}s$), usually expressed as a fraction of total pulmonary blood flow ($\dot{Q}T$). Calculation of the fraction requires determinations of the partial pressure of oxygen in mixed venous (pulmonary artery) blood (PvO_2), in systemic arterial blood (PaO_2), and in the inspired (PIO_2) and expired gas (PEO_2) along with the measurements of hemoglobin concentra-

tion and $PaCO_2$. From these data, the oxygen content of mixed venous (CvO_2), arterial (CaO_2), and pulmonary end-capillary blood ($Cc'O_2$) can be calculated† and then the shunt fraction estimated:

$$\frac{\dot{Q}s}{\dot{Q}T} = \frac{Cc'O_2 - CaO_2}{Cc'O_2 - CvO_2}$$

Such measurements and calculations are still limited in clinical practice, but they may be done more frequently with the increased availability of blood-gas analysis, pulmonary artery catheters, and programmable calculators.

In the usual clinical situation, the difference between alveolar ($PACO_2$) and arterial ($PaCO_2$) oxygen tension is taken as an indication of "virtual" shunting. This A-a gradient is subject to considerable misinterpretation.[44] For example, the A-a gradient and the apparent magnitude of shunting will be less when the patient is receiving less than 100 percent oxygen in the inspired gas (Fig. 13-2). Nevertheless, the concept of "virtual" shunt and the use of an isoshunt diagram in clinical practice is justified for estimating oxygen concentrations required to achieve a certain PaO_2 (verification of the accuracy of the estimate by blood-gas analysis is mandatory), for indicating progress in the patient's recovery, and for demonstrating the presence of problems other than shunting that may be contributing to the inadequate oxygenation of arterial blood.

THE CARDIOVASCULAR SYSTEM

The cardiovascular system functions as a means of transporting substances from one organ to another in the body. For example, it is

---

* Increased minute ventilation can compensate for a large right to left shunting of pulmonary blood flow in terms of carbon dioxide elimination. Oxygen uptake by blood perfusing ventilated alveoli is limited in amount by hemoglobin (Hb) saturation, since very little oxygen is carried by physical solution in blood. When arterial blood mixes with shunted venous blood, the PaO_2 and Hb saturation fall as oxygen is taken up by the unsaturated Hb in the shunted venous blood.

† Calculation of oxygen content is discussed and illustrated above, and is readily done for CaO_2 and CvO_2. The estimation of $Cc'O_2$ involves a number of assumptions and is based on the alveolar air equation:

$$PAO_2 = PIO_2 - PaCO_2 \left(\frac{PIO_2 - P\bar{E}O_2}{P\bar{E}O_2} \right)$$

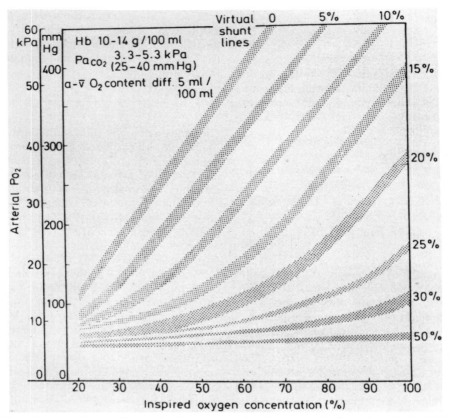

FIG. 13-2 An isoshunt diagram. The relationships between inspired oxygen concentration (abscissa) and arterial PO_2 (PaO_2) (ordinate) are shown for different percentages of right-to-left pulmonary shunting. If the degree of shunting is estimated, an inspired oxygen concentration can be chosen to produce a given PaO_2. If the relationship between the inspired oxygen concentration and PaO_2 is determined, the percentage of shunting can be estimated from this graph. (Redrawn by Nunn[44] from Benater SR, Hewlett AM, Nunn JF: The use of iso-shunt lines for control of oxygen therapy. Br J Anaesth 45:711, 1973.)

essential for the constant, continuous delivery of O_2 from the lung to all body tissues and for the conveyance of CO_2 from those tissues to the lung where it is eliminated. Probably the most precise indicator of satisfactory cardiovascular performance is the maintenance of efficient, effective, and integrated function of body organs and tissues (Table 13-11). Because of the effects of drugs and other variables, evaluation of individual organ function during anesthesia under clinical conditions has proved less practical and informative than the monitoring of various aspects of cardiovascular performance.

Monitoring of hemodynamics in the patient undergoing anesthesia and surgery is indicated for several reasons:

1. Anesthetic drugs alter cardiovascular functions.

2. Most accidents related to anesthesia and life support have premonitory signs, and cardiovascular changes are among the most prominent indicators of adverse, life-threatening incidents.

3. Surgery can result in acute and marked changes in hemodynamics as a result of body position, surgical manipulation, blood loss, and fluid loss and redistribution.

4. There is a prevalence of cardiovascular disease and of diseases affecting hemodynamics among surgical patients. The interactions of these disease states with anesthetic drugs and surgical procedures is not always

TABLE 13-11. Monitoring Organ Function and Perfusion

Organ or System	Monitor
Central nervous system	
Unanesthetized patient	Mentation, sensory and motor functions
Anesthetized or comatose patient	EEG, reflexes, pupils
Heart	ECG — ischemia, dysrhythmias Cardiac output vs preload (ventricular performance)
Kidney	Urine volume, specific gravity, composition
Skin	Color, capillary refill, temperature
Lung	Arterial blood gases, shunt

predictable. Appropriate monitoring techniques can indicate inappropriate or unexpected trends that often can be corrected.

5. Therapy of adverse hemodynamic changes often involves potent drugs with specific actions on the cardiovascular system. Monitoring techniques are essential for the selection of the most appropriate therapy and for the evaluation of its effectiveness and safety.

Hemodynamic monitoring of the patient during the perioperative period encompasses a large number of techniques differing in their degree of precision, accuracy, complexity, safety, and cost. The appropriateness and effectiveness of individual techniques will vary with the anesthesiologist and the clinical circumstances. Seldom is there only one right way to monitor a particular patient at a particular time in the perioperative course of events. In all cases, however, the objectives are the same, that is, to provide sufficient information in a form that can be collated and comprehended with sufficient speed by the anesthesiologist so that he or she can make a decision to act or withhold action.

The following discussion summarizes the indications and limitations of techniques currently used in clinical practice. Technical information underlying the instrumentation, descriptions of specific steps in the application of techniques, and interpretation of the data are omitted because they are well described elsewhere.[1,52,53]

ARTERIAL BLOOD PRESSURE

Arterial blood pressure remains the focal point of cardiovascular monitoring for a number of reasons. It is one of the traditional vital signs that can provide an indication of cardiovascular problems. It is easily and frequently measured along with heart rate and can be used to characterize the "usual state" of the patient against which alterations can be compared. It represents the potential for perfusion of all tissues. In the case of the brain and the heart, blood pressure along with local metabolic activity (i.e., autoregulation) are the primary determinants of cerebral and coronary blood flow.

But there are two important points to be emphasized and remembered: blood pressure is not equivalent to blood flow; blood pressure may be normal when cardiovascular function is very abnormal.

INDIRECT MEASUREMENT

Indirect measurement of arterial blood pressure is done with a sphygmomanometer, which measures the pressure required to occlude a major artery in an extremity. A pneumatic bladder enclosed in a cuff is positioned over the artery and inflated to a pressure greater than systolic blood pressure. The air in the bladder is slowly released and one of four basic techniques is used to detect the systolic (and in some cases the diastolic) blood pressure: oscillation of the cuff pressure; auscultation of Korotkoff sounds; ultrasonic detection of arterial wall motion under the cuff; or detection of blood flow distal to the sphygmomanometer cuff by palpation of a pulse, Doppler ultra sound, photoelectric plethysmography, or other means. The physical basis of each of these techniques is discussed elsewhere.[54] Auscultation of Korotkoff sounds is the most commonly used; the others are substituted when Korotkoff sounds are not easily heard or for purposes of convenience.

Many factors affect the accuracy of indirect blood pressure determinations (Table 13-12). The most common are the inaccuracy of

TABLE 13-12. Factors Affecting the Accuracy of Indirect Blood Pressure Measurements

Factor	Consequence
Hearing	Variable sensitivity to Korotkoff sounds
Stethoscope	Design and positioning determines intensity of sounds
Touch	Variable sensitivity to pulse palpation
Cuff size	Falsely high BP—too small or loose fitting cuff Falsely low BP—too large a cuff
Aneroid manometer	Inaccurate BP with improper calibration
Deflation of sphygmomanometer	Falsely low BP—too rapid deflation
Oscillometry	Imprecise detection of first and last oscillations, indicating systolic and diastolic pressures, respectively

aneroid manometers and the size and positioning of the blood pressure cuff. Aneroid manometers should be calibrated regularly against a mercury manometer. The width of the blood pressure cuff should be greater than 20 to 30 percent of the circumference of the limb; a cuff that is too wide relative to circumference of the arm will give falsely low pressures, and one that is too narrow will give incorrectly high estimates. The bladder should cover at least half of the circumference. The middle of the bladder should be positioned directly over the pulsating artery. In the auscultatory method, the stethoscope should be positioned directly over the pulsating artery under the most distal portion or just beyond the pneumatic cuff.

Noninvasive automatic devices controlled by microprocessors are being used more widely for blood pressure measurements in the routine practice of anesthesiology because of their convenience and especially because they free the hands of the anesthetist during busy times in the operation. Devices are available to measure systolic, diastolic, and mean arterial pressures utilizing pneumatic cuffs and various types of sensors. They have generally proven to be accurate and reliable, to provide more consistent readings than possible between different anesthetists, and to offer accurate estimates of mean blood pressure, the most important physiologically and the one needed in the calculation of hemodynamic variables (see below).

Even with the meticulous attention to details, considerable discrepancy can be observed between indirect and direct methods of blood pressure measurement. The greatest discrepancies have been noted in hypertension, obe-

sity, hypothermia, and shock. Both methods have their limitations as far as blood pressure measurements are concerned, but the direct method can provide other information useful in evaluating the overall hemodynamic status of the patient. Indirect measurement of blood pressure is usually sufficient for the patient who is hemodynamically stable in the preoperative period and who is not expected to experience marked instability for any reason during anesthesia and surgery.

DIRECT MEASUREMENT

Direct measurement of arterial blood pressure offers a number of advantages over sphygmomanometry that are especially useful to the anesthesiologist caring for hemodynamically unstable patients. Information is provided continuously and very conveniently on a beat-by-beat basis that facilitates the earliest possible recognition of adverse hemodynamic responses and unfavorable trends. Modern equipment for direct pressure measurement affords reliability and sustained accuracy over the full range of blood pressures encountered clinically. Visual analysis of the pulse-pressure versus time waveform on an oscilloscope or recorder can yield additional information about cardiovascular function (Table 13-13).

Direct measurement of arterial blood pressure requires arterial cannulation and the use of a pressure-measuring system. Both can affect the overall accuracy of the data, and at least certain features of each should be familiar to the anesthesiologist.

TABLE 13-13. **Information Derived from Visual Analysis of the Arterial Pressure**

Myocardial contractility
  The upstroke of the pulse pressure wave is dependent on left ventricular dP/dt.
  A steep upstroke indicates strong left ventricular contraction.

Stroke volume
  The area under the systolic ejection phase of the pulse pressure tracing (i.e., upstroke to dicrotic notch) is proportional to stroke volume

Systemic vascular resistance
  A low dicrotic notch and a steep downstroke indicates rapid diastolic runoff and a low SVR.

Heart rate, dysrhythmias, and their hemodynamic significance
  Knowledge of the sweep speed of the oscilloscope's beam or paper speed on the recorder permits an immediate estimate of heart rate and of sudden changes in rate and rhythm (especially useful with interruptions of ECG recording).
  A cardiotachometer can be triggered by the arterial pulse waveform.
  Dysrhythmia diagnosis is facilitated by relating the ECG to the arterial pulse waveform (e.g., bigeminy, junctional rhythm).
  The hemodynamic significance of rate and rhythm changes is indicated by alterations in blood pressure and pulse contour on a beat-to-beat basis.

Circulating blood volume
  Exaggerated beat-by-beat changes in blood pressure in relation to ventilation can indicate hypovolemia.
  During a single cycle of ventilation:
    Positive-pressure ventilation increases the stroke volume of the first beat or two and then decreases the stroke volume of subsequent beats.
    Spontaneous ventilation decreases the stroke volume of the first beat or two and increases stroke volume during expiration.

ARTERIAL CANNULATION

Arterial cannulation is an invasive technique that can be readily justified by its high yield of information and minimal discomfort and risk to the patient if properly done. Arterial cannulation not only offers the advantages of direct measurement of arterial blood pressure and pulse waveform analysis, but it facilitates the collection of arterial blood samples for gas, electrolyte, glucose, coagulation, and other types of analysis. When multiple samples are required for patient care, a single arterial cannulation is obviously preferable to multiple needle punctures in terms of greater reliability and convenience for the anesthetist and less trauma and discomfort to the patient. Indications for arterial cannulation in the surgical patient are listed in Table 13-14.

In most patients, arteries accessible for percutaneous cannulation include the radial, ulnar, brachial, axillary, dorsalis pedis, femoral, and superficial temporal. The radial artery is probably the most frequently used for intraoperative purposes because it is readily accessible, can be easily cannulated, supplies the hand (which normally has a collateral supply through the ulnar artery), and has been used

with few long-term, functionally significant complications when properly cared for.[55-59] Also, it is usually convenient to position the arm of the patient so that the arterial cannulation site is in the view of and accessible to the anesthesiologist intraoperatively. Contraindications to the use of a particular radial artery include the presence of an inadequate circulation to the hand and fingers (e.g., Raynaud's phenomenon), the lack of collateral circulation through the ulnar artery (abnormal Allen's test),* the presence of infection in the proximity of the cannulation site, and recent cannulation of the same radial artery or the brachial artery above it. Previous cannulation may have resulted in changes in the artery (e.g., thrombus formation, scarring with narrowing of the vessel) that may increase the risk of com-

---

* Abnormality of the Allen's test, the size and composition of the cannula, and the duration of radial artery cannulation up to 48 hours were found to be noncontributory to the development of abnormal radial artery blood flow in approximately 1,700 patients in one institution.[59] In the current litigious setting and in the face of previous evidence to the contrary, it is probably prudent to continue to perform the Allen's test, to be cautious about the choice of cannula, and to limit the duration of cannulation to the minimum necessary until these findings are repeated in other institutions and under other conditions.

TABLE 13-14. Indications for Arterial Cannulation in the Surgical Patient

Direct measurement of arterial pressure
    Cardiac surgery, especially with cardiopulmonary bypass
    Deliberate hypothermia
    Deliberate hypotension
    Intracranial operations
    Major vascular surgery — aorta, carotid, iliac, femoral arteries, vena cava
    Extensive surgery with prospect of sudden blood loss or marked shifts of body fluids
    Extensive trauma, especially with uncontrolled hemorrhage
    Thoracic or abdominal surgery with compression of the great vessels
    Noncardiac surgery in patients with significant cardiovascular disease and hemodynamic instability
    Cardiopulmonary resuscitation
    Inability to measure blood pressure indirectly (obesity, burns of the extremities)

Arterial blood sampling (repetitive)
    Blood gas analysis
        Pulmonary disease
        Lung surgery (one-lung ventilation)
        Airway surgery (apneic oxygenation)
        Major surgery (neural, cardiac, vascular, thoracic, abdominal)
    Severe metabolic derangements
        Acid – base evaluation
        Electrolyte determinations
        Glucose analysis
        Serum osmolarity measurement
    Heparin anticoagulation and protamine antagonism
        Cardiopulmonary bypass
        Arterial shunts (Gott shunt)

plications and may increase the discrepancy between arterial pressures measured at that site and central aortic pressure.

Should the radial arteries in both forearms prove unsatisfactory, alternative sites can be considered. The ulnar artery has the same relative contraindications and precautions as the radial. It may be the preferred vessel when the palmar arch is supplied primarily by the radial artery, as indicated by a rapid flush when compression of the radial artery is released after an abnormal Allen's test (i.e., lack of a palmar flush when the ulnar artery occlusion is released). The brachial artery is a larger diameter vessel and able to accommodate indwelling blood gas analyzing probes. Although some have reported few complications from brachial artery cannulation, there is reluctance to use this vessel because there is no collateral artery to provide circulation should the brachial artery become occluded. The axillary artery is of still larger diameter and has been used especially for placement of a central aortic cannula and for long-term cannulation (6 to 21 days).[61,62]

Cannulation of the dorsalis pedis artery is an easy and relatively safe alternative to the radial artery because of collateral circulation through the plantar vessels to the distal portions of the foot.[63] Plantar collateral circulation can be evaluated by occluding the dorsalis pedis artery, compressing the nail of the largest toe to blanch the nailbed, and observing capillary filling in the nailbed when pressure on the nail is released. The dorsalis pedis artery probably should not be used in patients with diabetes mellitus or peripheral vascular disease.

The femoral artery can be cannulated easily and there apparently has been a relatively low incidence of complications.[64] Cannulation of a femoral artery for monitoring purposes is indicated when it is necessary to evaluate arterial circulation to the lower half of the body (e.g., the use of circulatory bypass techniques while the descending aorta is clamped).

The superficial temporal artery has been cannulated for monitoring purposes, primarily in infants and children.

Techniques for cannulation of the radial artery and others are best learned from an experienced tutor. Skill is best developed by cannulating the arteries of patients with normal hemodynamics under the circumstances of elective surgery. Certainly, well-developed skills are essential if the techniques are to be applied in emergency situations and in patients with impaired cardiovascular function. The larger arteries (i.e., brachial, axillary, femoral) are easily cannulated by the Seldinger guide-wire technique, especially useful for the insertion of a longer cannula, which may be indicated by obesity, movement, or manipulation of the extremity, prolonged need for arterial cannulation, placement of a central aortic catheter for pulse wave contour analysis, or when peripheral vascular conditions render the pressure measurements in distal arteries suspect or unreliable.

The anesthesiologist should be aware of the potential complications of arterial cannulation and of the precautions to be taken. The principal complications at all sites are pain, trauma to the artery (e.g., dissection of the intima) and surrounding tissues (e.g., nerve), hematoma, infection, thrombosis, and distal embolization of air, clot, pieces of the cannula, and other debris. Central or proximal embolization is possible with a rapid flushing of the cannula with a large volume of fluid under high pressure.[65] Preventive measures for most of these complications are obvious, but a few deserve special mention. Skillful arterial cannulation obviously requires practice, but it is developed most rapidly and maintained at a high level by a thoughtful and deliberate approach. The accumulation of clot along the cannula can be minimized but not eliminated by using those made of the least thrombogenic material (e.g., Teflon), by using a nontapered, narrow-diameter cannula, by maintaining a continuous flushing of the cannula with an isotonic salt (no sugar) solution containing heparin (2 units/ml), and by limiting manipulation and movement of the cannula that can traumatize the arterial endothelium. Thrombosis of the more distal vessels (i.e., radial, ulnar, dorsalis pedis) is more common the longer the period of cannulation, but they almost always recanalize within a few weeks. Extreme care should be used in reinserting the metal needle stylet through a flexible cannula; some state that it should never be done because of the risks of puncturing the cannula and shearing off the tip in the artery. Meticulous care of the puncture site in the skin, the stopcocks, and so on is required to prevent infection. The lines, connectors, stopcocks, and flush solution must all be kept free of air bubbles.

Erroneous data and mistaken interpretations of data can be associated with the use of techniques involving arterial cannulation. Simultaneous direct blood pressure measurements will differ according to the site of measurement, degree of arterial constriction, and diameter of the cannula.[66] For example, systolic pressure is higher and diastolic pressure lower in the dorsalis pedis than in the brachial or radial arteries. Arterial spasm due to the use of vasoconstrictor drugs reduces the systolic pressure in the radial artery compared with the aorta. In general, the more distal the artery, the greater the vascular resistance in the vessels leading to the artery. The smaller the cannula, the greater the distortion of the pulse-pressure waveform and pressure measurements. The contour of the arterial pressure wave and the degree of correlation between direct and indirect measurements of arterial blood pressure varies with the functional status of the cardiovascular system. In most cases, the anesthesiologist is concerned more with trends than with absolute numbers, but he should be aware of the basis of apparent discrepancies in the values obtained by different methods and judge their significance for the patient accordingly.

Blood sampling from an indwelling arterial cannula may yield erroneous data because of technical failures. Sufficient blood should be withdrawn and discarded before taking a sample in order to minimize its contamination by old blood in the cannula and by the heparinized flush solution. Air bubbles must be eliminated promptly from samples intended for blood gas analysis, and the samples should be placed in ice until they are analyzed in order to reduce blood cell metabolism and gas diffusion through the walls of plastic syringes and liquid seals in glass syringes.

PRESSURE-MEASURING SYSTEMS

Pressure-measuring systems consist of a fluid-mechanical coupling, a pressure transducer, an amplifier and signal-processing unit, and one or more means of displaying the data. The anesthesiologist should understand the principles underlying the function of each system, should be able to calibrate the system both internally and against a mercury manometer, and should recognize the limitations and potential for inaccuracy in each system. Discussions of general principles of pressure measurement are available elsewhere,[67-69] and the manufacturer's representative should be consulted about the specific details of operation and the features of any particular device.

Obviously, the most important feature of the electromechanical system is how accurately it reflects the actual pressures and pulse wave occurring in the vascular system. The pressures displayed by the system can be compared with those simultaneously measured by a sphygmomanometer in the same patient. One method is to determine the return-to-flow pressure. The blood pressure cuff is placed above the site of arterial cannulation on an extremity and inflated until the pulse wave is eliminated. The cuff pressure is released slowly while watching the oscilloscope or recorder for the return of the first sign of a pulse wave, at which point the cuff pressure is noted as the "return-to-flow" systolic pressure. In most cases, there will be close agreement of systolic pressure determined by return-to-flow and by Korotkoff sounds, the latter being the most widely used clinically to describe the patient's usual blood pressure.

Direct pressure readings are commonly 10 to 20 mm Hg greater than those measured by return-to-flow, especially at higher blood pressures associated with systolic hypertension and atherosclerotic vascular disease. Discrepancies of this sort are usually attributable to the characteristics of the pressure transducer. Directly measured systolic pressures lower than those determined by sphygmomanometry and Korotkoff sounds are attributable to the use of compliant rather than rigid tubing to connect the arterial cannula to the transducer, to the presence of air bubbles in the connecting tubing or transducer dome, or to marked peripheral vascular constriction produced by intense sympathetic stimulation or vasopressor drugs.

An important step in the direct measurement and interpretation of intravascular pressure is to be certain that the transducer is placed at the appropriate level relative to the position of the patient. In the supine patient, the transducer diaphragm should be on the same level as the aortic root and atria of the heart (between the anterior and mid-axillary lines in most supine patients). It is especially important to remember that subsequent changes in the patient's position will affect the pressure readings, especially venous pressures, and it may be appropriate to reposition the transducer level accordingly. Some have suggested that if the patient is to be in a sitting position, the transducer should be raised to a higher level in order to more closely reflect brain perfusion pressures. Otherwise it is common practice to set the vascular pressure transducers at the level of the heart.

CENTRAL VENOUS PRESSURE

An anatomic definition of central venous pressure (CVP) is that pressure of blood measured in the vena cavae at their junction with the right atrium. In the normal subject lying in a supine position in the horizontal plane, the same mean pressure will exist in the right atrium, superior vena cava, and the inferior vena cava above the diaphragm. Phasic changes in the CVP occur normally as a result of right atrial contraction, opening and closing of the tricuspid valve, and as a result of ventilation. In the absence of certain disease states, phasic changes in the CVP are inconsequential; the mean CVP yields useful information about the hemodynamic status of the patient provided that factors affecting it are recognized and its limitations understood.

In the normal individual, CVP reflects the balances between blood volume, venous capacitance, and cardiac function. The CVP is elevated by increases in the circulating blood volume and decreases in venous capacitance or cardiac output. In the patient with normal cardiovascular and pulmonary function, the CVP is a useful monitor that should be used by the anesthesiologist in the following circumstances:

1. Surgical procedures in which large fluctuations of blood volume are anticipated (e.g., blood loss, transudation of fluid)

2. Hypovolemic or potentially hypovolemic patients (e.g., bowel obstruction, ascites, chronic hypertension)
3. Patients in shock (i.e., hemorrhage, anaphylaxis)
4. Severely traumatized patients

In the above circumstances, the trend of change in the CVP is usually more significant than the absolute pressure. Moreover, the CVP should be interpreted in the light of other indicators of cardiovascular function. For example, a declining arterial blood pressure and urine output may indicate cardiac failure in the presence of a rising CVP, or they may reflect hypovolemia with a low or falling CVP. In the latter case, a rapid infusion or fluid or blood may be given until a satisfactory arterial blood pressure is established or until the CVP rises to an abnormally high level (>15 mm Hg), at which point an inotropic drug may be indicated.

In patients with cardiac disease and abnormal ventricular function, the use of a Swan-Ganz catheter is usually indicated to monitor both right and left heart filling pressures. In the face of vena caval obstruction, pulmonary embolism, pulmonary hypertension, right ventricular failure, or cardiac temponade, it may be equally or more important to monitor the CVP than the left-sided filling pressures, and in some cases the Swan-Ganz catheter may be contraindicated. Obviously, the less expensive CVP catheter with its lesser risk of complications is preferable to the Swan-Ganz catheter when the latter is not indicated.

Observation of venous pressure waves on an oscilloscope or recorder is sometimes useful in the patient with cardiac disease. The *a* wave is absent in atrial fibrillation, is inconsistent in the presence of atrioventricular conduction block, and is very large (Cannon wave) if the atrium contracts against a closed tricuspid valve (e.g., junctional rhythm). Large *a* waves are also seen in the presence of tricuspid stenosis, right ventricular hypertrophy, pulmonic stenosis, and pulmonary hypertension. A large *v* wave is seen when there is tricuspid regurgitation. Similar changes are present in left atrial and pulmonary capillary wedge pressures associated with comparable functional derangements of the left atrium and ventricle.

It must be remembered that the CVP reflects primarily right heart function and is not a reliable indicator of left ventricular performance. Left ventricular failure and pulmonary edema can be present, especially on an acute basis, and the CVP may remain well within the normal range.[70]

Central venous cannulation is indicated for CVP monitoring and for a variety of other reasons (Table 13-15). It can be accomplished by way of a number of venous routes, and the techniques for each are best learned from a tutor. The choice of a particular site for central venous cannulation is determined by accessibility, convenience, success rate in directing the catheter to the central venous circulation, risk to the patient, and probable duration of use. Cannulation at any particular site is contraindicated by the presence of infection at the site and by the inclusion of the site in the surgical field.

The highest success rate of localizing the catheter in the superior vena cava or right atrium is achieved through the right internal jugular vein, which is a convenient and accessible route in most patients. There is a risk of cannulating the carotid artery, although this can be reduced to a minimum by careful adherence to proven techniques and especially the utilization of a small-caliber needle (22-gauge, 1.5-inch length) to localize the internal jugular vein prior to insertion of the larger bore catheter (Table 13-16 and Fig. 13-3). Relative contraindications to using the internal jugular route include heparinization of the patient at the time of cannulation, previous surgery of the

TABLE 13-15. Indications for Central Venous Cannulation

Central venous pressure monitoring (see text)
Lack of peripheral veins for cannulation
Intravenous administration of vasopressors, potassium, and other drugs likely to injure peripheral veins and tissues; also to reduce the delay in onset of drug action
Rapid infusion of blood and fluids
Removal of blood for later reinfusion (autologous transfusion)
Frequent unmixed venous blood sampling
Aspiration of air emboli
Hyperalimentation
Transvenous insertion of temporary pacing leads
Right heart catheterization studies
Insertion of a pulmonary artery catheter (Swan-Ganz)
    Pressure measurements
    Cardiac output determinations by thermodilution
    Pulmonary angiography
    Mixed venous blood sampling

TABLE 13-16. Sequence of Steps in Cannulating the Right Internal Jugular Vein

1. Patient's head lying flat (no pillow) and rotated completely to left.

2. Palpate lateral aspect of the medial head and medial aspect of the lateral head of the sternocleidomastoid muscle as it divides to insert on the sternum and clavicle. A triangle will be formed with the clavicle as its base and the apex located approximately 6 cm (3 average-sized fingerbreadths) above the clavicle. The apex in some people is higher than 3 fingerbreadths above the clavicle; in this case, the 6 cm distance is a more reliable guide than the muscular apex of the triangle. The presence of arterial pulsation within the triangle may contraindicate an attempt to cannulate the internal jugular vein at this lower level.
   (a) An alternative approach can be made at a higher level by palpating the carotid artery just below the angle of the mandible with the patient's head rotated less than completely to the left. The internal jugular vein will lie approximately 1 cm lateral to the carotid arterial pulse.
   (b) If the patient is to be anesthetized before cannulation of the internal jugular vein, it is useful to mark the skin (light markings to avoid tatooing by the needle) over the muscular landmarks while the patient is awake and able to tense the muscles.

3. Prepare the area with antiseptic (e.g., povidone-iodine, Betadine). Cover the surrounding area with a sterile drape and follow sterile technique until the procedure is completed. Infiltrate the skin and subcutaneous tissue at the apex of the triangle with a local anesthetic (0.5 percent lidocaine HCl).

4. Place the patient in an appropriate degree of head-down, legs-up position to distend the vein.

5. Verify the medial location of the carotid artery and the absence of arterial pulsations within the triangle. Starting at the apex direct the needle toward the middle third of the clavicle at a 30 degree angle to the skin and advance the needle while maintaining a slight negative pressure with the syringe plunger. Normally two "pops" will be felt: the first the carotid sheath and the second the vein wall. Using a 21-gauge 1.5-inch needle on a 5-ml syringe containing 1 ml of 0.5 percent lidocaine HCl, identify the internal jugular vein.

   If the vein is not identified when the full length of the needle is inserted, gradually withdraw it while maintaining negative pressure in the syringe; sometimes the needle will have penetrated the back wall of the vein. A Valsalva maneuver by the patient will distend the vein. If unsuccessful, redirect the needle more laterally; if unsuccessful, try a more medial direction with cautious awareness of the carotid artery.

   The color of the blood drawn into the syringe provides a clue to whether it is venous or arterial as long as two points are remembered.
   (a) The local anesthetic remaining in the syringe will make the original blood entering the syringe appear brighter red, but venous-colored blood will be evident as additional blood is withdrawn.
   (b) The PvO$_2$ may be elevated if the patient is breathing oxygen-enriched gases.

   The vein diameter is approximately the same as the patient's thumb; it should be possible to maintain a withdrawal of blood while advancing or withdrawing the needle a distance of 1 to 2 cm in a normal size adult male.

   If there is concern about the possibility of arterial puncture, three steps can be considered:
   (a) Remove the syringe from the needle and see whether there is a spurting flow of blood, from the needle left in the vessel, indicating arterial puncture. Absence of spurting blood does *not* guarantee that arterial cannulation has not occurred.
   (b) If there is an arterial cannula in the patient, ask an assistant to withdraw a sample of arterial blood into a syringe identical to that you are using to locate the vein. Comparing the color of blood in the two syringes held side by side and in the same angle to the source of light usually is sufficient to determine the difference between arterial and venous blood.
   (c) Determine the PO$_2$ of the blood withdrawn from the vessel in the neck.
   (d) Remove the needle, compress the vessel, and start over or choose an alternate site for venipuncture and cannulation.

6. If the vein is properly located, inject the local anesthetic-blood solution as the needle is withdrawn in order to anesthetize the track that will be followed when the larger needle-cannula is inserted.

7. Insert the CVP-size cannula in exactly the same direction that was followed by the localizing needle. Two methods are used to insert the CVP cannula:
   (a) An 18-gauge 1¾ inch cannula is inserted, a guide wire passed through it, the 1¾ inch cannula removed, and then the CVP cannula is passed over the guide wire into the vein (Seldinger technique). This technique requires that a dilator or dilating type cannula be used to penetrate the subcutaneous tissues and vein wall *after* a small 2 to 3 mm puncture of the skin has been made with a scalpel blade inserted *directly against* the guide wire. The Seldinger approach is used for insertion of a Swan-Ganz type catheter (see Table 13-21).
   (b) The large bore cannula of at least 5 inches in length, is inserted directly. The cannula can be over the needle or within the needle.

continued

TABLE 13-16 *(continued).* **Sequence of Steps in Cannulating the Right Internal Jugular Vein**

8. The success of central venous cannulation can be verified by (a) the lack of a spurting flow of blood, (b) easy withdrawal of venous-colored blood (a direct side-by-side comparison with arterial blood in a similar syringe should clearly demonstrate a difference in color), and (c) appropriate pressures and pressure wave forms for a CVP.

9. The cannula should be secured in place and the puncture site of the skin dressed with a sterile bandage. The site should be inspected periodically to detect evidence of hematoma formation and any change in the position of the cannula (i.e., to prevent dislodgement, kinking).

10. The external opening of the cannula should be closed by the operator's finger or by a cap to prevent venous air embolism. The patient should be returned to the normal supine or head-up position *only after* connecting the cannula to the pressure transducer or manometer in order to avoid the aspiration of air emboli through the cannula. It is also helpful to have the patient hold his breath in inspiration whenever the cannula is transiently open to air.

neck (e.g., thyroidectomy, carotid endarterectomy), distortion of anatomic relationships by tumor or trauma, and the inability to position the patient's head properly. Complications associated with internal jugular cannulation are those of any other route plus some specific ones (Table 13-17).

The availability of the J-wire guide for directing catheters past bends and branching of vessels has increased the success rate of localizing the catheter tip in the central circulation by way of the external jugular veins.[71,72] Cannulation of the external jugular vein avoids the

TABLE 13-17. Complications of Central Venous Cannulation

General
  Infection — local and systemic
  Tissue trauma — nerve, artery, vein injuries
  Hematoma and extravasation of infused substances
  Thrombophlebitis
  Catheter shearing and embolization
  Air embolism
  Perforation of vena cava or right atrium by catheter
    Mediastinal infusion of fluids
    Pericardial tamponade
    Hydrothorax, hemothorax
Specific sites
  Internal jugular cannulation
    Carotid artery puncture (hematoma, airway compression, arteriovenous fistula)
    Brachial plexus injury
    Thoracic duct perforation (left internal jugular vein cannulation)
    Pneumothorax
  Subclavian cannulation
    Subclavian artery puncture (hemothorax)
    Pneumothorax
  Femoral cannulation
    Femoral artery puncture (retroperitoneal hemorrhage)
    Femoral nerve injury
    Inferior vena cava perforation (retroperitoneal infusion of substances)
    Venous thrombosis and emboli

risks of inserting a needle deep into the neck. The high incidence of major complications has reduced the use of the subclavian vein by anesthesiologists. There is a low rate of success in reaching the central venous circulation by way of basilic and cephalic arm veins.[73] The femoral vein can be used providing the catheter is sufficiently long to reach the mediastinal level of the vena cava; the possibility of cannulating branches of the inferior vena cava is present.

Measurement of venous pressures can be done with a simple manometer filled with isotonic aqueous solution or with a pressure transducer system similar to that described for direct arterial pressure measurement (but with a higher gain to measure smaller changes and lower pressures). The recording of venous pressure waves requires a pressure transducer with a high-frequency response. Several technical points should be remembered:

1. Different units of pressure may be used; 1.36 cm H_2O equals 1 mm Hg or 0.74 mm Hg equals 1 cm H_2O. One kilopascal (kPa) equals 7.5 mm Hg or 10.2 cm H_2O.

2. The zero point of the manometer or transducer must be positioned exactly if low venous pressures are to be measured accurately and reproducibly; the right atrium is usually considered as the zero level, and it corresponds to the midaxillary line in the supine patient who has normal anatomy of the spine and thorax.

3. Changes in the CVP occur with ventilation because changes in intrathoracic pressure are readily transmitted through the pericardium and relatively thin-walled atrium and vena cavae. During spontaneous ventilation, inspiration lowers the CVP. Positive pressure ventilation and all forms of positive airway pressure raise the CVP as does coughing or any

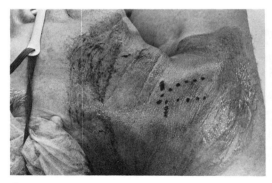
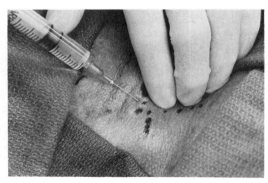

A   B

FIG. 13-3 Cannulation of the right internal jugular vein for insertion of a Swan-Ganz catheter. (A) Dotted lines on the skin of the neck indicate the lateral aspect of the medial head of the sternocleidomastoid muscle and also the medial aspect of the lateral head to form a triangle with the clavicle as its base. The apex of the triangle is slightly more than 5 cm above the clavicle along the medial head of the sternocleidomastoid muscle. The skin has been swabbed with Betadyne. The patient is breathing oxygen delivered by nasal prongs. (B) After applying sterile drapes, the anesthesiologist's fingers on the left hand are positioned along the medial head of the sternocleidomastoid muscle and the thumb and heel of his hand are resting on the mandible of the patient to encourage the patient to maintain leftward rotation of his head. A 1½ inch, 21-gauge ("finder") needle is inserted in the skin 5 cm above the clavicle along the medial head of the sternocleidomastoid muscle, and the needle is attached to an empty 5-ml syringe with the plunger withdrawn to create a vacuum into which blood will flow when the vein is entered.

Valsalva maneuver. (These CVP changes provide an indication of the central location of the CVP catheter tip, but do not prove it.) Changes in thoracic and mediastinal pressures as a result of the accumulation of air, fluid, and blood are also reflected in the CVP.

PULMONARY ARTERY PRESSURE

Availability of the balloon-tipped, flow-directed catheter (Swan-Ganz[74]) provides the anesthesiologist with an easy method of measuring pulmonary artery and left heart filling pressures in almost any patient. Swan-Ganz catheters are now produced with features that permit the measurement of central venous pressure (CVP) and pulmonary artery pressure (PAP) including diastolic (PAdP), systolic (PAsP), mean ($\overline{PAP}$), occluded (PAOP) or wedge (PAWP), or pulmonary capillary wedge pressure (PCWP). Samples of mixed venous blood can be obtained from the pulmonary artery (e.g., for measurements of PvO_2 and calcu-

lation intrapulmonary shunt) and to administer drugs into the central venous circulation or directly into the pulmonary artery (e.g., vasodilators). Most importantly, the inclusion of a thermistor permits the measurement of cardiac output (CO) by thermodilution and the calculation of systemic (SVR) and pulmonary (PVR) vascular resistances. The incorporation of bipolar electrical lead wires makes it possible either to monitor endocardial atrial and ventricular ECGs or to pace the heart with an external pacemaker. Catheters are also made for angiographic studies, oxyhemoglobin measurements, and right-sided cardiac catheterization of pediatric patients. These features can be utilized to great advantage by the anesthesiologist in the operating room and ICU for diagnostic, monitoring, therapeutic, and investigational purposes.

Data obtained with the aid of the Swan-Ganz catheter can be used to calculate hemodynamic variables of importance to the anesthesiologist. In addition to SVR and PVR, stroke volume, subendocardial coronary perfusion pressure, and several indices of cardiovascular performance can be estimated.

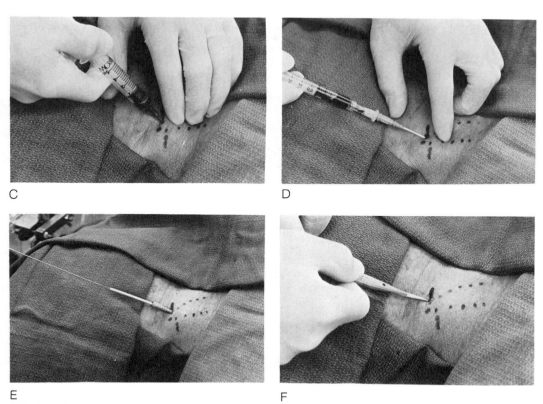

C   D

E   F

FIG. 13-3 (continued) (C) Venous blood is seen in the syringe indicating the location of the needle tip in the vein. The needle syringe unit will be withdrawn and replaced by a 1 ¾ inch, 18-gauge Teflon catheter-over-needle unit on a 3-ml syringe. The insertion of this unit will be at the same point on the skin and it will be inserted in exactly the same direction as the "finder" needle had been previously inserted to enter the internal jugular vein. (D) As blood is withdrawn into the syringe, the Teflon catheter-over-needle unit is advanced a few mm into the length of the jugular vein while blood is being withdrawn continuously. Once the tip of the Teflon catheter is inside the vein, the catheter is slid forward while the needle-syringe unit is held in a constant position. (E) A 0.9 mm × 40 cm flexible guidewire has been inserted through the 18-gauge Teflon catheter into the jugular vein. (F) A 3-mm incision in the skin is made with a scalpel blade directly in contact with the guidewire (hidden behind the blade) in order to facilitate insertion of the dilator-sheath unit. *(Figure continues on next page.)*

INDICATIONS

Indications for the preoperative insertion (intraoperative use) of a particular Swan-Ganz catheter are still evolving and differ among individual anesthesiologists. They are summarized in Table 13-18. Its potential usefulness to the anesthesiologist intraoperatively is illustrated in terms of differential diagnosis (e.g., see Table 13-19) and as a guide to therapy.

INTERPRETATION

Interpretation and application of information obtained with a Swan-Ganz catheter requires a good understanding of normal physiology (also see Ch. 33) as well as of individual disease states. Some generalizations and specific limitations should be remembered.

Normal hemodynamic values are shown in Table 13-20. In *normal* individuals the fol-

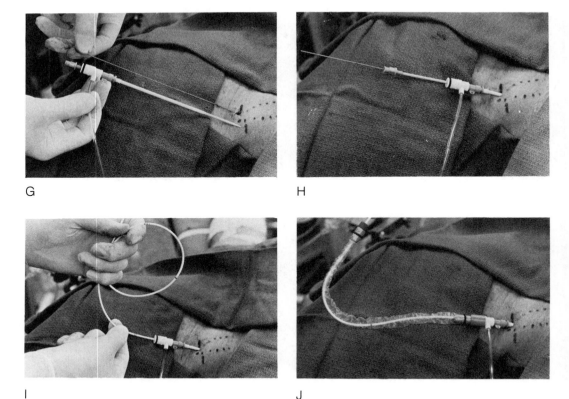

G   H

I   J

FIG. 13-3 (continued) (G) An 8-Fr dilator-sheath unit with a connector containing a side port for fluid infusion is aligned with the guidewire before insertion of the dilator. (H) The dilator sheath unit has been advanced into the jugular vein, the sheath is inserted to its full length except for approximately 1.5 cm, and the dilator and guidewire have been partially withdrawn. (I) A triple-lumen Swan-Ganz pulmonary artery catheter is being inserted through the side-arm connector and sheath into the internal jugular vein and, with continuous monitoring of the ECG and the venous pressure waves at the catheter tip (distal port), the balloon on the tip of the catheter is inflated and the catheter will be advanced to a wedge position in the pulmonary artery. Notice the 20-cm mark on the pulmonary artery catheter near the side-arm connector of the sheath. Other markings evident on the catheter are the four lighter markings indicating the 40-cm length and the single dark thicker marking indicating the 50-cm mark on the length of the catheter. (J) The catheter has been advanced into the wedge position at a distance of approximately 50 cm from the site of insertion. A sterile sleeve that was placed on the pulmonary artery catheter before its insertion has now been advanced in order to maintain sterility of the first 15 to 20 cm of the pulmonary artery catheter external to the patient. This will allow subsequent adjustments of the catheter so as to keep its tip in a proper position within the pulmonary artery.

lowing are true (~ approximates; = equals; ∞ is proportional to):

LAP ~ PAWP ~ PAdP ~ CVP
LAP ~ LVEDP
LVEDP ∞ LVEDV
LV performance ∞ LVEDV
LV output = RV output

In general, these variables tend to change in the same direction, and it is the degree of change rather than the absolute number that is usually more important. The RVEDP and CVP tend to be about 5 mm Hg lower than the LVEDP and its representatives. The important point is how closely they correlate as ventricular preload and afterload change. A close corre-

TABLE 13-18.   Indications for the Preoperative Insertion of a Swan-Ganz Catheter

Noncardiac surgery*
  Heart disease
    With suspicion or evidence of imparied left ventricular function (e.g., heart failure)
    Severe coronary artery disease, especially with evidence of left ventricular dysfunction on exertion or with angina
      pectoris
    Severe, uncontrolled systemic arterial hypertension, especially with left ventricular hypertrophy
    Pulmonary hypertension (cor pulmonale)
    Valvular disease
    Pericardial disease with evidence of tamponade
  Unstable circulation
    Massive trauma
    Extensive burns
    Hypotensive shock
    Sepsis
  Suspected or diagnosed pulmonary emboli
  Aortic surgery with anticipation of crossclamping
  Portal systemic shunt surgery; severe portal hypertension with cirrhosis
  Severe respiratory failure

Cardiac surgery†
  Coronary artery revascularization with
    Poor, left ventricular function: ejection fraction <0.4, left ventricular end-diastolic pressure (LVEDP) >18 mm Hg,
      regional hypokinesis, dyssynergy, or asynergy
    Recent myocardial infarction
    Complication of myocardial infarction (e.g., ventricular aneurysm, septal rupture, mitral valvular insufficiency and
      papillary muscle dysfunction)
    Extensive coronary obstruction (e.g., triple vessel disease) with evidence of impaired ventricular performance during
      ischemia (e.g., LVEDP increases by more than 10 mm Hg or is greater than 18 mm Hg after injection of contrast
      media into coronary arteries)
    Diffuse coronary atherosclerosis especially in distal vessels (anticipate impaired ventricular function after cardiopulmo-
      nary bypass due to poor myocardial preservation by cold hyperkalemic perfusion of coronary arteries and incom-
      plete revascularization)
    Valvular heart disease
  Mitral or aortic valvular replacement
  Pulmonary hypertension
  Hypertrophic obstructive cardiomyopathy, e.g., idiopathic hypertrophic subaortic stenosis (IHSS)
  Pericardiectomy with evidence of tamponade

* While major surgery involving significant blood and fluid replacement provides the strongest indication for use of the Swan-Ganz catheter in patients with the diseases listed, its use may also be advisable for some patients undergoing minor surgery while receiving a major anesthetic.

† The Swan-Ganz catheter is useful during cardiopulmonary bypass to detect elevations of pulmonary capillary pressure caused by the accumulation of blood in the absence of a functioning left ventricular vent. Elevated capillary hydrostatic pressure coupled with reduced oncotic pressure (i.e., hemodilution) can lead to pulmonary edema.

TABLE 13-19.   The Swan-Ganz Catheter in the Differential Diagnosis of Low Cardiac Output

Etiology of Low Cardiac Output	RAP or CVP	PAWP	PAdP vs PAWP
Hypovolemia	Low	Low	PAdP = PAWP
Left ventricular failure	Normal or high	High	PAdP = PAWP
Right ventricular failure	High	Normal or low	PAdP = PAWP
Pulmonary embolism	High	Normal or low	PAdP > PAWP
Pulmonary hypertension	High	Normal*	PAdP > PAWP
Cardiac tamponade	High	High	PAdP = PAWP

* In the absence of valvular disease.
  Abbreviations used: RAP = right atrial pressure, CVP = central venous pressure,
PAWP = pulmonary artery wedge pressure, PAdP = pulmonary artery diastolic pressure.

TABLE 13-20. Normal Pressures in the Cardiovascular Systems of Recumbent Adults

Location	Abbreviation	Pressure (mm Hg) Mean	Range
Central venous	CVP	6	1–10
Right atrium	RAP	4	−1–+8
Right ventricle			
Systolic	—	24	15–28
End-diastolic	RVEDP	4	0–8
Pulmonary artery			
Systolic	PAsP	24	15–28
Diastolic	PAdP	10	5–16
Mean	PAP	16	10–22
Pulmonary artery or capillary wedge or pulmonary artery occlusion pressure	PAWP or PCWP or PAOP	9	6–15
Left atrium	LAP	7	4–12
Left ventricle			
Systolic	—	130	90–140
End-diastolic	LVEDP	7	4–12
Brachial artery			
Systolic	sBP	130	90–140
Diastolic	dBP	70	60–90
Mean	BP or MAP	85	70–105

(Modified from Schlant RC, Sonnenblick EH, Gorlin R: Normal physiology of the cardiovascular system, The Heart. 5th Ed. Edited by Hurst JW. New York, McGraw-Hill, 1982, p 93.)

lation between CVP and PCWP changes produced by alterations of preload in patients with ischemic heart disease and normal left ventricular function (ejection fraction >0.5) has been shown, but there are two important reservations about these findings.[74a] First, in some cases there was a much greater change in PCWP than in CVP, and unless the relationship was determined for a particular patient under specific circumstances, a small change in CVP could be associated with a much larger change in PCWP.[74b] Second, changes in the compliance of the right and left ventricle may differ in degree and probably occur frequently in the patient with ischemic heart disease.[74c]

Thus, although some of these generalizations may be true in patients with certain cardiovascular diseases, they often must be verified in the particular patient; and it may prove worthwhile to do so. For example, it may be useful to record the PAWP and the PAdP simultaneously over the range of pressures encountered as time passes. If there is a close correlation, the PAdP can be used in place of the PCWP should it become impossible or undesirable to obtain wedge pressures because of bal-

loon malfunction or a change in the location of the catheter tip.

The generalizations clearly do not apply in certain disease states. For example, pulmonary diastolic hypertension (increased PVR) distorts the relationship of PAdP to PAWP and LAP. The presence of mitral stenosis or of a mitral valvular prosthesis creates a gradient between LAP and LVEDP. The proportionality between LVEDV and LVEDP is not linear under any condition and is markedly altered by changes in ventricular compliance (elastance) that are common in patients with heart disease, such as ↑compliance by nitroglycerin; ↓compliance by ischemia, sympathetic stimulation, or inotropic drugs (see Fig. 13-4).[75] Any left to right shunt (e.g., atrial or ventricular septal defect) will increase right ventricular output and thermodilution measurements of cardiac output while reducing left ventricular output. The application of positive pressure to the airway alters the intracardiac and pulmonary artery pressures. It is customary to make pressure measurements at the end-expiration to provide consistency. The use of positive end-expiratory pressure (PEEP) or continuous positive airway

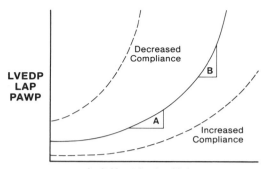

FIG. 13-4 Relationships between ventricular volume and pressure (elastance or compliance). At the lower portion of the curve (A) elastance is greater than at the upper portion (B) where a smaller increment in volume produces a larger increase in pressure. Examples of factors decreasing compliance include myocardial ischemia, positive end-expiratory pressure, pericardial tamponade, and inotropic drugs. Compliance is increased by correcting ischemia and by drugs such as nitroglycerin. LVEDP=left ventricular end-diastolic pressure; LAP=left atrial pressure; PAWP=pulmonary arterial wedge pressure.

pressure (CPAP) alters the pressure readings (e.g., PAWP may not correlate with LAP when PEEP > 10 cm H_2O). This has led to some controversy about the interpretation of pressure measurements. It would appear that a workable compromise involves following trends of pressure in relationship to other hemodynamic and ventilatory variables rather than focusing on the absolute values; assuming that measurements made under the actual clinical conditions are influencing cardiovascular performance in the manner expected; and most importantly, recognizing that changes in respiratory function and therapy will alter the measurements and probably cardiovascular function as well. Obviously, the effects of sudden large changes must be monitored closely and dealt with appropriately.

TECHNIQUE FOR INSERTION

Techniques for insertion of the Swan-Ganz catheter are best learned from an experienced tutor. The technique outlined in Table 13-21 has been sufficient and safe in our hands.[76] A few points are emphasized below in relation-

ship to minimizing the complications associated with the use of these catheters. Possible sites for insertion are the same as those for central venous cannulation, and again, the highest success rates are associated with the internal jugular route — especially the right internal jugular vein, which provides a straight path into the superior vena cava (Table 13-16 and 13-21 and Fig. 13-3 and 13-5). The limitations, complications, and contraindications related to each percutaneous cannulation site are essentially the same as described for central venous cannulation.

The curved tip containing an inflatable balloon can be used to advantage in directing the catheter to the right atrium (e.g., from a femoral vein) but adds the possibility of damaging veins, especially peripheral ones and those branching from the vena cava if it is inflated carelessly and inappropriately in relationship to the anatomy of the venous system. The balloon should always be inflated slowly and easily; no attempt should be made to inflate it against higher than normal resistance (as determined by the feel of inflating the balloon before its insertion into the body).[77]

COMPLICATIONS

Complications related to the insertion and maintenance of pulmonary artery catheters include the following[78]:

1. Complications related to central venous cannulation can occur (see Table 13-17). Because of the large-bore sheath (8F) required to insert a multilumen pulmonary artery catheter, the consequences of carotid artery cannulation with the dilator sheath are potentially severe, especially in a patient with carotid atherosclerosis, a coagulopathy, or who is or will be heparinized. Should the artery be cannulated, it is crucial *not to remove the sheath*, because it serves two important uses in minimizing the severity of the complication: (1) it occludes the hole in artery limiting the loss of blood and hematoma formation, and (2) it serves as a guide to the surgeon who will have to locate the carotid puncture site and do a primary closure of the hole. Because of the risks of reducing carotid blood flow, exerting pressure

(Text continues on page 450)

TABLE 13-21. **Sequence of Steps in the Insertion of a Swan-Ganz Catheter via the Right Internal Jugular Vein of an Average-Size Adult Patient**

1. Lidocaine (1 to 1.5 mg/kg) should be prepared for immediate intravenous injection in the event of significant dysrhythmias during the insertion procedure.

2. Place an 18-gauge 1¾ inch cannula into the right internal jugular vein as described in Table 13-16 (steps 1 to 7a). Verify the proper location of the cannula by the easy withdrawal of venous blood and the absence of arterial blood. This verification step is very important in minimizing the inadvertent insertion of the guide wire and introducer into extravascular tissues or the carotid artery. (See step no. 8 in Table 13-16.)

3. Insert a 0.9 mm × 40 cm guide wire flexible or J end first through the cannula. It should advance easily to a total distance of approximately 20 cm.

4. Remove the 1¾ inch cannula and with a No. 11 scalpel blade enlarge the cutaneous hole around the wire to a 3-mm slit to facilitate introduction of the dilator and sheath. It is important to insert the scalpel blade directly against the wire so that no strand of skin will obstruct the insertion of the dilator and sheath.

5. Place the dilator-sheath set over the wire but do not advance it into the skin until the external tip of the guide wire extends back beyond the length of the dilator where it can be grasped as needed to withdraw it from the patient. Insert the dilator-sheath set through the skin and subcutaneous tissues and into the vein while twisting (rotating) it back and forth to facilitate its penetration of the tissues. As the dilator-sheat set is advanced, withdraw the guide wire progressively to avoid its internal tip being advanced into the heart. When the sheath is inserted to an appropriate length (9 to 10 cm), remove the guidewire and verify proper placement of the sheath by the easy withdrawal of venous blood (from the dilator or sheath) and leave the syringe on the dilator or sheath to avoid the aspiration of air into the venous circulation. Aspiration of air into the vein is minimized by keeping the patient in a head-down position and by asking the patient to hold his breath at maximum inspiration. Some sheaths have a valve to minimize the risk of air embolism.

6. Prepare the Swan-Ganz catheter for insertion by (a) placing an "external sterility sheath" over the catheter, (b) inflating the 1.5 cc capacity balloon to check its configuration and for absence of leaks, (c) filling the CVP and PA channels with heparinized saline (2 units heparin per ml), and (d) checking the integrity of the electrical leads for the thermistor and pacing functions if these are in the catheter. With the pressure transducer open to the fluid-filled PA channel, the pressure tracing on the oscilloscope screen or writer should reflect vertical motion of the catheter tip.

7. Insert the Swan-Ganz catheter as follows (Fig. 13-3 and 13-5):
   (a) the curved tip of the catheter should be pointed to 11 or 12 o'clock as the catheter is inserted into the introducer sheath and internal jugular vein;
   (b) once the 20 cm mark reaches the hub of the sheath, the balloon should be inflated with 1.5 cc of air and a CVP tracing should be evident on the screen or recorder;
   (c) the catheter should then be advanced gradually as it passes through the right atrium (RA tracing usually evident after 25 to 30 cm of the catheter has been inserted), into the right ventricle (RV tracing at 30 to 35 cm and advanced into the pulmonary artery (PA tracing at 40 to 50 cm);
   (d) once a PA tracing is observed, the catheter should be advanced slowly to the wedge position (PAWP tracing 45 to 55 cm). Proper placement is indicated by a PA tracing when the balloon is deflated and a PAWP tracing when it is inflated. Frequently, the catheter will advance into a continuous wedge position as it becomes more compliant at body temperature and is subject to the continuous drag of flowing blood. Obviously, it will have to be withdrawn to the proper position.

8. With satisfactory positioning of the catheter in the pulmonary artery, the "external sterility sheath" can be connected to the introducer sheath and the sterility of an appropriate length (10 to 15 cm) of the external portion of the Swan-Ganz catheter can be maintained to allow its subsequent repositioning. Be sure to tape the distal end of the "external sterility sheath" to the catheter. Venous blood should be withdrawn from the side port of the introducer sheath (to remove air) and a continuous infusion of fluids through the side port should be maintained to minimize the clotting of blood within the introducer sheath.

9. The site of skin puncture should then be covered with a sterile dressing and the catheter secured so as to avoid kinking and dislodgement. The fluid-filled parts (PA, CVP, VIP) should be flushed intermittently with heparinized saline to prevent blood clotting and obstruction.

10. Some of the commonly encountered problems include:
    (a) Catheter enters the inferior vena cava instead of the right atrium (continuous CVP tracing as it is advanced)—withdraw the introducer sheath by 1 to 1.5 cm and repeat steps listed in item 7.
    (b) Catheter enters right atrium and ventricle but fails to enter pulmonary artery—often remedied by orienting curved tip of catheter toward 11 to 12 o'clock on insertion; may require different orientation; often facilitated by advancing the catheter from the right ventricle as the patient takes a deep inspiration, which increases the blood flow into the pulmonary artery.

continued

TABLE 13-21 *(continued).* **Sequence of Steps in the Insertion of a Swan-Ganz Catheter via the Right Internal Jugular Vein of an Average-Size Adult Patient**

(c) An excessive length of catheter is inserted (i.e., > 60 cm in adult) — coiling is likely, and this can be confirmed by portable anterior-posterior chest roentgenogram; the catheter should be withdrawn carefully and another attempt to insert it correctly should be made.

(d) Dysrhythmias, especially PVCs, can occur during passage of the catheter tip through the pulmonary outflow tract of the right ventricle. Usually these are transient and do not recur once the tip enters the pulmonary artery. If they are persistent and hemodynamically significant then (1) either advance the catheter into the pulmonary artery or withdraw it into a more proximal portion of the right ventricle, (2) administer an antiarrhythmic dose of lidocaine intravenously, and if the dysrhythmias persist or recur, (3) withdraw the catheter from the patient to examine the balloon and tip, and to reorient the curved tip before another attempt at insertion is made.

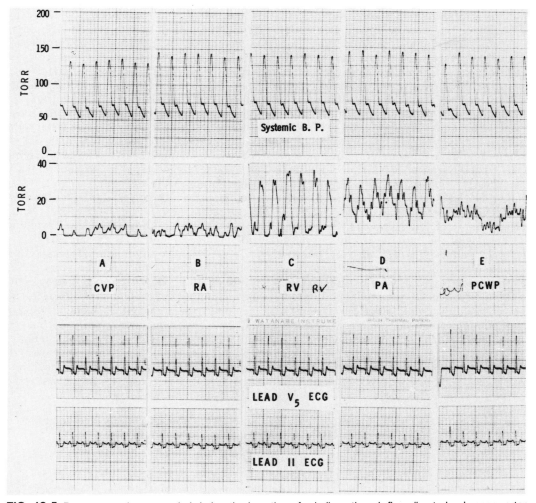

FIG. 13-5 Pressure tracings recorded during the insertion of a balloon-tipped, flow-directed pulmonary artery catheter (Swan-Ganz). The top tracing shows systemic blood pressure, the tracing beneath it shows pressures measured at the tip of the Swan-Ganz catheter as it passed through the superior vena cava, CVP; right atrium, RA; right ventricle, RV; pulmonary artery, PA; and into a wedge position, PCWP. The transient decrease in the PCWP occurred with spontaneous inspiration by the patient. Refer to Table 13-21 for details of catheter insertion.

over the puncture site to limit hematoma formation is inadvisable and may be only partially effective, since the blood can dissect inwardly in the soft tissues of the neck. The occurrence of carotid puncture often is a basis for canceling cardiac surgery with cardiopulmonary bypass. On the other hand, as long as the hole is closed without further complication, the situation is analogous to a combined carotid endarterectomy–coronary artery operation.

2. Perforation of the right atrium, right ventricle, or a pulmonary artery can result in hemopericardium, hemothorax, hemoptysis, or frank bleeding into the airway. Perforation of the right side of the heart and of the pulmonary artery is very unlikely to occur if the catheter is advanced gradually with the balloon inflated and without forcing its insertion. Coiling of the catheter in the heart or vessels should be avoided because its repeated abrasion of the endothelium could lead to erosion of the wall. Coiling is suspected when an unusually long length of catheter is inserted (i.e., greater than 60 cm from the internal jugular puncture site to the wedge position, see Table 13-22) and it can be verified by a standard anterior-posterior chest roentgenogram. Other clues to coiling are the recurrence of dysrhythmias and the apparent flipping of the catheter tip in and out of the right ventricle as indicated by pressure changes. Perforation of a small pulmonary artery can occur especially if the catheter tip is maintained in a continuous wedge position or if the vessel is ruptured by improper inflation of the balloon (i.e., overinflation or inflation against higher than normal resistance).[77]

3. Cardiac dysrhythmias of all types can occur due to contact of any part of the catheter with the wall of the heart, especially the intra-ventricular septum near the outflow track of the right ventricle in the area of the conducting system. Precautions include (1) electrocardiographic, and when appropriate for other purposes, continuous systemic arterial blood pressure monitoring during insertion of the catheter; (2) complete inflation of the balloon to shield the catheter tip when it enters the right ventricle; (3) efficient passage of the catheter through the ventricle and into the pulmonary artery (facilitated by orienting the curved tip of the catheter to 11 or 12 o'clock before inserting it into the right internal jugular vein and by having the patient take a deep inspiration as the catheter is advanced from the ventricle); (4) advancing the catheter into the pulmonary artery or withdrawing the catheter from the ventricle should dysrhythmias persist; (5) having intravenous lidocaine ready to administer rapidly; (6) having a functional defibrillator close at hand; (7) using a Swan-Ganz catheter with pacing leads in a patient with a high risk of developing complete heart block and (8) having an assistant experienced in cardiopulmonary resuscitation in the immediate vicinity. Dysrhythmias may also occur during withdrawal of the catheter after it has been used for some time. A smooth, steady withdrawal avoiding sudden forceful motions is probably best.

4. Pulmonary infarction can result from maintaining the catheter in a continuous wedge position. This can be prevented by limiting continuous inflation of the balloon to less than a few minutes; continuous monitoring of the PAP and immediately withdrawing the catheter should the pressure tracing change to that of the PAWP (the presence of a v wave in the PAWP tracing may lead to its being mistaken for a PAP tracing (Fig. 13-6); avoiding the

TABLE 13-22. Usual Distances from the Site of Percutaneous Venous Insertion of a Swan-Ganz Catheter to Various Locations in Adults

	Range of Distances (in cm) from Vein Puncture Site			
Location	Right Internal Jugular	Right Femoral	Right Antecubital	Left Antecubital
Junction vena cavae and right atrium	20	30	40	50
Right atrium	20–30	30–40	40–50	50–60
Right ventricle	30–40	40–50	50–60	60–70
Pulmonary artery	40–50	50–60	60–70	70–80
Pulmonary artery wedge position	45–55	55–65	65–75	75–85

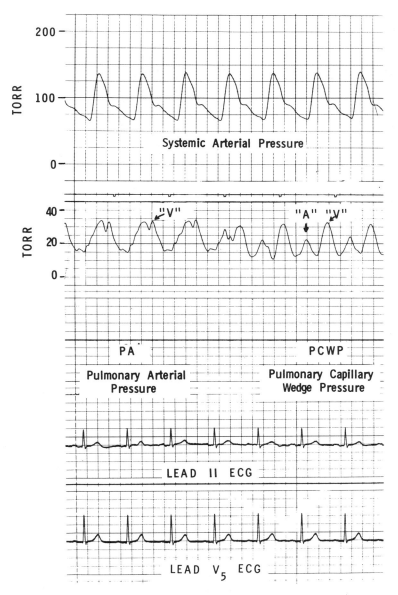

FIG. 13-6 An example of the occurrence of a *v* wave ("V") in both the pulmonary artery and pulmonary capillary wedge pressure tracings from a patient with impaired left ventricular function due to coronary artery disease. Note that the *v* wave in the PCWP tracing could be mistaken for a pulmonary arterial pressure tracing with the catheter in a continuous wedge position.

insertion of excessive lengths of catheter and coiling; and obtaining an anterior-posterior chest roentgenogram as soon as possible after insertion of the catheter (at least during the immediate postoperative period) and daily there-

after to rule out coiling and malpositioning of the catheter.

5. Significant obstruction of total pulmonary blood flow by inflation of the balloon is conceivable after pneumonectomy, in the pres-

ence of significant pulmonary embolism, and in a small patient.[79] This is another reason to observe the overall pattern of hemodynamic changes continuously and to inflate the balloon transiently for PAWP determination.

6. Thrombus formation begins to occur along the catheter immediately after its insertion. This appears to be of little consequence in the short term use of the catheter, but it may be a reason to avoid using it any longer than necessary. It results in a utilization of platelets[80] and theoretically could lead to embolization of the thrombus while the catheter is in position or during its removal. An attempt has been made to reduce the risk of these potential problems by bonding heparin to the surface of the catheter.

7. Infection along the length of the catheter can lead to thrombophlebitis, endocarditis, pulmonary vasculitis and interstitial infection. For this reason, insertion of the catheter should be done under sterile conditions, and prophylactic antibiotics may be indicated.[81,82]

In the intensive care setting, removal of the pulmonary artery catheter, and if necessary insertion of a new catheter through a different site, is recommended with evidence of sepsis, infection at the insertion site, and in the absence of these, no longer than 3 days after its insertion to minimize the risks of bacterial colonization on the catheter.[82]

8. Trauma to cardiac and vascular structures can occur during insertion and withdrawal of the catheter as a result of knotting of the catheter or retained air in the balloon. This is best prevented by avoiding coiling of the catheter and by avoiding kinking, which can obstruct the return of air from the balloon. Any unusual resistance encountered during removal of the catheter should be investigated (e.g., chest roentgenogram) before any further attempt to withdraw the catheter is made.[83]

9. Improper therapy based on misinterpretation of data obtained with the Swan-Ganz catheter. To minimize the incidence of obtaining incorrect data or of misinterpreting data the following procedures, among others, should be done: continuous display of the PAP tracing, continuous or frequent flushing of the catheter with a heparin solution and frequent verification of the catheter's tip location to prevent a continuous wedging in a pulmonary vessel,

TABLE 13-23. Relative Contraindications to the Insertion of a Swan-Ganz Catheter

Lack of experienced personnel*
Lack of suitable pressure monitoring equipment*
Presence of a recently inserted transvenous pacemaker†
Tricuspid or pulmonic valvular stenosis or prosthetic valve (mechanical valve is absolute contraindication)
Frequent ventricular dysrhythmias uncontrolled by antidysrhythmic drugs
Coagulopathy (relative contraindication to the use of internal jugular, subclavian, or femoral vein for insertion)
Bifascicular heart block, especially in combination with first-degree heart block; Mobitz type II second-degree heart block. Use Swan-Ganz catheter with biopolar pacing leads.
Inability to insert catheter into pulmonary artery because of pulmonary hypertension, pulmonic or tricuspid regurgitation, right to left shunt‡

* Virtually absolute contraindications.

† There is less risk of dislodging permanent pacing wires or entangling them with the Swan-Ganz catheter after the wires have been covered with tissue (scar, endothelium). The Swan-Ganz catheter should be inserted cautiously to avoid its coiling within the ventricle, and it should be removed as soon as possible when the patient's condition no longer warrants its use.

‡ The catheter tip should not be left in the right ventricle where it can contact the septum and cause dysrhythmias. A catheter coiled in the ventricle should be withdrawn as soon as the coiling is discovered or suspected and as carefully as possible to avoid entangling the chordae tendinae and papillary muscles.

regular checking of the function of the catheter and the pressure-measuring system; making therapeutic decisions in the light of an evaluation of the total patient and not relying just on a single monitoring device; and careful observation of the responses to therapy.

Contraindications to the insertion of a Swan-Ganz catheter (Table 13-23) are mostly relative to the benefits that may be derived from its use.

CARDIAC OUTPUT

Cardiac output is the volume of blood pumped into the systemic (or pulmonary) circulation each minute. It summarizes the overall performance of the cardiovascular system, but particularly the pumping function of the heart. It is the volume of blood available for tissue perfusion, although the actual blood flow to any specific tissue is regulated by several factors controlling resistance in the arterioles conveying blood to that tissue. Cardiac output is a useful clinical measure to help assess the overall status of the circulatory system.

Blood pressure, the most widely measured hemodynamic variable, is determined by two factors: cardiac output and systemic vascular resistance:

$$BP = CO \times SVR$$

This relationship is important on two counts: if cardiac output and blood pressure are known, the systemic vascular resistance can be calculated (Table 13-24); and it is apparent that blood pressure can be in the normal range even with a low cardiac output, if vascular resistance is sufficiently high. A patient with a very high vascular resistance and an abnormally low cardiac output does not survive very long in that state because tissues and organs are not being perfused adequately even if blood pressure is normal. On that basis, determinations of cardiac output have considerable clinical significance.

INDICATIONS

Indications for measurements of cardiac output in patients undergoing anesthesia and surgery are essentially the same as those listed in Table 13-18. Anytime an assessment of ventricular performance would be useful in diagnosis and therapy, the measurement of cardiac output in relationship to preload (e.g., PAWP) and systemic vascular resistance (i.e., afterload) is indicated.

It is important to note the high frequency at which unexpectedly low cardiac outputs and high vascular resistances are found during the perioperative period when incidental measurements are made in patients whose hemodynamic status otherwise appears satisfactory. The significance of such unexpected findings awaits greater clinical experience and formal studies of the impact of such measurements on the overall results of patient care.

Clearly, cardiac output determinations have become a mainstay in the therapeutic management of the hemodynamically unstable patient in the operating room and intensive care unit.[84-86] The analysis of cardiovascular function and particularly left ventricular performance, in relation to cardiac filling pressures, cardiac output, and systemic vascular resistance, has simplified the therapeutic management of such patients. For example, is hypotension following cardiopulmonary bypass a result of inadequate blood volume, poor myocardial contractility, or low systemic vascular resistance? Under anesthesia produced by nitrous oxide and narcotic analgesics, is a hyper-

TABLE 13-24. Hemodynamic Values for Normal Recumbent Adults

Variable	Abbreviation	Formula	Units	Range
Cardiac output (70 kg, 1.7 m², male)	CO	*	L/min	5–6
Cardiac index	CI	$= \dfrac{CO}{BSA\dagger}$	L/min/m²	2.8–4.2
Heart rate	HR	*	bpm	60–90
Stroke volume	SV	$= \dfrac{CO}{HR} \times 1{,}000$	ml/beat	60–90
Stroke index	SI	$= \dfrac{SV}{BSA\dagger}$	ml/beat/m²	40–65
LV stroke work index	LVSWI	$= \dfrac{1.36\ BP - PAWP}{100} \times SI$	g·m/m²	45–60
RV stroke work index	RVSWI	$= \dfrac{1.36\ PAP - CVP}{100} \times SI$	g·m/m²	5–10
Total resistances				
Systemic vascular (Total peripheral)	SVR (TPR)	$= \dfrac{BP - CVP}{CO} \times 80$	dynes-sec/cm⁵	900–1,400
Pulmonary vascular	PVR	$= \dfrac{PAP - PAWP}{CO} \times 80$	dynes-sec/cm⁵	150–250

* Determine by measurement.

† BSA = body surface area in square meters (m²).

tensive episode better treated with a myocardial depressant such as halothane or with a vasodilating drug such as sodium nitroprusside? In the treatment of cardiac failure with an infusion of catecholamine, is there an undesirable increase in vascular resistance that will impede the pumping of blood by the heart and limit perfusion of vital organs such as the kidney and liver? What conditions of ventricular preload and vascular resistance are best for optimal cardiac performance? (also see Ch. 33.)

METHODS

Methods of measuring cardiac output include thermodilution, dye dilution, the Fick technique, and analysis of the aortic pulse contour.[87-89] The principles underlying each of these techniques are discussed in the references cited along with the details of their application.

Thermodilution has become the most widely used technique in clinical practice for a number of reasons. It can be accomplished with the thermodilution-type Swan-Ganz catheter, and the catheter is usually needed for pressure measurements in the same patients who would benefit from cardiac output determinations. Multiple determinations can be made at frequent intervals. The indicator is a small volume of 5 percent dextrose in water at room temperature or chilled in ice. There is no need for the withdrawal and reinfusion of arterial blood. There is no recirculation of the indicator to confound computations of cardiac output. The measurement is easily made with a portable and compact, though expensive, computer. (Computer costs will probably lessen as catheter sales increase.) With good technique, the measurements by thermodilution are reproducible and correlate closely with those obtained by more traditional methods.

There are several limitations of the thermodilution technique. It measures right heart output and therefore is invalid in the presence of intracardiac and pulmonary-systemic shunts (e.g., atrial and ventricular septal defects, patent ductus arteriosus); it requires the insertion of a Swan-Ganz catheter, which is not always possible or desirable; the speed of injec-

tion and the temperature of the thermal indicator solution should be constant for reproducible results; measurements are affected by ventilation and should be made at end-inspiration for consistency; rapid infusions of fluids and blood, especially when cold, can affect the measurements of cardiac output by thermodilution.

The principle of cardiac output determination by thermodilution is similar to that of other indicator dilution techniques. That is, a known quantity of the indicator is injected at one point, and its concentration is measured at a more distant point after it has been thoroughly mixed with the blood volume that dilutes it. Knowing the initial quantity and measuring the final concentration permits calculation of the dilution volume. In the case of thermodilution, a cold solution is diluted by warm blood; the amount of "cold" injected is known, and the change of temperature over time in the blood passing from the injection site (CVP port of the Swan-Ganz catheter) to the catheter-thermistor site in the pulmonary artery is a measure of the dilution of the "cold" bolus.

VENTRICULAR PERFORMANCE CURVES

Cardiac function in the clinical setting is most easily defined by constructing ventricular performance curves that relate an estimate of ventricular stroke work to an estimate of ventricular end-diastolic volume. This relationship is based on the Frank-Starling law of the heart. It is relatively easy to determine the relationship in the operating room and ICU. Sequential measurements of cardiac output by thermodilution are related to pulmonary arterial wedge pressure which can be varied systematically by tilting the patient (or raising and lowering the legs) so as to increase or decrease the venous return of blood to the heart. The procedure is safe and the consequences of the manipulations readily reversible by repositioning the patient in almost all cases. Ventricular performance curves thus constructed are not only useful in terms of quantitative diagnosis, but they facilitate the selection and the evaluation of cardiovascular therapy.

DERIVED HEMODYNAMIC VARIABLE AND INDICES

With pressure measurements and cardiac output determinations in hand, it is possible to calculate a number of other estimates of cardiovascular performance. These are summarized in Table 13-24. Calculations can be facilitated with a pocket calculator or a computer (programmable calculator). Computers are becoming more common in the operating room suite and intensive care units, and they can easily be programmed to perform these simple calculations.

OTHER MEASURES OF CARDIOVASCULAR FUNCTION

A number of other techniques for assessing cardiac function are employed in clinical research. Their use in patient care outside the investigational setting is currently very limited but, with further refinements, clinical applications will likely develop, especially for those that are noninvasive. Systolic time intervals,[90] echocardiography,[91-93] cardiokymography,[94] radioisotopes in combination with scanning devices[95a] and nuclear magnetic resonance (NMR) are examples of noninvasive methods.[54]

Mixed venous blood oxygen saturation ($S\bar{v}O_2$) is determined by pulmonary and cardiac function and by tissue perfusion and oxygen consumption.[96] In normal adults $S\bar{v}O_2$ averages 75 percent with a range of 68 to 77 percent considered acceptable. Increases in $S\bar{v}O_2$ above this level are uncommon (e.g., left-to-right shunt secondary to sepsis, decreased oxygen utilization secondary to hypothermia or cyanide toxicity). A more common cause is a wedged pulmonary artery catheter (from which mixed venous blood is obtained) beyond which blood stagnates and absorbs oxygen from surrounding alveoli. Decreases in $S\bar{v}O_2$ can result from decreased oxygen transfer in the lung, decreased oxygen transport to tissue, and increased oxygen consumption (e.g., shivering).[97] Because oxygen utilization is less likely to change than its delivery under stable

anesthetic conditions, $S\bar{v}O_2$ can serve as a minute-to-minute indicator of the adequacy of ventilation and cardiac output.[96-98] A sudden decrease of $S\bar{v}O_2$ to below 60 percent warrants investigation. With normal and stable body temperature, inspired oxygen tension and ventilatory conditions, a fall in cardiac output is the most likely cause and it should be measured. Persistent mixed venous oxygen tensions of less than 60 percent indicate cardiac decompensation, below 50 percent are associated with the progressive development of acidosis, under 30 percent compromise CNS function leading to unconsciousness, and less than 20 percent have been followed by permanent neurologic sequelae. Pulmonary oximetry's place in monitoring during anesthesia and intensive care of the hemodynamically unstable patient remains to be determined. Its usefulness lies in its function as a continuous early warning of deteriorating cardiopulmonary function.

In addition to new techniques, modifications and new uses of existing methods may prove useful to the anesthesiologist in the operating room. As for most of the modern sophisticated monitoring techniques, new developments in cardiovascular monitoring are likely to occur primarily in the care of patients undergoing anesthesia and surgery for heart disease. Of current interest is the estimation of myocardial oxygen supply and demand.

Direct measurements of total and regional coronary blood flow (CBF) are largely confined to the research setting. Recognition of the important factors determining CBF has led to the development of some indicators of the potential for coronary perfusion, although each index has its limitations.[99] For example, CBF depends on the coronary perfusion pressure. Also, coronary perfusion, especially in the subendocardium, occurs mostly during diastole when the intracavitary pressure transmitted to the coronary capillaries is lowest. Thus, two indices of the potential for coronary perfusion are as follows:

$$CPP = dBP - LVEDP$$

where CPP = coronary perfusion pressure, dBP = diastolic arterial blood pressure, and LVEDP = left ventricular diastolic pressure, which can be estimated by the PAWP in the absence of certain types of congenital and valvular heart disease; and

$$DPTI = (dBP - LAP) \times d_t$$

where DPTI = diastolic pressure time index, dBP = diastolic arterial blood pressure, LAP = left atrial pressure for which the PAWP can be substituted, and d_t = the diastolic time.

It should be noted that increases in left ventricular filling pressures (LVEDP, LAP, PAWP) will decrease CPP and DPTI and at the same time increase myocardial oxygen demand. Similarly, tachycardia reduces diastolic time and DPTI and increases oxygen utilization by the heart. Most importantly, it has to be recognized that coronary perfusion in the presence of coronary artery obstruction is determined primarily by the resistance at the individual obstructions rather than by LVEDP. Thus, the above indices represent the potential for total coronary perfusion and do not indicate the sufficiency of perfusion of any particular areas of the myocardium, especially those dependent on blood flow through partially obstructed vessels.

Estimates of myocardial oxygen demand are also based on the knowledge of the most important factors that determine it; systolic blood pressure (sBP), LVEDP, heart rate, and contractility. A series of indices of demand have been proposed because no one index has been developed to include all four factors.[100]

The rate of pressure product (RPP) is the product of heart rate and systolic blood pressure:

$$RPP = sBP \times HR$$

The RPP correlates with myocardial oxygen consumption during exercise and bears a fairly constant relationship to the onset of angina pectoris in any one patient with ischemic heart disease. If the RPP for the development of angina or ischemic changes in the ECG is known for a particular patient, the anesthesiologist should attempt to maintain a lower RPP during the perioperative period. In the absence of specific information, it is desirable to keep the RPP at less than 15,000 (e.g., HR <100 bpm, sBP <150 mm Hg). There is controversy about the usefulness of the RPP because an increase in heart rate may be more detrimental than an increase in blood pressure. Increased heart rate

increases oxygen demand and reduces its supply (i.e., less diastolic perfusion time). Increased systolic blood pressure increases oxygen demand but also increases mean and often diastolic blood pressure so that coronary perfusion pressure and oxygen supply tend to increase.

The tension time index (TTI) is the product of heart rate and area under the systolic portion of the aortic blood pressure curve. It can be calculated as

$$TTI = sBP \times Ts$$

where sBP = mean systolic blood pressure, and Ts = duration of systole. The mean systolic blood pressure is not readily determined, and the correlation of TTI with direct measurements of oxygen consumption is not uniformly consistent.

The endocardial viability ration (EVR) has been suggested as an index of subendocardial ischemia under certain conditions. It can be represented as

$$EVR = \frac{DPTI}{TTI} = \frac{\text{oxygen supply}}{\text{oxygen demand}}$$

A normal EVR is above 1.0. Its usefulness in patients with coronary artery obstructions is questionable, since perfusion through the obstructed vessel is determined primarily by resistance at the site of partial obstruction.

RENAL FUNCTION (Also See Ch. 35)

Monitoring renal function intraoperatively is important for two reasons: (1) renal function is intimately linked to the hemodynamic status of the patient and the volume, specific gravity, and composition of urine are sensitive indicators of hypovolemia and deficiencies of cardiovascular performance; and (2) the kidneys are vulnerable to damage from a variety of causes and renal failure accounts for a significant portion of the postoperative morbidity and mortality in critically ill patients.

TABLE 13-25. Indications for the Preoperative Insertion of Urinary Bladder Catheter and Monitoring of Urine Volume, Specific Gravity, and Composition

Hypovolemia (e.g., dehydration, hemorrhage) existing preoperatively or anticipated intraoperatively
Major trauma
Anticipation of the need for transfusion of large volumes of blood
Brain surgery, especially with deliberate dehydration
Extracorporeal circulation
Cardiac surgery
Aortic or renal vascular surgery
Renal disease
Obstructive jaundice, major biliary tract surgery
Sepsis and therapy with nephrotoxic antibiotics
Lengthy or extensive surgery especially in elderly and critically ill patients
Complicated obstetrics (e.g., abruptio placentae)

(Modified from Mazze RI: Critical care of the patient with acute renal failure. Anesthesiology 47:138, 1977.)

The primary means of monitoring renal function intraoperatively involves the collection of urine, which usually necessitates the insertion of a urinary bladder catheter. As with almost any other monitoring device, there are risks associated with bladder catheterization, especially the risk of a urinary tract infection and the associated fever, which presents problems of differential diagnosis and antibacterial therapy that occur during the postoperative period. Obviously, the decision to insert a catheter should be justified by the benefits of monitoring renal function (and by the potential risks of failing to do so). Indications for urinary bladder catheterization prior to surgery are listed in Table 13-25.[101]

The major problem faced by the anesthesiologist in terms of renal function is oliguria. It is widely held that a urine flow rate of <0.5 ml/kg/hr during the perioperative period represents oliguria and should be investigated. It is essential first to rule out mechanical problems in the transfer of urine from the bladder to the urometer (e.g., obstruction of the catheter by mucus plugs, tissue, clots; kinking or disconnection of the tubing; and impairment of gravity drainage by a steep head-down position). Once mechanical problems have been eliminated as the cause of a low recovery of urine, the anesthesiologist is faced with the differential diagnosis of oliguria. This is discussed in detail in Chapters 35 & 45. However, it is worth noting here that the differential diagnosis is facilitated by laboratory analysis of the specific gravity and composition of urine, especially in relation to plasma (e.g., see Table 13-26). Differential diagnosis is also aided by the use of hemodynamic monitoring techniques to evaluate the adequacy of fluid and blood replacement and to determine cardiovascular performance.[101,102]

The anesthesiologist may gain some useful information about nonrenal disorders by observing the appearance of the urine and by making some simple tests of its composition. For example, a pink to port-wine coloration of urine is indicative of hemolysis that may result from cardiopulmonary bypass or from the transfusion of incompatible blood (also see Chs. 39 & 41). Testing the urine from a diabetic patient for glucose and ketones is one way to evaluate the patient's need for insulin. Cloudy urine may indicate a high protein content reflecting myoglobinuria in the traumatized patient, renal damage in the patient with acute tubular necrosis, or the presence of bacteria from a urinary tract infection. Appropriate testing of the urine at the direction of the anes-

TABLE 13-26. Differential Diagnosis of Oliguria

Measure	Physiological Oliguria*	Prenal Oliguria†	Acute Tubular Necrosis
Urinary sodium	<10 mEq/L	<25 mEq/L	>25 mEq/L
Urinary specific gravity	>1.024	>1.015	1.010–1.015
Urine/Plasma osmolality	>2.25	>1.8	<1.1
Urine/Plasma urea	>100	>20	<10
Urine/Plasma creatinine	>60	>30	<10

* Due to the action of antidiuretic hormone.
† Due to poor perfusion of the kidneys.
(Modified from Mazze RI: Critical care of the patient with acute renal failure. Anesthesiology 47:138, 1977.)

TABLE 13-27.   Causes of Body Temperature Changes Intraoperatively

Exposure (skin, operative site, especially open thorax or abdomen)
Mechanical devices (e.g., thermal blankets, heat lamps)
Intravenously administered fluids, blood products
Irrigating solutions, wet packs
Chemical reactions (e.g., polymerization of bone cement — methylmethacrylate)
Alterations of body temperature regulation (e.g., anesthetic effects on the hypothalamus, muscle relaxants prevent shivering)
Deliberate hypothermia, extracorporeal circulation
Disease states (e.g., malignant hyperthermia, thyrotoxicosis, infection)

thesiologist can lead to the early initiation of the appropriate therapy and enhance the possibilities of preserving renal function.

BODY TEMPERATURE

It is common for body temperature to change during anesthesia and surgery for many reasons (Table 13-27). A decrease of 2° or 3°C is usually tolerated without serious adverse consequences except for postoperative shivering, which increases oxygen demand and patient discomfort. There is greater concern about body temperature 2° or 3°C above normal and about temperatures below 34°C (Table 13-28). Because of the high risk of morbidity and mortality associated with above-normal intraoperative temperature and because it is induced by certain anesthetic drugs, the detection of malignant hyperthermia is of special importance to anesthesiologists. For these reasons, it has become standard practice to monitor body temperature in all patients undergoing general anesthesia except for the briefest minor surgical procedures.

Certain patients are especially at risk for significant changes in body temperature. Infants and young children have a large body surface relative to their body mass; as a result they are vulnerable to both hypothermia and hyperthermia from external causes (also see Ch. 49). Their relatively high minute ventilation adds to this vulnerability. Patients with a personal or family history of malignant hyperpyrexia are obviously at unusual risk, perhaps even when the suspected causes (e.g., succinylcholine, halothane) are avoided. Patients undergoing prolonged operations are at risk of hypothermia because of their prolonged ventilation with dry gases through an endotracheal tube; patients undergoing extensive abdominal or thoracic surgery easily become hypothermic because of the exposure of large surface areas in the operative field and because of the inefficiency of warming blankets placed under them.

There are a number of body sites at which body temperature can be monitored (Table 13-29).[54] They differ in the precision with which they reflect the temperature of the body core and in the complications of improper placement of the temperature probe. In most cases, however, it is the direction and rate of change rather than the precise degree of temperature that is of concern to the anesthesiologist.

There are a number of devices including the standard thermometer to measure body temperature.[54,103] Liquid-crystal thermometers are simple and convenient for the measurement of skin temperature, which does not reflect body core temperature under many conditions (Table 13-29). The temperature probes

TABLE 13-28.   Consequences of Hyperthermia and Hypothermia

Hyperthermia (Fever)	Hypothermia
Increased oxygen demand	Decreased oxygen availability
Respiratory and metabolic acidosis	Slowing of metabolically dependent process
Increased ventilatory work	Decreased drug biotransformation
Increased cardiac work	Impaired renal transport processes
Hypovolemia due to evaporation	Altered membrane excitability
Hypoglycemia	Cardiac rate and rhythm changes, CNS depression, coma
Malignant hyperthermia	Shivering
Death	Sympathetic nervous system stimulation, hyperglycemia

TABLE 13-29. Sites of Body Temperature Monitoring

Skin	Varies with subcutaneous blood flow, sweating, radiation and conduction of heat to/from extracorporeal objects
Axilla	Varies with blood flow
Tympanic membrane	Closely approximates temperature of blood perfusing the brain when probe is against tympanic membrane; discrepancies arise when probe is located away from membrane or impacted in cerumen, which acts as an insulator; risks of membrane perforation and hemorrhage
Nasopharyngeal	Reflects temperature of blood going to brain; nasal probes can cause epistaxis
Oropharyngeal and upper esophagus	Reflects temperature of respiratory gases
Lower esophagus (20 cm below pharyngoesophageal junction)	Closely approximates temperature of aortic blood (core temperature)
Rectum	Varies with blood flow, fecal mass acts as an insulator
Urinary bladder[104]	Catheter with thermistor can be used to measure core temperature
Pulmonary artery (Swan-Ganz thermodilution catheter)	Measures the temperature of blood in the body core except with pericardial irrigation during cardiac operations
Muscle	Requires special probe; varies with blood flow

most commonly used in modern operating rooms are thermistors made of semiconductive elements in which electrical resistance varies with temperature. Others are thermocouples in which voltage produced by an electromotive force between two different metals depends on the temperature difference between the probe end of the thermocouple and a standard "cold" junction. Although they are relatively sophisticated and sturdy devices, they occasionally malfunction. The wise anesthesiologist regularly evaluates their function in order to minimize the occurrence of spurious readings. And when unexpected and extreme temperature readings are made, the anesthetist should verify their accuracy by another means.

invaluable to the management of anesthetized and critically ill patients. It is essential that the anesthesiologist understand the laboratory procedures and methods in order to recognize the potential sources of errors. It is important for the laboratory to function efficiently; accurate results should be produced in a minimum time to permit the anesthesiologist to identify problems and recognize trends in time to take corrective actions that will minimize the morbidity and mortality of patients under his or her care. Obviously, the accuracy of the results is of primary importance. The anesthesiologist should be alert to the possibility of technical errors, equipment malfunction, and spurious results (e.g., the interchange of samples from different patients). The anesthesiologist should always attempt to correlate the biochemical data with that derived from physiologic monitoring.

THE ANESTHESIA LABORATORY[105]

It is common for anesthesia departments to operate a clinical biochemistry laboratory in close proximity to the operating rooms for rapid determinations of blood gases, Hct and Hb, electrolytes (K^+, Na^+, Ca^{2+}), glucose, osmolality, coagulation studies, and so forth. The information provided by these analyses can be

REFERENCES

1. Saidman LJ, Smith NT (Editors): Monitoring in Anesthesia. 2nd Ed. Boston, Butterworth, 1984
2. Gravenstein JS, Newbower RS, Ream AK, et al (eds): An Integrated Approach to Monitoring. Boston, Butterworth, 1983

3. Gravenstein JS, Newbower RS, Ream AK, et al (eds): Essential Noninvasive Monitoring. New York, Grune & Stratton, 1980

4. Gravenstein JS, Newbower RS, Ream AK, et al (eds): Monitoring Surgical Patients in the Operating Room. Springfield, Ill, Charles C Thomas, 1979

5. Laver MB (ed): Symposium on Monitoring. Anesthesiology 45:113, 1976

6. Bruner JMR: Fundamental concepts of electrical safety. ASA Refresher Courses Anesthesiol 2:11, 1974

7. Ausems ME, Hug CC Jr, de Lange S: Variable rate infusion of alfentanil as a supplement to nitrous oxide anesthesia for general surgery. Anesth Analg 62:982, 1983

8. McPherson RW, Harne BJ: Hemodynamic responses without EEG signs of arousal in patients receiving high dose fentanyl. Anesthesiology 59:A314, 1983

9. Hug CC Jr, Moldenhauer CC: Pharmacokinetics of fentanyl infusions in cardiac surgical patients. Anesthesiology 57:A45, 1982

10. Eger EI II: Anesthetic Uptake and Action. Baltimore, Williams & Wilkins, 1974

11. Quasha AL, Eger EI II, Tinker JH: Determinations and applications of MAC. Anesthesiology 53:315, 1980

12. Ausems ME, Hug CC Jr: Plasma concentrations of alfentanil required to supplement nitrous oxide anesthesia for lower abdominal surgery. Br J Anaesth 55:191s, 1983

13. Scott JC, Ponganis KV, Stanski DR: EEG quantitation of narcotic effect: The comparative pharmacodynamics of fentanyl and alfentanil. Anesthesiology 62:234, 1985

14. Hug CC Jr: Lipid solubility, pharmacokinetics and the EEG: Are you better off today than you were (four) years ago? Anesthesiology 62:221, 1985

15. Murphy MR, Hug CC Jr: The anesthetic potency of fentanyl in terms of its reduction of enflurane MAC. Anesthesiology 57:485, 1982

16. Mainzer J Jr: Awareness, muscle relaxants, and balanced anesthesia. Can Anaesth Soc J 26:386, 1979

17. Editorial: On being aware. Br J Anaesth 51:711, 1979

18. Bogetz MS, Katz JA: Recall of surgery for major trauma. Anesthesiology 61:6, 1984

19. Blacher RS: Awareness during surgery. Anesthesiology 61:1, 1984

20. Levy WJ, Shapiro HM, Maruchak G, et al: Automated EEG processing for intraoperative monitoring: A comparison of techniques. Anesthesiology 53:223, 1980

21. Levy WJ, Grundy BL, Smith NT: Monitoring the electroencephalogram and evoked potentials during anesthesia, Monitoring in Anesthesia. 2nd Ed. Edited by Saidman LJ, Smith NT. Boston, Butterworth, 1984, pp 227–267

22. Stockard J, Bickford R: The neurophysiology of anaesthesia, A Basis and Practice of Neuroanaesthesia. Edited by Gordon E. Amsterdam, Excerpta Medica, 1975, pp 1–46

23. Shapiro HM: Monitoring in neurosurgical anesthesia, Monitoring in Anesthesia. Edited by Saidman LJ, Smith NT. Boston, Butterworth, 1984, pp 269–309

24. Clark DL, Rosner BS: Neurophysiologic effects of general anesthetics: 1. Electroencephalogram and sensory evoked responses in man. Anesthesiology 38:564, 1973

25. Smith NT, Dec-Silver H, Sanford TJ, et al: EEGs during high-dose fentanyl-, sufentanil-, or morphine-oxygen anesthesia. Anesth Analg 63:386, 1984

26. Jones TH, Morawetz RB, Cromwell RM, et al: Thresholds of focal cerebral ischemia in awake monkey. J Neurosurg 54:773, 1981

27. Rampil IJ, Holzer JA, Quest DO, et al: Prognostic value of computerized EEG analysis during carotid endarterectomy. Anesth Analg 62:186, 1983

28. Barash PG, Katz JD, Kopriva CJ, et al: Assessment of cerebral function during cardiopulmonary bypass. Heart Lung 8:280, 1979

29. Slogoff S, Girgis KZ, Keats AS: Etiologic factors in neuropsychiatric complications associated with cardiopulmonary bypass. Anesth Analg 61:903, 1982

30. Levy WJ: Quantitative analysis of EEG changes during hypothermia. Anesthesiology 60:291, 1984

31. Grundy BL, Sanderson AC, Webster MW, et al: Hemiparesis following carotid endarterectomy: Comparison of monitoring methods. Anesthesiology 55:462, 1981

32. Rampil IJ, Sasse FJ, Smith NT, et al: Spectral edge frequency—A new correlate of anesthetic depth. Anesthesiology 53:s12, 1980

33. Levy WJ: Intraoperative EEG patterns: Implications for EEG monitoring. Anesthesiology 60:430, 1984

34. Chiappa KH, Ropper AH: Evoked potentials in clinical practice. N Engl J Med 306:1140, 1205, 1982

35. Bunegin L, Albin MS, Helsel P, et al: Changes in somatosensory evoked responses and cerebral blood flow following induced hypotension. Anesthesiology 53:s46, 1980

36. Lindsey RL: A simple solution for determining shunt flow during carotid endarterectomy. Anesthesiology 61:215, 1984

37. Hill DW: Electrode system for the measurement of blood-gas tensions, content and saturation, Scientific Foundations of Anaesthesia. 3rd Ed. Edited by Scurr C, Feldman S. Chicago, Year Book, 1982, pp 96–108

38. Shapiro BA, Harrison RA, Walton JR: Clinical Application of Blood Gases. 3rd Ed. Chicago, Year Book, 1982

39. Kelman GR, Nunn JF: Nomograms for correction of blood PO_2, P_{CO_2}, pH and base excess for time and temperature. J Appl Physiol 21:1484, 1966

40. Severinghaus JW: Blood gas calculator. J Appl Physiol 21:1108, 1966

41. Ream AK, Reitz BA, Silverberg GD: Temperature correction of PCO_2 and pH in estimating acid-base status: An example of the emperor's new clothes? Anesthesiology 56:41, 1982

42. White FN: A comparative physiological approach to hypothermia. J Thorac Cardiovasc Surg 82:821, 1981

43. Foster RB, Zaidan JR, Mullins R, et al: Effect of $PaCO_2$ management during CPB on post CPB cardiac performance. Anesthesiology 61:A262, 1984

44. Nunn JF: Applied Respiratory Physiology. 2nd Ed. London, Butterworth, 1977

45. Dripps RD, Eckenhoff JE, Vandam LD: Introduction to Anesthesia. The Principles of Safe Practice. 6th Edition Philadelphia, WB Saunders, 1982, pp 264–269

46. Benumof JL: Monitoring respiratory function during anesthesia, Monitoring in Anesthesia. 2nd edition. Edited by Saidman LJ, Smith NT. Boston, Butterworth, 1984, pp 35–77

47. Special symposium: Transcutaneous O_2 and CO_2 monitoring in the adult and neonate. Crit Care Med 9:689, 1981

48. Mazze RI: Therapeutic misadventures with oxygen delivery systems: The need for continuous in-line oxygen monitors. Anesth Analg 51:787, 1972

49. Smalhout B, Kalenda ZA: Atlas of Capnography. 2nd Ed. Vol. 1, Netherlands, Kerckebosch-Zeist, 1981

50. Fink BR: The Human Larynx: A Functional Study. New York, Raven Press, 1975

51. Suter PM, Schlobohm RM: Determination of functional residual capacity during mechanical ventilation. Anesthesiology 41:605, 1974

52. Scurr C, Feldman S (eds): Scientific Foundations of Anaesthesia. 3rd Ed. Chicago, Year Book, 1982

53. Prys-Roberts C (ed): The Circulation in Anaesthesia: Applied Physiology and Pharmacology. Oxford, Blackwell Scientific Publications, 1980

54. Reitan JA, Barash PG: Noninvasive monitoring, Monitoring in Anesthesia. 2nd Ed. Edited by Saidman LJ, Smith NT. New York, Butterworth, 1984, pp 117–191

55. Mandel MA, Dauchot PJ: Radial artery cannulation in 1,000 patients: Precautions and complications. J Hand Surg 2:482, 1977

56. Bedford RF: Wrist circumference predicts the risk of radial-arterial occlusion after cannulation. Anesthesiology 48:377, 1978

57. Bedford RF: Long-term radial artery cannulation: Effects on subsequent vessel function. Crit Care Med 6:64, 1978

58. Mangano DT, Hickey RF: Ischemic injury following uncomplicated radial artery catheterization. Anesth Analg 58:55, 1979

59. Slogoff S, Keats AS, Arlund C: On the safety of radial artery cannulation. Anesthesiology 59:42, 1983

60. Barnes RW, Foster EJ, Janssen GA, et al: Safety of brachial artery catheters as monitors in the intensive care unit — Prospective evaluation with the Doppler ultrasonic velocity detector. Anesthesiology 44:260, 1976

61. Prys-Roberts C: Monitoring of the cardiovascular system, Monitoring in Anesthesia. Edited by Saidman LJ, Smith NT. New York, Wiley, 1978, pp 53–83

62. Adler DC, Byron-Brown CW: Use of the axillary artery for intravascular monitoring. Crit Care Med 1:148, 1973

63. Youngberg JA, Miller ED: Evaluation of percutaneous cannulation of the dorsalis pedis artery. Anesthesiology 44:80, 1976

64. Ersoz CJ, Hedden M, Lain L: Prolonged femoral artery catheterization for intensive care. Anesth Analg 49:160, 1970

65. Lowenstein E, Little JW, Lo HH: Prevention of cerebral embolization from flushing radial-artery cannulas. N Engl J Med 285:1414, 1971

66. O'Rourke MF, Yaginuma T: Wave reflections and the arterial pulse. Arch Intern Med 144:366, 1984

67. Cliffe P: Transducers for the measurement of pressure, Scientific Foundations of Anaesthesia. 3rd Ed. Edited by Scurr C, Feldman S. Chicago, Year Book, 1982, pp 40–52

68. Gardner RM: Direct blood pressure measurement — Dynamic response requirements. Anesthesiology 54:227, 1981

69. Shinozaki T, Deane RS, Mazuzan JE: The dynamic responses of liquid-filled catheter systems for direct measurements of blood pressure. Anesthesiology 53:498, 1980

70. Civetta JM, Gabel JC, Laver MB: Disparate ventricular function in surgical patients. Surg Forum 22:136, 1971

71. Blitt CD, Wright WA, Petty WC, et al: Central

venous catheterization via the external jugular vein: A technique employing the J-wire. JAMA 229:817, 1984

72. Blitt CD, Carlson GL, Wright WA, et al: J-wire versus straight wire for central venous system cannulation via the external jugular vein. Anesth Analg 61:536, 1982

73. Webre DR, Arens JF: Use of cephalic and basilic veins for introduction of central venous catheters. Anesthesiology 38:389, 1973

74. Swan HJC, Ganz W, Forrester JS, et al: Catheterization of the heart in man with the use of a flow directed balloon tipped catheter. N Engl J Med 283:447, 1970

74a. Mangano DT: Monitoring pulmonary arterial pressure in coronary artery disease. Anesthesiology 53:364, 1980

74b. Lowenstein E, Teplick R: To (PA) catheterize or not to (PA) catheterize — That is the question. Anesthesiology 53:61, 1980

74c. Kaplan JA, Wells PH: Early diagnosis of myocardial ischemia using the pulmonary arterial catheter. Anesth Analg 60:789, 1981.

75. Sibbald WJ, Calvin J, Driedger AA: Right and left ventricular preload and diastolic ventricular compliance: Implications for therapy in critically ill patients, *Critical Care. State of the Art.* Vol. 3. Society of Critical Care Medicine, Fullerton, California 1982, pp III(F):1–33

76. Waller JL, Zaidan JR, Kaplan JA, et al: Hemodynamic responses to preoperative vascular cannulation in patients with coronary artery disease. Anesthesiology 56:219, 1982

77. McDonald DH, Zaidan JR: Pressure–volume relationships of the pulmonary artery catheter balloon. Anesthesiology 59:240, 1983

78. Benumof JL: Complications of pulmonary vascular pressure monitoring. Semin Anesth 2:153, 1983

79. Berry AJ, Geer RT, Marshall BE: Alteration of pulmonary blood flow by pulmonary-artery occluded pressure measurement. Anesthesiology 51:164, 1979

80. Kim YL, Richman KA, Marshall BE: Thrombocytopenia associated with Swan-Ganz catheterization in patients. Anesthesiology 53:261, 1980

81. Nagle DM, Levy JH, Waller JL, et al: An improved technique for contamination reduction during central venous cannulation. Anesthesiology 61:A100, 1984

82. Applefield JJ, Caruthers TE, Reno DJ, et al: Assessment of the sterility of long-term cardiac catheterization using the thermodilution Swan-Ganz catheter. Chest 74:377, 1978

83. Fibuch EE, Tuohy GF: Intracardiac knotting of a flow-directed balloon-tipped catheter. Anesth Analg 59:217, 1980

84. Hug CC Jr: Management of hemodynamic instability complicated by hypotension. ASA Refresher Courses Anesthesiol 13:(in press), 1985

85. Barash PG, Chen Y, Kitahata LM, et al: The hemodynamic tracking system: A method of data management and guide for cardiovascular therapy. Anesth Analg 59:169, 1980

86. Forrester JS, Waters DD: Hospital treatment of congestive heart failure. Management according to hemodynamic profile. Ann J Med 65:173, 1978

87. English JB, Hodges MR, Sentker C, et al: Comparison of aortic pulse-wave contour analysis and thermodilution methods of measuring cardiac output during anesthesia in the dog. Anesthesiology 52:56, 1980

88. Ganz W, Swan HJC: Measurement of blood flow by thermodilution. Am J Cardiol 29:241, 1972

89. Guyton AC, Jones CE, Coleman TG: Circulatory Physiology: Cardiac Output and Its Regulation. 2nd Ed. Philadelphia. WB Saunders, 1973

90. Lewis RP, Rittgers SE, Forester WF, et al: A critical review of the systolic time intervals. Circulation 56:146, 1977

91. Beaupre PN, Kremer PF, Cahalan MK, et al: Intraoperative detection of changes in left ventricular segmental wall motion by transesophageal two-dimensional echocardiography. Am Heart J 107:1021, 1984

92. Smith JS, Benefiel DJ, Lurz FW, et al: Detection of intraoperative myocardial ischemia: ECG vs 2-D transesophageal echocardiography. Anesthesiology 61:A158, 1984

93. Glenski JA, Cucchiara RF, Michenfelder JD: Detection of venous air embolism in dog with transcutaneous O_2 and transesophageal echocardiography. Anesthesiology 61:A160, 1984

94. Bellows WH, Bode RH, Levy JH, et al: Noninvasive detection of periinduction ischemic ventricular dysfunction by cardiokymography in humans: Preliminary experience. Anesthesiology 60:155, 1984

95. Pitt B, Strauss HW: Evaluation of ventricular function by radioisotopic techniques. N Engl J Med 296:1097, 1977

95a. Casarella WJ, Berger HJ: Magnetic resonance imaging of the heart and great vessels, The Heart. 6th ed. Edited by Hurst JW. New York, McGraw-Hill, 1985 (in press)

96. Kandel G, Aberman A: Mixed venous oxygen saturation. Its role in the assessment of the critically ill patient. Arch Intern Med 143:1400, 1983

97. Divertie MB, McMichan JC: Continuous monitoring of mixed venous oxygen saturation. Chest 85:423, 1984

98. Waller JL, Kaplan JA, Bauman DI, et al: Clinical evaluation of a new fiberoptic catheter oxim

eter during cardiac surgery. Anesth Analg 61:676, 1982

99. Klocke FJ, Ellis AK, Orlick AE: Sympathetic influences on coronary perfusion and evolving concepts of driving pressure, resistance, and transmural flow regulation. Anesthesiology 52:1, 1980

100. Ream AK: Cardiovascular physiology: Application to clinical problems, Acute Cardiovascular Management: Anesthesia and Intensive Care. Edited by Ream AK, Fogdall RP. Philadelphia, JB Lippincott, 1982, pp 9–44

101. Mazze RI: Critical care of the patient with acute renal failure. Anesthesiology 47:138, 1977 acute renal failure. Anesthesiology 47:138, 1977

102. Bastron RD, Deutsch S: Anesthesia and the Kidney. New York, Grune & Stratton, 1976

103. Cliffe P: The measurement of temperature, Scientific Foundations of Anaesthesia. 3rd Ed. Edited by Scurr C, Feldman S. Chicago, Year Book, 1982, pp 76–80

104. Lilly JK, Boland JP, Zekan S: Urinary bladder temperature monitoring: a new index of body core temperature. Crit Care Med 8:742, 1980

105. Gabel JC, Fallon KD: Monitoring of body chemistry during anesthesia, Monitoring in Anesthesia. 2nd Ed. Edited by Saidman LJ, Smith NT. Boston, Butterworth, 1984, pp 19–34

14

The Electrocardiogram and Anesthesia*

Joel A. Kaplan, M.D.
Daniel M. Thys, M.D.

INTRODUCTION

The electrocardiogram (ECG) is currently used as a routine monitor during anesthesia and surgery. Cannard, Dripps and associates[1] showed the value of the ECG in diagnosing rhythm disturbances during anesthesia back in 1960. Standard limb lead II was used at that time and is still often used to diagnose dysrhythmias, since its electrical axis parallels the electrical axis of the heart and the P wave is usually easily observed. In recent years, coronary artery disease has become the number one health problem in the United States. Patients coming for all types of surgical procedures have significant coronary artery disease, and in these patients, the ECG should be used

to identify myocardial ischemia as well as to recognize dysrhythmias. As many patients are now coming to surgery with pacemakers in place, the ECG enables the physician to evaluate the function of the pacemaker during the surgical procedure. The major uses of the ECG during the perioperative period may be divided into its role during the preoperative, intraoperative, and postoperative periods.

PREOPERATIVE DIAGNOSTIC USES

1. Rate and rhythm disturbances[2] — Bradycardias and tachycardias can be diagnosed as to their site of origin, possible etiologies, and clinical importance. Supraventricular rhythms can be separated from ventricular rhythms and decisions about therapeutic interventions made preoperatively.

2. Ischemic heart disease[3] — Previous my-

* Parts of this chapter are reproduced with modification from Kaplan JA (Editor): Cardiac Anesthesia. New York, Grune & Stratton, 1979, by permission of the publisher.

465

ocardial infarction or myocardial ischemia can be diagnosed from the QRS complex and the ST segments of the ECG. Acute changes indicating ischemia must always be sought during the preoperative period.

3. Chamber enlargement[4] — Atrial and ventricular hypertrophy can easily be diagnosed from the preoperative ECG. Specific chamber enlargements tend to be associated with certain diseases, such as left ventricular hypertrophy with hypertension and left atrial hypertrophy with mitral stenosis.

4. Heart block[5] — Both sinoatrial (SA) and atrioventricular (AV) conduction blocks can be diagnosed. Especially important are combinations of bundle branch blocks of the conduction system. First-degree, second-degree, and third-degree heart block, as well as different types of hemiblocks, can be diagnosed and may even lead to insertion of a pacemaker during the preoperative period.

5. Electrolyte and/or drug effects[6,7] — Such effects can frequently be diagnosed from the preoperative ECG. For example, a tentative diagnosis of hypokalemia and digitalis effect may be important in the anesthetic management of the patient.

6. Pericardial disease[8] — Occasionally pericardial disease may be diagnosed from the preoperative ECG, as pericarditis and pericardial effusions are associated with characteristic ECG abnormalities.

INTRAOPERATIVE USES

1. Dysrhythmia detection[9] is still the most important use of the intraoperative ECG. The ability to separate supraventricular from ventricular dysrhythmias and to assess therapeutic interventions are extremely important uses of the ECG. Common dysrhythmias, such as wandering atrial pacemaker or atrioventricular (AV) dissociation under halogenated anesthetics, may explain hemodynamic changes that occur during the anesthetic procedure.

2. Ischemia detection[10] has become much more important, since we now often anesthetize patients with severe coronary artery disease. Differentiation of inferior wall ischemia

from anterior or lateral wall ischemia is now possible during the intraoperative period.

3. Electrolyte changes frequently occur during anesthesia and mechanical ventilation.[11] Significant changes in potassium as well as calcium levels occur and can be diagnosed with the ECG.

4. Pacemaker function requires continuous evaluation during surgical procedures in patients with permanent pacemakers.[12] This is especially important when the surgical procedure will be carried out near the pacemaker wires or pacemaker unit or when the electrocautery will be used during surgery.

POSTOPERATIVE USES

1. Detection of significant dysrhythmias, with associated changes in blood gases or electrolytes that may be a result of the anesthetic procedure.[13]

2. Diagnosis of myocardial ischemia or infarction that may occur during the postoperative period.[14]

BASIC REQUIREMENTS OF ECG MONITORING

Although monitoring of the ECG has become routine intraoperatively, particular problems pertain to its use in the surgical environment. During surgery, the ECG is read off the oscilloscope and may be recorded if indicated. All operating rooms in which cardiac surgery is performed should have permanent ECG recording capabilities, and portable recorders should be available to all other operating rooms for interesting diagnostic problems. It would be ideal to have a single-channel ECG recorder on all operating room oscilloscope monitors. The recorder is needed to make accurate diagnoses of complex dysrhythmias as well as to permit precise evaluation of changes in the P wave, QRS complex, ST segment, and T wave. In addition, a recorder is frequently needed to ensure that no artifacts are being seen on the oscilloscope. It is preferable to have the recorder make the tracing directly from the patient without going through the additional filtering circuits of the oscilloscope. The presence of a written record of the dysrhythmia is far preferable to the storage, nonfade oscilloscopes that have been employed on some operating room monitors. The ability to store the tracing on the oscilloscope adds little to the capability of diagnosis in the operating room. It certainly does not provide written documentation and a legal record, both of which are provided by a written ECG trace when added to the patient's hospital record. The ECG recorder in the operating room should meet all the standards of accepted cardiology ECG recorders, including types of paper, paper speeds, and markers.

ARTIFACTS ON THE OSCILLOSCOPE

Artifacts on the oscilloscope can be a major problem, as they can lead to incorrect diagnosis during the intraoperative period. The ECG may simulate dysrhythmias under the following conditions:

1. Tremors of various types, as when the patient is awake and shivering in the operating room
2. Hiccoughing or movements of the diaphragm
3. Artifacts in the ECG machine
4. Poor ECG connections
5. Interference from other electrical appa-

ratus, especially the electrocautery or heart–lung machine
6. Interference from contact with other persons

The ECG may produce several types of artifacts as a result of either malfunction or improper adjustment.[15] Loose electrodes may simulate many types of dysrhythmias. Broken electrode wires, as well as hypothermia with shivering, have been reported to produce an ECG pattern easily mistaken for atrial flutter.[16] Artifacts produced by the roller pumps on the heart–lung machine can also create an ECG pattern that resembles atrial flutter (Fig. 14-1).

The biggest electrical problem with ECG monitoring in the operating room is the electrocautery. When the cautery is used, the standard ECG is totally lost as a result of electrical interference. This interference is a combination of radiofrequency current (800 to 2,000 kHz), AC-line frequency (60 Hz), and low-frequency current (0.1 to 10 Hz). Doss et al.[17] have shown that it is possible to modify the ECG preamplifiers so that they will function well in the presence of the electrocautery. It is surprising that this has not been done to more monitoring units designed for use in the operating room.

In addition to the above causes of ECG changes that may occur during surgery, purely mechanical factors can also affect the ECG.[18] Respiratory variation can affect the height of the QRS complex, which is most marked in leads III and AVF. This is due to either a shift of the mediastinum with respirations or a change in volume of the heart with the respiratory effects on venous return. Studies have shown

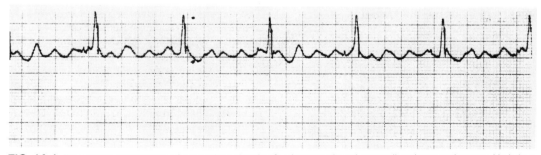

FIG. 14-1 The electrocardiogram of the patient shortly after he was placed on cardiopulmonary bypass. He is in a regular sinus rhythm; however, the ECG appears to show atrial flutter because of an artifact created by the roller pump on the heart–lung machine.

that increases in the ventricular end-diastolic volume lead to increased height of the QRS complex, and that hemorrhage leads to a decreased height of the QRS complex.[19]

The use of ECG telemetry has been tried in a few institutions up to the present time. Most authorities believe that it is not necessary in the modern operating room setting. The advantages of having no hard wires are balanced against disadvantages with technical problems and limitations in capabilities and modifications. However, there are some instances in which it could be extremely useful, such as during neurodiagnostic radiologic procedures [e.g., pneumoencephalography or computed tomography (CT scan)]. In these cases, access to the patient is not very good; wires are totally in the way, easily twisted, and dislodged; and telemetry may be a useful method of monitoring.

The computer has been increasingly employed in the ECG diagnosis of dysrhythmias by cardiologists.[20] However, its intraoperative use as part of a routine monitoring system is still in the future. There are many difficulties with electronic interpretation of the ECG, especially in the area of dysrhythmia analysis when external interference is a common event. The P wave is especially difficult to analyze, since in most leads it has a low amplitude that may be only 50 to 70 percent of the level of external noise. Short periods of time, such as 5 to 10 seconds, are usually sampled, and complex dysrhythmias usually detected with long rhythm strips may be misdiagnosed. The present availability and economics of this computer technology make it primarily a research tool. However, developments in computer design and refinements of programming during the next decade may permit effective use of these techniques in the operating room.

ECG LEAD SYSTEMS

The usual ECG lead systems employed intraoperatively consist of either three, four, or five electrodes. All systems have one electrode on each arm and one on the left leg. The four-wire system has an additional electrode that serves as the ground which is placed on the right leg. In a five-wire system, the fifth electrode is placed on the precordium and is used specifically in the diagnosis of ischemia. The following are the best leads for diagnosing dysrhythmias[21]:

1. V_1 uses the four limb electrodes; the fifth electrode is placed in the fourth intercostal space to the right of the sternum. This lead shows a good atrial deflection and QRS complex and is probably the best surface lead from which to make specific rhythm diagnoses.

2. MCL_1 (modified chest lead I) is a popular lead for cardiac monitoring, dysrhythmia detection, and conduction disturbance monitoring in the coronary care unit.[22] The MCL_1 lead is really a modified V_1 lead. However, it is a bipolar lead with the positive electrode to the right of the sternum in the fourth intercostal space (V_1 position), while the negative electrode is placed near the left shoulder or beneath the left clavicle (Fig. 14-2). This lead system can be set up by placing the left arm electrode beneath the left clavicle and the left leg electrode in the V_1 position and by setting the lead selector switch on lead III.

3. Lead II is the third choice for dysrhythmia detection. It shows a good atrial deflection, but not necessarily a good QRS complex. Overall, this is probably still the most commonly used lead intraoperatively. It allows not only for dysrhythmia detection but for the observation of inferior wall myocardial ischemia as well.

4. CB_5 is a new lead described by Bazaral and Norfleet[23] that permits dysrhythmia detection and observation of anterolateral ischemia. The negative electrode is placed on the right scapula on the back, while the positive electrode is put in the V_5 position. The CB_5 lead has a large P wave, aiding in rhythm diagnosis, and a QRS complex and ST segment similar to that in lead V_5 for ischemia detection.

5. Unipolar or bipolar esophageal leads have been used to record atrial complexes and to diagnose dysrhythmias. The active electrodes are placed in the esophagus as part of an esophageal stethoscope arrangement, and the posterior surface of the left ventricle (LV) and AV junction can be monitored (Fig. 14-3). Kates et al.[24] recently compared the efficacy and

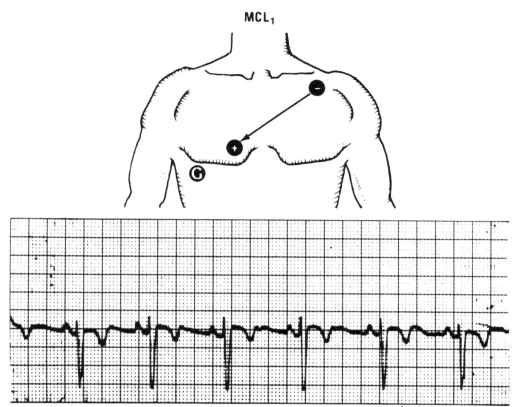

FIG. 14-2 The electrode position and ECG tracing of a typical MCL₁ lead are demonstrated. (Hampton AG: Monitoring and dysrhythmia recognition in advanced life support. American Heart Association Advanced Life Support Course.)

safety of the esophageal ECG with a conventional ECG (leads II and V_5) for the detection of dysrhythmias during anesthesia. Using an intraatrial ECG as the standard, the correct diagnosis was made from leads II and V_5 in 53.8 percent and 42.3 percent of cases, respectively (no significant difference), whereas 100 percent of the dysrhythmias were properly diagnosed from the esophageal ECG lead (see Table 14-1). With the esophageal ECG, P waves could be distinctly recognized and the temporal relationships between atrial and ventricular depolarization could be clearly seen. By contrast, indistinct P waves on standard lead II and precordial lead V_5 resulted in incorrect diagnosis of dysrhythmias, and in two patients dysrhythmias were totally missed (Figs. 14-4 and 14-5).

6. Intracardiac electrocardiography has also been used for diagnostic purposes, since it is relatively easy to obtain these traces. In the past, a long central venous pressure (CVP) cath-

eter was filled with hypertonic saline and advanced into the cardiac chambers. The catheter was attached to the V lead of the ECG by an alligator clip in order to read the tracing. When the catheter reached the superior vena cava, the ECG tracing looked like a normal-lead AVR with inverted P, QRS, and T waves. In the high right atrium, the P wave was large and deeply inverted, in mid-atrium the P wave was biphasic, and in the low atrium it was upright. When the ventricle was entered, the QRS complex became very large. Recently, multipurpose pulmonary artery catheters with both atrial and ventricular ECG and/or pacing electrodes have become available.[25] These catheters permit monitoring of bipolar atrial or ventricular ECGs and diagnosis of complex dysrhythmias using any of the five electrodes placed on the catheter (Fig. 14-6). In addition, the ECG signal from the catheter provides an electrical spike that is relatively insensitive to electrocautery

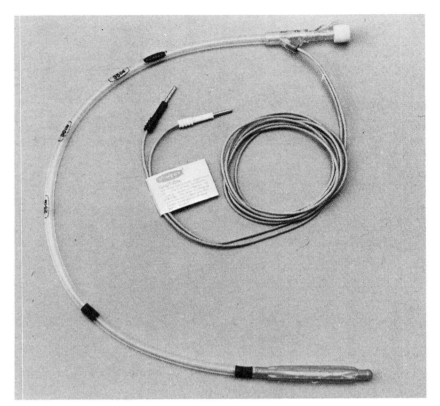

FIG. 14-3 New disposable transesophageal electrocardiographic probe.

TABLE 14-1. Comparison of Esophageal ECG and Standard ECG for Correct Diagnosis of Dysrhythmia

| Dysrhythmia | No. | Correct Diagnosis | | |
		V_5	II	Esophageal
Sinus bradycardia	4	4	4	4
Sinus tachycardia	1	1	1	1
1° heart block	1	0	0	1
2° heart block	2	0	0	2
3° heart block	4	0	1	4
Frequent premature ventricular contractions	2	2	2	2
Frequent premature atrial contractions	5	2	3	5
Atrial flutter	2	0	0	2
Atrial fibrillation	3	2	2	3
Paroxysmal atrial tachycardia	1	0	0	1
Nodal rhythm	1	0	0	1
% correct	—	42.3	53.8	100

(Kates RA: Esophageal lead for intraoperative electrocardiographic monitoring. Anesth Analg 61:781, 1982.)

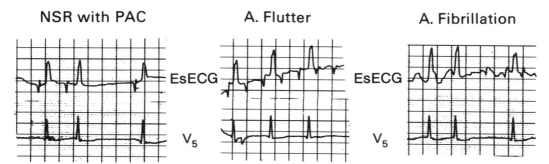

FIG. 14-4 Dysrhythmia progression in one patient is shown. Esophageal ECG (EsECG) distinctly reflects changes in atrial rhythm from normal sinus rhythm (NSR) with one premature atrial contraction (PAC), to atrial flutter (A. Flutter), and atrial fibrillation (A. Fibrillation). Lack of information about atrial activity from lead V₅ made definitive diagnosis impossible.

interference and useful for intraaortic balloon pump triggering.[26]

7. A further diagnostic ECG step is to record the bundle of His electrogram using an intracardiac catheter.[27] This part of electrical conduction in the heart is so rapid that it does not appear on the standard ECG. This technique may be used to localize heart blocks to certain areas of the conduction system or to diagnose the mechanism of complex dysrhythmias (Fig. 14-7).

DYSRHYTHMIA DETECTION

Dysrhythmia detection has been and still is the most important use of the ECG during and after surgery. Intraoperative dysrhythmias were reported during the early 1900s, but the

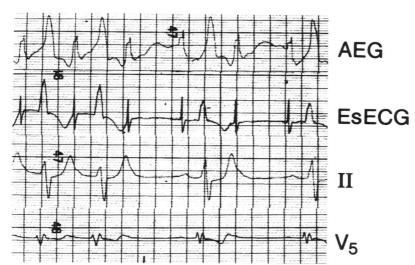

FIG. 14-5 Clear identification of P waves in esophageal ECG (EsECG) and intraatrial electrogram (AEG) allows for correct diagnosis of first-degree heart block and left bundle branch block progressing to second-degree heart block, Mobitz type II. P waves are practically lost in downslope of preceding T waves in leads II and V₅, resulting in incorrect diagnosis of sinus bradycardia rather than of second-degree heart block.

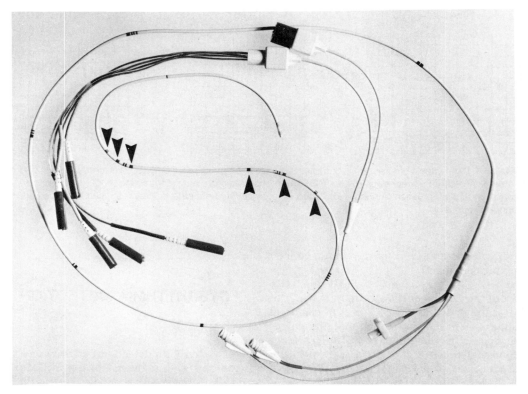

FIG. 14-6 A multipurpose Swan-Ganz catheter with both atrial and ventricular ECG or pacing electrodes is demonstrated. There are three atrial electrodes (right arrows) and two ventricular electrodes plus a wire stiffener (left arrows). This catheter can be used to diagnose complex dysrhythmias or for atrial, ventricular, or atrioventricular sequential pacing.

first large series of ECG studies during anesthesia was reported in 1936 by Kurtz et al.[28] In more than 100 patients, these workers found that sinus dysrhythmias, premature ventricular contractions (PVCs), and downward displacement of the pacemaker site predominated. In more recent studies by Katz and Bigger[9] the incidence of intraoperative dysrhythmias has been found to vary from 16 to 62 percent. Bertrand et al.[29] studied 100 patients, using continuous electromagnetic tape recording during surgery, and reported an 84 percent incidence of supraventricular and ventricular dysrhythmias. Dysrhythmias were most common at times of endotracheal intubation and extubation. Patients with preexisting cardiac disease had a higher incidence of ventricular dysrhythmias than did patients without known heart disease (60 percent versus 37 percent). Twenty-four of 25 patients with heart disease

had a rhythm disturbance during surgery. In a further study of patients undergoing cardiac surgery, Angelini et al.[13] reported that in 29 of 50 patients (58 percent) having valve surgery, and in 35 of 78 patients (45 percent) undergoing coronary revascularization, significant postoperative dysrhythmias developed. These dysrhythmias tended to correlate with the severity of the heart disease, led to a prolonged hospital stay, and were responsible for up to 80 percent of the surgical mortality in the series.

The following factors have been shown to be possible contributors to the etiology of dysrhythmias during the perioperative period:

1. Anesthetic agents—Halogenated hydrocarbons such as halothane or enflurane have been shown to produce dysrhythmias, probably by a reentrant mechanism.[30] In addition, these agents, especially halothane, have been shown to sensitize the myocardium to

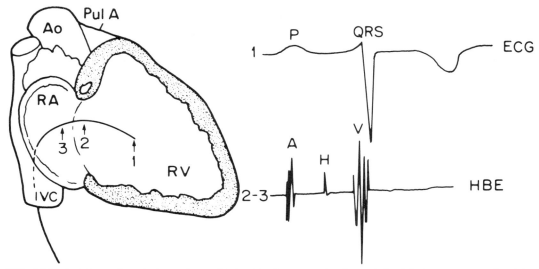

FIG. 14-7 An intracardiac electrocardiographic lead is shown coming through the inferior vena cava, the right atrium, and across the tricuspid valve, with the tip in the right ventricle. A normal ECG is shown as well as the intracavitary His bundle ECG. The His bundle electrocardiogram (HBE) demonstrates normal A, H, and V waves (Akhtar M: Clinical use of His bundle electrocardiography. Am Heart J 91:520, 1976.)

both endogenous and exogenous catechol-amines. Such drugs as cocaine and ketamine, which block the reuptake of norepinephrine, can facilitate the development of epinephrine-induced dysrhythmias.[31]

2. Abnormal arterial blood gases or electrolytes — Edwards et al.[11] showed that hyperventilation to a $PaCO_2$ of 30 or 20 mm Hg lowered a normal serum potassium to 3.64 or 3.12 mEq/L, respectively. If serum and total-body potassium start at low levels, it is possible to decrease the serum potassium to the 2 mEq/L range by hyperventilation and thus precipitate severe cardiac dysrhythmias. Alterations of blood gases or electrolytes may lead to dysrhythmias either by producing reentrant mechanisms or by altering phase 4 depolarization of conduction fibers.

3. Endotracheal intubation — This may be the most common cause of dysrhythmias during surgery. These dysrhythmias are occasionally associated with severe hypertension.[32] Several investigators (e.g., Stoelting[33]) have emphasized the hemodynamic alterations that may occur during endotracheal intubation (also see Ch. 16).

4. Reflexes — Vagal stimulation may produce sinus bradycardias and permit ventricu-lar escape mechanisms to occur. In addition, specific reflexes such as the oculocardiac reflex can produce severe rhythm disturbances during surgery.[9]

5. Central nervous system stimulation[34] — Many ECG abnormalities have been reported with intracranial pathology, especially subarachnoid hemorrhage, including changes in QT intervals, development of Q waves, ST-segment changes, and the occurrence of U waves. The mechanism of these dysrhythmias appears to be due to changes in the autonomic nervous system.

6. Location of surgery — Dental surgery is often associated with dysrhythmias, since profound stimulation of both the sympathetic and parasympathetic nervous systems often occurs.[35] Junctional rhythms commonly occur and may be due to stimulation of the autonomic nervous system via the 5th cranial nerve.

7. Preexisting cardiac disease — Studies by Angelini et al.[13] have shown that patients with known cardiac disease have a much higher incidence of dysrhythmias during anesthesia than do patients without known cardiac disease.[13]

8. The insertion of catheters or wires in

the heart—Dysrhythmias may be induced by the placement of a Swan-Ganz catheter, often leading to premature ventricular contractions (Fig. 14-8).

Dysrhythmias may also be attenuated or eliminated by general anesthesia.[36] This could be due to relief of anxiety and loss of sympathetic stimulation, to an antidysrhythmic property of the anesthethic agent itself, or to the correction of abnormalities of respiration, blood gases, and electrolytes.

The diagnosis and treatment of important intraoperative dysrhythmias can be simplified by using the following six questions as a checklist when looking at a rhythm strip or oscilloscope and attempting to decide whether treatment is necessary[37]:

1. What is the heart rate?
2. Is the rhythm regular?
3. Is there one P wave for each QRS complex?
4. Is the QRS complex normal?
5. Is the rhythm dangerous?
6. Does the rhythm require treatment?

The following are common intraoperative dysrhythmias that require diagnosis and treatment and to which the six key questions should be applied.

JUNCTIONAL RHYTHM

The cardiac impulse arises in the AV junctional tissue and travels down into the ventricles in the normal fashion. In addition, it may travel retrograde into the atrium (the P wave may be distorted). There are three varieties of this rhythm.[38]

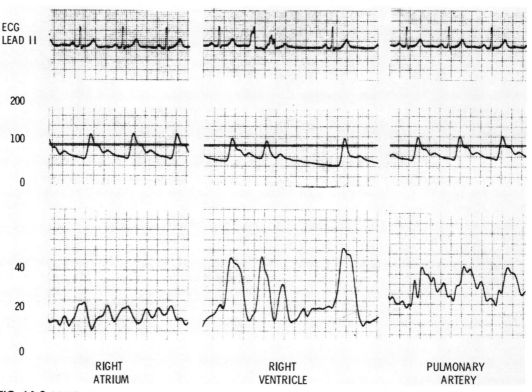

FIG. 14-8 Multifocal premature ventricular contractions are demonstrated on lead II of the ECG. These occurred with passage of the Swan-Ganz catheter from the right atrium into the right ventricle and then disappeared upon entrance of the catheter into the pulmonary artery. The arterial tracing demonstrates the systemic hemodynamic effects of these premature contractions.

1. High-nodal rhythm—The impulse reaches the atrium before the ventricle; therefore, the P wave precedes the QRS but has a shortened P-R interval (less than 0.1 second).
2. Mid-nodal rhythm—The impulse arrives in the atrium and the ventricle at the same time, and the P wave is lost in the QRS. ˌ
3. Low-nodal rhythm—The impulse reaches the ventricle first and then the atrium so that the P wave follows the QRS complex.

Characteristics of AV junctional rhythms include the following:
   a. Heart rate—variable, 40 to 180 beats/min: Nodal bradycardia to nodal tachycardia.
   b. Rhythm—regular.
   c. P:QRS—1:1, but appears variable, depending on the location of the P wave.
   d. QRS complex—normal, unless altered by the P wave.
   e. Significance—junctional rhythms are common under anesthesia (about 20 percent of cases), especially with halogenated anesthetic agents. The junctional rhythm frequently decreases blood pressure and cardiac output by about 15 percent, but it can decrease it by up to 30 percent in patients with heart disease (Fig. 14-9).[39]
   f. Treatment—usually no treatment is re-quired, and the rhythm reverts spontaneously. If hypotension and poor perfusion are associated with the rhythm, treatment is indicated. Atropine, ephedrine, or isoproterenol can be used in an effort to increase the activity of the sinoatrial (SA) node so it will take over as the pacemaker. A small dose of succinylcholine (10 mg IV) may cause a nodal rhythm to revert to a sinus rhythm during anesthesia with halothane or enflurane.[40] This probably works as a result of the effect of succinylcholine as a sympathetic ganglionic stimulator. In some cases, propranolol may correct the rhythm disturbance if it is due to sympathetic stimulation.

PREMATURE ATRIAL CONTRACTIONS

Premature atrial contractions (PACs) arise from an atrial focus other than the SA node, making them ectopic. They are recognized by a premature, abnormally shaped P wave and usually by a normal QRS complex. They tend to reset the SA node and to cause a slight pause, but not a full compensatory pause. Occasionally, PACs may find part of the ventricular con-

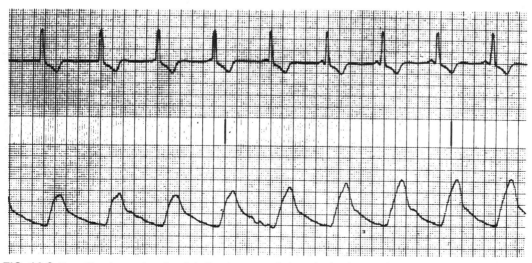

FIG. 14-9 Transition from a junctional rhythm to a normal sinus rhythm is associated with an increase in blood pressure.

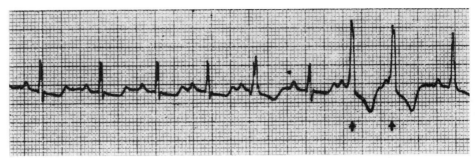

FIG. 14-10 An ECG tracing with multiple premature atrial contractions is demonstrated. The fourth beat shows no aberration, while the fifth beat shows partial aberration and the seventh and eighth beats, with arrows, show marked aberration.

duction system refractory. In that case, they will travel down an aberrant pathway and create an abnormal QRS complex. They are then called PACs with ventricular aberration and can very easily be confused with premature ventricular contractions (PVCs). Since the recovery period of the right ventricular (RV) conduction system outlasts that of the left, the most common form of aberration appears as a right bundle branch block (RBBB). Helpful points in separating a PAC with aberration from a PVC are (1) a preceding P wave, usually abnormally shaped; (2) a QRS complex with RBBB configuration; (3) an rSR' in V_1; and (4) initial vector forces identical to the preceding beat but usually the opposite with a PVC (Fig. 14-10). Other characteristics of PACs are as follows:

1. Heart rate—variable, depending on frequency of PACs.
2. Rhythm—irregular.
3. P : QRS—usually 1 : 1, the P waves have various shapes and may even be lost in the QRS

or T waves. Occasionally, the P wave will be so early as to find the ventricle refractory, and a nonconducted beat will occur.

4. QRS complex—usually normal unless there is ventricular aberration.
5. Significance—usually not dangerous, but very frequent PACs can lead to other supraventricular tachydysrhythmias or be a sign of digitalis intoxication.
6. Treatment—usually none. Rarely, digitalis, propranolol, or verapamil are needed when the dysrhythmia is causing poor hemodynamic function.

SINUS BRADYCARDIA

The discharge site in sinus bradycardia is the SA node, but at a slower-than-normal rate (Fig. 14-11). Occasionally, other pacemaker

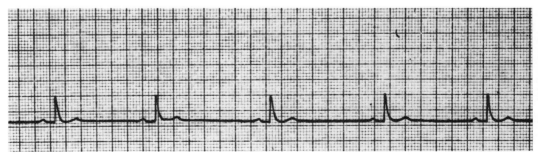

FIG. 14-11 A sinus bradycardia with an intrinsic rate of about 45 beats/min is demonstrated. It can also be noticed that the patient has a mild sinus dysrhythmia with variations in heart rate associated with respirations.

sites will try to take over and cause escape beats, such as PVCs. The characteristics of sinus bradycardia are as follows:

1. Heart rate—40 to 60 beats/min. In patients receiving propranolol chronically, this dysrhythmia should be redefined to be a heart rate <50 beats/min.[41]
2. Rhythm—regular, except for premature ventricular escape beats, which occasionally occur.
3. P:QRS—1:1.
4. QRS complex—normal.
5. Significance—this is the goal for patients treated with β-adrenergic blockers for ischemic heart disease. It may also be seen with acute inferior myocardial infarction and with many drugs, including narcotics and neostigmine. It is of little significance unless peripheral perfusion is decreased in association with hypotension or premature escape beats occur. A sinus bradycardia may be part of the so-called sick sinus syndrome, in which sinus node dysfunction can precipitate bradycardias, heart block, tachydysrhythmias, or alternating bradytachydysrhythmias.[42]
6. Treatment—usually none. Atropine is indicated if the bradycardia is associated with hypotension or escape beats. Rarely, isoproterenol or a pacemaker are necessary.

SINUS TACHYCARDIA

The discharge site in sinus tachycardia is the SA node, but at a faster-than-normal rate (Fig. 14-12). This is a very common dysrhythmia during and after surgery. Determining its etiology is frequently a problem, since there are many diverse causes, such as pain, light anesthesia, hypovolemia, fever, emotion, heart failure, and hyperthyroidism, to name just a few. Its characteristics are as follows:

1. Heart rate—above 100 beats/min. The top sinus node rate is 150 to 170 beats/min, which may be seen with a severe episode of hyperpyrexia.
2. Rhythm—regular.
3. P:QRS—1:1.
4. QRS complex—normal. There may be associated ST-segment depression with severe increases in heart rate and resulting myocardial ischemia.
5. Significance—prolonged tachycardias in patients with underlying heart disease can precipitate congestive heart failure (CHF) due to the increased myocardial work required. The tachycardia decreases coronary perfusion time, which can cause secondary ST-T wave changes and precipitate angina pectoris in patients with coronary artery disease. A major diagnostic problem is encountered when the heart rate is 150 beats/min, since this is a common rate for either a sinus tachycardia, paroxysmal atrial tachycardia (PAT), or atrial flutter with a 2:1 block.[43] These three dysrhythmias can sometimes be separated by using carotid sinus massage, intravenous administration of edrophonium, or atrial or esophageal ECG leads in order to get a better look at the P waves on the ECG.
6. Treatment — the underlying disorder should be treated. While determining the cause, the use of propranolol may be necessary in patients with ischemic heart disease

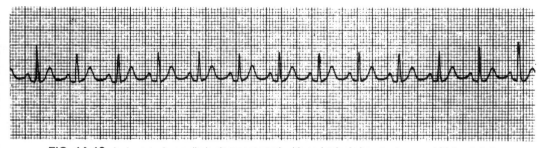

FIG. 14-12 A sinus tachycardia is demonstrated with an intrinsic heart rate over 100 beats/min.

in whom ST-segment changes develop, in order to prevent further myocardial ischemia.

PAROXYSMAL ATRIAL TACHYCARDIA

This dysrhythmia is a run of rapidly repeated supraventricular premature beats arising from a site other than the SA node. It is frequently seen in patients with Wolff-Parkinson-White (WPW) syndrome, in which an abnormal conduction pathway is present through the bundle of Kent (Fig. 14-13). The characteristics of PAT are as follows:

1. Heart rate—150 to 250 beats/min.
2. Rhythm—usually regular.
3. P:QRS—1:1; P waves often abnormal and may be difficult to see.
4. QRS complex—normal; ST-T wave depression is common.
5. Significance—may occur under anesthesia when precipitated by changes in the autonomic nervous system, by drug effects, or by volume shifts, and can produce severe hemodynamic deterioration.[44] PAT can be seen in 5 percent of normal young adults and in many patients with WPW. At times, the PAT may be associated with AV block due to the fast atrial rate and slow AV conduction. PAT with 2:1 block represents digitalis intoxication in many patients.
6. Treatment—this dysrhythmia often must be treated because of its rapid rate and associated poor hemodynamic function. The following steps can be taken to treat this dysrhythmia[45]:
    a. Vagal maneuvers such as carotid sinus massage, which should only be applied to one side.
    b. Verapamil, 5 to 10 mg IV, terminates AV nodal reentry successfully in about 90 percent of cases and has become the drug of choice.[46] However, it should be avoided in patients with known WPW, since it may lead to increased conduction through the abnormal pathway.
    c. Propranolol in 0.5-mg IV bolus doses.
    d. Edrophonium (Tensilon) in 5- to 10-mg IV bolus doses.
    e. Phenylephrine—if the patient is hypotensive, 100 μg IV bolus doses can be used in an effort to increase the blood pressure and achieve a reflex vagal slowing of the heart rate.
    f. Intravenous digitalization with one of the short-acting digitalis preparations: Ouabain 0.25 to 0.5 mg IV or digoxin 0.5 to 1.0 mg IV[47].
    g. Rapid overdrive pacing, in an effort to capture the ectopic focus;[48]
    h. Cardioversion with appropriate synchronization.[49]

ATRIAL FLUTTER

Atrial flutter represents a faster discharge from an irritable focus in the atria than does a rapid atrial tachycardia. Since it is so fast, this

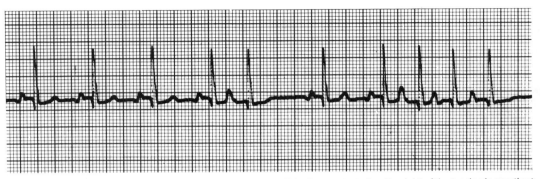

FIG. 14-13 A short run of paroxysmal atrial tachycardia (PAT) is demonstrated on the right of the tracing in a patient with an underlying normal sinus rhythm. The heart rate during the tachycardia is about 150 beats/min. The P waves are difficult to see, since they are buried in the previous T wave.

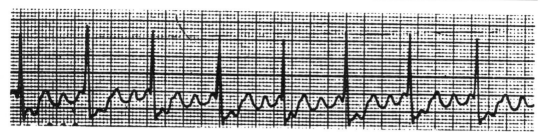

FIG. 14-14 Classic sawtoothed flutter waves (F waves) are seen in this patient with atrial flutter.

dysrhythmia is usually associated with AV block. Classic sawtoothed flutter waves (F waves) are usually present (Fig. 14-14). The characteristics of atrial flutter are as follows:

1. Heart rate—atrial rate 250 to 350 beats/min; with a ventricular rate of about 150 beats/min.
2. Rhythm—atrial rhythm is regular; the ventricular rhythm may be regular if a fixed AV block is present or irregular if a variable block exists.
3. P:QRS—usually 2:1 block with an atrial rate of 300 and ventricular rate of 150, but may vary between 2:1 and 8:1. F waves are best seen in leads V_1 or II or the esophageal lead.
4. QRS complex—normal; T waves are lost in the F waves.
5. Significance—associated with severe heart disease.
6. Treatment:
   a. The initial treatment of choice is synchronous direct-current (DC) cardioversion using very low voltage (10 to 40 watt-sec), which is effective in more than 90 percent of cases.[50]
   b. Rapid atrial pacing effectively terminates atrial flutter in many patients and results in a return to sinus rhythm or atrial fibrillation with a slow ventricular rate.[51]
   c. Verapamil 5 to 10 mg IV.[46]
   d. Digitalis, with or without propranolol.

ATRIAL FIBRILLATION

Atrial fibrillation is an excessively rapid and irregular atrial focus with no P waves appearing on the ECG, but, instead, a fine fibrillatory activity called f waves. This is the most irregular rhythm; it is called irregularly irregular and may be associated with a pulse deficit (Fig. 14-15). The characteristics are as follows:

1. Heart rate—atrial rate 350 to 500 beats/min and a ventricular rate between 60 and 170 beats/min.
2. Rhythm—irregularly irregular.
3. P:QRS—P wave is absent and replaced by f waves or no obvious atrial activity at all.
4. QRS complex—normal.
5. Significance—associated with severe heart disease.
6. Treatment—digitalis is usually used to slow

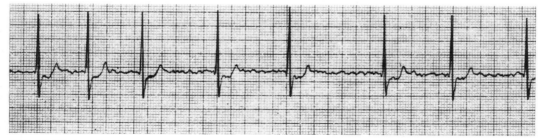

FIG. 14-15 Atrial fibrillation with fine fibrillatory activity is demonstrated. The irregularly irregular pattern of the QRS complexes should be noted.

the ventricular response, and propranolol or verapamil is added if necessary. Cardioversion is often used to reestablish sinus rhythm in patients with a recent onset of atrial fibrillation.

PREMATURE VENTRICULAR CONTRACTIONS

Premature ventricular contractions are premature ectopic beats arising from a focus below the AV junction and are one of the most common dysrhythmias seen in anesthesia and in patients with cardiac disease. Identification of PVCs is made on the basis of the following characteristics: premature, wide QRS complex, an ST segment that slopes in the opposite direction, and a compensatory pause. Usually no P wave is associated with these beats (Fig. 14-16). PVCs are characterized by:

1. Heart rate—depends on the frequency of PVCs.
2. Rhythm—irregular.
3. P:QRS—no P waves are seen with the PVCs.
4. QRS complex—wide and bizarre with a width of >0.12 seconds.
5. Significance—potentially a very dangerous dysrhythmia that can proceed to ventricular tachycardia or fibrillation. The most dangerous forms are multiple PVCs, multifocal PVCs, coupled PVCs, short runs of PVCs (three or more in a row is generally considered ventricular tachycardia), or the R-on-T phenomenon in which the PVCs are near the vulnerable period on the ECG.[52]
6. Treatment—the first step is to correct any underlying abnormalities such as low potassium or arterial oxygen tension. Then lidocaine is usually the treatment of choice with an initial bolus dose of 1.5 mg/kg IV. Recurrent PVCs can be treated with a lidocaine infusion of 1 to 4 mg/min; or additional therapy can be supplied with propranolol, bretylium, procainamide, quinidine, verapamil, disopyramide, atropine, or overdrive pacing.

VENTRICULAR TACHYCARDIA

Ventricular tachycardia is characterized by a run of rapidly repeated ectopic beats that arise from the ventricle, and are potentially life threatening. Diagnostic criteria include the presence of fusion beats, capture beats, and AV dissociation (Fig. 14-17).[53] The characteristics of ventricular tachycardia are as follows:

1. Heart rate—100 to 200 beats/min.
2. Rhythm—usually regular, but may be irregular if the ventricular tachycardia is paroxysmal.
3. P:QRS—no fixed relationship, since ventricular tachycardia is a form of AV dissociation in which the P waves can be seen marching through the QRS complex.
4. QRS complex—wide, >0.12 seconds in width.

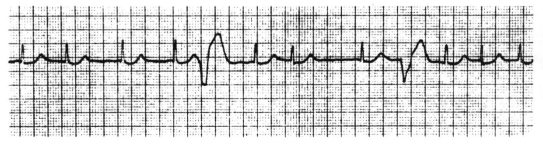

FIG. 14-16 Premature ventricular contractions (PVCs) are identified by the fact that they are premature, have a wide QRS complex, and an ST segment that slopes in the opposite direction. They may also have a compensatory pause.

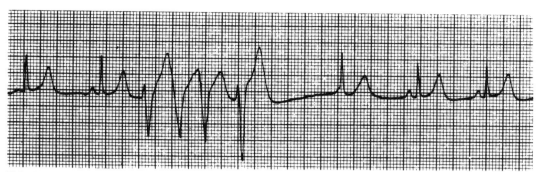

FIG. 14-17 Three or more premature ventricular contractions (PVCs) in a row is defined as a run of ventricular tachycardia. A fusion beat, capture beat, or AV dissociation seen on the trace helps make the specific diagnosis of ventricular tachycardia.

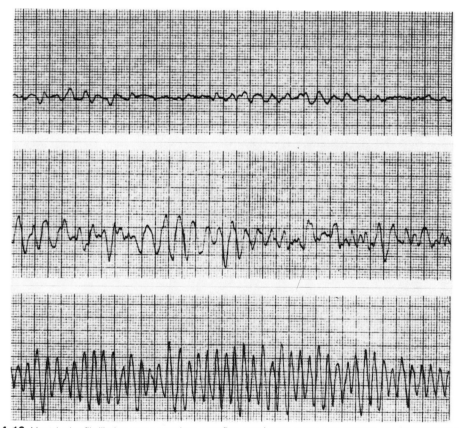

FIG. 14-18 Ventricular fibrillation can occur in a very fine, moderate, or coarse pattern, as demonstrated on the ECGs.

5. Significance—acute onset is life threatening and requires immediate treatment.
6. Treatment—lidocaine and/or immediate cardioversion is usually required. Recurrent episodes may require therapy with any or all the drugs listed under the treatment of PVCs.

VENTRICULAR FIBRILLATION

The ventricle is discharged in a completely chaotic asynchronous fashion without effective cardiac output. No clear-cut ventricular complex is seen on the ECG (Fig. 14-18). The characteristics are as follows:

1. Heart rate—rapid and grossly disorganized.
2. Rhythm—totally irregular.
3. P:QRS—none are seen.
4. QRS complex—not present.
5. Significance—there is no effective cardiac output, and life must be sustained by artificial means, such as external cardiac massage.
6. Treatment—cardiopulmonary resuscitation must be initiated immediately and then defibrillation performed as rapidly as possible. External defibrillation should be performed with a DC defibrillator, using 200 to 400 watt-sec.[54] Supportive pharmacologic therapy may include propranolol, bretylium, or lidocaine. In some instances, epinephrine is used to coarsen the fibrillation in an attempt to defibrillate the patient.[52]

ASYSTOLE

During asystole, no ventricular activity is present (Fig. 14-19). Asystole is the second most common rhythm disorder (after ventricular fibrillation) during cardiac arrests. The characteristics are as follows:

1. Heart rate—none present.
2. Rhythm—straight line on the ECG.
3. P:QRS—none present.
4. QRS complex—absent.
5. Significance—difficult to treat and an attempt should be made to convert it to ventricular fibrillation.
6. Treatment—maintain cardiopulmonary resuscitation (CPR) while administering calcium chloride, isoproterenol, epinephrine, or sodium bicarbonate and, if necessary, insert a transvenous pacemaker.

CONDUCTION ABNORMALITIES

Three types of conduction system block are possible: sinoatrial block, intraventricular conduction block, and atrioventricular heart block. Bundle of His electrograms have greatly improved the understanding of conduction through the heart.[55] In SA block, the block occurs at the sinus node. Since atrial excitation is not initiated, P waves are not found on the ECG. The next beat can be a normal sinus beat,

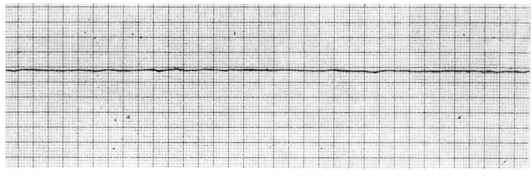

FIG. 14-19 Asystole is diagnosed by the straight line on the ECG. It must be ascertained that this is not an ECG strip taken with a lead or cable disconnected from the patient.

a nodal escape beat, or a ventricular escape beat.

The second type of block is an intraventricular conduction disturbance, which is usually classified as either a LBBB, RBBB, or hemiblock.[56]

The LBBB is the most serious of these conduction disturbances. Impulses reach the ventricles exclusively through the right bundle branch, hence the wide QRS complex of more than 0.12 seconds and a wide-notched R wave seen in leads I, AVL, and V_6. The most important leads to study in bundle branch blocks are I, V_1, and V_6. The pattern of LBBB in V_6 is similar to LV hypertrophy, but exaggerated. A LBBB pattern is always associated with significant cardiac disease (Fig. 14-20).

In a RBBB, the QRS complex exceeds 0.11 seconds, and leads V_1 to V_3 have broad rSR' complexes, while leads I and V_6 have wide S waves. A RBBB may be of no clinical significance, as opposed to the LBBB. However, it is frequently associated with chronic lung disease or atrial-septal defects (Fig. 14-21).

Hemiblock is a term used when one of two divisions of the left bundle is blocked, since if both divisions are blocked a complete LBBB exists. Even though hemiblocks are a form of intraventricular block, the QRS complex is not prolonged. Marriott's criteria for left anterior hemiblock[56] are as follows (Fig. 14-22): (1) left axis deviation (usually −60°); (2) a small Q in lead I and aVL, small R in II, III, and aVF; (3) a normal QRS duration; (4) a late intrinsicoid deflection in aVL (>0.045 sec); and (5) an increased QRS voltage in limb leads. By contrast, the criteria for a left posterior hemiblock are as follows (Fig. 14-23): (1) right axis deviation (usually +120°); (2) a small R in lead I and aVL, small Q in II, III, and aVF; (3) a normal QRS duration; (4) a late intrinsicoid deflection in aVF (>0.045 sec); (5) an increased QRS voltage in limb leads; and (6) no evidence of RV hypertrophy. The hemiblocks can occur by themselves but are often associated with a RBBB to form a bilateral bundle branch block. Patients with RBBB and a left anterior hemiblock progress to complete heart block only 10 percent of

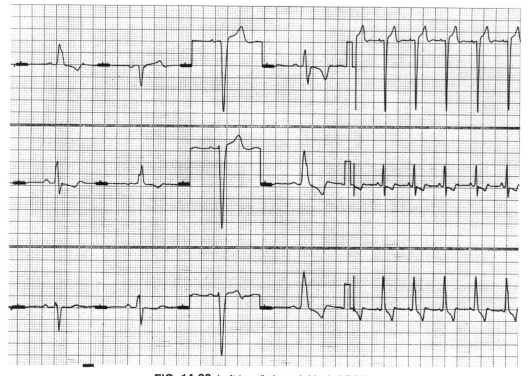

FIG. 14-20 Left bundle branch block (LBBB).

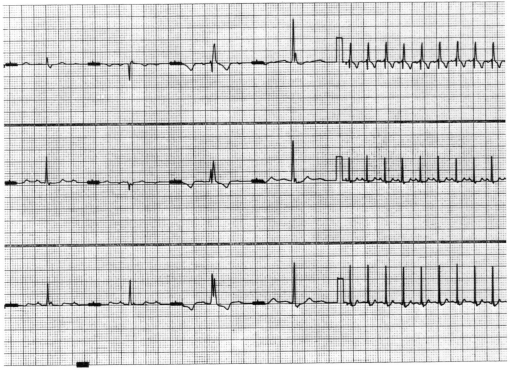

FIG. 14-21 Right bundle branch block (RBBB).

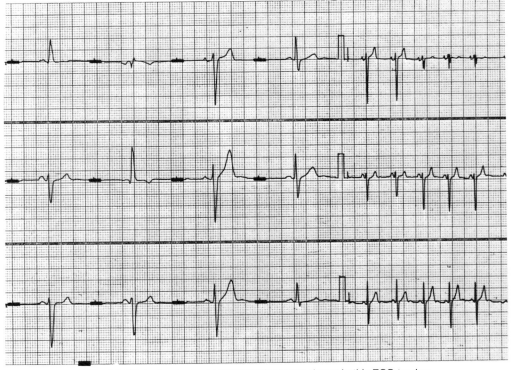

FIG. 14-22 Left anterior hemiblock criteria are shown in this ECG tracing.

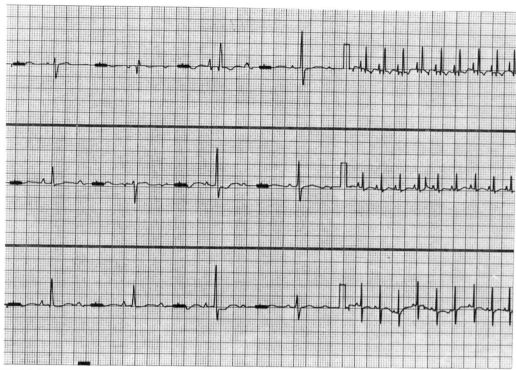

FIG. 14-23 Left posterior hemiblock in association with biatrial enlargement and nonspecific ST- and T-wave abnormalities.

the time, while patients with RBBB and a left posterior hemiblock usually proceed to complete heart block (Fig. 14-24).

The third type of heart block is an AV heart block, or AV block, which may be either incomplete or complete.[57] First- and second-degree AV blocks are usually considered incomplete, while a third-degree AV block is considered to be complete heart block. First-degree AV block is often found in normal hearts but is also associated with coronary artery disease or digitalis administration. It is characterized by a PR interval longer than 0.21 seconds. All atrial impulses progress through the AV node to the Purkinje system. This form of heart block ordinarily requires no treatment (Fig. 14-25).

Second-degree AV block is associated with the conduction of some, but not all, of the atrial impulses to the AV node and into the Purkinje system. It is further subdivided into two specific types.[58] Mobitz type 1, or Wenckebach block, is characterized by progressive length-

ening of the PR interval until an impulse is not conducted and the beat is dropped (Fig. 14-26). This form of block is relatively benign and often reversible and does not require a pacemaker. It may be caused by digitalis toxicity or myocardial infarction and is usually transient in nature. The Mobitz type 1 block reflects disease of the AV node. The other form of second-degree heart block is a Mobitz type 2 block, which reflects disease of the His bundle Purkinje tissues. In this, the less common and more serious form of second-degree heart block, dropped beats occur without any progressive lengthening of the PR interval. This type of block has a serious prognosis, since it frequently progresses to complete heart block and may require pacemaker insertion prior to major surgical procedures (Fig. 14-27).

Third-degree AV block, also called complete heart block, occurs when all electrical activity from the atria fails to progress into the Purkinje system. The atrial and ventricular contractions have no relationship to each

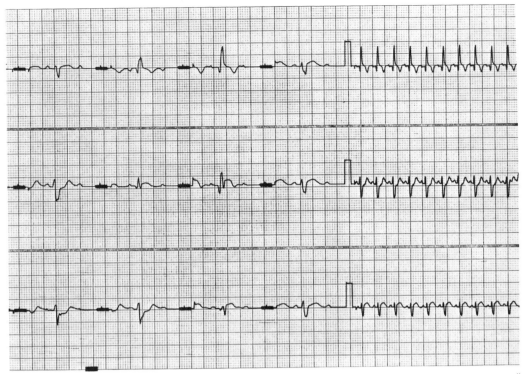

FIG. 14-24 Right bundle branch block (RBBB) and left anterior hemiblock in a patient with a recent myocardial infarction.

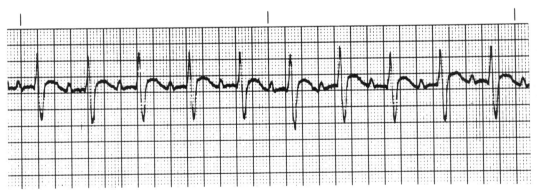

FIG. 14-25 First-degree heart block is diagnosed by the presence of a PR interval of longer than 0.21 seconds.

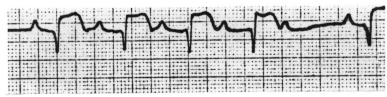

FIG. 14-26 Mobitz type 1 (or Wenckebach) block is diagnosed by the progressive lengthening of the PR interval until an impulse is not conducted and a dropped beat occurs.

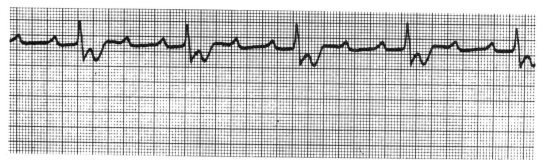

FIG. 14-27 Mobitz type 2 second-degree heart block is demonstrated in which dropped beats occur without a progressive lengthening of the PR interval.

other, although each can regularly contract. The ventricular rate will be approximately 40 beats/min. The QRS complex may be normal if the pacemaker site is in the AV node, but it is usually widened to longer than 0.12 seconds when the pacer site is located in the ventricle. The heart rate is usually too slow to maintain adequate cardiac output, and syncope or Stokes-Adams syndrome may occur, as well as heart failure. These patients usually require insertion of either a transvenous endocardial or epicardial pacemaker to increase their heart rate and cardiac output (Fig. 14-28).

MYOCARDIAL ISCHEMIA

Electrocardiographic monitoring of myocardial ischemia is a relatively new intraoperative technique. Early studies of intraoperative

ECG monitoring did not even mention the use of the ECG for the diagnosis of ischemia, but only its role in the diagnosis of dysrhythmias.[1] In recent years, coronary artery disease has been recognized as the most common major health problem in the United States. All types of surgical procedures are being performed on patients with coronary artery disease, many of whom have a history of acute myocardial infarctions or angina pectoris. In these patients, the ECG should be used to identify myocardial ischemia during the stresses of anesthesia and surgery, as well as for dysrhythmia detection. Until recently, the older ECG lead systems and monitors designed primarily for dysrhythmia detection have been the only ones available in the operating room. These have frequently been inadequate for the diagnosis and recording of subtle ST-segment changes that occur with early myocardial ischemia. The most obvious deficiency has been the lack of flexibility in selecting the appropriate leads for diagnosing myocardial ischemia.

In 1931, precordial leads were first noted to have a greater sensitivity in detecting ST-seg-

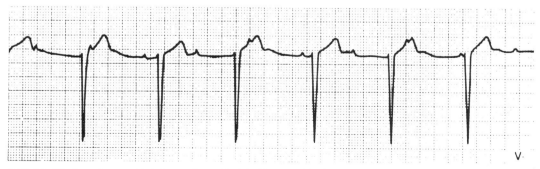

FIG. 14-28 Complete, or third-degree, heart block is diagnosed by the total dissociation between the atrial and the ventricular complexes with a ventricular rate of about 40 beats/min.

ment depression of ischemic origin than the standard leads. Since then, a number of lead systems have been developed to monitor myocardial ischemia and have been studied extensively during exercise stress testing. Blackburn[59] performed many studies of the lead systems and found the most sensitive exploring electrode to be at the V_5 chest position. He showed that 89 percent of the ST-segment information contained in a conventional 12-lead ECG was found in lead V_5. It was not until 1976, however, that any monitoring for ischemia during anesthesia was advocated. Dalton[60] recommended placing a sterile spinal needle in the V_4 or V_5 position after the skin was prepared for cardiac surgery. Kaplan and King[10] first reported that a multiple-lead ECG system, including a V_5 lead, should be used for all patients with coronary artery disease undergoing either cardiac or noncardiac surgery. The multiple-lead system consists of four disposable ECG pads placed on the extremities and a fifth pad

placed in the V_5 position and covered with a small piece of Steri-drape (Fig. 14-29). The V_5 lead does not interfere with the majority of surgery and can be placed before the induction of anesthesia and monitored during the entire operative procedure. Using the five electrodes, seven different ECG leads can be observed (leads I, II, III, AVR, AVL, AVF, and V_5) (Fig. 14-30). All seven leads are observed before the start of anesthesia and are recorded for later reference. In patients with known cardiac disease, two leads (V_5, II) are simultaneously displayed using two different ECG amplifier circuits (Fig. 14-31). This permits observation of the anterior lateral wall (V_5 lead) and of the inferior wall (lead II) of the heart at the same time. Robertson et al.[61] have shown that there is good correlation between the site of the coronary artery obstruction and the lead in which ischemia is detected. ST-segment changes in leads II, III, and AVF correspond to disease of the right coronary artery; ischemic changes in

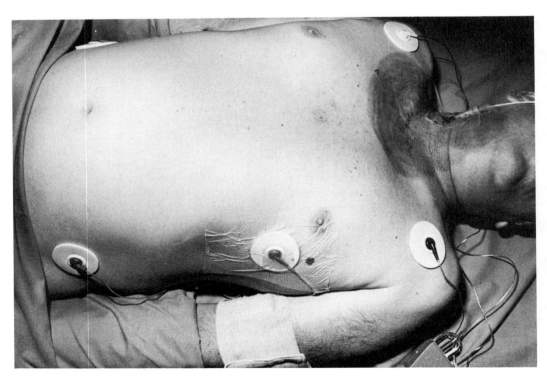

FIG. 14-29 The five disposable ECG pads are demonstrated. One pad is placed on each extremity, and the fifth pad is placed in the V_5 position and covered with a small piece of Steri-drape.

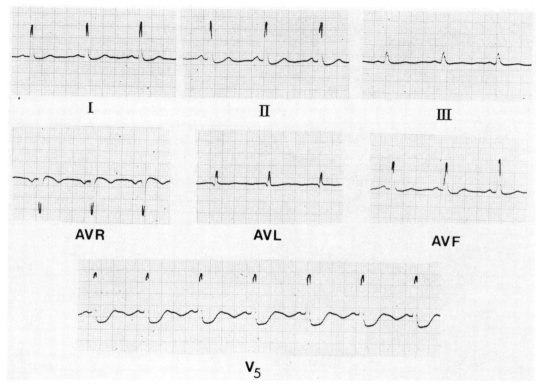

FIG. 14-30 The seven different ECG leads that can be observed and recorded during surgery when using the five-electrode system are shown. (Kaplan JA: The precordial electrocardiographic lead (V_5) in patients with coronary artery disease. Anesthesiology 45:570, 1976.)

V_4 to V_6 indicate disease of the left anterior descending or circumflex coronary artery (Fig. 14-32).[62]

Whenever possible, the five-electrode system including the true V_5 lead is preferred. However, some operating room ECG systems still have only three or four electrode wires. A modification of the V_5 lead can be readily used in those cases, as is frequently done during exercise stress testing.[63,64] The most popular modified leads during stress testing have been the CM_5 or CS_5 bipolar leads, in which the negative electrode is at the upper sternum in CM_5 or under the right clavicle in CS_5, with the positive electrode at the V_5 position. These leads are more convenient than V_5 because they require fewer wires. They are good leads for the detection of ischemia, but Froelicher et al.[65] have shown they are not as good as V_5. In the operating room, the right arm electrode can be placed just below the clavicle on the right shoulder, and the left arm electrode placed in the V_5 position, while the left leg lead is left in its usual place. Then lead I can be selected to observe the anterior heart wall (a modified CS_5) and lead II for the inferior wall (Fig. 14-33).

Myocardial ischemia is diagnosed by changes in the ST segment and T wave of the ECG.[66] Significant myocardial ischemia is defined as >1 mm of horizontal or downsloping ST-segment depression measured from a point 0.06 seconds from the J point. Increased magnitude of ST-segment depression probably denotes an increased degree of ischemia. All ST-segment elevations of >1 mm are considered indicative of significant transmural myocardial ischemia (Fig. 14-34). It is crucial that the ECG monitor or oscilloscope not introduce any type of artifact or distortion into the ST segments or the T waves of the ECG when it is being used for

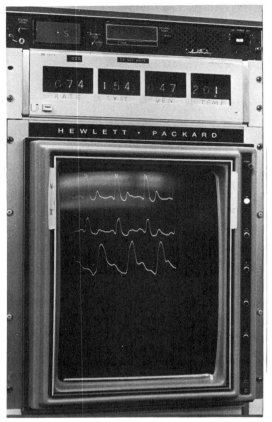

FIG. 14-31 A simultaneous display of lead V_5 (top) and lead II (bottom) is shown. Also demonstrated are the arterial trace and digital readouts.

is susceptible to baseline wandering caused by respirations and movement. As more filtration is added, up to 4 Hz, the baseline becomes more stable, but the ECG complex becomes more distorted. The P and T waves may decrease in amplitude, but the main problem with this mode is changes in the ST segment. An isoelectric ST segment may be elevated or depressed, resembling ischemic changes. In addition, elevated or depressed ST segments may also be shifted toward the isoelectric line, hiding ongoing myocardial ischemia (Fig. 14-35).

The ST segments and T waves can be affected by many factors other than myocardial ischemia. These other factors produce the nonspecific ST-T wave changes. Drugs that can affect the ST segments include digitalis, diuretics, and reserpine.[6] Hypokalemia or glucose can affect the ST segment by altering the membrane–potassium relationship. The ST segments may appear to be depressed by the T_a wave of atrial repolarization and to be altered by conduction disturbances such as LBBB or WPW syndrome.

Another problem has been that when the size of the oscilloscope tracing is increased on some monitoring equipment, an obvious resolution problem appears. As the size of the tracing is increased, the stair-step effect of the electronic beam on the oscilloscope is much more obvious and can even resemble the horizontal ST-segment changes of myocardial ischemia. Manufacturers will have to be made more aware of the fact that the ST segments are critical and should be kept entirely normal when making their electronic modifications on modern operating room monitors.

Computerized ST-segment analyzers are now available for use during exercise stress testing.[67,68] They can analyze 10 to 20 heartbeats and produce a histogram and digital readout of ST-segment level, ST index, ST slope, and ST interval. These computations are still controversial with regard to their usefulness in diagnosing myocardial ischemia. Kotrly et al.[69] recently reported a case in which an ST-segment trend line was displayed by a modified microcomputer-based ECG and provided an early indication of myocardial ischemia before ST-segment depression could be clearly observed on the standard V_5 lead. Their example

the diagnosis of myocardial ischemia. This has been a problem with many of the oscilloscopes now in use in operating rooms.[15] The low-frequency filters of the ECG circuitry have been the main source of the problem. The diagnostic mode on some monitors filters frequencies below 0.1 Hz. A second mode that is frequently available is called the monitor mode, and this filters all frequencies below 4 Hz. The diagnostic mode should be used when trying to diagnose ST-segment changes but, unfortunately, it

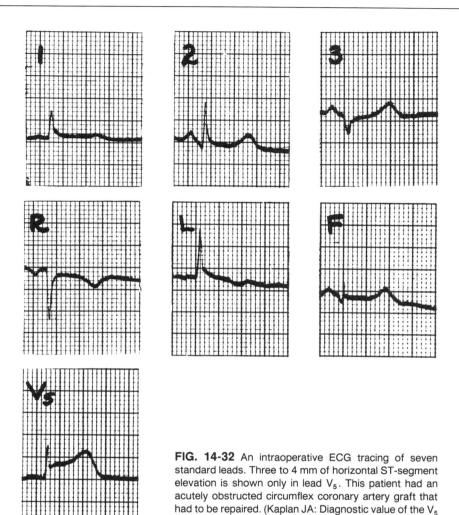

FIG. 14-32 An intraoperative ECG tracing of seven standard leads. Three to 4 mm of horizontal ST-segment elevation is shown only in lead V_5. This patient had an acutely obstructed circumflex coronary artery graft that had to be repaired. (Kaplan JA: Diagnostic value of the V_5 precordial lead. Anesth Analg 57:364, 1978.)

illustrates that these instruments can at times be of intraoperative value. However, they are useless when the electrocautery is switched on, since they must then reset themselves and count 10 to 20 beats before they can give the next reading.

Electrocardiographic mapping techniques have been developed in an effort to define the size of the area of ischemia that has occurred in humans and animals. This is important, since an ischemic area or even a necrotic area is not fixed in size at its initial onset, but may be

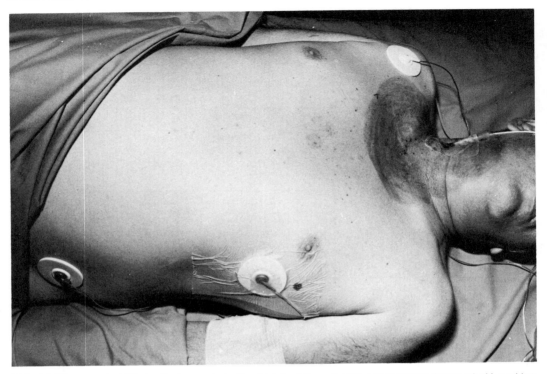

FIG. 14-33 A modified CS$_5$ lead is demonstrated in which the left arm lead has been moved down to the V$_5$ position. Lead I can then be turned on to measure from the right arm to the V$_5$ position (CS$_5$), and lead II can be used to look at the inferior wall.

modified by therapeutic interventions in either a positive or negative direction. In order to measure the areas of ischemia and evaluate therapeutic interventions, Muller, Maroko, and Braunwald[70,71] have developed a series of mapping techniques. These techniques have evolved from epicardial ST-segment mapping, to epicardial QRS mapping, to precordial ST mapping, and, finally, to precordial QRS mapping. The epicardial techniques were first used experimentally in animals and then compared with precordial techniques in animals and are now being applied in patients. A good correlation has been shown between the epicardial and precordial mapping techniques. Epicardial ST-segment mapping has been used to evaluate most potential therapeutic interventions in dogs with acute myocardial ischemia. In this model, known as the Maroko dog model, an

occlusion is placed on the left anterior descending coronary artery of the dog and the ST-segment elevation at multiple epicardial sites is determined after the occlusion (Fig. 14-36).[72] The procedure is then repeated in the presence of the specific intervention under study and the mean ST-segment elevations compared in the treatment and control groups. Hillis and Braunwald[73] summarized all the data on interventions obtained by this technique. They divided therapeutic interventions into those that increase myocardial injury either by increasing MVO$_2$ or decreasing myocardial oxygen supply (e.g., isoproterenol) and those that decrease myocardial injury either by decreasing MVO$_2$ or increasing myocardial oxygen supply (e.g., nitroglycerin).

The greatest clinical application of these techniques has been in precordial ST-segment

(*Text continues on page 496*)

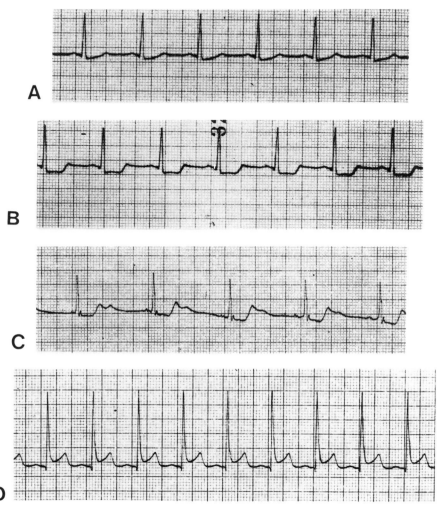

FIG. 14-34 Significant myocardial ischemia is defined as >1 mm of horizontal or downsloping ST-segment depression, or as an ST-segment elevation >1 mm. ST-segment changes of myocardial ischemia are demonstrated. (A) J-point depression and upsloping ST-segment depression of possible ischemia. (B) Horizontal ST-segment depression of ischemia. (C) Downsloping ST-segment depression of ischemia. (D) ST-segment elevation of ischemia.

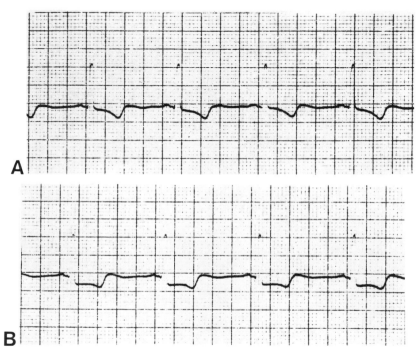

FIG. 14-35 An artifact on the ECG can be demonstrated by switching from the diagnostic filter mode (A) to the monitoring filter mode (B). Significant changes in the ST segments can be produced by altering these filters, as demonstrated.

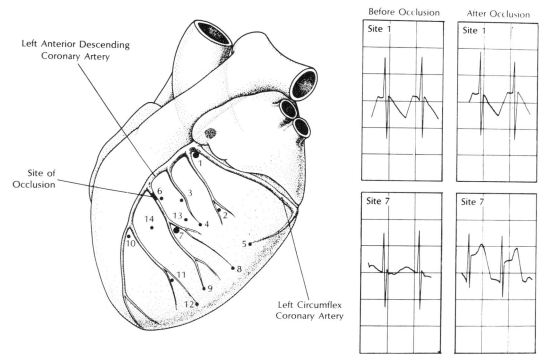

FIG. 14-36 The Maroko dog model is demonstrated. A branch of the left anterior descending coronary artery is occluded and epicardial ST-segment mapping is performed. An affected site, site 7, which became ischemic, is demonstrated as well as an unaffected site, site 1. (Figure by R. Ingle from Braunwald E, Maroko R: Protection of the ischemic myocardium, The Myocardium: Failure and Infarction. Edited by Braunwald E. New York, HP Publishing Co., 1974. Reproduced with permission.)

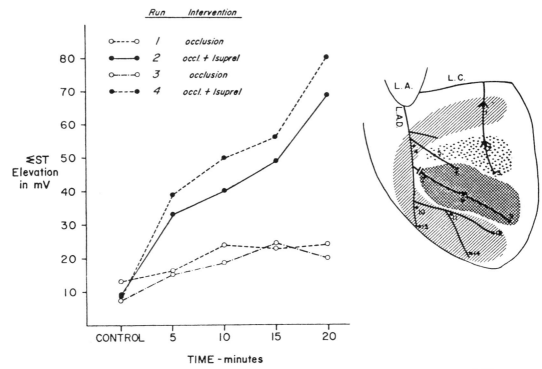

FIG. 14-37 Pharmacologic interventions have also been shown to be able to increase an area of ST-segment elevation. Infusion of isoproterenol increased the severity of myocardial ischemia, as reflected in the sum of the ST-segment elevation recorded after coronary occlusion. After occlusion, the sum ranged from 15 to 25 mV while, after occlusion and Isuprel, it ranged from 40 to 80 mV. (Figure by R. Ingle from Braunwald E, Maroko R: Protection of the ischemic myocardium, The Myocardium: Failure and Infarction. Edited by Braunwald E. New York, HP Publishing Co., 1974. Reproduced with permission.)

mapping. A 35-lead electrode blanket was developed by Maroko to record precordial maps in patients with acute myocardial infarctions. Interventions such as propranolol, aortic counterpulsation, nitroglycerin, and oxygen have been shown to reduce ST-segment elevation (Fig. 14-37).[74]

There are many limitations and controversies associated with ST-segment mapping techniques. The greatest limitation is that they can only be used in patients with anterior or lateral wall ischemia. In addition, they cannot be used in patients with intraventricular conduction defects, since these markedly affect the ST segment. The areas of controversy involve validation of this method in relationship to other techniques that measure infarct size, as well as questions about the technical limitations and electrophysiology involved in the technique.[75-77]

REFERENCES

1. Cannard TH, Dripps RD, Helwig J, et al: The ECG during anesthesia and surgery. Anesthesiology 21:194, 1960
2. Cranefield PF, Wit AL, Hoffman BF: Genesis of cardiac arrhythmias. Circulation 47:109, 1973
3. Benchimol A, Harris CL, Desser KB, et al: Resting ECG in major coronary artery disease. JAMA 224:1489, 1973
4. Hurst JW: The Heart. 4th Ed. New York, McGraw-Hill, 1978
5. Rooney S, Goldiner P, Muss E: Relationship of right bundle branch block and marked left axis deviation to complete heart block during general anesthesia. Anesthesiology 44:64, 1976

6. Surawicz B, Lasseter KC: Effect of drugs on the ECG. Prog Cardiovasc Dis 13:26, 1970

7. Surawicz B: Relationship between ECG and electrolytes. Am Heart J 73:814, 1967

8. Spodick DH: Acute pericardial tamponade, pathologic physiology, diagnosis and management. Prog Cardiovasc Dis 10:64, 1967

9. Katz RL, Bigger JT: Cardiac arrhythmias during anesthesia and operation. Anesthesiology 33:193, 1970

10. Kaplan JA, King SB: The precordial electrocardiographic lead (V_5) in patients who have coronary artery disease. Anesthesiology 45:570, 1976

11. Edwards R, Winnie AL, Ramamurthy S: Acute hypocapnic hypokalemia: An iatrogenic anesthetic complication. Anesth Analg 56:786, 1977

12. Zaidan JR: Pacemakers. Anesthesiology 60:319, 1984

13. Angelini L, Feldman MI, Lufschonowski R, et al: Cardiac arrhythmias during and after heart surgery: Diagnosis and management. Prog Cardiovasc Dis 16:469, 1974

14. Kennedy FB, Ticzon AR, Duffy FC, et al: Disappearance of ECG pattern of inferior wall myocardial infarction after aortocoronary bypass surgery. J Thorac Cardiovasc Surg 74:585, 1977

15. Arbeit SR, Rubin IL, Gross H: Dangers in interpreting the ECG from the oscilloscope monitor. JAMA 211:453, 1970

16. Borrello G: ECG artifacts simulating atrial flutter. JAMA 223:439, 1973

17. Doss JD, McCabe CW, Weiss GK: Noise free ECG data during electrosurgical procedures. Anesth Analg 52:156, 1973

18. Goldberg E: Mechanical factors and the ECG. Am Heart J 93:629, 1977

19. Voukydis PC: Effect of intracardiac blood on the ECG. N Engl J Med 291:612, 1974

20. Caceres CA, Hochberg HM: Performance of the computer and physician in the analysis of the electrocardiogram. Am Heart J 79:439, 1970

21. Schamroth L: How to approach an arrhythmia. Circulation 47:420, 1973

22. Hampton AG: Monitoring and dysrhythmia recognition in advanced life support. American Heart Association Advanced Life Support Course.

23. Bazaral MG, Norfleet EA: Comparison of CB_5 and V_5 leads for intraoperative electrocardiographic monitoring. Anesth Analg 60:849, 1981

24. Kates RA, Zaidan JR, Kaplan JA: Esophageal lead for intraoperative electrocardiographic monitoring. Anesth Analg 61:781, 1982

25. Mantel JA, Massing GK, James TN, et al: A multipurpose catheter for electrocardiographic and hemodynamic monitoring plus atrial pacing. Chest 72:285, 1977

26. Lichtenthal PR, Wade L, Collins JT: Multipur-

pose pulmonary artery catheter. Ann Thorac Surg 36:493, 1983

27. Aktar M, Damato AN: Clinical uses of His bundle electrocardiography. Part I. Am Heart J 91:520, 1976

28. Kurtz CM, Bennett JH, Shapiro HH: ECG studies during surgical anesthesia. JAMA 106:434, 1936

29. Bertrand CA, Steiner NV, Jameson AG, et al: Disturbances of cardiac rhythm during anesthesia and surgery. JAMA 216:1615, 1971

30. Atlee JL, Rusy BF: Ventricular conduction times and AV nodal conductivity during enflurane anesthesia in dogs. Anesthesiology 47:498, 1977

31. Koehntop DE, Liao JC, Van Bergen FH: Effects of pharmacologic alterations of adrenergic mechanisms by cocaine, tropolone, aminophylline, and ketamine on epinephrine-induced arrhythmias during halothane-nitrous oxide anesthesia. Anesthesiology 46:83, 1977

32. Fox EJ, Sklar GS, Hill CH, et al: Complications related to the pressor response to endotracheal intubation. Anesthesiology 47:524, 1977

33. Stoelting RK: Circulatory changes during direct laryngoscopy and tracheal intubation: Influence of duration of laryngoscopy with and without prior lidocaine. Anesthesiology 47:381, 1977

34. Smith M, Ray CT: Cardiac arrhythmias, increased intracranial pressure, and the autonomic nervous system. Chest 61:125, 1972

35. Alexander JP: Dysrhythmia and oral surgery. Br J Anesth 43:773, 1971

36. Borg DE: Paradox of cardiac arrhythmias in anaesthesia. Br J Anaesth 41:709, 1969

37. Kaplan JA: Electrocardiographic monitoring, Cardiac Anesthesia. Edited by Kaplan JA. New York, Grune & Stratton, 1979, pp 117–166

38. Scherlag BJ, Lazzara R, Helfant RH: Differentiation of "AV junctional rhythms." Circulation 48:304, 1973

39. Haldemann G, Schoer H: Haemodynamic effects of transient atrioventricular dissociation in general anesthesia. Br J Anaesth 44:159, 1972

40. Galindo A, Wyte SR, Wetherhold JW: Junctional rhythm induced by halothane anesthesia — Treatment with succinylcholine. Anesthesiology 37:261, 1972

41. Kaplan JA, Dunbar RW, Bland JW, et al: Propranolol and cardiac surgery: A problem for the anesthesiologist? Anesth Analg 54:571, 1975

42. Slapa WJ: The sick sinus syndrome. Am Heart J 92:648, 1976

43. Moe GK, Mendez C: Physiologic basis of premature beats and sustained tachycardia. N Engl J Med 288:250, 1973

44. Sprague DH, Mandel SD: Paroxysmal supraventricular tachycardia during anesthesia. Anesthesiology 46:75, 1977

45. Chung EK: Tachyarrhythmias in Wolff-Parkin-

son-White syndrome: Antiarrhythmia therapy. JAMA 237:376, 1977

46. Rinkenberger RL, Prystowsky EN, Heger JJ: Effects of intravenous and chronic oral verapamil administration in patients with supraventricular tachyarrhythmias. Circulation 62:996, 1980

47. Zipes DP: Specific arrhythmias, diagnosis and treatment, Heart Disease. Edited by Braunwald E. Philadelphia, WB Saunders, 1984, p 709

48. Escher DJW, Furman S: Emergency treatment of cardiac arrhythmias: Emphasis on use of electrical pacing. JAMA 214:2028, 1970

49. Kleiger RE: Cardioversion of paroxysmal arrhythmias. JAMA 213:107, 1970

50. Glassman E: Direct current cardioversion. Am Heart J 82:128, 1971

51. Camm J, Ward D, Spunell R: Response of atrial flutter to overdrive atrial pacing and intravenous disopyramide phosphate, singly and in combination. Br Heart J 44:240, 1980

52. Cranefield PF: Ventricular fibrillation. N Engl J Med 289:732, 1973

53. Pietras RJ, Mautner R, Denes P, et al: Chronic recurrent right and left ventricular tachycardia: Comparison of clinical, hemodynamic and angiographic findings. Am J Cardiol 40:32, 1977

54. Geddes LA, Tacker WA, Rosborough J, et al: The electrical dose for ventricular defibrillation with electrodes applied directly to the heart. J Thorac Cardiovasc Surg 68:593, 1974

55. Hecht HH, Kossman EC, Childers RW, et al: Atrioventricular and intraventricular conduction: Revised nomenclature and concepts. Am J Cardiol 31:232, 1973

56. Marriott HJL: Practical Electrocardiography. 7th Ed. Baltimore, Williams & Wilkins, 1983

57. Kastor JA: Atrioventricular block. N Engl J Med 292:462, 572, 1976

58. Wynands JE: Anesthesia for patients with heart block and artificial cardiac pacemakers. Anesth Analg 55:626, 1976

59. Blackburn H: The exercise electrocardiogram: Technological, procedural, and conceptual development, Measurements in Exercise Electrocardiography. Edited by Blackburn H. Springfield, Ill, Charles C Thomas, 1967

60. Dalton B: A precordial ECG lead for chest operations. Anesth Analg 55:740, 1976

61. Robertson D, Kostuk WJ, Ahuja SP: The localization of coronary artery stenosis by 12 lead ECG response to graded exercise test. Am Heart J 91:437, 1976

62. Kaplan JA, Dunbar RW, Hatcher CR: Diagnostic value of the V_5 precordial electrocardiographic lead. Anesth Analg 57:364, 1978

63. Ellestad MH: Stress-testing: Principles and Practice. Philadelphia, FA Davis, 1975

64. Fortuin NJ, Weiss JL: Exercise stress testing. Circulation 56:699, 1976

65. Froelicher VF, Wolthius R, Keiser N, et al: A comparison of two bipolar exercise ECG leads to lead V_5. Chest 70:611, 1976

66. Kattus AA: Exercise ECG: Recognition of the ischemic response, false positive and negative pattern. Am J Cardiol 33:721, 1976

67. Scheffield GT, Holt JH, Lester FM: On-line analysis of the exercise electrocardiogram. Circulation 40:935, 1969

68. Roy WL, Edelist G, Gilbert B: Myocardial ischemia during non-cardiac surgical procedures in patients with coronary artery disease. Anesthesiology 51:393, 1979

69. Kotrly KJ, Kotter GS, Montana D, et al: Intraoperative detection of myocardial ischemia with an ST segment trend monitoring system. Anesth Analg 63:343, 1984

70. Muller JE, Maroko PR, Braunwald E: Precordial ECG mapping: A technique to assess the efficacy of interventions designed to limit infarct size. Circulation 57:1, 1978

71. Muller JE, Maroko PR, Braunwald E: Evaluation of precordial ECG mapping as a means of assessing change in myocardial ischemic injury. Circulation 52:16, 1975

72. Maroko PR, Kjekshus JK, Sobel BE, et al: Factors influencing infarct size following experimental coronary artery occlusion. Circulation 43:67, 1971

73. Hillis LD, Braunwald E: Myocardial ischemia. N Engl J Med 296:971, 1977

74. Madias JE, Madias NE, Hood WB: Precordial ST segment mapping. Effects of oxygen inhalation on ischemic injury in patients with acute myocardial infarction. Circulation 53:411, 1976

75. Holland RP, Brooks H: TQ-ST segment mapping: Critical review and analysis of current concepts. Am J Cardiol 40:110, 1977

76. Surawicz B: The disputed ST segment mapping: Is the technique ready for wide application in practice? Am J Cardiol 40:137, 1977

77. Fozzard HA, Da Gupta DS: ST segment potential and mapping: Theory and experiment. Circulation 54:533, 1976

15

Diagnosis and Treatment of Intraoperative Cardiac Dysrhythmias

Mark C. Rogers, M.D.

INTRODUCTION

Analysis of cardiac dysrhythmias intraoperatively requires appropriate monitoring and an understanding of the physiologic factors predisposing to the development of those dysrhythmias. This chapter proposes how the anesthesiologist can detect, analyze, and treat most significant cardiac dysrhythmias. (Also see Ch. 14 for a description of the fundamentals of the ECG.) Unlike other monographs written by nonanesthesiologists, however, this chapter does not attempt to explain very rare dysrhythmias unlikely to be of clinical importance during the perioperative period. Rather, explanations for clinical situations are provided in which dysrhythmias occur in a reproducible fashion during the perioperative period. All of this must begin, however, with appropriate electrocardiographic (ECG) monitoring of the patient.

INTRAOPERATIVE DYSRHYTHMIA MONITORING

Much of the focus of ECG monitoring during anesthesia has been directed toward the detection of myocardial ischemia. In particular, monitoring of V_5 has been recommended because this is a convenient way to monitor cardiac ischemia.[1-3] Nevertheless, it is important to reflect that patients cared for in coronary care units (CCUs) are rarely if ever monitored exclusively with V_5.

The reason for this is simple. While ischemia is a great risk factor for cardiac catastrophe, it is not the mechanism by which cardiovascular collapse ultimately occurs. Cardiovascular collapse is more likely to occur from cardiac dysrhythmias than from any other single event in either the CCU or the operating room. To monitor cardiac dysrhythmias, however, monitoring for ST segment elevation or depression

499

is not appropriate. Rather, the patient should be monitored for detection of P waves and for analysis of QRS form. Without P waves, the relationship between atrial and ventricular activity cannot be detected. Lead V_5 is a poor lead for the detection of P waves. In a similar fashion, it is necessary to analyze QRS form. One of the common misconceptions is that wide and bizarre QRS complexes automatically mean ventricular premature beats with ventricular dysrhythmias. In fact, there may be many kinds of atrial premature beats and atrial dysrhythmias in which abnormalities of QRS form are commonplace. The ability to detect patterns indicative of right bundle branch block (RBBB) and left bundle branch block (LBBB) is absolutely integral to the ability to analyze dysrhythmias. For this reason, lead systems other than V_5 should be available for the evaluation of patients at risk for cardiac dysrhythmias during anesthesia. In this regard, several ECG leads are commonly monitored;

these should include some modification of standard lead II, which is very useful for detecting P waves, as well as an anterior precordial chest lead, generally a modified V_1 or a mid-clavicular lead system as detailed in Figure 15-1. Making the assumption that these are the leads being monitored, this review analyzes the physiologic conditions responsible for generating atrial and ventricular dysrhythmias, the treatments appropriate for these dysrhythmias, and unusual surgical–anesthetic interactions likely to produce dysrhythmias of interest to the anesthesiologist.

SIMPLE DYSRHYTHMIAS

While most anesthesiologists like to focus on complex ventricular dysrhythmias, the dysrhythmias that generally occur during anes-

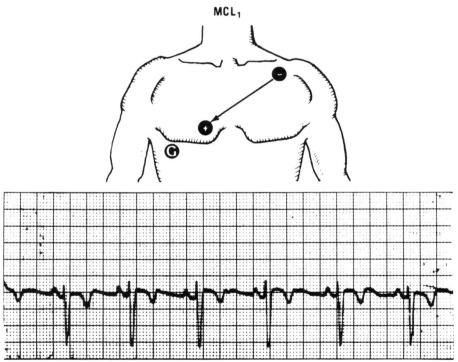

FIG. 15-1 The electrode position in an ECG tracing of a typical MCL₁ lead demonstrated. (Hampton AG: Monitoring and dysrhythmia recognition and advanced life support. American Heart Association Advanced Life Support Course.)

thesia are premature atrial beats, bradycardias, nodal rhythms, and simple premature ventricular contractions (PVCs). More than 15 years ago, a Holter monitoring study done on 154 patients undergoing anesthesia indicated that 195 dysrhythmias were detected in 95 patients.[4] Of these dysrhythmias, nodal rhythm was most common, occurring in 63 patients, while wandering pacemaker was the next most frequent cause, occurring in 43 patients. The hemodynamic significance of these bradydysrhythmias and nodal rhythms should not be underestimated, particularly in patients with heart disease. For example, while a normal atrial contraction preceding ventricular contraction is responsible for approximately 15 percent of cardiac output in the normal patient, in a patient with heart disease this may account for as much as 40 percent of cardiac output.[5-7] Clearly, the sinus node slowing that results in nodal rhythms and wandering atrial pacemakers seen so frequently under anesthesia is an important concept that should be viewed as having potential hemodynamic significance, meriting analysis of the factors responsible for its frequency under anesthesia. Furthermore, if one looks at the predisposing physiologic factors responsible for the generation of atrial dysrhythmias, slow heart rate, long PR intervals, and multiple reentry pathways all set up the circumstances for ectopic beats in the atrium and the ventricle. Sinus bradycardia and nodal rhythms can produce all these circumstances.

Table 15-1 lists the factors that predispose toward sinus bradycardia under anesthesia. The combination of anesthetic agents, vagal response, and decreased temperature (general or local in the right atrium) can cause sinus bradycardia, nodal rhythms, and serious cardiac dysrhythmias. With regard to anesthetic agents, inhaled anesthetics clearly depress sinus node activity (also see Ch. 20). As can be seen in Figure 15-2, the cardiac action potential characteristically shown in the ventricle has four phases of depolarization. Phase 0 is the fast upstroke phase, phase 1 is the beginning of recovery, phase 2 is the plateau period, phase 3 is the more slopelike recovery period, and phase 4 is the area in which spontaneous depolarization can occur. In the atrium, and in particular in the sinus node, these phases are shortened, so that the atrial action potential is different from the ventricular action potential. As shown in Figure 15-3, anesthetic agents themselves slow the response of the atrium by altering the slope of phase 4 depolarization, resulting in bradycardia. There appears to be a relationship between the effects of anesthetic agents and calcium flux,[8] which is one of the reasons why bradycardia is so common even with hypotension during anesthesia.

Further reasons why bradycardia develops result from what I like to term vagal responses. These vagal responses can be reflex induced or pharmacologically induced. As an example, there are many vagal responses associated with the upper airway in which endotracheal intubation or reflex manipulation of the airway or bronchus is likely to result in bradycardia (also see Ch. 16). Once these occur, the setting of anesthetic interactions and vagal responses is likely to generate the rhythm known as *isorhythmic AV dissociation*.[9] This rhythm, very familiar to the anesthesiologist, is one in which the P wave appears to march in and out of the QRS complex. It is also associated with fluctuations in the arterial blood pressure as the P wave synchronizes prior to the QRS to produce

TABLE 15-1. Factors That Cause Sinus Bradycardia Under Anesthesia

Intrinsic to the patient
    Sick sinus syndrome
    Increased intracranial pressure
    Nonanesthetic drug related (i.e., propranolol, digoxin)
Vagal responses
    Reflex stimulation of nasopharynx, lateral rectus, bronchus, peritoneum, etc.
    Acetylcholine-related drugs, such as muscle relaxants (succinylcholine), neostigmine
Direct anesthetic agent related
    Inhalational (halothane, ethrane, isoflurane)
    Narcotic (fentanyl, morphine)

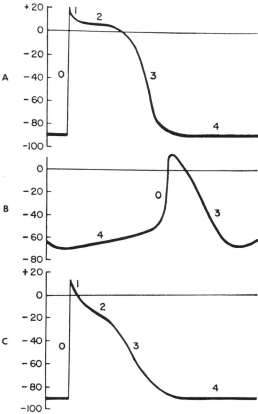

FIG. 15-2 Typical action potential in millivolts recorded from cells in the ventricle (A), sinoatrial node (B), and atrium (C). Sweep velocity in B is one-half of that in A or C. (Hoffman BF, Cranefield PF: Electrophysiology of the Heart, New York, McGraw-Hill, 1960.)

sia drugs that cause vagal bradycardia include succinylcholine, as well as any of a host of anesthetic-related drugs such as neostigmine (also see Ch. 27).[10] All these physiologic and pharmacologic factors have the potential to produce profound bradycardias under anesthesia and to exacerbate situations providing for hemodynamic instability. As described in Table 15-1, hypothermia is also such a predisposing factor to bradycardia (also see Ch. 57). This is commonly known to the anesthesiologist in the form of the bradycardias associated with deep hypothermia during cardiopulmonary bypass but actually has been documented to occur merely from the injection of iced saline into the right atrium during thermodilution cardiac output measurements (also see Ch. 13).[11-14]

SICK SINUS SYNDROME

An impulse originating in the sinus node that is blocked before it can depolarize the atrium is referred to as sinoatrial (SA) block. When this is repetitive, it is referred to as a sinus pause (see Fig. 15-4). These conditions occur frequently in elderly patients. In the absence of drug therapy, sinus block is part of the sick sinus syndrome.[15] This syndrome is defined by severe sinus bradycardia and by sinus pause of arrest with escape. It frequently leads to atrial fibrillation. Most patients with sick sinus syndrome are elderly and have coronary artery disease. While it can be mild, producing syncope, it is a frequent symptom and requires permanent pacemaker implantation.

Sick sinus syndrome is an important condition for anesthesiologists to recognize. Elderly patients with sinus bradycardia and/or unexplained syncope should be fully evaluated before surgery is undertaken. If sudden intraoperative long sinus pause or sinus arrest is noted, a pacemaker should be inserted. With elderly patients increasingly presenting for surgery (also see Ch. 50), anesthesiologists should become more aware of sick sinus syndrome and of the possibility that the triad of advanced age, heart disease, and anesthetics may interact to produce this syndrome in the operating room.

a normal cardiac output, as well as hypotension, when the P wave marches through and ultimately follows the QRS, decreasing cardiac output. The interaction of vagal response and arterial baroreceptor response regulates the relationship of the P wave to the QRS and is thought to be responsible for the phasic fluctuations of arterial blood pressure seen under halothane, enflurane, and isoflurane anesthesia. The bradycardias associated with morphine and fentanyl are thought to be due to direct actions on the sinus node in addition to CNS effects.[3] These are not as well understood as the inhaled anesthetic effects. Non-anesthe-

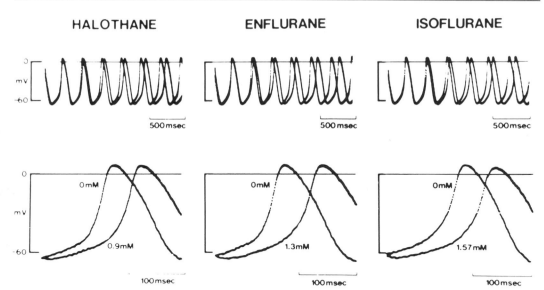

FIG. 15-3 The effect of halothane, enflurane, and isoflurane on the action potentials of spontaneously active fibers in the guinea pig SA node region. The action potential tracings of the control and after 5 minutes of exposure to anesthetics (2 MAC) are superimposed at two different speeds and magnifications (Adapted from Bosnijak ZJ, Kampine JP: Effects of halothane, enflurane, and isoflurane on the SA node. Anesthesiology 58:314, 1983.)

PREMATURE ATRIAL BEATS

Premature atrial beats occur frequently in healthy patients and in patients undergoing anesthesia. A premature atrial beat is easily recognized when it occurs with a P wave early in the cycle followed by a QRS complex (Fig. 15-5). Simple atrial premature beats can in themselves be significant hemodynamic events even in simple form, since they have the potential to generate serious cardiac dysrhythmias, such as atrial fibrillation. In fact, most serious atrial dysrhythmias do not occur spontaneously but rather only in response to a setting in which premature atrial beats initiate multiple reentry pathways and paroxysmal atrial tachycardia (PAT) or atrial fibrillation. As a result, it pays to be alert to the development of premature atrial beats and to be aware

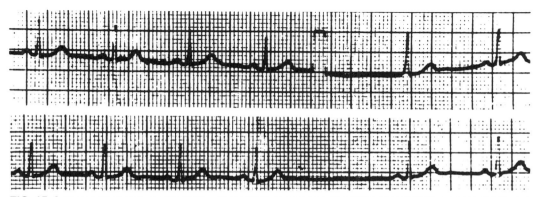

FIG. 15-4 Sinoatrial disease manifested by sinoatrial block and dropping of the expected sinus generated P wave. (Lamb LE: Electrocardiography and Vector Cardiography. Philadelphia, WB Saunders, 1965.)

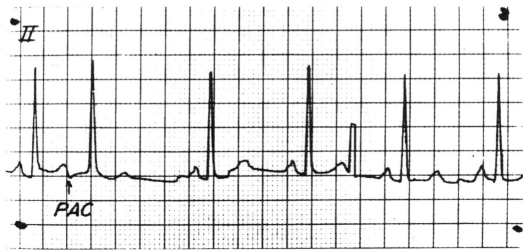

FIG. 15-5 Premature atrial complex (indicated by arrow) and lack of compensatory pause. (Adapted from Shoemaker WC, Thompson WL, Holbrook PR: Textbook of Critical Care. Philadelphia, WB Saunders, 1984.)

that simple premature atrial beats do not merely signify an early P wave with a normal QRS. On the contrary, there are many other possibilities. Atrial premature beats may occur early enough in the cardiac cycle to be blocked at the atrioventricular (AV) node, thereby preventing their conductance to the ventricle. This is sometimes difficult to detect unless the lead system is appropriate — which is why we have emphasized the need for multiple lead systems, including lead II. Furthermore, if multiple premature atrial beats occur, constantly interrupting the sinus cycle and resetting it, it is impossible to distinguish these multiple irregular beats from the setting of atrial fibrillation if the only monitoring device is an esophageal stethoscope. For this reason, I consider ECG monitoring mandatory for every patient undergoing anesthesia. Since "unexpected" hemodynamic disasters are likely to be the end product of a number of physiologic events, which include abnormalities of heart rates and rhythm, the need to monitor the ECG continually and effectively is clear. This becomes even more apparent when one looks into the situation regarding atrial premature beats with bizarre QRS complexes.

As alluded to earlier, analysis of QRS form is absolutely indispensable for the interpreta-

tion of cardiac rhythm. The concept that wide and bizarre QRS complexes automatically mean ventricular premature beats or ventricular dysrhythmias is both erroneous and dangerous. It makes a big difference to the sophistication of anesthetic care if you are anesthetizing a 6-year-old undergoing a tonsillectomy, for whom the monitor shows the development of wide bizarre QRS complexes, if you can be reassured that this rhythm is atrial rather than ventricular (also see Ch. 52). Atrial dysrhythmias in a patient undergoing tonsillectomy would not be unusual and might result from reflex vagal stimulation in the nasopharynx. Ventricular dysrhythmias, on the other hand, might be very serious and reflect either hypoxia or severe intraoperative problems. As a result, analysis of QRS form is extremely important, since premature atrial beats conducted through the AV node may be blocked in the bundle branches and may produce a wide and bizarre QRS complex that does not have to be a PVC. It may mean a premature atrial contraction conducted with aberration. Furthermore, 90 percent of premature atrial contractions (PACs) conducted with aberration have a RBBB pattern; analysis of QRS form is critical for characterization of dysrhythmias.[6] A wide and bizarre QRS complex that sticks out like a

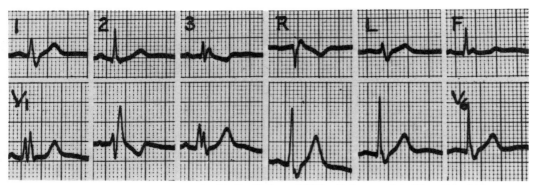

FIG. 15-6 Right bundle branch block with wide S_1, M-shaped QRS with large upright R^1 and V_1. (Marriott HJL: Practical Electrocardiography. 7th edition. © 1983 The Williams & Wilkins Co, Baltimore.)

sore thumb may or may not be a PVC—only through evaluation of QRS form is it possible to tell which one is a PAC and which a PVC. The characteristic rSR′ pattern in V_1 or any right precordial lead that documents a RBBB pattern (Figure 15-6) is a very reassuring sign that the wide and bizarre QRS complex is a PAC conducted with a RBBB pattern, diminishing the likelihood of a hypoxic or catastrophic event.

What is true for one PAC (Fig. 15-7) is also true for multiple PACs or for a change in heart rate. The concept that a series of wide bizarre QRS complexes is proof positive of a sudden burst of ventricular tachycardia is incorrect; it may in fact represent only a rate-dependent RBBB pattern as the heart rate suddenly speeds up (see Fig. 15-8). It is also true that in settings of atrial fibrillation, short intervals in the irregu-

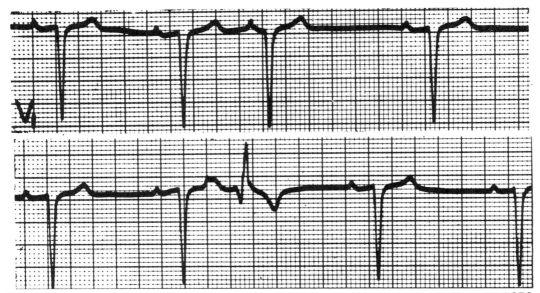

FIG. 15-7 Atrial premature beats. In upper tracing, the third beat is an atrial premature beat with a normal QRS complex. In the lower tracing, the atrial premature beat occurs earlier and the P wave of this beat is included in the previous T wave. Because of the early conductance of this beat, it has a right bundle branch pattern. (Adapted from Marriott HJL: Practical Electrocardiography. © 1977 The Williams and Wilkins Co, Baltimore.)

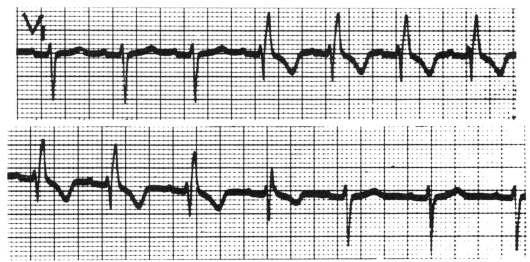

FIG. 15-8 Rate-dependent intermittent right bundle branch block pattern. Fourth beat has a right bundle branch block pattern, despite the fact that it is normally conducted and the reason is that there is an acceleration in the underlying rate from 98 to 102. (Marriott HJL: Practical Electrocardiography. © 1977 The Williams and Wilkins Co, Baltimore.)

lar rhythm are associated with bizarre QRS complexes generally of the RBBB pattern; they do not mean that the rhythm is ventricular tachycardia. These physiologic principles demonstrate that PACs can be (1) simple with a defined P wave and QRS occurring at a short interval, (2) associated with a blocked P wave with no QRS but a resetting of the sinus node, or (3) associated with a block in the bundle branches generally of a RBBB configuration (see Table 15-2). Furthermore, these findings can occur multiple times in a row, resulting in what appeared to be rather complex and sophisticated dysrhythmias susceptible to simple analysis once the underlying physiology is understood. All of this is predicated on the ability to monitor the patient adequately for both the presence of P waves and the analysis of QRS form.

TABLE 15-2. ECG Forms of Premature Atrial Contractions

1. Early P wave, normal QRS
2. Early P wave blocked in AV node
3. Early P wave, blocked in bundle branches, wide QRS with high likelihood of right bundle branch block

PREMATURE VENTRICULAR BEATS

The transition between premature atrial beats and premature ventricular beats following discussion of ventricular conduction abnormalities is a logical way to approach the subject of intraoperative dysrhythmias. While everyone knows that a PVC sticks out like a sore thumb, it is now apparent that not everything that sticks out like a sore thumb is a premature ventricular beat. Wide bizarre QRS complexes may be premature atrial beats. Suspicion of premature ventricular beats is enhanced when they do not have a RBBB form, although it should be stated without reservation that a PVC can have any form. Nevertheless, a bizarre QRS without classic RBBB form should alert the anesthesiologist to suspect a premature ventricular beat or a ventricular rhythm.

One of the ways of distinguishing premature ventricular beats from premature atrial beats relates to the concept of compensatory pause.[16] Compensatory pause deals with the long interval following a premature ventricular beat (Fig. 15-9). Stated simply, premature ven-

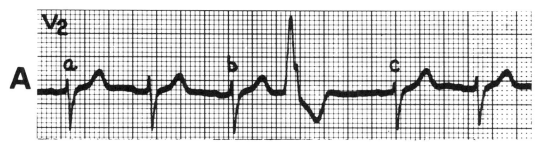

FIG. 15-9 A PVC with a compensatory pause outline. The time from a to b, which is two sinocycles is exactly equal to the time between b and c. (Marriott HJL: Practical Electrocardiography. Baltimore, © 1977 The Williams and Wilkins Co, Baltimore.)

tricular beats do not commonly have the opportunity to be conducted retrograde through the AV node, to enter the atrium, and to depolarize the sinus node. As a result, the sinus node continues through at a regular interval during the premature ventricular beat. The effect is that a premature ventricular beat starts off with a short interval following the normal sinus cycle, but then the P wave of the next sinus cycle is undisturbed and the succeeding sinus cycle occurs on time. The sinus rhythm is never reset, as contrasted with an atrial premature beat. Comparison of an atrial premature beat with a premature ventricular beat is shown in Table 15-3. The atrial premature beat has one short cycle and one normal cycle, whereas the premature ventricular beat has one short cycle followed by an abnormally long one. This very long cycle consists of the time from the PVC to the next sinus cycle, which is unseen, and then a complete normal sinus cycle. This total of a short QRS to unseen P wave followed by a normal P-P interval results in an extra long interval referred to as the compensatory pause. In summary, the premature ventricular beat does

TABLE 15-3. Comparison of Premature Atrial Contractions and Premature Ventricular Contractions

PAC	PVC
Resets sinus node, no compensatory pause	Does not reset sinus node, compensatory pause
Most have normal QRS, some have no QRS (blocked), some have RBBB pattern	Wide and bizarre patterns seen in any shape

not reset the sinus cycle, the shape of the P wave may be untouched and normal or may be unobserved, the QRS form is bizarre and widened and not likely to have right bundle branch block, and the timing is such that it has a compensatory pause.

Since many patients have PVCs throughout their lives, the clinician must determine when a PVC is serious and requires treatment (Table 15-4). All PVCs are potentially serious, of course, because they can initiate ventricular fibrillation. Treatment of PVCs is based on a mathematical likelihood of initiating ventricular fibrillation, which is related to their frequency, to when they occur in the cardiac cycle, and to the clinical setting in which they occur. Frequent PVCs, generally defined as six or more per minute, are likely to have an increased likelihood of initiating ventricular fibrillation and should be treated. Likewise, multifocal PVCs, defined as PVCs arising from two different foci or having two different reentry pathways (so that the QRS form of PVCs varies in a given lead) also carry a high risk of initiating ventricular fibrillation, hence require treatment. In addition, three PVCs in a row and perhaps even two PVCs in a row may be construed as a short burst of ventricular tachycardia, requiring treatment. Finally, the concept that a PVC that occurs on the preceding T wave of the ECG (vulnerable period) is very serious is the most important concept to be communicated.[3]

The T wave of the ECG represents the repolarization period during phase 3 of the preceding action potential. A PVC that occurs during this cycle is likely to find some of the

TABLE 15-4. When to Treat a Premature Ventricular Contraction

1. High frequency (> 6/minute)
2. Three or more in a row (ventricular tachycardia)
3. Multifocal (different QRS forms)
4. Vulnerable period (PVC on T wave)

ventricle repolarized and some of the ventricle not repolarized. As a result, the PVC can find available multiple reentry pathways in the ventricle likely to generate ventricular fibrillation. It is the frequency with which this is likely to occur that has led to the description of the descending limb of the T wave as the vulnerable period. It is crucial not to be encouraged by the fact that a PVC occurring in a patient during this period does not initiate ventricular fibrillation. Rather, it is a mathematical relationship—a repeat of the same PVC 15 seconds later could very well result in ventricular fibrillation. It is, therefore, extremely important to be aggressive about treating a patient in whom PVCs are found to fall on the descending limit of the T wave.

Still, patients have been observed for years with premature ventricular beats. Cardiologists are more comfortable about PVCs and have called into question some of the rules of treating ventricular premature beats in ambulatory patients. The key point is that none of these ambulatory patients is under the stress of anesthesia and surgery. For this reason, it is still advisable for anesthesiologists to use criteria for treating PVCs under the stress of anesthesia and surgery more liberally than the more relaxed criteria now recommended by some of our cardiology colleagues. It is better to treat PVCs unnecessarily than to have PVCs generate into ventricular fibrillation.

The treatment of PVCs intraoperatively is still most effectively accomplished by lidocaine. A bolus of 1.0 to 1.5 mg/kg followed as necessary by the administration of a continuous infusion of 20 to 40 μg/kg/min is usually all that is required. Occasionally there may be unusual circumstances such as profound bradycardias, which allow escape ventricular beats, or drug-related PVCs, such as those seen with digitalis intoxication (these concepts will be discussed separately).

PAROXYSMAL ATRIAL TACHYCARDIA

This dysrhythmia is actually a combination term for a number of supraventricular tachycardias previously identified as arising independently in the atrium or the AV node.[17] Paroxysmal atrial tachycardia (PAT) is defined as a supraventricular rhythm at a rate of approximately 170 to 250 beats/min that may be transient or that may last for days. It may occur in patients with a wide variety of underlying conditions ranging from atrial septal defect, to thyrotoxicosis, to Wolff-Parkinson-White syndrome, to mitral valve prolapse. Generally, the ventricular rate is quite regular and is conducted from the atrium in a 1:1 relationship in patients who have normal AV conduction. Nevertheless, the ventricular rate may be slower than the atrial rate due to AV block as the ventricular rate increases toward 250 beats/min or as AV node function is decreased by disease or by the use of certain drugs. By itself, this rhythm is not definitive of heart disease and may be induced by combinations of factors, such as caffeine, stress, alcohol, or drugs such as catecholamines. Whereas it was originally anticipated that this rhythm was the result of an ectopic focus other than sinus node, it is now generally perceived that there are multiple pathways through the AV node and that the rhythm is a circus rhythm involving the upper AV node and the atrium. This is why many authorities combine nodal tachycardia and atrial tachycardia in the diagnosis of PAT. Generally, the ventricular rate during PAT is regular and of normal QRS configuration (Fig. 15-10). At faster rates, however, the QRS may be wide with the RBBB pattern, and it may be difficult to diagnose PAT in a setting in which it may be confused with ventricular tachycardia (Fig. 15-11).

Many concepts are used in treating PAT. Among the oldest is altering autonomic tone to the heart by maneuvers such as carotid massage. Other therapies include electrical countershock, overdrive pacing, or drug administration. Intravenous digoxin is a classic approach to drug therapy of PAT, and many anesthesiologists also have found the parasympathetic drug, neostigmine, of use intraoperatively. Propranolol and, most recently, verapa-

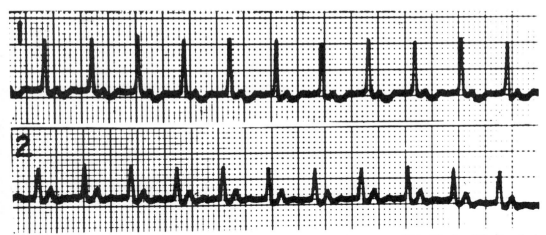

FIG. 15-10 Atrial tachycardia with visible P waves, which in this case follow each QRS. (Marriott HJL: Practical Electrocardiography. © 1977 The Williams & Wilkins Co, Baltimore.)

mil have been used successfully for the treatment of this dysrhythmia. Verapamil,[18] in particular, has been found extremely effective in the setting of PAT and is now commonly used in many operating rooms.

Variations of this dysrhythmia include PAT with block when the rapid supraventricular rate is accompanied by variable AV block, usually second degree and usually at 2 : 1 conduction. This dysrhythmia is dangerous and is generally seen in the setting of digitalis intoxication or hypokalemia. It is commonly treated by withholding digoxin and giving potassium intravenously under cautious supervision. In this setting, digitalis is commonly contraindicated for fear that the converted rhythm will degenerate into ventricular fibrillation.

ATRIAL FLUTTER

Atrial flutter (Fig. 15-12) is a regular atrial rate faster than that of PAT and generally between 250 and 350 beats/min. It is thought to

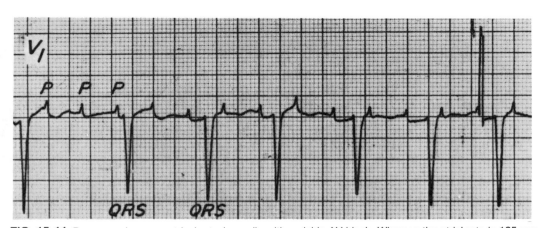

FIG. 15-11 Paroxysmal supraventricular tachycardia with variable AV block. Whereas the atrial rate is 185 per minute, there is both 3 : 1 and 2 : 1 AV block present. (Shoemaker WC, Thompson WL, Holbrook PR: Textbook of Critical Care. Philadelphia, WB Saunders, 1984.)

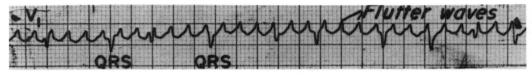

FIG. 15-12 Atrial flutter with a flutter rate of 375 per minute and characteristic saw tooth in configuration. As is expected with this fast atrial rate, the ventricular response is slow with a variable AV block ranging from 2:1 to 6:1. (Shoemaker WC, Thompson WL, Holbrook PR: Textbook of Critical Care. Philadelphia, WB Saunders, 1984.)

be a circus rhythm intrinsic to the atrium; because of the fast rate, it is very rarely associated with 1:1 conduction to the ventricles. Frequently, there is significant AV block, and AV conduction ratios of 1:1 to 3:1 are common with ventricular rates of 150 beats/min.

Atrial flutter is seen in patients with underlying heart disease such as rheumatic heart disease with enlarged atria; it is not commonly a manifestation of digitalis toxicity. The classic atrial rate is in the sawtooth pattern of atrial activity. These flutter waves are most commonly seen in leads 2, 3, AVF, and V_1. The degree of block may vary and can change quite rapidly. One of the common problems associated with atrial flutter is that some drugs that are used for treatment of supraventricular dysrhythmias, such as quinidine, may be contraindicated early in the course of this condition. The reason is that the vagolytic action of these drugs will actually increase ventricular rate before converting the rhythm. This may actually lower cardiac output unless the patient is treated with digitalis first. Regardless, atrial flutter is another dysrhythmia for which there has been significant success with verapamil as well as with electric countershock, generally responding to relatively low energy levels of 10 to 25 watt-sec. It may also be treated with digitalis, which does not necessarily convert the atrial flutter to sinus rhythm but slows down the ventricular response to an acceptable level. Propranolol has been used for the same reason.

ATRIAL FIBRILLATION

Atrial fibrillation (Fig. 15-13) is a very common dysrhythmia generally seen in patients with heart disease and with enlarged atria. It is rarely seen in healthy patients and can be thought of as being associated with coronary, rheumatic, and hypertensive heart disease. It is sometimes seen in an intermittent pattern but, because of its association with enlarged atria, it is frequently stable in patients for many years at a time. Because of the lack of atrial contribution to ventricular filling seen with normal P-wave pattern, atrial fibrillation is sometimes associated with a low cardiac output despite the rapid heart rate.

The mechanism for the fibrillation is probably abnormal atrial pathology with widely diffuse abnormalities in diastolic resting potentials and heterogeneous conduction velocities.[3,6,7] These abnormalities present opportunities for reentry pathways that begin with ectopic atrial beats. The atrial fibrillation itself may be very rapid rates of 400 to 800 beats/min or may even be invisible, as the atrial fibrillation may be very "fine." At times it may resemble atrial flutter with 4–5–6 beats having a sawtooth pattern, but then it degenerates into atrial fibrillation.

Because of the rapid atrial rate, 1:1 conduction cannot exist—by definition all such patients have some degree of AV block. As a result, the ventricular response is "irregularly irregular" with no apparent frequent cycle length of the RR intervals. Nevertheless, studies of the RR interval indicate that there are frequency distributions that have been used as documentation of the existence of multiple pathways through the AV node and that the RR intervals tend to fall along the conduction times of these multiple pathways. It is of note that aberrant conduction with the RBBB (as described with PACs) also occurs with the very early cycle lengths seen in some of the beats during atrial fibrillation. This is referred to as the Ashman phenomenon. Since there are ab-

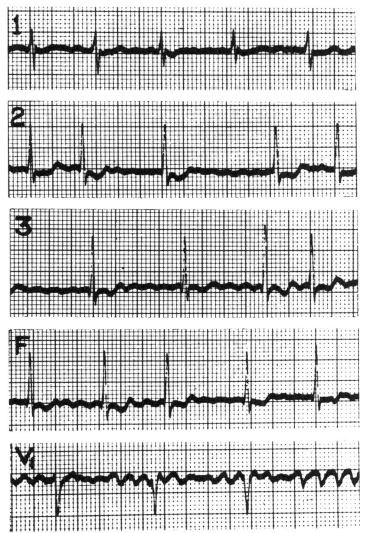

FIG. 15-13 Atrial fibrillation with the irregularly irregular flutter waves visible in all leads. Note the totally irregular response to the ventricular complexes. (Marriott HJL: Practical Electrocardiography. © 1977 The Williams & Wilkins Co, Baltimore.)

normalities of ventricular conduction, it is sometimes difficult to diagnose PVCs and aberrantly conducted supraventricular beats in the setting of atrial fibrillation.

Therapy in atrial fibrillation is related to some extent to the underlying disease state. If there is a recent onset of atrial fibrillation, that cardioversion to sinus rhythm probably will result in a stable normal sinus rate. On the other hand, chronic atrial fibrillation is not sus-

ceptible to cardioversion in that the patient reverts to atrial fibrillation very rapidly. It is more appropriate to try to control the ventricular response, and digitalis controls the ventricular rate by decreasing AV conduction in a well known manner. Propranolol has been used similarly in this setting with a good deal of success, but digitalis remains the most commonly used agent.

Since most patients with atrial fibrillation

are being treated with digitalis, digitalis toxicity must be recognized in this setting. One mechanism relates to advanced AV block and the slowing of ventricular rate to 40 or 50 beats/min. This case should raise significant concern that the patient is overdigitalized. Similarly, if the ventricular rate becomes regular, the possibility of digitalis producing advanced AV block with a subsidiary pacemaker producing a regular rate despite the fact the atrium remains in fibrillation also must be suspected. Frequent PVCs, particularly multifocal PVCs, are also suggestive of digitalis toxicity. Particular attention must be paid in these patients to the possibility of hypokalemia and the possible interaction of digitalis and muscle relaxants, such as succinylcholine, to produce ventricular dysrhythmias.[8] Propranolol and verapamil also have been used to decrease conduction through the AV node for acute control of the ventricular rate during atrial fibrillation.

ventricular QRS configuration is bizarre and prolonged. Generally the rate is greater than 140 beats/min in most patients, although relatively slow rates have also been observed. One way of distinguishing ventricular tachycardia from atrial tachycardia is as follows: if a rhythm with a wide bizarre QRS complex dominating is periodically interrupted with a normal QRS that appears to be conducted, then the underlying rhythm must be ventricular and the conducted atrial beat (Dressler beat) is considered diagnostic of underlying ventricular tachycardia.[6,18] Similarly, fusion beats suggest a diagnosis of ventricular tachycardia. Further diagnostic criteria may involve the use of esophageal or atrial leads in order to distinguish P waves in this setting. Regardless, it is important to recognize that most commonly this is a life-threatening and very severe dysrhythmia generally requiring immediate treatment, including electrical countershock or such antidysrhythmic agents as lidocaine.

VENTRICULAR TACHYCARDIA

Ventricular tachycardia (Fig. 15-14) is a rhythm defined as three or more PVC episodes in a row that generally degenerates rapidly into ventricular fibrillation.[17] Occasionally it may last for days, but it is always viewed as a dysrhythmia associated with severe heart disease, particularly myocardial ischemia, and it is considered life threatening. Ventricular conduction occurs through ventricular muscle, and

ATRIOVENTRICULAR BLOCK

Atrioventricular block implies some abnormality in the conduction between the atrium and the ventricle, but the block may be within the AV node itself, in the bundle of His, or in the bundle branches. Block at any of these sites may result in partial or total AV block.

Commonly, AV block is divided into first-, second-, and third-degree block in order to dis-

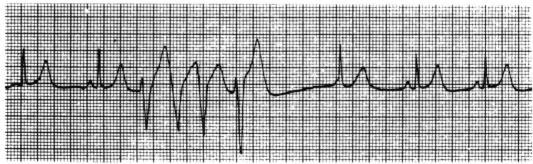

FIG. 15-14 Three or more premature ventricular contractions in a row is defined by a run of ventricular tachycardia. Some authorities would even stipulate that two PVCs in a row is ventricular tachycardia. (Courtesy of Joel Kaplan, M.D.)

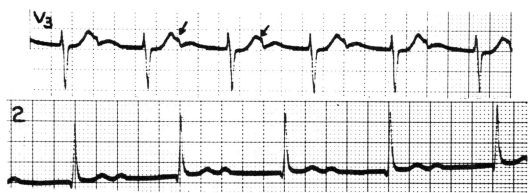

FIG. 15-15 Two examples of first degree AV block with very long PR intervals. The P waves are indicated by the arrows and the PR interval is about 0.46 seconds. (Adapted from Marriott HJL: Practical Electrocardiography. © 1977 Williams & Wilkins Co, Baltimore.)

tinguish whether all the beats are conducted with delay (first degree), some of the beats are conducted (second degree), or none of the beats is conducted (third degree).

First-degree AV block (Fig. 15-15) is a simple delay in conduction between the atrium and the ventricle generally thought to occur within the AV node that results in a prolonged PR interval. By itself it is not necessarily dangerous, but in certain clinical settings it may set up multiple reentry pathways through the AV node. When this happens, atrial dysrhythmias or more severe block may develop subsequently.

Second-degree AV block is defined as conduction of some, but not every, atrial impulse to the ventricles. It is commonly divided into two types of block: Mobitz type I and Mobitz type II. Mobitz type I is referred to as Wenckebach (Fig. 15-16) and is characterized by a PR interval that progressively prolongs for 2, 3, 4,

or even 5 beats before a P wave is not conducted. Physiologically, the site is always within the AV node and this contrasts sharply with Mobitz type II block.[6,7,16]

Mobitz type II block (Fig. 15-17) is the sudden dropping out of a QRS that is expected to follow a P wave.[19] No PR interval prolongations occur before the block beat, and generally every third, fourth, or fifth beat is not conducted to the ventricle. It is generally thought that Mobitz type II block occurs, not in the AV node, but in the His bundle and even more frequently in the bundle branches from bilateral bundle branch block. Mobitz type II block is generally thought to be a serious form of AV conduction delay and generally warrants pacemaker capability during anesthesia.

Third-degree or complete AV block (Fig. 15-18) means that no atrial beats are conducted to the ventricle. While in older patients with heart disease this is very serious, particularly

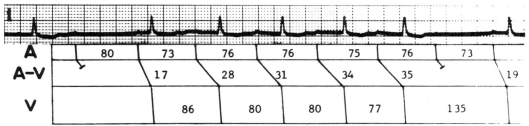

A	80	73	76	76	75	76	73
A–V		17	28	31	34	35	19
V		86	80	80	77	135	

FIG. 15-16 Mobitz Type I–Wenkebach block. The progressive prolongation of the PR interval is seen not only in the tracing but also in the delineation of the intervals in hundredths of a second in the ladder gram listed below. (Marriott HJL: Practical Electrocardiography. © 1977 The Williams & Wilkins Co, Baltimore.)

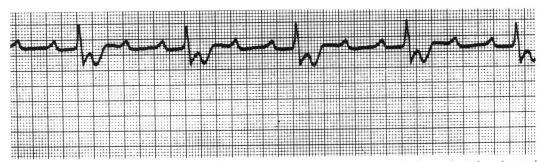

FIG. 15-17 Mobitz Type II second degree block in which P waves which are expected to be conducted are dropped suddenly without a progressive PR interval prolongation. (Courtesy of Joel Kaplan, M.D.)

when the ventricular rate is very low and there is a possibility for low cardiac output, this is not always the case. Some patients are born with third-degree heart block and do not have any problems for many years. Nevertheless, with the exception of congenital heart block, older patients with third-degree heart block are candidates for pacemakers prior to surgery as are patients with Mobitz type II block.

them wisely. I consider lidocaine, propranolol, verapamil, and digitalis the hallmarks of antidysrhythmic drug therapy for the anesthesiologist. For completeness, pertinent information on both bretylium and on diphenylhydantoin is described in this section. Finally, while I do not review pacing in its entirety, new developments in emergency atrial pacing available to the anesthesiologist through the use of the esophagus as an atrial pacing site are highlighted (also see Ch. 28).

ANTIDYSRHYTHMIC THERAPY

The number of drugs used as antidysrhythmics is constantly increasing. Even so, the anesthesiologist probably should be familiar with only a few therapies and should use

LIDOCAINE

This drug has been available for treatment of dysrhythmias for 20 years and is the most commonly used agent in the treatment of ventricular dysrhythmias, particularly premature ventricular beats. Lidocaine has little effect on the atrium, on the sinus node or AV node, or on atrial fibers and is very rarely used in the

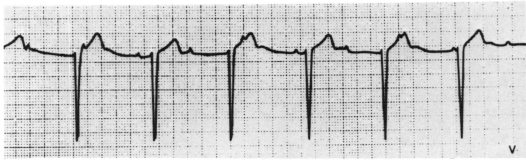

FIG. 15-18 Complete or third degree heart block indicating complete disassociation between atrial and ventricular complexes. (Courtesy of Joel Kaplan, M.D.)

setting of atrial dysrhythmias. It tends to work by an increase in refractory period or a decrease in spontaneous depolarization of ventricular fibers and is, therefore, used for ventricular dysrhythmias. It is primarily metabolized in the liver (also see Ch. 29) and is relatively short acting following an initial bolus, unless it is continued in an intravenous drip or infusion. Lidocaine is commonly administered as an intravenous bolus of 1.0 to 1.5 mg/kg, followed by an intravenous infusion of 20 to 40 μg/kg/min. Periodically, an intravenous bolus is used above the infusion rate, as long as the infusion rate does not exceed these limits. One beneficial effect of lidocaine is this fact that there is little change in ventricular performance or peripheral motor tone at the level of lidocaine, which appears to be clinically useful in suppressing ventricular dysrhythmias. Unfortunately, even at low doses, lidocaine stimulates the CNS, which can cause seizures. High levels in particular have been shown to do this, and toxic levels have also been shown to depress ventricular function. As a result, intravenous administration should not exceed 5 mg/kg in a short period of time.

PROPRANOLOL

This is the most commonly used β-adrenergic blocking drug available as an antidysrhythmic. It is commonly used intravenously intraoperatively and is a nonspecific β_1- and β_2-adrenergic receptor blocker.[20] In addition, it has no clinically significant intrinsic sympathomimetic activity. As a result of its β-blocking actions, propranolol decreases automaticity and the rate of phase IV spontaneous depolarization. It results in a mild decrease in heart rate and is particularly effective in the setting of stress—be it exercise, emotion, or surgery. Since it works directly on membranes and increases permeability of potassium, propranolol also has membrane-stabilizing activity and is thought to be quinidine-like in this property.

In the operating room, the most frequent indication for the use of propranolol is for the control of sinus rate. This occurs during stimulation such as laryngoscopy and endotracheal intubation, as well as surgical stimulation during the incision. The use of propranolol in this setting decreases heart rate and contractility, which may result in an increase in oxygen consumption producing myocardial ischemia in patients who are unable to respond appropriately. It is this combination of properties of controlling heart rate and of controlling contractility to lower myocardial oxygen consumption that makes propranolol such a potent drug to use intraoperatively. Its property to decrease AV node conduction means that it can be used along with digitalis in fast atrial dysrhythmias such as atrial flutter and fibrillation to control ventricular response. Similarly, it can be used in the Wolff-Parkinson-White syndrome and in the setting of ventricular dysrhythmias in combination with agents such as quinidine or procainamide. Despite its excellent antidysrhythmic property, its potential for decreasing ventricular contractility means that propranolol must be used carefully. Doses of 0.5 to 1 mg can be given intravenously every few moments while the patient is carefully monitored as an effective way to give the agent. The reasons for concern are that the sinus-slowing effect may produce profound bradycardias and that the beneficial effects of propranolol in slowing AV conduction may ultimately produce profound AV block. Furthermore, the drug's property of decreasing contractility may be dangerous in patients with poor left ventricular (LV) function. For this reason, its use should be avoided if possible in patients with sick sinus syndrome, with advanced AV block, or with poor LV function. In addition to its decreasing contractility and the potential for bradycardia, propranolol also has the potential to produce hypoglycemia, which may be important in certain patients under anesthesia. Finally, propranolol can provoke bronchospasm in patients with asthma or chronic obstructive pulmonary disease.

BRETYLIUM

Bretylium has been available for about 10 to 15 years for the treatment of severe life-threatening ventricular dysrhythmias. The primary site of action of bretylium appears to be on the sympathetic nervous system, where it inhibits the release of norepinephrine from adrenergic nerve terminals. In addition, bretylium has membrane effects such that it increases action potential duration as well as the effective refractory period in the ventricular conducting system. The net result is to increase the threshold for ventricular fibrillation. Bretylium should be reserved for the treatment of life-threatening ventricular dysrhythmias that have not responded to therapeutic doses of more common antidysrhythmic drugs such as lidocaine. It is also used to treat multifocal PVCs, ventricular tachycardia, and ventricular fibrillation. When administered intravenously, it is given in a dose of 5.0 to 10.0 mg/kg infused slowly over a period of 10 to 20 minutes. The dose may be repeated at 30-minute intervals to a maximum cumulative dose of 30 mg/kg. For more prolonged use, 5.0 to 10.0 mg/kg may be given every 6 to 8 hours; alternatively, an intravenous infusion at 1.0 to 2.0 mg/min may be used.

The classically recognized adverse side effect of bretylium is hypotension due to its effect on the sympathetic nervous system. Frequently, the hypotensive episode is preceded by a brief period of mild hypertension due to transient release of catecholamines. The incidence of hypotension is reported in about 40 percent of patients receiving the drug following myocardial infarction.

DIPHENYLHYDANTOIN

Diphenylhydantoin as an antidysrhythmic agent is the same drug used for seizures. It is particularly useful in the treatment of dysrhythmias due to digitalis toxicity. In particular, it is useful for the treatment of certain specific digitoxic rhythms such as multifocal PVCs, ventricular tachycardia, and paroxysmal supraventricular tachycardia with AV block. It is not effective for profound sinus bradycardia or for sinus arrest produced by digitalis, which are treated with a pacemaker. Diphenylhydantoin is also used in the treatment of ventricular premature beats of many causes but is largely ineffective with supraventricular dysrhythmias.

The method of intravenous injection of this drug is by slow injection of approximately 100 mg every 5 minutes. This can be repeated, and the total dose required for dysrhythmia control is usually less than 5.0 to 10.0 mg/kg. Some patients have required 1,000 mg IV. Since the drug solution has a pH of 11 and may cause phlebitis, it is often given through a central venous line and flushed immediately with intravenous fluid. Rapid administration of the drug has produced respiratory arrest, hypotension, and death. These side effects appear to be related to the speed of injection rather than to total dose administered.

Diphenylhydantoin is metabolized almost entirely in the liver. One-half the drug is eliminated every day. Continuous intravenous infusion of diphenylhydantoin is unusual, particularly since it is not an extremely effective antidysrhythmic. Central nervous system toxicity, evidenced by nystagmus, ataxia, and other cerebellar signs, occurs at high levels of the drug. Since these signs are difficult to see under anesthesia, it is intellectually useful but practically difficult to use serum levels. Therapeutic blood levels are 10 to 20 μg/ml, and signs of CNS side effects begin at the upper limit of the therapeutic range.

DIGITALIS

The most commonly employed form of digitalis, digoxin, shares virtually all the electrophysiologic properties of this class of drugs. It decreases pacemaker function in the AV node but makes the ventricular Purkinje system a more active pacemaker. It decreases AV conduction and shortens the effective refractory period of the ventricle while increasing the effective refractory period of the AV node. On the ECG, it slows atrial rate, prolongs PR interval, increases conduction time across the AV node as denoted by His bundle recordings, and produces the classic down-sloped appearance of the ST segment. It is used widely for the purpose of increasing ventricular contractility, thought to be a cardiac membrane ATPase-related function. The net effect is that the intracellular calcium electrolyte changes produced by digitalis-induced alteration in the membrane ATPase improve cardiac contractility but increase the likelihood of cardiac dysrhythmias. In addition to the cardiac contractility effect, it is also used because of its property of decreasing AV conduction and of slowing the ventricular response to atrial dysrhythmias such as PAT or atrial fibrillation.

Intraoperatively, digitalis is generally given intravenously in response to rapid supraventricular dysrhythmias or to a need for a cardiac contractility agent. Digitalis has a rapid onset when given intravenously and works within a matter of several moments. Because of its rapid onset and the tremendous amount of information known about it, digitalis is used during emergency situations in preference to other digitalis agents, such as ouabain, which may have more rapid onset but which are not readily available and the doses of which are not commonly known.

The drug is largely excreted by the kidney and requires no hepatic metabolism prior to excretion. During the past decade, it has been possible to monitor digitalis levels in humans; a range of 1.2 ± 0.4 for ng/ml is generally accepted as the appropriate plasma concentration in adults, although it is somewhat higher in infants and children.[21]

The major antidysrhythmic use of digitalis is in the treatment of supraventricular dysrhythmias. While digitalis does have the ability under certain circumstances to cardiovert some supraventricular dysrhythmias, depending on the physiologic state and timing of the dysrhythmias, its major purpose is to hinder AV conduction and permit a more physiologic ventricular rate than can be seen in certain dysrhythmias, such as atrial flutter. Controlling the ventricular response is often all that is needed to stabilize a hemodynamically unstable supraventricular tachycardia.

The major problem with digitalis is that it can be extremely toxic, particularly in certain intraoperative situations. Digitalis toxicity is manifested by ventricular premature beats, ventricular dysrhythmias, prolonged AV conduction, slow responses to atrial tachycardias such as atrial fibrillation, and the potential for complete AV block with slow ventricular rates arising from subsidiary pacemakers. Virtually any dysrhythmia could be attributable to digitalis toxicity.

Since the mechanism of the effect and toxicity of digitalis relates to alterations in sodium, potassium, and calcium flux across the cell membrane, it is understandable why the potential for muscle relaxants to interact with digitalis is widely known. In fact, case reports in the literature document the fact that in patients who were not considered digitalis toxic preoperatively, dysrhythmia suggestive of digitalis toxicity may develop following administration of drugs such as succinylcholine, which rapidly alter intracellular potassium (also see Ch. 27). This is very important to the anesthesiologist in evaluating the advisability of proceeding with nonemergency surgery in patients on digitalis therapy. Classic cases generally involve elderly patients who are unable to give a coherent history of their digitalis usage (also see Ch. 50). In patients in atrial fibrillation, fast ventricular responses (in excess of 90 to 100 beats/min) probably indicate that the patient has not been taking adequate digoxin. Conversely, very slow ventricular responses (less than 70 beats/min) may indicate that the patient has been taking excessive amounts of digoxin and is not ready for anything less than emergency surgery. For emergencies, the use of diphenylhydantoin for the treatment of ventricular dysrhythmias associated with digitalis has been discussed previously. It should be emphasized, however, that digoxin toxicity resulting in severe bradycardia is not treatable by diphenylhydantoin and emergency pacemaker therapy may be indicated.

EMERGENCY TREATMENT OF DYSRHYTHMIAS BY PACEMAKER INSERTION

While every anesthesiologist has long been aware that certain dysrhythmias such as third-degree heart block may require pacemaker insertion during the perioperative period and that transvenous pacemaker insertion may be indicated in certain crises in the operating room, this is often difficult to arrange. Furthermore, it is not always necessary when the dysrhythmia is a bradycardia of supraventricular origin, as in the sick sinus syndrome. These bradydysrhythmias appear quite frequently and may be the sudden result of the interaction of cardiovascular drugs, an aging sinus node, and anesthetic agents.

The potential exists for esophageal pacing of the atrium in patients with sinus bradycardia or nodal bradycardia. Since the esophagus sits directly posterior to the left atrium, it is possible to pace from this site as has been shown in the cardiac catheterization laboratory. Recently, Backofen et al.[22] found this to be a very effective means of treating bradycardia in patients with sick sinus syndrome or with propranolol-induced bradycardia intraoperatively. It should be emphasized, however, that it is not always possible to pace the ventricle from this site under current technological conditions; attempts to do so by increasing electrical voltage beyond that recommended for atrial pacing may result in episodes of ventricular fibrillation. This is because the ventricle is quite distant from the esophagus and also because it is always important to avoid timing a high electrical current that will coincide with the vulnerable period of the T wave and thereby initiate ventricular fibrillation. Regardless, atrial pacing through the esophagus clearly has a role in the treatment of bradycardias that develop intraoperatively.

ANESTHETIC – SURGERY – DYSRHYTHMIA INTERACTIONS

While it is clear that certain settings such as coronary artery bypass surgery are likely to produce a high frequency of cardiac dysrhythmias, it is also true that other conditions increase the likelihood of dysrhythmias under anesthesia and surgery. This section comments specifically on two such situations. These are CNS-induced dysrhythmias and drug interactions that relate to ventricular acetylcholine receptors.

CNS-INDUCED ECG CHANGES

Thirty years ago, it was recognized that patients with CNS injury developed bizarre T waves and ventricular dysrhythmias.[23] At first it was not clear why this was the case, since these patients were known not to have heart disease. But it is now apparent that one of the mechanisms by which these dysrhythmias occur is through alterations in sympathetic innervation to the heart.[24]

The heart apparently receives definitive innervation from the right stellate ganglion and different innervation from the left stellate ganglion. Both ganglia innervate the ventricular myocardium, but the areas that are innervated are not entirely the same (Fig. 15-19). Most of the heart receives dual innervation, but a portion of the anterior and largely right ventricle receives innervation from the right stellate ganglion, while the posterior and lateral ventriculum myocardium is innervated by the left stellate ganglion.[25,26] Conditions in which the right or left stellate ganglia themselves are altered have different effects on the heart; for example, the right stellate ganglion is more likely to produce sinus bradycardia by alteration and sympathetic innervation to the sinus node located in the right atrium.

The areas represented by the right and left stellate ganglia also exist in the right and left hypothalamus. That means that there are areas in the right hypothalamus responsible for the sympathetic outflow of the right stellate ganglia and that similar areas exist on the left side for the left stellate ganglia. Central nervous system lesions produced by trauma or during surgery may actually result in differential sympathetic tone flowing through the right and left stellate ganglia to the ventricular myocardium. This may result in areas of prolonged recovery in certain areas of the myocardium as compared with other areas and may set up the mechanism both for T-wave changes and for dysrhythmias.

For the anesthesiologist, this is extremely important. Bizarre T waves do not mean that patients undergoing CNS surgery have suffered myocardial infarcts from poor anesthetic care. Likewise, the sudden development of ventricular dysrhythmias in the same patients may be

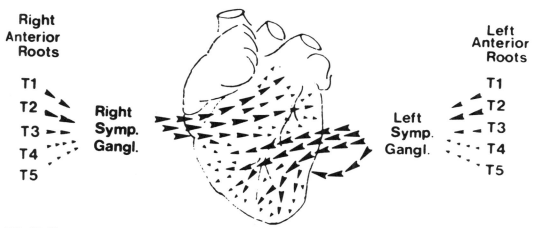

FIG. 15-19 Sympathetic innervation of the heart. Distribution of upper thoracic anterior roots to the myocardium of a dog. Please note that there are areas that have representation from right and left ganglia but there are other areas which have only innervation from the right or left side. (Adapted from Randall WC: Neural Regulation of the Heart. New York, Oxford University Press, 1977.)

the result of direct CNS alteration rather than hypoxia or hypocarbia. These effects occur not only during surgery, but for hours and days afterward. Ventricular dysrhythmias also may occur from CNS trauma such as head injury or stroke, independent of surgery.[3,23]

Regardless of the mechanism, the classic division of anesthesia into subspecialties such as cardiac and neuroanesthesia obscures the fact that neurologic patients undergoing CNS procedures are at great risk for the development of hemodynamic alterations and cardiac dysrhythmias from CNS-induced sympathetic changes. What is required in such cases is ECG monitoring as well as the ability to distinguish true ischemia from ST segment alteration induced by the CNS surgery. Anesthesiologists should be alert to this problem and should understand this mechanism in order to be able to deal with the dysrhythmias so commonly seen in these patients.

ACETYLCHOLINE RECEPTORS IN THE VENTRICLE

Anesthesiologists currently in practice have generally been taught that sympathetic node innervates both the atrium and the ventricle but that parasympathetic innervation of the heart exists only in the atrium and perhaps through the AV node to the His bundle. The classic physiology and pharmacology textbooks used in the medical schools stated that acetylcholine (ACh) receptors do not exist in the ventricle and that parasympathetic innervation of the heart is nonexistent in the ventricle. New evidence suggests that this is not the case[27,28] shedding new light on the concept that certain reflex- and drug-induced changes commonly seen by anesthesiologists may be due to activation or alterations in these ACh receptors. In fact, at least two types of ACh receptors are found in the ventricle. Type I receptors are vagal, while type II receptors are not blocked by atropine. As a result, it is possible that ACh may produce significant inotropic effects in the ventricle. Furthermore, histochemical studies of cholinergic receptors in the heart along with electrophysiologic studies in the ventricle document that ACh has profound effects on automaticity and action potential duration in the ventricle. Although still a developing research area, it underscores the fact that large numbers of the dysrhythmias seen with muscle relaxants and muscle relaxant reversal as well as hemodynamic fluctuations in response to these drugs are not fully understood.[10] The potential exists for the interaction of muscle relaxant drugs and of ACh receptors in the ventricle muscle and in the Purkinje system.

SUMMARY

Anesthesiologists are becoming increasingly sophisticated about the monitoring, detection, and treatment of dysrhythmias intraoperatively. It has also become clear that there are situations in which the combination of surgery, patient medications, and anesthetic drugs creates unique circumstances likely to provoke dysrhythmias. This offers the opportunity for the anesthesiologist to become involved, not only in the patient care aspects of dysrhythmia management, but also in the understanding of why dysrhythmias are such a frequent event under anesthesia.

REFERENCES

1. Stevenson RL, Rogers MC: Electrocardiographic change during anesthesia. Semin Anesthesiol 1:207, 1982
2. Bazaral MG, Norfleet EA: Comparison of CB$_5$ and V$_5$ leads for intraoperative electrocardiographic monitoring. Anesth Analg 60:849, 1981
3. Rogers MC: Anesthetic management of patients with heart disease. Modern Concepts Cardiovasc Dis 52:29, 1983
4. Kuner J: Cardiac arrhythmias during anesthesia. Dis Chest 52:580, 1967
5. Marriott HJL: Practical Electrocardiography. 6th Ed. Baltimore, Williams & Wilkins, 1977
6. Helfant RH: Bellet's Essentials of Cardiac Arrhythmias. 2nd Ed. Chicago, WB Saunders, 1979
7. Boba A: Significant effects on the blood pressure of an apparently trivial atrial dysrhythmia. Anesthesiology 48:282, 1978
8. Bosnijak ZJ, Kampine JP: Effects of halothane, enflurane, and isoflurane on the SA node. Anesthesiology 58:314, 1983
9. Levy MN: Role of the baroreceptor reflexes in cardiac arrhythmias, Neural Mechanisms in Cardiac Arrhythmias. Edited by PJ Schwartz, AM Brown, A Malliani, A Zanchetti. New York, Raven Press, 1978
10. Edwards RP, Miller RD, Roizen MF, et al: Cardiac responses to impiramine and pancuronium during anesthesia with halothane or enflurane. Anesthesiology 50:421, 1979
11. Trevino A, Razi B, Beller BM: The characteristic electrocardiogram of accidental hypothermia. Arch Intern Med 127:470, 1971
12. Clements SD, Hurst JW: Diagnostic value of electrocardiographic abnormalities observed in subjects accidentally exposed to cold. Am J Cardiol 29:729, 1972
13. Nishikawa T, Dohi S: Slowing of heart rate during cardiac output measurement by thermodilution. Anesthesiology 57:538, 1982
14. Todd MM: Atrial fibrillation induced by the right atrial injection of cold fluids during thermodilution cardiac output determination: A case report. Anesthesiology 59:253, 1983
15. Chung EK: Sick sinus syndrome: Current views. Modern Concepts Cardiovasc Dis 49:61, 67, 1980
16. Chung EK: Principles of Cardiac Arrhythmias. 2nd Ed. Baltimore, Williams & Wilkins, 1977
17. Moe GK, Mendez C: Physiologic basis of premature beats and sustained tachycardias. N Engl J Med 288:250, 1973
18. Singh BN, Ellrodt G, Peter CT: Verapamil: A review of its pharmacological properties and therapeutic use. Drugs 15:169, 1978
19. Zipes DP: Second-degree atrioventricular block. Circulation 60:465, 1979
20. Schwartz AJ, Wollman H: Anesthetic considerations for patients on chronic drug therapy: L-Dopa, monoamine oxidase inhibitors, tricyclic antidepressants and propranolol. Refresher Courses Anesthesiol 4:99, 1976
21. Rogers MC, Willerson JT, Goldblatt A, et al: Digoxin studies in the human fetus, neonate and infant. N Engl J Med 287:1010, 1972
22. Backofen JE, Schauble JF, Rogers MC: Transesophageal pacing for bradycardia. Anesthesiology 61:777, 1984
23. Burch GE: The EKG, the heart, and the CNS and autonomic nervous system, Neural Mechanisms in Cardiac Arrhythmias. Edited by PJ Schwartz, AM Brown, A Malliani, A Zanchetti. New York, Raven Press, 1978
24. Rogers MC, Abildskov JA, Preston JB: Neurogenic ECG changes in critically ill patients: An experimental model. Crit Care Med 1:192, 1973
25. Rogers MC, Battit G, McPeek B, et al: Lateralization of sympathetic control of the human sinus node: ECG changes of stellate ganglion block. Anesthesiology 48:139, 1978
26. Schwartz PJ, Stone HL: Unilateral stellectomy and sudden death, Neural Mechanisms in Cardiac Arrhythmias. Edited by PJ Schwartz, AM

Brown, A Malliani, A Zanchetti. New York, Raven Press, 1978

27. Jacobowitz D, Cooper T, Barner HB: Histochemical and chemical studies of the localization of adrenergic and cholinergic nerves in normal and denervated cat hearts. Circ Res 20:289, 1967

28. Kent KM, Epstein SE, Cooper T, et al: Cholinergic innervation of the canine and human ventricular conducting system. Circulation 50:948, 1974

29. Higgins CB, Vatner SF, Braunwald E: Parasympathetic control of the heart. Pharmacol Rev 25:119, 1973

1

16

Endotracheal Intubation

Robert K. Stoelting, M.D.

INTRODUCTION

Endotracheal intubation is the translaryngeal placement of a tube into the trachea via the nose (nasotracheal intubation) or mouth (orotracheal intubation). In 1880 Sir William Macewen, a Scottish surgeon, was the first to perform endotracheal intubation without resorting to tracheostomy.[1] In 1895, Kirstein became the first to perform endotracheal intubation with the aid of a laryngoscope.[2] But the credit for developing the scientific principles of direct laryngoscopy and endotracheal intubation belongs to the American otolaryngologist, Dr. Chevalier Jackson.[3] In 1913, Jackson described the use of his U-shaped laryngoscope to facilitate placement of a tracheal tube, which then served as a conduit for administration of inhaled anesthetics and oxygen. The same year, Janeway introduced an L-shaped laryngoscope with batteries in the handle.[4] Dorrance described the use of an inflatable cuff on the endotracheal tube in 1910.[5] It was during World War I that blind nasotracheal intubation was popularized by Rowbotham and Magill.[6]

Today, endotracheal intubation is an integral part of the anesthesiologist's contribution to patient care. Continued improvement in equipment and use of neuromuscular blockers combined with the technical skills of the anesthesiologist have made endotracheal intubation a safe and common practice in modern-day anesthesia.

ANATOMY OF THE LARYNX

The larynx is a boxlike structure anterior to the bodies of the 4th, 5th, and 6th cervical vertebrae. Its primary function is to guard the entrance to the respiratory tract. Structurally, the larynx is composed of nine articulating cartilages, three of which are paired (arytenoid, corniculate, and cuneiform cartilages) and three of which are unpaired (thyroid, cricoid, and epiglottic cartilage). The major skeleton of the larynx is formed anteriorly by the thyroid cartilage, and the posterior wall consists of the arytenoid and cricoid cartilages. The two laminae of the thyroid cartilage meet in the midline, forming the thyroid notch. The upper border of this fusion projects forward as the laryngeal prominence (Adam's apple), identifying the position of the larynx. The cricoid cartilage is a complete ring with its broad aspect posteriorly. The epiglottic cartilage overhangs the laryngeal inlet like a door. The upper rounded border of the epiglottis projects into the pharynx, while the lower stalk is attached to the thyroid laminae.

The thyrohyoid, cricothyroid, and cricotracheal ligaments or membranes stabilize and connect the cricoid and thyroid cartilages. The vocal ligaments are attached to the angles of the thyroid cartilage anteriorly and to the arytenoid cartilage posteriorly. The vocal ligaments form the framework of the vocal cords. The vocal cords apear as pale white structures due to the absence of a submucosa with the usual network of blood vessels. The triangular fissure between the vocal cords is known as the glottic opening. This represents the narrowest part of the laryngeal cavity in adults. In children less than about 10 years of age, the narrowest part of the larynx is usually at the cricoid cartilage.

The nine intrinsic muscles (four paired and one unpaired) of the larynx are classified as (1) abductors of the vocal cords, (2) adductors of the vocal cords, and (3) regulators of vocal cord tension. The posterior cricoarytenoid muscles are the only abductors of the vocal cords. They create the glottic opening by rotating the arytenoid cartilages so that the vocal processes move laterally. The lateral cricoarytenoid muscles adduct the vocal cords and close the glottis by rotating the arytenoid cartilages in the reverse direction. The cricothyroid muscles tense the vocal cords by increasing the distance between the vocal process of the arytenoid cartilage and thyroid cartilage.

The entire motor and sensory supply to the larynx is derived bilaterally from two branches of the vagus nerve: the superior laryngeal and the recurrent laryngeal nerves. The superior laryngeal nerves divide into smaller external branches and larger internal branches at the level of the cornu of the hyoid bone. The external branches supply motor fibers to the cricothyroid muscles, which serve as the tensors of the vocal cords. The internal branches provide sensory innervation to the epiglottis, base of the tongue and interior of the larynx down to the vocal cords. The recurrent laryngeal nerves provide motor innervation to all the muscles of the larynx except the cricothyroid muscles.

PREOPERATIVE EVALUATION OF THE PATIENT

Preoperative patient evaluation determines the route (oral or nasal) and method (awake or anesthetized) for endotracheal intubation. Examination includes an assessment of anatomic or pathologic factors that may make endotracheal intubation difficult, a thorough dental inspection, and evaluation of temporomandibular joint function and cervical spine mobility. A written note in the patient's medical record documents pertinent findings related to anesthesia management of the airway.

If nasotracheal intubation is planned, the patency of the nares is evaluated by asking the patient to breathe through each naris while the examiner occludes the other. This examination is supplemented by direct questioning about previous nasal trauma, pathology, or difficulty breathing through the nose.

Anatomic characteristics that impair alignment of the oral, pharyngeal, and laryngeal axes (Fig. 16-1) and make visualization of the glottis by direct laryngoscopy difficult include a short muscular neck with a full set of teeth, a receding mandible, protruding maxillary incisor teeth, poor mandibular mobility, and a long high-arched palate associated with a long narrow mouth.[7]

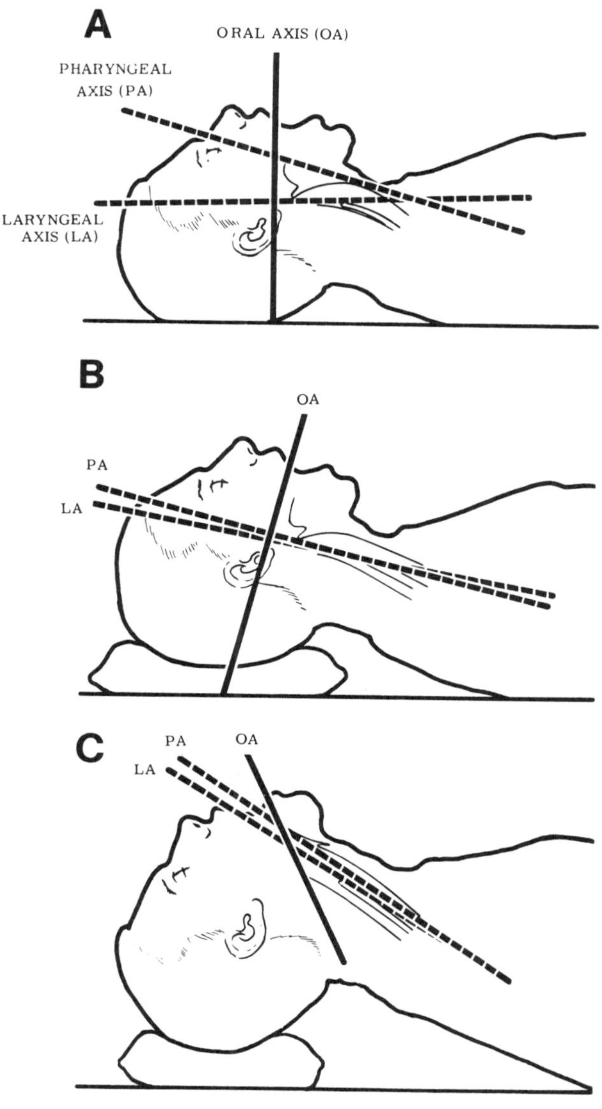

A

ORAL AXIS (OA)

PHARYNGEAL AXIS (PA)

LARYNGEAL AXIS (LA)

B

OA

PA

LA

C

PA   OA

LA

FIG. 16-1 Schematic diagram demonstrating head position for endotracheal intubation. (A) Successful direct laryngoscopy for exposure of the glottic opening requires alignment of the oral, pharyngeal, and laryngeal axes. (B) Elevation of the head about 10 cm with pads under the occiput with the shoulders remaining on the table aligns the laryngeal and pharyngeal axes. (C) Subsequent head extension at the atlanto-occipital joint serves to create the shortest distance and most nearly straight line from the incisor teeth to glottic opening.

The dental state must be appraised before direct laryngoscopy is attempted. If orotracheal intubation might involve a high risk of dental injury, it is best to advise the patient of that possibility preoperatively, or the anesthesiologist should consider nasotracheal intubation — either blind or with the aid of a fiberoptic laryngoscope. The preoperative dental examination includes several important observations and steps[8]:

Presence of loose teeth. Newly erupted deciduous teeth or permanent teeth initially have little support because the roots are only partially formed. Deciduous teeth begin to erupt at about 6 months of age and permanent teeth start at about 6 years of age. As a permanent tooth erupts, the root portion of the overlying deciduous tooth undergoes resolution such that just before exfoliation it may be held in place only by fibrous tissue. Children 6 to 12 years of age are considered to be in the mixed dentition stage. In adults, loosening of teeth most likely reflects peridontal disease that results in loss of bony support.

Existence and position of dental crowns and bridges. An individual crown (cap) is affixed to an underlying natural tooth and is difficult to detect, particularly if it is porcelain. A fixed bridge fills a gap between one or more missing permanent teeth, and prosthetic (often porcelain) appliances are attached to the bridge. Crowns and fixed bridges are not removable and are vulnerable to injury by a laryngoscope blade or bite block.

Removable bridges or dentures. These prostheses may be removed preoperatively or left in place until after anesthesia induction so as to facilitate a mask fit.

Preexisting dental abnormalities. The position of missing teeth and chips or fractures (especially on maxillary incisors) must be noted in the written preanesthetic note. Otherwise, subsequent discovery of these defects may be falsely attributed to damage incurred during endotracheal intubation.

Proclination. Loosening and fracture of anterior maxillary teeth is an ever-present danger during orotracheal intubation. Protruding maxillary incisors are particularly susceptible to levering effects of the laryngoscope blade.

The mandibular opening can be evaluated by having the patient open his or her mouth as widely as possible. Normal opening in an adult is in the range of 40 mm (at least two fingerbreadths).[9] Any form of arthritis (degenerative or rheumatoid) may limit mandibular mobility. The temporomandibular joint can be evaluated by placing the index finger just anterior to the targus and instructing the patient to open the mouth maximally. One should feel the initial rotational (hinge action) and secondary transitional movement (forward gliding) of the condylar head. Arthritis usually interferes with the forward gliding of the condylar head. If only the first phase of opening is present, difficulty may be experienced in opening the mouth wide enough to accomplish direct laryngoscopy for endotracheal intubation.

Mobility of cervical vertebrae, as demonstrated by flexion and extension of the head, is essential for proper positioning and ease of naso- or orotracheal intubation. The normal range of flexion–extension of the head varies from 165 to 90 degrees, with range decreasing approximately 20 percent by 75 years of age.[4] Patients may be unaware preoperatively of impaired motion of their cervical vertebrae since the head may be extended to some degree at the lower cervical vertebrae with the aid of bending the back in the lumbar area.

INDICATIONS FOR OROTRACHEAL INTUBATION

Orotracheal intubation may be considered for every patient receiving general anesthesia. Specific indications for endotracheal intubation in the surgical patient receiving general anesthesia are several (Table 16-1).

Aspiration of vomitus, blood, or secretions into the lungs is minimized by placement of a tracheal tube and inflation of the cuff to provide a seal between tracheal mucosa and tube. Protection of the lungs with a cuffed tracheal tube is mandatory in patients who have recently ingested food or in whom intestinal obstruction is present. Tracheal tubes of less than 5.0-mm internal diameter rarely have cuffs; selection of a proper-sized uncuffed tube for pediatric patients, who have small tracheas,

TABLE 16-1. Indications for Orotracheal Intubation

Provide patent upper airway
Prevent aspiration of gastric contents
Facilitate tracheal suctioning
Positive-pressure ventilation of the lungs
    Thoracotomy
    Neuromuscular blockade
    Prolonged need for controlled ventilation
Adverse operative position
    Sitting
    Prone
    Lateral
    Extreme lithotomy or head-down
Operative site near or involving upper airway
Airway maintenance by mask difficult
Disease involving upper airway

usually results in a sufficient seal to provide acceptable protection against aspiration.[10] Any patient requiring frequent tracheal suction can best be managed with an endotracheal tube in place.

Operations in which positive-pressure ventilation of the lungs is required (thoracotomy, neuromuscular blockade) or when prolonged controlled ventilation of the lungs is necessary are most reliably managed with the aid of an endotracheal tube. Without an endotracheal tube, upper airway pressure greater than 25 cm H_2O may force air through a relaxed cricopharyngeal sphincter. When neuromuscular blockade is incomplete or partial airway obstruction exists, even less pressure may force some gas into the stomach. Gastric distention from air impedes spontaneous ventilation and increases the incidence of regurgitation or vomiting.

Operations performed in other than the supine position require an endotracheal tube. Maintenance of a patent upper airway or delivery of positive-pressure ventilation of the lungs is not reliable without an endotracheal tube when the patient is in the prone, lateral, or sitting position. Steep head-down or lithotomy position may displace abdominal contents against the diaphragm, resulting in compromised ventilation or an increased hazard of aspiration. Operations about the head, neck, or upper airway require a tracheal tube for both airway maintenance and/or removal of anesthetic equipment from the operative site.

Prolonged application of a face mask may result in tissue ischemia. Although maintenance of an acceptable mask fit on an edentulous patient can be difficult, tracheal intubation usually is technically easy. Various anatomic characteristics (receding mandible, large tongue, short neck, large facial features) make mask placement difficult and airway obstruction likely. Although tracheal intubation is indicated, exposure of the glottic opening may be technically difficult due to the adverse anatomic characteristics.

The presence of a paralyzed vocal cord, supraglottic or subglottic tumor, or external compression of the airway requires placement of a tracheal tube to ensure a patent airway during anesthesia and operation.

TECHNIQUES FOR OROTRACHEAL INTUBATION

Orotracheal intubation under direct vision in an anesthetized patient is routinely chosen unless specific circumstances dictate otherwise. This is a technique that requires training and experience to make it safe, effective, and atraumatic. Equipment for endotracheal intubation varies and often depends on personal preferences but always includes proper-sized endotracheal tube(s), functioning laryngoscope, appropriate anesthetic drugs and neuromuscular blockers, suction, and facilities to provide positive-pressure ventilation of the lungs with oxygen. If a cuffed endotracheal tube is chosen, the cuff is checked for airtightness.

ANESTHESIA FOR ENDOTRACHEAL INTUBATION

A popular and safe approach in most patients is to produce anesthesia with an intravenous injection of barbiturate or similar rapid-acting drug (e.g., etomidate, benzodiazepine), followed by succinylcholine to provide skeletal muscle relaxation. With the use of this drug combination, direct laryngoscopy may be initiated about 60 seconds following administration of succinylcholine. Oxygen administration prior to laryngoscopy (preoxygenation) minimizes the risk of the development of arterial hypoxemia during the apneic period required for placement of the tracheal tube. An alternative approach is administration of a volatile anesthetic for several minutes to achieve an anesthetic depth for laryngoscopy similar to that which will be necessary for surgery. Intubation of the trachea may then be accomplished utilizing the muscle relaxation produced by the volatile anesthetic, but most often succinylcholine is administered as well. In some cases, intubation of the trachea is facilitated with skeletal muscle relaxation provided by a nondepolarizing muscle relaxant.

HEAD POSITION FOR OROTRACHEAL INTUBATION

Successful direct laryngoscopy requires aligning the oral, pharyngeal, and laryngeal axes such that the passageway from the incisor teeth to glottis is most nearly a straight line (Fig. 16-1). Elevating the head about 10 cm with pads under the occiput (shoulders remaining on the table) and head extension at the atlanto-occipital joint serves to align these axes most nearly into a straight line. This posture is described as the "sniffing position." Full extension of the head, without elevation of the occiput, increases the lips to glottis distance, rotates the larynx anteriorly, and may necessitate leverage on the maxillary teeth or gums with the laryngoscope blade to expose the larynx. A frequently forgotten but important element in successful intubation of the trachea is adjustment of the table to a height such that the patient's face is at the level of the anesthesiologist's xiphoid cartilage. If not opened by the head extension, the mouth may be manually opened by depressing the mandible with the right thumb while stabilizing the head by counter pressure on the maxillary teeth. Simultaneously, the lower lip is rolled away with the right index finger.

USE OF THE LARYNGOSCOPE

A laryngoscope is a device used for visualizing the larynx directly, usually for purposes of endotracheal intubation. It consists of a handle that contains batteries and a blade fitted with a bulb that lights automatically when the blade and handle are at right angles to each other, the position in which the instrument is used. Fiberoptic illumination can be adapted to the laryngoscope and, unlike battery models,

provides a long-term and high-intensity light source. The blades are detachable from the handle, interchangeable, and of various lengths and sizes to correspond to patient size. The size of the blade, which varies from 0 (smallest) to 4 (largest), is marked on the side of the blade adjacent to its point of attachment to the handle. The three basic types of blades are the curved blade (MacIntosh), the straight blade (Jackson or Wisconsin), and the straight blade with curved tip (Miller) (Fig. 16-2).[5,6] Each of these blades has a closed side for keeping the tongue out of the line of sight and an open side for visualization of the larynx and for ease of removal of the blade from the oropharynx once the endotracheal tube is in place.

The laryngoscope is held in the left hand (near the junction between the handle and blade) whether the anesthesiologist is right- or left-handed and is inserted on the right side of the patient's mouth so as to avoid the incisor teeth and deflect the tongue away from the lumen of the blade. The laryngoscope handle must be maintained perpendicular to the plane of the patient's body after placing the blade in the mouth. Gentleness and avoidance of pressure on the teeth or gums are essential — a protective shield over the maxillary incisors may prevent damage. The anesthesiologist should never lever the handle toward himself or herself. The epiglottis is visualized. The next step depends on the type of laryngoscope blade used.

CURVED BLADE (MACINTOSH)

The distal end (tip) of the blade is advanced into the space between the base of the tongue and the pharyngeal surface of the epiglottis (vallecula) (Fig. 16-3A). Subsequent forward and upward movement of the blade (exerted along the axis of the handle, not by pulling back on the handle) stretches the hypoepiglottic ligament causing the epiglottis to move upward. The glottic opening is exposed. Insertion of the blade too far into the mouth prevents elevation of the epiglottis and subsequent exposure of the glottic opening may be limited.

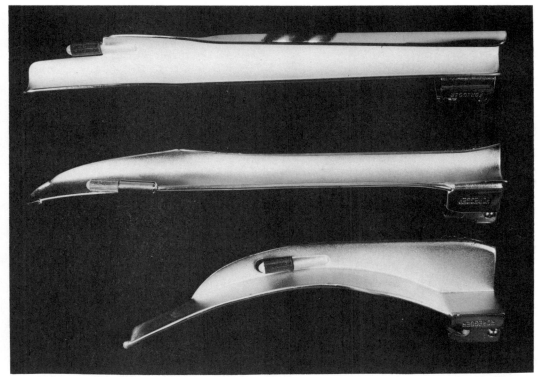

FIG. 16-2 Examples of the most frequently used detachable laryngoscope blades, which can be used interchangeably on the same handle. The uppermost blade is the straight or Jackson-Wisconsin design. The middle blade incorporates a curved distal tip (Miller). The lowermost blade is the curved or MacIntosh blade. All three blades are available in lengths appropriate for neonates and adults.

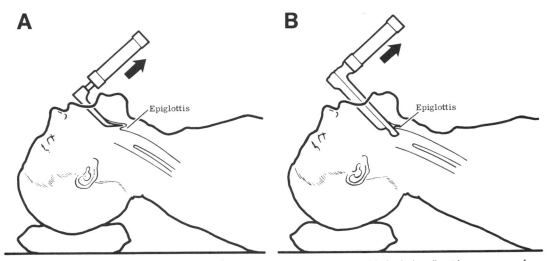

FIG. 16-3 Schematic diagram depicting proper position of the laryngoscope blade during direct laryngoscopy for exposure of the glottic opening. (A) The distal end of the curved blade is advanced into the space between the base of the tongue and pharyngeal surface of the epiglottis (vallecula). (B) The distal end of the straight blade (Jackson-Wisconsin or Miller) is advanced beneath the laryngeal surface of the epiglottis. Regardless of blade design, forward and upward movement exerted along the axis of the laryngoscope blade, as denoted by the arrows, serves to elevate the epiglottis and expose the glottic opening.

529

STRAIGHT BLADE (JACKSON–WISCONSIN) OR STRAIGHT BLADE WITH CURVED TIP (MILLER)

The distal end (tip) of the blade is advanced beneath the laryngeal surface of the epiglottis (Fig. 16-3B). Subsequent forward and upward movement of the blade (exerted along the axis of the handle, not by pulling back on the handle) elevates the epiglottis and exposes the glottic opening. Depression or lateral movement of the thyroid cartilage externally on the neck with the right hand may facilitate exposure of the glottic opening. This maneuver is especially helpful when the epiglottis is floppy and tends to double back on itself. Too deep insertion of the blade may result in elevation of the entire larynx and exposure of the esophagus.

CHOICE OF LARYNGOSCOPE BLADE

The choice of laryngoscope blade is often based on personal preference. Advantages cited for the straight blade include greater exposure of the glottic opening permitting observation of the tube as it passes through the glottic opening and less need for a stylet to direct the tube into an anterior larynx. Some recommend routine use of a stylet when a curved blade is used. Advantages cited for the curved blade include less trauma to teeth and more room for passage of the tracheal tube through the oropharynx, less bruising of the epiglottis since the blade tip should not touch this structure, and decreased incidence of coughing and laryngospasm. The last theoretical advantage of the curved blade relates to the sensory innervation of the laryngeal surface of the epiglottis by the superior laryngeal nerves and the pharyngeal surface by the glossopharyngeal nerves. Stimulation of the laryngeal surface of the epiglottis is alleged to predispose to laryngospasm and coughing. The frequent use of neuromuscular blockers during endotracheal intubation largely negates this theoretical advantage.

ENDOTRACHEAL TUBE SIZE, LENGTH, AND DESIGN

Various types of endotracheal tubes are shown in Figure 16-4. Endotracheal tube sizes are specified according to internal diameter (ID), which is marked on each tube (Table 16-2). Knowledge of tracheal anatomy is important in selecting the proper diameter and length of tracheal tube (Table 16-3). Tracheal tubes are available in 0.5-mm internal diameter increments. Tube size may also be designated in French units (external diameter in millimeters times 3, which approximates the circumference of the external tube). Most adult tracheas (after 14 years of age) readily accept a cuffed 8.0- to 9.0-mm internal diameter tube. The tube also has lengthwise centimeter markings starting at the distal tracheal end to permit accurate determination of tube length inserted past the nares or lips. The letters I.T. (implantation tested) or Z-79 (Committee Z-79 on Anesthesia Equipment of the USA Standards Institute) on a tube indicate that the tube material has been determined to be free of any tissue irritant or toxicity properties. Tube material should contain a radiopaque stripe to demonstrate position of the tube in vivo and should be transparent to permit visualization of secretions or blockage of airflow as by cessation of breath fogging. Plastic has proved the most satisfactory material and transparent, smooth-walled tubes made of polyvinylchloride or similar plastics have become the standard for orotracheal or nasotracheal intubation. These tubes are sterile, disposable, and nontoxic to mucous membranes and also soften at body temperature to conform to the contour of the airway. Discarding the tube after a single use removes all question about the need for an ideal method of resterilization.

Most endotracheal tubes have a single curve such that maximal pressure is exerted on the arytenoid cartilages and the anterior tracheal wall. In an attempt to minimize these sites of pressure, an anatomically shaped tube (Lindholm tube) incorporating a second curve (S-shaped) has been introduced (Fig. 16-5).[13] Indeed, fewer pressure-induced lesions at these sites were found in the tracheas of patients in-

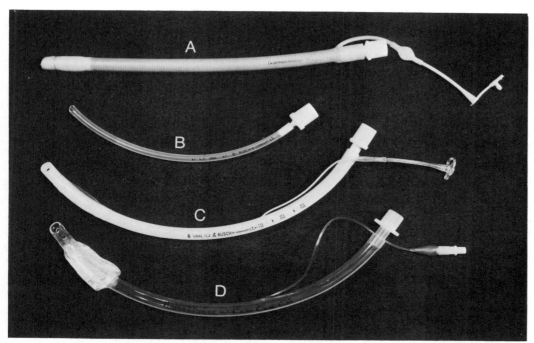

FIG. 16-4 Various types of endotracheal tubes. Tube A is an armored or anode tube with a built-in spiral wire to minimize the opportunity of collapse or kinking. Tubes B, C, and D are made of smooth plastic and are recommended for single use. Tube B is uncuffed and is a size appropriate for a child. Tubes C and D are appropriate for adult patients. Tube C is equipped with a built-in high-pressure, low-residual-volume cuff. Tube D is constructed to incorporate a low-pressure high-residual-volume cuff. Numbers and letters visible on tubes B, C, and D denote tube diameter, length from tracheal end, and confirmation that the tubes have been tested for tissue compatibility (I.T. or Z-79).

TABLE 16-2. **Average Dimensions of Endotracheal Tubes Based on Patient Age**

Age	Internal Diameter (mm)	French Unit	Distance Inserted from Lips to Place Distal End in the Mid-trachea (cm)*
Premature	2.5	10–12	10
Full term	3.0	12–14	11
1–6 months	3.5	16	11
6–12 months	4.0	18	12
2 years	4.5	20	13
4 years	5.0	22	14
6 years	5.5	24	15–16
8 years	6.5	26	16–17
10 years	7.0	28	17–18
12 years	7.5	30	18–20
14 years and over	8.0–9.0	32–36	20–24

* Add 2 to 3 cm for nasal tubes.

TABLE 16-3. Anatomy of the Trachea (Average Dimensions)

	Adult		Child (6 years of age)	Infant
	Male	Female		
Diameter of the trachea (mm)	20	15	8	5
Length of the trachea (cm)	14	12	8	6
Distance from upper teeth to carina (cm)	28	24	17	13

tubated with this S-shaped tube as compared with the single-curve tube.[14] The incidence of sore throat, however, was not decreased by the use of an S-shaped tube.[15] Finally, regardless of trachea tube shape, use of a small-diameter tube relative to the patient's trachea and avoiding extension of the head when the tube is in place may reduce the damage produced on the anterior tracheal wall by the distal end of the tube.[16]

ENDOTRACHEAL TUBE CUFF

Cuffs or balloons near the tracheal end of the tube are built into the structure of the tube. The cuff is inflated with air to create a seal against the underlying tracheal mucosa. This seal facilitates positive-pressure ventilation of the lungs and prevents pulmonary aspiration. Cuffs are classified as low residual volume

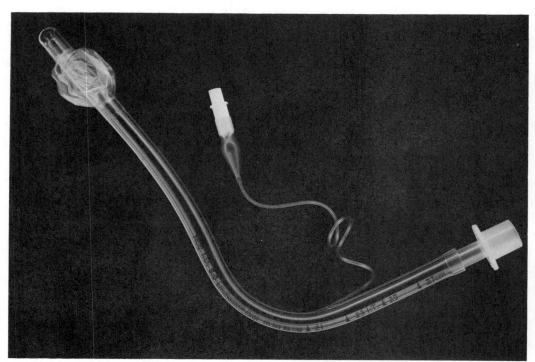

FIG. 16-5 An anatomically shaped endotracheal tube incorporating a second curve to provide an S shape was introduced by Lindholm.[13] In contrast to conventional single curve tubes, this S-shaped Lindholm endotracheal tube should minimize pressure transmitted by the tube to the arytenoid cartilages and anterior tracheal wall.

(high pressure) or high residual volume (low pressure).[17] Residual volume is the volume of air that can be withdrawn from the cuff after it has been inflated to just produce a no-leak seal against the tracheal mucosa.

Low residual volume cuffs must be inflated to high intraluminal cuff pressures (180 to 250 mm Hg) before they expand sufficiently to create a seal between the tube and tracheal mucosa. This high cuff pressure is partially transmitted to the underlying tracheal mucosa. Sensing devices placed in the anterior tracheal wall reveal that tracheal wall pressure may exceed 100 to 200 mm Hg.[18] Ischemia may occur whenever the pressure on the tracheal mucosa (tracheal wall pressure) exceeds capillary arteriolar pressure (about 32 mm Hg). Small increments of air (1 ml) added to the cuff above that necessary to achieve a no-leak seal may result in further marked increases in tracheal wall pressure. These cuffs may also inflate asymmetrically, deforming the trachea and eventually producing tracheal dilation.

Tracheal wall changes at low residual volume cuff sites show a consistent pattern of damage.[19] Initially, mucosa beneath the cuff becomes inflamed, followed after 3 to 5 days by the appearance of ulcers overlying cartilaginous rings. Ulcers usually develop first on the more rigid anterior tracheal wall. The exposed cartilaginous rings may subsequently become infected, contributing to destruction of the tracheal wall. With continued cuff inflation, the infected cartilaginous rings may soften and disappear. This is accompanied by expansion of the trachea at the cuff site visible on standard roentgenograms or tantalum tracheograms.[20] Continued pressure from the inflated cuff may result in posterior erosion into the esophagus or anterior erosion into the innominate artery. Following extubation of the trachea, the tracheal segment may persist as an area of tracheomalacia or become a circumferential scar with resulting tracheal stenosis.[21]

High residual volume cuffs inflate symmetrically, adapting to tracheal wall contour and developing low intraluminal cuff pressure at no-leak inflation volumes. The resulting tracheal wall pressure has been found to equal peak airway pressure (15 to 30 mm Hg) during positive-pressure ventilation of the lungs.[22]

Furthermore, additional air (1 ml) entering these cuffs after the minimal occlusive volume results in small (6 to 25 mm Hg) increases in tracheal wall pressure, providing some margin of safety in the event of inadvertent overinflation of the cuff. Thus, tracheal mucosa ischemia and tracheal dilation would seem less likely with high residual volume cuffs. Indeed, high residual volume cuffs decrease but do not prevent tracheal injury observed at the cuff site.[22]

The intracuff pressure should be controlled at a level sufficient to prevent aspiration yet low enough to permit capillary blood flow in the area contacted by the cuff. Maintaining intracuff pressure in high residual volume thin-walled cuffs (cuff thickness 0.1 mm or less) between 17 and 23 mm Hg during either spontaneous or controlled ventilation of the lungs prevents pulmonary aspiration and should still permit adequate capillary mucosal blood flow.[23] Compared with thin cuffs, thick-walled cuffs (0.25 mm and greater) form larger channels or folds when inflated in the trachea and may not prevent aspiration with intracuff pressures in this range. For this reason, high-residual-volume thin-walled cuffs are recommended.

The intraluminal pressure of both high and low residual volume cuffs may be increased by temperature changes as the air used to inflate the cuffs warms to body temperature and by diffusion of anesthetic gases (particularly nitrous oxide) into the air-filled cuff.[24] Inflation of the cuff with the gas mixture delivered from the anesthesia machine negates this latter effect.

Periodic monitoring of the intraluminal cuff pressure and readjustments to prevent excessive pressures may be achieved with an aneroid pressure gauge and a syringe connected to the endotracheal tube cuff via a standard three-way stopcock. Intracuff pressure at no-leak or minimal occlusive volume in high residual volume cuffs is a reasonable guide to tracheal wall pressure. Similar measurements, however, may not reliably reflect tracheal wall pressure exerted by low residual volume cuffs. Nevertheless, there is probably no period of tracheal intubation that does not produce some laryngotracheal damage. Ciliary denudation has been found to occur predominantly over the tracheal rings and underlying cuff site with only 2 hours of intubation and tracheal wall pressures of less than 25 mm Hg.[22] Tracheal intubation with cuff inflation for 72 hours is often sufficient to cause wide exposure of several cartilage rings.

LUBRICANTS AND TRACHEAL SPRAY

Lubricants containing a local anesthetic are often placed on the tracheal end of the tube. Such lubrication, however, is probably not essential for easy passage of the tube through the already mucus-lubricated glottic opening. The hazards of an allergic or irritant response to the local anesthetic and/or lubricant must be considered.[25] Tracheal spray of local anesthetic (lidocaine) just before intubation of the trachea decreases the duration of circulatory responses to tracheal intubation and permits early toleration of the tube with less anesthetic drug.[26]

PLACEMENT OF THE ENDOTRACHEAL TUBE

The glottic opening is recognized by its triangular shape and the pale white vocal cords (Fig. 16-6).[27] The endotracheal tube is held in the right hand like a pencil and introduced on the right side of the patient's mouth with the built in curve directed anteriorly. Attempts to insert the tube in the midline of the mouth and then down the lumen of the laryngoscope blade usually obscures vision of the glottic opening. The tube is advanced past the vocal cords until the cuff just disappears or with an uncuffed tube a distance predicted to place the distal end of the tube midway between the vocal cords and carina (Table 16-3). At this point, the laryngoscope blade is withdrawn or readjusted to facilitate placement of an esophageal stethoscope. Then the high residual volume cuff should be inflated with air to just a no-leak volume during positive-pressure ventilation of the lungs and a bite block placed between the premolar and molar teeth. Central placement of the bite block may result in impaction or dislodgement of monorooted incisor teeth if forceful closure occurs. Distention of the small pilot balloon attached to the inflation tube leading to the tracheal cuff confirms cuff inflation. Distention of the pilot balloon, however, may be misleading if the inflating tube between the balloon and the cuff is obstructed. Insertion of the tube into the trachea is confirmed by equal chest and air movement bilaterally. Noting the depth of insertion as determined by the centimeter markings on the endotracheal tube at the lips is useful in predicting a mid-tracheal position of the distal end of the tube (Table 16-3). For example, insertion of a tracheal tube about 22 cm beyond the lips of an adult should reliably place the distal end of the tube in the

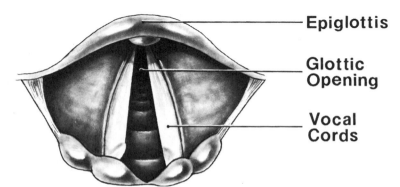

Epiglottis

Glottic Opening

Vocal Cords

FIG. 16-6 Schematic view of glottic opening during direct laryngoscopy when the epiglottis is elevated with a curved or straight laryngoscope blade. The glottic opening is recognized by its triangular shape and the pale white vocal cords. (Stoelting RK, Miller RD: Basics of Anesthesia. Churchill Livingstone, New York, 1984.)

mid-trachea. Furthermore, if a cuffed tube is properly placed in the mid-trachea, the anesthesiologist can easily detect, by external palpation, cuff distention in the suprasternal notch during rapid inflation of the cuff. Finally, the tracheal tube is secured in position with tape placed around the tube and applied above and below the lips extending over the cheeks.

Anatomic problems leading to difficult visualization of the glottic opening may be overcome occasionally with a stylet placed in the tube to facilitate directing the tube anteriorly. When properly shaped, the tracheal end of the tube should resemble a "hockey stick." Rotating the patient's head to the left, retracting the mouth to the right and placing the laryngoscope blade between the molar teeth provides the shortest distance to the glottic opening and may be an effective solution to mechanical problems.

When orotracheal intubation under direct vision during general anesthesia is impossible (due to adverse anatomic characteristics) or unsafe due to recent food ingestion, bowel obstruction, or upper airways disease, other approaches may be considered, such as awake intubation, nasotracheal intubation, intubation using a fiberoptic laryngoscope, or retrograde intubation.

cent lidocaine. It is helpful to reduce secretions with an anticholinergic. When nasotracheal intubation is planned, cocaine (1 to 2 ml of 4 to 5 percent) is also used to constrict and anesthetize the nasal mucosa. This is accomplished by inserting into the selected naris cocaine-containing pledgets attached to applicators. Spray devices are usually less satisfactory, since they may provide topical anesthesia for only the anterior portion of the nasal cavity. Furthermore, advancement of the pledgets into the nasopharynx confirms patency and illustrates the direction the nasotracheal tube should follow through the naris. If cocaine is not available, constriction but not anesthesia of the nasal mucosa can be produced with topical phenylephrine.

The superior laryngeal nerve may be blocked as it penetrates the thyrohyoid membrane near the cornu of the hyoid bone. The needle is inserted caudad to the hyoid and 2 to 3 ml of 2 percent lidocaine deposited just below the greater cornu.[29]

Injection of 2 to 3 ml of 2 to 4 percent lidocaine into the lumen of the trachea will anesthetize the trachea and larynx below the vocal cords. The cricothyroid or cricotracheal membrane is pierced with a needle attached to a syringe, correct placement is confirmed by aspiration of air, and the lidocaine is injected rapidly at end-exhalation to enable subsequent inhalation and cough to distribute the local anesthetic along the trachea and against the inferior aspects of the vocal cords.

AWAKE INTUBATION

Local analgesia for awake intubation of the trachea may include topical spray, superior laryngeal nerve blocks, and transtracheal injection of a local anesthetic. This combination permits painless direct laryngoscopy and endotracheal intubation without coughing. When vomiting is a hazard, only topical spray is generally recommended to avoid anesthetization of either the larynx or trachea.[28]

The lips, tongue, palate, and pharynx should be sprayed with 3 to 5 ml of 2 to 4 per-

NASOTRACHEAL INTUBATION

Nasotracheal intubation is performed electively for intraoral operations, when anatomic abnormalities or disease of the upper airway make direct laryngoscopy difficult or impossible and occasionally when long-term mechanical ventilation of the lungs is anticipated. Advantages cited for nasotracheal intubation include more stable tube fixation, less chance for tube kinking, greater comfort in an awake patient, and fewer oropharyngeal secretions. Awake blind nasotracheal intubation is usually reserved for situations in which direct laryngoscopy or ventilation of the lungs would be impossible or induction of anesthesia before endotracheal intubation would be hazardous. When vomiting is not a hazard and ventilation of the lungs can be maintained by mask but direct laryngoscopy is impossible, anesthesia may be safely produced before blind nasotracheal intubation. Otherwise, nasotracheal intubation is accomplished under direct laryngoscopy with anesthesia and frequently with neuromuscular blockade.

tube is then advanced along the floor of the nose (in the direction determined earlier with cocaine-soaked pledgets) into the oropharynx and aligned with the glottic opening by listening to exhaled air passing from the proximal end of the tube. The tube is advanced as long as breath sounds are maximal. The anesthesiologist must keep an ear close to the tube connector to readily detect change in breath sounds. Ideally, the tube is swiftly passed through the glottic opening just before inhalation, since the glottic opening is largest during inhalation and the risk of vocal cord trauma is thus minimized. The technique of passing the tube at the moment of an explosive cough is often successful. Successful placement of the tube in the trachea is confirmed by continued breathing through the tube.

TECHNIQUE FOR AWAKE BLIND NASOTRACHEAL INTUBATION

To ensure maximum patient comfort and nasal patency and to minimize the chance of epistaxis, the nasal mucosa is anesthetized and constricted with cocaine. Topical anesthesia of the tongue and pharynx, superior laryngeal nerve block and transtracheal anesthesia may be performed to improve patient comfort. Conversely, local anesthesia of the upper airway, larynx, and trachea may be distressing to an awake patient and may impair protective reflexes should vomiting occur. Either naris may be chosen, depending on history and examination, but the right is preferable because the bevel of most nasotracheal tubes when introduced through the right naris will face the flat nasal septum, reducing damage to the turbinates. In an adult, a 7.0 to 7.5 mm ID tracheal tube is usually adequate. Single curved nasal and oral tracheal tubes may be used interchangeably.

The occiput should be elevated about 10 cm and a well-curved and generously lubricated nasotracheal tube is introduced into the selected naris. Extension of the head at the atlanto-occipital joint helps lift the epiglottis away from the posterior pharyngeal wall. The

BLIND NASOTRACHEAL INTUBATION DURING ANESTHESIA

Nasotracheal intubation during general anesthesia is acceptable when vomiting is not a hazard and ventilation of the lungs can be maintained via an anesthesia face mask. Cocaine or phenylephrine is applied to the nasal mucosa to provide vasoconstriction. No additional anesthesia is necessary, but transtracheal anesthesia may be performed to prevent coughing when the tube enters the trachea. Anesthesia is produced with intravenous or inhalation drugs, taking care to avoid deep anesthesia, as maintenance of spontaneous ventilation of the lungs is essential to identify the glottic opening. Occasionally, carbon dioxide or doxapram may be used to stimulate ventilation. Anesthesia with intravenous ketamine 2 to 3 mg/kg followed by transtracheal anesthesia (prevents subsequent laryngospasm) may also be used, advantages being maintenance of the airway and spontaneous ventilation.[30] After appropriate anesthesia, the tracheal tube is introduced through the nose and directed toward the glottic opening in the same manner as described for awake blind nastracheal intubation.

DIAGNOSIS AND CORRECTIVE MANEUVERS WHEN THE NASOTRACHEAL TUBE DOES NOT ENTER THE LARYNX

A common problem is for the tube to impinge in the sulcus between the base of the tongue and epiglottis or on the anterior commissure of the glottic opening. Observation of the neck reveals a bulge in the mid-line just above the thyroid cartilage. The remedy is to divert the tube more posterior by increased flexion of the head. Conversely, passage into the esophagus, manifested by easy advancement to the full length of the tube, loss of breath sounds, and continued phonation in the awake patient is corrected by diverting the tube more anterior by increased extension of the head. Lateral displacement into the pyriform sinus is manifested by loss of breath sounds, resistance to further tube advancement, and bulging in the neck lateral to the laryngeal prominence. Withdrawing the tube 2 to 3 cm and rotation 45 to 90 degrees in the opposite direction serves to orient the tube to the midline. Alternatively, the thyroid cartilage may be manually and externally displaced to align the glottic opening with the tracheal tube.

Excessive force should never be used to pass a tube through the nasopharynx. If the nasotracheal tube has an excessive curve, advancement beyond the level of the vocal cords may be impossible because the tip impinges against the anterior wall of the larynx. If hyperflexion of the head does not resolve this problem, a less curved tube may be substituted. Nasotracheal intubation under direct vision demonstrates the maneuvers that are necessary to produce appropriate deflections of the tube when blind intubation of the trachea is necessary.

NASOTRACHEAL INTUBATION WITH DIRECT VISION OF THE GLOTTIS

After application of cocaine or phenylephrine to the nasal mucosa, anesthesia is produced with intravenous or inhaled anesthetics most often combined with succinylcholine to produce skeletal muscle relaxation. After the nasotracheal tube has entered the oropharynx, the glottic opening is visualized by direct laryngoscopy. The tracheal tube is guided into the larynx under vision by manually advancing at the nasal end or the tube may be grasped in the orpharynx with intubating forceps (Magill type) and directed so that pressure on the nasal end causes the tube to pass between the vocal cords. Again, the right naris is usually preferred because a left nasotracheal tube is clumsy to advance under direct vision with the anesthesiologist's left hand holding the laryngoscope.

COMPLICATIONS PECULIAR TO NASOTRACHEAL INTUBATION

A summary of these complications is shown in Table 16-4. Epistaxis may follow avulsion of nasal mucosa covering the turbinates. Proper shrinkage of the nasal mucosa with cocaine or phenylephrine and use of small, generously lubricated tracheal tubes should minimize this complication. Should bleeding occur, the nasotracheal tube should be left in place to provide a tamponade effect. In some instances, the tube may be withdrawn so that only the cuff remains in the naris and subsequent cuff inflation tamponades the bleeding site. Perforation and dissection of the posterior pharyngeal wall creating a false passage may occur especially if force is used to advance the tracheal tube through the nasopharynx. Pharyngeal tonsils (adenoids) may be prominent, especially in children, producing resistance to passage through the nasopharynx or bleeding if they are traumatized. Again, gentle advance-

TABLE 16-4. Complications Peculiar to Nasotracheal Intubation

Epistaxis
Trauma to posterior pharyngeal wall
Dislodgement of pharyngeal tonsils (adenoids)
Pressure necrosis
Auditory tube obstruction
Maxillary sinusitis
Bacteremia

ment and avoidance of excessive force should minimize this hazard. When pharyngeal tonsils are prominent, all nasotracheal intubations probably should be performed under direct vision so as to prevent carrying a dislodged piece of tonsil into the trachea with the tube.

Necrosis of the external naris reflects excessive pressure from the nasotracheal tube and may be minimized by proper fixation of the tube and, obviously, the earliest extubation of the trachea consistent with patient safety.[31] Ulceration of the inferior turbinate may be more likely when a large tracheal tube is placed.[32] Auditory tube obstruction by the nasotracheal tube may impair hearing. Maxillary sinusitis resulting from impaired drainage due to obstruction by the nasotracheal tube may be manifested by facial pain, nasal stuffiness, purulent secretions, or fever.[33]

Bacteremia may occur following nasotracheal intubation, reflecting the entrance of normal upper-airway flora into the circulation via traumatized nasal mucosa or the transport of flora from the nose into the trachea by the tube and the subsequent entrance into the circulation via the vascular tracheal mucosa.[34] When nasotracheal intubation is necessary in patients with heart disease, prophylactic antibiotics may be indicated.

TECHNIQUE FOR FIBEROPTIC LARYNGOSCOPY

Endotracheal intubation using a flexible fiberoptic laryngoscope (fiberscope) has been described[35-37] (also see Ch. 52). The fiberscope is lubricated to allow easy passage through an appropriate-sized endotracheal tube (about 8 mm internal diameter) and the tip is treated with an antifogging solution to assure a clear view during laryngoscopy. The pediatric fiberoptic bronchoscope has a diameter of 3.5 to 4.8 mm, permitting its passage through tracheal tubes as small as 5-mm internal diameter.[37] After topical anesthesia as described for awake nasotracheal intubation, with or without intravenous analgesia, the endotracheal tube is passed through the naris into the oropharynx. The transnasal approach is usually preferred because the tongue is less likely to interfere and the patient cannot bite down. Fiberoptic intubation of the trachea is best done in an awake patient, who can then assist the anesthesiologist by swallowing secretions, phonating, or panting. Oxygen can be insufflated via the suction port if it is deemed important to administer supplemental oxygen. Even high-frequency jet ventilation has been described using the suction port.[38]

The fiberscope is advanced through the tracheal tube until the epiglottis is visualized. After the fiberscope is passed between the vocal cords, the endotracheal tube is advanced using the fiberscope as a guide. The endotracheal tube is positioned proximal to the carina by direct vision. Oral intubation of the trachea is accomplished in a similar manner by placing the fiberscope behind the base of the tongue with the fingers or with limited traction using a laryngoscope blade. It is important to have an assistant monitor the patient's vital signs and ventilation during fiberoptic intubation of the trachea.

Appreciation of the following points will increase success with the fiberscope[36]:

1. Secretions obscure the view; therefore, an anticholinergic in the preoperative medication is helpful.
2. The epiglottis is surprisingly high in the oropharynx.
3. In contrast to the stretched appearance with direct laryngoscopy, the pyriform sinuses are relaxed and can resemble the pathway to the glottis.
4. It is essential that the fiberscope be kept in the midline to avoid entering the pyriform sinus.
5. The optics of the fiberscope exaggerate the depth of the vocal cords, which may not be seen until the false vocal cords are passed.
6. A helpful sign that the fiberscope is properly positioned is the glow seen over the anterior neck from transillumination of the larynx and trachea as the fiberscope tip passes through the glottic opening. This is not seen when the fiberscope is passed posteriorly into the esophagus.

Any anatomic problem that makes successful direct laryngoscopy doubtful is an indication for fiberoptic intubation of the trachea (Table 16-5).[37] In addition to its use for difficult tracheal intubations, the fiberscope may be passed through an endotracheal tube to diagnose accidental endobronchial intubation or the cause of tube obstruction (kinks, secretions) during anesthesia. Also, proper placement of double-lumen endobronchial tubes may be confirmed if the tube lumen is sufficient to permit passage of the fiberscope. Verification of tube position in the midtrachea or appropriate bronchus using the fiberscope is rapid and avoids both the delay and expense of obtaining a radiograph of the chest.

The use of an oral Airway Intubator with or without a special anesthetic face mask incorporating a diaphragm opening for passage of a tracheal tube has been proposed as a simplified technique to the more traditional approach for fiberoptic intubation of the trachea (Fig. 16-7).[39] The Airway Intubator is a plastic oropharyngeal airway with a cylindric passage that permits passage of the tracheal tube containing the fiberscope. This airway can be placed in awake patients following appropriate topical anesthesia. Conversely, the combination of the special anesthetic face mask with the Airway Intubator permits unhurried use of the fiberscope in unconscious patients during mechanical ventilation of the lungs.

RETROGRADE INTUBATION

Retrograde intubation of the trachea is accomplished by passing a plastic catheter through a needle (17-gauge intracath) previously placed through the cricothyroid membrane.[40] The catheter is directed cephalad and brought out the mouth or naris. An endotracheal tube is threaded over the plastic catheter and directed through the glottic opening using the catheter as a guide. This technique is probably best considered only when other approaches such as nasotracheal intubation or use of the fiberoptic laryngoscope have proved unsuccessful.

TABLE 16-5. Indications for Fiberoptic Intubation of the Trachea

Laryngeal–pharyngeal pathology
  Tumor
  Partial surgical resection
  Acromegaly
  Abscess
  Cystic hydroma
Tracheal pathology
  Mediastinal mass
  Subglottic stenosis
Congenital–developmental pathology
  Mandibular hypoplasia
  Mandibulofacial dysostosis
  Klippel-Feil
  Airway hemangioma
  Craniofacial synostosis
Immobile neck
  Arthritis
  Kyphoscoliosis
  Cervical traction
Morbid obesity

(Modified from Watson CS: Fiberoptic bronchoscopy for anesthesia. Anesth Rev 9:17, 1982.)

ENDOTRACHEAL INTUBATION IN CHILDREN
(Also See Ch. 49)

ANATOMIC DIFFERENCES FROM ADULTS

Because newborns and children are anatomically different from adults, their tracheas may be more difficult to intubate than adults.[41] These differences result in difficulty aligning the oral, pharyngeal and tracheal axes and elevating the epiglottis to expose the anterior glottic opening. For example, the newborn head and tongue are large and the neck is short. The larynx is more cephalad than in the adult — the

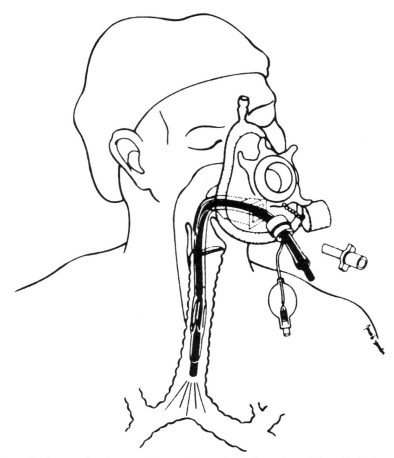

FIG. 16-7 Schematic diagram showing use of the oral Airway Intubator and special anesthetic face mask incorporating a diaphragm. The endotracheal tube and flexible fiberoptic laryngoscope are introduced through the diaphragm of the face mask and directed toward the glottic opening via the oral Airway Intubator. After the endotracheal tube is positioned in the mid-trachea, the fiberoptic laryngoscope is removed and the face mask with diaphragm is removed over the endotracheal tube before the tube is connected to the anesthetic breathing system. Removal of the oral Airway Intubator is optional. (Rogers SN, Benumof JL: New and easy techniques for fiberoptic endoscopy-aided tracheal intubation. Anesthesiology 59:569, 1983.)

lower border of the cricoid cartilage is opposite the 4th cervical vertebra at birth and opposite the 5th cervical vertebra after 6 years of age. The epiglottis is U-shaped and stiff. Furthermore, the cricoid cartilage is the narrowest point in the larynx, and a tracheal tube that passes through the glottic opening may resist subsequent advancement at this site. Also, excessive traction with the laryngoscope blade may angulate the trachea, producing the same problem.

ENDOTRACHEAL TUBE SIZE AND LENGTH

Selection of the appropriate tracheal tube size and length is critical in children, as the margin for error is small (Tables 16-2 and 16-3). Excessive tracheal tube size is responsible for unnecessary laryngotracheal trauma, which may be manifest as laryngeal edema when the tube is removed. Likewise, the short glottis-to-carina distance in children necessitates careful calculation of correct tube length. Ideally, the distal end of the tracheal tube should be located midway between the glottic opening and carina to minimize the hazards of accidental endobronchial intubation or extubation. One must be aware that head flexion or changes from the supine to head-down position may shift the carina upward, thereby converting a tracheal tube placement to an endobronchial intubation, and that head extension may place the tube in the pharynx.

Recommended tube size and distance of insertion are summarized in Table 16-2. In children 2 to 14 years of age, proper tube size may be predicted using the following formulas, recognizing that these are provided only as a guide:

1. Internal diameter (mm) for children less than 6.5 years of age = age in years/3 + 3.5 (ref. 42)
2. Internal diameter (mm) for children over 6.5 years of age = age in years/4 + 4.5 (ref. 42)
3. French catheter size (units) = 18 + age in years (ref. 44)

An endotracheal tube one size above and below the calculated size should be available with the final choice made when the glottic opening is visualized and the tube is inserted into the trachea. Cuffed tubes are probably not necessary in children under 5 years of age because the narrow subglottic tracheal diameter ensures an adequate seal and prevents aspiration.[10]

A formula may be used as a guide to predict proper tube length for ideal tube placement in the trachea. This formula may be useful in children up to about 14 years of age. Nasotracheal tubes should be about 20 percent longer.

Orotracheal tube length for mid-trachea placement (cm) = age in years/2 (ref. 44)

Resistance to breathing is a consideration for the small lumen tubes and connectors necessary in children. Narrow curved endotracheal tube connectors should be avoided, as they increase airway resistance and impede passage of a suction catheter. A connector with a lumen as large as or larger than the endotracheal tube should always be employed. When increased airway resistance is a concern, the best approach is placement of a proper-sized (not the largest possible) tracheal tube and controlled ventilation of the lungs to prevent increased work of breathing.

METHOD OF ENDOTRACHEAL INTUBATION

Complications of endotracheal intubation in children have been minimized by employing single-use polyvinylchloride sterile tracheal tubes of appropriate size that have been inserted with minimal trauma. Orotracheal intubation is routinely chosen for short-term endotracheal tube placement. Awake intubation of the trachea in the newborn is preferable. This is accomplished with the head elevated on a padded ring while an assistant immobilizes and extends the head and depresses the shoulders. Two-week-old healthy infants are sufficiently strong to vigorously resist awake intubation of the trachea, and anesthesia may be produced before direct laryngoscopy. A straight laryngoscope blade may provide better exposure of the glottic opening than the curved blade especially in children less than 3 years of age.

The route of tube placement when intubation of the trachea is likely to be prolonged beyond 12 hours is unsettled. Orotracheal intubation permits use of a large internal diameter tube and easier suctioning; however, nasotracheal intubation permits more stable tube fixation with decreased chance of accidental extubation.

The tracheal tube must be securely fixed to prevent tube movement, which may result in accidental slippage of the tube into a mainstem bronchus or into the pharynx. Benzoin applied to the skin and tube at the lips or nose facilitates fixation with tape. For prolonged intubation of the trachea, covering the benzoin-prepared skin with Elastoplast and then suturing the tube to the Elastoplast may be considered. A sand bag behind the occiput may help maintain the head in a neutral position.

EXTUBATION OF THE TRACHEA

Extubation of the trachea following general anesthesia is ideally accomplished while the patient is still adequately anesthetized to diminish coughing and laryngospasm. This assumes that adequate ventilation of the lungs is present or can be maintained without the endotracheal tube and that vomiting is not a likely hazard. Suctioning of the pharynx should be performed prior to extubation of the trachea so that secretions proximal to the cuff do not drain into the trachea when the cuff is deflated. Unless secretions are audible in the endotracheal tube or the lungs, suction through the tube is not advised because of the risk of introducing bacteria into the trachea. The cuff is then deflated and the tube removed. Some prefer pressure on the reservoir bag as the tube is removed so that the lungs will be inflated and initial gas flow will be outward. This maneuver may also facilitate a cough and expulsion of any aspirated material. Laryngospasm and vomiting are the most serious immediate hazards; therefore, oxygen, succinylcholine, equipment for reintubation of the trachea, and suction must be immediately available.

When vomiting is a hazard at the conclusion of anesthesia, the endotracheal tube must be left in place until protective laryngeal reflexes have returned. However, patients occasionally "cough" vigorously when allowed to awaken with an endotracheal tube in place. This response is often referred to as "bucking" and represents a modified cough, as the glottic opening cannot close. Coughing and associated contraction of abdominal and chest muscles, allowed to persist, may strain recently placed sutures, produce arterial hypoxemia if breath-holding occurs, and increase intracranial pressure. Furthermore, laryngeal trauma is more likely when the arytenoid cartilages attempt to close forceably around the endotracheal tube. Vigorous reaction to the tracheal tube ("bucking") signals the return of the cough reflex, and at this point either the tracheal tube must be removed or further sedation instituted to permit tolerance of the tracheal tube. Lidocaine 1 mg/kg administered intravenously over about 2 minutes before extubation of the trachea may prevent coughing, hypertension, and tachycardia associated with removal of the tracheal tube.[45]

COMPLICATIONS OF ENDOTRACHEAL INTUBATION

The complications of endotracheal intubation rarely occur. Even this low incidence may be reduced by skillful techniques, appropriate use of anesthetic drugs, and neuromuscular blockers, as well as an understanding of the causes of these complications. Certainly, the benefits of a properly placed and patent endotracheal tube far exceed the risks of intubation of the trachea. Complications may be categorized as those that occur during direct laryngoscopy and endotracheal intubation, while the endotracheal tube is in place, and following extubation of the trachea—either immediately or after a delay (Table 16-6).[46]

COMPLICATIONS DURING DIRECT LARYNGOSCOPY AND ENDOTRACHEAL INTUBATION

Trauma related to direct laryngoscopy may occur anywhere from the lips to the glottis, but dental trauma is the most serious and frequent complication. Avoidance of pressure on teeth from the laryngoscope blade will minimize the hazard of dental trauma. Tooth protectors may protect vulnerable natural teeth (maxillary incisors) or fragile dental prostheses from chipping or fracture by the laryngoscope blade. Should injury occur, immediate expert dental advice is necessary, and a notation describing the circumstances surrounding the injury should be placed in the patient's medical

TABLE 16-6.   Complications of Endotracheal Intubation

Complications during direct laryngoscopy and endotracheal intubation
    Dental and oral soft tissue trauma
    Hypertension and tachycardia
    Cardiac dysrhythmias
    Aspiration of gastric contents
Complications while the endotracheal tube is in place
    Tracheal tube obstruction
    Endobronchial intubation
    Esophageal intubation
    Accidental extubation
    Increased resistance to breathing
    Aspiration of gastric contents
    "Bucking"
    Bronchospasm
    Tracheal mucosa ischemia
Immediate and delayed complications following intubation
    Laryngospasm
    Aspiration of gastric contents
    Pharyngitis (sore throat)
    Laryngitis
    Laryngeal or subglottic edema
    Laryngeal ulceration with or without granuloma formation
    Tracheitis
    Tracheal stenosis
    Introduction of bacteria into the lungs
    Vocal cord paralysis — unilateral or bilateral
    Arytenoid cartilage dislocation

(Modified from Blanc BF, Tremblay NAG: The complications of tracheal intubation. A new classification with a review of the literature. Anesth Analg 53:202, 1974.)

record. A dislodged tooth must be recovered; if the search is unsuccessful, appropriate thoracic and abdominal radiographs should be taken. A displaced tooth should be placed in saline, as reimplantation may be possible.[47]

Hypertension and tachycardia frequently accompany laryngoscopy and endotracheal intubation. The increases in blood pressure are accompanied by corresponding elevations of the circulating concentration of norepinephrine.[48] Similar circulatory changes accompany the use of either a straight or curved laryngoscope blade.[49] Limiting the duration of direct laryngoscopy to about 15 seconds and immediately preceding placement of the tube in the trachea with laryngotracheal lidocaine spray 2 mg/kg of a 4 percent solution minimizes the magnitude and duration of these responses.[50] Laryngotracheal lidocaine produces almost immediate topical anesthesia such that a 3- to 5-minute delay between application and placement of the tracheal tube is not necessary.

The transient circulatory responses evoked by direct laryngoscopy and endotracheal intubation are probably innocuous in patients with a normal circulatory system. Overzealous use of deep anesthesia, local anesthetics, depressant drugs, or vasodilators in an attempt to prevent circulatory changes caused by direct laryngoscopy and intubation of the trachea may ultimately introduce more hazard than the response they were intended to attenuate. Circulatory responses to direct laryngoscopy, however, may be exaggerated in patients with preexisting hypertension. Furthermore, these responses may jeopardize tissue viability in patients with coronary artery disease, valvular heart disease, or elevated intracranial pressure. Pharmacologic attempts to attenuate circulatory responses are indicated in these high-risk patients in whom direct laryngoscopy cannot be predictably accomplished within less than 15 seconds. Approaches that have been reported to attenuate the blood pressure response evoked by direct laryngoscopy include intravenous administration of (1) lidocaine 1.5 mg/kg 90 seconds before the start of laryngoscopy, (2) nitroprusside 1 to 2 μg/kg 15 seconds before starting laryngoscopy, and (3) fentanyl 8 μg/kg 2 to 4 minutes before starting laryngoscopy.[51-54]

Cardiac dysrhythmias apart from sinus tachycardia or bradycardia occur in 5 to 15 percent of patients undergoing endotracheal intubation under light anesthesia.[55] These dysrhythmias are rarely serious or prolonged, especially if adequate oxygenation is maintained. Ventilation of the lungs with oxygen for 1 minute before initiating laryngoscopy maintains the PaO$_2$ above awake levels for at least 2 to 3 minutes of apnea in most adults.[55]

COMPLICATIONS WHILE THE ENDOTRACHEAL TUBE IS IN PLACE

Obstruction of the endotracheal tube may result from secretions, blood, or a foreign body in the tube; from kinking; from inward collapse of the tube lumen by pressure on the inflated cuff; from migration of a slip-on cuff over the tip of the tube; and from asymmetrical cuff inflation forcing the tube against the tracheal wall. Passage of a fiberoptic laryngoscope through the endotracheal tube may facilitate rapid diagnosis when obstruction is not relieved by deflating the cuff or passing a suction catheter through the tube.

Inadvertent endobronchial intubation will be minimized by calculating the proper tube length for every patient and then noting the cm marking on the tube at the point of fixation (Tables 16-2 and 16-3). Ideally, the distal tip of the tracheal tube should be midway between the glottis and carina. Since the suprasternal notch is midway between the glottis and carina, proper tracheal tube position may be confirmed by external palpation in the suprasternal notch and detection of cuff distention during rapid inflation. Auscultation to determine equal air entry, visual confirmation of equal and bilateral chest movement (particularly upper chest), and a radiograph of the chest are also helpful in confirming proper tube placement. The trachea may move cephalad with head flexion, lateral rotation of the head, or the head-down position, converting a tracheal tube to an endobronchial tube. This is especially likely if the tube was placed near the carina with the head in a neutral position. Hyperextension of the head may place the distal end of the tracheal tube in the pharynx. Accurate interpretation of tube placement on a radiograph of the chest requires knowledge of head position at the time the picture was taken. Radiographs of the chest of adult patients demonstrated in average 1.9-cm movement of the distal end of the tracheal tube with both flexion and extension of the head from the neutral position.[56] Lateral head rotation moved the tube 0.7 cm away from the carina.

Esophageal placement of the endotracheal tube is accompanied by a characteristic bubbly sound and by auscultation of gastric air entry with attempted positive-pressure ventilation of the lungs. Should esophageal intubation occur, the tube should be disconnected from the anesthetic system to avoid further gastric distention. If regurgitation is a consideration, one may leave the tube in the esophagus and inflate the cuff. Following tracheal intubation, the stomach should be decompressed and the esophageal tube removed.

Accidental extubation of the trachea, which is most likely in young patients, may be minimized by proper fixation of the endotracheal tube and maintenance of the head in a neutral position. Narrow endotracheal tubes and connectors cause turbulent air flow, increasing the work of breathing; if extreme, arterial hypoxemia and hypercarbia result. Secretions of blood may pool above the endotracheal tube cuff only to enter the trachea if the cuff is deflated. Vigorous attempts ("bucking") by the patient to dislodge the tracheal tube may decrease lung volumes, with subsequent arterial hypoxemia. Bronchospasm has been attributed to placement of the tracheal tube in a lightly anesthetized patient.

The inflated tracheal tube cuff may transmit excessive pressure to tracheal mucosa and impair capillary blood flow. Ischemia of the tracheal mucosa is minimal with high residual volume cuffs, but low residual volume cuffs may exert tracheal wall pressures above 100 mm Hg.[17]

IMMEDIATE AND DELAYED COMPLICATIONS FOLLOWING EXTUBATION OF THE TRACHEA (Also See Chs. 52 & 63)

Laryngospasm is reflex closure of the glottic opening due to contraction of the laryngeal muscles resulting in total cessation of gas flow into or from the lungs. Two conditions are usually present in order for laryngospasm to occur. First, the level of anesthesia is inadequate at the time of extubation of the trachea. Laryngospasm rarely occurs in fully conscious or surgically anesthetized patients. Second, there must be irritation of the larynx by secretions or vomitus, hence the importance of adequate pharyngeal suctioning before extubation of the trachea. Laryngospasm may or may not be preceded by laryngeal stridor, characterized as a crowing sound with inhalation. There is no respiratory sound with laryngospasm, since there is no gas flow through the upper airway. The diagnosis of laryngospasm is aided by a high index of suspicion and signs of upper airway obstruction evidenced by inward collapse of the patient's thorax accompanied by protrusion of the abdomen with each inspiratory effort. Although laryngoscopy will confirm the existence of laryngospasm, it is not an appropriate maneuver because it consumes valuable time and is not therapeutic. It is virtually impossible to force a tube through a closed glottic opening without producing serious trauma. Initial treatment of laryngospasm is delivery of oxygen under positive pressure via an anesthetic face mask. Simultaneously, forward displacement of the patient's mandible by placing the index and middle fingers of each hand at the temporomandibular joint is applied by the anesthesiologist. This maneuver has the added advantage that it pulls the tongue forward off the posterior pharyngeal wall, thereby correcting airway obstruction from this cause. This forward mandible displacement can be performed while delivering oxygen via the mask on the patient's face. If laryngospasm persists despite oxygen and forward mandible displacement, succinylcholine 0.5 to 1.0 mg/kg should be administered intravenously. Sublingual or another vascular intramuscular injec-

tion site for succinylcholine is an alternative if an intravenous route is not available.

Aspiration is most likely to occur in the debilitated patient or in the presence of gastrointestinal obstruction. There is evidence that prolonged intubation of the trachea (8 hours or more) may impair the ability of the larynx to sense foreign material for several hours after extubation even though the patient is fully awake (Fig. 16-8).[57] Recovery of normal reflex function in some patients does not occur until 4 to 8 hours following extubation of the trachea.

Some denudation of pharyngeal and laryngeal epithelium is inevitable with endotracheal intubation. A number of studies have attempted to determine the incidence of phar-

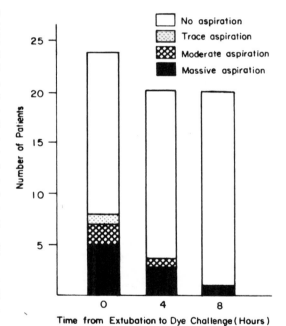

FIG. 16-8 The number of patients who aspirated radiopaque dye administered orally immediately after extubation of the trachea (0 hours, 4 hours, and 8 hours) was determined. All patients were alert and awake at the time of extubation of the trachea. The tracheas of these patients had been previously intubated for 8 to 28 hours (average 11.8 hours) during and after cardiac operations. Aspiration was significantly less in the 8-hour group compared with the immediately challenged group ($P < 0.05$). (Burgess GE, Cooper JR, Marino RJ, et al: Laryngeal competence after tracheal extubation. Anesthesiology 51:73, 1979.)

**TABLE 16-7.   Influence of Cuff and Lubricant on
Postoperative Sore Throat***

Cuff Tracheal Contact Length (mm)	Incidence of Sore Throat (%)		
	No Lubricant	Surgilube	Lidocaine
20	12	16	24
29	30	20	30
29	26	30	38
37	26	30	58*

* $p < 0.05$ vs. all other groups.
(Modified from Loeser EA, Kaminsky A, Diaz A, et al: The influence of endotracheal tube cuff design and cuff lubrication on postoperative sore throat. Anesthesiology 58:376, 1983.)

yngitis (sore throat) after endotracheal intubation. The incidence ranges from 5.7 percent to as high as 90 percent.[58,59] The incidence of sore throat is 15 to 22 percent in the absence of tracheal intubation.[60,61] Direct questioning about symptoms of sore throat results in a higher incidence of this complication than basing the incidence on complaints volunteered by the patient.[62] The cuff tracheal contact area influences the incidence of sore throat.[25,63,64] For example, when the cuff tracheal contact area was 20 mm, the incidence of sore throat was 12 percent versus 26 percent when the contact area was 37 mm (Table 16-7).[25] In this same study, the incidence of sore throat was further increased by the use of lidocaine ointment on the tracheal tube (Table 16-7).[25] Conversely, others have failed to demonstrate an association between the use of tracheal tube lubricant and the occurrence of sore throat (Table 16-8).[65] Females manifest sore throat more often than males possibly because of the thinner mucosal

**TABLE 16-8.   Influence of Lubricant
on Incidence of Postoperative Sore
Throat**

	Sore Throat (%)
No tube (N = 38)	21
Dry tube (N = 22)	45
Normal saline (N = 19)	42
Water-soluble jelly (N = 20)	45
Lidocaine jelly (N = 27)	41
Lidocaine ointment (N = 34)	50

N = number of patients.
(Modified from Stock MC, Downs JB: Lubrication of tracheal tubes to prevent sore throat from intubation. Anesthesiology 57:418, 1982.)

covering over the posterior vocal cords. The use of succinylcholine may contribute to an increased incidence of sore throat 24 to 30 hours following extubation of the trachea (Table 16-9).[66] Presumably, peripharyngeal muscles are damaged by succinylcholine, resulting in patient complaints of a sore throat. The mechanism is not different from the skeletal muscle myalgias that often follow administration of succinylcholine. The incidence of sore throat was not influenced by the duration of intubation of the trachea, age of the patient, type of operation, or intracuff pressure.[64] Regardless of the mechanism, sore throat almost always disappears within 48 to 72 hours without any specific therapy. In severe cases, a local anesthetic containing mouthwash may provide temporary symptomatic relief. Sore throat is a minor side effect and should not influence the decision to perform intubation of the trachea.

Laryngitis occurs in about 3 percent of patients and is manifested by hoarseness and a tight feeling in the throat.[67] Recovery is usually spontaneous without any treatment.

Symptomatic laryngeal or subglottic edema is most likely in children because a small amount of laryngeal swelling greatly reduces the lumen of the larynx.[69] For example, 1 mm of edema in a newborn infant reduces the cross-sectional area of the larynx 65 percent. The same amount of edema produces only slight hoarseness in an adult. In addition, the cricoid cartilage prevents any external expansion when edema occurs. The most likely causes of edema in children are mechanical injury (traumatic intubation of the trachea, oversized tracheal tube) or infection (unsterile endotracheal tube or a recent or preexisting

TABLE 16-9. Succinylcholine-Induced Postoperative Sore Throat

Muscle Relaxant	Incidence 24 to 30 hours postoperatively	
	Sore Throat (%)	Myalgia (%)
None (N = 21)	10	5
SCh bolus (1 mg/kg) (N = 22)	68	68
dTc (0.05 mg/kg) SCh (1.5 mg/kg) (N = 20)	45	50
SCh infusion (36 ± 17 mg) (N = 20)	50	30

Abbreviations used: SCh = succinylcholine, dTc = *d*-tubocurarine, N = number of patients.

(Modified from Capan LM, Bruce DL, Patel KP, et al: Succinylcholine-induced postoperative sore throat. Anesthesiology 59:202, 1983.)

upper respiratory infection). Prolonged periods of tracheal intubation do not seem to increase the incidence and/or severity of mucosal edema proportionally.[69] Although some recommend prophylactic administration of methylprednisolone before extubation of the trachea, there is no prospective study to support the efficacy of this treatment.[69] Red rubber tubes are more irritating to the tracheal mucosa than are polyvinylchloride and silicone tubes. It must be recognized that even with adequate precautions and flawless techniques mucosal edema may still occur.

Laryngeal ulceration with or without granuloma formation, typically occurs on the posterior portion of the vocal cords overlying the rigid projection of the arytenoid cartilage known as the vocal process.[70] This initial contact ulcer is most likely produced by the endotracheal tube moving on the thin mucoperichondrial covering that overlies the vocal processes. Hyperextension of the head, as during thyroid operations, may increase the pressure exerted on the vocal processes by the tracheal tube. Excessive head movement or inadequate depression of laryngeal reflexes by anesthetic drugs may also accentuate damage when the arytenoid cartilages scrape the endotracheal tube. Often the cause of ulceration is unrelated to the endotracheal tube and remains unknown. Preoperative respiratory infections seem to exacerbate the laryngeal reaction by constantly bathing the ulcerated mucosa with bacteria. Granulation tissue tends to cover the ulcerated area resulting in a sessile granuloma. Subsequently, the ulcer base narrows by fibrosis until pedunculation occurs.

Granuloma of the larynx following endotracheal intubation is rare (1 in every 10,000 to 20,000 intubations) and has been described only in adults.[71] There is no correlation between the incidence of granuloma formation and the duration of tracheal intubation, suggesting that tube material (red rubber more than polyvinylchloride) and host factors are more important.[69] Use of an S-shaped tube reduced the incidence of hoarseness and granuloma formation following intubation of the trachea lasting 1 to 2 days.[14] The greater incidence of granuloma formation in females may reflect the fact that the mucosal layer covering the vocal processes of the arytenoid cartilages is twice as thick in males as in females. Granulomas are bilateral in about one-half of reported cases. Bilateral ulcerations may heal by side-to-side adhesions, resulting in a laryngeal web or stenosis.[72] Postintubation granulomas usually require 14 to 21 days to develop but may appear in as little as 72 hours.[73] Persistent hoarseness is the most common symptom and alone or in combination with sore throat, pain, or fullness in the laryngotracheal area, or unexplained upper airway obstruction is an indication for indirect laryngoscopy. If an ulceration is observed, strict vocal rest should permit healing without granuloma formation. Surgical removal of the pedunculated granuloma under direct laryngoscopy followed by absolute vocal rest may be required.

During prolonged intubation of the trachea, the route used for tracheal tube insertion may influence the incidence and type of laryngeal injury. In patients intubated an average 6.7 days, laryngeal injury (vocal cord ulceration and cratering) following extubation of the trachea was more frequent and severe after oral than nasal tracheal intubation.[74] This may reflect the use of smaller tracheal tubes for nasal intubation and better stability so that nasotracheal tube movement is less likely with changes in head position.

Ulceration of the tracheal mucosa may occur at the anterior tracheal wall where the distal tip of the endotracheal tube has abraded the epithelium. The curve of the tracheal tube is such that pressures as high as 90 mm Hg may be exerted on the area of contact of the distal tip of the tube with the anterior tracheal wall. Tracheitis with substernal discomfort and persistent coughing may be a manifestation of this tracheal tube-induced injury.

The endotracheal tube cuff may exert excessive pressure on the tracheal wall (capillary pressure at the arterial end is about 30 mm Hg), producing mucosa ischemia. This may progress to destruction of cartilaginous rings and subsequent circumferential constricting scar formation and tracheal stenosis. Other causative factors to consider include duration of intubation of the trachea (greater than 48 hours), high ventilator pressures with tracheal tube movement, bacterial infection, and persistent systemic hypotension. Tracheal stenosis becomes symptomatic when the adult tracheal lumen is reduced to less than 5 mm. Some patients may be managed with dilitation but surgical resection of the stenotic tracheal segment may be necessary. These hazards are minimized by use of high residual volume cuffs which, when properly used, do not produce excessive tracheal wall pressures.

A relationship between endotracheal intubation and pulmonary complications (pneumonia) has never been proved. More important are the preoperative pulmonary status and the operative procedure. Nevertheless, oropharyngeal bacteria not ordinarily present in the trachea may be introduced into the trachea with an endotracheal tube; indeed bacteremia has been observed after nasotracheal (not orotracheal) intubation.[34] Good oral hygiene may reduce tracheal contamination, especially in patients with carious teeth.

Unilateral and bilateral vocal cord paralyses have been reported after short-term endotracheal intubation for operations not about the larynx.[67,75,76] The mechanism is unknown. Irregular tracheal cuff inflation compressing a branch of the recurrent laryngeal nerve between the cuff and thyroid cartilage has been implicated.[68,77] When paralysis is unilateral, the left vocal cord is affected twice as frequently as the right. Males are affected approximately seven times more frequently than females.[78] Asymptomatic laryngeal nerve palsy may even predate tracheal intubation. In such patients, any edema from instrumentation might produce hoarseness with a subsequent diagnosis of recurrent laryngeal nerve palsy and wrongful implication of the tracheal tube as the etiology.[79]

Arytenoid cartilage dislocation is a rare complication that has been attributed to inserting the laryngoscope blade too far behind the cricoid cartilage with resulting arytenoid cartilage dislocation during elevation of the blade.[80] A weak voice following extubation of the trachea after prolonged intubation has been reported due to dislocation of unilateral arytenoid cartilage.[81] Treatment is reduction and cricoarytenoid arthrodesis.

DELIBERATE ENDOBRONCHIAL INTUBATION

Endobronchial intubation (also see Ch. 40) serves to provide separate airways to healthy and diseased lung or to improve intrathoracic operating conditions during lung resection by providing a nonventilated quiet lung. Specific indications for selective lung ventilation or suction include lung abscess, bronchiectasis, or bronchopleural fistula. Selective lung ventilation may be accomplished with a double-lumen endobronchial tube that permits isolated but simultaneous ventilation of both lungs. It should be remembered that the carina to right upper lobe bronchus distance is about 1.5 cm compared with about 5 cm on the left. Proper endobronchial tube position is confirmed by auscultation, by a radiograph of the chest, or by passing a fiberoptic laryngoscope through the tube. Auscultation for breath sounds in the axillary regions minimizes the possibility that an examiner will confuse them with transmitted breath sounds.

The need for one-lung ventilation must be weighed against the risk of arterial hypoxemia. The magnitude of intrapulmonary shunt will be influenced by the level of activity of hypoxic pulmonary vasoconstriction and the degree of surgical retraction. Intrapulmonary shunting occurs regardless of ventilation patterns, and efforts to improve arterial oxygenation by raising intraalveolar pressure in the ventilated lung may act to divert blood flow to the unventilated lung.[82] Arterial hypoxemia left uncorrected by high inspired oxygen concentrations has been documented during anesthesia delivered through a double-lumen tube with collapse of the nondependent (operated) lung.[83] Patients undergoing similar operations with conventional endotracheal tubes manifested less intrapulmonary shunting and maintained satisfactory arterial oxygen partial pressures breathing high inspired oxygen concentra-

tions. This suggests that the partially inflated upper lung contributed to their oxygenation during the surgical procedure. When arterial hypoxemia persists despite inhalation of 100 percent oxygen, it is acceptable to cautiously apply positive end-expiratory pressure (PEEP) to the nonventilated lung in an attempt to divert blood flow from this to the ventilated lung. Arterial oxygenation would be best maintained by deferring unilateral ventilation until circulation to the nonventilated lung has been surgically interrupted. The $PaCO_2$ does not change greatly during one-lung ventilation.[84]

The Carlens double-lumen tube is introduced under direct vision using a rotational motion and advanced down the trachea with the tip pointed to enter the left main-stem bronchus until the rubber hook engages the carina (Fig. 16-9).[85] The left lung is ventilated through the tube lumen, which lies in the bronchus, and the right lung is ventilated through the lumen, which opens above the carina. Disadvantages of the Carlens tube include increased airway resistance and difficulty suctioning thick secretions through the small lumens of the tube (6 to 8 mm). The small

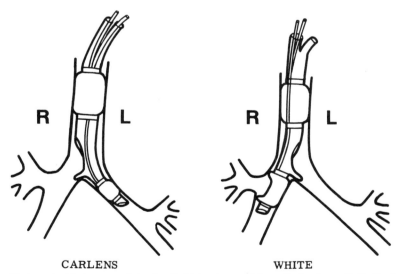

CARLENS   WHITE

FIG. 16-9 The Carlens double-lumen endotracheal tube is advanced down the trachea with the tip directed to enter the left mainstem bronchus until the rubber hook engages the carina. Inflation of the tracheal and left mainstem bronchus cuffs effectively isolates the lungs and permits selective ventilation. The White tube is advanced with the distal end directed to enter the right mainstem bronchus until the rubber hook engages the carina. Inflation of the cuffs isolates the lungs. Ventilation of the right upper lobe is accomplished via an opening in the portion of the tube opposite the right mainstem bronchus.

lumen size may make it difficult or impossible to pass a fiberoptic laryngoscope to confirm proper tube placement. Furthermore, this tube must be withdrawn into the trachea during a left pneumonectomy.

The White double-lumen tube (Fig. 16-9) is designed for introduction into the right mainstem bronchus.[86] The lumen of the tube in the bronchus carries a cuff surrounding a rectangular slot in the tube so the right upper lobe bronchus can be ventilated. A rubber hook on the tube engages the carina.

The Robertshaw double-lumen tube was designed for maximum lumen size to offset the disadvantages of the Carlens tube.[87] Both left- and right-sided bronchial models are available. Left-sided tubes have a tip angled at 45 degrees to enter the left mainstem bronchus while the tip of the right-sided tube is angled at 20 degrees to enter the right mainstem bronchus. Neither tube has a carinal hook. Single-use (disposable) Robertshaw endobronchial tubes are available.

Use of a right-sided endobronchial tube introduces the risk of inadequate ventilation of the right upper lobe. In order to avoid this complication, it is acceptable to utilize a left-sided tube for all operations requiring one-lung anesthesia. If clamping of the left mainstem bronchus is necessary, the tube can be withdrawn into the trachea.

REFERENCES

1. Macewen W: Clinical observations on the introduction of tracheal tubes by the mouth instead of performing tracheotomy or laryngotomy. Br Med J 2:163, 1880
2. Kirstein A: Autoskopie des larynx and der trachea. Berl Klin Wochenschr 32:475, 1895
3. Jackson C: The technique of insertion of intratracheal insufflation tubes. Surg Gynecol Obstet 17:507, 1913
4. Janeway HH: Intratracheal anesthesia from the standpoint of the nose, throat and oral surgery with a description of a new instrument for catheterizing the trachea. Laryngoscope 23:1082, 1913
5. Dorrance GM: On the treatment of traumatic injuries of the lungs and pleurae. Surg Gynecol Obstet 11:160, 1910
6. Rowbotham ES, Magill I: Anaesthetics in the plastic surgery of the face and jaws. Proc R Soc Med 14:17, 1921
7. Cass NM, James NR, Lines V: Difficult direct laryngoscopy complicating intubation for anesthesia. Br. Med J 1:488, 1956
8. Wright RB, Manfield FFV: Damage to teeth during the administration of general anesthesia. Anesth Analg 53:405, 1974
9. Block C, Brechner VL: Unusual problems in airway management. II. The influence of the temporomandibular joint, the mandible, and associated structures on endotracheal intubation. Anesth Analg 50:114, 1971
10. Goitein KJ, Rein AJJT, Gornstein A: Incidence of aspiration in endotracheally intubated infants and children. Crit Care Med 12:19, 1984
11. MacIntost RR: New laryngoscope. Lancet 1:205, 1943
12. Miller RA: A new laryngoscope. Anesthesiology 2:317, 1941
13. Lindholm CE: Prolonged endotracheal intubation. Acta Anaesth Scand (suppl) 13:1, 1969
14. Alexopoulos C, Larsson SG, Lindholm CE: The conformity of an anatomically shaped endotracheal tube to the shape of the airway. Acta Anaesthesiol Scand 27:235, 1983
15. Loeser EA, Machin R, Colley J, et al: Postoperative sore throat—importance of endotracheal tube conformity versus cuff design. Anesthesiology 49:1430, 1978
16. Benumof JL, Berryhill RE, Maruschak GF, et al: Tracheal wall pressure caused by endotracheal tube tip. Anesthesiology 51:S193, 1979
17. Carroll R, Hedden M, Safar P: Intratracheal cuffs. Performance characteristics. Anesthesiology 31:275, 1969
18. Knowlson GTG, Bassett HFM: The pressures exerted on the trachea by endotracheal inflatable cuffs. Br J Anaesth 42:834, 1970
19. Cooper JD, Grillo HC: Analysis of problems related to cuffs on intratracheal tubes. Chest 62:215, 1972
20. Dunn CR, Dunn DL, Moser KM: Determinants of tracheal injury by cuffed tracheostomy tubes. Chest 65:128, 1974
21. Andrews MJ, Pearson FG: Incidence and pathogenesis of tracheal injury following cuffed tube tracheostomy and assisted ventilation: Analysis of a two year prospective study. Ann Surg 173:249, 1971
22. Klainer AS, Turndorf H, Wen-Hsien WU, et al: Surface alterations due to endotracheal intubation. Am J Med 58: 674, 1975
23. Bernhard AV, Cottrell JE, Sivakumaran C, et al:

Adjustment of intracuff pressure to prevent aspiration. Anesthesiology 50:363, 1979

24. Stanley TH: Effects of anesthetic gases on endotracheal tube cuff gas volumes. Anesth Analg 53:480, 1974
25. Loeser EA, Kaminsky A, Diaz A, et al: The influence of endotracheal tube cuff design and cuff lubrication on postoperative sore throat. Anesthesiology 58:376, 1983
26. Stoelting RK, Peterson C: Circulatory changes during anesthetic induction: Impact of d-tubocurarine pretreatment, thiamylal, succinylcholine, laryngoscope and tracheal lidocaine. Anesth Analg 55:77, 1976
27. Stoelting RK, Miller RD: Airway management, Basics of Anesthesia. Edited by Stoelting RK, Miller RD. New York, Churchill Livingstone, 1984, pp 153–165
28. Walts LF: Anesthesia of the larynx in the patient with a full stomach. JAMA 192:121, 1965
29. Wycoff CC: Aspiration during induction of anesthesia. Anesth Analg 38:5, 1959
30. Defalque RJ: Ketamine for blind nasal intubation. Anesth Analg 50:984, 1971
31. Zwillich C, Pierson DJ: Nasal necrosis: A complication of nasotracheal intubation. Chest 64:376, 1973
32. Sherry KM: Ulceration of the inferior turbinate: A complication of prolonged nasotracheal intubation. Anesthesiology 59:148, 1983
33. Arens JF, LeJeune FE, Webre DR: Maxillary sinusitis, a complication of nasotracheal intubation. Anesthesiology 40:415, 1974
34. Berry FA, Blenkenbaker WL, Ball CG: A comparison of bacteremia occurring with nasotracheal and orotracheal intubation. Anesth Analg 52:873, 1973
35. Davis NJ: A new fiberoptic laryngoscope for nasal intubation. Anesth Analg 52:807, 1973
36. Raj PP, Forestner J, Watson TD, et al: Techniques for fiberoptic laryngoscopy in anesthesia. Anesth Analg 53:708, 1974
37. Watson CB: Fiberoptic bronchoscopy for anesthesia. Anesthesiol Rev 9:17, 1982
38. Heifetz M, DeMyttenaeres D, Lemer J: Intermittent positive pressure inflation during fiberoptic bronchoscopy. Chest 72:480, 1977
39. Rogers SN, Benumof JL: New and easy techniques for fiberoptic endoscopy-aided tracheal intubation. Anesthesiology 59:569, 1983
40. Powell WF, Ozdil T: A translaryngeal guide for tracheal intubation. Anesth Analg 46:231, 1967
41. Eckenhoff JE: Some anatomic considerations of the infant larynx influencing endotracheal anesthesia. Anesthesiology 12:401, 1951
42. Penlington GN: Endotracheal tube sizes for children (letter). Anaesthesia 29:494, 1974

43. Cole F: Correspondence. Anesthesiology 14:506, 1953
44. Levine J: Endotracheal tube in children. Anaesthesia 13:40, 1958
45. Bidwai AV, Bidwai VA, Rogers CR, et al: Blood pressure and pulse rate responses to endotracheal extubation with and without prior injection of lidocaine. Anesthesiology 57:171, 1979
46. Blanc VF, Tremblay NAG: The complications of tracheal intubation. A new classification with a review of the literature. Anesth Analg 53:202, 1974
47. Lind GL, Spiegel EH, Munson ES: Treatment of traumatic tooth avulsion. Anesth Analg 61:469, 1982
48. Derbyshire DR, Chmielewski A, Fell D, et al: Plasma catecholamine responses to tracheal intubation. Br J Anaesth 55:855; 1983
49. Takeshima K, Noda K, Higaki M: Cardiovascular response to rapid anesthesia induction and endotracheal intubation. Anesth Analg 43:201, 1964
50. Stoelting RK: Blood pressure and heart rate changes during short duration laryngoscopy for tracheal intubation. Influence of viscous or intravenous lidocaine. Anesth Analg 57:197, 1978
51. Stoelting RK: Circulatory changes during direct laryngoscopy and tracheal intubation: Influence of duration of laryngoscopy with or without prior lidocaine. Anesthesiology 47:381, 1977
52. Stoelting RK: Attenuation of blood pressure response to laryngoscopy and tracheal intubation with sodium nitroprusside. Anesth Analg 58:116, 1979
53. Martin DE, Rosenberg H, Aukburg SJ, et al: Low-dose fentanyl blunts circulatory responses to tracheal intubation. Anesth Analg 61:680, 1982
54. Gibbs JM: The effects of endotracheal intubation on cardiac rate and rhythm. NZ Med J 66:465, 1967
55. Cole WL, Stoelting VK: Blood gases during intubation following two types of oxygenation. Anesth Analg 50:68, 1971
56. Conrardy PA, Goodman LR, Lainge F, et al: Alteration of endotracheal tube position. Flexion and extension of the neck. Crit Care Med 4:8, 1976
57. Burgess GE, Cooper JR, Marino RJ, et al: Laryngeal competence after tracheal extubation. Anesthesiology 51:73, 1979
58. Hartsell CJ, Stephen CR: Incidence of sore throat following endotracheal intubation. Can Anaesth Soc J 11:307, 1964
59. Loeser EA, Stanley TH, Jordan W, Machin R: Postoperative sore throat: Influence of tracheal tube lubrication versus cuff design. Can Anaesth Soc J 27:156, 1980
60. Loeser EA, Orr DL, Bennett GM, Stanley TH: Endotracheal tube cuff design and postoperative sore throat. Anesthesiology 45:684, 1976

61. Jensen PJ, Hommelgaard P, Sondergaard P, Eriksen S: Sore throat after operation: influence of tracheal intubation, intracuff pressure and type of cuff. Br J Anaesth 54:453, 1982
62. Winkel E, Knudsen J: Effect of the incidence of postoperative sore throat of 1 percent cinchocaine jelly for endotracheal intubation. Anesth Analg 50:92, 1971
63. Loeser EA, Machin R, Colley J, et al: Postoperative sore throat-importance of endotracheal tube conformity versus cuff design. Anesthesiology 49:430, 1978
64. Loeser EA, Bennett GM, Orr DL, Stanley TH: Reduction of postoperative sore throat with new endotracheal tube cuffs. Anesthesiology 52:257, 1980
65. Stock MC, Downs JB: Lubrication of tracheal tubes to prevent sore throat from intubation. Anesthesiology 57:418, 1982
66. Capan LM, Bruce DL, Patel KP, Turndorf H: Succinylcholine-induced postoperative sore throat. Anesthesiology 59:202, 1983
67. Holley HS, Gildea JE: Vocal cord paralysis after tracheal intubation. JAMA 215:281, 1971
68. McGovern FH, Fitz-Hugh GS, Edgemon LJ: The hazards of endotracheal intubation. Ann Otol Rhinol Laryngol 80:556, 1971
69. Bishop MJ, Weymuller EA, Fink RB: Laryngeal effects of prolonged intubation. Anesth Analg 63:335, 1984
70. Jackson C: Contact ulcer granuloma and other laryngeal complications of endotracheal anesthesia. Anesthesiology 14:425, 1953
71. Snow JC, Harano M, Balogy K: Postintubation granuloma of the larynx. Anesth Analg 45:425, 1966
72. Hawkins DB, Luxford WM: Laryngeal stenosis from endotracheal intubation. Ann Otol Rhinol Laryngol 89:454, 1980
73. Fine J, Finestone SC: An unusual complication of endotracheal intubation: Report of a case. Anesth Analg 52:204, 1973
74. Dubick MN, Wright BD: Comparison of laryngeal pathology following long term oral and nasal endotracheal intubations. Anesth Analg 57:663, 1978
75. Stenqvist O, Sonander H, Nilsson K: Small endotracheal tubes. Br J Anaesth 51:375, 1979
76. Hahn FW, Martin JT, Lillie JC: Vocal cord paralysis with endotracheal intubation. Arch Otolaryngol 92:226, 1970
77. Ellis PDM, Pallister WK: Recurrent laryngeal nerve palsy and endotracheal intubation. J Laryngol Otol 89:823, 1975
78. Cook WR: A comparison of idiopathic laryngeal paralysis in man and horse. J Laryngol Otol 89:819, 1970
79. Ellis PDM: Letter to the Editor. Anesthesiology 16:374, 1977
80. Jaffe BF: Postoperative hoarseness. Am J Surg 123:432, 1972
81. Prasertwanitch Y, Schwartz JJH, Vandam LD: Arytenoid cartilage dislocation following prolonged endotracheal intubation. Anesthesiology 41:516, 1974
82. Khanam T, Branthwaite MA: Arterial oxygenation during one-lung anesthesia (2). Anaesthesia 28:280, 1973
83. Tarhan S, Lundborg RO: Carlens endobronchial catheter versus regular endotracheal tube during thoracic surgery. A comparison of blood gas tensions and pulmonary shunting. Can Anaesth Soc J 18:595, 1971
84. Kerr J, Smith AC, Prys-Roberts C, et al: Observations during endobronchial anesthesia. I: Ventilation and carbon dioxide clearance. Br J Anaesth 45:159, 1973
85. Bjork VO, Carlens E: The prevention of spread during pulmonary resection by the use of a double lumen catheter. J Thorac Surg 20:151, 1950
86. White GMJ: A new double-lumen tube. Br J Anaesth 32:232, 1960
87. Robertshaw FL: Low resistance double lumen endobronchial tubes. Br J Anaesth 34:576, 1962

17

Anesthetic Depth and MAC

David J. Cullen, M.D.

INTRODUCTION

General anesthesia may be defined as that state in which the body is insensible to pain and possibly to other stimuli as well. For the anesthesiologist to detect that the patient feels pain or other sensations, the responses to noxious stimuli must be observed. Thus, some method to assess depth of anesthesia must be introduced. Attempts to assess anesthetic depth and potency first appeared in an 1847 monograph on diethyl ether by John Snow.[1] Snow and subsequent clinicians analyzed the inspired,[2] mixed expired,[3] arterial,[4] and even venous anesthetic concentrations that yielded specific signs of central nervous system (CNS) depression, which included abolition of movement in response to surgical simulation,[1-3] loss of the righting reflex,[2] attainment of a given level of electroencephalographic suppression,[4] and achievement of certain changes in pupillary diameter, eye movement, respiration, and muscle tone.[5]

In 1963 Merkel and Eger[6] described the minimum alveolar concentration of anesthetic at 1 atmosphere required to abolish movement in 50 percent of patients or animals in response to a noxious stimulus — abbreviated MAC — as an index of anesthetic potency that facilitated comparison of the pharmacologic properties of several anesthetic agents. Unlike previous estimates of anesthetic potency, MAC emphasized measurement of the alveolar anesthetic partial pressure at equilibrium, which means the inspired and alveolar concentrations were equal. Also the alveolar and brain partial pressures should be the same at equilibrium. Therefore, MAC represented anesthetic activity at the anesthetic site of action. Unlike clinical signs, which relied on side effects and varied from one drug to another, MAC could be applied to all inhaled anesthetics.[7] Thus, MAC has become the most widely accepted measure by which potencies of different anesthetics are compared.

DEFINITION

MAC 1.0 was initially defined as the "minimal alveolar concentration of anesthetic required to keep a dog from responding by gross purposeful movement to a painful stimulus."[6] Anesthetic dose could then be expressed as MAC multiples, such as 1.5 MAC or 3.0 MAC. MAC for humans was defined as the alveolar anesthetic concentration at which 50 percent of patients moved in response to a surgical incision.[8] These early studies revealed that MAC was remarkably consistent in both animals and in humans and that beyond a certain point, an increase in stimulus intensity (supramaximal stimulation) did not increase MAC.

MAC is defined in terms of percent of 1 atmosphere and as such is an alveolar anesthetic partial pressure (i.e., MAC would be the same at sea level or on top of Mount Everest). Because partial pressures of anesthetics will be equal in all body tissues (e.g., alveolus, blood, and brain) at equilibrium, MAC should, at equilibrium, represent the anesthetic partial pressure—not the concentration—at the anesthetic site of action (e.g., the brain). The consistency of MAC for animals and humans, the relative ease of its measurement, and its predictable relationship with the partial pressure of anesthetic at the site of action have established MAC as the most widely accepted measure of anesthetic potency.[9]

TECHNICAL ASPECTS OF OBTAINING MAC IN ANIMALS AND HUMANS

MAC differs slightly for animals and humans. An animal is anesthetized with the anesthetic to be studied in oxygen, and the trachea is intubated usually without succinylcholine. A predetermined end-tidal anesthetic concentration is obtained and held constant for at least 15 minutes to equilibrate alveolus, blood, and brain. The animal is then stimulated with either a tail clamp (full-length hemostat applied close to the base of the tail and clamped a full-rachet lock) or subcutaneous electrical current (50 volts at 50 cps for 10 msec). If no movement occurs in response to stimulation, the end-tidal ("alveolar") anesthetic concentration is lowered to 80 or 90 percent of the initial concentration and the stimulus is repeated after allowing 15 minutes for reequilibration. If, however, a positive response to stimulation is obtained initially, the end-tidal anesthetic concentration is increased 10 to 20 percent, and the process of reequilibration for 15 minutes (followed by stimulus application) is repeated. MAC 1.0 is the concentration midway between that which allows and that which prevents movement. The narrower the brackets (e.g., 10 percent versus 20 percent step changes in anesthetic concentration), the more precise (and time-consuming) will be the determination (Fig. 17-1).

The standard stimulus applied to humans is a surgical skin incision, although electrical currents passed through subcutaneous tissues have also been used[8] (application via 20-gauge needles in the forearm, of 30 to 45 volts AC with a 1.2-msec pulse at 50 cycles/sec for less than 60 seconds). Since a patient is normally incised only once, the bracketing technique used in animals cannot be applied to a single subject. In all other respects, the determination of MAC is the same. Anesthesia is induced with the anesthetic in oxygen. No premedication is given and no other anesthetic agents are administered. A preselected end-tidal anesthetic is held constant for 15 minutes before skin incision. During and immediately after incision, the patient is observed for movement or for lack of movement. Several such patient studies are accomplished over a range of end-tidal anesthetic concentrations that permit and prevent movement. Patients may then be taken in groups of four or more, starting with those having the lowest end-tidal (alveolar) concentration (Fig. 17-2). The percentage of patients moving within each group is plotted against the average end-tidal concentration for the group. A visual line of best fit through these points yields the concentration at which 50 percent of patients respond, i.e., MAC (Fig. 17-3). A more rigorous analysis yields the same value for MAC and adds one element, an estimate of the variance of MAC (i.e., standard deviation).[10,11] Thus, the determination of MAC has three components: the measurement of end-tidal an-

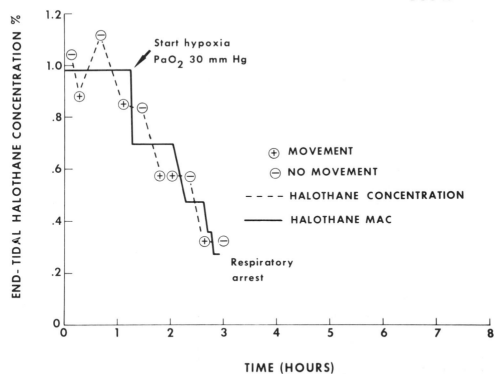

DETERMINATION OF MAC DURING NORMOCAPNIC HYPOXIA

DOG 18

FIG. 17-1 Determination of MAC during normocapnic hypoxia: After control MAC was determined, halothane concentration (dashed line) was maintained at a level where movement previously had occurred in response to the tail clamp (+). Hypoxia to a PaO₂ of 30 mm Hg was then induced and no movement occurred after tail clamping (−). When halothane concentration was lowered to 0.6 percent, movement occurred (+). Thus, MAC was bracketed midway between 0.8 and 0.6 percent (solid line). As each movement response converted to no movement, halothane concentration was lowered further. Less than 2 hours after hypoxia, respiratory arrest occurred, and MAC was defined as midway between the concentration at respiratory arrest and the previous concentration at which there had been no movement. (Cullen DJ, Eger EI II: The effects of hypoxia and isovolemic anemia on the halothane requirement (MAC) in dogs. I. The effect of hypoxia. Anesthesiology 32:28, 1970.)

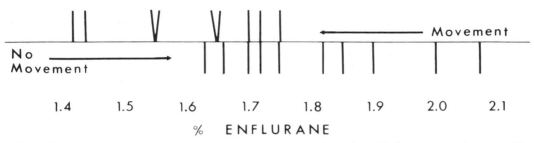

FIG. 17-2 End-tidal enflurane concentrations are plotted on the horizontal axis. Patient response (movement) to surgical incision is expressed as an upward deflection, and lack of response (no movement), as a downward deflection. (Gion H, Saidman LJ: The minimum alveolar concentration of enflurane in man. Anesthesiology 35:361, 1971.)

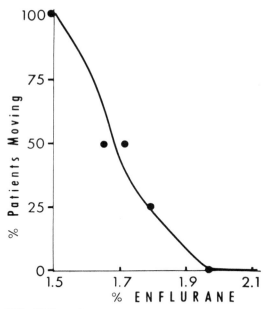

FIG. 17-3 MAC determined from data in Figure 17-2. Starting with the lowest end-tidal enflurane concentrations, subjects were taken in groups of four. The percentage of patients moving within each group was plotted against that group's mean end-tidal enflurane concentration. MAC is the enflurane concentration corresponding to the 50 percent point on the vertical axis, i.e., 1.68 percent. (Gion H, Saidman LJ: The minimum alveolar concentration of enflurane in man. Anesthesiology 35:361, 1971.)

esthetic concentration, an applied noxious stimulus, and a defined response.

In early animal studies, variability in MAC decreased as stimulus intensity increased, and certain stimuli appeared to be supramaximal.[12] Simultaneous application of two different supramaximal stimuli did not increase MAC above that seen with a single supramaximal stimulus. A skin incision was not quite a supramaximal stimulus in dogs. Because the tail clamp was simply applied and because MAC did not change with the application of a more intense stimulus, tail clamping was chosen as the standard noxious stimulus required to determine MAC. Skin incision remains the standard stimulus in humans.

A positive response is considered to be "gross purposeful muscular movement,"[12] usually of the head or extremities. Head movement does not include a twitch or grimace, but only a jerking or twisting motion.[12] Extremity movements are most common; motion of the torso without motion of the head or extremity is rare. Coughing, swallowing, and chewing are not considered positive responses.

The concept of MAC assumes that end-tidal, alveolar, arterial, and brain anesthetic partial pressures are equal after 15 minutes of equilibration. This assumption may be incorrect, but any dysequilibrium is usually small. End-tidal gas partial pressure in normal unanesthetized humans reasonably approximates the "ideal" alveolar partial pressure.[13] Anesthesia may enhance the ventilation/perfusion ratio inequalities that exist even in normal patients, and thus some degree of alveolar-to-arterial partial pressure gradient must result.[14,15] Decreasing the inspired-to-alveolar (end-tidal) anesthetic partial-pressure difference minimizes this potential error[15] (i.e. with poorly soluble anesthetics, with normal ventilation (V) and cardiac output (Q), as opposed to hypoventilation or increased cardiac output, and/or after prior equilibration at a higher anesthetic partial pressure) (Fig. 17-4).

Several factors may produce a difference between the end-tidal and arterial anesthetic partial pressures.[16] Contamination of end-tidal samples by gas from nonperfused alveoli (alveolar deadspace) or from poorly perfused alveoli (severe V/Q abnormalities) increases the end-tidal partial pressure by contributing anesthetic partial pressures that approach those in inspired gas. The greater the difference between inspired and "true" alveolar (normally ventilated and perfused alveoli) partial pressures, the greater the error introduced by this contamination. A slower emptying of the ventilated, nonperfused portion of the lung exaggerates the error (the difference between end-tidal and arterial partial pressures). Finally, significant amounts of very soluble gases will dissolve in the airway tissues during inhalation and are released during expiration. The contribution of this gas to the end-tidal sample will erroneously increase the estimate of the arterial anesthetic partial pressure.

The technique for determination of MAC described above also assumes that equilibration for 15 minutes produces equality of arterial and brain partial pressures. This is based on the following equation[17]:

$$t = \frac{\lambda \cdot VT}{CBF} \cdot \log_e \frac{1}{0.05}$$

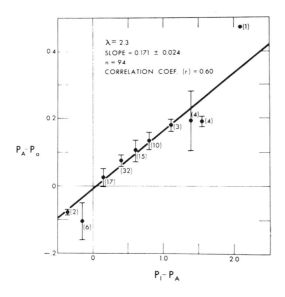

TABLE 17-1. Anesthetic Brain/Blood Partition Coefficient at 37° ± 0.5°C

Anesthetic	Brain/Blood partition coefficient
Nitrous oxide	1.06
Ethylene	1.2
Xenon	
White matter	1.2
Gray matter	0.74
Chloroform	1.0
Diethyl ether	1.14
Fluroxene	1.43
Methoxyflurane	
White matter	2.34
Gray matter	1.7
Halothane	2.6
Enflurane	1.42 (calculated)
Isoflurane	2.5 (calculated)

FIG. 17-4 The relationship between halothane end-tidal (P_A) to arterial (P_a) partial pressure difference and inspired (P_I) to end-tidal difference is depicted. The halothane blood/gas partition coefficient is assumed to equal 2.3. Differences are expressed as a percentage of 1 atm. Data are from 94 sets of samples (i.e., 3×94 values) in 17 young, healthy human volunteers. Values were grouped by 0.25 percent segments of the P_A-P_I difference. Bars indicate standard errors of the mean. The data suggest that there is a 5:1 relationship between P_I-P_A and P_A-P_a; that is, if $P_I = 2$ percent and $P_A = 1$ percent, then $P_a = 0.8$ percent. (Eger EI II, Bahlman SH: Is the end-tidal anesthetic partial pressure an accurate measure of the arterial anesthetic partial pressure? Anesthesiology 35:301, 1971.)

where t is the time to 95 percent blood–brain equilibration in minutes, λ is the anesthetic brain–blood partition coefficient (Table 17-1), CBF is cerebral blood flow (44 ml/100 g tissue/min), and VT is the volume of brain tissue. A lower brain tissue solubility or a greater tissue blood flow, as achieved by hypoventilation or anesthesia itself,[18] will accelerate equilibration.[19,20] Hypoventilation, particularly with relatively insoluble agents, may slightly delay equilibration.[21] In any case, the time to equilibration is probably shorter than that implied above because gray matter (presumably the part of the brain important to the anesthetic process) has a blood flow 1.5 to 2.0 times mean cerebral blood flow.[18]

FACTORS THAT HAVE LITTLE OR NO EFFECT ON MAC

TYPE OF STIMULATION

MAC is unaffected by type of stimulation, provided a supramaximal stimulus is applied.[12]

DURATION OF ANESTHESIA

Gregory et al.[22] and Eger[23] found no difference in MAC in humans for the separate stimuli of two herniorrhaphy incisions performed at different times during the same anesthesia. Halothane MAC in dogs is constant for up to 500 minutes of anesthesia.[12] Yet acute[24] and chronic[25,26] tolerance to N_2O-induced analgesia have been described. Mice can be made tolerant to nitrous oxide with cross-tolerance to cyclopropane and isoflurane.[27,28] These changes in murine anesthetic requirement are generally small, that is, 10 to 20 percent. In addition, the development of acute tolerance is

TABLE 17-2. Anesthetic Potency (MAC) of Various Anesthetics in Different Species (and Classes) of Animals*

Anesthetic	Human	Monkey Java	Monkey Stump-tail	Dog	Horse	Cat	Rabbit	Rat	Mouse	Toad	Newt	Goldfish
Halothane	0.73[a] 0.74[k,l] 0.77[o]	1.15[b]	0.89[c]	0.86[d] 0.87[c,m]	0.88[e]	0.82[f] 1.14[c]	0.82[g]	1.11[h,†] 1.13[n,†] 1.17[p,†]		0.67[l]		0.76[l]
Enflurane	1.68[q]	1.84[b]		2.2[r] 2.06[t]	2.12[s]	1.2[l]						
Isoflurane	1.15[u]	1.28[b]		1.28[v]	1.31[s]	1.63[v]		1.38[h,†]				
Methoxyflurane	0.16[o]			0.23[w] 0.24[m]		0.23[l]		0.27[p,†]		0.22[l]		0.13[l]
Cyclopropane	9.2[o]			15.9[m] 17.5[w] 20.6[d]		19.7[f]		20.5[†]		9.0[l]		
Fluroxene	3.4[x]			6.0[w] 6.57[m]				4.22[y]				
Ethylene	67[a]											
Diethyl ether	1.92[o]			3.04[w] 3.29[m]		2.1[l]		132[y]	3.2[z]	1.64[l]		2.20[l]
Nitrous oxide	105[aa]		200[c]	188[w] 222[c]		255[c]		136[y]	150[bb] 146[cc]	82.2[l]		
Chloroform				0.77[r]					0.78[z]			
Sulfur hexafluoride									530[cc] 540[bb]		193[cc]	0.63[l]
Carbon tetrafluoride				2,600[r]					2,290[cc]			
Xenon	71[dd]								95[bb]			
Argon				119[w]					1,520[bb] 1,640[cc]		1,690[cc]	

[a] Ref. 92; [b] ref. 168; [c] ref. 34; [d] ref. 60; [e] ref. 135; [f] ref. 164; [g] ref. 35; [h] ref. 32; [i] ref. 174; [j] ref. 59; [k] ref. 8; [l] ref. 38; [m] ref. 61; [n] ref. 132; [o] ref. 93; [p] ref. 172; [q] ref. 33; [r] ref. 169; [s] ref. 175; [t] ref. 36; [u] ref. 96; [v] ref. 170; [w] ref. 171; [x] ref. 171; [y] ref. 71; [z] ref. 103; [aa] ref. 2; [bb] ref. 104; [cc] ref. 173; [dd] ref. 99; [ee] ref. 100.

*All values are expressed as a percentage of 1 atm. The observed variance in MAC among species is in part due to variations in the technique used in measuring MAC as well as to some variability in the ages, temperatures, and circadian cycles of the subjects tested. The stimulus used to obtain MAC in humans was either a surgical incision or electrical pulse, and in the dog and horse, either a tail clamp or electrical pulse. Monkeys, cats, rabbits, and rats were tested with a tail clamp. The stimulus in mice and newts was a rotating chamber, and the end point was loss of righting reflex. Toads were stimulated with a clamp to the lower extremity. Goldfish were electrically stimulated. End-tidal anesthetic concentrations were measured in humans, monkey, dog, horse, cat, and rabbit (and in rat where indicated; by †), while in all other subjects, inspired anesthetic concentration was used.

complete after 10 min of anesthesia,[27] while chronic tolerance does not develop for several days.[28]

CIRCADIAN RHYTHMS

MAC varies slightly (±10 percent) in the same animal when measured at different times.[12] Circadian rhythms may play some role in this observed variation.[29-31] MAC increases 10 to 14 percent from the mean during the "dark" phase of circadian cycle in the rat, which is the period of greatest metabolic activity in that species.[31]

INTRASPECIES AND INTERSPECIES VARIATIONS

The standard deviation obtained from analysis of MAC values from several animals of a given species is usually less than 10 percent of the MAC value itself.[12] This variation is only slightly greater than that observed (7 percent) for different determinations in a single animal.[12] Different species or classes of animals (e.g., amphibians versus mammals) do not show large variations in MAC; MAC values for a given anesthetic remain within a twofold range (Table 17-2).[23,32-37]

SEX

Unpublished work from two laboratories indicates that MAC is not different between the sexes in humans or rats.[23] However, MAC in female mice may be slightly higher than MAC in male mice (EI Eger, II, unpublished data).

HYPOCARBIA AND HYPERCARBIA

Reducing $PaCO_2$ from 42 to 14 mm Hg (pH 7.7) does not alter halothane MAC in dogs.[12] Bridges and Eger[38] reported no difference in halothane MAC in humans with normocapnia ($PaCO_2 = 38$ mm Hg) versus hypocapnia ($PaCO_2 = 21$ mm Hg). Extreme hypocapnia ($PaCO_2 = 10$ mm Hg) in dogs does not affect MAC for halothane administered in oxygen but slightly (10 percent) reduces MAC for halothane in air,[39] possibly due to cerebral hypoxia secondary to cerebral vasoconstriction in the presence of a reduced blood–oxygen content and PaO_2. Increasing $PaCO_2$ from 15 to 95 mm Hg (arterial and cerebrospinal fluid pH = 7.6 to 7.10) does not affect halothane MAC in dogs.[40] $PaCO_2$ levels greater than 95 mm Hg associated with arterial and cerebrospinal fluid pH less than 7.10 are, however, increasingly anesthetic[40]; 1.0 MAC anesthesia is produced by a $PaCO_2$ of approximately 245 mm Hg (cerebrospinal fluid pH less than 6.90) (Fig. 17-5). The degree of CO_2 narcosis correlates with cisternal cerebrospinal fluid pH, but not with pHa, $PaCO_2$, or $P_{CSF}CO_2$.

METABOLIC ACIDOSIS

In dogs, intravenous infusion of 60 to 80 mEq of ammonium chloride[12] decreased halothane MAC from 0.90 to 0.73 percent. End-tidal PCO_2 was held constant, while at the same time arterial pH fell from 7.38 to 7.20. This modest change in MAC cannot be attributed to such a small change in pH and may have resulted from the increase in ammonia.[12] Infusion of hydrochloric acid in dogs sufficient to lower pH_a from 7.34 to 6.90 was associated with a decrease in halothane MAC of less than 15 percent.[40] An alternative explanation for the small decrease in MAC following ammonium chloride infusion is that such an infusion may have decreased the sodium concentration in cerebrospinal fluid, which may decrease the magnitude of nerve action potential and thereby decrease MAC (see section on electrolytes).

METABOLIC ALKALOSIS

Eisele et al.[40] determined halothane MAC in dogs and then concomitantly increased $PaCO_2$ and infused 30 mEq/kg of sodium bicar-

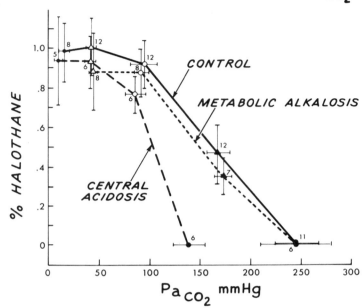

FIG. 17-5 Halothane requirement (MAC) in the dog may be affected by increasing $PaCO_2$. Three groups were studied. All dogs were anesthetized with some combination of carbon dioxide and halothane in oxygen. The control group received no other treatment. The central acidosis group was hyperventilated prior to the experiment for several hours ($PaCO_2 \leq 10$ mm Hg) and received intravenous hydrochloric acid to reduce cerebrospinal fluid bicarbonate from 23 to 13 mEq/L. The metabolic alkalosis group received 30 mEq/kg sodium bicarbonate intravenously. Number of dogs is given beside each point. Note that at a $PaCO_2$ of 245 mm Hg, carbon dioxide becomes "anesthetizing," and that by reducing the cerebrospinal fluid buffer, base $PaCO_2$ becomes "anesthetizing" at 130 mm Hg. In both instances, cerebrospinal fluid pH is about 6.80. Note also the lack of effect of bicarbonate administration (metabolic alkalosis). (Eisele JH, Eger EI II, Muallem M: Narcotic properties of carbon dioxide in the dog. Anesthesiology 28:856, 1967.)

bonate. The infusion of bicarbonate limited the decrease in pH_a, increasing the $PaCO_2$. Because carbon dioxide and not bicarbonate readily crosses the blood–brain barrier, the cerebrospinal fluid pH was far more affected. Not surprisingly the associated changes in MAC associated with changes in cerebrospinal fluid pH were identical to those seen in the absence of bicarbonate infusion.

THYROID FUNCTION

Guedel[41,42] believed that anesthetic requirement correlates with metabolic activity. Although MAC and cerebral oxygen consump-

tion ($CMRO_2$) decrease with increasing age or decreasing body temperature, anesthetic requirement is not proportional to whole-body oxygen consumption (VO_2). Doubling whole-body VO_2 (grossly hypothyroid to hyperthyroid) in dogs was found to cause only a 20 percent increase in halothane MAC.[43] Similarly, Munson et al.[44] were unable to demonstrate a significant effect of hypothyroidism or hyperthyroidism on cyclopropane MAC in rats, despite marked alterations in basal metabolic requirements. Whole-body metabolic changes induced by changes in thyroid function may have less effect on MAC than do age or temperature because $CMRO_2$ is not affected by thyroid function.[44] Neither acute (2 or 10 mg/kg intravenously) nor chronic (10 mg/kg/day orally for 10 days) administration of propranolol or isoproterenol affects halothane MAC in dogs.[45]

MAGNESIUM

In 1906 Meltzer and Auer[46] reported that intravenous administration of magnesium salt in animals produces sedation followed by paralysis and respiratory arrest. Peck and Meltzer[47] proposed in 1916 that magnesium has a definite, albeit limited, role as an adjunct to general anesthesia. Subsequently, however, the anesthetic effect of magnesium was shown to be cerebral hypoxia due to progressive cardiac and respiratory depression.[48] Magnesium-induced peripheral neuromuscular blockade occurs at a lower serum magnesium concentration than does the central sedative effect, and humans remain conscious when skeletal muscle function is depressed.[49,50] Aldrete[51] concluded that although magnesium does depress nerve tissue, the amount of magnesium that crosses the blood–brain barrier is insufficient to produce narcosis.

BROMINE

The production of bromine by halothane biodegradation may result in postoperative sedation.[52,53] Sedation from bromine alone can occur at serum levels of 6 mEq/L, and toxicity may occur at concentrations greater than 10 mEq/L.[52] Increases in serum bromine concentrations (2.4 to 4.2 mEq/L) were found for 9 days following anesthesia in 7 volunteers given 6 MAC-hr of halothane.[52] The findings of Tinker et al.[53] in patients given halothane are in agreement. However, bromine production does not significantly affect halothane MAC. Although the half-life is long (12 to 25 days), the peak serum bromine levels require 2 days to develop.[52,53] Bromine levels at the end of anesthesia average only 0.5 mEq/L.[52]

FACTORS THAT DECREASE MAC

HYPOXIA

The lower limit of PaO_2 in normal humans compatible with consciousness is between 25 and 35 mm Hg.[54] The mechanism by which such severe hypoxia produces narcosis is unknown. Halothane MAC in dogs may not be affected until PaO_2 falls below 30 mm Hg.[12] Cullen et al.[55-57] demonstrated that halothane MAC in dogs was unaffected by a PaO_2 between 38 and 500 mm Hg. Below 38 mm Hg, hypoxia was found to induce progressive narcosis.[55] At a PaO_2 of 38 mm Hg, MAC was still 80 percent of control, whereas a PaO_2 of approximately 28 mm Hg decreased MAC to 40 percent of control. A metabolic acidosis indicating anaerobic metabolism always accompanied this decrease in PaO_2 and MAC.[55] A decrease in oxygen content during normocapnic hypoxia (pHa = 7.29) decreased MAC more than during hypocapnic hypoxia (pHa = 7.39), possibly because the Bohr effect produced a higher oxygen content at the same PaO_2 during hypocapnia. The effects of hypoxic-induced lactic acidosis could not be differentiated from those of decreased oxygen content.[55] This finding differed from the data reported by Eisele et al.[40] for severe metabolic acidosis without hypoxemia. This apparent conflict may be related to the differing effects of endogenously produced metabolic acidosis (secondary to hypoxia) and exogenously administered acidosis (hydrochloric acid infusion). The former would likely reduce cerebrospinal fluid pH whereas the latter would not. However, in a subsequent study, Cullen et al.[56] did not find a consistently quantitative correlation between hypoxia-induced decreases in halothane MAC in dogs and cerebral extracellular fluid PO_2, PCO_2, or pH obtained with cortical surface electrodes, although hypoxia induced major reductions in CSF HCO_3 and cerebral extracellular fluid pH.

ANEMIA

The effect of hypoxia on MAC might be related to a decrease in either PaO_2, arterial

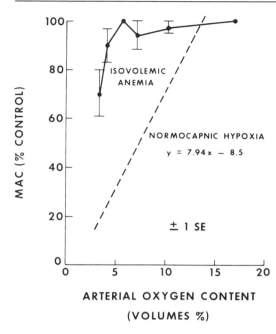

FIG. 17-6 The decrease in MAC with hypoxemia-induced decreasing oxygen content (dashed regression line) in dogs does not occur with anemia-induced decreasing oxygen content (solid line) until the oxygen content is decreased to levels that are nearly fatal. (Cullen DJ, Eger EI II: The effects of hypoxia and isovolemic anemia on the halothane requirement (MAC) of dogs. III. The effects of acute isovolemic anemia. Anesthesiology 32:46, 1970.)

oxygen content, or both. To distinguish between these possibilities, Cullen and Eger[57] measured MAC before and after imposition of graded isovolemic anemia in dogs. Halothane MAC was unchanged until arterial oxygen content decreased below 4.3 ml of oxygen/100 ml of blood. Unlike the hypoxic models, this model showed no evidence of metabolic acidosis (Fig. 17-6).

HYPOTENSION

That hypotension may reduce anesthetic requirement was evaluated by Tanifuji and Eger[58] in three groups of dogs. In the first group,

mean arterial pressure (MAP) was reduced to between 40 and 50 mm Hg. Halothane MAC decreased by 20 percent after the first hour; no further reduction in MAC occurred during the ensuing 3 hours of hypotension. Neither arterial nor cerebrospinal fluid lactate and pyruvate concentrations were affected, and PH_a declined minimally. In the second group, MAP was gradually and successively reduced to 40 to 50 mm Hg, 30 to 40 mm Hg, and 20 to 30 mm Hg. MAC decreased by 30 to 50 percent at the lower two pressure ranges (Fig. 17-7). In the third group, MAP was rapidly decreased to 20 to 30 mm Hg. MAC decreased by 75 to 85 percent, a significantly greater decrease than occurred with the slower three-stage pressure reduction imposed in the second group. MAC returned to control levels (i.e., there was hysteresis) when blood pressure was restored to normal in group I but not in groups II and III (Fig. 17-7). The implication of the hysteresis is that neural function is impaired and not readily reversible by profound hypotension. Perhaps a MAP below 40 to 50 mm Hg should be deliberately sought (i.e., induced hypotension) only in essential situations.

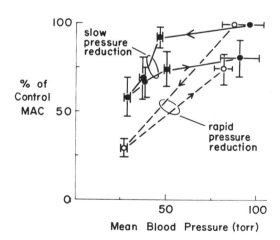

FIG. 17-7 Halothane requirement in dogs is expressed as a percentage of control MAC with a stepwise reduction of mean arterial pressure (filled circles, continuous lines) or an immediate reduction to that same pressure (open circles, dashed lines). Arrows indicate the sequence of pressure changes. The decrease in MAC was significantly greater ($P < 0.05$) with rapidly established hypotension. (Tanifuji Y, Eger EI II: Effect of arterial hypotension on anesthetic requirement in dogs. Br J Anaesth 48:947, 1976.)

HYPOTHERMIA

Hypothermia decreases MAC in a rectilinear fashion.[59-62] The absolute decrease may differ among anesthetics as a function of their lipid solubilities or the change in lipid solubility with temperature. MACs for halothane, methoxyflurane, and isoflurane decrease by about 50 percent when temperature is reduced from 37° to 27°C,[60-62] while the decrease with cyclopropane is only about 20 percent[60,61] for the same temperature change.

LITHIUM

Mannisto and Saarnivaara[63] reported that lithium enhances morphine analgesia in mice. Y Tanifuji and EI Eger II (unpublished data) have found administration of lithium to decrease MAC.

CALCIUM

The anesthetic potency of halothane and cyclopropane in cats varies directly with calcium ion concentrations in cerebrospinal fluid.[64] Very high calcium ion concentrations in cerebrospinal fluid may produce a state resembling general anesthesia.[65]

SODIUM, POTASSIUM, AND OSMOLALITY

Tanifuji and Eger[66] studied the effects of hyperkalemia, hypernatremia, and hyperosmolality and hypo-osmolality on halothane MAC in dogs. Hyperkalemia neither altered the concentration of cerebrospinal fluid potassium nor affected MAC. Hypernatremia proportionally increased the concentration of cerebrospinal fluid sodium and osmolality and increased halothane MAC by 43 percent. Serum hyperosmolality increased cerebrospinal fluid osmolality without consistently al-

tering the concentration of cerebrospinal fluid sodium or MAC. Serum and cerebrospinal fluid hypo-osmolality diluted cerebrospinal fluid sodium and reduced halothane MAC by 24 percent. Thus, changes in serum electrolytes or osmolality appear to alter anesthetic requirement only if associated with changes in brain sodium concentration (Fig. 17-8).

NARCOTICS

Narcotics reduce anesthetic requirement. Seevers et al.[67] reported in 1934 that dogs premedicated with morphine and scopolamine required far less cyclopropane to achieve a given plane of anesthesia. Subsequent investigations in animals[68,69] have confirmed this conclusion. Hoffman and DiFazio[68] demonstrated a log dose-related reduction in cyclopropane requirement for morphine and meperidine in rats. Unlike morphine and meperidine, pentazocine demonstrated a *ceiling effect,* i.e., above 20 mg/kg little additional reduction in anes-

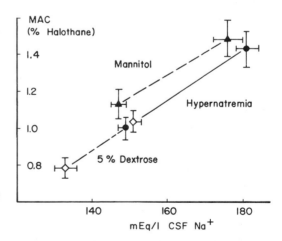

FIG. 17-8 Cerebrospinal fluid sodium concentration was altered by intravenous administration of mannitol, hypertonic saline, or 5 percent dextrose. Halothane requirement (MAC) in dogs increased with increasing cerebrospinal fluid sodium and decreased with decreasing sodium. (Tanifuji Y, Eger EI II: Brain sodium, potassium, and osmolality: Effects on anesthetic requirement. Anesth Analg 57:404, 1978.

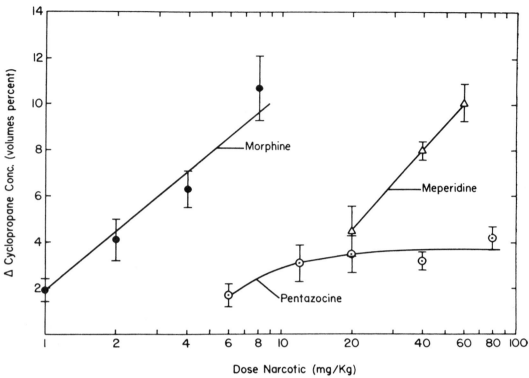

FIG. 17-9 Morphine and meperidine each produce a progressive, log dose-related reduction of cyclopropane requirement in rats. A ceiling effect is demonstrated for pentazocine. Brackets show the standard error of the differences. (Hoffman JC, DiFazio CA: The anesthesia-sparing effect of pentazocine, meperidine, and morphine. Arch Int Pharmacodyn 186:261, 1970.)

thetic requirement occurred (Fig. 17-9). In 1957, Taylor et al.[70] administered 10 mg of morphine intravenously to patients 10 minutes before induction of ether anesthesia: the arterial blood ether concentration necessary to produce a predetermined level of electroencephalographic suppression decreased approximately 15 percent. Numerous clinical studies since 1957 have shown similar results.[8,71–73]

Tolerance to morphine occurs with chronic use, and this tolerance extends to other depressants. Han et al.[69] studied morphine-addicted dogs and found halothane MAC to increase linearly during the course of addiction. Also, morphine was found to have a decreasing effect on halothane MAC as the animals became tolerant. Similarly, rats made tolerant to morphine exhibit a decreased analgesic response to nitrous oxide.[74]

Using a continuous infusion of fentanyl in dogs, enflurane[75] and isoflurane[76] MACs were reduced by fentanyl. As the fentanyl concentration increased, there was less incremental reduction in MAC, until a plateau was reached. MAC was reduced a maximum of 65 to 67 percent despite increasing fentanyl concentrations threefold, indicating a ceiling effect to this concentration–response relationship. Thus, there is little to be gained in terms of depressing somatic responses to noxious stimulation by increasing doses of fentanyl. On the other hand, sufentanil, which is more potent than fentanyl, reduced halothane MAC by 90 percent.[77] Naloxone completely reversed the analgesic and respiratory depression. A plateau or ceiling effect was not observed until nearly complete anesthesia, which is very different from studies with fentanyl.

NALOXONE

Studies in mice and rats suggested that naloxone antagonized both analgesia induced by nitrous oxide[25,78,79] and anesthesia produced by cyclopropane, enflurane, halothane,[80] or barbiturate.[81] However, studies by other investigators failed to confirm a significant effect of naloxone on anesthesia with halothane in rats,[82,83] nitrous oxide in mice,[84] and barbiturates in patients.[85] The importance of these findings lies in the hypothesis that anesthesia might in part be attributable to the release of endogenous morphine-like substances.[78] Therefore, although the analgesic component of general anesthesia might result from release of endogenous morphine-like substances, the failure to demonstrate a significant increase in halothane MAC by the administration of naloxone suggested that the analgesic component is not vital to production of general anesthesia.[86] In contrast, Arndt and Freye[87] found that continuous perfusion of the fourth cerebral ventricle of the dog with naloxone antagonized the hypnotic effects of halothane, as evidenced by reversal of electroencephalographic suppression and by an increase in responsiveness to stimulation.[87] Nitrous-oxide-induced analgesia has been reversed with naloxone in human subjects.[88] These reports are thus conflicting, and the importance of endogenous morphine-like receptors in the maintenance of the analgesic and hypnotic components of general anesthesia remains unsettled.

KETAMINE

Intramuscular injection of ketamine, 50 mg/kg, decreases halothane MAC in rats by 56 percent 1 to 2 hours after injection, and 14 percent after 5 to 6 hours.[89]

SEDATIVES AND TRANQUILIZERS

Nonnarcotic premedicants also decrease anesthetic requirement. Barbital (150 mg/kg) given to dogs 30 minutes prior to anesthesia decreases cyclopropane requirement 49 to 67 percent, while 250 mg/kg decreases anesthetic requirement 66 to 77 percent.[90] Premedication with 30 mg/kg amobarbital decreases the cyclopropane requirement in dogs 42 to 59 percent, while 45 mg/kg causes a 66 to 70 percent reduction.[90] Chlorpromazine, 50 mg given intramuscularly 1 hour before anesthesia, decreased the ether concentration needed to produce a specific level of electroencephalographic suppression in patients by 13 percent while the intravenous administration of pentobarbital 200 mg 10 minutes prior to anesthesia caused a 27 percent reduction.[70] Halothane MAC in humans is only 0.43 to 0.48 percent 15 to 30 minutes after the intravenous administration of diazepam, 0.2 to 0.5 mg/kg.[72,91] Since halothane MAC in unpremedicated patients is approximately 0.75 percent,[8,38,92,93] this represents a significant reduction in anesthetic requirement. The higher dose of diazepam significantly was found to depress ventilation without causing an additional decrease in MAC.[73] Hydroxyzine, 2 mg/kg intravenously, reduced halothane MAC in volunteers by 24 percent (0.95 to 0.72 percent).[72]

Phencyclidine (2 mg/kg) decreased cyclopropane MAC 32 percent.[94] Since naloxone pretreatment failed to alter the effect of PCP on decreasing cyclopropane MAC, an interaction of PCP with opiate mechanisms is unlikely.

CANNABIS

Delta-9-tetrahydrocannabinal, 1.0 and 2.0 mg/kg injected intraperitoneally 2 hours prior to cyclopropane anesthesia in rats, decreases MAC by 12 and 25 percent, respectively.[95]

OTHER INHALATIONAL ANESTHETICS

The effects of combinations of inhaled anesthetics are cumulative[4,8,71,96-99] and generally are additive (Fig. 17-10),[92,100] although some combinations are synergistic[101] or even antagonistic.[102,103] In patients, nitrous oxide lowers the blood concentration of diethyl ether required to produce a given level of electroen-

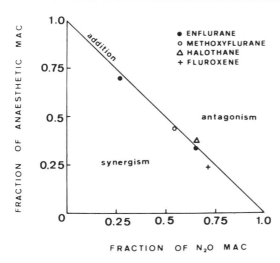

FIG. 17-10 The vertical axis represents the fraction of MAC in patients for four anesthetics. The value 1.0 represents 1 MAC of 1.68 percent enflurane, 0.76 percent halothane, 0.16 percent methoxyflurane, or 3.4 percent fluroxene. The horizontal axis represents MAC fraction of nitrous oxide; in this case, 1 MAC represents 101 percent nitrous oxide. The straight line connecting the 1.0 MAC points represents the line of simple addition. Points falling to the left of the line would represent synergism, while those to the right, antagonism. Note that the values obtained with all four anesthetics fall very near the line of simple addition. (Torri G, Damia G, Fabiani ML: Effect of nitrous oxide on the anesthetic requirement of enflurane. Br J Anaesth 46:468,1974.)

cephalographic suppression.[4] Similarly, 70 percent nitrous oxide decreases halothane MAC by 61 percent[8] and isoflurane MAC by 60 percent.[96] Seventy-seven percent nitrous oxide decreases fluroxene requirement from 3.4 to 0.8 percent, a 76 percent reduction.[71] Sixty percent nitrous oxide decreases methoxyflurane MAC by 56 percent.[97] Enflurane MAC in the presence of 30 percent nitrous oxide is 1.17 percent and is only 0.5 percent when 70 percent nitrous oxide is concomitantly administered.[98] Presuming additivity, these data consistently suggest that MAC for nitrous oxide equals 105 to 110 percent of 1 atmosphere (atm). Under hyperbaric conditions, nitrous oxide MAC in humans is 105 percent of 1 atm, supporting the data obtained by extrapolation.[104]

The combination of halothane plus xenon[100] or halothane plus ethylene[92] also appears to be additive. However, not all inhaled anesthetics may be additive. Low concentrations of nitrous oxide or ethylene plus cyclopropane appear to produce antagonistic effects,[102,103] whereas cyclopropane plus isoflurane are synergistic.[101] Sulfur hexafluoride (SF6) plus nitrous oxide and argon plus nitrous oxide are additive in mice, but argon plus SF6 are less than additive (i.e., exhibit antagonism).[99] These results cannot be explained.

CHOLINESTERASE INHIBITORS

Physostigmine and neostigmine decrease halothane MAC in dogs in a dose-dependent fashion.[105] Physostigmine, unlike neostigmine, transiently (within the first 30 minutes after intravenous injection) increases anesthetic requirement. The clinical significance of these findings is unclear because the effect on MAC was small and the doses used were at least 10 times greater than those used clinically.

LOCAL ANESTHETICS

Local anesthetics have been used systemically to supplement general anesthesia for more than 25 years.[106–108] Lidocaine linearly reduces cyclopropane MAC in rats up to blood lidocaine concentrations of 1.0 $\mu g/ml$.[109] Higher concentrations decrease anesthetic requirement slightly more, with a maximal reduction of 42 percent.[109] In humans, a plasma lidocaine concentration of 3.2 $\mu g/ml$ plus 70 percent nitrous oxide equals 1.0 MAC.[110] In dogs, plasma lidocaine concentrations of less than 1.0 $\mu g/ml$ cause little or no decrease in halothane MAC.[110,111] Higher concentrations decrease MAC; a 45 percent reduction occurs at a lidocaine level of 11.6 $\mu g/ml$.[110] In dogs, lidocaine arterial plasma concentrations of 1.0 to 3.5 $\mu g/ml$ produce dose-related decreases in enflurane MAC of up to 37 percent[111] (Fig. 17-11). These alterations in anesthetic require-

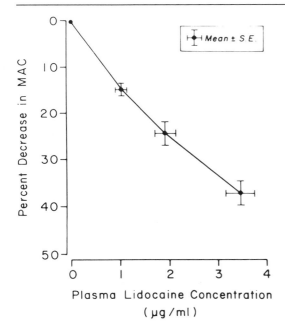

FIG. 17-11 Enflurane MAC in dogs decreases as a function of plasma lidocaine concentration. (Himes RS Jr, Munson ES, Embro WJ: Enflurane requirement and ventilatory response to carbon dioxide during lidocaine infusion in dogs. Anesthesiology 51:131, 1979.)

ment may result from blockade of nociceptive impulses by suppression of spinal cord neurons.[112]

PREGNANCY

Selye[113] was the first to note that steroids such as progesterone exhibit anesthetic activity. Large daily intravenous doses of progesterone can induce sleep in women.[114] Pregnancy in sheep is associated with reductions in MAC of 32 percent for methoxyflurane, 25 percent for halothane, and 40 percent for isoflurane.[115] Plasma progesterone increases 10- to 20-fold during late pregnancy in ewes.[116] Pregnancy in rats also decreases halothane MAC,[117] but the reductions do not correlate with changes in progesterone levels.[118] Thus progesterone changes apparently are not entirely responsible for pregnancy-associated reductions in MAC.

TRANSCUTANEOUS CRANIAL ELECTRICAL STIMULATION

The effect of transcutaneous cranial electrical stimulation (TCES) was studied in 90 patients in whom urologic procedures were about to be performed using a thigh clamp rather than a surgical incision as the stimulus.[119] Compared with nitrous oxide alone, TCES plus N_2O increased analgesic potency by almost 40 percent, or 0.4 atm. Analgesia following the stimulus was also prolonged. However, since the stimulus was not intense enough to cause major cardiovascular or respiratory changes, it is not equivalent to a skin incision, the standard in humans.

PANCURONIUM

Halothane MAC in 18 patients was compared with halothane MAC after intravenous administration of pancuronium 0.1 mg/kg in 17 patients in whom a limb was isolated to prevent the total muscle relaxant effect of pancuronium.[120] Halothane MAC was 25 percent less in patients given pancuronium than in the control group. Perhaps very small quantities of nondepolarizing muscle relaxant crossed the blood–brain barrier to block neural synapses. In addition, patients may be relatively deafferentiated in that there is far less muscle spindle afferent input to the reticular activating system.

VERAPAMIL

Verapamil, 0.5 mg/kg, was infused over 10 minutes to achieve a pharmacologic effect on heart rate (40 percent increase in the P-R interval). MAC decreased 25 percent and there was no clinically significant neuromuscular blockade present.[121] Verapamil is supplied as a racemic mixture of both the D- and L-stereoisomers. The D form has local anesthetic effects blocking the fast sodium channel, while the L form is the slow calcium channel blocker. Hence, the authors postulate that the D-isomer is responsible for reducing MAC. It would be prudent to decrease the halothane concentration in the presence of verapamil, both because MAC is decreased, and to minimize hemodynamic effects.

FACTORS RELATED TO CENTRAL SYMPATHETIC ACTIVITY

Drugs that interfere with central neurotransmitter release may decrease MAC. A dose-related reduction in halothane MAC in dogs has been demonstrated after acute and chronic administration of α-methyldopa and reserpine—drugs that reduce both central and peripheral catecholamines and serotonin.[122] Guanethidine reduces norepinephrine peripherally, but not centrally, and does not affect MAC (Fig. 17-12). Conversely, pretreatment with a monoamine oxidase inhibitor (iproniazid) slightly but significantly increases the cyclopropane requirement in rats.[123] Iproniazid increases intracellular levels of catecholamines and serotonin by interfering with their degradation. Selective blockade of nerve terminals containing catecholamine and serotonin in rat brain slightly decreases halothane requirement. Acute intravenous administration of d-amphetamine in dogs during halothane anesthesia increases MAC up to 96 percent.[124] In contrast, chronic treatment with d-amphetamine decreases halothane MAC by 22 percent.[124] The fact that acute administration of d-amphetamine increases norepinephrine release in central nervous system (CNS) nerve terminals, whereas chronic administration depletes CNS norepinephrine, further supports the hypothesis that increases in the release of CNS catecholamines cause anesthetic requirement to increase.[125] This hypothesis is still further supported by the finding that the increase

in halothane MAC in dogs secondary to acute d-amphetamine administration could be partially blocked by pretreatment with large doses of reserpine or α-methyl-p-tyrosine (an inhibitor of norepinephrine synthesis).[125] Pretreatment with parachlorophenylalanine, a serotonin depleter, did not affect halothane MAC.[125] This result conflicts with an earlier finding in rats by Mueller et al.[123]

Halothane MAC in dogs increases in a dose-dependent fashion following administration of 2 to 4 mg/kg of cocaine.[126] Cocaine inhibits catecholamine reuptake in CNS nerve terminals, thereby increasing extracellular catecholamine concentrations.

Moderate intravenous doses of L-Dopa reduce halothane MAC in dogs.[127] Larger doses (50 mg/kg) transiently increase MAC but reduce it 3 hours later. Chronic pretreatment with L-Dopa does not consistently alter anesthetic requirement.[127] Levodopa is a precursor of CNS dopamine and norepinephrine. The increase in dopamine is greater than that of norepinephrine.[128] Because dopamine is an inhibitory neurotransmitter[129] (as opposed to norepinephrine, which is excitatory), smaller doses of L-Dopa may reduce MAC by increasing central dopamine concentrations, and large doses of L-Dopa may cause central excitement by displacing norepinephrine from the adrenergic neurons.

Both cyclopropane and halothane selectively increase catecholamines[130] and serotonin[131] in discrete areas of rat brain, suggesting that these anesthetics depress neurotransmitter release at highly specific CNS sites. Stereotactic electrolytic destruction of these specific brain sites in rats decreases MAC for both halothane and cyclopropane by up to 35 percent.[132]

HYPERTENSION

More than 25 years ago investigators reported potentiation of chloral-induced and barbiturate-induced CNS depression following administration of large doses of epinephrine.[133,134] Conversely, Westfall[135] had found epinephrine to antagonize pentobarbital anesthesia. The effects of various inotropes and vasopressors on

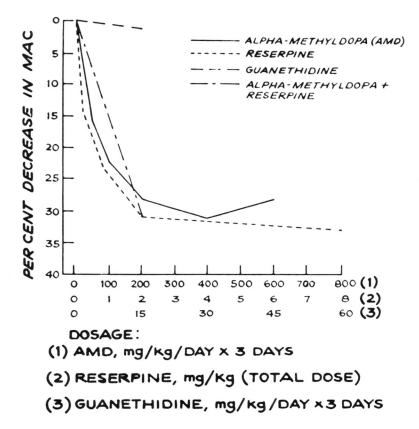

FIG. 17-12 Halothane requirement (MAC) in dogs decreased with α-methyldopa or reserpine alone or in combination. Note that guanethidine, which does not enter the CNS, had no effect on MAC. (Miller RD, Way WL, Eger EI II: The effects of alpha-methyldopa, reserpine, guanethidine, and iproniazid on minimum alveolar anesthetic requirement (MAC). Anesthesiology 29:1153, 1968.)

halothane MAC have been evaluated in dogs.[12,136] Only infusion of ephedrine increased MAC significantly (50 percent), although the increase with mephentermine (21 percent) approached statistical significance. Phenylephrine, metaraminol, methoxamine, norepinephrine, and epinephrine did not alter MAC. MAP was increased 50 to 100 percent in all cases. These results support the hypothesis that anesthetic requirement is increased by release of central catecholamines: ephedrine and mephentermine cause a central release of norepinephrine (ephedrine to a greater degree than mephentermine), whereas metaraminol, phenylephrine, methoxamine, norepinephrine, and epinephrine cause only a peripheral release and, therefore, exert only peripheral ef-

fects in the dose administered. These results also indicate that arterial hypertension per se does not affect MAC.

CLONIDINE

Clonidine is a potent central analgesic in animals that is 10 times more potent than morphine but is not reversed by naloxone. However, naloxone has been said to reverse the antihypertensive effects of clonidine. Since it produces profound sedation when administered acutely, clonidine might modify the anesthetic requirement. Tolazoline, an α-adrenergic antagonist, should reverse any clonidine-induced changes in anesthetic requirement for halothane if the mechanism of action is by α-adrenergic stimulation. In dogs, 5 μg/kg of clonidine decreased halothane MAC maximally 42 percent after 2.3 hours, while clonidine 20 μg/kg reduced halothane MAC 48 percent after 2.6 hours.[137] There was no significant effect on blood pressure during halothane anesthesia. Tolazoline alone did not significantly alter halothane MAC, but it immediately reversed the clonidine-induced decrease in halothane MAC. Bloor and Flacke suggest that clonidine acts on a presynaptic α_2-receptor that inhibits the release of norepinephrine and decreases norepinephrine turnover. Chronic administration of clonidine (50 μg/kg 3 × per day) in rats reduced halothane MAC by only 14.5 percent.[138] Perhaps this demonstrates a rapid development of tolerance in both the sedative and analgesic effects of clonidine.

probit transformation described by Litchfield and Wilcoxon[11] to analyze their data, they concluded that halothane requirement decreases with increasing age, that is, MAC for infants less than 24 months old was 1.18 percent; for children 25 to 48 months old, 1.07 percent; and for adults, 0.94 percent. Hypotension was more frequent at MAC in infants than in adults, implying a smaller cardiovascular margin of safety in the infant group. Stevens et al.[96] determined isoflurane MAC both with and without nitrous oxide in three patient populations grouped by age (Fig. 17-13). Their results agree with those of both Gregory et al.[22] and Nicodemus et al.,[141] that is, isoflurane requirement decreases with age. Addition of 70 percent nitrous oxide decreased isoflurane requirement by 57 to 65 percent regardless of age. Recently, MAC for 12 neonates, 0 to 31 days of age, and for 12 infants, 1 to 6 months of age, were studied because previous reports suggested that infants below the age of 6 months had the highest MAC levels of any age group. Halothane MAC in neo-

FACTORS THAT INCREASE MAC

YOUNG AGE

In 1937, Guedel[41] observed that anesthetic requirement decreases with age. Fifteen years later, Deming[139] demonstrated that infants require higher blood cyclopropane concentrations than adults to achieve a similar level of electroencephalographic suppression. Gregory et al.[22] determined MAC for halothane in eight groups of patients defined by age. MAC was greatest (1.1 percent) in the newborn (0 to 6 months) and smallest 0.64 percent) in the elderly (72 to 91 years). This decrease in anesthetic requirement with age parallels several physiologic variables that also decrease with age, namely, cerebral blood flow, cerebral oxygen consumption, and neuronal density.[22,140] Nicodemus et al.[141] measured MAC in three groups of pediatric patients. Using the log dose-

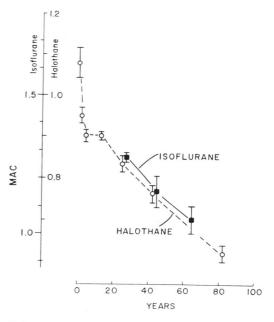

FIG. 17-13 MAC for halothane[22] and isoflurane decreases with increasing age. (Modified from Stevens WC, Dolan WM, Giffons RT, et al: Minimum alveolar concentrations (MAC) of isoflurane with and without nitrous oxide in patients of various ages. Anesthesiology 42:197, 1975.)

nates was only 0.87 percent, significantly less than that of infants whose MAC was 1.2 percent.[142]

peratures greater than 42°C, MAC decreased (Fig. 17-14). Death occurred at a mean temperature of 45°C.

HYPERTHERMIA

Steffey and Eger[143] evaluated the effect of hyperthermia on halothane requirement in dogs. MAC increased linearly 8 percent per degree centigrade (from 37.3° to 40.7°C). At tem-

ALCOHOL

Standard textbooks[144] and clinical reports[145] since 1937 have suggested that alcoholic subjects require larger doses of inhalation anesthetics than do nonalcoholic subjects.

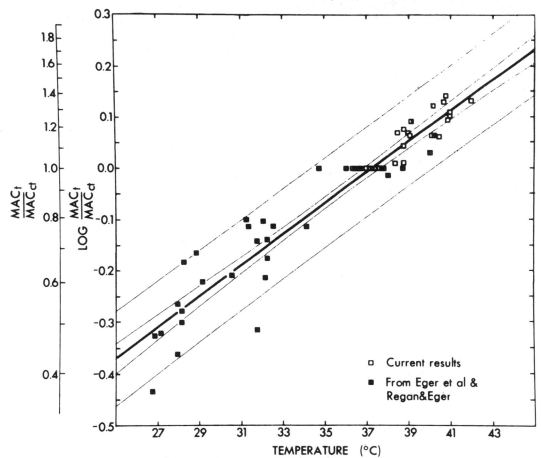

FIG. 17-14 An increase in esophageal temperatures from 26° to 42°C causes a rectilinear increase in halothane MAC in dogs. Hypothermic data are from Eger et al.[60] and Regan and Eger,[61] while hyperthermic data are from Steffey and Eger.[143] MAC values are plotted as fractional changes from normothermic values (control or MAC CT) on logarithmic (right y axis) and arithmetic (left y axis) coordinates. Ninety-five percent confidence limits are shown. (Steffey EP, Eger EI II: Hyperthermia and halothane MAC in the dog. Anesthesiology 41:392, 1974.)

Animal[146-149] and human[150-152] studies have provided qualitative and quantitative evidence that support these clinical impressions. Chronic ingestion of alcohol produces a 30 to 45 percent increase in MAC for isoflurane[148] or halothane.[149-152] As might be expected from its depressant effects, acute administration of alcohol decreases anesthetic requirement.[148,149,153]

MAC AND PHARMACOLOGIC PRINCIPLES

MAC is defined by a quantal dose (concentration)–response curve. As such, it differs from the two other kinds of dose–response curves, namely, graded and ordered.[10,154-156] Graded responses are those that can be measured precisely on a continuous scale, such as body temperature, pulse rate, and intravascular pressure. Ordered responses are qualitative in nature, wherein x is known to be greater than y and y greater than z, but the difference cannot be quantitated, that is, the precise scale is in doubt. Guedel's signs of anesthetic depth are an example of ordered responses. Quantal responses are counts of the number of "yes" or "no" observations, wherein the subject may only respond in one of two ways. Thus, a quantal "dose–response curve" is in fact a cumulative frequency distribution. MAC fits this description.

MAC provides one measure of anesthetic potency. The quantal dose–response relationships that define MAC are not depth-of-anesthesia dose–response curves. MAC represents one point in a presumed continuum of anesthetic depth. Other end points define different levels of anesthetic depth, for example, MAC awake[157] in the sub-MAC range, MAC for endotracheal intubation,[158,159] and MAC-BAR in the supra-MAC range.[160]

Yakaitis et al. showed that halothane[158] and enflurane[159] MAC for successful endotracheal intubation in children appear to be about 30 percent higher than MAC for incision. The log dose–response curve plotting enflurane and halothane is parallel, indicating that in regard to anesthetizing the upper airway, the potency differential between the two agents is fairly uniform (Fig. 17-15). However, the length

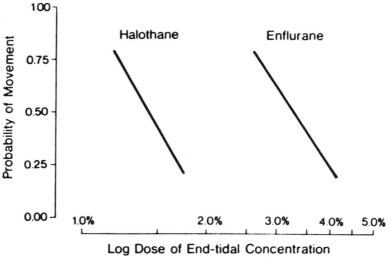

FIG. 17-15 Comparative plots of log dose-response curves for halothane and enflurane. Corrected to barometric conditions at sea level, MAC$_{EI}$ values for halothane and enflurane are 1.33 and 2.93 percent, respectively. (Yakaitis RW, Blitt CD, Angiulo JP: End-tidal enflurane concentration for endotracheal intubation. Anesthesiology 50:59, 1979.)

TABLE 17-3. Five Well-Defined End Points Describing Alveolar Anesthetic Concentration and the Response of the Patient*

Anesthetic	Awake MAC[157] % Alveolar Concentration	% of MAC	MAC[6,9,12] % Alveolar Concentration	% of MAC	ED$_{95}$[9] % Alveolar Concentration	% of MAC	MAC EI$_{50}$[158,159] % of MAC Corrected for Age	MAC-BAR[160] % of MAC Corrected for Age
Halothane	0.41	55	0.74	100	0.90	122	133	145
Methoxyflurane	0.081	51	0.16	100	0.22	138	—	—
Ether	1.41	73	1.92	100	2.22	116	—	—
Fluroxene	2.2	65	3.4	100	3.57	105	—	—
Enflurane	—	—	1.68	100	—	—	139	160
Nitrous oxide†	65–86	59–78	105	100	—	—	—	—

* References given as superscripts.
† El Eger II, personal communication.

of time required to achieve an end-tidal enflurane concentration of 2.9 percent is longer than for halothane because the 4 to 5 percent inspired enflurane concentration that can be administered is proportionally less relative to enflurane MAC than the amount of halothane that can be administered relative to its MAC. Since enflurane produces CNS excitation at 2.5 percent alveolar concentration, which is less than that achieved in these patients, these investigators noted movements in 15 of 17 patients studied with end-tidal enflurane concentrations of 2.9 percent or more. If hyperventilation were used with enflurane to hasten induction of anesthesia, the likelihood of central excitation would be even greater. Presumably, if enflurane were combined with nitrous oxide, the need for higher concentrations would be obviated, but intubation of the trachea would be performed with less than 100 percent oxygen having been given. Therefore, halothane can be used with hyperventilation and with 100 percent oxygen to achieve an end-tidal concentration for endotracheal intubation faster and with more safety. It is therefore more suitable when intubation of the trachea is planned without the use of muscle relaxants.

Roizen et al. determined the MAC-BAR (anesthetic concentration that blocks the adrenergic response) in surgical patients.[160] These doses of anesthetic were all considerably higher than MAC itself, but within the clinical range. In most patients, the adrenergic response could be decreased or completely ablated, resulting in a relatively stress-free state of anesthesia. Prevention of the stress response may be important to myocardial protection. Thus, several responses can be elicited for varying doses of halothane and enflurane that elaborate the MAC concept. If anesthesia is administered simply to render a patient immobile to surgery, then MAC alone defines that goal. If, however, prevention of respiratory reflexes or of adrenergic responses is important, then considerably higher doses of inhaled anesthetic are required and their quantitation has begun. These additional responses generally occur at similar percentages of MAC for various anesthetics (Table 17-3). The constant relationship of MAC to these concentrations associated with the indices of anesthetic depth suggests that the

dose (alveolar concentration)–response (anesthetic depth) curves for different anesthetics are indeed roughly parallel. The importance of such a parallel relationship lies in the fact that a shift of one point (e.g., MAC) may be used to indicate a shift in the whole curve (rather than an alteration in the slope of the curve).[154] Comparisons between anesthetics defined only by MAC also assume greater significance, since the comparisons could also apply equally to other indices of depth.[154]

The use of MAC fractions or MAC multiples for purposes of comparing physiologic side effects of anesthetics (e.g., circulatory depression, respiratory depression, and neuromuscular block) has been generally accepted.[161-166] By determining the concentration required to produce unacceptable circulatory or respiratory depression and by relating those concentrations to MAC, the margin of safety of any anesthetic can be determined.[6,60,167]

SUMMARY

From the discovery of the first anesthetics, the need for measurement of potency was apparent. Early concepts emphasized inspired anesthetic concentration or concentrations in arterial or venous blood. Perhaps the major contribution of MAC was to emphasize alveolar (end-tidal) anesthetic partial pressure, which at equilibrium represents the partial pressure at the anesthetic site of action (the brain). MAC has gained wide acceptance and has become the primary index of anesthetic potency. There are several reasons for this. First, the end point—abolition of movement in response to a surgical incision—is the basic element of clinical anesthesia and as such is of obvious importance to all clinicians. Second, MAC applies equally to all inhaled anesthetics, unlike clinical signs of anesthesia such as pupillary dilatation or respiratory depression, which vary from drug to drug. Third, MAC is remarkably and easily reproducible in the laboratory, making it attractive to those involved in research.

The uses of MAC are many. It permits definition of the therapeutic index of various anesthetics with respect to vital organ depression. MAC may be used to quantitate the effect of age, body temperature, drugs, and other factors on anesthetic requirements, thereby serving as a clinical guide to the delivery of anesthesia. The ultimate clinical criterion remains each patient's unique response to the balance between anesthetic depression and surgical stimulation. Finally, MAC may be used as a tool in research attempting to define the mechanism of anesthesia (also see Ch. 18).

REFERENCES

1. Snow J: On the Inhalation of the Vapour of Ether in Surgical Operations Containing a Description of the Various Stages of Etherization and a Statement of the Result of Nearly Eight Operations in which Ether has been Employed in St. George's and University College Hospitals, London, John Churchill, 1847
2. Robbins BH: Preliminary studies of the anesthetic activity of fluorinated hydrocarbons. J Pharmacol Exp Ther 86:197, 1946
3. Haggard HW: The absorption, distribution, and elimination of ethyl ether. J Biol Chem 59:783, 1924
4. Faulconer A: Correlation of concentrations of ether in arterial blood with electroencephalographic patterns occurring during ether–oxygen and during nitrous oxide, oxygen and ether anesthesia of human surgical patients. Anesthesiology 13:361, 1952
5. Guedel AE: Inhalation Anesthesia: A Fundamental Guide. New York, Macmillan, 1937, pp 14–60
6. Merkel G, Eger EI II: A comparative study of halothane and halopropane anesthesia. Anesthesiology 24:346, 1963
7. Cullen DJ, Eger EI II, Stevens WC, et al: Clinical signs of anesthesia. Anesthesiology 36:21, 1972
8. Saidman LJ, Eger EI II: Effect of nitrous oxide and of narcotic premedication on the alveolar concentration of halothane required for anesthesia. Anesthesiology 25:302, 1964
9. DeJong RH, Eger EI II: MAC expanded: AD_{50} and AD_{95} values of common inhalation anesthetics in man. Anesthesiology 42:384, 1975
10. Waud DR: On biological assays involving quantal responses. J Pharmacol Exp Ther 183:577, 1972
11. Litchfield JT, Wilcoxon F: A simplified method of evaluating dose-effect experiments. J Pharmacol Exp Ther 96:99, 1949
12. Eger EI II, Saidman LJ, Brandstater B: Minimum alveolar anesthetic concentration: A standard of anesthetic potency. Anesthesiology 26:756, 1965
13. Nunn JF: Applied Respiratory Physiology. Second edition. London, Butterworths, 1977, p 214
14. Eger EI II, Babad, AA, Regan MJ, et al: Delayed approach of arterial to alveolar nitrous oxide partial pressures in dog and in man. Anesthesiology 27:288, 1966
15. Eger EI II, Bahlman SH: Is the end-tidal anesthetic partial pressure an accurate measure of the arterial anesthetic partial pressure? Anesthesiology 35:301, 1971
16. Eger EI II, Severinghaus JW: Effect of uneven pulmonary distribution of blood and gas on induction with inhalation anesthetics. Anesthesiology 25:620, 1964
17. Larson CP, Eger EI II, Severinghaus JW: The solubility of halothane in blood and tissue homogenates. Anesthesiology 23:349, 1962
18. Smith AL, Wollman H: Cerebral blood flow and metabolism: Effects of anesthetic drugs and techniques. Anesthesiology 36:378, 1972
19. Eger EI II: Anesthetic Uptake and Action. Baltimore, Williams & Wilkins, 1974, pp 122–123
20. Eger EI II, Larson CP: Anesthetic solubility in blood and tissues: Values and significance. Br J Anaesth 36:140, 1964
21. Munson ES, Bowers DL: Effects of hyperventilation on the rate of cerebral anesthetic equilibration. Anesthesiology 28:377, 1967
22. Gregory GA, Eger EI II, Munson ES: The relationship between age and halothane requirement in man. Anesthesiology 30:488, 1969
23. Eger EI II: Anesthetic Uptake and Action. Baltimore, Williams & Wilkins, 1974, p 5
24. Whitwam JG, Morgan M, Hall GM, et al: Pain during continuous nitrous oxide administration. Br J Anaesth 48:425, 1976
25. Berkowitz BA, Finck AD, Ngai SH: Nitrous oxide analgesia: Reversal by naloxone and development of tolerance. J Pharmacol Exp Ther 203:539, 1977
26. Kripke BJ, Hechtman HB: Nitrous oxide for pen-

tazocine addiction and for intractable pain: Report of case. Anesth Analg 51:520, 1972

27. Smith RA, Winter PM, Smith M, et al: Rapidly developing tolerance to acute exposures to anesthetic agents. Anesthesiology 50:496, 1979

28. Smith RA, Winter PM, Smith M, et al: Tolerance to and dependence on inhalational anesthetics. Anesthesiology 50:505, 1979

29. Matthews JH, Marte E, Halberg F: A circadian susceptibility–resistance cycle to Fluothane in male B$_1$ mice. Can Anaesth Soc J 11:280, 1964

30. Matthews JH, Marte E, Halbert F: Fluothane toxicity in mice studied by indirect periodicity analysis, Toxicity of Anesthetics. Edited by Fink BR. Baltimore, Williams & Wilkins, 1968, pp 197–208

31. Munson ES, Martucci RW, Smith RE: Circadian variations in anesthetic requirement and toxicity in rats. Anesthesiology 32:507, 1970

32. White PF, Johnston RR, Eger EI II: Determination of anesthetic requirement in rats. Anesthesiology 40:52, 1974

33. Gion H, Saidman LJ: The minimum alveolar concentration of enflurane in man. Anesthesiology 35:361, 1971

34. Steffey EP, Gillespie JR, Berry JD, et al: Anesthetic potency (MAC) of nitrous oxide in the dog, cat, and stump-tail monkey. J Appl Physiol 36:530, 1974

35. Davis NL, Nunnally RL, Malinin TI: Determination of the minimum alveolar concentration (MAC) of halothane in the white New Zealand rabbit. Br J Anaesth 47:341, 1975

36. Steffey EP, Howland D: Potency of enflurane in dogs: Comparison with halothane and isoflurane. Am J Vet Res 39:573, 1978

37. Steffey EP: Enflurane and isoflurane anesthesia: A summary of laboratory and clinical investigations in horses. J Am Vet Med Assoc 172:367, 1978

38. Bridges BE, Eger EI II: The effect of hypocapnia on the level of halothane anethesia in man. Anesthesiology 27:634, 1966

39. Cullen DJ, Eger EI II: The effect of extreme hypocapnia on the anesthetic requirement (MAC) of dogs. Br J Anaesth 43:339, 1971

40. Eisele JH, Eger EI II, Muallem M: Narcotic properties of carbon dioxide in the dog. Anesthesiology 28:856, 1967

41. Guedel AE: Inhalation Anesthesia: A Fundamental Guide. New York, Macmillan, 1937, pp 61–62

42. Guedel AE: Metabolism and reflex irritability in anesthesia. JAMA 83:1736, 1924

43. Babad AA, Eger EI II: The effects of hyperthyroidism and hypothyroidism on halothane and oxygen requirements in dogs. Anesthesiology 29:1087, 1968

44. Munson ES, Hoffman JC, DiFazio CA: The effects of acute hypothyroidism and hyperthyroidism on cyclopropane requirement (MAC) in rats. Anesthesiology 29:1094, 1968

45. Tanifuji Y, Eger EI II: Effect of isoproterenol and propranolol on halothane MAC in dogs. Anesth Analg 55:383, 1976

46. Meltzer SJ, Auer J: Physiological and pharmacological studies of magnesium salts. Am J Physiol 15:387, 1906

47. Peck CH, Meltzer SJ: Anesthesia in human beings by intravenous injection of magnesium sulphate. JAMA 67:1131, 1916

48. Aldrete JA, Barnes DR, Aikawa JK: Does magnesium produce anesthesia? Anesth Analg 47:428, 1968

49. Somjen G, Hilmy M. Stephen CR: Failure to anesthetize human subjects by intravenous administration of magnesium sulfate. J Pharmacol Exp Ther 154:652, 1966

50. Hilmy MI, Somjen GG: Distribution and tissue uptake of magnesium related to its pharmacological effects. Am J Physiol 214:406, 1968

51. Aldrete JA: Clinical implications of magnesium therapy. The Anesthesiologist, Mother and Newborn. Edited by Shnider SM, Moya F. Baltimore, Williams & Wilkins, 1974, pp 128–135

52. Johnstone RE, Kennell EM, Behar MG, et al: Increased serum bromide concentration after halothane anesthesia in man. Anesthesiology 42:598, 1975

53. Tinker JH, Gandolfi AJ, Van Dyke RA: Elevation of plasma bromide levels in patients following halothane anesthesia: Time correlation with total halothane dosage. Anesthesiology 44:194, 1976

54. Nunn JF: Applied Respiratory Physiology. Second edition. London, Butterworths, 1977, pp 416–419

55. Cullen DJ, Eger EI II: The effects of hypoxia and isovolemic anemia on the halothane requirement (MAC) of dogs. I. The effect of hypoxia. Anesthesiology 32:28, 1970

56. Cullen DJ, Cotev S, Severinghaus JW, et al: The effects of hypoxia and isovolemic anemia on the halothane requirement (MAC) of dogs. II. The effects of acute hypoxia on halothane requirement and cerebral-surface PO$_2$, PCO$_2$, pH and HCO$_3$. Anesthesiology 32:35, 1970

57. Cullen DJ, Eger EI II: The effects of hypoxia and isovolemic anemia on the halothane requirement (MAC) of dogs. III. The effects of acute isovolemic anemia. Anesthesiology 32:46, 1970

58. Tanifuji Y, Eger EI II: Effect of arterial hypotension on anesthetic requirement in dogs. Br J Anaesth 48:947, 1976

59. Cherkin A, Catchpool JF: Temperature

dependence of anesthesia in goldfish. Science 144:1460, 1964

60. Eger EI II, Saidman LJ, Brandstater B: Temperature dependence of halothane and cyclopropane anesthesia in dogs: Correlation with some theories of anesthetic action. Anesthesiology 26:764, 1965

61. Regan MJ, Eger EI II: Effect of hypothermia in dogs on anesthetizing and apneic doses of inhalation agents. Determination of the anesthetic index (apnea/MAC). Anesthesiology 28:689, 1967

62. Vitez TS, White PF, Eger EI II: Effects of hypothermia on halothane MAC and isoflurane MAC in the rat. Anesthesiology 41:80, 1974

63. Mannisto PT, Saarnivaara L: Effect of lithium and rubidium on the sleeping time caused by various intravenous anesthetics in the mouse. Br J Anaesth 48:185, 1976

64. Johnson ER, Crout JR: Calcium ion concentration in cerebrospinal fluid and anesthetic potency. Abstracts of Scientific Papers, Annual Meeting of the American Society of Anesthesiologists, 1970, p 1

65. Feldberg W, Sherwood SL: Effects of calcium and potassium injected into the cerebral ventricles of the cat. J Physiol (Lond) 139:408, 1957

66. Tanifuji Y, Eger EI II: Brain sodium, potassium, and osmolality: Effects on anesthetic requirement. Anesth Analg 57:404, 1978

67. Seevers MH, Meek WJ, Rovenstine EA, et al: A study of cyclopropane anesthesia with especial reference to gas concentrations, respiratory and electrocardiographic changes. J Pharmacol Exp Ther 51:1, 1934

68. Hoffman JC, DiFazio CA: The anesthesia-sparing effect of pentazocine, meperidine, and morphine. Arch Int Pharmacodyn 186:261, 1970

69. Han YJ, Shiwaku Y, Deery A, et al: Effects of chronic morphine addiction and naloxone on halothane MAC in dogs. Abstracts of Scientific Papers, Annual Meeting of the American Society of Anesthesiologists, 1977, pp 737–738

70. Taylor HE, Doerr JC, Gharib A, et al: Effect of preanesthetic medication on ether content of arterial blood required for surgical anesthesia. Anesthesiology 18:849, 1957

71. Munson ES, Saidman LJ, Eger EI II: Effect of nitrous oxide and morphine on the minimum anesthetic concentration of fluroxene. Anesthesiology 26:134, 1965

72. Tsunoda Y, Hattori Y, Takatsuka E, et al: Effects of hydroxyzine, diazepam, and pentazocine on halothane minimum alveolar anesthetic concentration. Anesth Analg 52:390, 1973

73. Woodruff RE, Bartee RM, Steffenson JL: The effect of fentanyl, droperidol and Innovar[R] on MAC and respiratory depression. Abstracts of

Scientific Papers, Annual Meeting of the American Society of Anesthesiologists, 1977, pp 739–740

74. Berkowitz BA, Finck AD, Hynes MD, et al: Tolerance to nitrous oxide analgesia in rats and mice. Anesthesiology 51:309, 1979

75. Murphy MR, Hug CC Jr: The anesthetic potency of fentanyl in terms of its reduction of enflurane MAC. Anesthesiology 57:485, 1982

76. Murphy MR, Hug CC Jr: Efficacy of fentanyl in reducing isoflurane MAC. Antagonism by naloxone and nalbuphine. Anesthesiology 59:A338, 1983

77. Hecker BR, Lake CL, DiFazio CA, et al: The decrease of the minimum alveolar anesthetic concentration produced by sufentanil in rats. Anesth Analg 62:987, 1983

78. Berkowitz BA, Finck AD, Ngai SH: Nitrous oxide analgesia and its reversal by narcotic antagonists. Pharmacologist 18:177, 1976 (abst)

79. Berkowitz BA, Ngai SH, Finck AD: Nitrous oxide "analgesia." Resemblance to opiate action. Science 194:967, 1976

80. Finck AD, Ngai SH, Berkowitz BA: Antagonism of general anesthesia by naloxone in the rat. Anesthesiology 46:241, 1977

81. Furst Z, Foldes FF, Knoll J: The influence of naloxone on barbiturate anesthesia and toxicity in the rat. Life Sci 20:921, 1977

82. Harper MH, Winter PM, Johnson BH, et al: Naloxone does not antagonize general anesthesia in the rat. Anesthesiology 49:3, 1978

83. Bennett PB: Naloxone fails to antagonize the righting response in rats anesthetized with halothane. Anesthesiology 49:9, 1978

84. Smith RA, Wilson M, Miller KW: Naloxone has no effect on nitrous oxide anesthesia. Anesthesiology 49:6, 1978

85. Duncalf D, Nagashima H, Duncalf RM: Naloxone fails to antagonize thiopental anesthesia. Anesth Analg 57:558, 1978

86. Goldstein A: Enkephalins, opiate receptors, and general anesthesia (editorial). Anesthesiology 49:1, 1978

87. Arndt JO, Freye E: Perfusion of naloxone through the fourth cerebral ventricle reverses the circulatory and hypnotic effects of halothane in dogs. Anesthesiology 51:58, 1979

88. Chapman CR, Benedetti C: Nitrous oxide effects on cerebral evoked potential to pain: Partial reversal with a narcotic antagonist. Anesthesiology 51:135, 1979

89. White PF, Johnston RR, Pudwill CR: Interaction of ketamine and halothane in rats. Anesthesiology 42:179, 1975

90. Robbins BH, Baxter JH Jr, Fitzhugh OG: Studies of cyclopropane. V. The effect of morphine, barbital, and amytal upon the concentration of cy-

clopropane in the blood required for anesthesia and respiratory arrest. J Pharmacol Exp Ther 65:136, 1939

91. Perisho JA, Buechel DR, Miller RD: The effect of diazepam (Valium^R) on minimum alveolar anaesthetic requirement (MAC) in man. Can Anaesth Soc J 18:536, 1971

92. Miller RD, Wahrenbrock EA, Schroeder CF, et al: Ethylene–halothane anesthesia: Addition or synergism? Anesthesiology 31:301, 1969

93. Saidman LJ, Eger EI II, Munson ES, et al: Minimum alveolar concentrations on methoxyflurane, halothane, ether and cyclopropane in man: Correlation with theories of anesthesia. Anesthesiology 28:994, 1967

94. Raja SN, Moscicki JC, Woodside JR Jr, et al: The effect of acute phencyclidine administration on cyclopropane requirement (MAC) in rats. Anesthesiology 56:275, 1982

95. Vitez TS, Way WL, Miller RD, et al: Effects of delta-9-tetrahydrocannabinol on cyclopropane MAC in the rat. Anesthesiology 38:525, 1973

96. Stevens WC, Dolan WM, Gibbons RT, et al: Minimum alveolar concentrations (MAC) of isoflurane with and without nitrous oxide in patients of various ages. Anesthesiology 42:197, 1975

97. Stoelting RK: The effect of nitrous oxide on the minimum alveolar concentration of methoxyflurane needed for anesthesia. Anesthesiology 34:353, 1971

98. Torri G, Damia G, Fabiani ML: Effect of nitrous oxide on the anesthetic requirement of enflurane. Br J Anaesth 46:468, 1974

99. Clarke RF, Daniels S, Harrison CB, et al: Potency of mixtures of general anesthetic agents. Br J Anaesth 50:979, 1978

100. Cullen SC, Eger EI II, Cullen BF, et al: Observations on the anesthetic effect of the combination of xenon and halothane. Anesthesiology 31:305, 1969

101. DiFazio CA, Hurt D, Burney RG, et al: Unusual observations in anesthetic additivity. Abstracts of Scientific Papers, Annual Meeting of the American Society of Anesthesiologists, 1977, pp 619–620

102. DiFazio CA, Brown RE: Additive effects of combined anesthetics. Fed Proc 28:475, 1969 (abst)

103. DiFazio CA, Brown RE, Ball CG, et al: Additive effects of anesthetics and theories of anesthesia. Anesthesiology 36:57, 1972

104. Winter PM, Hornbein TF, Smith G, et al: Hyperbaric nitrous oxide anesthesia in man: Determination of anesthetic potency (MAC) and cardiorespiratory effects. Abstracts of Scientific Papers, Annual Meeting of the American Society of Anesthesiologists, 1972, pp 103–104

105. Horrigan RW: Physostigmine and anesthetic requirement for halothane in dogs. Anesth Analg 47:180, 1978

106. De Clive-Lowe SG, Desmond J, North J: Intravenous lignocaine anaesthesia. Anaesthesia 13:138, 1954

107. Steinhaus JE, Howland DE: Intravenously administered lidocaine as a supplement to nitrous oxide–thiobarbiturate anesthesia. Anesth Analg 37:40, 1958

108. Phillips OC, Lyons WB, Harris LC, et al: Intravenous lidocaine as an adjunct to general anesthesia: A clinical evaluation. Anesth Analg 39:317, 1960

109. DiFazio CA, Niederlehner JR, Burney RG: The anesthetic potency of lidocaine in the rat. Anesth Analg 55:818, 1976

110. Himes RS, DiFazio CA, Burney RG: Effects of lidocaine on the anesthetic requirements for nitrous oxide and halothane. Anesthesiology 47:437, 1977

111. Himes RS Jr, Munson ES, Embro WJ: Enflurane requirement and ventilatory response to carbon dioxide during lidocaine infusion in dogs. Anesthesiology 51:131, 1979

112. Dohi S, Kitahata LM, Toyooka H, et al: An analgesic action of intravenously administered lidocaine on dorsal-horn neurons responding to noxious thermal stimulation. Anesthesiology 51:123, 1979

113. Selye H: Studies concerning the anesthetic action of steroid hormones. J Pharmacol Exp Ther 73:127, 1941

114. Merryman W, Boiman R, Barnes L, et al: Progesterone "anesthesia" in human subjects (correspondence). J Clin Endocrinol Metab 14:1567, 1954

115. Palahniuk RJ, Shnider SM, Eger EI II: Pregnancy decreases the requirement for inhaled anesthetic agents. Anesthesiology 41:82, 1974

116. Stabenfeldt GH, Drost M, Franti CE: Peripheral plasma progesterone levels in the ewe during pregnancy and parturition. Endocrinology 90:144, 1972

117. Strout CD, Nahrwold ML, Wolf JW, et al: Halothane requirement during pregnancy and lactation in rats. Anesthesiology 55:322, 1981

118. Grota LJ, Eik-Nes KB: Plasma progesterone concentrations during pregnancy and lactation in the rat. J Reprod Fertil 13:83, 1967

119. Stanley TH, Cazalaa JA, Limoge A, et al: Transcutaneous cranial electrical stimulation increases the potency of nitrous oxide in humans. Anesthesiology 57:293, 1982

120. Forbes AR, Cohen NH, Eger EI II: Pancuronium reduces halothane requirement in man. Anesth Analg 58:497, 1977

121. Maze M, Mason DM Jr, Kates RE: Verapamil decreases MAC for halothane in dogs. Anesthesiology 59:327, 1983
122. Miller RD, Way WL, Eger EI II: The effects of alpha-methyldopa, reserpine, guanethidine, and iproniazid on minimum alveolar anesthetic requirement (MAC). Anesthesiology 29:1153, 1968
123. Mueller RA, Smith RD, Spruill WA, et al: Central monoaminergic neuronal effects on minimum alveolar concentrations (MAC) of halothane and cyclopropane in rats. Anesthesiology 42:143, 1975
124. Johnston RR, Way WL, Miller RD: Alteration of anesthetic requirement by amphetamine. Anesthesiology 36:357, 1972
125. Johnston RR, Way WL, Miller RD: The effect of CNS catecholamine-depleting drugs on dextroamphetamine-induced evaluation of halothane MAC. Anesthesiology 41:57, 1974
126. Stoelting RK, Creasser CW, Martz RC: Effect of cocaine administration on halothane MAC in dogs. Anesth Analg 54:422, 1975
127. Johnston RR, White PF, Way WL, et al: The effect of levodopa on halothane anesthetic requirements. Anesth Analg 54:178, 1975
128. Everett GM, Borcherding JW: L-dopa: Effect on concentrations of dopamine, norepinephrine, and serotonin in brain of mice. Science 168:849, 1970
129. Hornykiewicz O: Dopamine (3-hydroxytyramine) and brain function. Pharmacol Rev 18:925, 1966
130. Roizen MF, Kopin IJ, Thoa NB, et al: The effect of two anesthetic agents on norepinephrine and dopamine in discrete brain nuclei, fiber tracts and terminal regions of the rat. Brain Res 110:515, 1976
131. Roizen MF, Kopin IJ, Palkovitz M, et al: The effect of two diverse inhalation anesthetic agents on serotonin in discrete regions of the rat brain. Exp Brain Res 24:203, 1975
132. Roizen MF, White PF, Eger EI II, et al: Effects of ablation of serotonin or norepinephrine brainstem areas on halothane and cyclopropane MACs in rats. Anesthesiology 49:252, 1978
133. Lamson PD, Greig ME, Williams L: Potentiation by epinephrine of the anesthetic effect in chloral and barbiturate anesthesia. J Pharmacol Exp Ther 106:219, 1952
134. Milosevic MP: The action of sympathomimetic amines on intravenous anesthesia in rats. Arch Int Pharmacodyn 106:437, 1956
135. Westfall BA: Pyruvic acid antagonism to barbiturate depression. J Pharmacol Exp Ther 87:33, 1946
136. Steffey EP, Eger EI II: The effect of seven vasopressors on halothane MAC in dogs. Br J Anaesth 47:435, 1975
137. Bloor BC, Flacke WE: Reduction in halothane anesthetic requirement by clonidine, an alpha-adrenergic agonist. Anesth Analg 61:741, 1982
138. Kaukinen S, Pyykko K: The potentiation of halothane anesthesia by clonidine. Acta Anaesth Scand 23:107, 1979
139. Deming MN: Agents and techniques for induction of anesthesia in infants and young children. Anesth Analg 31:113, 1952
140. Kety SS: Human cerebral blood flow and oxygen consumption as related to aging. J Chronic Dis 3:478, 1956
141. Nicodemus HF, Nassiri-Rahimi C, Bachman L, et al: Median effective doses (ED_{50}) of halothane in adults and children. Anesthesiology 31:344, 1969
142. Lerman J, Robinson SL, Willis MM, et al: Anesthetic requirements for halothane in young children, 0–1 month and 1–6 months of age. Anesthesiology 59:421, 1983
143. Steffey EP, Eger EI II: Hyperthermia and halothane MAC in the dog. Anesthesiology 41:392, 1974
144. Sollman T: A Manual of Pharmacology and Its Applications to Therapeutics and Toxicology. Philadelphia, WB Saunders, 1937
145. Keilty SR: Anesthesia for the alcoholic patient. Anesth Analg 48:659, 1969
146. Abreu BE, Emerson GA: Susceptibility to ether anesthesia of mice habituated to alcohol, morphine or cocaine. Anesth Analg 18:294, 1939
147. Lee PK, Cho MH, Dobkin AB: Effects of alcoholism, morphinism, and barbiturate resistance on induction and maintenance of general anesthesia. Can Anaesth Soc J 11:354, 1964
148. Johnstone RE, Kulp RA, Smith TC: Effects of acute and chronic ethanol administration on isoflurane requirement in mice. Anesth Analg 54:277, 1975
149. Orkin LR, Chien-Hsu C: Addiction, alcoholism and anesthesia. South Med J 70:1172, 1977
150. Tammisto T, Takki S: Nitrous oxide–oxygen-relaxant anesthesia in alcoholics: A retrospective study. Acta Anaesthesiol Scand (suppl) 53:68, 1973
151. Han YJ: Why do chronic alcoholics require more anesthesia? Anesthesiology 30:341, 1969
152. Barber RE: Anesthetic requirement in alcoholic patients. Abstracts of Scientific Papers, Annual Meeting of the American Society of Anesthesiologists, 1978, pp 623–624
153. Parikh RK: Effect of acute ethanol administration on halothane requirement in rats. Br J Anaesth 48:1126, 1976
154. Waud BE, Waud DR: On dose-response curves

and anesthetics (editorial). Anesthesiology 33:1, 1970

155. Eger EI II: MAC and dose-response curves (correspondence). Anesthesiology 34:202, 1971

156. Waud BE, Waud DR: MAC and dose-dependent curves (correspondence). Anesthesiology 34:203, 1971

157. Stoelting RK, Longnecker DE, Eger EI II: Minimum alveolar concentrations in man on awakening from methoxyflurane, halothane, ether and fluroxene anesthesia: MAC awake. Anesthesiology 33:5, 1970

158. Yakaitis RW, Blitt CD, Angiulo JP: End-tidal halothane concentration for endotracheal intubation. Anesthesiology 47:386, 1977

159. Yakaitis RW, Blitt CD, Angiulo JP: End-tidal enflurane concentration for endotracheal intubation. Anesthesiology 50:59, 1979

160. Roizen MF, Horrigan RW, Frazer BM: Anesthetic doses blocking adrenergic (stress) and cardiovascular responses to incision—MAC-BAR. Anesthesiology 54:390, 1981

161. Munson ES, Larson CP, Babad AA, et al: The effects of halothane, fluroxene and cyclopropane on ventilation: A comparative study in man. Anesthesiology 27:716, 1966

162. Larson CP, Eger EI II, Muallem M, et al: Effects of diethyl ether and methoxyflurane on ventilation. II. A comparative study in man. Anesthesiology 30:174, 1969

163. Eger EI II, Smith NT, Cullen DJ, et al: A comparison of the cardiovascular effects of halothane, fluroxene, ether and cyclopropane in man: A resume. Anesthesiology 34:25, 1971

164. Brown BR, Crout JR: A comparative study of the effects of the five general anesthetics on myocardial contractility. I. Isometric conditions. Anesthesiology 34:236, 1971

165. Merin RG, Kumazawa T, Luka NL: Enflurane depresses myocardial function, perfusion, and metabolism in the dog. Anesthesiology 45:501, 1976

166. Miller RD, Way WL, Dolan WM, et al: Comparative neuromuscular effects of pancuronium, gallamine, and succinylcholine during Forane and halothane anesthesia in man. Anesthesiology 35:509, 1971

167. Wolfson B, Hetrick WD, Lake CL, et al: Anesthetic indices—Further data. Anesthesiology 48:187, 1978

168. Tinker JH, Sharbrough FW, Michenfelder JD: Anterior shift of the dominant EEG rhythm during anesthesia in the Java monkey: Correlation with anesthetic potency. Anesthesiology 46:252, 1977

169. Eger EI II, Lundgren C, Miller SL, et al: Anesthetic potencies of sulfur hexafluoride, carbon tetrafluoride, chloroform and Ethrane in dogs: Correlation with the hydrate and lipid theories of anesthetic action. Anesthesiology 30:129, 1969

170. Steffey EP, Howland D Jr: Isoflurane potency in the dog and cat. Am J Vet Res 38:1833, 1977

171. Eger EI II, Brandstater B, Saidman LJ, et al: Equipotent alveolar concentration of methoxyflurane, halothane, diethyl ether, fluroxene, cyclopropane, xenon and nitrous oxide in the dog. Anesthesiology 26:771, 1965

172. Waizer PR, Baez S, Orkin LR: A method for determining minimum alveolar concentration of anesthetic in the rat. Anesthesiology 39:394, 1973

173. Miller KW, Paton WDM, Smith EB, et al: Physicochemical approaches to the mode of action of general anesthetics. Anesthesiology 36:339, 1972

174. Shim CY, Andersen NB: The effects of oxygen on minimal anesthetic requirements in the toad. Anesthesiology 34:333, 1971

175. Steffey EP, Howland D, Giri S, et al: Enflurane, halothane and isoflurane potency in horses. Am J Vet Res 38:1037, 1977

176. Eger EI II: Uptake, distribution, and elimination of inhaled anesthetics. In: Scientific Foundations of Anethesia. Edited by Scurr C, Feldman S. Philadelphia, FA Davis, 1970, p 342

18

How Do Inhaled Anesthetics Work?

Donald D. Koblin, M.D., Ph.D.
Edmond I. Eger II, M.D.

INTRODUCTION

Although currently popular inhaled anesthetics include nitrous oxide, halothane, isoflurane, and enflurane, a far greater variety of inhaled agents can produce anesthesia (Fig. 18-1). The properties of these anesthetics vary considerably. For example, cyclopropane and ether are no longer widely used because of their explosiveness and flammability. Halothane is nonflammable but possesses a permanent dipole moment, can form hydrogen bonds, and is metabolized by the liver. Xenon, an anesthetic more potent than nitrous oxide in humans,[1] is essentially inert and undergoes no known transformation in the body. The molecular size of inhaled anesthetics may differ by a factor of about 10.

The structural diversity of the inhaled anesthetics suggests that they do not interact directly with a single specific receptor site. However, some correlations of the potencies of anesthetics with their physicochemical properties do suggest a common (unitary) mechanism of general anesthetic action. An example is the striking relationship between anesthetic potency and lipid solubility (see later section on the physicochemical nature of the site of anesthetic action). Although such correlations do not provide a detailed mechanism of anesthesia, they have been helpful in defining the environment in which anesthetics act.

Any molecular hypothesis of anesthesia must explain the effects of anesthetics on the whole organism. For instance, since anesthetic administration can rapidly induce unconsciousness and awakening can quickly occur following the discontinuation of anesthesia, physical or biochemical changes important to the mechanism of anesthesia must occur within seconds. Similarly, physical or biochemical alterations caused by anesthetics are meaningful only at clinical doses and not at high anesthetic levels. High levels may pro-

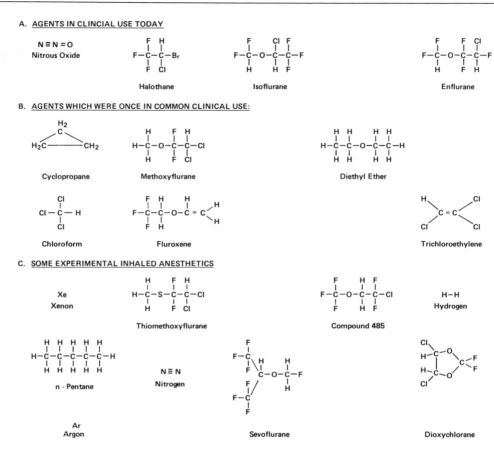

FIG. 18-1 Chemical structures of various inhaled anesthetics. Note that several resonance structures may exist for nitrous oxide.[402]

duce toxic effects unrelated to the mechanism by which inhaled anesthetics act. Furthermore, anesthetic requirement does not change with increasing duration of anesthesia,[2,3] except perhaps for a small hyperacute tolerance that is complete within 10 to 30 minutes of the start of anesthesia.[4] Thus, any physical or biochemical change causally related to anesthesia should be stable for a period of hours or days.

Finally, the mechanism(s) by which inhaled anesthetics act may overlap the mechanism(s) of action of local anesthetics (Ch. 29), of intravenous narcotic (Ch. 23) and nonnarcotic (Ch. 24) anesthetics, and even of alcohols. This chapter considers only the inhaled agents.

MEASUREMENT OF ANESTHETIC POTENCIES

An exploration of the mechanism(s) by which anesthetics act requires a knowledge of relative anesthetic potencies for each of the agents. The best estimate of anesthetic potency is MAC — the minimum alveolar concentration (at 1 atmosphere) of an agent that produces immobility in 50 percent of those subjects exposed to a noxious stimulus (also see Ch. 17).

For determination of MAC in humans, the stimulus is a surgical skin incision. In animals, the noxious stimulus is usually produced by clamping the tail or by passing an electrical current through subcutaneous electrodes. The advantage of measuring the alveolar concentration is that after a short period of equilibration, this concentration directly represents the partial pressure of anesthetic in the central nervous system and is independent of the uptake and distribution of the agent to other tissues.[5] Another advantage of MAC is its consistency for a given animal or species or between different species or classes of animals.[6] This consistency makes it possible to discern small changes in anesthetic requirement that may provide a clue as to how anesthetics act.

The anesthetic concentration that abolishes the righting reflex in 50 percent of the animals is often used to measure anesthetic potencies in smaller animals, that is, it is an anesthetic ED_{50}.[7] Since the inspired rather than the alveolar concentrations are measured, the method applies best to rapidly equilibrating (poorly blood-soluble) agents. Only with equilibration can it be assumed that the partial pressure of the inspired gas equals that at the site of action. The use of small animals and inspired

TABLE 18-1. Ratios of Anesthetic Potencies*

| Anesthetic | (Tail-clamp ED_{50})/ (Righting-Reflex ED_{50}) | |
	Mouse	Rat
Halothane	1.67	1.74
Enflurane	1.91	—
Isoflurane	2.10	2.41
Chloroform	1.61	—
Cyclopropane	1.97	—
Nitrous oxide	>1.82	—
Methoxyflurane	1.63–2.08	—
Diethyl ether	—	1.25

* Values are taken from references 8, 9, and 10.

concentrations facilitates work with agents at very high pressures, (i.e., tens or hundreds of atmospheres). The anesthetic ED_{50} in the mouse, as determined by the rolling response (i.e., the righting reflex), correlates closely with MAC in humans over a 500-fold range in anesthetic requirements (Fig. 18-2).

It must be noted, however, that the tail-clamp ED_{50} (MAC) and the righting-reflex ED_{50} are not identical. The tail-clamp ED_{50} is higher than the righting-reflex ED_{50}, and the ratio of these measurements averages approximately 1.8 (Table 18-1).[8-10] This ratio varies slightly with the anesthetic examined, implying that the righting reflex is depressed, at least in part, by a different mechanism from that which depresses the response to application of a tail clamp.[8,10] Thus, the relative potencies of inhaled anesthetics may depend on the end point measured.

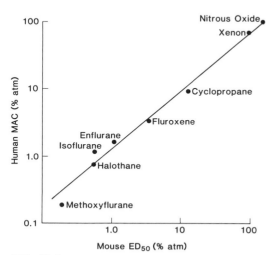

FIG. 18-2 A close correlation exists between the minimum alveolar concentrations (MAC) of various anesthetics preventing a response to surgical incision in humans and the inspired dose of an anesthetic (ED_{50}) required to abolish the righting reflex in the mouse. Values are taken from refs. 6, 9, and 403.

ALTERATIONS IN ANESTHETIC REQUIREMENT PERTINENT TO THEORIES OF NARCOSIS

EFFECTS OF TEMPERATURE

In mammals, MAC decreases with decreasing body temperatures (from 41°C to 26°C) for all anesthetics, but the reduction per degree decrease in body temperature varies from agent to agent.[11-14] The decrease in MAC varies from 2 percent per degree for cyclopropane to 5 percent per degree for halothane. Similar decreases in requirement with decreasing temperature are seen in fish[15] and toads.[16]

EFFECTS OF PRESSURE

The application of increasing hydrostatic pressures progressively increases the anesthetic dose required to bring about unresponsiveness, a phenomenon termed the *pressure reversal of anesthesia*.[17-20] In experiments with mammals, pressure is increased by the addition of helium, since helium does not produce anesthesia.[21] At a total pressure of 100 atmospheres, a 30 to 60 percent increase in the partial pressure of nitrous oxide, isoflurane, argon, or nitrogen is required to abolish the righting reflex.[19,20,22,23]

EFFECTS OF AGE

Older patients are more susceptible to central nervous system (CNS) depression by inhaled anesthetics. In humans, halothane MAC is maximal in infants 1 to 6 months of age, with a value of 1.20 percent atm,[24] and decreases to 0.64 percent atm in patients with a mean age of 81 years.[25] In mice, the righting-reflex ED_{50} for nitrous oxide progressively decreases with age from 1.48 to 1.09 atm.[26] Comparison of mice and humans over similar life-spans shows the decrease in anesthetic requirement of mice to parallel that clinically seen in humans (Fig. 18-3). These effects of pressure, temperature, and aging may be used to test the various models of general anesthetic action.

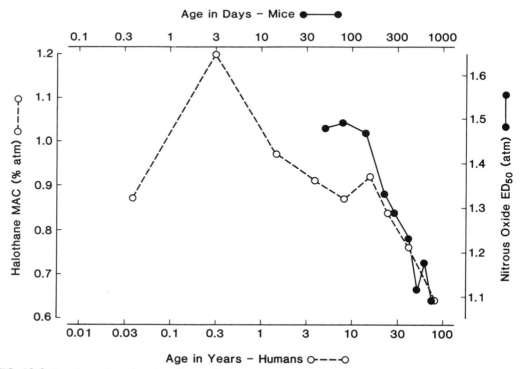

FIG. 18-3 Age-dependent alterations in anesthetic requirement in humans and mice over similar life-spans. Data for halothane in humans are taken from refs. 24 and 25. Data for nitrous oxide in mice are from ref. 26.

EFFECTS OF SODIUM CONCENTRATION

Hypernatremia increases sodium proportionately in cerebrospinal fluid and increases halothane MAC in dogs by as much as 43 percent.[27] Conversely, hyponatremia dilutes cerebrospinal fluid sodium and reduces halothane MAC.[27] These results may be pertinent to theories of anesthetic action at the opiate receptor, since alterations in sodium concentration can affect the binding properties of opiate receptors.[28]

ACTION OF INHALED ANESTHETICS IN THE CENTRAL NERVOUS SYSTEM

BRAIN

General anesthetics may act by altering neuronal activity in selected regions of the central nervous system. Since the brainstem reticular formation plays a role in altering the state of consciousness and alertness and in regulating motor activity,[29] this structure is thought to be an important site of anesthetic action. An initial study by French et al.[30] found that ether blocked conduction of auditory-evoked potentials in the ascending reticular activating system. Later experiments confirmed the reversible disruption of the midbrain reticular system with anesthetizing concentrations of various inhaled agents.[31-34] However, other studies showed that the effect of anesthesia on evoked and spontaneous nervous activity in the reticular formation is variable and that it can be increased, unchanged, or decreased, depending on the agent and the neuronal unit examined.[32,35-39] These experiments suggest that the anesthetic-induced disruption of nervous activity in the reticular formation depends on the specific interaction of a general

anesthetic with specific structures within each neuronal unit. Moreover, consciousness cannot simply be equated with activity in the reticular formation, since gross lesions in the reticular formation can completely abolish the arousal reaction of the electroencephalogram while animals remain behaviorally awake.[40]

General anesthetics interrupt transmission in the central nervous system at sites other than the reticular formation. Anesthetizing doses of inhaled agents depress excitatory transmission in the cerebral cortex,[41,42] olfactory cortex,[43] and hippocampus.[44] General anesthetics reduce the sensitivity of neurons in several brain regions to iontophoretically applied putative neurotransmitters. The excitatory effects of iontophoretically applied acetylcholine are depressed by ether in the caudate nucleus[45] and by halothane, but not by methoxyflurane, in single cortical neurons.[46] Ether and methoxyflurane depress the excitatory effects of L-glutamate applied to olfactory cortex neurons.[47] In addition to blocking excitatory effects, halothane prolongs the γ-aminobutyric acid(GABA)-induced inhibition of mitral cells in the olfactory cortex[48] and increases the duration of inhibitory postsynaptic currents in the olfactory cortex by two- to threefold.[49] Inhaled agents may also enhance excitation. Acetylcholine-induced firing in the olfactory cortex is augmented by ether, methoxyflurane, and halothane.[50] Halothane may potentiate the efficiency of synaptic transmission through the cuneate nucleus,[51] although others have found depression[52] or little alteration[34] of activity of cuneate neurons with inhaled anesthetics.

SPINAL CORD

Transmission through the spinal cord is markedly depressed by general anesthetics. The monosynaptic excitatory postsynaptic potentials recorded in the ventral root are blocked by ether, halothane, cyclopropane, chloroform, methoxyflurane, trichloroethylene, and nitrous oxide.[53-56] The effect may be on specific laminae of the spinal cord.[55,57] Wide dynamic range neurons in the dorsal horn are mainly associated with lamina V and exhibit, with halothane, a dose-dependent decrease in spontaneous and evoked discharge frequencies in the spinal cord-transected cat.[58] In addition to a direct action on spinal neurons, inhaled agents may depress activity by activating the descending inhibition system from the brain.[59] Blockade of spinal cord transmission may also occur through enhanced presynaptic inhibition.[60]

SUMMARY

Thus, inhaled anesthetics interrupt transmission in many areas of the central nervous system, and anesthesia may not selectively influence one specific region. Although the most common action of anesthetics is to depress excitatory transmission, instances are known in which clinical concentrations of anesthetics have essentially no effect, prolong inhibitory transmission, or even potentiate excitatory transmission. Considering the complexity of the human brain, which consists of approximately 20 billion neurons, each having thousands of synapses,[61] the variable nature of the effects of general anesthetics is not surprising. Attempts to reduce this complexity and to increase our understanding of general anesthetic action have led to experiments on isolated neuronal preparations.

INTERRUPTION OF NEURONAL TRANSMISSION BY INHALED ANESTHETICS

AXONAL VERSUS SYNAPTIC TRANSMISSION

Anesthetizing concentrations of inhaled agents block synaptic transmission but have a comparatively smaller effect on peripheral receptors or axonal transmission. The concentration of ether or chloroform that reduces the amplitude of the action potential in sympathetic nerve axons by one-half is three to five times the concentration that reduces synaptic transmission by one-half.[62] Anesthetizing concentrations of ether, halothane, and methoxyflurane do not alter compound action potentials recorded from the saphenous branch of the femoral nerve, nor do these concentrations alter cutaneous receptor responses to touch or to movement of hair.[63] Anesthetic concentrations close to 1.0 MAC do not alter either the compound action potential of lateral olfactory tract fibers[43] or the electrical excitability of afferent fibers to the hippocampus.[44] Such concentrations do produce a 50 to 100 percent blockade of postsynaptic potentials. In these areas of the brain, compound action potentials in presynaptic fibers are little affected until concentrations of 2.0 MAC are obtained. At halothane concentrations of 0.75 to 1.5 percent atmospheres, there is a marked depression in synaptic transmission through the stellate ganglion, whereas axonal transmission is essentially unaltered.[64] These findings are consistent with the idea that general anesthetics selectively block synaptic transmission in the central nervous system.

Nevertheless, at near-clinical concentrations, inhaled anesthetics partially block transmission through axons of vertebrates[65-67] and invertebrates.[68-72] By decreasing the amplitude or duration of the membrane depolarization above threshold, even partial blockade by anesthetics can markedly alter the amount of transmitter secreted[73] and thereby influence synaptic transmission. That is, an apparent effect at the synapse may simply reflect depression of axonal transmission.

The diameter of an axon may influence its susceptibility to anesthetics.[74] For local anesthetics, it has been traditionally taught (and is now disputed) that small nerve fibers are blocked at lower concentrations than are large nerve fibers. For inhaled agents, only one careful study has related diameter of the axon to anesthetic potency. In the squid axon, the effect of n-hexane, n-heptane, and n-octane on the rate of action potential decline was found to be inversely proportional to the square of axon diameter.[75]

The frequency at which axons transmit impulses may also alter anesthetic potency. At impulse frequencies of 0.1 to 10 cps (Hz), a given concentration of a volatile anesthetic produces a constant level of action potential block.[76,77] However, at frequencies above 10 Hz, conduction block by halothane, methoxyflurane, and diethyl ether progressively increases, that is, it is use-dependent.[77]

Moreover, the branch points of axons exhibit a further increase in sensitivity to high-frequency conduction block.[78] This increased sensitivity may play a role in the mechanism of anesthesia, since even in the absence of frank conduction block, partial or complete block can exist at axonal branches.[78]

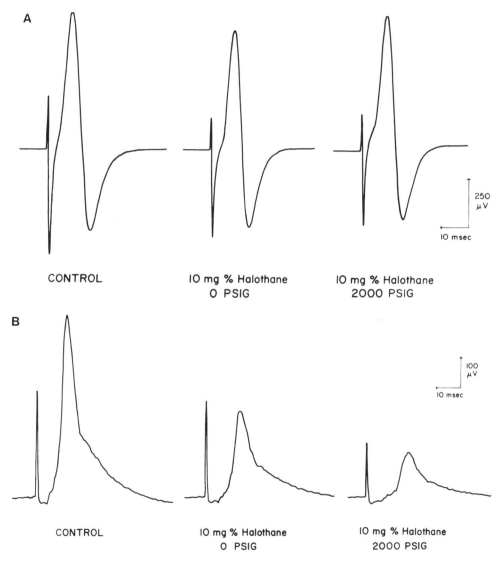

FIG. 18-4 (A) Halothane reduces the amplitude of the action potential measured in the preganglionic nerve from the superior cervical ganglion of the rat. The effect is reversed by the application of 2,000 psig (136 atm). (B) Recordings of the postganglionic action potential show that halothane depresses synaptic transmission, and that high pressures add to this effect. (Kendig JJ, Trudell JR, Cohen EN: Effects of pressure and anesthetics on conduction and synaptic transmisson. J Pharmacol Exp Ther 195:216, 1975. © 1975 The Williams & Wilkins Co., Baltimore.)

Conversely, anesthetics change the frequency pattern of firing activity in isolated neurons. This alteration in frequency of neuronal activity occurs both in autoactive neurons[79] and in neurons responding to external stimuli.[80,81]

Since high pressures antagonize anesthesia in the intact animal, the effects of pressure on axonal conduction and synaptic transmission in the presence of anesthetics may provide a clue to the cellular site of anesthetic action. Compression of the isolated superior cervical ganglion of the rat by pressures of approximately 100 atmospheres reverses the depression of the compound action potential amplitudes in rat preganglionic sympathetic nerves treated with halothane or methoxyflurane at concentrations greater than 1.0 MAC[82] (Fig. 18-4A). By contrast, pressure alone depresses synaptic transmission[83] and adds to the depressant effects of anesthetics[82] (Fig. 18-4B). Similarly, pressure at least partially reverses the effects of gaseous agents on action potentials in single axons.[65,84,85] These results in isolated model systems imply that conduction block is a possible mechanism of anesthesia, rather than blockade of excitatory synaptic transmission. This inference assumes, however, that pressure produces its antagonism by acting at the same site at which the anesthetics produce their effect—an assumption that may be in error (see later section on volume expansion by inhaled anesthetics).

SYNAPSES

Anesthetics may disrupt normal synaptic transmission by interfering with the release of neurotransmitter from the presynaptic nerve terminals into the synaptic cleft, by altering the binding of neurotransmitter to receptor sites on the postsynaptic membrane, or by influencing the ionic conductance change that follows activation of the postsynaptic receptor by neurotransmitter.[86]

PRESYNAPTIC ACTION

Intracellular recordings from lumbosacral motor neurons suggest a presynaptic site of diethyl ether action.[56] Ether decreases monosynaptic excitatory postsynaptic potentials evoked by impulses in single Ia afferent fibers but does not affect the postsynaptic potential change produced by one transmitter quantum.[56] These findings imply that ether presynaptically depresses excitatory transmitter release without altering the chemosensitivity of the postsynaptic membrane. Ether may decrease the number of synaptic vesicles attached to the presynaptic membrane.[87,88]

Halothane decreases the release of norepinephrine from the guinea pig vas deferens secondary to hypogastric nerve stimulation.[89] Similarly, halothane depresses the electrically stimulated, but not the norepinephrine-induced, contractile response of the saphenous vein of the dog.[90] Halothane also inhibits norepinephrine output evoked by activation of sympathetic nerve terminals in the heart[91] and in the adrenal medulla.[92,93] Cyclopropane inhibits agonist-induced release of catecholamines from the adrenal medulla but has no effect on spontaneous release.[94] The decrease in catecholamine output from the adrenal medulla caused by inhaled anesthetics may be related to decreased uptake of catecholamines into chromaffin granules, disruption of chromaffin granules,[95] or inhibition of exocytosis.[93] In rat brain striatal slices, halothane decreases the release of dopamine following the application of a nicotinic agonist.[96] These alterations in catecholamine release imply a presynaptic effect.

Inhaled anesthetics also decrease acetylcholine release from the brain,[97] but whether this results from a direct presynaptic action or a general decrease in activity is unknown. By contrast, inhaled agents may also promote the release of transmitters from certain CNS sites; halothane increases the release of GABA in the dorsal raphe nucleus of the cat.[98] In the isolated guinea pig ileum preparation, ether and chloroform decrease acetylcholine output at all rates of stimulation,[99] whereas the gaseous anesthetics increase both spontaneous and electrically evoked release of acetylcholine.[100,101]

These increases in acetylcholine output are not reversed by adding helium to a total pressure of 136 atmospheres (Fig. 18-5), a pressure that reverses their anesthetic effect in vivo.

POSTSYNAPTIC ACTION

Evidence is also available for postsynaptic effects of anesthetics in certain preparations. Postsynaptic sites of anesthetic action may be studied by iontophoretic application of putative neurotransmitters thought to act directly on postsynaptic membrane receptors. Concentrations of methoxyflurane and ether, but not halothane, that depress synaptic transmission in the olfactory cortex also depress the sensitivity of the cortical neurons to L-glutamate.[47] Halothane does, however, depress the excitatory response of dorsal horn neurons to glutamate.[55]

An opposite yet still postsynaptic effect on cortical neurons is produced by these same volatile agents; that is, the anesthetics augment, in a dose-related fashion, the cortical neuron firing induced by iontophoretic application of acetylcholine.[50] A postsynaptic anesthetic action may be implied by the ability of halothane to block discharges elicited by the application of a nicotinic agonist to the hamster stellate ganglion, although halothane does not block the discharges elicited by a muscarinic agonist.[102] General anesthetics can alter the postsynaptic response at the neuromuscular junction. The ability of volatile anesthetics to depress the carbachol-induced depolarization at the end-plate region of the guinea pig lumbrical muscles closely correlates with their anesthetic potencies in humans.[103] At the neuromuscular junction, a spontaneously secreted quantum of acetylcholine generates a miniature end-plate current (MEPC) and a miniature end-plate potential (MEPP). Volatile agents decrease the amplitude of MEPPs and inhibit the suxamethonium-induced depolarization of muscle end-plate.[104] The rate of the MEPC decay is increased by halothane, enflurane, ether, and chloroform[105,106] (Fig. 18-6). The time constant of the MEPC decay and its amplitude are essentially determined by the number of ions and the amount of charge transferred across the postsynaptic membrane. The increase in channel closing rate caused by the volatile agents[107,108] decreases the amplitude of the postsynaptic response (the MEPP), thereby depressing synaptic transmission (Fig. 18-6). In sum, inhaled anesthetics appear to depress the postsynaptic response to some (but not all) neurotransmitters and may alter the decay of the postsynaptic response.

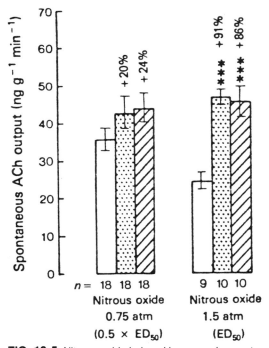

FIG. 18-5 Nitrous oxide-induced increases in spontaneous acetylcholine (ACh) output from guinea pig ileum are not reversed by the application of high pressures. Open columns = controls; stipled columns = effects of nitrous oxide; hatched columns = effects of nitrous oxide plus helium to pressures of 136 atm. Mean values are shown ±SE. Gaseous agents also increase the electrically evoked acetylcholine output. (Halliday DJX, Little HJ, Paton WDM: The effects of inert gases and other general anesthetics on the release of acetylcholine from the guniea pig ileum. Br J Pharmacol 67:229, 1979.)

MONOSYNAPTIC VERSUS POLYSYNAPTIC PATHWAYS

If anesthetics act by blocking synaptic transmission, it might be assumed that polysynaptic pathways would be more susceptible

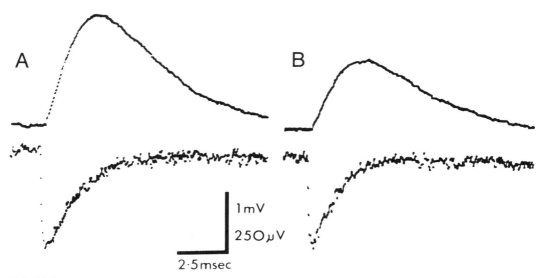

1mV

250µV

2·5msec

FIG. 18-6 Halothane (1 mM) reduces the amplitude of miniature end-plate potentials (upper traces) by reducing the time constant of decay of miniature end-plate currents (lower traces). Records are shown in control solution (A) and in 1 mM halothane (B). (Gage PW, Hamill OP: Effects of several inhalation anesthetics on the kinetics of postsynaptic conductance changes in mouse diaphragm. Br J Pharmacol 57:263, 1976.)

to anesthetic blockade than monosynaptic pathways, as the probability of blockade could increase with the number of synaptic connections.[109] However, inhaled agents depress equally monosynaptic and polysynaptic responses recorded from the ventral root of the spinal cord[53,56] and may even depress the monosynaptic reflex to a greater extent.[110] Thus, the safety factor for transmission during anesthesia along a chain of neurons does not seem to be a function of synaptic chain length. This finding may be owing to the variable sensitivities of different synapses to anesthetics, or to a combination of the depressing effects of anesthetics on excitatory and inhibitory pathways. In addition, the output of a given neuron depends on its input from hundreds or thousands of other neurons, and anesthetics could disrupt normal synaptic transmission by altering the summation of the potential changes produced by these converging inputs. Thus, a single synapse in effect may act as a polysynaptic pathway.

NEUROTRANSMITTERS

Anesthetics do not affect synaptic transmission by depleting neurotransmitters. Neither halothane nor enflurane alters acetylcholine concentrations in the brain.[111] However, these agents do decrease acetylcholine turnover rate, and the magnitude of this decrease varies with the region of the brain examined.[111] Ether also reduces the turnover rate of acetylcholine.[112] This decrease in turnover rate by volatile agents may result from an inhibition of acetylcholine release or simply from a decrease in activity. For nitrous oxide, brain acetylcholine levels and turnover rate have been reported not to change[112] and acetylcholine synthesis has been found to decrease.[113]

Halothane and cyclopropane do not alter norepinephrine or dopamine in most brain regions but may increase norepinephrine content in the nucleus accumbens, locus ceruleus, and central gray catecholamine areas.[114] Whole brain levels of serotonin and dopamine increase during enflurane anesthesia,[115] and discrete brain regions have increased serotonin levels after halothane or cyclopropane anesthesia.[116] Halothane and ether promote an increase in dopamine metabolism in several brain regions.[117]

Halothane treatment of rat cerebral cortex slices inhibits the catabolism and increases the content of the inhibitory transmitter GABA but does not affect the uptake or release of GABA.[118] If this accumulation of GABA in inhibitory neurons were associated with an increase in inhibitory activity, the resulting decrease in synaptic transmission could give rise to the anesthetic state (the GABA theory of anesthesia).[119] However, halothane does not cause an increase in GABA levels in all cellular systems.[120]

Although anesthesia does not deplete brain neurotransmitters, a change in neurotransmitter availability significantly influences anesthetic requirement. Drugs that decrease central levels of norepinephrine and dopamine result in a dose-related decrease in halothane MAC,[16,121–124] whereas agents that elevate central norepinephrine levels increase anesthetic requirement.[121,122,125] Clonidine, an α-adrenergic agonist that probably reduces release of norepinephrine by activating the inhibitory presynaptic receptors, can reduce halothane MAC by almost 50 percent.[126,127] The ablation of certain norepinephrine-rich and serotonin-rich brainstem areas produces a lower MAC value in rats than in sham-operated littermate controls.[128] However, since gross depletions in central monoamine levels cause at most a 35 percent reduction in MAC, other factors besides central monoamine levels must be the primary determinants of anesthetic requirement.

In summary, inhaled anesthetics probably act on synaptic regions, including small-diameter afferent axons at the nerve terminal. General anesthetics depress synaptic transmission in isolated neuronal systems and may have both pre- and postsynaptic effects. Clinical concentrations of inhaled agents can depress, leave unchanged, or enhance presynaptic transmitter release and postsynaptic membrane excitation. The effect depends on the preparation, the particular neurotransmitter, and the anesthetic examined. Furthermore, since high pressure further depresses synaptic transmission, synaptic regions may not be the site of pressure-anesthetic antagonism. Anesthetizing concentrations of inhaled agents have little or no effect on peripheral receptors or transmission in large axons, but partially block conduction in small-diameter axons. This partial conduction block is antagonized by high pressure.

PHYSICOCHEMICAL NATURE OF THE SITE OF ANESTHETIC ACTION

The preceding sections suggested that anesthetics may act at several gross (e.g., spinal cord versus reticular activating system) or microscopic (e.g., presynaptic versus postsynaptic) sites to produce the anesthetic state. The varied nature of these sites, however, does not preclude a unique action at a molecular level. For instance, depression of presynaptic transmitter release and blockade of current flow through the postsynaptic membrane may arise from an anesthetic perturbation at an identical molecular site, even though the geographic locations of these sites differ. The thought that all inhaled anesthetics have a common mode of action on a specific molecular structure is called the unitary theory of narcosis. The nature of this presumed common site has been explored by correlating the physical properties of anesthetics with their potencies. The rationale behind this approach is that the best correlation between anesthetic potency and a physical property will suggest the nature of the anesthetic site of action. For example, the correlation of MAC and lipid solubility indicates that the site of action is hydrophobic. Note that the correlations that depend on forces exerted between anesthetic molecules (e.g., the boiling point of an anesthetic) are not important to the study of anesthetic mechanisms, as such inter-

TABLE 18-2. Oil/Gas Partition Coefficients and Potencies of Inhaled Anesthetics in Dogs, Humans, and Mice*

Anesthetic	Oil/Gas Partition Coefficient (37°C)	Dogs MAC (atm)	Dogs MAC × Oil/Gas (atm)	Humans MAC (atm)	Humans MAC × Oil/Gas (atm)	Mice Righting-Reflex ED50 (atm)	Mice Righting-Reflex ED50 × Oil/Gas (atm)
Thiomethoxyflurane	7,230[a]	0.00035[a]	2.53				
Methoxyflurane	970[b]	0.0023[c]	2.23	0.0016[d]	1.55	0.0023[e]	2.23
Dioxychlorane	1,286[f]	0.0011[f]	1.41			0.0033[g]	4.24
Chloroform	265[b]	0.0077[h]	2.08			0.00357[i]	0.95
Halothane	224[b]	0.0087[c]	1.95	0.0074[d]	1.66	0.00645[i]	1.45
Enflurane	96.5[j]	0.0267[l]	2.58	0.0168[d]	1.62	0.0123[i]	1.19
Isoflurane	90.8[j]	0.0141[l]	1.28	0.0115[d]	1.04	0.00663[i]	0.60
Compound 485[j]	25.8[j]	0.125[l]	3.23				
Hoechst compound[j] ($HFClCOCHFCF_3$)	96.6[j]	0.0224[j]	2.16				
Iso-Indoklon	27.0[k]	0.0460[k]	1.24			0.0265[k]	0.72
Aliflurane	124[l]	0.0184[l]	2.28				
Ether	65[b]	0.0304[c]	1.98	0.0192[d]	1.25	0.032[d]	2.08
Fluroxene	47.7[b]	0.0599[c]	2.86	0.034[d]	1.62	0.0345[m]	1.65
Cyclopropane	11.8[b]	0.175[c]	2.06	0.092[d]	1.09	0.142[i]	1.68
Xenon	1.9[b]	1.19[c]	2.26	0.71[d]	1.35	0.95[n]	1.80
Ethylene	1.26[b]			0.67[o]	0.84	1.30[m]	1.64
Nitrous oxide	1.4[b*]	1.88[c]	2.63	1.04[o]	1.46	1.54[i]	2.16
Krypton	0.5[b]					4.5[i]	2.25
Sulfur hexafluoride	0.293[b]	4.9[h]	1.44			5.4[i]	1.58
Argon	0.15[b]					15.2[n]	2.28
Hexafluoroethane	0.126[b]					17.7[n]	2.23
Carbon tetrafluoride	0.073[b]	26[h]	1.90			18.7[p]	1.36
Nitrogen	0.072[b]	>43.5[h]				34.3[p]	2.47
Mean ± SE			2.12 ± 0.13		1.35 ± 0.09		1.82 ± 0.18

[a] Ref. 404; [b] ref. 19; [c] ref. 406; [d] ref. 409; [e] ref. 6; [f] ref. 9; [g] ref. 405; [h] ref. 134; [i] ref. 8; [j] ref. 148; [k] ref. 151; [l] ref. 7; [m] ref. 403; [n] ref. 407; [o] ref. 130; [p] ref. 408.

* This value has been disputed.[410]

molecular forces cannot be representative of a single site of action. That is, such correlations are defined by the interaction of each anesthetic with itself rather than with a common site.

HYDROPHOBIC SITE: THE MEYER-OVERTON RULE

The physical property that correlates best with anesthetic potency is lipid solubility[74,129-134] (see Table 18-2 and Fig. 18-7). This correlation is termed the Meyer-Overton rule, after its two discoverers. The product of the anesthetizing partial pressure of an inhaled agent and its olive oil/gas partition coefficient varies little over approximately a 100,000-fold range of anesthetizing partial pressures (Table 18-2, Fig. 18-7). In order for the correlation to be perfect, this product would have to be the same for all anesthetics for a given animal. Within a given species, the product of anesthetizing partial pressure and oil/gas partition coefficient varies only slightly. The product tends to be somewhat lower in humans (1.35 ± 0.09 atmospheres) than in dogs (2.12 ± 0.13 atmospheres) or mice (1.82 ± 0.18 atmospheres for righting-reflex ED_{50}) (Table 18-2). The amazing closeness of this correlation implies a unitary molecular site of action and suggests that anesthesia results when a specific number of anesthetic molecules occupy a crucial hydrophobic region in the central nervous system. No other corre-

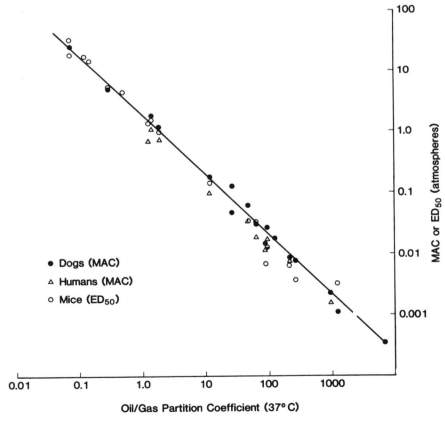

FIG. 18-7 Correlation of MAC in humans and dogs and the righting-reflex ED_{50} in mice with lipid solubility (i.e., the oil/gas partition coefficient). Values are taken from Table 18-2. The line drawn through the points represents the best linear fit to the data and has a correlation coefficient of −0.991.

lation employing the complete spectrum of inhaled agents approaches the excellent fit of that observed between anesthetic potency and lipid solubility.[135-139] This finding has led most investigators to look for the molecular basis of anesthetic action in cellular hydrophobic regions.

FURTHER CHARACTERIZATION OF THE HYDROPHOBIC SITE OF ANESTHETIC ACTION

The correlation of potency to solubility in olive oil (see Fig. 18-7 and Table 18-2) suggests that olive oil closely mimics the anesthetic site of action, and that anesthesia occurs when a critical anesthetic concentration is attained at that site. However, since olive oil is a mixture of oils and is not very well characterized from a physicochemical point of view, attempts have been made to examine anesthetic solubility in simpler solvents in order to better define the nature of the site of anesthetic action. A pure solvent may be characterized by its solubility parameter, which is a measure of the intermolecular forces in that solvent.[130] Anesthetic potency correlates best with solubility in solvents having solubility parameters of about 8 to 11 (calories cm^{-3})$^{1/2}$.[130,140,141] These values are representative of a solvent such as benzene and again imply a hydrophobic site of anesthetic action.

Franks and Lieb[142,143] have stated that an even better correlation between anesthetic potency and solubility is obtained when octanol, having a solubility parameter of approximately 10 (calories cm^{-3})$^{1/2}$, is used as the model solvent. These workers suggest that the anesthetic site of action has both polar and apolar characteristics. However, the improved correlation using octanol as the model solvent resulted from the inclusion of alcohols in the analyses.[142] For the inhaled anesthetics, the correlations between anesthetic potency and solubility in olive oil and octanol are essentially equivalent, implying either a hydrophobic or amphophilic site of anesthetic action.

ADDITIVE EFFECTS OF INHALED ANESTHETICS

The Meyer-Overton rule postulates that it is the number of molecules dissolved at the site of anesthetic action, and not the types of molecules present, that causes anesthesia. Thus 0.5 MAC of one agent and 0.5 MAC of another agent should have the same effect as 1.0 MAC of either agent. In general, this prediction has been confirmed[1,144-147] with only a few minor exceptions. A slight antagonism is reported for ethylene–nitrous oxide and cyclopropane–nitrous oxide mixtures in rats, but this may arise from errors in the extrapolations made to estimate the potencies of nitrous oxide and ethylene.[145] The slight antagonism also noted for mixtures of sulfur hexafluoride with carbon tetrafluoride or argon may be due to specific pulmonary effects associated with the breathing of sulfur hexafluoride at high pressures.[146] The addition of compound 485 (Fig. 18-1) produced a nonlinear decrease in the fraction of isoflurane MAC required to produce anesthesia,[148] indicating that the effect of compound 485 and isoflurane may be antagonistic. Such an antagonism might result from the convulsive activity of compound 485.[148] Overall, however, the evidence to date is consistent with an additive effect of anesthetics.

APPARENT EXCEPTIONS TO THE MEYER-OVERTON RULE

MINOR DEVIATIONS

In spite of the close correlation between lipid solubility and anesthetic potency, minor deviations from this correlation do exist. For example, enflurane and isoflurane are structural isomers having approximately the same oil/gas partition coefficient, yet anesthetic requirement for enflurane is 45 to 90 percent greater than that for isoflurane (Table 18-2). These differences in anesthetic requirements for agents having similar oil/gas partition coefficients suggest that the potency of an agent may depend on factors other than lipid solubility. One of these factors may be the convulsive properties of an agent. The possession of convulsant properties (e.g., as seen with enflurane) may oppose the anesthetic properties and increase anesthetic requirement.

CONVULSANT GASES

Another apparent exception to the Meyer-Overton rule is the ability of certain lipid-soluble compounds to produce convulsions. Indeed, complete halogenation (or full halogenation of the end methyl groups) of alkanes and ethers tends to decrease the anesthetic potencies of these agents and to enhance convulsant activity.[149,150] For flurothyl ($CF_3CH_2OCH_2CF_3$), convulsions are produced in 50 percent of mice at a concentration of 0.122 percent atmospheres.[151] However, higher concentrations of flurothyl have an anesthetic effect, and an ED_{50} for loss of righting reflex is obtained at a flurothyl concentration of 1.22 percent atmospheres.[151] The product of the oil/gas partition coefficient of flurothyl (46.9) and the righting-reflex ED_{50} in mice is 0.57 atmospheres, a value that is close to but somewhat lower than the value for conventional anesthetics (Table 18-2). Similarly, there is a biphasic pattern to the convulsive properties of enflurane in cats, with maximal seizure activity occurring between 3 and 4 percent atm enflurane and less seizure activity occurring both above and below this range of concentrations.[152]

Compound 485 (Fig. 18-1) possesses completely halogenated methyl groups and is a structural isomer of enflurane and isoflurane. It occasionally produced convulsions in dogs at concentrations near 6 percent atmospheres.[148] As an isomer of enflurane and isoflurane, it was predicted to have similar potency and solubility characteristics; however, its MAC was found to be 12.5 percent atmospheres. This high value was balanced by a low oil/gas partition coefficient of 25.8 (approximately four times lower than the value for isoflurane or enflurane), again yielding a product (3.23 atm) similar to but slightly greater than that for other inhaled agents[148] (Table 18-2).

Oxygen is a convulsant gas at low pressures, with higher pressures producing a state very similar to anesthesia.[153] The product of its ED_{50} in mice (5.3 atmospheres) and the oil/gas partition coefficient for oxygen is 0.70 atmospheres, a value that is also comparable to that for other anesthetics (Table 18-2).

Thus, the convulsant gases provide minor deviations from, but not marked exceptions to, the correlation between anesthetic potency and lipid solubility. These minor deviations may be explained by the following observations. Convulsant halogenated ethers may have different physical properties from the anesthetic halogenated ethers, since the convulsants are characterized by a low solubility parameter.[154] For example, flurothyl has a solubility parameter of 6.9, whereas the anesthetic halogenated ethers have values of approximately 8.0.[154] Furthermore, halogenated compounds that are anesthetics and convulsants may have different effects on synaptic transmission. Anesthetic agents block the excitatory glutamate response but not inhibitory transmission mediated by GABA at the crab neuromuscular junction, whereas convulsant agents block inhibitory but not excitatory transmission.[155] (However, both inhaled anesthetics and convulsants have a depressant effect on the postsynaptic action of acetylcholine.[156,157]) Anesthetics and convulsants may exhibit differential solubilities in subregions of the membrane, with each membrane subregion characterized by a particular solubility parameter, and may thereby provide a nonsteric mechanism for their different physiologic effects.[158]

CUTOFF EFFECT

The highly lipid-soluble n-decane is non-anesthetic in animals, even though lower paraffin homologs such as n-pentane cause anesthesia.[159] Similarly, n-pentane is more potent in suppressing conduction in an isolated nerve than is its more lipid-soluble homolog n-octane.[75,160] This decrease in anesthetic potency in the higher members of a homologous series is known as the *cutoff effect* and is a characteristic that is not compatible with the Meyer-

Overton rule. One postulate is that this phenomenon occurs because n-decane is too large to fit into the anesthetic site.[159] Alternatively, the cutoff in potency with higher alkane homologs may be owing to limited solubilities of these compounds at the anesthetic site of action (e.g., membrane).[133,161,162] Any unitary theory of narcosis involving a single hydrophobic site of action must eventually explain why such lipid-soluble compounds are not anesthetics.

HYDROPHILIC SITE

Some investigators believe that the anesthetic site of action is not necessarily hydrophobic. For example, both Pauling[163] and Miller[164] suggested that anesthesia might be caused by the ability of anesthetics to precipitate the formation of hydrates (this is the "hydrate theory of anesthesia"). However, the correlation between the ability of anesthetics to form hydrates and their potency is relatively poor.[130,134] Because of this, the unitary hydrate theory of anesthesia no longer holds water.

Another hypothesis is that inhaled anesthetics act by disrupting hydrogen bonds.[165,166] This seems unlikely, however, since chloroform and deuterated chloroform[167] and halothane and deuterated halothane[168] have different hydrogen bonding properties and yet have essentially identical anesthetic potencies.

Although it is improbable that inhaled agents act solely in a hydrophilic region, their binding may alter water structure near the anesthetic site of action.[169-171] Such an alteration in water structure could contribute to neuronal dysfunction (e.g., by altering the membrane penetration or membrane transport of current-carrying hydrated ions).[172] Also, certain theoretical and experimental considerations imply that the anesthetic binding site has both polar and nonpolar characteristics.[133,142,173,174] Spectroscopic studies of the intact brain imply a brain anesthetic environment with both polar

and lipophilic components.[175,176] However, these measurements do not necessarily represent the binding of anesthetics to their active site(s), and most probably a large percentage of the spectroscopic signal intensity is derived from binding to inactive sites.

VOLUME EXPANSION BY INHALED ANESTHETICS

Although the Meyer-Overton rule postulates that anesthesia occurs when a sufficient number of anesthetic molecules dissolve at a certain site, it does not explain why anesthesia results. Mullins[140] took the lipid solubility correlation one step further and hypothesized that anesthesia occurs when the absorption of anesthetic molecules expands the volume of a hydrophobic region beyond a critical amount (critical volume hypothesis). Such an expansion might produce anesthesia by obstructing ion channels or by altering the electrical properties of a membrane.[177] The influence of anesthetics on membrane properties and membrane dimensions is discussed further in later sections of this chapter.

The volume expansion hypothesis of anesthetic action suggested several experiments. One prediction of the hypothesis was that anesthetizing partial pressures of inhaled agents should produce a consistent volume expansion in a model hydrophobic system. Indeed, anesthetizing doses of inhaled agents cause hydrophobic solvents to undergo a significant increase in volume.[178,179] The hypothesis also predicts that anesthesia should be reversed by compressing the volume of the expanded hydrophobic region. High pressures do reverse anesthetic effects in vivo.[18,20,180] In addition, the critical volume theory is consistent with the observations that helium and neon, agents having low lipid solubilities, are not anesthetics. It also explains why hydrogen is not as potent as its lipid solubility-anesthetic potency correlation would predict; that is, the expansion caused by these agents is counterbalanced by the compression resulting from their high pressures.[180-183]

The critical volume model also suggests that a decrease in body temperature should antagonize the effect of anesthesia by contracting the volume of the expanded hydrophobic region. However, MAC does not increase but rather decreases as temperature decreases.[11,14] Although this fact seemingly contradicts the critical volume hypothesis, it should be noted that this prediction is complicated by the increased partitioning of anesthetics into nonpolar solvents at decreased temperatures[184,185] and the uncertainty of the effects of temperature per se on the organism.

Several other arguments may be raised against the critical volume hypothesis. If all inhaled agents at MAC cause an equal volume increase, (1) the degree of pressure reversal for a given total pressure should be the same for all agents, and (2) the increase in anesthetic requirement should be rectilinearly related to the total pressure. However, the degree of pressure reversal differs for certain agents, and the anesthetic requirements of argon and nitrogen increase in a curvilinear fashion with increases in pressure.[22] For other inhaled anesthetics, the relationship between pressure and anesthetic requirement at total pressure above 100 atmospheres is nonlinear.[182] Although there is some question concerning the degree of this nonlinearity,[141] a nonlinear pressure antagonism suggests that anesthetics and pressure may act at different sites[186] and that the main effect of pressure may be to increase the general level of CNS excitability. Indeed, in the absence of anesthetics, high pressures produce tremors and convulsions.[181,182] These results have led to a *multisite expansion hypothesis*,[187] which holds that general anesthesia results from expansion of several hydrophobic molecular sites, each having somewhat different physical properties.

The fact that not all lipid-soluble compounds are anesthetics poses another difficulty for the critical volume hypothesis. There is no immediate explanation of why these nonanesthetics should not expand the suspected crucial hydrophobic sites. In summary, the critical volume hypothesis is probably an oversimplified view of the way in which anesthetics act.

THE MEMBRANE AS THE SITE OF ANESTHETIC ACTION

The activity immediately underlying transmission of nervous impulses occurs principally at the surface of nerves. Since inhaled agents disrupt this transmission, synaptic and axonal membranes are usually assumed to be the primary sites of anesthetic action. A membrane site of action is also consistent with the hydrophobic theories of anesthesia, since cellular membranes consist largely of hydrophobic components.

Electrophysiologic studies reveal the effects of anesthetics on the flow of ions through excitable membranes. In isolated axons, the conduction of the nervous impulse requires the sequential flow of sodium and potassium ions through selective transmembrane channels. Excitation produces a rapid increase in sodium conductance to a peak (the activation process) followed by a slower decline in sodium conductance to zero (the inactivation process). Inhaled anesthetics (albeit at relatively high concentrations) decrease the magnitude of the sodium current and speed up (shorten) the inactivation and activation processes associated with the flow of sodium and potassium ions through membranes.[70-72,76,160] The magnitude of the steady-state inactivation is a function of voltage, and the curve relating these two parameters is shifted in the hyperpolarizing direction by inhaled agents. This effect is opposed by the application of high pressure.[85] In addition, the gating currents (i.e., the membrane-bound charges or dipoles that move under the influence of a transmembrane electric field to promote the opening of ion channels) are decreased by general anesthetics.[188] Inhaled agents directly hyperpolarize spinal neurons and hippocampal pyramidal cells[189] and yet may also depolarize isolated axons,[68] both changes being attributed to alterations in potassium permeability. With recent advances in technology, electrophysiologic recordings of single membrane channels can now be obtained. These recordings show that halothane decreases the time that a channel spends in the open state.[190] All these above facts point to a membrane site of anesthetic action.

For reasons primarily related to the importance of the membrane to the conduction process, the cytoplasm is thought to play a relatively minor role in the short-term conduction of nervous impulses. Nevertheless, anesthetics could act indirectly at a cytoplasmic membrane site. For example, anesthetics might depress the ion-accumulating activity of mitochondria, thus altering the cytoplasmic levels of free ions (e.g., calcium), which could in turn influence the conductance properties of excitable membranes and alter the presynaptic release of neurotransmitters.[191] Indeed, inhaled agents do inhibit mitochondrial activity and brain metabolism,[192-195] but they do not diminish the content of energy-rich substances (e.g., ATP) in the brain. The failure of high pressure to reverse the halothane-induced depression of mitochondrial respiration[196] goes against a mitochondrial site of anesthetic action.

Reversible depolymerization of cytoplasmic microtubules and microfilaments has been suggested as a mechanism of anesthetic action —the *microtubular theory of anesthesia*. Although some inhaled agents depolymerize microtubules,[197] others do not.[198] Nor does colchicine block membrane excitation,[199] except at very high concentrations (100 times greater than the concentration required to disrupt microtubules) at which levels it probably acts as a channel blocker.[200] Moreover, high pressures also depolymerize microtubules;[201] thus, if microtubules were the site of anesthetic action, high pressure should augment rather than antagonize the effect of anesthetics.

The above discussion suggests that anesthesia results from an association of inhaled agents with plasma membranes of nerves. Which components of the membrane are altered by the anesthetics? Biologic membranes consist of a cholesterol–phospholipid bilayer matrix having peripheral proteins weakly bound to the exterior hydrophilic membrane and integral proteins deeply embedded in, or passing through, the lipid bilayer[202] (Fig. 18-8A). Synaptic plasma membranes that are relatively free from other cellular contaminants are approximately 50 percent lipid and 50 percent protein by weight.[203] Anesthetics could act on the nonpolar interior of the lipid bilayer, at hydrophobic pockets in membrane proteins, or at the hydrophobic interface between intrinsic membrane proteins and the lipid matrix (Fig. 18-8A).

Attempts to better understand the penetration of inhaled agents into, and their interaction with, membrane sites have led to an examination of isolated membrane components. These experiments were greatly aided by the discovery that phospholipids dispersed in an aqueous medium spontaneously form bilayers comprising the surface of spherical structures (liposomes). These phospholipid bilayers act as a permeability barrier to ions and are similar to those found in biomembranes.[204] Liposomes have been extensively employed as model systems for the study of interactions between anesthetics and membrane lipids. In contrast, membrane proteins are difficult to isolate and purify, although recent advances have resulted in the partial biochemical characterization of certain protein ionophores thought to permit the passage (tunneling) of ions through membranes during excitation.[205] Thus, most experiments that examine anesthetic–protein interactions employ soluble proteins as model systems. Such proteins are easy to prepare in reasonable quantities but may not mimic precisely the natural proteins responsible for ion translocation.

INTERACTION OF INHALED ANESTHETICS WITH MEMBRANE LIPIDS

BINDING OF ANESTHETICS TO MEMBRANE LIPIDS

The solubility of gaseous and volatile agents in phospholipid bilayers correlates with their anesthetic potency.[133,161,206-208] This correlation is at least as good as that obtained when olive oil is the model solvent.[208] Although incorporation of cholesterol into phospholipid membranes decreases the partitioning of inhaled agents, the more soluble agents tending to have a greater decrease in partition coefficient,[208-210] a good correlation remains between anesthetic potency and membrane solubility. The degree of saturation of lipid acyl chains[161] or the length of the lipid acyl chains[206,210] has little effect on the partition coefficient. On the other hand, a decrease in temperature increases the partition coefficients of all agents, with the exception of carbon tetrafluoride.[133,208] Partitioning of inhaled anesthetics in lipid bilayers may increase as anesthetic concentrations increase.[211] At anesthetic concentrations close to 1.0 MAC, one anesthetic molecule binds to approximately every 25 phospholipid molecules.

High pressures may eject anesthetic molecules from phospholipid bilayers, and each 100 atmospheres of pressure may displace approximately 9 percent of anesthetic molecules.[212] However, other theoretical predictions indicate that this displacement is too small to explain the pressure reversal of anesthesia.[180] Although hyperbaric pressures have little effect on the partitioning of a barbiturate[213] or of a small spin-labeled molecule[214,215] into lipid bilayers, the analogous experiments for inhaled anesthetics remain to be performed.

The interaction with membrane lipids is a dynamic process, and anesthetic molecules rapidly exchange between the membrane and aqueous phases.[216-219] Anesthetics may penetrate all depths of the lipid bilayer.[216] They may accumulate in the center of the bilayer[220,221] or may preferentially lodge at the polar head group-aqueous interface of a phospholipid membrane.[222] Thus, the precise location at which anesthetics bind in the lipid bilayer is not known with certainty and may depend in part on the individual characteristics of the anesthetic or lipid examined.

EFFECTS ON MEMBRANE PERMEABILITY

Liposomes prepared in a salt solution containing radioactive ions entrap such ions. The untrapped ions exterior to the liposomes can be removed, and the subsequent flux of ions from the interior to the exterior can be measured. Inhaled agents increase the cation permeability of liposomes in a dose-related manner.[223,224] These anesthetic-induced increases in cation permeability occur both in the presence of ionophores that facilitate the transport of ions through membranes and in the absence of ionophores.[223,224] Although all agents increase cation permeability, the magnitude of the increase depends on the lipid composition of the liposome and on the anesthetic examined.[223] The anesthetic-induced increases in cation permeability are reversed by the application of high pressures (approximately 100 atmospheres).[223] This reversibility parallels the antagonism observed between anesthesia and pressure in vivo.

In bimolecular (black) lipid membranes, halothane increases membrane conductance,[225] and chloroform increases permeability to organic cations and anions.[226] Similarly, chloroform increases the movement of organic ions across the intact squid axon membrane.[188] Such alterations in ion permeability may be secondary to alterations in membrane surface charge by the inhaled agents[227] (e.g., a greater positive membrane surface charge would tend to concentrate more anions at the surface). General anesthetics increase the flow of protons across lipid vesicles.[228] Bangham suggested that anesthetics may act by increasing proton permeability across synaptic vesicles, collapsing the pH gradient required for retainment of catecholamines in their charged form and thereby depressing neurotransmission by releasing catecholamines from synaptic storage vesicles.[229] However, this hypothesis would only partly explain anesthesia, namely, that although depletion of catecholamines lowers anesthetic requirement, it does not of itself produce anesthesia (see the previous section on neurotransmitters).

ALTERATIONS IN MEMBRANE DIMENSION

Inhaled agents increase the lateral pressure of lipid monolayers in a manner that parallels their anesthetic potency.[230,231] This finding is consistent with the notion that anesthetics might exert pressure on the ionic channels needed for impulse transmission—a variation of the volume expansion theory of anesthesia—and thereby inhibit their opening or accelerate their closure. Such an expansion may also explain the ability of inhaled agents to protect erythrocytes from hypotonic hemolysis.[232] Indeed, direct microscopic visualization of the red blood cell surface shows an area of expansion ranging from 0.13 to 0.62 percent for halothane, methoxyflurane, ether, fluroxene, and isoflurane at concentrations of one to four times MAC.[233] However, long chain alcohols that are not anesthetics also expand red cell surface area, thereby casting uncertainty on the role of membrane area expansion in anesthesia.[233]

The degree of membrane expansion has been debated. Seeman[74] initially calculated that anesthetics swell biomembranes (but not lipid membranes) approximately 10 times more than the volume of anesthetic molecules in the biomembrane phase and postulated that this was secondary to alterations in membrane protein conformation. However, Trudell[234] pointed out that this calculation included the probably false assumption that biomembrane thickness expands at the same rate as surface area. After corrections are made for alterations in biomembrane thickness with expansion of surface area the estimated volume expansion produced by anesthetics is approximately the same as that occupied by the anesthetic molecules.[234] Precise measurements show a contraction of total volume when inhaled agents are dissolved in water[235-237] and an expansion of model lipid membranes[235,237] and of red cell membranes[238] by 0.1 to 0.4 percent at concentrations near 1.0 MAC.

Anesthetics may thicken the membrane bilayer. The finding of an inverse relationship between the thickness and conductance of bimolecular lipid membranes led to the suggestion that an anesthetic-induced increase in bilayer thickness destabilizes the open channels formed during electrical excitation.[239,240] Similarly, the alterations in the steady-state sodium inactivation curve by anesthetics may be owing to an increase in axonal membrane thickness.[241] Pentane does thicken nerve membranes, but only after producing an irreversible

blockade of neuronal conduction.[242,243] Although spectroscopic measurements support the concept of an anesthetic-induced increase in lipid-bilayer width in certain experiments,[244,245] other studies found no alterations[221,246,247] and even a decrease[248] in bilayer thickness by anesthetics. Thus, the effects, if present, of anesthetics on membrane thickness are probably small; it is unknown whether changes in membrane thickness play a role in anesthesia.

According to the critical volume hypothesis, an increase in pressure or a decrease in temperature should reverse anesthesia, because these processes compress membranes. However, a decrease in body temperature consistently increases anesthetic potency. This apparent contradiction is partly resolved by the finding of an increased partitioning of anesthetics into membranes at lower temperatures. Moreover, the expansion of membranes by anesthetics and an increase in temperature may not be equivalent.[133] For example, anesthetics may expand membranes without changing thickness, and a decrease in temperature may cause a net contraction with an increase in membrane thickness.[235]

ALTERATIONS IN MEMBRANE PHYSICAL STATE

Further studies of the molecular changes occurring on the insertion of anesthetic molecules into lipid membranes led to the suggestion that anesthetics increase the mobility of membrane components (the fluidization theory of anesthesia). Inhaled agents cause a dose-related increase in the mobility of fatty acid chains in a phospholipid bilayer.[249-253] High pressure reverses this "fluidization" of the bilayer,[254,255] a finding consistent with the previously described pressure reversal of anesthesia.

The ability of an anesthetic to fluidize a lipid bilayer depends on the structure of the agent examined and on the composition of the lipid bilayer.[133] Lipid bilayers are most readily fluidized by a given partial pressure of anesthetic when the liposomes contain about 30 percent cholesterol and about 10 percent of an acidic phospholipid.[256] Whether this fluidization occurs at clinical concentrations is in dispute.[142,211,246] Nevertheless, anesthetizing doses of agents seem to increase the fluidity of most cholesterol-containing bilayers.[257] However, the same may not be true for biologic membranes. In red blood cell membranes[258] and synaptic membranes,[259] the disordering (fluidizing) effects of anesthetics may depend on the depth in the bilayer at which fluidization is measured. The fluidity of synaptic membranes *decreases* at clinical concentrations of halothane.[260]

Even a small change in lipid fluidity may profoundly change membrane function: a 2 percent change in the fluidity structural parameter may produce a 20 percent change in liposome cation permeability.[224] Anesthesia might result from such changes in permeability. The permeability changes might be induced indirectly on physiologic ionophores: the ion-transporting properties of several membrane proteins depend in part on the physical state of their neighboring lipids.[261] The increased decay rate of postsynaptic currents caused by inhaled agents may result from an increased fluidity of the postsynaptic membrane. The increased fluidity may promote a more rapid relaxation (i.e., return to the closed configuration) of the proteins involved in the conductance change occurring after acetylcholine activation.[108,262] Similarly, the speeding up of sodium current inactivation in isolated axons has been attributed to an anesthetic-induced increase in the mobility of the lipids surrounding the channels.[70] However, incompatible with this hypothesis is the fact that hypothermia (which lessens mobility of membrane lipids) can potentiate nerve blockade by halothane,[263] and that volatile agents cannot alter the kinetics of gating currents in an axonal membrane.[188]

Liposomes composed of a single type of phospholipid undergo a *phase transition*, i.e., a sudden conversion of the lipids from a solid or gel phase to a liquid or fluid phase, as temperature slowly increases past a critical point.[264] Dipalmitoylphosphatidylcholine, a lecithin molecule possessing two saturated fatty acid chains 16 carbon atoms in length, undergoes a major transition at 41°C.[264] Inhaled agents decrease the phase-transition temperature of phosphatidylcholines,[206,265-269] and high pressures reverse this effect.[212,266,268] The charge of the lipid bilayer determines the decrease in phase transition temperature by anesthetics. Methoxyflurane depresses the transition temperature of dipalmitoylphosphatidic acid bilayers (which are negatively charged) by 10°C, whereas the same concentration of methoxyflurane decreases the transition temperature of dipalmitoylphosphatidylcholine (DPPC) bilayers, which have an overall neutral charge, only 1.5°C.[270] High pressures (100 atmospheres) almost completely antagonize the 10°C depression in transition temperature of methoxyflurane–phosphatidic acid bilayers, but increase the transition temperature of phosphatidic acid bilayers only 1.5°C in the absence of anesthetic. These differences might be accounted for if high pressures extrude anesthetic molecules from the lipid phase in these charged bilayers.[270] According to one hypothesis, lipids surrounding an excitable membrane channel are normally exclusively in the more rigid gel phase, thereby helping maintain patency of the channel. Adding anesthetic may fluidize these lipids, impair the surrounding structural support, and allow the channel to close (the phase transition theory of anesthesia).[271] However, if a major phase transition is important in the production of anesthesia, one would predict a discontinuity in the relationship between temperature and MAC. However, there is no such discontinuity.[11]

Since neuronal membranes consist of several types of phospholipids having different fatty acid compositions, a lateral phase separation may exist; that is, neuronal membrane lipids may exist in both fluid and gel forms. The conversion from one form to another may permit the expansion or contraction of the membrane with greater ease than would be required if the membrane were purely fluid or gel.[272] The gel and liquid phases differ in density, and their interconversion supposedly permits an expansion or contraction of other membrane constituents at a minimal energy cost. Figure 18-8 illustrates the importance of this concept to the effect of an anesthetic on nerve transmission. A globular protein that possesses a closed ionic channel spans the lipid bilayer of the resting neuronal membrane. The surrounding

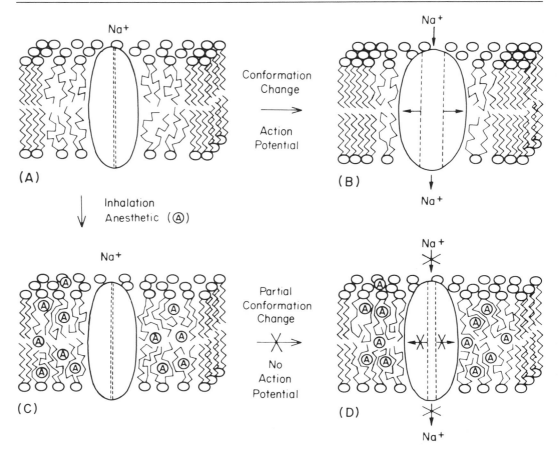

FIG. 18-8 (A) This representation of a neuronal membrane contains an integral membrane protein (the oval structure) that spans the phospholipid bilayer. The membrane protein has an ionic channel in the closed configuration. The small circles depict the phosphate head groups, and the zigzag lines depict fatty acid chains. On the left and right edges of the bilayer segment are regions in which the fatty acid chains are highly ordered. The phospholipids surrounding the intrinsic protein are disordered. (B) After a stimulus is received, the membrane protein expands (i.e., it undergoes a conformational change) and permits passage of ions through the channel. This expansion is accomplished by converting some high-volume fluid-phase lipids into the low-volume solid phase. (C) Anesthetic molecules invade both solid and fluid phases and convert much of the solid to a fluid phase. (D) After a stimulus is received, the membrane protein is unable to expand and open its channel, because the high-volume fluid-phase lipids cannot be converted into the low-volume solid-phase lipids in the presence of the anesthetic. The compression of the fluid phase without conversion is thought to require more lateral pressure than is immediately available. (Trudell JR: A unitary theory of anesthesia based on lateral phase separations in nerve membranes. Anesthesiology 46:5, 1977.)

lipids are in a disordered (fluid) state (Fig. 18-8A). During membrane excitation, a change in protein conformation opens the channel. This volume expansion of the protein is accomplished by converting a fraction of the high-volume fluid phase lipids to low-volume solid-phase lipids (Fig. 18-8B). Because anesthetic molecules in the membrane sustain fluidity (Fig. 18-8C) and block formation of the low-vol-

ume solid phase, the protein cannot change its conformation to the open channel state (Fig. 18-8D). Support for this hypothesis comes from the finding that general anesthetics disrupt lateral-phase separations in model membranes composed of two types of phospholipids and that these effects are partially reversed by the application of high pressure.[273]

The interconversions permitted by lateral

phase separations are thought to permit an energy-efficient way to expand or contract membranes. That is, less energy may be necessary to reduce membrane lipid volume through a phase change and conversion of fluid lipids to solid lipids than through compression of the lipids without a phase change. However, some simple calculations do not support this idea. If one assumes an ideal compression, less energy is required to alter the volume of DPPC through compression than through a phase change.* However, correction for nonideality may give an opposite result, a result that may confirm the original notion that reducing volume by compression is more "expensive" than by a phase change. In addition, since a lateral compression is being considered, the energy required to compress the lipids should be calculated on the two-dimensional level, a calculation that remains to be performed.

Both the *fluidization* and *lateral-phase separation* theories suggest that anesthetics may act by making membranes more disordered or fluid, and that the expansion in the membrane that accompanies this anesthetic perturbation

---

* For DPPC, the measured volume change (ΔV) that occurs by going through the phase transition is 0.035 ml/g, and the measured energy change associated with the transition is 8,400 cal/mole.[266] The energy required to compress DPPC by 0.035 ml/g can be approximated. The compressibility for DPPC is assumed to be about the same as for olive oil, 6×10^{-5} atm^{-1} (i.e., the volume decreases by 6×10^{-5} of the original volume for each atmosphere increase in pressure). Also, 1 g of DPPC is assumed to occupy about 1 ml. The pressure (P) needed to be applied to this 1 ml (1 g) of DPPC to change the volume by 0.035 ml is as follows:

$$P = \frac{0.035}{6 \times 10^{-5} \text{atm}^{-1}} = 583 \text{ atm}$$

Assuming ideality, the energy involved in this process is PΔV:

$$
\begin{aligned}
P\Delta V &= (583 \text{ atm}) (0.035 \text{ ml}) \\
&= 20.4 \text{ atm-cm}^3 \frac{(10^6 \text{ dynes/cm}^2)}{\text{atm}} \\
&= 2.04 \times 10^7 \text{ dynes-cm} \\
&= 2.04 \times 10^7 \text{ erg} \frac{(1 \text{ cal})}{(4.2 \times 10^7 \text{ erg})} \\
&= \frac{0.49 \text{ cal}}{\text{g DPPC}} \cdot \frac{(750 \text{ g DPPC})}{\text{mole DPPC}} = 367 \text{ cal/mole DPPC}
\end{aligned}
$$

According to these calculations, 23 times less energy is required to change the volume of DPPC by compressing it than by having it go through the phase change.

---

can be counterbalanced by applying high pressures. These theories are compromised by the fact that an increase in temperature also increases membrane fluidity and therefore should augment anesthesia. However, an increase in body temperature decreases anesthetic potency. Furthermore, these theories imply that an age-dependent increase in membrane disorder should accompany the decrease in anesthetic requirement with age (Fig. 18-3). In contrast, the fluidity of synaptic membranes tends to decrease[274,275] or remain unchanged[276] with age.

Another difficulty in relating the above work on artificial lipid membranes to anesthetic action is the significant difference between such membranes and neuronal membranes. In fact, halothane may have a biphasic effect on mammalian synaptic plasma membranes, increasing the ordering (decreasing fluidity) of these membranes at low (anesthetizing) halothane concentrations and increasing the fluidity at higher concentrations.[260] Moreover, low halothane concentrations produce an ordering only in synaptic plasma membranes and not in myelin or mitochondrial membranes.[260] This finding is more consistent with the effect of temperature on anesthetic requirement but implies that at very high anesthetic concentrations patients should awaken!

THE INTERACTION OF INHALED AGENTS WITH PROTEINS

Few of the neuronal membrane proteins that permit the translocation of ions during membrane excitation have been isolated. Little information is available on the interaction of anesthetics with these membrane proteins, and most experiments have employed other soluble proteins as model systems for the study of anesthetic effects.

Distinct anesthetic binding sites have been identified in myoglobin,[219,277,278] hemoglobin,[278-280] β-lactoglobulin,[281,282] adenylate kinase,[283] serum albumin,[284,285] and serum lipoproteins.[286] Anesthetics move rapidly between soluble proteins and the surrounding aqueous solvent,[219,278] although the exchange between plasma proteins and membranes may be relatively slow (milliseconds) on a molecular scale.[287] A binding site can be occupied by more than one anesthetic molecule.[282] A protein may contain considerable nonspecific as well as specific binding sites for anesthetics,[219] and not all nonpolar regions of a protein may act as binding sites.[283] Cooperative protein motions may be required to allow for passage of an anesthetic to its binding site.[278] Conversely, the binding of inhaled agents to proteins may give rise to conformational changes,[279-281] and these perturbations may be transmitted to a part of the protein molecule relatively distant from the anesthetic binding site.[280,288] The perturbation of β-lactoglobulin[281] and hemoglobin[280] caused by an anesthetic is related to the lipid solubility and potency of that anesthetic. Such conformational changes may expand the protein and disrupt the association of water molecules at the protein surface.[285]

The interaction of inhaled agents with enzymes may be reflected indirectly in changes in enzyme activity. Anesthetics inhibit the enzyme-induced luminescence output of light-emitting organisms, and application of high pressure reverses this inhibition.[289] Anesthetics may depress luminescence (1) by binding to areas near the active site of the enzyme luciferase, thus interfering with the normal access of the substrate, or (2) by acting at a second site to alter the binding of the enzyme cofactor.[290,291] The ability of inhaled agents to depress luminescence intensity parallels their lipid solubility,[292] and thermodynamic arguments suggest that anesthetic binding to a hydrophobic site results in inactivation by inducing a major conformational change of the enzyme structure. Inhaled anesthetics bind to the photoprotein aequorin, but with conflicting results, i.e. reports suggest both a subsequent decrease[293] and an increase[294] of light emission.

Anesthetics do not affect all enzyme systems. Glycolytic enzymes are not influenced even by high doses of anesthetics.[295] Only concentrations much higher than MAC alter ATPase isolated from brain tissue.[296,297] Serum cholinesterase activity is unchanged by saturated solutions of volatile agents.[298] High anesthetic concentrations are required to inhibit acetylcholinesterase activity,[296,298] and this inhibition does not bear a constant relationship to anesthetic potency.[298] Although intravenous agents appear to decrease the phosphorylation of brain proteins by a protein kinase, inhaled agents have no effect.[299]

Inhaled agents affect various enzymes in different ways. The anesthetic inhibition of glutamate dehydrogenase activity is related to the lipid solubility of the agent, and the decreased activity probably results from a conformational change that prevents the enzyme subunits from associating into an active form.[295] Inhaled agents may inhibit glucose phosphorylation in brain by converting mitochondrial hexokinase from its more active particulate form to a less active soluble form.[300] Halothane alters the affinity of pterin cofactor for tyrosine hydroxylase[301] and thus alters its activity. The depression of cardiac sarcoplasmic reticulum Ca^{+2}-ATPase by halothane can be antagonized by calcium.[302] Nitrous oxide inactivates the vitamin B_{12}-dependent enzyme methionine synthetase by oxidizing the cobalt atom of the vitamin B_{12} molecule.[303,304] However, even trace levels of nitrous oxide can cause inactivation, and other inhaled anesthetics do not produce inactivation.[305]

Most studies demonstrate an increase in brain cAMP content during anesthesia,[306-309] although this has not always been found[310,311] and may depend somewhat on experimental conditions. cAMP has received considerable attention because of its possible role as a second messenger in altering neurotransmission. Its increase with anesthesia probably results, at least in part, from an anesthetic-induced activation of adenylate cyclase[312] and inhibition of phosphodiesterase.[307] In contrast to the activation of adenylate cyclase in brain, inhaled agents decrease adenylate cyclase activity in the heart[313] and bladder.[314] Although catecholamines may regulate adenylate cyclase activity, inhaled anesthetics do not alter the binding properties of myocardial β-adrenergic receptors.[315]

Inhaled anesthetics can also alter the activity of enzymes involved in lipid synthesis and degradation, and thereby alter membrane lipid composition. Anesthetics enhance the activity of neuronal membrane-bound neuraminidase,[316-318] increasing the release of sialic acid from the surface of neurons. Similarly, halothane increases the activity of sphingomyelinase in synaptic plasma membranes and stimulates sphingomyelin degradation.[319] Inhaled agents inhibit the turnover of phosphatidic acid and phosphatidylinositol in synaptosomes,[320] inhibit the incorporation of serine into phospholipid,[321] and may decrease the synthesis of phosphatidylethanolamine.[322] Halothane (but not enflurane, chloroform, or ether) at high concentrations promotes the hydrolysis of lecithin bilayers by the enzyme phospholipase A_2.[323] Although some of the above effects may be due to a direct anesthetic–enzyme interaction, an indirect effect on enzyme activity secondary to perturbation of membrane lipids remains possible.

Other studies indicate a linkage between membrane lipids and membrane proteins. The ability of halothane to alter protein conformational state in neuronal membranes correlates with the halothane-induced alteration in lipid physical state.[324] Incorporation of a peptide into phosphatidic acid bilayers promotes the formation of domains of peptide-bound phospholipids in a matrix of a bilayer of unbound phosphatidic acid.[325] Methoxyflurane disrupts this peptide-induced lateral-phase separation, thus producing a homogeneously dispersed phase, presumably by lowering the packing density and increasing the surface area per phospholipid. This effect is antagonized by high pressure.[325]

A few studies have examined the influence of anesthetics on the properties of protein ionophores involved in the membrane translocation of ions. Inhaled anesthetics inhibit the light-induced proton uptake of retinal rod outer segment membranes, presumably by altering the conformational changes of the rhodopsin molecule that normally occur during excitation.[326] Volatile agents stabilize the membrane-bound acetylcholine receptor protein in a conformational form that binds agonists with high affinity and may be associated with a desensitized and thus inactive state of the acetylcholine receptor–ionophore complex.[327,328] In support of these findings, anesthetics increase the binding of acetylcholine to its receptor.[329,330] In addition, pressure decreases the binding.[329,330]

Such observations on isolated proteins have led to the postulate that general anesthetics inactivate proteins essential for CNS function by combining with hydrophobic regions of protein molecules and inducing a conformational change in the molecules.[143,331,332] This conformational change is thought to be due to an unfolding of the molecule, accompanied by an increase in volume.[331] Alternatively, anesthetics may alter electron mobility and prevent the dipole-related protein conformational responses required for neuronal transmission.[333] Although some convincing thermodynamic arguments exist, these protein perturbation hypotheses do not offer a distinct mechanism by which anesthetics produce inactivation. A clearer picture may develop with an increased understanding of the structure and function of membrane proteins.

ACTION OF INHALED ANESTHETICS AT THE OPIATE RECEPTOR

During the late 1970s, two reports suggested that naloxone, a narcotic antagonist, partially reversed the action of inhalational anesthetics either when given intravenously[334] or when perfused through the fourth (but not the third) cerebral ventricle.[335] The investigators hypothesized that anesthetics may act by releasing endogenous opiate-like substances (the endorphin-release theory of anesthesia). However, replication of these studies showed that the antagonistic effect of naloxone could be explained by a minor shift in the anesthetic dose–response curve.[336] Anesthetic requirement, as measured by lack of response to a noxious stimulus[336-339] or by the ability to abolish the righting reflex[340-343] was altered no more than a few percent by narcotic antagonists, even at doses of naloxone as high as 250 mg/kg.[336] Similarly, naloxone did not alter cerebral oxygen consumption during halothane anesthesia, whereas cerebral oxygen consumption increased when narcotic anesthesia was reversed by a narcotic antagonist.[344] In isolated preparations, naloxone did not antagonize the depression of spinal cord activity[345] nor the inhibition of contractions of guinea pig ileum[342,346] produced by inhaled agents. Exposure of rats to 80 percent nitrous oxide for 18 hours did not alter levels of met-enkephalin in brain regions associated with nociceptive pathways.[347] In humans, anesthesia does not increase opioid peptides in cerebrospinal fluid, and thus any contribution of the endorphin system to the production of general anesthesia does not appear to require the release of β-endorphin.[348] The administration of nitrous oxide during labor is accompanied by β-endorphin release into the bloodstream, but the levels of β-endorphin do not inversely correlate with the intensity of the pain.[349] Isoflurane–nitrous oxide anesthesia has no effect on plasma β-endorphin immunoreactivity in humans.[350] The ability of high doses of naloxone to decrease halothane-induced sleep times in rats[343] and to reverse the halothane-induced depression of the baroreceptor reflex in the dog[351] probably results from a general increase in central nervous system excitation and not by pharmacologic competition for opiate receptors.

Nevertheless, other experiments indicate a possible role for opiate receptors in anesthesia or analgesia. β-endorphin administered into the cerebral ventricles of rats causes a sequence of behavioral and electroencephalographic responses similar to those produced with general anesthesia, and naloxone reverses these effects.[352] Naloxone partially antagonizes the analgesic effect of nitrous oxide in mice (as measured by the writhing response),[353] and antagonizes nitrous oxide- but not halothane- or ether-produced analgesia in the rat (as measured by the tail flick).[342,354] In humans, reports of the action of naloxone have varied. Naloxone antagonized nitrous oxide-induced analgesia, as measured by cerebral evoked potential response to painful electrical shocks to tooth pulp[355] and ischemic pain produced by a tourniquet.[356] However, naloxone had no effect on dental postoperative pain[357] and even enhanced the analgesic action of nitrous oxide.[358]

Studies on isolated brain membranes have provided some evidence for interaction of inhaled agents with the opiate receptor. Nitrous oxide[359] and ether[28] decrease the specific binding of naloxone to brain tissue. Although both anesthetics and the convulsant flurothyl decrease naloxone binding, the effects of the anesthetic and the convulsant agents are modulated differently by altering the sodium concentration or pH of the suspension.[28] Methoxyflurane decreases the binding affinity of agonists for various subtypes (mu, kappa, delta, sigma) of opiate receptors,[360] but the binding of dihydromorphine (indicative of mu receptors) is not altered by halothane, ether, or nitrous oxide.[342,360] Studies with a leucine enkephalin analogue indicate a possible dual mechanism of anesthetic action: one having an opiate receptor-specific mechanism that is reversible by opiate antagonist, and the other having a nonspecific mechanism related to lipid solubility that is reversible with the application of high pressure.[361]

Thus, evidence to date concerning general anesthetic–opiate receptor interaction is inconclusive. Although anesthetics may produce analgesia by release of endogenous opiate-like compounds (or an increase in sensitivity to their effects), the evidence to date does not indicate that a simple action on or through an opiate receptor mediates the predominant effects of general anesthetics.[362]

USE OF ANIMAL MODELS: ATTEMPTS TO RELATE SUSTAINED ALTERATIONS IN ANESTHETIC POTENCY WITH NEUROCHEMICAL COMPOSITION

One approach to the mechanism of anesthetic action relates alterations in anesthetic requirement with biochemical and biophysical changes occurring in the central nervous system. A correlation between changes in anesthetic requirement and a structural change in the nervous system might indicate the critical properties of the anesthetic site of action and how anesthetics affect that site.

TOLERANCE STUDIES

CHRONIC TOLERANCE

General anesthetic requirement can be increased by the chronic exposure of mice to subanesthetic levels of nitrous oxide.[363-366] The maximal increase in nitrous oxide ED_{50} for mice placed under 40 to 70 percent nitrous oxide is approximately 0.25 atm and occurs after 2 weeks of exposure. Tolerance disappears within 6 days of removing the mice from the subanesthetic environment.[363,365] Animals tolerant to nitrous oxide are also more tolerant to cyclopropane and isoflurane.[364] Auto- and cross-tolerance may occur after multiple exposures to volatile agents.[367]

Tolerance to nitrous oxide might result from an alteration in synaptic membrane lipid composition so that the physical state of the membrane is returned to that present prior to nitrous oxide exposure. Indeed, in simple cellular systems, exposure to anesthetics can increase synthesis of saturated fatty acids,[368] increase cholesterol content and membrane order,[369] and alter membrane glucolipids.[370] However, no significant alterations in membrane order or in the composition of synaptic membrane fatty acid, phospholipid, or cholesterol occur in animals tolerant to nitrous oxide.[363,365]

Animals become tolerant to the analgesic effects of nitrous oxide after exposure to 75 percent nitrous oxide for approximately 18 hours.[354,371] Also, a patient was reported to develop tolerance to analgesic concentrations of nitrous oxide.[372] Prolonged exposure to nitrous oxide decreases brainstem opiate receptor density by about 20 percent and may account for tolerance to the analgesic action of nitrous oxide.[373]

The need of chronic alcoholic patients for increased doses of general anesthetic agents is a long-established clinical impression.[374-376] The MAC for inhaled anesthetics is increased by approximately 30 percent in mice,[377] rats,[378] cats,[379] and humans[380] following chronic administration of ethanol. Furthermore, animals made tolerant to nitrous oxide are also tolerant to the hypnotic effects of ethanol.[381] Although the mechanism of cross-tolerance is unknown, an increase in synaptic plasma membrane rigidity and a decreased partitioning of inhaled agents into synaptic membranes of ethanol-tolerant animals have been suggested.[382]

ACUTE TOLERANCE

In humans, a tolerance to the analgesic effects of nitrous oxide is seen in some patients within 10 to 60 minutes of administration.[357,383] Similarly, tolerance to nitrous oxide and ethylene anesthesia is observed in mice within approximately 10 minutes.[4] Rapid tolerance to the effects of nitrous oxide is also manifested on the electroencephalogram,[32,384] on cerebrocortical responses to electrical stimuli applied to the forepaw of the rat,[42] and on blockade of sympathetic ganglia.[385] However, no clue has been found concerning the molecular mechanism behind this phenomenon.

Associated with this rapidly developing tolerance is a withdrawal syndrome after exposure to nitrous oxide, ethylene, cyclopropane, and diethyl ether.[386] Exposure to nitrous oxide at partial pressures greater than 0.9 atm for 15 to 30 minutes produces a withdrawal syndrome in mice.[387] Most mice stimulated by gentle raising by the tail convulse 15 minutes after removal from the anesthetic environment.[387] This syndrome may be related to the emergence delirium seen in some patients after general anesthesia. Although arguments have been made for cholinergic involvement[388] and for[389] and against[390] involvement of endogenous opiates, the mechanistic basis of this withdrawal syndrome remains to be explored.

GENETIC STUDIES

One method of producing two groups of animals having different anesthetic requirements makes use of the fact that anesthetic requirement varies slightly among animals of a given species and that members resistant and vulnerable to anesthesia may be found in a normal population. Mice can be selected from a normal population with consistently high and consistently low nitrous oxide requirements.[391] Offspring from parents having consistently high nitrous oxide requirements also have high requirements (HI mice), whereas offspring from parents having low requirements similarly have low requirements (LO mice).[391] Selection of the offspring having the highest and lowest nitrous oxide requirements and repeating the process of breeding, testing for nitrous oxide requirement, and selection through 15 generations have produced two lines of mice having nitrous oxide requirements that are ap-

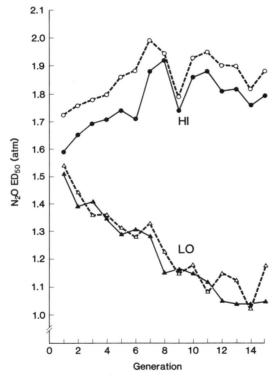

FIG. 18-9 Nitrous oxide righting-reflex ED_{50} values for male (closed symbols) and female (open symbols) offspring of mice selectively bred for resistance (HI group, circles) or susceptibility (LO group, triangles) to nitrous oxide anesthesia. The anesthetic requirements for HI and LO mice became progressively more separated over 15 generations of selective breeding. Standard errors about most points are less than 0.03 atmosphere. Values for generations 1 through 10 are taken from refs. 9 and 391.

proximately 0.7 atmospheres apart[9,391] (Fig. 18-9). The nitrous oxide righting-reflex ED_{50} value for the population extremes of these HI and LO mice (i.e., those selected as breeders to produce the following generations) have nitrous oxide requirements approximately 1 atmosphere apart.[9] The HI mice also have a higher anesthetic requirement for other inhaled anesthetics, but the separation in righting-reflex ED_{50} values between the two lines is inversely related to the lipid solubility of the anesthetic.[9] HI and LO mice are also differentially sensitive to ethanol[9] and to barbiturates,[392] but the magnitude of the difference in CNS sensitivity between the two lines varies among barbiturates.[392] HI mice are more susceptible to the convulsant effects of high-pressure helium, flurothyl, pentylenetetrazole, strychnine, bicuculline, and picrotoxin than are LO mice. This higher nitrous oxide requirement might be explained, at least in part, by a generalized increase in CNS excitability.[393] Nitrous oxide ED_{50} values of offspring produced by cross-mating animals of the HI and LO lines approximate the average value of the parents, implying that the genetic control of resistance or susceptibility probably involves many genes.[394] For both lines of mice, the nitrous oxide requirement declines with age, the HI mice having a greater age-related decrease in requirement.[26]

The discovery of the structural changes in the central nervous system that produce these differences in nitrous oxide requirement could provide an important insight into the mechanism of anesthetic action. When the possibility that HI and LO mice differed in synaptic membrane composition was examined, no differences could be found in synaptic membrane fatty acid, phospholipid, or cholesterol composition.[391] HI mice do have a higher brain catecholamine content than LO mice (DD Koblin, MF Roizen, BM Frazer, NT Nelson, EI Eger II, CR Bainton, and FW Lurz: unpublished observations). If catecholamine levels are important in explaining the separation in anesthetic requirement between the HI and LO lines, the offspring produced by cross-mating HI and LO mice should have intermediate levels of catecholamines in the brain, and such catecholamines would be expected to decrease to a greater extent in the HI mice than in the LO mice with age. These experiments have not yet been performed.

Mice selectively bred for sensitivity (long-sleep mice) or resistance (short-sleep mice) to the hypnotic effects of alcohol also have a differential sensitivity to certain[395] but not all[396,397] inhaled anesthetics. However, the differential effect between short-sleep and long-sleep mice is greater for alcohol than for inhaled agents. The greater anesthetic requirement of the short-sleep mice is not associated with a different synaptic membrane phospholipid, fatty acid, or cholesterol composition.[395] Conversely, gross alterations in the lipid composition of CNS myelin in the quaking mouse (an autosomal recessive mutant deficient in CNS myelin) have little or no influence on anesthetic requirement.[398]

Strains of *Drosophila melanogaster* that are resistant and sensitive to ether have also been obtained. Such strains are also resistant and sensitive to halothane and chloroform.[399] Resistance to halothane appears to be a sex-linked recessive trait, and resistance to chloroform an incompletely dominant autosomal trait. These two strains have different fatty acid and diglyceride content in the phosphatidylethanolamine fraction but not in the phosphatidylcholine fraction.[400] However, these analyses were performed on lipids extracted from whole organism, and it is uncertain how such lipid alterations might relate to the mechanism of anesthesia.

DIETARY STUDIES

Mice fed diets of different fatty acid composition from birth have large alterations in certain synaptic membrane fatty acid components.[401] However, these alterations have essentially no influence on anesthetic requirement.[401] Nevertheless, the diets of different fatty acid content do not alter synaptic membrane phospholipid or cholesterol composition. The possible effect of dietary alterations in synaptic membrane phospholipids and cholesterol on anesthetic potency remains to be examined.

CONCLUSIONS

Inhaled anesthetics disrupt neuronal transmission in many areas of the central nervous system. They either enhance inhibitory effects or depress excitatory transmission through synaptic regions or small-diameter axons at the nerve terminal. Both pre- and postsynaptic actions have been found. Regardless of the macroscopic site of action, anesthetics almost certainly exert their effect by interacting with neuronal membranes. The excellent correlation between lipid or membrane bilayer solubility and anesthetic potency suggests that anesthetics have a hydrophobic or amphipathic site of action. Anesthetics cause conformational perturbations in both membrane lipids and proteins, but it is presently uncertain how these perturbations might lead to the anesthetic state. Experiments to date reveal no relationship between anesthetic potency and brain lipid composition. Future advances in anesthetic mechanisms will go hand in hand with an increased knowledge of synaptic transmission in selective regions of the central nervous system, a better understanding of membrane proteins and membrane lipids in synaptic processes, and an ability to relate biophysical and biochemical changes in synaptic regions to alterations in anesthetic requirement.

REFERENCES

1. Cullen SC, Eger EI II, Cullen BF, et al: Observations on the anesthetic effect of the combination of xenon and halothane. Anesthesiology 31:305, 1969
2. Eger EI II, Saidman LJ, Brandstater B: Minimum alveolar anesthetic concentration: a standard of anesthetic potency. Anesthesiology 26:756, 1965

3. Murphy MR, Hug CC: The anesthetic potency of fentanyl in terms of its reduction of enflurane MAC. Anesthesiology 57:485, 1982

4. Smith RA, Winter PM, Smith M, et al: Rapidly developing tolerance to acute exposures to anesthetic agents. Anesthesiology 50:496, 1979

5. Eger EI II: Anesthetic Uptake and Action. Baltimore, Williams & Wilkins, 1974

6. Quasha AL, Eger EI II, Tinker JH: Determination and applications of MAC. Anesthesiology 53:315, 1980

7. Miller KW, Paton WDM, Smith EB: The anaesthetic pressures of certain fluorine-containing gases. Br J Anaesth 39:910, 1967

8. Deady JE, Koblin DD, Eger EI II, et al: Anesthetic potencies and the unitary theory of narcosis. Anesth Analg 60:380, 1981

9. Koblin DD, Deady JE, Eger EI II: Potencies of inhaled anesthetics and alcohol in mice selectively bred for resistance and susceptibility to nitrous oxide anesthesia. Anesthesiology 56:18, 1982

10. Kissin I, Morgan PL, Smith LR: Anesthetic potencies of isoflurane, halothane, and diethyl ether for various end points of anesthesia. Anesthesiology 58:88, 1983

11. Regan MJ, Eger EI II: Effect of hypothermia in dogs on anesthetizing and apneic doses of inhalation agents. Anesthesiology 28:689, 1967

12. Hoffman JC, DiFazio CA: The anesthetic-sparing effect of pentazocine, meperidine, and morphine. Arch Int Pharmacodyn Ther 186:261, 1970

13. Steffey EP, Eger EI II: Hyperthermia and halothane MAC in the dog. Anesthesiology 41:392, 1974

14. Vitez TS, White PF, Eger EI II: Effects of hypothermia on halothane MAC and isoflurane MAC in the rat. Anesthesiology 41:80, 1974

15. Cherkin A, Catchpool JF: Temperature dependence of anesthesia in goldfish. Science 144:1460, 1964

16. Shim CY, Anderson NB: The effect of oxygen on minimal anesthetic requirements in the toad. Anesthesiology 34:333, 1971

17. Lever MJ, Miller KW, Paton WDM, et al: Pressure reversal of anesthesia. Nature 231:368, 1971

18. Halsey MJ, Wardley-Smith B: Pressure reversal of narcosis produced by anesthetics, narcotics and tranquilizers. Nature 257:811, 1975

19. Kent DW, Halsey MJ, Eger EI II, et al: Isoflurane anesthesia and pressure antagonism in mice. Anesth Analg 56:97, 1977

20. Miller KW, Wilson MW: The pressure reversal of a variety of anesthetic agents in mice. Anesthesiology 48:104, 1978

21. Miller KW: The pressure reversal of anesthesia and the critical volume hypothesis, Progress in Anesthesiology, vol 1. Edited by Fink BR. New York, Raven Press, 1975, pp 341–351.

22. Smith RA, Smith M, Eger EI II, et al: Nonlinear antagonism of anesthesia in mice by pressure. Anesth Analg 58:19, 1979

23. Halsey MJ, Eger EI II, Kent DW, et al: High-pressure studies of anesthesia, Progress in Anesthesiology, vol 1: Molecular Mechanisms of Anesthesia. Edited by Fink BR. Raven Press, New York, 1975, pp 353–361

24. Lerman J, Robinson S, Willis MM, et al: Anesthetic requirements for halothane in young children 0–1 month and 1–6 months of age. Anesthesiology 59:421, 1983

25. Gregory GA, Eger EI II, Munson ES: The relationship between age and halothane requirement in man. Anesthesiology 30:488, 1969

26. Koblin DD, Lurz FW, Eger EI II: Age-dependent alterations in nitrous oxide requirement in mice. Anesthesiology 58:428, 1983

27. Tanifuji Y, Eger EI II: Brain sodium, potassium, and osmolality: Effects on anesthetic requirement. Anesth Analg 57:404, 1978

28. LaBella FS: Opiate radioreceptor assay distinguishes between anesthetics and convulsants: The effect of pH. Brain Res 241:378, 1982

29. Siegel JM: Behavioral functions of the reticular formation. Brain Res Rev 1:69, 1979

30. French JD, Verzeano M, Magoun HW: A neural basis of the anesthetic state. Arch Neurol Psychiatry 69:519, 1953

31. Rosner BS, Clark DL: Neurophysiologic effects of general anesthetics:II. Sequential regional actions in the brain. Anesthesiology 39:59, 1973

32. Mori K, Winters WD: Neural background of sleep and anesthesia. Int Anesthesiol Clin 13:67, 1975

33. Winters WD: Effects of drugs on the electrical activity of the brain: Anesthetics. Annu Rev Pharmacol Toxicol 16:413, 1976

34. Angel A: Effect of anaesthetics on nervous pathways, General Anaesthesia. Edited by Gray TC, Nunn JF, Utting JE. London, Butterworth, 1980, pp 117–139

35. Darbinjan TM, Golovchinsky VB, Plehotkina SI: The effects of anesthetics on reticular and cortical activity. Anesthesiology 34:219, 1971

36. Kikuchi H, Kitahata LM, Collins JG, et al: Halothane-induced changes in neuronal activity of cells of the nucleus reticularis gigantocellularis of the cat. Anesth Analg 59:897, 1980

37. Dubois MY, Sato S, Chassy J, et al: Effects of enflurane on brainstem auditory evoked responses in humans. Anesth Analg 61:898, 1982

38. Thornton C, Heneghan CPH, James MFM, et al:

Effects of halothane or enflurane with controlled ventilation on auditory evoked potentials. Br J Anaesth 56:315, 1984

39. Shimoji K, Fujioka H, Ebata T: Anesthetics block excitation with various effects on inhibition in MRF neurons. Brain Res 295:190, 1984

40. Richards CD: In search of the mechanisms of anesthesia. Trends Neurochem Sci 3:9, 1980

41. Rabe LS, Moreno L, Rigor BM, et al: Effects of halothane on evoked field potentials recorded from cortical and subcortical nuclei. Neuropharmacology 19:813, 1980

42. Angel A, Gratton DA: The effect of anaesthetic agents on cerebral cortical responses in the rat. Br J Pharmacol 76:541, 1982

43. Richards CD, Russel WJ, Smaje JC: The action of ether and methoxyflurane on synaptic transmission in isolated preparations of the mammalian cortex. J Physiol (Lond) 248:121, 1975

44. Richards CD, White AE: Actions of volatile anaesthetics on synaptic transmission in the dentate gyrus. J Physiol (Lond) 252:241, 1975

45. Bloom FE, Costa E, Salmoiraghi GC: Anesthesia and the responsiveness of individual neurons of the caudate nucleus of the cat to acetylcholine, norepinephrine and dopamine administered by microelectrophoresis. J Pharmacol Exp Ther 150:244, 1965

46. Crawford JM: Anesthetic agents and the chemical sensitivity of cortical neurones. Neuropharmacology 9:31, 1970

47. Richards CD, Smaje JC: Anaesthetics depress the sensitivity of cortical neurones to L-glutamate. Br J Pharmacol 58:347, 1976

48. Nicoll RA: The effects of anaesthetics on synaptic excitation and inhibition in the olfactory bulb. J Physiol (Lond) 223:803, 1972

49. Scholfield CN: Potentiation of inhibition by general anesthetics in neurones of the olfactory cortex in vitro. Pflugers Arch 383:249, 1980

50. Smaje JC: General anesthetics and the acetylcholine-sensitivity of cortical neurones. Br J Pharmacol 58:359, 1976

51. Morris ME: Synaptic facilitation by general anesthetics, Progress in Anesthesiology, vol 2: Molecular Mechanisms of Anesthesia. Edited by Fink BR. New York, Raven Press, 1980, pp 463–468

52. Galindo A: Effects of procaine, pentobarbital and halothane on synaptic transmission in the central nervous system. J Pharmacol Exp Ther 169:185, 1969

53. de Jong RH, Robles R, Corbin RW, et al: Effect of inhalation anesthetics on monosynaptic and polysynaptic transmission in the spinal cord. J Pharmacol Exp Ther 162:326, 1968

54. Richens A: The action of general anaesthetic agents on root responses of the frog isolated spinal cord. Br J Pharmacol 36:294, 1969

55. Heavner J: Jamming spinal sensory input: Effects of anesthetic and analgesic drugs in the spinal cord dorsal horn. Pain 1:239, 1975

56. Zorychta E, Capek R: Depression of spinal monosynaptic transmission by diethyl ether: Quantal analysis of unitary synaptic potentials. J Pharmacol Exp Ther 207:825, 1978

57. Kitahata LM, Ghazi-Saidi K, Yamashita M, et al: The depressant effect of halothane and sodium thiopental on the spontaneous and evoked activity of dorsal horn cells: Laminal specificity, time course and dose dependence. J Pharmacol Exp Ther 195:515, 1975

58. Namiki A, Collins JG, Kitahata LM, et al: Effects of halothane on spinal neuronal responses to graded noxious heat stimulation in the cat. Anesthesiology 53:475, 1980

59. Komatsu T, Shingu K, Tomemori N, et al: Nitrous-oxide activates the supraspinal pain inhibition system. Acta Anaesthesiol Scand 25:519, 1981

60. Chin JH, Crankshaw DP, Kendig JJ: Changes in the dorsal root potential with diazepam, and with the analgesics aspirin, nitrous oxide, morphine and meperidine. Neuropharmacology 13:305, 1974

61. Eccles JC: The Understanding of the Brain. New York, McGraw-Hill, 1977

62. Larrabee MG, Posternak JM: Selective action of anesthetics on synapses and axons in mammalian sympathetic ganglia. J Neurophysiol 15:91, 1952

63. de Jong RH, Nace RA: Nerve impulse conduction and cutaneous receptor responses during general anesthesia. Anesthesiology 28:851, 1967

64. Bosnjak ZJ, Seagard JL, Wu A, et al: The effects of halothane on sympathetic ganglionic transmission. Anesthesiology 57:473, 1982

65. Roth SH, Smith RA, Paton WDM: Pressure antagonism of anaesthetic-induced conduction failure in frog peripheral nerve. Br J Anaesth 48:621, 1976

66. Kendig JJ, Cohen EN: Pressure antagonism to nerve conduction block by anesthetic agents. Anesthesiology 47:6, 1977

67. Nishino T, Shirahata M, Yonezawa T, et al: Comparison of changes in the hypoglossal and the phrenic nerve activity in reponse to increasing depth of anesthesia in cats. Anesthesiology 60:19, 1984

68. Shrivastav BB, Narahashi T, Kitz RJ, et al: Mode of action of trichloroethylene on squid axon membranes. J Pharmacol Exp Ther 199:179, 1976

69. Kendig JJ, Schneider TM, Cohen EN: Anes-

thetics inhibit pressure-induced repetitive impulse generation. J Appl Physiol 45:747, 1978

70. Bean BP, Shrager P, Goldstein DA: Modification of sodium and potassium channel gating kinetics by ether and halothane. J Gen Physiol 77:233, 1981

71. Haydon DA, Urban BW: The action of hydrocarbons and carbon tetrachloride on the sodium current of the squid axon. J Physiol (Lond) 338:435, 1983

72. Haydon DA, Urban BW: The effects of some inhalation anesthetics on the sodium current of the squid giant axon. J Physiol (Lond) 341:429, 1983

73. Datyner NB, Gage PW: Secretion of acetylcholine in response to graded depolarization of motor nerve terminals. J Physiol (Paris) 78:412, 1982

74. Seeman P: The membrane actions of anesthetics and tranquilizers. Pharmacol Rev 24:583, 1972

75. Haydon DA, Hendry BM: Nerve impulse blockage in squid axons by n-alkanes: The effect of axon diameter. J Physiol (Lond) 333:393, 1982

76. Kendig JJ, Courtney KR, Cohen EN: Anesthetics: Molecular correlates of voltage- and frequency-dependent sodium channel block in nerve. J Pharmacol Exp Ther 210:446, 1979

77. Strichartz G: Use-dependent conduction block produced by volatile general anesthetic agents. Acta Anaesthesiol Scand 24:402, 1980

78. Grossman Y, Kendig JJ: General anesthetic block of a bifurcating axon. Brain Res 245:148, 1982

79. Parmentier JL, Shrivastav BB, Bennett PB, et al: Effect of interaction of volatile anesthetics and high hydrostatic pressure on central neurons. Undersea Biomed Res 6:75, 1979

80. Parmentier JL, Bennett PB: Hydrostatic pressure does not antagonize halothane effects on single neurons of *Aplysia californica*. Anesthesiology 53:9, 1980

81. Roth SH: Membrane and cellular actions of anesthetic agents. Fed Proc 39:1595, 1980

82. Kendig JJ, Trudell JR, Cohen EN: Effects of pressure and anesthetics on conduction and synaptic transmission. J Pharmacol Exp Ther 195:216, 1975

83. Ashford MLJ, MacDonald AG, Wann KT: The effects of hydrostatic pressure on the spontaneous release of transmitter at the frog neuromuscular junction. J Physiol (Lond) 333:531, 1982

84. Bryant HJ, Blankenship JE: Action potentials in single axons: Effects of hyperbaric air and hydrostatic pressure. J Appl Physiol 47:561, 1979

85. Kendig JJ: Nitrogen narcosis and pressure reversal of anesthetic effects in node of Ranvier. Am J Physiol 246:C91, 1984

86. Richards CD: The action of anesthetics on synaptic transmission. Gen Pharmacol 9:287, 1978

87. Hajos F, Csillag A, Kalman M: The effect of pentobarbital, chloralhydrate, ether, and protoveratrine on the distribution of synaptic vesicles in rat cortical synaptosomes. Exp Brain Res 33:91, 1978

88. Jones DG: Recent perspectives on the organization of central synapses. Anesth Analg 62:1100, 1983

89. Roizen MF, Thoa NB, Moss J, et al: Inhibition by halothane of release of norepinephrine, but not of dopamine-beta-hydroxylase, from guinea-pig vas deferens. Eur J Pharmacol 31:313, 1975

90. Muldoon SM, Vanhoutte PM, Lorenz RR, et al: Venomotor changes caused by halothane acting on sympathetic nerves. Anesthesiology 43:41, 1975

91. Gothert M, Duhrsen U, Rieckesmann JM: Ethanol, anesthetics and other lipophilic drugs preferentially inhibit 5-hydroxytryptamine- and acetylcholine-induced noradrenaline release from sympathetic nerves. Arch Int Pharmacodyn Ther 242:196, 1979

92. Gothert M, Dorn W, Loewenstein I: Inhibition of catecholamine release from the adrenal medulla by halothane. Naunyn Schmiedebergs Arch Pharmacol 294:239, 1976

93. Sumikawa K, Matsumoto T, Ishizaka N, et al: Mechanism of the differential effects of halothane on the nicotinic- and muscarinic-receptor mediated responses of the dog adrenal medulla. Anesthesiology 57:444, 1982

94. Sumikawa K, Amakata Y, Kashimoto T, et al: Effects of cyclopropane on catecholamine release from bovine adrenal medulla. Anesthesiology 53:49, 1980

95. Sumikawa K, Amakata Y, Yoshikawa K, et al: Catecholamine uptake and release in isolated chromaffin granules exposed to halothane. Anesthesiology 53:385, 1980

96. Westfall TC, DiFazio CA, Saunders J: Local anesthetic- and halothane-induced alteration of the stimulation-induced release of ^{3}H-dopamine from rat striatal slices. Anesthesiology 48:118, 1978

97. Pepeu G: The release of acetylcholine from the brain: An approach to the study of the central cholinergic mechanisms. Prog Neurobiol 2:257, 1973

98. Soubrie P, Blas C, Ferron A, et al: Chlordiazepoxide reduces *in vivo* serotonin release in the basal ganglia of *Encephale isole* but not anesthetized cats: Evidence for a dorsal raphe site of action. J Pharmacol Exp Ther 226:526, 1983

99. Speden RN: The effect of some volatile anesthetics on transmurally stimulated guinea-pig ileum. Br J Pharmacol Chemother 25:104, 1965

100. Little HJ, Paton WDM: The effects of high-pressure helium and nitrogen on the release of acetylcholine from the guinea-pig ileum. Br J Pharmacol 67:221, 1979

101. Halliday DJX, Little HJ, Paton WDM: The effects of inert gases and other general anesthetics on the release of acetylcholine from the guinea-pig ileum. Br J Pharmacol 67:229, 1979

102. Christ D: Effects of halothane on ganglionic discharges. J Pharmacol Exp Ther 200:336, 1977

103. Waud BE, Waud DR: Comparison of the effects of general anesthetics on the end-plate of skeletal muscle. Anesthesiology 43:540, 1975

104. Kennedy RD, Galindo AD: Comparative site of action of various anesthestic agents at the mammalian myoneural junction. Br J Anaesth 47:533, 1975

105. Gage PW, Hamill O: General anesthetics: Depression consistent with increased membrane fluidity. Neurosci Lett 1:61, 1975

106. Gage PW, Hamill O: Effects of several inhalation anaesthetics on the kinetics of postsynaptic conductance changes in mouse diaphragm. Br J Pharmacol 57:263, 1976

107. Gage PW, Hamill O, Van Helden D: Dual effects of ether on end-plate currents. J Physiol (Lond) 287:353, 1979

108. Gage PW, Hamill OP: Effects of anesthetics on ion channels in synapses. Int Rev Physiol 25:1, 1981

109. James B: The toad in the hole: An hypothesis to explain the action of anaesthetics. Br J Anaesth 52:359, 1980

110. Sugai N, Maruyama H, Goto K: Effect of nitrous oxide alone or its combination with fentanyl on spinal reflexes in cats. Br J Anaesth 54:567, 1982

111. Ngai SH, Cheney DL, Finck AD: Acetylcholine concentrations and turnover in rat brain structures during anesthesia with halothane, enflurane, and ketamine. Anesthesiology 48:4, 1978

112. Cheney DL, Ngai SH: Effects of anesthetics and related drugs on the acetylcholine turnover rate in various structures of the rat brain, Progress in Anesthesiology, vol 2: Molecular Mechanisms of Anesthesia. Edited by Fink BR. New York, Raven Press, 1980, pp 189–198

113. Gibson GE, Duffy TE: Impaired synthesis of acetylcholine by mild hypoxic hypoxia or nitrous oxide. J Neurochem 36:28, 1981

114. Roizen MF, Kopin IJ, Thoa NB, et al: The effect of two anesthetic agents on norepinephrine and dopamine in discrete brain nuclei, fiber tracts, and terminal regions of the rat. Brain Res 110:515, 1976

115. Rosenberg PH, Klinge E: Some effects of enflurane anesthesia on biogenic amines in the brain and plasma of rats. Br J Anaesth 46:708, 1974

116. Roizen MF, Kopin IJ, Palkovits M, et al: The effect of two diverse inhalation anesthetic agents on serotonin in discrete regions of the rat brain. Exp Brain Res 24:203, 1975

117. Westerink BHC, Lejeune B, Korf J, et al: On the significance of regional dopamine metabolism in the rat brain for the classification of centrally acting drugs. Eur J Pharmacol 42:179, 1977

118. Cheng SC, Brunner EA: Inhibition of GABA metabolism in rat brain slices by halothane. Anesthesiology 55:26, 1981

119. Cheng SC, Brunner EA: Effect of anesthetic agents on synaptosomal GABA disposal. Anesthesiology 55:34, 1981

120. Nahrwold ML, Hess WH, Bethell DR: Halothane and gamma-aminobutyric acid in cultured cells of nervous system origin. Brain Res Bull (suppl 2), 5:477, 1980

121. Miller RD, Way WL, Eger EI II: The effects of alpha-methyldopa, reserpine, guanethidine, and iproniazid on minimum alveolar anesthetic requirement (MAC). Anesthesiology 29:1153, 1968

122. Johnston RR, Way WL, Miller RD: The effect of CNS catecholamine-depleting drugs on dextroamphetamine-induced elevation of halothane MAC. Anesthesiology 41:57, 1974

123. Mueller RA, Smith RD, Spruill WA, et al: Central monoaminergic neuronal effects on minimum alveolar concentrations (MAC) of halothane and cyclopropane in rats. Anesthesiology 42:143, 1975

124. Raja SN, Moscicki JC, Woodside JR, et al: The effect of acute phencyclidine administration on cyclopropane requirement (MAC) in rats. Anesthesiology 56:275, 1982

125. Johnston RR, White PF, Eger EI II: Comparative effects of dextroamphetamine and reserpine on halothane and cyclopropane anesthetic requirements. Anesth Analg 54:655, 1975

126. Kaukinen S, Pyykko K: The potentiation of halothane anesthesia by clonidine. Acta Anaesthiol Scand 23:107, 1979

127. Bloor BC, Flacke WE: Reduction in halothane anesthetic requirement by clonidine, an alpha adrenergic agonist. Anesth Analg 61:741, 1982

128. Roizen MF, White PF, Eger EI II, Brownstein M: Effects of ablation of serotonin or norepinephrine brainstem areas on halothane and cyclopropane MACs in rats. Anesthesiology 49:252, 1978

129. Meyer KH: Contributions to the theory of narcosis. Trans Faraday Soc 33:1062, 1937

130. Miller KW, Paton WDM, Smith EB, et al: Physicochemical approaches to the mode of action of general anesthetics. Anesthesiology 36:339, 1972

131. Koblin DD, Eger EI II: Theories of narcosis. N Engl J Med 301:1222, 1979

132. Roth SH: Mechanisms of anaesthesia: A review. Can Anaesth Soc J 27:433, 1980

133. Janoff AS, Miller KW: A critical assessment of the lipid theories of general anesthetic action, Biological Membranes. Edited by Chapman D. London, Academic Press, 1982, pp 417–476

134. Eger EI II, Lundgren C, Miller SL, et al: Anesthetic potencies of sulfur hexafluoride, chloroform, and Ethrane in dogs. Anesthesiology 30:129, 1969

135. Miller JC, Miller KW: Approaches to the mechanisms of action of general anesthetics, MTP International Review of Science, Biochemistry Series 1, vol 12. Edited by Blaschko HKF. London, Butterworth, 1975, pp 33–76

136. Kaufman RD: Biophysical mechanisms of anesthetic action. Anesthesiology 46:49, 1977

137. Richards CD: Anesthetics and membranes. Int Rev Biochem 19:157, 1978

138. Wardley-Smith B, Halsey MJ: Recent molecular theories of general anesthesia. Br J Anaesth 51:619, 1979

139. Burnie JP: Molecular mechanisms of general anaesthesia. Anaesthesia 36:1027, 1981

140. Mullins LJ: Some physical mechanisms in narcosis. Chem Rev 54:289, 1954

141. Miller KW, Wilson MW, Smith RA: Pressure resolves two sites of action of inert gases. Mol Pharmacol 14:950, 1978

142. Franks NP, Lieb WR: Where do general anesthetics act? Nature 274:339, 1978

143. Franks NP, Lieb WR: Molecular mechanisms of general anesthesia. Nature 300:487, 1982

144. Miller RD, Wahrenbrock EA, Schroeder CF, et al: Ethylene–halothane anesthesia. Anesthesiology 31:301, 1969

145. DiFazio CA, Brown RE, Ball CG, et al: Additive effects of anesthetics and theories of anesthesia. Anesthesiology 36:57, 1972

146. Clarke RF, Daniels S, Harrison CB, et al: Potency of mixtures of general anesthetic agents. Br J Anaesth 50:979, 1978

147. Eger EI II: MAC, Nitrous Oxide/N$_2$O. Edited by Eger EI II. New York, Elsevier, 1985, pp 57–67

148. Koblin DD, Eger EI II, Johnson BH, et al: Minimum alveolar concentrations and oil/gas partition coefficients of four anesthetic isomers. Anesthesiology 54:314, 1981

149. Rudo FG, Krantz JC: Anesthetic molecules. Br J Anaesth 46:181, 1974

150. Burns THS, Hall JM, Bracken A, et al: Fluorine compounds in anaesthesia (9). Examination of six aliphatic compounds and four ethers. Anaesthesia 37:278, 1982

151. Koblin DD, Eger EI II, Johnson BH, et al: Are convulsant gases also anesthetics? Anesth Analg 60:464, 1981

152. Stevens JE, Fujinaga M, Oshima E, et al: The biphasic pattern of the convulsive property of enflurane in cats. Br J Anaesth 56:395, 1984

153. Smith RA, Paton WDM: The anesthetic effect of oxygen. Anesth Analg 55:734, 1976

154. Cohen S, Goldschmid A, Shtacher G, et al: The inhalation convulsants: a pharmacodynamic approach. Mol Pharmacol 11:379, 1975

155. Richter J, Landau EM, Cohen S: Anaesthetic and convulsant ethers act on different sites at the crab neuromuscular junction *in vitro*. Nature 266:70, 1977

156. Landau EM, Richter J, Cohen S: The mean conductance and open-time of the acetylcholine receptor channels can be independently modified by some anesthetic and convulsant ethers. Mol Pharmacol 16:1075, 1979

157. Gage PW, Sah P: Postsynaptic effects of some central stimulants at the neuromuscular junction. Br J Pharmacol 75:493, 1982

158. Landau EM, Richter J, Cohen S: Differential solubilities in subregions of the membrane: A nonsteric mechanism of drug specificity. J Med Chem 22:325, 1979

159. Mullins LJ: Anesthetics, Handbook of Neurochemistry, vol 6. Edited by Laitha A. New York, Plenum Press, 1971, pp 395–421

160. Haydon DA, Requena J, Urban BW: Some effects of aliphatic hydrocarbons on the electrical capacity and ionic currents of the squid axon membrane. J Physiol (Lond) 309:229, 1980

161. Janoff AS, Pringle MJ, Miller KW: Correlation of general anesthetic potency with solubility in membranes. Biochim Biophys Acta 649:125, 1981

162. Pringle MJ, Brown KB, Miller KW: Can the lipid theories of anesthesia account for the cutoff in anesthetic potency in homologous series of alcohols? Mol Pharmacol 19:49, 1981

163. Pauling L: A molecular theory of general anesthesia. Science 134:15, 1961

164. Miller SL: A theory of gaseous anesthetics. Proc Natl Acad Sci USA 47:1515, 1961

165. Yokono S, Shieh DD, Goto H, et al: Hydrogen bonding and anesthetic potency. J Med Chem 25:873, 1982

166. Hobza P, Sandorfy C: Quantum chemical and statistical thermodynamic investigations of anesthetic activity. 3. The interaction between CH_4, $CHCl_3$, CH_2Cl_2, $CHCl_3$, CCl_4, and an OH—O hydrogen bond. Can J Chem 62:606, 1984

167. Wood S, Wardley-Smith B, Halsey MJ, et al: Hydrogen bonding in mechanisms of anesthesia tested with chloroform and deuterated chloroform. Br J Anaesth 54:387, 1982

168. Vulliemoz Y, Triner L, Verosky M, et al: Deuterated halothane—Anesthetic potency, anticon-

vulsant activity, and effect on cerebellar cyclic guanosine 3′,5′-monophosphate. Anesth Analg 63:495, 1984

169. Suezaki Y, Kaneshina S, Ueda I: Statistical mechanics of pressure-anesthetic antagonism on the phase transition of phospholipid membranes: Interfacial water hypothesis. J Colloid Interface Sci 93:225, 1983

170. Hunt GRA, Jones IC: A^{1}H-NMR investigation of the effects of ethanol and general anesthetics on ion channels and membrane fusion using unilamellar phospholipid membranes. Biochim Biophys Acta 736:1, 1983

171. Shibata A, Suezaki Y, Kamaya H, et al: Adsorption of inhalation anesthetics on air/water interface and the effect of water structure. Biochim Biophys Acta 646:126, 1981

172. Yoshida T, Okabayashi H, Takahashi K, et al: A proton nuclear magnetic resonance study on the release of bound water by inhalation anesthetic in water-in-oil emulsion. Biochim Biophys Acta 772:102, 1984

173. Hansch C, Vittoria A, Silipo C, et al: Partition coefficients and the structure activity relationship of the anesthetic gases. J Med Chem 18:546, 1975

174. Katz Y, Simon SA: Physical parameters of the anesthetic site. Biochim Biophys Acta 471:1, 1977

175. Caughey JM, Lumb WV, Caughey WS: Detection and characterization of nitrous oxide sites in the brain of a dog under halothane–N_2O anesthesia by infrared spectroscopy. Biochem Biophys Res Commun 78:897, 1977

176. Wyrwicz AM, Pszenny MH, Schofield JC, et al: Noninvasive observations of fluorinated anesthetics in rabbit brain by fluorine-19 nuclear magnetic resonance. Science 222:428, 1983

177. Volgyesi GA: The mechanism of anesthesia: A new hypothesis based on the effects on electrical properties of a model membrane: Preliminary studies. Can Anaesth Soc J 25:173, 1978

178. Miller KW: Inert gas narcosis, the high pressure neurological syndrome, and the critical volume hypothesis. Science 185:867, 1974

179. Mori T, Matubayasi N, Ueda I: Membrane expansion and inhalational anesthetics. Mean excess volume hypothesis. Mol Pharmacol 25:123, 1984

180. Miller KW, Paton WDM, Smith RA, et al: The pressure reversal of anesthesia and the critical volume hypothesis. Mol Pharmacol 9:131, 1973

181. Halsey MJ: Effects of high pressure on the central nervous system. Physiol Rev 62:1341, 1982

182. Brauer RW, Hogan PM, Hugon M, et al: Patterns of interaction of effects of light metabolically inert gases with those of hydrostatic pressure as

such—A review. Undersea Biomed Res 9:353, 1982

183. Smith RA, Dodson BA, Miller KW: The interaction between pressure and anaesthetics. Philos Trans R Soc Lond [Biol] 304:69, 1984

184. Allott PR, Steward A, Flook V, et al: Variation with temperature of the solubilities of inhaled anesthetics in water, oil, and biological media. Br J Anaesth 45:294, 1973

185. White DC, Halsey MJ: Effects of changes in temperature and pressure during experimental anaesthesia. Br J Anaesth 46:196, 1976

186. Halsey MJ, Wardley-Smith B: Non-anaesthetic steroids ameliorate the high pressure neurological syndrome in rats. Neuropharmacology 22:103, 1983

187. Halsey MJ, Wardley-Smith B, Green CJ: Pressure reversal of anesthesia—A multisite expansion hypothesis. Br J Anaesth 50:1091, 1978

188. Fernandez JM, Bezanilla F, Taylor RE: Effect of chloroform on charge movement in the nerve membrane. Nature 297:150, 1982

189. Nicoll RA, Madison DV: General anesthetics hyperpolarize neurons in the vertebrate central nervous system. Science 217:1055, 1982

190. Lechleiter J, Moffett S, Gruener R: Effects of halothane on the acetylcholine receptor channel in cultured *Xenopus* myocytes. Biophys J 45:15, 1984

191. Krnjevic K: Central actions of general anesthetics, Molecular Mechanisms of General Anesthesia. Edited by Halsey MJ, Millar RA, Sutton JA Edinburgh. Churchill Livingstone, 1974, pp 65–89

192. Biebuyck JF: Effects of anaesthetic agents on metabolic pathways: Fuel utilization and supply during anaesthesia. Br J Anaesth 45:263, 1973

193. Brunner EA, Cheng SC, Berman ML: Effects of anesthesia on intermediary metabolism. Annu Rev Med 26:391, 1975

194. Rottenberg H: Uncoupling of oxidative phosphorylation in rat liver mitochondria by general anesthetics. Proc Natl Acad Sci USA 80:3313, 1983

195. Hawkins RA, Biebuyck JF: Regional brain function during graded halothane anesthesia, Progress in Anesthesiology, vol 2. Molecular Mechanisms of Anesthesia. Edited by Fink BR. New York, Raven Press, 1980, pp 145–156

196. Cohen PJ: Effect of hydrostatic pressure on halothane-induced depression of mitochondrial respiration. Life Sci 32:1647, 1983

197. Allison AC, Nunn JF: Effects of general anesthetics on microtubules. Lancet 2:1326, 1968

198. Saubermann AJ, Gallagher ML: Mechanisms of general anesthesia: Failure of pentobarbital and

halothane to depolymerize microtubules in mouse optic nerve. Anesthesiology 38:25, 1973

199. Hinkley RE, Green LS: Effects of halothane and colchicine on microtubules and electrical activity of rabbit vagus nerves. J Neurobiol 2:97, 1971

200. Chang DC: A voltage-clamp study of the effects of colchicine on the squid giant axon. J Cell Physiol 115:260, 1983

201. Salmon ED: Pressure-induced depolymerization of brain microtubules in vitro. Science 189:884, 1975

202. Unwin N, Henderson R: Structure of proteins in biological membranes. Sci Am 250(2):78, 1984

203. Breckenridge WC, Gombos G, Morgan IG: The lipid composition of adult rat brain synaptosomal plasma membranes. Biochim Biophys Acta 266:695, 1972

204. Bangham AD: Liposome Letters. London, Academic Press, 1983

205. Catterall WA: The molecular basis of neuronal excitability. Science 223:653, 1984

206. Kamaya H, Kaneshina S, Ueda I: Partition equilibrium of inhalation anesthetics and alcohols between water and membranes of phospholipids with varying acyl chain-lengths. Biochim Biophys Acta 646:135, 1981

207. Katz Y: Solubility of noble gases in phospholipid membranes. A potential probe for function and structure. Biochim Biophys Acta 647:119, 1981

208. Smith RA, Porter EG, Miller KW: The solubility of anesthetic gases in lipid bilayers. Biochim Biophys Acta 645:327, 1981

209. Miller KW, Hammond L, Porter EG: The solubility of hydrocarbon gases in lipid bilayers. Chem Phys Lipids 20:229, 1977

210. Simon SA, McIntosh TJ, Bennett PB, et al: Interaction of halothane with lipid bilayers. Mol Pharmacol 16:163, 1979

211. Lieb WR, Kovalycrik M, Mendelsohn R: Do clinical levels of general anesthetics affect lipid bilayers? Evidence from Raman scattering. Biochim Biophys Acta 688:388, 1982

212. Kaneshina S, Kamaya H, Ueda I: Thermodynamics of pressure-anesthetic antagonism on the phase transition of lipid membranes: Displacement of anesthetic molecules. J Colloid Interface Sci 93:215,1983

213. Miller KW, Wu SCT: The dependence of the lipid bilayer membrane: buffer partition coefficient of pentobarbitone on pH and lipid composition. Br J Pharmacol 61:57, 1977

214. Trudell JR, Hubbell WL, Cohen EN, et al: Pressure reversal of anesthesia: The extent of small molecule exclusion from spin-labeled phospholipid model membranes. Anesthesiology 38:207, 1973

215. Boggs JM, Roth SH, Yoong T, et al: Site and mechanism of anesthetic action. II. Pressure effect on the nerve conduction-blocking activity of a spin label anesthetic. Mol Pharmacol 12:136, 1976

216. Trudell JR, Hubbell WL: Localization of molecular halothane in phospholipid bilayer model nerve membranes. Anesthesiology 44:202, 1976

217. Koehler LS, Fossel ET, Koehler KA: Halothane fluorine-19 nuclear magnetic resonance in dipalmitoylphosphatidylcholine liposomes. Biochemistry 16:3700, 1977

218. Kaneshina S, Lin HC, Ueda I: Anisotropic solubilisation of an inhalation anesthetic, methoxyflurane, into the interfacial region of cationic surfactant micelles. Biochim Biophys Acta 647:223, 1981

219. Miller KW, Reo NV, Schoot Uiterkamp AJM, et al: Xenon NMR: Chemical shifts of a general anesthetic in common solvents, proteins, and membranes. Proc Natl Acad Sci USA 78:4946, 1981

220. McIntosh TJ, Costello MJ: Effects of n-alkanes on the morphology of lipid bilayers. A freeze-fracture and negative-stain analysis. Biochim Biophys Acta 645:318, 1981

221. White SH, King GI, Cain JE: Location of hexane in lipid bilayers determined by neutron diffraction. Nature 290:161, 1981

222. Yokono S, Shieh DS, Ueda I: Interfacial preference of anesthetic action upon the phase transition of phospholipid bilayers and partition equilibrium of inhalation anesthetics between membrane and deuterium oxide. Biochim Biophys Acta 645:237, 1981

223. Johnson SM, Miller KW, Bangham AD: The opposing effects of pressure and general anaesthetics on the cation permeability of liposomes of varying lipid composition. Biochim Biophys Acta 307:42, 1973

224. Pang KY, Chang TL, Miller KW: On the coupling between anesthetic-induced membrane lipid fluidization and cation permeability in lipid vesicles. Mol Pharmacol 15:729, 1979

225. Dluzewski AR, Halsey MJ: Clinical concentrations of halothane increase the conductance of black lipid membranes, Progress in Anesthesiology, vol 2: Molecular Mechanisms of Anesthesia. Edited by Fink BR. New York, Raven Press, 1980, pp 405–409

226. Reyes J, Latorre R: Effect of the anesthetics benzyl alcohol and chloroform on bilayers made from monolayers. Biophys J 28:259, 1979

227. Okuda C: The effects of volatile anesthetics on the binding of 1-anilino-8-napthalene sulfonate to biological membranes and lipid vesicles: The role of cholesterol. J Biochem (Tokyo) 92:357, 1982

228. Cafiso DS, Hubbell WL: Electrogenic H^+/OH^- movement across phospholipid vesicles measured by spin-labeled hydrophobic ions. Biophys J 44:49, 1983

229. Bangham AD, Mason WT: Anesthetics may act by collapsing pH gradients. Anesthesiology 53:135, 1980

230. Clements JA, Wilson KM: The affinity of narcotic agents for interfacial films. Proc Natl Acad Sci USA 48:1008, 1962

231. Ueda I, Shieh DD, Eyring H: Anesthetic interactions with a model cell membrane. Anesthesiology 41:217, 1974

232. Seeman P, Roth SH: General anesthetics expand cell membranes at surgical concentrations. Biochim Biophys Acta 255:171, 1972

233. Bull MH, Brailsford JD, Bull BS: Erythrocyte membrane expansion due to the volatile anesthetics, the 1-alkanols, and benzyl alcohol. Anesthesiology 57:399, 1982

234. Trudell JR: The membrane volume occupied by anesthetic molecules: A reinterpretation of the erythrocyte expansion data. Biochim Biophys Acta 470: 509, 1977

235. Kita Y, Bennett LJ, Miller KW: The partial molar volumes of anesthetics in lipid bilayers. Biochim Biophys Acta 647:130, 1981

236. Matubayasi N, Ueda I: Is membrane expansion relevant to anesthesia? Mean excess volume. Anesthesiology 59:541, 1983

237. Mori T, Matubayasi N, Ueda I: Membrane expansion and inhalation anesthetics. Mean excess volume hypothesis. Mol Pharmacol 25:123, 1984

238. Franks NP, Lieb WR: Is membrane expansion relevant to anaesthesia? Nature 292:248, 1981

239. Haydon DA, Hendry BM, Levinson SR, et al: The molecular mechanism of anesthesia. Nature 268:356, 1977

240. Haydon DA, Hendry BM, Levinson SR, et al: Anesthesia by the n-alkanes. Biochim Biophys Acta 470:17, 1977

241. Haydon DA, Kimura JE: Some effects of n-pentane on the sodium and potassium currents of the squid giant axon. J Physiol (Lond) 312:57, 1981

242. Padron R, Mateu L, Requena J: A dynamic x-ray diffraction study of anesthetic action. Thickening of the myelin membrane by n-pentane. Biochim Biophys Acta 552:535, 1979

243. Padron R. Mateu L, Requena J: A dynamic x-ray diffraction study of anesthesia action. Changes in myelin structure and electrical activity recorded simultaneously from frog sciatic nerves treated with n-alkanes. Biochim Biophys Acta 602:221, 1980

244. Lea EJA: Effect of n-alkanes on membranes in lipid–water systems. Int J Biol Macromol 1:185, 1979

245. McIntosh TJ, Simon SA, MacDonald RC: The organization of n-alkanes in lipid bilayers. Biochim Biophys Acta 597:445, 1980

246. Franks NP, Lieb WR: The structure of lipid bilayers and the effects of general anaesthetics. An x-ray and neutron diffraction study. J Mol Biol 133:469, 1979

247. Cornell BA, Separovic F: Membrane thickness and acyl chain length. Biochim Biophys Acta 733:189, 1983

248. Yoshida T, Mori T, Ueda I: Giant planar lipid bilayer. I. Capacitance and its biphasic response to inhalation anesthetics. J Colloid Interface Sci 96:39, 1983

249. Trudell JR, Hubbell WL, Cohen EN: The effect of two inhalation anaesthetics on the order of spin-labeled phospholipid vesicles. Biochim Biophys Acta 291:321, 1973

250. Kendig JJ, Trudell JR, Cohen EN: Halothane stereoisomers: Lack of stereospecificity in two model systems. Anesthesiology 39:518, 1973

251. Chin JH, Trudell JR, Cohen EN: The compression-ordering and solubility-disordering effects of high pressure gases on phospholipid bilayers. Life Sci 18:489, 1976

252. Vanderkooi JM, Landesberg R, Selick H, et al: Interaction of general anesthetics with phospholipid vesicles and biological membranes. Biochim Biophys Acta 464:1, 1977

253. Puskin JS, Martin T: Effects of anesthetics on divalent cation binding and fluidity of phosphatidylserine vesicles. Mol Pharmacol 14:454, 1978

254. Trudell JR, Hubbell WL, Cohen EN: Pressure reversal of inhalation anesthetic-induced disorder in spin-labeled phospholipid vesicles. Biochim Biophys Acta 291:328, 1973

255. Mastrangelo CJ, Trudell JR, Cohen EN: Antagonism of membrane compression effects by high pressure gas mixtures in a phospholipid bilayer system. Life Sci 22:239, 1978

256. Miller KW, Pang KY: General anesthetics can selectively perturb lipid bilayer membranes. Nature 263:253, 1976

257. Mastrangelo CJ, Trudell JR, Edmunds HN, et al: Effect of clinical concentrations of halothane on phospholipid-cholesterol membrane fluidity. Mol Pharmacol 14:463, 1978

258. Finch ED, Kiesow LA: Pressure, anesthetics, and membrane structure: A spin-probe study. Undersea Biomed Res 6:41, 1979

259. Lenaz G, Curatola G, Mazzanti L, et al: Spin label studies on the effect of anesthetics in synaptic membranes. J Neurochem 32:1689, 1979

260. Rosenberg PH: Effects of halothane, lidocaine,

and 5-hydroxytryptamine on fluidity of synaptic membranes, myelin membranes, and synaptic mitochondrial membranes. Naunyn Schmiedebergs Arch Pharmacol 307:199, 1979

261. Miller C: Integral membrane channels: Studies in model membranes. Physiol Rev 63:1209, 1983

262. Lechleiter J, Gruener R: Halothane shortens acetylcholine channel kinetics without affecting conductance. Proc Natl Acad Sci USA 81:2929, 1984

263. Rosenberg PH, Heavner JE: Temperature dependent nerve-blocking concentration of lidocaine and halothane. Acta Anaesthesiol Scand 24:314, 1980

264. Chapman D: Phase transitions and fluidity characteristics of lipids and cell membranes. Q Rev Biophys 8:185, 1975

265. Hill MW: The effect of anaesthetic-like molecules on the phase transition in smectic mesophases of dipalmitoyllecithin. I. The normal alcohols up to C=9 and three inhalation anesthetics. Biochim Biophys Acta 356:117, 1974

266. MacDonald AG: A dilatometric investigation of the effects of general anesthetics, alcohols, and hydrostatic pressure on the phase transition in smectic mesophases of dipalmitoyl phosphatidylcholine. Biochim Biophys Acta 507:26, 1978

267. Mountcastle DB, Biltonen RL, Halsey MJ: Effects of anesthetics and pressure on the thermotropic behavior of multilamellar dipalmitoyl phosphatidylcholine liposomes. Proc Natl Acad Sci USA 75:4906, 1978

268. MacNaughton W, MacDonald AG: Effects of gaseous anaesthetics and inert gases on the phase transition in smectic mesophases of dipalmitoylphosphatidylcholine. Biochim Biophys Acta 597:193, 1980

269. Jacobs RE, White SH: Behavior of hexane dissolved in dimyristoylphosphatidylcholine bilayers: An NMR and calorimetric study. J Am Chem Soc 106:915, 1984

270. Galla HJ, Trudell JR: Asymmetric antagonistic effects of an inhalation anesthetic and high pressure on the phase transition temperature of dipalmitoyl phosphatidic acid bilayers. Biochim Biophys Acta 599:336, 1980

271. Lee AG: Model for action of local anesthetics. Nature 262:545, 1976

272. Trudell JR: A unitary theory of anesthesia based on lateral phase separations in nerve membranes. Anesthesiology 46:5, 1977

273. Trudell JR, Payan DG, Chin JH, et al: The antagonistic effect of an inhalation anesthetic and high pressure on the phase diagram of mixed dipalmitoyl-dimyristoylphosphatidyl-

choline bilayers. Proc Natl Acad Sci USA 72:210, 1975

274. Calderini G, Bonetti AC, Battistella A, et al: Biochemical changes of rat membranes with aging. Neurochem Res 8:483, 1983

275. Nagy K, Simon P, Nagy IZ: Spin label studies on synaptosomal membranes of rat brain cortex during aging. Biochem Biophys Res Commun 117:688, 1983

276. Armbrecht HJ, Wood WG, Wise RW, et al: Ethanol-induced disordering of membranes from different age groups of C57BL/6NNYA mice. J Pharmacol Exp Ther 226:387, 1983

277. Schoenborn BP: Binding of anesthetics to protein: An x-ray crystallographic investigation. Fed Proc 27:888, 1968

278. Tilton RF Jr, Kuntz ID Jr: Nuclear magnetic resonance studies of Xenon-129 with myoglobin and hemoglobin. Biochemistry 21:6850, 1982

279. Laasberg LH, Hedley-Whyte J: Optical rotary dispersion of hemoglobin and polypeptides. Effect of halothane. J Biol Chem 246:4886, 1971

280. Halsey MJ, Brown FF, Richards RE: Perturbations of model protein systems as a basis for the central and peripheral mechanisms of general anesthesia, Molecular Interactions and Activity in Proteins. CIBA Foundation Symposium 60. Amsterdam, Excerpta Medica, 1978, pp 123–136.

281. Balasubramanian D, Wetlaufer DB: Reversible alteration of the structure of globular proteins by anesthetic agents. Proc Natl Acad Sci USA 55:762, 1966

282. Wishnia A, Pinder TW: Hydrophobic interactions in proteins. The alkane binding site of beta-lactoglobulins A and B. Biochemistry 5:1534, 1966

283. Sachsenheimer W, Pai EF, Schulz GE, et al: Halothane binds in the adenine-specific niche of crystalline adenylate kinase. FEBS Lett 79:310, 1977

284. Mashimo T, Suezaki Y, Ueda I: Anesthetic–protein interaction: Suppression of dye binding and limitation of applicability of the Scatchard plot. Physiol Chem Phys 14:543, 1982

285. Ueda I, Mashimo T: Anesthetics expand partial molal volume of lipid-free protein dissolved in water: Electrostriction hypothesis. Physiol Chem Phys 14:157, 1982

286. Stone WL: Hydrophobic interaction of alkanes with liposomes and lipoproteins. J Biol Chem 250:4368, 1975

287. Wyrwicz AM, Li Y, Schofield JC, Burt CT: Multiple environments of fluorinated anesthetics in intact tissues observed with ^{19}F-NMR spectroscopy. FEBS Lett 162:334, 1983

288. Brown FF, Halsey MJ: Interactions of anesthetics with proteins, Progress in Anesthesiology, Vol 2: Molecular Mechanisms of Anesthesia, Edited by Fink BR. New York, Raven Press, 1980, p 385

289. Johnson FH, Eyring H, Stover BJ: Reaction rate theory in bioluminescence and other life phenomena. Annu Rev Biophys Bioeng 6:111, 1977

290. Middleton AJ, Smith EB: General anaesthetics and bacterial luminescence. II. The effect of diethyl ether on the *in vitro* light emission of *Vibrio fisheri*. Proc R Soc Lond [Biol] 193:173, 1976

291. White DC, Wardley-Smith B, Adey G: The site of action of anesthetics on bacterial luminescence. Life Sci 12:453, 1973

292. Ueda I, Kamaya H: Kinetic and thermodynamic aspects of the mechanism of general anesthesia in a model system of firefly luminescence *in vitro*. Anesthesiology 38:425, 1973

293. Kamaya H, Ueda I, Eyring H: Reversible and irreversible inhibition by anesthetics of the calcium-induced luminescence of aequorin. Proc Natl Acad Sci USA 74:5534, 1977

294. Baker FF, Schapira AHV: Anaesthetics increase light emission from aequorin at constant ionized calcium. Nature 284:168, 1980

295. Brammal A, Beard DJ, Hulands GH: Inhalation anaesthetics and their interaction *in vitro* with glutamate dehydrogenase and other enzymes. Br J Anaesth 46:643, 1974

296. Maheshwari UR, Chan SL, Trevor A: Reversible inhibition of mammalian brain acetylcholinesterase and sodium potassium-stimulated adenosine triphosphatase by cyclopropane. Biochem Pharmacol 24:663, 1975

297. Levitt JD: The effects of halothane and enflurane on rat brain synaptosomal sodium-potassium-activated adenosine triphosphatase. Anesthesiology 42:267, 1975

298. Braswell LM, Kitz RJ: The effect *in vitro* of volatile anesthetics on the activity of cholinesterases. J Neurochem 29:665, 1977

299. Strombom U, Forn J, Dolphin AC, et al: Regulation of the state of phosphorylation of specific neuronal proteins in mouse brain by *in vivo* administration of anesthetic and convulsant agents. Proc Natl Acad Sci USA 76:4687, 1979

300. Bielicki L, Krieglstein J: The effect of anesthesia on brain mitochondrial hexokinase. Naunyn Schmiedebergs Arch Pharmacol 298:229, 1977

301. Masserano JM, Weiner N: The rapid activation of adrenal tyrosine hydroxylase by decapitation and its relationship to a cyclic AMP-phosphorylating mechanism. Mol Pharmacol 16:513, 1979

302. Malinconico SM, McCarl RL: Effect of halothane on cardiac sarcoplasmic reticulum Ca^{+2}-ATPase at low calcium concentrations. Mol Pharmacol 22:8, 1982

303. Koblin DD, Waskell L, Watson JE, et al: Nitrous oxide inactivates methionine synthetase in human liver. Anesth Analg 61:75, 1982

304. Nunn JF, Chanarin I: Interaction of nitrous oxide and vitamin B_{12}, Nitrous oxide/N_2O. Edited by Eger EI II. New York, Elsevier, 1985, pp 211–233

305. Koblin DD, Watson JE, Deady JE, et al: Inactivation of methionine synthetase by nitrous oxide in mice. Anesthesiology 54:318, 1981

306. Dedrick DF, Scherer YD, Biebuyck JF: Use of a rapid brain-sampling technique in a physiologic preparation: Effects of morphine, ketamine, and halothane on tissue energy intermediates. Anesthesiology 42:651, 1975

307. Triner L, Vulliemoz Y, Verosky M, et al: Action of volatile anesthetics on cyclic nucleotides in the brain, Progress in Anesthesiology, vol 2: Molecular Mechanims of Anesthesia. Edited by Fink BR. New York, Raven Press, 1980, p 229

308. Kant GJ, Muller TW, Lanox RH, et al: *In vivo* effects of pentobarbital and halothane anesthesia on levels of adenosine 3',5'-monophosphate and guanosine 3',5'-monophosphate in rat brain regions and pituitary. Biochem Pharmacol 29:1891, 1980

309. MacMurdo SD, Nemoto EM, Nikki P, et al: Brain cyclic-AMP and possible mechanisms of cerebrovascular dilation by anesthetics in rats. Anesthesiology 55:435, 1981

310. Nahrwold ML, Lust WD, Passonneau JV: Halothane-induced alterations of cyclic nucleotide concentrations in three regions of the mouse nervous system. Anesthesiology 47:423, 1977

311. Divakaran P, Rigor BM, Wiggens RC: Brain cyclic nucleotide responses to anesthesia with halothane delivered in air or purified oxygen. J Neurochem 35:514, 1980

312. Woo SY, Verosky M, Vulliemoz Y, et al: Dopamine-sensitive adenylate cyclase activity in the rat caudate nucleus during exposure to halothane and enflurane. Anesthesiology 51:27, 1979

313. Bernstein KJ, Verosky M, Triner L: Halothane inhibition of canine myocardial adenylate cyclase-modulation by endogenous factors. Anesth Analg 63:285, 1984

314. Levine SD, Weber H, Schlondorff D: Inhibition of adenylate cyclase by general anesthetics in toad urinary bladder. Am J Physiol 237:F372, 1979

315. Bernstein KJ, Gangat Y, Verosky M, et al: Halo-

thane effect on beta-adrenergic receptors in canine myocardium. Anesth Analg 60:401, 1981

316. Sandhoff K, Schraven J, Nowoczek G: Effect of xenon, nitrous oxide, and halothane on membrane-bound sialidase from calf brain. FEBS Lett 62:284, 1976

317. Sandhoff K, Pallmann B: Membrane-bound neuraminidase from calf-brain: Regulation of oligosialoganglioside degradation by membrane fluidity and membrane components. Proc Natl Acad Sci USA 75:122, 1978

318. Knight PR, Nahrwold ML, Rosenberg A: Sialic acid release by *Vibrio cholerae* sialidase (neuraminidase) from the outer surface of neural cells is greatly raised by halothane. J Neurochem 30:1645, 1978

319. Pellkofer R, Sandhoff K: Halothane increases membrane fluidity and stimulates sphingomyelin degradation by membrane-bound neutral sphingomyelinase of synaptosomal plasma membranes from calf brain already at clinical concentrations. J Neurochem 34:988, 1980

320. Miller JC: Anesthetics and phospholipid metabolism, Progress in Anesthesiology, vol 1: Molecular Mechanisms of Anesthesia. Edited by Fink BR. New York, Raven Press, 1975, p 439

321. Paton WDM, Wing DR: Effects of halothane on the incorporation of ^{14}C-serine into phospholipid in the guinea-pig ileum. Br J Pharmacol 72:393, 1981

322. Tam SW, Choy PC: Differential effects of anesthetics on phosphatidylethanolamine biosynthesis in hamster tissue. Biochim Biophys Acta 754:111, 1983

323. Upreti GC, Rainier S, Jain MK: Intrinsic differences in the perturbing ability of alkanols in bilayer: Action of phospholipase A$_2$ on the alkanol-modified phospholipid bilayer. J Membr Biol 55:97, 1980

324. Grof P, Belagyi J: The effect of anaesthetics on protein conformation in membranes as studied by the spin-labelling technique. Biochim Biophys Acta 734:319, 1983

325. Galla HJ, Trudell JR: Perturbation of peptide-induced lateral phase separations in phosphatidic acid bilayers by the inhalation anesthetic methoxyflurane. Mol Pharmacol 19:432, 1981

326. Mashimo T, Tashiro C, Yoshira I: Effects of volatile anesthetics on light-induced proton uptake of rhodopsin in bovine rod outer segment disk membrane. Anesthesiology 61:439, 1984

327. Young AP, Sigman DS: Allosteric effects of volatile anesthetics on the membrane bound acetylcholine receptor protein. I. Stabilization of the high affinity state. Mol Pharmacol 20:498, 1981

328. Young AP, Sigman DS: Conformational effects of volatile anesthetics on the membrane-bound acetylcholine receptor protein: Facilitation of the agonist-induced affinity conversion. Biochemistry 22:2155, 1983

329. Sauter JF, Braswell LM, Miller KW: Action of anesthetics and high pressure on cholinergic membranes, Progress in Anesthesiology, vol 2: Molecular Mechanisms of Anesthesia. Edited by Fink BR. Raven Press, New York, 1980, pp 199–207

330. Sauter JF, Braswell, L, Wankowicz P, et al: The effects of high pressures of inert gases on cholinergic receptor binding and function, Underwater Physiology, Vol VII. Edited by Bachrach AJ, Matzen MM. Bethesda, Md, Undersea Medical Society, 1981, p 629

331. Eyring H, Woodbury JW, D'Arrigo JS: A molecular mechanism of general anesthesia. Anesthesiology 38:415, 1973

332. LaBella FS: Is there a general anesthesia receptor? Can J Physiol Pharmacol 59:432, 1981

333. Hameroff SR, Watt RC: Do anesthetics act by altering electron mobility? Anesth Analg 62:936, 1983

334. Finck AD, Ngai SH, Berkowitz BA: Antagonism of general anesthesia by naloxone in the rat. Anesthesiology 46:241, 1977

335. Arndt JO, Freye E: Perfusion of naloxone through the fourth cerebral ventricle reverses the circulatory and hypnotic effect of halothane in dogs. Anesthesiology 51:58, 1979

336. Harper MH, Winter PM, Johnson BH, et al: Naloxone does not antagonize general anesthesia in the rat. Anesthesiology 49:3, 1978

337. Pace NL, Wong KC: Failure of naloxone and naltrexone to antagonize halothane anesthesia in the dog. Anesth Analg 58:36, 1979

338. MacLeod BA, Ping FC, Jenkins LC: The absence of antagonism by naloxone during halothane/nitrous oxide anesthesia in man. Can Anaesth Soc J 27:29, 1980

339. Tay AL, Tseng CK, Pace NL, et al: Failure of narcotic antagonist to alter electropuncture modification of halothane anesthesia in the dog. Can Anaesth Soc J 29:231, 1982

340. Smith RA, Wilson M, Miller KW: Naloxone has no effect on nitrous oxide anesthesia. Anesthesiology 49:6, 1978

341. Bennett PB: Naloxone fails to antagonize the righting response in rats anesthetized with halothane. Anesthesiology 49:9, 1978

342. Lawrence D, Livingston A: Opiate-like analgesic activity in general anesthetics. Br J Pharmacol 73:435, 1981

343. Kraynack BJ, Gintautas JG: Naloxone: Analeptic action unrelated to opiate receptor antagonism? Anesthesiology 56:251, 1982

344. Artru AA, Steen PA, Michenfelder JD: Cerebral metabolic effects of naloxone administered with anesthetic and subanesthetic concentrations of halothane in the dog. Anesthesiology 52:217, 1980

345. Shingu K, Osawa M, Omatsu Y, et al: Naloxone does not antagonize the anesthetic-induced nociceptor-driven spinal cord response in spinal cats. Acta Anaesthesiol Scand 25:526, 1981

346. Shiwaku S, Nagashima H, Duncalf RM, et al: Naloxone fails to antagonize halothane-induced depression of the longitudinal muscle of the guinea pig ileum. Anesth Analg 58:93, 1979

347. Morris B, Livingston A: Effects of nitrous oxide exposure on met-enkephalin levels in discrete areas of rat brain. Neurosci Lett 45:11, 1984

348. Way WL, Hosobuchi Y, Johnson BH, et al: Anesthesia does not increase opioid peptides in cerebrospinal fluid of humans. Anesthesiology 60:43, 1984

349. Thomas TA, Fletcher JE, Hill RG: Influence of medication, pain and progress in labour on plasma beta-endorphin-like immunoreactivity. Br J Anaesth 54:401, 1982

350. Subaiya L, Rege A, Weng JT, et al: The influence of isoflurane on plasma beta-endorphin immunoreactivity. Anesth Analg 63:278, 1984

351. Freye E, Hartung E, Schenk GK: Naloxone reverses the hypnotic effect and the depressed baroreceptor reflex of halothane anesthesia in the dog. Can Anaesth Soc J 30:235, 1983

352. Havlicek V, LaBella FS, Pinsky C, et al: Beta-endorphin induces general anesthesia by an interaction with opiate receptors. Can Soc Anaesth J 27:535, 1980

353. Berkowitz BA, Ngai SH, Finck AD: Nitrous oxide "analgesia": resemblence to opiate action. Science 194:967, 1976

354. Berkowitz BA, Finck AD, Ngai SH: Nitrous oxide analgesia: Reversal by naloxone and development of tolerance. J Pharmacol Exp Ther 203:539, 1977

355. Chapman CR, Bendetti C: Nitrous oxide effects on cerebral evoked potential to pain: Partial reversal with a narcotic antagonist. Anesthesiology 51:135, 1979

356. Yang JC, Clark WC, Ngai SH: Antagonism of nitrous oxide analgesia by naloxone in man. Anesthesiology 52:414, 1980

357. Levine JD, Gordon NC, Fields HL: Naloxone fails to antagonize nitrous oxide analgesia for clinical pain. Pain 13:165, 1982

358. Gillman MA, Kok L, Lichtigfeld FJ: Paradoxical effect of naloxone on nitrous oxide analgesia in man. Eur J Pharmacol 61:175, 1980

359. Daras C, Cantrill RC, Gillman MA: [^{3}H]-Naloxone displacement: Evidence for nitrous oxide as

opioid receptor agonist. Eur J Pharmacol 89:177, 1983

360. Inoki R, Kim SY, Maeda S, et al: Effect of inhalational anesthetics on the opioid receptors in the rat brain. Life Sci (Suppl I), 33:223, 1983

361. Dodson BA, Miller KW: Evidence for a dual mechanism in the anesthetic action of an opiate peptide. Anesthesiology 59:A531, 1983

362. Yaksh TL, Howe JR: Opiate receptors and their definition by antagonists. Anesthesiology 56:246, 1982

363. Koblin DD, Dong DE, Eger EI II: Tolerance of mice to nitrous oxide. J Pharmacol Exp Ther 211:317, 1979

364. Smith RA, Winter PM, Smith M, et al: Tolerance to and dependence on inhalational anesthetics. Anesthesiology 50:505, 1979

365. Koblin DD, Eger EI II, Smith RA, et al: Chronic exposure of mice to subanesthetic doses of nitrous oxide, Progress in Anesthesiology, vol 2: Molecular Mechanisms of Anesthesia. Edited by Fink BR. New York, Raven Press, 1980, pp 157–164

366. Koblin DD, Deady JE, Nelson NT, et al: Mice tolerant to nitrous oxide are not tolerant to barbiturates. Anesth Analg 60:138, 1981

367. Chalon J, Tank CK, Roberts C, et al: Murine auto- and cross-tolerance to volatile anesthetics. Can Anaesth Soc J 30:230, 1983

368. Nandini-Kishore SG, Kitajama Y, Thompson GA Jr: Membrane fluidizing effects of the general anesthetic methoxyflurane elicit an acclimation response in *Tetrahymena*. Biochim Biophys Acta 471:157, 1977

369. Koblin DD, Wang HH: Chronic exposure to inhaled anesthetics increases cholesterol content in *Acholeplasma laidlawii*. Biochim Biophys Acta 649:717, 1981

370. Christiansson A, Gutman H, Wieslander A, et al: Effects of anesthetics on water permeability and lipid metabolism in *Acholeplasma laidlawii* membranes. Biochim Biophys Acta 645:24, 1981

371. Berkowitz BA, Finck AD, Hynes MD, et al: Tolerance to nitrous oxide analgesia in rats and mice. Anesthesiology 51:309, 1979

372. Kripke BJ, Hechtman HB: Nitrous oxide for pentazocine addiction and for intractable pain: Report of a case. Anesth Analg 51:520, 1972

373. Ngai SH, Finck AD: Prolonged exposure to nitrous oxide decreases opiate receptor density in rat brainstem. Anesthesiology 57:26, 1982

374. Han YH: Why do chronic alcoholics require more anesthesia? Anesthesiology 30:341, 1969

375. Tammisto T, Tigerstedt I: The need for halothane supplementation of N_2O–O_2-relaxant anesthesia in chronic alcoholics. Acta Anaesthesiol Scand 21:17, 1977

376. Bruce DL: Alcoholism and anesthesia. Anesth Analg 62:84, 1983

377. Johnstone RE, Kulp RA, Smith TC: Effects of acute and chronic ethanol administration on isoflurane requirement in mice. Anesth Analg 54:277, 1975

378. Harper MH, Johnson BH, Eger EI II, et al: Cross tolerance between alcohol and cyclopropane in rats. Anesth Analg 59:545, 1980

379. Orkin LR, Chen CH: The effect of alcohol on the MAC with halothane in the cat. Abstracts of Scientific Papers, American Society of Anesthesiologists Annual Meeting, 1977, pp 735–736

380. Barber RE: Anesthetic requirement in alcoholic patients. Abstracts of Scientific Papers, American Society of Anesthesiologists Annual Meeting, 1978, pp 623–624

381. Koblin DD, Deady JE, Dong DE, et al: Mice tolerant to nitrous oxide are also tolerant to alcohol. J Pharmacol Exp Ther 213:309, 1980

382. Rubin E, Rottenberg H: Ethanol and biological membranes: Injury and adaptation. Pharmacol Biochem Behav (suppl 1), 18:7, 1983

383. Whitwam JG, Morgan M, Hall GM, et al: Pain during continuous nitrous oxide administration. Br J Anaesth 48:425, 1976

384. Stevens JE, Oshima E, Mori K: Effects of nitrous oxide on the epileptogenic property of enflurane in cats. Br J Anaesth 55:145, 1983

385. Sauter JF: Electrophysiological activity of a mammalian sympathetic ganglion under hyperbaric nitrous oxide. Neuropharmacology 18:71, 1979

386. Smith RA, Winter PM, Smith M, et al: Convulsions in mice after anesthesia. Anesthesiology 50:501, 1979

387. Harper MH, Winter PM, Johnson BH, et al: Withdrawal convulsions in mice following nitrous oxide. Anesth Analg 59:19, 1980

388. Rupreht J, Dworacek B, Ducardus R, et al: The involvement of the central cholinergic and endorphinergic systems in the nitrous oxide withdrawal syndrome in mice. Anesthesiology 58:524, 1983

389. Manson HJ, Dyke G, Melling J, et al: The effect of naloxone and morphine on convulsions in mice following withdrawal from nitrous oxide. Can Anaesth Soc J 30:28, 1983

390. Milne B, Cervenko FW, Jhamandas KH: Physical dependence of nitrous oxide in mice: Resemblance to alcohol but not to opiate withdrawal. Can Anaesth Soc J 28:46, 1983

391. Koblin DD, Dong DE, Deady JE, et al: Selective breeding alters murine resistance to nitrous oxide without alteration in synaptic membrane lipid composition. Anesthesiology 52:401, 1980

392. Koblin DD, Lurz FW, O'Connor B, et al: Potencies of barbiturates in mice selectively bred for resistance or susceptibility to nitrous oxide anesthesia. Anesth Analg 63:35, 1984

393. Koblin DD, O'Connor B, Deady JE, et al: Potencies of convulsant drugs in mice selectively bred for resistance and susceptibility to nitrous oxide anesthesia. Anesthesiology 56:25, 1982

394. Koblin DD, Eger EI II: Cross-mating of mice selectively bred for resistance and susceptibility to nitrous oxide anesthesia: Potencies of nitrous oxide in the offspring. Anesth Analg 60:646, 1981

395. Koblin DD, Deady JE: Anaesthetic requirement in mice selectively bred for differences in ethanol sensitivity. Br J Anaesth 53:5, 1981

396. Erwin VG, Heston WDW, McClearn G, et al: Effect of hypnotics on mice genetically selected for sensitivity to ethanol. Pharmacol Biochem Behav 4:679, 1976

397. Baker R, Melchior C, Deitrich R: The effect of halothane on mice selectively bred for differential sensitivity to alcohol. Pharmacol Biochem Behav 12:691, 1980

398. Koblin DD: Anesthetic requirement in the quaking mouse. Anesthesiology 54:17, 1981

399. Gamo S, Ogaki M, Nakashima-Tanaka E: Strain differences in minimum anesthetic concentrations in *Drosophila melanogaster*. Anesthesiology 54:289, 1981

400. Gamo S, Nakashima-Tanaka E, Ogaki M: Alteration in molecular species of phosphatidylethanolamine between anesthetic resistant and sensitive strains of *Drosophila melanogaster*. Life Sci 30:401, 1982

401. Koblin DD, Dong DE, Deady JE, et al: Alteration of synaptic membrane fatty acid composition and anesthetic requirement. J Pharmacol Exp Ther 212:546, 1980

402. Jones K: Nitrous oxide, Comprehensive Inorganic Chemistry, vol 2. Edited by Bailar JC. London, Pergamon Press, 1973, pp 316–323

403. Smith RA, Koblin DD, Smith M, et al: The anesthetic potency of volatile agents in mice. Abstracts of Scientific Papers. 1978 ASA meeting, p 617

404. Tanifuji Y, Eger EI II, Terrell RC: Some characteristics of an exceptionally potent inhaled anesthetic: Thiomethoxyflurane. Anesth Analg 56:387, 1977

405. Eger EI II, Koblin DD, Collins PA: Dioxychlorane: A challenge to the correlation of anesthetic potency and lipid solubility. Anesth Analg 60:201, 1981

406. Eger EI II, Brandstater B, Saidman LJ, et al: Equipotent alveolar concentrations of methoxyflu-

rane, halothane, diethylether, fluroxene, cyclopropane, xenon, and nitrous oxide in the dog. Anesthesiology 26:771, 1965

407. Munson ES, Schick LM, Chapin JC, et al: Determination of the minimum alveolar concentration (MAC) of Aliflurane in dogs. Anesthesiology 51:545, 1979

408. Hornbein TF, Eger EI II, Winter PM, et al: The minimum alveolar concentration of nitrous oxide in man. Anesth Analg 61:553, 1982

409. Uyeno ET, Denson DD, Simon RL Jr, et al: Bioassay of fluorinated volatile anesthetics. Proc West Pharmacol Soc 20:357, 1977

410. Cooper JB, Joseph DM: A new value for the solubility of nitrous oxide in olive oil. Anesthesiology 55:720, 1981

19

Uptake and Distribution of Inhaled Anesthetics

Edmond I. Eger II, M.D.

INTRODUCTION

To produce a brain anesthetic concentration sufficient for surgery requires proper manipulation of anesthetic delivery to the patient. Proper manipulation also requires that the concentration delivered not produce excessive depression. Thus, knowledge of the factors governing the relationship between the delivered and brain (or heart or muscle) concentrations is indispensable to the optimum conduct of anesthesia. It is these factors that are the substance of anesthetic uptake and distribution.

THE INSPIRED TO ALVEOLAR ANESTHETIC RELATIONSHIP

Of the steps between delivered and brain anesthetic partial pressures, none is more pivotal than that between the inspired and alveolar gases. By use of high inflow rates (and hence conversion to a nonrebreathing system), the anesthetist can precisely control the partial pressure of anesthetic inspired. The alveolar partial pressure governs the partial pressure of anesthetic in all body tissues: all must approach and ultimately equal the alveolar partial pressure.

THE EFFECT OF VENTILATION

Two factors determine the rate at which the alveolar concentration of anesthetic (FA) rises toward the concentration being inspired (FI): the inspired concentration (discussed in the section on the concentration effect) and the alveolar ventilation. The effect of ventilation is a powerful one. If unopposed, on induction ventilation rapidly increases the alveolar concentration (i.e., FA/FI quickly approaches 1). This is seen with preoxygenation to achieve nitrogen washout: normally a 95 percent or greater washout of nitrogen occurs in 2 minutes or less when a nonrebreathing (or high inflow rate) system is used.

The rapid washout of nitrogen or washin of oxygen is not mimicked by the inhaled anesthetics. The solubility of anesthetics is far higher than that of nitrogen, and the higher solubility causes the transfer of substantial quantities of anesthetic to the blood passing through the lung. This uptake opposes the effect of ventilation to increase the alveolar anesthetic concentration. At low inspired concentrations, the FA/FI ratio is ultimately determined by the balance between the delivery of anesthetic by ventilation and its removal by uptake. The relationship is a simple one. For example, if uptake removes 1/3 of the inspired anesthetic molecules the FA/FI ratio will equal 2/3; if uptake removes 3/4 of the inspired molecules, the FA/FI ratio will equal 1/4.

ANESTHETIC UPTAKE FACTORS

Anesthetic uptake itself is the product of three factors: solubility (λ), cardiac output ($\dot{Q}$), and the alveolar to venous partial pressure difference (PA − Pv).[1] That is

$$\text{Uptake} = \lambda \cdot \dot{Q} \cdot (\text{PA} - \text{Pv})/\text{BP} \qquad (1)$$

where BP is the barometric pressure. Being a product rather than a sum means that if any component of uptake approaches zero, uptake must approach zero and the effect of ventilation to drive the alveolar concentrations rapidly upward will be unopposed. Thus, if the solubility is small (as in the case of nitrogen), the cardiac output approaches zero (profound myocardial depression or death), or the alveolar to venous difference becomes inconsequential (as might occur after an extraordinarily long anesthetic), then uptake would be minimal and FA/FI would equal 1.

SOLUBILITY

The blood/gas partition coefficient, or "blood solubility," describes the relative affinity of anesthetic for two phases and therefore how the anesthetic will *partition* itself between

the two phases when equilibrium has been achieved. For example, enflurane has a blood/gas partition coefficient of 1.9, indicating that at equilibrium the concentration in blood will be 1.9 times the concentration in the gas (alveolar) phase. Remember that "equilibrium" means that no difference in partial pressure exists — that is, the blood/gas partition coefficient of 1.9 does *not* indicate that the partial pressure in blood will be 1.9 times that in the gas phase. The partition coefficient may be thought of in one other way: it indicates the relative capacity of the two phases. Thus, a value of 1.9 means that each milliliter of blood can hold 1.9 times as much enflurane as 1 ml of alveolar gas.

A larger blood/gas partition coefficient will produce a greater uptake, hence a lower FA/FI ratio. Since the anesthetic partial pressure in all tissues approaches that in the alveoli, the development of an adequate brain anesthetic partial pressure may be delayed in the case of highly blood-soluble agents such as ether or methoxyflurance (Table 19-1).[1] Even the moderate solubility of isoflurane, enflurane, or halothane would slow induction of anesthesia with these agents were it not for our use of anesthetic overpressure. That is, the uptake of anesthetic can be compensated for by delivering a far higher concentration than we hope to achieve in the alveoli. For example, on induction of anesthesia, we may use 3 to 4 percent halothane to produce an alveolar concentration of 1 percent.

CARDIAC OUTPUT

The effect of altering cardiac output is intuitively obvious. The passage of more blood through the lungs will remove more anesthetic and thereby lower the alveolar anesthetic concentration. To the beginning student of uptake and distribution, this may appear to produce a conflict. It would seem that if more agent were taken up and delivered more rapidly to the tissues, the tissue anesthetic partial pressure would rise more rapidly. In one sense this *is* true: an increase in cardiac output does hasten the equilibration of tissue anesthetic partial pressure with the partial pressure in arterial blood. What this reasoning ignores is the fact

TABLE 19-1.   Partition Coefficients at 37°C

Anesthetic	Blood / Gas	Brain / Blood	Liver / Blood	Kidney / Blood	Muscle / Blood	Fat / Blood
Cyclopropane	0.4–4.6	1.1	1.2	0.6	1.2	13
Nitrous oxide	0.47	1.1	0.8	—	1.2	2.3
Isoflurane	1.4	2.6	2.5	—	4.0	45
Enflurane	1.8	1.4	2.1	—	1.7	36
Halothane	2.3	2.9	2.6	1.6	3.5	60
Diethyl ether	12	1.1	1.0	1.1	1.0	3.7
Methoxyflurane	12	2.0	1.9	0.9	1.3	49

(Adapted from Eger EI II: Anesthetic Uptake and Action. Baltimore, Williams & Wilkins, 1974. © 1974 EI Eger II, M.D.)

that the anesthetic partial pressure in arterial blood is lower than it would be if cardiac output were normal.

The effect of a change in cardiac output is analogous to the effect of a change in solubility. Since doubling solubility doubled the capacity of the same volume of blood to hold anesthetic, doubling cardiac output also would double capacity, but in this case by increasing the volume of blood exposed to anesthetic.

THE ALVEOLAR TO VENOUS ANESTHETIC GRADIENT

The alveolar to venous anesthetic partial pressure difference results from tissue uptake of anesthetic. Were there no tissue uptake, the venous blood returning to the lungs would contain as much anesthetic as it had when it left the lungs as arterial blood. That is, the alveolar (equals arterial) to venous partial pressure difference would be zero. The presumption that alveolar and arterial anesthetic partial pressures are equal is reasonable in normal patients who have no barrier to diffusion of anesthetic from alveoli to pulmonary capillary blood and who do not have ventilation/perfusion ratio abnormalities. Later we shall consider the effect of ventilation/perfusion ratio abnormalities on anesthetic uptake.

The factors that determine the fraction of anesthetic removed from blood traversing a given tissue parallel those factors that govern uptake at the lungs: tissue solubility, tissue blood flow, and arterial to tissue anesthetic partial pressure difference. Again, uptake is the

product of these three factors. If any one factor approaches zero, uptake by that tissue becomes inconsequential. The succeeding paragraphs discuss the characteristics of each of these factors and then how uptake by individual tissues can be summed to give the venous component of the alveolar to venous anesthetic partial pressure difference.

Blood/gas partition coefficients span a range of values extending from 0.47 for nitrous oxide to 12 for methoxyflurane (Table 19-1). In contrast, tissue/blood partition coefficients (i.e., "tissue solubility") for lean tissues are close to 1, ranging from slightly less than 1 to a maximum of 4 (Table 19-1). That is, different lean tissues do not have greatly different capacities per milliliter of tissue. Put another way, a given anesthetic has roughly the same affinity for lean tissues and blood. As with blood/gas partition coefficients, tissue/blood partition coefficients define the concentration ratio of anesthetic at equilibrium. For example, a halothane brain/blood partition coefficient of 2.9 means that 1 ml of brain can hold 2.9 times more halothane than 1 ml of blood having the same halothane partial pressure.

Lean tissues differ in terms of their perfusion per gram — that is, the volume of tissue relative to the blood passing that tissue. A larger volume of tissue relative to flow confers a greater capacity to hold anesthetic. This has two implications. First, the large tissue capacity increases the transfer of anesthetic from blood to tissue. Second, it takes longer to fill up a tissue that has a large capacity; that is, it will take longer for the tissue to equilibrate with the anesthetic partial pressure being delivered in arterial blood. In other words, a large tissue volume relative to blood flow will sustain the arterial to tissue anesthetic partial pressure difference (hence uptake) for a longer time. Brain tissue, with its high perfusion per gram, will equilibrate rapidly. Muscle, with about one-twentieth the perfusion of brain, will take about 20 times longer to equilibrate. Uptake of anesthetic by muscle will continue long after uptake by brain has ceased.

Fat has a tissue/blood coefficient significantly greater than 1 (Table 19-1). Fat/blood coefficients range from 2.3 (nitrous oxide) to 60 (halothane). That is, each milliliter of fat tissue will contain 2.3 times more nitrous oxide or 60 times more halothane than 1 ml of blood having the same nitrous oxide or halothane partial pressure. This enormous capacity of fat for anesthetic means that most of the anesthetic contained in the blood perfusing fat will be transferred to the fat. Even so, the anesthetic partial pressure in that tissue will rise very slowly. Both the large capacity of fat and the low perfusion per milliliter of tissue prolong the time required to narrow the anesthetic partial pressure difference between arterial blood and fat.

TISSUE GROUPS

The algebraic sum of anesthetic uptake by individual tissues determines the alveolar to venous partial pressure difference and hence uptake at the lungs. It is not necessary to analyze the effect of individual tissues to arrive at the algebraic sum. Rather, we can group tissues in terms of their perfusion and solubility characteristics, that is, in terms of those features that define the duration of a substantial arterial to tissue anesthetic partial pressure difference. Four tissue groups have been determined by such analysis (Table 19-2).[1]

The vessel-rich group (VRG) is composed of the brain, heart, splanchnic bed (including liver), kidney, and endocrine glands. These organs make up less than 10 percent of the body weight but receive 75 percent of the cardiac output. This high perfusion confers several features. Access to a large flow of blood permits the VRG to take up a relatively large volume of anesthetic in the earliest moments of induction. However, the small volume of tissue relative to perfusion produces a rapid equilibration of this tissue group with the anesthetic delivered in arterial blood. The time to half-equilibration (i.e., the time at which the VRG anesthetic partial pressure equals half that in arterial blood) varies from about 1 minute for nitrous oxide to 3 minutes for halothane or enflurane. The longer time to equilibration with halothane or enflurane results from their higher tissue/blood partition coefficients (Table 19-1). Equilibration of the VRG with the anesthetic partial pressure in arterial blood is more than 90 percent complete in 3 to 10 minutes. Thus, after 10 minutes, uptake by the VRG is too small (i.e., the arterial to VRG anesthetic partial pressure difference is too small) to influence the alveolar concentration significantly. Uptake after 10 minutes is principally determined by the muscle group.

Muscle and skin, which make up the muscle group (MG), have similar blood flow and solubility (lean tissue) characteristics. The lower perfusion (about 3 ml blood per 100 ml tissue per minute) sets this group apart from the VRG (75 ml per 100 ml per minute). Although about one-half the body bulk is muscle and skin, this volume receives only 1 L/min blood flow at rest. The large bulk relative to perfusion means that during induction, most of the anesthetic delivered to the MG is removed from the MG blood flow. The time to half-equilibration ranges from 20 to 25 minutes (nitrous oxide) to

TABLE 19-2. Tissue Group Characteristics

	VRG (Vessel Rich)	MG (Muscle)	FG (Fat)	VPG (Vessel Poor)
Percentage body mass	10	50	20	20
Perfusion as percentage of cardiac output	75	19	6	0

(Adapted from Eger EI II: Anesthetic Uptake and Action. Baltimore, Williams & Wilkins, 1974. © 1974 EI Eger II, M.D.)

70 to 90 minutes (enflurane or halothane). Thus, long after equilibration of the VRG has taken place, muscle continues to take up substantial amounts of anesthetic. This tissue approaches equilibration within 1 to 4 hours.

Once equilibration of muscle is complete, only fat (i.e., the fat group, or FG) continues to serve as an effective depot for uptake. Fat occupies one-fifth of the body bulk and receives a blood flow of about 300 ml/min. That is, the perfusion per 100 ml of fat nearly equals the perfusion per 100 ml of resting muscle. Fat differs from muscle in its higher affinity for anesthetic, a property that greatly lengthens the time over which it absorbs anesthetic. The half-time to equilibration of fat ranges from 70 to 80 minutes for nitrous oxide to 19 to 32 *hours* for enflurane and halothane, respectively. It is apparent that equilibration with fat will not occur during the course of an ordinary halothane or enflurane anesthetic.

One tissue group, the vessel-poor group (VPG), remains to be defined. This group is composed of ligaments, tendons, bone, and cartilage—those lean tissues that have little or no perfusion. The absence of a significant blood flow means that this tissue group does not participate in the uptake process despite the fact that it makes up one-fifth of the body mass.

SYNTHESIS OF THE FACTORS GOVERNING THE RISE OF THE FA/FI RATIO

We may now consider the combined impact of ventilation, solubility, and the distribution of blood flow on the development of the alveolar anesthetic partial pressure. The initial rate of rise of FA/FI is rapid for all agents regardless of their solubility (Fig. 19-1).[2-4] The rapidity with which this upswing occurs results from the absence of an alveolar to venous anesthetic partial pressure difference (there is no anesthetic present in the lung to create a gradient), hence the absence of uptake in the first moment of induction. Thus, the effect of ventilation to generate a sudden rise in FA/FI is unopposed. Obviously, the delivery of more and more anesthetic to the alveoli by ventilation produces a progressively greater alveolar to venous partial pressure difference. The increasing uptake that ensues will increasingly oppose the effect of ventilation to drive the alveolar concentration upward. Ultimately a rough balance is struck between the input by ventilation and removal by uptake. The height of the FA/FI ratio at which the balance is struck depends on the solubility factor in the uptake

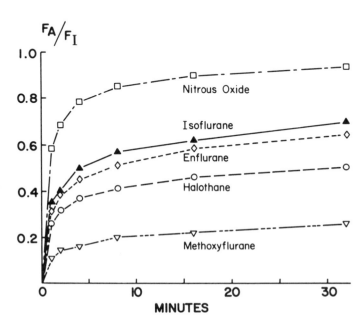

FIG. 19-1 The rise in alveolar (FA) anesthetic concentration toward the inspired (FI) concentration is most rapid with the least soluble anesthetic, nitrous oxide, and slowest with the most soluble anesthetic, diethyl ether. All data are from human studies.[2,3] (Eger EI II: Isoflurane (Forane[R]), A Reference and Compendium. Madison, Wisc, Ohio Medical Products, 1981.)

equation [equation (1)]. A higher solubility produces a greater uptake for a given alveolar to venous partial pressure difference. The initial rapid rise in F_A/F_I will therefore be halted at a lower level with a more soluble agent. This results in the first "knee" in the curve — higher for nitrous oxide than for isoflurane, higher for isoflurane than for enflurane, higher for enflurane than for halothane, and higher for halothane than for ether.

The balance struck between ventilation and uptake does not remain constant. F_A/F_I continues to rise, albeit at a slower rate than seen in the first minute. This rise results from the progressive decrease in uptake by the vessel-rich group, a decrease to an inconsequential amount after 10 minutes. Thus, by about 10 minutes the three-quarters of the cardiac output that is returning to the lungs (i.e., the blood from the VRG) contains nearly as much anesthetic as it had when it left the lungs. The consequent rise in venous anesthetic partial pressure decreases the alveolar to venous partial pressure difference and therefore uptake — allowing ventilation to drive the alveolar concentration upward to the second knee at 10 to 15 minutes.

With the termination of effective uptake by the VRG, muscle and fat become the principal determinants of tissue uptake. The slow rate of change of the anesthetic partial pressure difference between arterial blood and muscle or fat produces the relatively stable terminal portion of each curve shown in Figure 19-1. In fact, this terminal portion gradually ascends as muscle and, to a lesser extent, fat progressively equilibrate with the arterial anesthetic partial pressure. Were the graphs extended for several hours, a third knee would be found, indicating equilibration of the muscle group. Uptake after that point would principally depend on the partial pressure gradient between arterial blood and fat.

THE CONCENTRATION EFFECT

The above analysis ignores the impact of the "concentration effect" on F_A/F_I. The inspired anesthetic concentration influences both the alveolar concentration that may be attained and the rate at which that concentration may be attained.[5,6] Increasing the inspired concentration accelerates the rate of rise. At an inspired concentration of 100 percent, the rate of rise is extremely rapid, since it is dictated solely by the rate at which ventilation washes gas into the lung. That is, at 100 percent in-

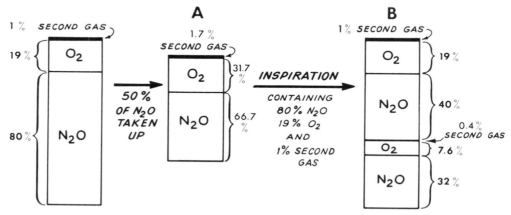

FIG. 19-2 The rectangle to the left represents a lung filled with 80 percent nitrous oxide plus 1 percent of a second gas. Uptake of half the nitrous oxide (A) does not halve the concentration of nitrous oxide and the reduction in volume concentrates and thereby increases the concentration of the second gas. Restoration of the lung volume (B) by addition of gas at the same concentration as that contained in the left-most rectangle will increase the nitrous oxide concentration and will add to the amount of the second gas present in the lung. (Stoelting RK, Eger EI II: An additional explanation for the second gas effect: A concentrating effect. Anesthesiology 30:273, 1969.)

spired concentration, uptake no longer limits the level to which F_A/F_I may rise. The cause of this extreme effect is readily perceived. At 100 percent inspired concentration, the uptake of anesthetic creates a void that draws gas down the trachea. This additional "inspiration" replaces the gas that is taken up. Since the concentration of the replacement gas is 100 percent, uptake cannot modify the alveolar concentration.

The concentration effect results from two factors: a concentrating effect and an augmentation of inspired ventilation.[7] Both effects are illustrated in Figure 19-2. The first rectangle represents a lung containing 80 percent nitrous oxide. If one-half of this gas is taken up, the residual 40 volumes of nitrous oxide exists in a total of 60 volumes, yielding a concentration of 67 percent (Fig. 19-2A). That is, uptake of one-half the nitrous oxide does not halve the concentration because the remaining gases are "concentrated" in a smaller volume. If the void created by uptake is filled by drawing more gas into the lungs (and augmentation of inspired ventilation), the final concentration equals 72 percent (Fig. 19-2B).

The impact of the concentration effect of F_A/F_I may be thought of as identical to the impact of a change in solubility.[8] As the inspired concentration increases, the effective solubility decreases. That is, at 50 percent inspired nitrous oxide, F_A/F_I rises as rapidly as the F_A/F_I of an anesthetic given at 1 percent that equals one-half the solubility of nitrous oxide. Seventy-five percent inspired nitrous oxide acts like an anesthetic given at 1 percent that has one-quarter the solubility of nitrous oxide.

THE SECOND GAS EFFECT

The factors governing the concentration effect also influence the concentration of any gas given concomitantly.[7,9] This second gas effect applies to halothane or enflurane when administered with nitrous oxide. The loss of volume associated with the uptake of nitrous oxide concentrates the halothane or enflurane (Fig. 19-2A). Replacement of the gas taken up by an increase in inspired ventilation will aug-

ment the amount of halothane or enflurane present in the lung (Fig. 19-2B).

Both the concentration effect and second gas effect were demonstrated by the following experiments.[9] In dogs given 0.5 percent halothane in either 10 percent nitrous oxide or 70 percent nitrous oxide, the F_A/F_I for nitrous oxide rose more rapidly when 70 percent nitrous oxide was inspired than when 10 percent was inspired (the concentration effect — see Fig. 19-3). Similarly, the F_A/F_I ratio for halo-

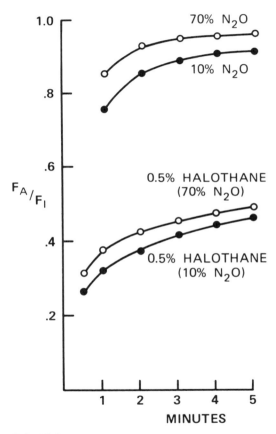

FIG. 19-3 In dogs, administration of 70 percent nitrous oxide produces a more rapid rise in F_A/F_I of nitrous oxide than does administration of 10 percent (concentration effect, upper two curves). The F_A/F_I for 0.5 percent halothane rises more rapidly when given with 70 percent nitrous oxide than when given with 10 percent (second gas effect, lower two curves). (Epstein RM, Rackow H, Salanitre E, et al: Influence of the concentration effect on the uptake of gas mixtures: The second gas effect. Anesthesiology 25:364, 1964.)

thane rose more rapidly when 70 percent nitrous oxide was inspired than when 10 percent was inspired (second gas effect).

FACTORS MODIFYING THE RATE OF RISE OF FA/FI

Alteration of those factors governing the rate of delivery of anesthetic to the lungs or its removal from the lungs will alter the alveolar concentration of anesthetic. We have seen the importance of differences in solubility (Fig. 19-1). The succeeding sections examine the impact of differences in ventilation and circulation as well as the interaction of these differences with such factors as solubility.

THE EFFECT OF VENTILATORY CHANGES

By augmenting the delivery of anesthetic to the lungs, an increase in ventilation accelerates the rate of rise of F_A/F_I (Fig. 19-4).[1,10] A change in ventilation produces a greater relative change in F_A/F_I with a more soluble anesthetic. As shown in Figure 19-4, an increase in ventilation from 2 to 8 L/min triples the ether concentration at 10 minutes, only doubles the halothane concentration, and scarcely affects the nitrous oxide concentration.

The impact of solubility may be explained as follows. With a poorly soluble agent such as nitrous oxide, the rate of rise of F_A/F_I is rapid even with hypoventilation. Since F_A normally cannot exceed F_I, there is little room for an augmentation of ventilation to increase F_A/F_I. With a highly soluble agent such as ether or methoxyflurane, most of the anesthetic delivered to the lungs is taken up. That is, if the uptake at 2 L/min ventilation equaled X, the uptake at 4 L/min would approach 2 X. Thus, if cardiac output is held constant, ventilation of 4

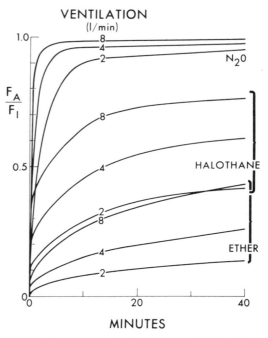

FIG. 19-4 The F_A/F_I ratio rises more rapidly if ventilation is increased. Solubility modifies this impact of ventilation: the effect on the anesthetizing partial pressure is greatest with the most soluble anesthetic (ether) and least with the least soluble anesthetic (nitrous oxide). (Eger EI II: Anesthetic Uptake and Action. Baltimore, Williams & Wilkins, 1974. © 1974 EI Eger II, M.D.)

L/min produces an arterial ether concentration nearly twice the concentration produced by a ventilation of 2 L/min. Since arterial and alveolar concentrations are in equilibrium, our example suggests that doubling ventilation must nearly double the anesthetic concentration in lung or blood.

These observations imply that imposed alterations in ventilation (e.g., an increase produced by conversion from spontaneous to controlled ventilation) produces greater changes in anesthetic effect with more soluble agents. Since such effects include both anesthetic depth and depression of circulation, greater caution must be exercised when ventilation is augmented during anesthesia produced with a highly soluble agent.

Anesthetics themselves may alter ventilation and thereby alter their own uptake.[11,12] Modern potent agents such as halothane, enflu-

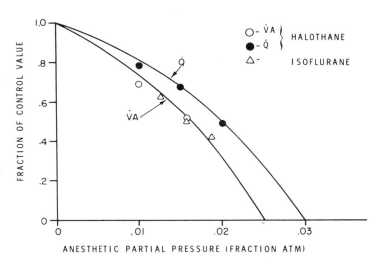

FIG. 19-5 Alveolar ventilation ($\dot{V}_A$) and cardiac output ($\dot{Q}$) are expressed as a percentage of awake values. These data for halothane and isoflurane are taken from human studies.[12,13] (Munson ES, Eger EI II, Bowers DL: Effects of anesthetic-depressed ventilation and cardiac output on anesthetic uptake. Anesthesiology 38:251, 1973.)

rane, or isoflurane all are profound respiratory depressants whose depression of ventilation is inversely related to anesthetic dose (Fig. 19-5).[13-15] At some dose, all the inhaled anesthetics probably produce apnea—a feature that must limit the maximum alveolar concentration that can be obtained if ventilation is spontaneous.

Thus, administration of an anesthetic concentration that produces significant respiratory depression progressively decreases delivery of anesthetic to the alveoli.[11,16] That is, doubling the inspired concentration does not double the alveolar concentration attained at a given point in time. At high inspired concentrations, further increases in inspired concentration produce little absolute change in the alveolar concentration (Fig. 19-6). Anesthetics can thereby exert a negative feedback effect on their own alveolar concentration, an effect that

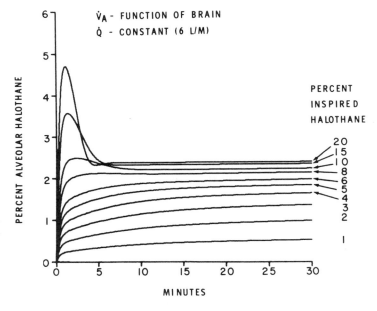

FIG. 19-6 An increase in inspired halothane concentration does not produce a proportional increase in the alveolar concentration because of the progressively greater depression of ventilation that occurs as alveolar halothane is increased. The initial "overshoot" seen with 10 to 20 percent inspired halothane results from the delay in the transfer of alveolar halothane partial pressure to the brain. (Munson ES, Eger EI II, Bowers DL: Effects of anesthetic-depressed ventilation and cardiac output on anesthetic uptake. Anesthesiology 38: 251, 1973.)

increases the safety of spontaneous ventilation by limiting the maximum concentration attained in the alveoli.

THE EFFECT OF CHANGES IN CARDIAC OUTPUT

The discussion in the previous section assumed a constant cardiac output and examined the effect of changes in ventilation. In this section the reverse process is discussed. An increase in cardiac output augments uptake and thereby hinders the rise in F_A/F_I.[1,17] As with a change in ventilation, a change in cardiac output scarcely affects the alveolar concentration of a poorly soluble agent; the alveolar concentration of a highly soluble agent will be much more influenced (Fig. 19-7). The reason for the impact of a change in solubility is similar to that which explains the effect of a change in ventilation. A decrease in cardiac output can do little to increase the F_A/F_I ratio of a poorly soluble agent, since the rate of rise is rapid at any cardiac output. In contrast, nearly all of a highly soluble agent will be taken up, and a halving of blood flow through the lungs must concentrate the arterial (equals alveolar) anesthetic (partial pressure), nearly doubling it in the case of an extremely soluble agent.

This effect of solubility suggests that conditions that lower cardiac output (e.g., shock) may produce unexpectedly high alveolar anesthetic concentrations if highly soluble agents are used. The higher F_A/F_I ratio should be anticipated and the inspired anesthetic concentration lowered accordingly to avoid further depression of circulation. Shock presents a two-pronged problem: an increase in ventilation usually accompanies the circulatory depression. Both factors accelerate the rise in F_A/F_I, perhaps accounting for the heavy reliance placed on the use of nitrous oxide in patients in shock. In contrast to methoxyflurane or halothane, the alveolar concentration of nitrous oxide would be little influenced by the associated cardiorespiratory changes.

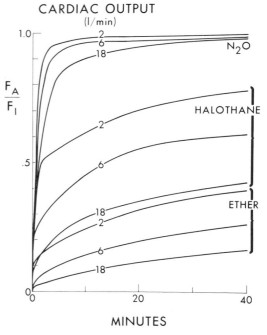

CARDIAC OUTPUT
(l/min)

MINUTES

FIG. 19-7 If unopposed by a concomitant increase in ventilation, an increase in cardiac output will decrease alveolar anesthetic concentration by augmenting uptake. The resulting alveolar anesthetic change is greatest with the most soluble anesthetic. (Eger EI II: Anesthetic Uptake and Action. Baltimore, Williams & Wilkins, 1974. © 1974 EI Eger II, M.D.)

Anesthetics also affect circulation. Usually they depress cardiac output (Fig. 19-5),[18,19] although stimulation may occur with some agents (e.g., ether or fluroxene). In contrast to the negative feedback that results from respiratory depression, circulatory depression produces a positive feedback: depression decreases uptake, thereby increasing the alveolar concentration, which in turn further decreases uptake. A potentially lethal acceleration of the rise in F_A/F_I results from the depression of cardiac output (Fig. 19-8).[11,12,16] The impact of this acceleration becomes more significant with increasing anesthetic solubility. High inspired concentrations of agents such as enflurane or halothane should be administered with considerable caution, particularly if ventilation is controlled.

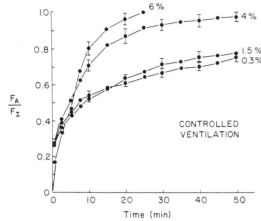

FIG. 19-8 Dogs given a constant ventilation demonstrate different rates of rise of FA/FI. The rates of rise depend on the inspired halothane concentration. The two higher concentrations accelerated the rate of rise by depressing cardiac output and thereby decreasing uptake. (Gibbons RT, Steffey EP, Eger EI II: The effect of spontaneous versus controlled ventilation on the rate of rise of alveolar halothane concentration in dogs. Anesth Analg 56:32, 1977.)

THE EFFECT OF CONCOMITANT CHANGES IN VENTILATION AND PERFUSION

Consideration of the effects of ventilatory and circulatory alterations generally presumed only one of these variables to be changed while the other was held constant. In fact, both may change concomitantly. If both ventilation and cardiac output increase proportionately, an intuitive expectation might be that FA/FI would be little altered. After all, uptake equals the product of solubility, cardiac output, and the alveolar to venous anesthetic partial pressure difference [eq. (1)]. In the absence of other changes, doubling cardiac output will double uptake, and this should balance exactly the influence of doubling of ventilation on FA/FI. That is, a doubling of both delivery of anesthetic to the lungs and removal of anesthetic from the lungs should produce no net change in the alveolar concentration.

The above reasoning ignores one other factor in the uptake equation. By accelerating the rate at which tissue equilibration occurs, an increase in cardiac output accelerates the narrowing of the alveolar to venous partial pressure difference.[20] This accelerated narrowing of the alveolar to venous partial pressure difference reduces the impact of the increase in cardiac output on uptake. Thus, a proportional increase in ventilation and cardiac output will increase the rate at which FA/FI will rise.

The magnitude of the acceleration of rise in FA/FI will depend in part on distribution of the increase in cardiac output. If the increase is distributed proportionately to all tissues (i.e., if a doubling of output doubles flow to all tissues), the increase is fairly small (Fig. 19-9).[20,21] Thus, conditions such as hyperthermia or thyrotoxicosis would only slightly influence the development of an anesthetizing anesthetic concentration through their influence on FA/FI. However, if the increase in cardiac output is diverted to the VRG, a greater effect is seen.[20,22] Perfusion of the VRG normally is high and results in rapid equilibration. Further increases in perfusion only hasten the rate of equilibration. Since blood returning from the VRG soon has the same partial pressure it had when it left the lungs, it cannot remove more anesthetic from the lungs. Thus, after a few seconds or minutes, the increase in ventilation will not be matched, even in part, by an increase in uptake. The result will be a considerable acceleration in the rise in FA/FI. This effect may be seen in a comparison of the FA/FI curves for children and adults (Fig. 19-10). Children (especially infants) have a relatively greater perfusion of the VRG and consequently show a significantly faster rise in FA/FI.[22] A clinical result of this accelerated rise is the more rapid development of anesthesia in young patients. The higher perfusion of the brain further accelerates the development of anesthesia.

VENTILATION/PERFUSION RATIO ABNORMALITIES

To this point it has been assumed that alveolar and arterial anesthetic partial pressures are equal; that is, the alveolar gases completely

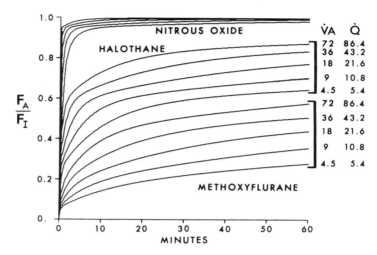

FIG. 19-9 Proportional increases in alveolar ventilation ($\dot{V}_A$) and cardiac output ($\dot{Q}$) will increase the rate at which FA/FI rises. As indicated, the effect is relatively small if the increase in cardiac output is distributed proportionately to all tissues (i.e., if $\dot{Q}$ is doubled, then all tissue blood flows are doubled). The greatest effect occurs with the most soluble anesthetic. (Eger EI II, Bahlman SH, Munson ES: Effect of age on the rate of increase of alveolar anesthetic concentration. Anesthesiology 35:365, 1971.)

equilibrate with the blood passing through the lungs. To some extent this assumption is incorrect, but the usual deviation from complete equilibration is small. Diseases such as emphysema, atelectasis, or congenital cardiac defects increase the deviation. The associated ventilation/perfusion ratio abnormality will do two things: increase the alveolar (end-tidal) anesthetic partial pressure, and decrease the arterial anesthetic partial pressure (i.e., a partial pressure difference will appear between alveolar gas and arterial blood). The relative change depends on the solubility of the anesthetic. With a poorly soluble agent, the end-tidal concentration is slightly increased, but the arterial partial pressure is significantly reduced. The opposite occurs with a highly soluble anesthetic.[23]

The considerable decrease in the arterial anesthetic partial pressure that occurs with poorly soluble agents may be explained as follows. Ventilation/perfusion ratio abnormalities increase ventilation relative to perfusion of some alveoli, while in other alveoli the reverse occurs. With a poorly soluble anesthetic, an in-

crease in ventilation relative to perfusion does not appreciably increase alveolar or arterial anesthetic partial pressure issuing from those alveoli (see the effect for nitrous oxide in Fig. 19-4). However, when ventilation decreases relative to perfusion, a significant effect can occur, particularly when ventilation is absent, as in a segment of atelectatic lung. Blood emerges from that segment with no additional anesthetic. Such anesthetic-deficient blood then mixes with the blood from the ventilated segments containing a normal complement of anesthetic. The mixture produces an arterial anesthetic partial pressure that is considerably below normal.

With highly soluble agents, a different situation results from similar ventilation/perfusion ratio abnormalities. In alveoli receiving more ventilation relative to perfusion, the anesthetic partial pressure rises to a higher level than usual (see Fig. 19-4 for the effect on diethyl ether). That is, blood issuing from these alveoli has an increased anesthetic content that is nearly proportional to the increased ventilation. Assuming that overall (total) venti-

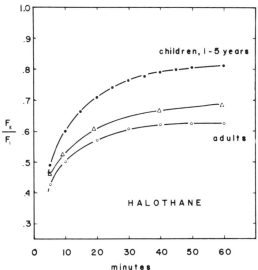

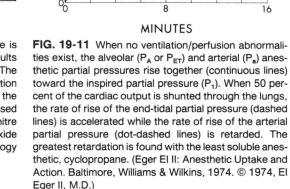

FIG. 19-10 The alveolar rate of rise of halothane is more rapid in children (uppermost curve) than adults (lower two curves, each from separate studies). The difference probably results from the greater ventilation and perfusion per kilogram of tissue in children and the fact that a disproportionate amount of the increased perfusion is devoted to the vessel-rich group. (Salanitre E, Rackow H: The pulmonary exchange of nitrous oxide and halothane in infants and children. Anesthesiology 30:388, 1969.)

FIG. 19-11 When no ventilation/perfusion abnormalities exist, the alveolar (P_A or P_{ET}) and arterial (P_a) anesthetic partial pressures rise together (continuous lines) toward the inspired partial pressure (P_1). When 50 percent of the cardiac output is shunted through the lungs, the rate of rise of the end-tidal partial pressure (dashed lines) is accelerated while the rate of rise of the arterial partial pressure (dot-dashed lines) is retarded. The greatest retardation is found with the least soluble anesthetic, cyclopropane. (Eger EI II: Anesthetic Uptake and Action. Baltimore, Williams & Wilkins, 1974. © 1974, EI Eger II, M.D.)

lation remains normal, this increase in the anesthetic contained by blood from the relatively hyperventilated alveoli will compensate for the lack of anesthetic uptake in unventilated alveoli.

These effects are illustrated in Figure 19-11 for a condition that may be iatrogenically produced: endobronchial intubation. Since all ventilation is now directed to the intubated lung, this lung will be hyperventilated relative to perfusion. FA/FI for this lung will be slightly increased (relative to the increase obtained in the absence of endobronchial intubation) with the poorly soluble cyclopropane and greatly increased with the highly soluble ether. The increase with ether will compensate for the absence of uptake from the unventilated lung—a compensatory mechanism not available with

cyclopropane. The result is that the arterial partial pressure of cyclopropane is well below normal, while the arterial partial pressure of ether is scarcely changed.

These concepts have been confirmed experimentally by comparing the rate of arterial anesthetic rise with and without endobronchial intubation in dogs.[24] Endobronchial intubation significantly slowed the arterial rate of rise of cyclopropane but did not influence the rise with methoxyflurane. An intermediate result was obtained with halothane (Fig. 19-12). These data suggest that in the presence of ventilation/perfusion ratio abnormalities, the anesthetic effect of agents such as cyclopropane or nitrous oxide may be delayed, whereas the effect of ether or methoxyflurane will be unaffected.

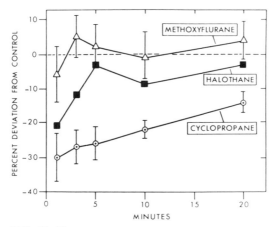

FIG. 19-12 In dogs when only the right lung was ventilated, the rise of the very soluble anesthetic, methoxyflurane, in arterial blood was normal (i.e., did not deviate from control) while the rise for the poorly soluble anesthetic, cyclopropane, was significantly slowed. (Stoelting RK, Longnecker DE: Effect of right-to-left shunt on rate of increase in arterial anesthetic concentration. Anesthesiology 36:352, 1972.)

PERCUTANEOUS ANESTHETIC LOSS

Thus far we have ignored two possible avenues by which anesthetics may be lost: transcutaneous movement and metabolism. Probably neither is a major determinant of anesthetic uptake during the course of a clinical anesthetic. Although transcutaneous movement occurs, the movement is small.[25,26] The greatest loss per alveolar anesthetic percent occurs with nitrous oxide. Loss of nitrous oxide might equal 5 to 10 ml/min with an alveolar concentration of 70 percent.

METABOLISM OF ANESTHETIC

Loss of anesthetic by biodegradation is also probably limited. However, some evidence suggests that anesthetic metabolism may be important with agents that undergo extensive biodegradation. Berman et al.[27] found phenobarbital pretreatment in rats to decrease the

arterial level of methoxyflurane. However, three reasons suggest that agents such as halothane, isoflurane, or enflurane are less likely to be affected. First, they are not metabolized as readily as methoxyflurane.[28] Second, anesthetizing concentrations appear to saturate the enzymes responsible for anesthetic metabolism.[29] Third, halothane, enflurane, and isoflurane are less soluble than methoxyflurane. The lower solubility means that relatively fewer molecules reach the liver. The combined effect of these factors remains to be determined, but it appears that metabolism is not a major determinant of F_A/F_I during anesthesia.

THE EFFECT OF NITROUS OXIDE ON CLOSED GAS SPACES

VOLUME CHANGES IN HIGHLY COMPLIANT SPACES

Thus far we have not discussed a third avenue for gas transfer-movement of nitrous oxide into closed gas spaces. Although this transfer does not influence F_A/F_I, it may have important functional consequences. There are two types of closed gas spaces in the body: compliant and noncompliant. Compliant spaces, such as bowel gas, pneumothorax, or pneumoperitoneum, are subject to changes in volume secondary to the transfer of nitrous oxide into these spaces.[30] These spaces normally contain nitrogen (from air), a gas whose low solubility (blood/gas partition coefficient = 0.015) limits its removal by blood. Thus, the entrance of nitrous oxide (whose solubility permits it to be carried by blood in substantial quantities) is not countered by an equal loss. The result is an increase in volume. The theoretical limit to the increase in volume is a function of the alveolar nitrous oxide concentration, since it is this concentration that is ultimately achieved in the closed gas space. That is, at equilibrium the partial pressure of nitrous oxide in the closed gas space must equal its partial pressure in the alveoli. An alveolar concentration of 50 percent might double the gas space volume, while a 75 percent concentration might produce a fourfold increase.

These theoretical limits may be approached when equilibrium is rapidly achieved, as with a pneumothorax or with gas emboli. Administration of 75 percent nitrous oxide in the presence of a pneumothorax may double the pneumothorax volume in 10 minutes and triple it by 30 minutes (Fig. 19-13).[30] This increase in volume may seriously impair cardiorespiratory function,[31] and the use of nitrous oxide is contraindicated in the presence of a significant pneumothorax.

A still more rapid expansion of volume occurs when air inadvertently enters the blood stream in a patient anesthetized with nitrous oxide. Expansion may be complete in seconds rather than in minutes. Munson and Merrick[32] demonstrated that the lethal volume of an air embolus was decreased in animals breathing nitrous oxide as opposed to air (Fig. 19-14). The difference could be entirely explained by expansion of the embolus in the animals breathing nitrous oxide, that is, the pre-

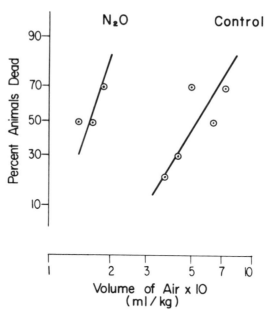

FIG. 19-14 Fifty percent of rabbits breathing oxygen were killed by an air embolus equaling 0.55 ml/kg. If the inspired gas mixture contained 75 percent nitrous oxide, only 0.16 ml/kg were required to kill one-half the animals. (Munson ES, Merrick HC: Effect of nitrous oxide on venous air embolism. Anesthesiology 27:783, 1966.)

dicted total volume of air plus nitrous oxide in the embolus equaled the volume of air needed to produce death in animals breathing only air. These studies suggest caution in the use of nitrous oxide for procedures where air embolization is a risk (e.g., posterior fossae craniotomies, laparoscopy). They also suggest that if air embolization is suspected, an immediate part of therapy should be the discontinuation of nitrous oxide. On the other hand, a nitrous oxide challenge may be used to test whether air embolization has occurred.[33]

The endotracheal tube cuff normally is filled with air. It, too, is susceptible to expansion by nitrous oxide.[34] The presence of 75 percent nitrous oxide surrounding such a cuff can double or triple the volume of the cuff. The result may be an unwanted increase in pressure exerted on the tracheal mucosa. Similarly, nitrous oxide may expand the cuffs of balloon-tipped (e.g., Swan-Ganz) catheters[35,36] when the balloons are inflated with air. The expansion is rapid, and a doubling of volume may occur within 10 minutes.

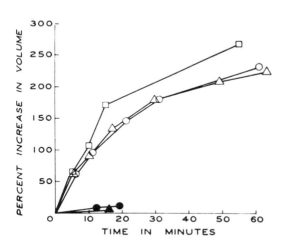

FIG. 19-13 The volume of a pneumothorax created by air injection is little affected when oxygen subsequently is breathed (filled triangle and circles). However, if 75 percent nitrous oxide is breathed, the volume doubles in 10 minutes and triples in a half-hour (open circles, squares, and triangles). (Eger EI II, Saidman LJ: Hazards of nitrous oxide anesthesia in bowel obstruction and pneumothorax. Anesthesiology 26:61, 1965.)

PRESSURE CHANGES IN POORLY COMPLIANT SPACES

Pressure can be produced by the entrance of nitrous oxide into gas cavities surrounded by poorly compliant walls. Unwanted increases in intraocular pressure may be imposed by nitrous oxide administration after intravitreal sulfur hexafluoride injection.[37] Other examples include the gas space created by pneumoencephalography and the natural gas space in the middle ear. Pressures in the head or middle ear may rise by 20 to 50 mmHg due to the ingress of nitrous oxide at a faster rate than air can be removed.[38,39] Recognition of this problem has decreased the use of nitrous oxide for pneumoencephalography, or for tympanoplasty, where the increased pressure may displace the graft. Increase in middle ear pressure may cause adverse postoperative effects on hearing.[40] The capacity of nitrous oxide to expand the gas in the middle ear also has been used to elevate an adherent atelectic tympanic membrane off the promontory and ossicles.[41]

WASHIN OF THE CIRCUIT

To begin anesthesia, anesthetic must be "washed into" the volume of the circuit. At inflow rates of 1 to 5 L/min and a circuit volume of 7 L (3 L bag, 2 L carbon dioxide absorber, and 2 L in corrugated hoses and fittings), the washin of the circuit is 75 to 100 percent complete in 10 minutes (Fig. 19-15). Higher inflow rates produce a more rapid rise in the inspired concentration, suggesting that induction can be accelerated and made more predictable by the use of high flow rates.

ANESTHETIC LOSS TO PLASTIC AND SODA LIME

Uptake of anesthetic by several depots also constitutes a hindrance to the development of an adequate inspired anesthetic concentration. The rubber or plastic components of the circuit may remove agent.[42] This is a significant problem in the case of methoxyflurane (rubber/gas

ANESTHETIC CIRCUITRY
(Also See Ch. 5)

The previous discussions generally have considered that the alveolar anesthetic concentration (F_A) was moving toward a constant inspired anesthetic concentration (F_I). In practice, the inspired concentration usually is not constant because a nonrebreathing system is not used. The rebreathing that results from the use of an anesthetic circuit causes the inspired concentration to be less than that in the gas delivered from the anesthetic machine. The inspired concentration thus is influenced by the delivered concentration, by the need to "wash in" the circuit, and by the depletion of anesthetic in rebreathed gases produced by uptake of anesthetic.

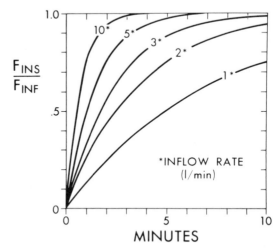

FIG. 19-15 The rate at which the inspired anesthetic concentration (F_{INS}) rises toward the inflowing concentration (F_{INF}) is determined by the inflow rate and circuit volume. In the case illustrated here, the circuit volume is 7 L. (Eger EI II: Anesthetic Uptake and Action. Baltimore, Williams & Wilkins, 1974. © 1974 EI Eger II, M.D.)

partition coefficient of 630) but has a relatively minor influence on halothane (a coefficient of 120), enflurane (74), isoflurane (62), or nitrous oxide (1.2).[43] Similarly, uptake by soda lime is small unless the soda lime becomes dry, in which case substantial amounts may be absorbed.[44] Dry soda lime may slow induction by this mechanism and subsequently may also supply halothane.[45,46]

THE EFFECT OF REBREATHING

Inspired gas actually consists of two gases: that delivered from the anesthetic machine and that previously exhaled by the patient and subsequently rebreathed. Since the patient has removed (i.e., taken up) anesthetic from the rebreathed gas, the amount taken up and the amount rebreathed will influence the inspired anesthetic concentration. An increase in uptake or rebreathing will lower the inspired concentration of a highly soluble gas more than the inspired concentration of a poorly soluble gas. This effect of uptake can be diminished by decreasing rebreathing. Rebreathing is reduced by increasing the inflow rate. With a ventilation of 5 L/min, rebreathing can essentially be abolished by the use of a 5 L/min inflow rate.[47]

High inflow rates (i.e., 5 L/min or greater) have the advantage of increasing the predictability of the inspired anesthetic concentration. They have the disadvantage of being wasteful and of increasing the tendency toward atmospheric pollution. They also may result in drier inspired gas and greater difficulty in estimating ventilation from excursions of the rebreathing bag.

THE LOW FLOW OR CLOSED CIRCLE TECHNIQUE

These disadvantages of high inflow rates have led to a small but increasing application of closed-circuit anesthesia.[48] Administration of closed-circuit anesthesia has two requirements. First, if nitrous oxide is used, oxygen concentration must be measured and inflow adjusted to ensure adequacy of the inspired oxygen partial pressure. Second, there must be some gauge by which anesthetic is delivered from the machine. Ultimately this delivery is dictated by the response of the patient, but an initial estimate of the amount of anesthetic needed may be made from a special formula that suggests that uptake decreases as a function of the square root of time.

Originally noted by Severinghaus,[49] application of the square root of time formula requires that anesthetic uptake for the first minute of anesthesia (U_1) be calculated. Uptake at subsequent times (U_1) is obtained as

$$U_1 = U_1/(t)^{1/2} \qquad (2)$$

Uptake during the first minute may be estimated from the formula for uptake given earlier in equation (1). Thus

$$U_1 = \lambda \cdot \dot{Q} \cdot (A - v)/BP \qquad (3)$$

The individual components are either known or can be easily estimated. For example, blood solubility (λ) for enflurane is 1.9. Cardiac output ($\dot{Q}$) in a normal adult is about 5,000 ml/min. During the first minute of anesthesia, the venous anesthetic partial pressure (v) is zero or low, so that $(A - v)/BP$ reduces to A/BP. We may assume that A/BP is the alveolar concentration that we want to achieve. Since the minimal alveolar concentration (MAC) of enflurane with 60 percent nitrous oxide is about 0.8 percent enflurane and since we need something modestly in excess of MAC—say 1.2 percent—A/BP equals 0.012. Thus $U_1 = 1.9 \cdot 5000 \cdot 0.012$, or 114 ml/min. After 9 minutes of anesthesia, this reduces to $114/3 = 38$ ml/min; after 25 minutes, it is $114/5 = 23$ ml/min, and so on. Flow through the vaporizer then must be adjusted to give the above output; for example, a 23 ml/min enflurane output at 20°C and 1 atm pressure would require a flow through a copper kettle of 78 ml/min (about 3.3 times as much as the amount of vapor desired; for halothane or isoflurane the factor is about 2 times).

These calculations form a rough guide to the volume of anesthetic that must be delivered to sustain a given alveolar concentration. In practice the volumes vary considerably,[50] in part as a function of variables such as body weight, fat-free body mass, and body surface area.[51] The estimate of the volume of anesthetic to be delivered should be modified by a knowledge of any factors that might alter anesthetic requirement. Thus, the amount of anesthetic needed would be reduced by hypothermia, advanced age, or shock. The patient's response ultimately must govern the amount of anesthetic delivered: movement, hypertension, or tachycardia might indicate an increased need; hypotension might indicate a decreased need.

RECOVERY FROM ANESTHESIA

GENERAL PRINCIPLES

Nearly all the factors that governed the rate at which the alveolar anesthetic concentration rose on induction apply to recovery. Thus, the immediate decline is extremely rapid, since the washout of the functional residual capacity by ventilation is as rapid as the washin. It should be recalled that only 2 minutes are required to eliminate 95 to 98 percent of nitrogen from the lungs when pure oxygen is breathed.

Nitrogen, however, is a poorly soluble gas relative to the inhaled anesthetics. As ventilation sweeps anesthetic from the alveoli, an anesthetic partial pressure gradient develops from the returning venous blood to that in the alveoli. This gradient drives anesthetic into the alveoli, thereby opposing the tendency of ventilation to lower the alveolar concentration. The effectiveness of the venous to alveolar gradient in opposing the tendency of ventilation to decrease the alveolar anesthetic partial pressure is in part determined by the solubility of the anesthetic. A highly soluble agent such as methoxyflurane will be more effective than a poorly soluble agent such as nitrous oxide because a greater reserve exists in blood for the highly soluble agent. That is, far more methoxyflurane is available at a given partial

pressure for transfer to the alveoli. Thus, the fall in the alveolar partial pressure of methoxyflurane is slower than the fall with halothane, and the latter in turn decreases less rapidly than does nitrous oxide. The rate at which recovery occurs is similarly affected: it is rapid with nitrous oxide and may be slow with methoxyflurane.

DIFFERENCES BETWEEN INDUCTION AND RECOVERY

Recovery differs from induction in two crucial ways. First, on induction, the effect of solubility to hinder the rise in alveolar anesthetic concentration could be overcome by increasing the inspired anesthetic concentration (i.e., by the application of "overpressure"). No such luxury is available during recovery: the inspired concentration cannot be reduced below zero. Second, on induction, all the tissues initially have the same anesthetic partial pressure — zero. On recovery, the tissue partial pressures are variable. The VRG has a pressure that usually equals that required for anesthesia. That is, the VRG has come to equilibrium with the alveolar anesthetic partial pressure. The muscle group may or may not have the same partial pressure as that found in the alveoli. A long anesthetic (2 to 4 hours) might permit equilibrium to be approached, but a shorter case would not. The high capacity of fat for all anesthetics except nitrous oxide precludes equilibration of the fat group with the alveolar anesthetic partial pressure with hours or even days of anesthesia.

The failure of muscle and fat to equilibrate with the alveolar anesthetic partial pressure means that these tissues initially cannot contribute to the transfer of anesthetic back to the lungs. In fact, as long as an anesthetic partial pressure gradient exists between arterial blood and that in a tissue, that tissue will continue to take up anesthetic. Thus, for the first several hours of recovery from halothane anesthesia, fat continues to take up halothane and by so doing accelerates the rate of recovery. Only after the alveolar (equals arterial) anesthetic partial pressure falls below that in a tissue can the tissue contribute anesthetic to the alveoli.

The failure of several tissues to reach equilibration with the alveolar anesthetic partial pressure means that the rate of decrease of alveolar anesthetic on recovery is more rapid than the rate of increase on induction. The difference between the rates for induction and recovery depends in part on the duration of anesthesia (Fig. 19-16).[52,53] A longer anesthetic puts more anesthetic into the slowly filling muscle and fat depots. Obviously, these reservoirs can supply more anesthetic to the blood returning to the lungs when they are filled than when they are empty.

Solubility influences the effect of duration of anesthesia on the rate at which the alveolar anesthetic partial pressure declines.[53] The decline of the partial pressure of a poorly soluble agent such as nitrous oxide is rapid in any anesthetic, and thus the acceleration imparted by a less-than-complete tissue equilibration cannot significantly alter the rate of recovery. The approach to equilibration becomes important with halothane and even more so with methoxyflurane (Fig. 19-16). A rapid recovery may follow a short methoxyflurane anesthetic but may occur slowly after a prolonged anes-

thetic. This is one of the reasons why nitrous oxide is usually a component of an inhaled (or for that matter, an injected) anesthetic regimen. The rapid elimination of this component permits at least a portion of recovery to be rapid.

Recovery from anesthesia results from the elimination of anesthetic from the brain. This requires both that the arterial partial pressure of anesthetic decrease and that the decrease in arterial partial pressure be reflected in a decrease in the brain partial pressure of anesthetic. The high blood flow to brain combined with the limited brain/blood partition coefficient should ensure the second of these requirements. However, using nuclear magnetic resonance techniques, Wyrwicz et al.[54] have found that substantial amounts of halothane or a breakdown product of halothane remains in the brain of rabbits for as long as 98 hours after the administration of 1 percent halothane for 30 minutes.

This finding has been interpreted by others as probably indicating the continued presence of depressant levels of halothane in the brain. The interpretation has been extrapolated to apply to all currently available inhaled anesthetics (i.e., enflurane and isoflurane).

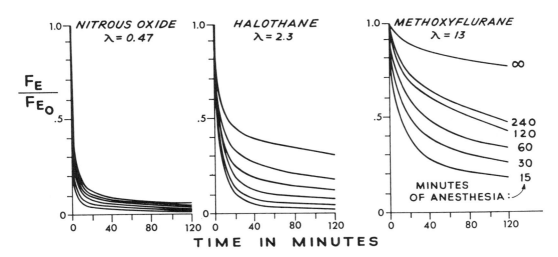

FIG. 19-16 Both solubility and duration of anesthesia affect the fall of the alveolar concentration (F_E) from the alveolar concentration immediately preceeding the cessation of anesthetic administration (F_{E_O}). A longer anesthetic slows the fall as does a greater solubility. (Stoelting RK, Eger EI II: The effects of ventilation and anesthetic solubility on recovery from anesthesia: An in vivo and analog analysis before and after equilibration. Anesthesiology 30:290, 1969.)

Such an interpretation is not likely to be correct for halothane or for other anesthetics. It would imply that large quantities of halothane (and other anesthetics) are bound to high-affinity sites in the brain. No such sites have thus far been discovered, and measurements of halothane solubility do not suggest the existence of such sites.[55] Autoradiographic studies indicate that 90 percent of the halothane introduced into the gray matter of the brain of monkeys by a brief anesthetizing exposure disappears from the brain within 20 minutes after exposure.[56] Thus, it appears that the findings of Wyrwicz and co-workers indicate the prolonged presence in the brain of halothane metabolites rather than of halothane itself.

METABOLISM

The saturation of the enzymes responsible for the metabolism of anesthetics probably prevents metabolism from significantly altering the rate at which the alveolar anesthetic partial pressure rises. This limitation does not exist on recovery, and metabolism may be an important determinant of the rate at which the alveolar anesthetic partial pressure declines. The importance of metabolism to recovery is implied by results from Munson et al.,[57] who showed that contrary to what might be predicted from their respective solubilities, the alveolar washout of halothane is more rapid than that of enflurane. This agrees with the relative ease with which these two agents are metabolized: 15 to 20 percent of the halothane taken up during the course of an ordinary anesthetic can be recovered as urinary metabolites.[58] Only 2 to 3 percent of enflurane can be recovered as urinary metabolites.[59] Thus, there are two major routes by which halothane can be eliminated: the lung and the liver. With enflurane, elimination via the liver is relatively minor and explains why Munson et al. found a more rapid fall in alveolar halothane.[57]

Cahalan et al.[60] have confirmed the results of Munson's group. In addition, Cahalan and associates found that higher initial concentrations of enflurane and halothane did not alter the results. They also found that the metabolism of halothane may equal as much as 45 percent of the halothane taken up.

DIFFUSION HYPOXIA

The uptake of large volumes of nitrous oxide on induction of anesthesia gives rise to the concentration and second gas effects. On recovery from anesthesia, the outpouring of large volumes of nitrous oxide can produce what Fink called "diffusion anoxia."[61] These volumes may cause hypoxia (Fig. 19-17) in two ways. First, they may directly affect oxygenation by displacing oxygen.[61–63] Second, by diluting alveolar carbon dioxide they may decrease respiratory drive and hence ventilation.[63] Both effects require that large volumes of nitrous oxide be released into the alveoli. Since large volumes of nitrous oxide are released only during the first 5 to 10 minutes of recovery, this is the period of greatest concern. This concern is enhanced by the fact that the first 5 to 10 minutes of recovery also may be the time of greatest respiratory depression. For these reasons many anesthetists administer 100 percent oxygen for the first 5 to 10 minutes of recovery. This procedure may be particularly indicated in patients with preexisting lung disease or when postoperative respiratory depression is anticipated (e.g., after a nitrous oxide-narcotic anesthetic).

THE ANESTHETIC CIRCUIT

The anesthetic circuit may limit the rate of recovery just as it limited induction. If the patient is not disconnected from the circuit on cessation of anesthetic delivery, the patient may continue to inspire anesthetic. To reduce the inspired level to zero or near zero, several factors must be taken into account. The anesthetic within the circuit must be washed out. In addition, the rubber or plastic components of the circuit and the soda lime within the circuit will have absorbed anesthetic that can be re-

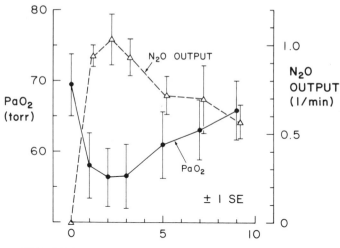

FIG. 19-17 At time zero the inspired gas was changed from 21 percent oxygen/79 percent nitrous oxide to 21 percent/79 percent nitrogen. Arterial oxygen subsequently fell in association with the outpouring of nitrous oxide. (Adapted from Sheffer L, Steffenson JL, Birth AA: Nitrous oxide-induced diffusion hypoxia in patients breathing spontaneously. Anesthesiology 37:436, 1972.)

leased back into the gas phase,[64] and this too must be washed out. Finally, the patient's exhaled air contains anesthetic that cannot be rebreathed if the inspired anesthetic concentration is to approach zero. The effect of each of these factors to raise the inspired anesthetic concentration can be negated by the use of high inflow rates of oxygen, that is, 5 L/min or greater.

REFERENCES

1. Eger EI II: Anesthetic Uptake and Action. Baltimore, Williams & Wilkins, 1974
2. Cromwell TH, Eger EI II, Stevens WC, Dolan WM: Forane uptake, excretion, and blood solubility in man. Anesthesiology 35:401, 1971
3. Munson ES, Eger EI II, Tham MK, et al: Increase in anesthetic uptake, excretion, and blood solubility in man after eating. Anesth Analg 57:224, 1978
4. Eger EI II: Isoflurane (Forane^R). A compendium and reference. Madison Wisc, Ohio Medical Products, 1981
5. Eger EI II: Application of a mathematical model of gas uptake, Uptake and Distribution of Anesthetic Agents. Edited by Papper EM, Kitz RJ. New York, McGraw-Hill, 1963, pp 88–103
6. Eger EI II: Effect of inspired anesthetic concentration on the rate of rise of alveolar concentration. Anesthesiology 24:153, 1963
7. Stoelting RK, Eger EI II: An additional explanation for the second gas effect: A concentrating effect. Anesthesiology 30:273, 1969
8. Eger EI II, Smith RA, Koblin DD: The concentration effect can be mimicked by a decrease in blood solubility. Anesthesiology 49:282, 1978
9. Epstein RM, Rackow H, Salnitre E, et al: Influence of the concentration effect on the uptake of anesthetic mixtures: The second gas effect. Anesthesiology 25:364, 1964
10. Yamamura H, Wakasugi B, Okuma Y, et al: The effects of ventilation on the absorption and elimination of inhalation anesthetics. Anaesthesia 18:427, 1963
11. Munson ES, Eger EI II, Bowers DL: Effects of anesthetic-depressed ventilation and cardiac output on anesthetic uptake. Anesthesiology 38:251, 1973
12. Fukui Y, Smith NT: Interactions among ventilation, the circulation, and the uptake and distribution of halothane—Use of a hybrid computer multiple model: I. The basic model. Anesthesiology 54:107, 1981
13. Munson ES, Larson CP Jr, Babad AA, et al: The effects of halothane, fluroxene and cyclopropane on ventilation: A comparative study in man. Anesthesiology 27:716, 1966
14. Fourcade HE, Stevens WC, Larson CP Jr, et al: Ventilatory effects of Forane—A new inhaled anesthetic. Anesthesiology 35:26, 1971

15. Calverley RK, Smith NT, Jones CW, et al: Ventilatory and cardiovascular effects of enflurane anesthesia during spontaneous ventilation in man. Anesth Analg 57:610, 1978
16. Gibbons RT, Steffey EP, Eger EI II: The effect of spontaneous versus controlled ventilation on the rate of rise of alveolar halothane concentration in dogs. Anesth Analg 56:32, 1977
17. Yamamura H: The effect of ventilation and blood volume on the uptake and elimination of inhalation anesthetic agents, Progress in Anaesthesiology, Proceedings of the Fourth World Congress of Anesthesiologists. Amsterdam, Excerpta Medica International Congress Series 200, 1968, pp 394–399
18. Eger EI II, Smith NT, Stoelting RK, et al: Cardiovascular effects of halothane in man. Anesthesiology 32:396, 1970
19. Calverley RK, Smith NT, Eger EI II: Cardiovascular effects of enflurane anesthesia during controlled ventilation in man. Anesth Analg 57:619, 1978
20. Eger EI II, Bahlman SH, Munson ES: Effect of age on the rate of increase of alveolar anesthetic concentration. Anesthesiology 35:365, 1971
21. Wahrenbrock EA, Eger EI II, Lavaruso RB, et al: Anesthetic uptake of mice and men (and whales). Anesthesiology 40:19, 1974
22. Salanitre E, Rackow H: The pulmonary exchange of nitrous oxide and halothane in infants and children. Anesthesiology 30:388, 1969
23. Eger EI II, Severinghaus JW: Effect of uneven pulmonary distribution of blood and gas on induction with inhalation anesthetics. Anesthesiology 25:620, 1964
24. Stoelting RK, Longnecker DE: Effect of right-to-left shunt on rate of increase in arterial anesthetic concentration. Anesthesiology 36:352, 1972
25. Stoelting RK, Eger EI II: Percutaneous loss of nitrous oxide, cyclopropane, ether and halothane in man. Anesthesiology 30:278, 1969
26. Cullen BG, Eger EI II: Diffusion of nitrous oxide, cyclopropane, and halothane through human skin and amniotic membrane. Anesthesiology 36:168, 1972
27. Berman ML, Lowe HJ, Hagler KT, et al: Uptake and elimination of methoxyflurane as influenced by enzyme induction in the rat. Anesthesiology 38:352, 1973
28. Halsey MJ, Sawyer DC, Eger EI II, et al: Hepatic metabolism of halothane, methoxyflurane, cyclopropane, Ethrane and Forane in miniature swine. Anesthesiology 35:43, 1971
29. Sawyer DC, Eger EI II, Bahlman SH, et al: Concentration dependence of hepatic halothane metabolism. Anesthesiology 34:230, 1971
30. Eger EI II, Saidman LJ: Hazards of nitrous oxide anesthesia in bowel obstruction and pneumothorax. Anesthesiology 26:61, 1965
31. Hunter AR: Problems of anesthesia in artificial pneumothorax. Proc R Soc Med 48:765, 1955
32. Munson ES, Merrick HC: Effect of nitrous oxide on venous air embolism. Anesthesiology 27:783, 1966
33. Shapiro HM, Yoachim J, Marshall LF: Nitrous oxide challenge for detection of residual intravascular pulmonary gas following venous air embolism. Anesth Analg 61:304, 1982
34. Stanley TH, Kawamura R, Graves C: Effects of nitrous oxide on volume and pressure of endotracheal tube cuffs. Anesthesiology 41:256, 1974
35. Kaplan R, Abramowitz MD, Epstein BS: Nitrous oxide and air-filled balloon-tipped catheters. Anesthesiology 55:71, 1981
36. Eisenkraft JB, Eger EI II: Nitrous oxide anesthesia may double the balloon gas volume of Swan-Ganz catheters. Mt Sinai J Med 49:430, 1982
37. Wolf GL, Capuano C, Hartung J: Nitrous oxide increases intraocular pressure after intravitreal sulfur hexafluoride injection. Anesthesiology 59:547, 1983
38. Thomsen KA, Terkildsen LK, Arnfred J: Middle ear pressure variations during anesthesia. Arch Otolaryngol 82:609, 1965
39. Saidman LJ, Eger EI II: Change in cerebrospinal fluid pressure during pneumoencephalography under nitrous oxide anesthesia. Anesthesiology 26:67, 1965
40. Waun JE, Sweitzer RS, Hamilton WK: Effect of nitrous oxide in middle ear mechanics and hearing acuity. Anesthesiology 28:846, 1967
41. Graham MD, Knight PR: Atelectative tympanic membrane reversal by nitrous oxide supplemented general anesthesia and polyethylene ventilation tube insertion. A preliminary report. Laryngoscope 41:1469, 1981
42. Eger EI II, Larson CP Jr, Severinghaus JW: The solubility of halothane in rubber, soda lime and various plastics. Anesthesiology 23:365, 1962
43. Titel JH, Lowe HJ: Rubber–gas partition coefficients. Anesthesiology 29:1215, 1968
44. Titel JH, Lowe HJ, Elam JO, et al: Quantitative closed-circuit halothane anesthesia. Anesth Analg 47:560, 1968
45. Grodin WK, Epstein MAF, Epstein RA: Mechanisms of halothane adsorption by dry soda-lime. Br J Anaesth 54:561, 1982
46. Grodin WK, Epstein RA: Halothane adsorption complicating the use of soda-lime to humidify anaesthetic gases. Br J Anaesth 54:555, 1982
47. Harper M, Eger EI II: A comparison of the efficiency of three anesthesia circle systems. Anesth Analg 55:724, 1976

48. Aldrete JA, Lowe HJ, Virtue RW: Low Flow and Closed System Anesthesia. New York, Grune & Stratton, 1979
49. Severinghaus JW: The rate of uptake of nitrous oxide in man. J Clin Invest 33:1183, 1954
50. Ross JAS, Wloch RT, White DC, et al: Servo-controlled closed-circuit anaesthesia. Br J Anaesth 55:1053, 1983
51. O'Callaghan AC, Hawes DW, Ross JAS, et al: Uptake of isoflurane during clinical anaesthesia. Br J Anaesth 55:1061, 1983
52. Mapleson WW: Quantitative prediction of anesthetic concentrations, Uptake and Distribution of Anesthetic Agents. Edited by Papper EM, Kitz RJ. New York, McGraw-Hill, 1963, pp 104–119
53. Stoelting RK, Eger EI II: The effects of ventilation and anesthetic solubility on recovery from anesthesia: An in vivo and analog analysis before and after equilibration. Anesthesiology 30:290, 1969
54. Wyrwicz AM, Pszenny MH, Schofield C, et al: Noninvasive observations of fluorinated anesthetics in rabbit brain by fluorine-19 nuclear magnetic resonance. Science 222:428, 1983
55. Larson CP Jr, Eger EI II, Severinghaus JW: The solubility of halothane in blood and tissue homogenates. Anesthesiology 23:349, 1962
56. Cohen EN, Chow KL, Mathers L: Autoradiographic distribution of volatile anesthetics within the brain. Anesthesiology 37:324, 1972
57. Munson ES, Eger EI II, Tham MK, et al: Increase in anesthetic uptake, excretion and blood solubility in man after eating. Anesth Analg 57:224, 1978
58. Rehder K, Forbes J, Alter H, et al: Halothane biotransformation in man: A quantitative study. Anesthesiology 28:711, 1967
59. Chase RE, Holaday DA, Fiserova-Bergerova V, et al: The biotransformation of Ethrane in man. Anesthesiology 35:262, 1971
60. Cahalan MK, Johnson BH, Eger EI II: Relationship of concentrations of halothane and enflurane to their metabolism and elimination in man. Anesthesiology 54:3, 1981
61. Fink BR: Diffusion anoxia. Anesthesiology 16:511, 1955
62. Sheffer L, Steffenson JL, Birch AA: Nitrous-oxide-induced diffusion hypoxia in patients breathing spontaneously. Anesthesiology 37:436, 1972
63. Rackow H, Salanitre E, Frumin MH: Dilution of alveolar gases during nitrous oxide excretion in man. J Appl Physiol 16:723, 1961
64. Eger EI II, Brandstater B: Solubility of methoxyflurane in rubber. Anesthesiology 24:679, 1963

20

Circulatory Pharmacology of Inhaled Anesthetics

Robert F. Hickey, M.D.
Edmond I. Eger II, M.D.

INTRODUCTION

The search for the ideal inhaled anesthetic has led to the development of agents with properties that differ markedly from those possessed by older agents. Included in these differences are the circulatory effects of modern anesthetics. Older agents, such as nitrous oxide, ether, and cyclopropane, tended to support the circulation by increasing sympathetic activity, by less directly depressing the heart, and/or by producing contraction of peripheral vessels. As anesthesiologists took a more active role in controlling the circulation through pharmacologic or physiologic means, they became progressively less fearful of the cardiovascular depression inherent in anesthesia and in fact made use of such depression. The modern anesthetics both engender and reflect this attitude. In the present chapter we contrast the circulatory properties of old and new inhaled agents. These contrasts provide insight into the breadth and limitations imposed by anesthesia.

HUMAN VOLUNTEER STUDIES

Studies in human volunteers permit the isolation of anesthetic effects from those of disease, surgery, and concomitant pharmacologic and physiologic interventions. These studies are therefore more likely to reveal the untainted effects of anesthesia, but these effects may be modified by the milieu of clinical practice, which is explored in a later section of this chapter. First we consider the circulatory changes that result from anesthesia when $PaCO_2$ is maintained normal by controlled ventilation.

ARTERIAL BLOOD PRESSURE

The modern anesthetics, halothane,[1,2] enflurane,[3] and isoflurane,[4] all decrease mean arterial blood pressure in direct proportion to their concentration. At 2.0 minimal alveolar anesthetic concentration (MAC), mean arterial pressure is approximately 50 percent of the control (awake) value (Fig. 20-1). By contrast, many older anesthetics (diethyl ether,[5] fluroxene,[6] and cyclopropane[7,8]) have little effect on arterial pressure even at concentrations above 3.0 MAC.

CARDIAC OUTPUT

Halothane[1,2] and enflurane[3] reduce cardiac output, and this effect parallels their effect on arterial pressure (Fig. 20-2). Similarly, the older anesthetics, cyclopropane,[7,8] diethyl ether,[5] and fluroxene,[6] which do not reduce arterial pressure, also do not change cardiac output. The exception to this dichotomy is isoflurane, which has little effect on cardiac output but profoundly reduces mean arterial pressure.

Figure 20-2 provides potentially misleading information. Enflurane appears similar to halothane in its effect on cardiac output but in fact differs significantly. In volunteers given 2.0 MAC enflurane, a progressive decrease in cardiac output and blood pressure to unacceptable levels occurs but no such progression is evident with halothane, even at 2.4 MAC. In the steady state, fluroxene either does not change or increases cardiac output.[6] However, an acute increase in fluroxene concentration temporarily decreases cardiac output. A similar effect is seen with diethyl ether.[5] This response indicates an underlying capacity of these agents to cause cardiovascular depression and suggests

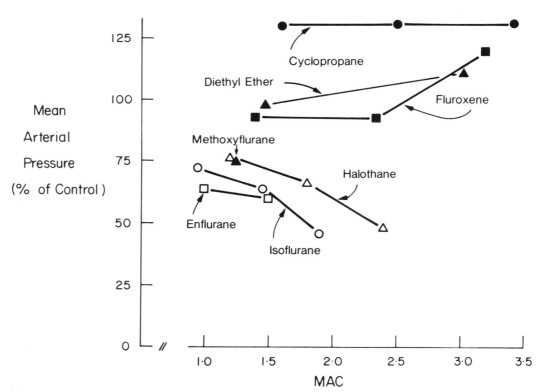

FIG. 20-1 Halothane, isoflurane, enflurane, and methoxyflurane decrease mean arterial pressure in a dose-related fashion. Arterial pressure is unchanged with diethyl ether and lower concentrations of fluroxene. It is increased with cyclopropane and at the highest concentration of fluroxene studied. In this figure and subsequent ones, control values are those obtained prior to induction of anesthesia. Ventilation is controlled and $PaCO_2$ is normal.

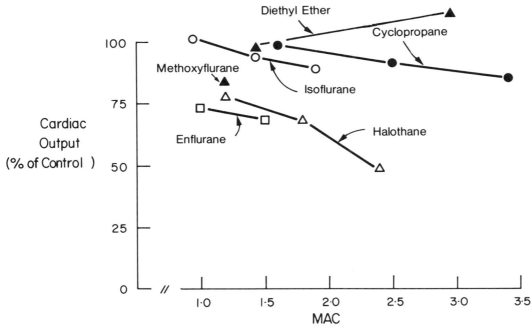

FIG. 20-2 Cardiac output is depressed by enflurane, halothane, and methoxyflurane. Isoflurane, cyclopropane, and diethyl ether have little effect on cardiac output.

that in the steady state these anesthetics permit or cause a compensatory circulatory stimulation that masks the underlying depressant effect.

SYSTEMIC VASCULAR RESISTANCE (Fig. 20-3)

This calculated variable is obtained by dividing systemic perfusion pressure (mean arterial minus right atrial pressure) by cardiac output. Systemic vascular resistance (SVR) is increased by cyclopropane,[7,8] is not changed by diethyl ether[5] or halothane[1,2] and is reduced by fluroxene,[6] enflurane,[3] and isoflurane[4] (Fig. 20-3). The largest reduction in SVR is caused by isoflurane[4] (50 percent reduction at 1.9 MAC).

All inhaled anesthetics reduce resistance to flow to the brain and the skin. An earlier impression that halothane is a profound vasodilator resulted from studies done during spontaneous ventilation where the associated respiratory depression and consequently elevated

PaCO$_2$ contributed significantly to the vasodilation. Cyclopropane is the only potent inhaled anesthetic that significantly increases SVR in all anesthetic levels. Cyclopropane increases resistance by several mechanisms: it directly causes contraction of vessels; it increases the sensitivity of vessel musculature to norepinephrine; and it also increases sympathetic outflow.[9]

HEART RATE

Inhaled anesthetics change heart rate by altering rate of sinus node depolarization, by changing myocardial conduction times, or by shifting autonomic nervous system activity. The bradycardia sometimes seen with halothane may result from a direct depression of atrial rate. Halothane at 0.5 to 1.5 MAC decreases the contractile rate of isolated rat atria.[10]

Fluroxene, diethyl ether, methoxyflurane, isoflurane, and enflurane all increase heart

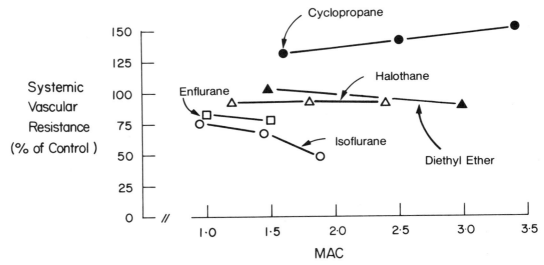

FIG. 20-3 Cyclopropane increases, halothane and diethyl ether do not change, and enflurane and isoflurane reduce systemic vascular resistance.

rate in human volunteers (Fig. 20-4). An anesthetic-induced reduction in arterial blood pressure would tend to increase heart rate by withdrawal of baroreceptor stimulation. Many of the volatile anesthetics studied inhibit the baroreflex control of heart rate in humans. This inhibition is almost complete for halothane[11] and enflurane.[12] Methoxyflurane, by contrast, does not alter the sensitivity of the baroreflex control of heart rate.[13] Isoflurane is intermediate in its effect, diminishing the baroreflex sensitivity 70 and 42 percent of control at 1.0 and 1.5 MAC, respectively.[14]

The effect of anesthesia on heart rate and arterial blood pressure also must be considered in the context of preanesthesia values for these

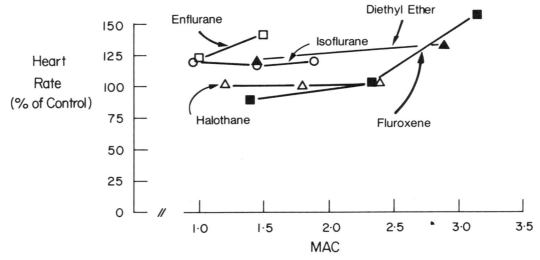

FIG. 20-4 Heart rate is unchanged with halothane, is concentration dependent with fluroxene and is increased with enflurane, isoflurane, and diethyl ether.

variables. Anesthesia abolished the tachycardia, hypertension, and increased cardiac output produced by excitement; excitement is ultimately abolished, and heart rate, pressure, and output decrease may not be harmed. In contrast, if preanesthetic parasympathetic activity is enhanced, anesthesia may increase pulse rate and pressure. This hypothesis has been supported by Roizen et al.,[15] who measured the changes in heart rate, blood pressure, rate–pressure product, and plasma norepinephrine content that occurred with induction of anesthesia in elective ASA I or II adult patients. Anesthesia produced by halothane, enflurane, morphine, or spinal anesthesia tended to decrease high systemic pressure and heart rates and to increase low systemic pressure and heart rates.

RIGHT ATRIAL PRESSURE

All inhaled anesthetics tend to increase right atrial pressures in a dose-related fashion (Fig. 20-5). The changes are related both to a depression of myocardial function and to an anesthetic effect on peripheral vasculature. In vitro, halothane, enflurane, and isoflurane produce comparable myocardial depression; yet right atrial pressure is less at similar doses of isoflurane and enflurane. Vasodilation may account for this finding. Certainly the right atrial pressure increases produced by cyclopropane are in part explained by the direct constriction of veins caused by cyclopropane. Nitrous oxide similarly may cause vasoconstriction.

PULMONARY ARTERY OCCLUDED PRESSURE

In patients with coronary artery disease anesthetized with halothane[16] or isoflurane[17] at concentrations of about 1.0 MAC, pulmonary artery occluded pressure (PAOP) decreases slightly.

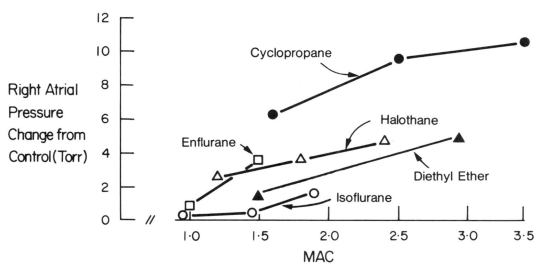

FIG. 20-5 All anesthetics depicted increase right atrial pressure in a dose-dependent fashion. Cyclopropane, enflurane, and halothane induce the greatest increases.

MYOCARDIAL EFFECTS

MYOCARDIAL FUNCTION

At some concentration, all inhaled anesthetics depress myocardial contractibility. This is clearly seen in in vitro studies in which direct myocardial depressant properties of the anesthetics are not obscured by homeostatic mechanisms and/or the capacity of the anesthetics to cause peripheral vasodilation or stimulate sympathetic activity. Brown and Crout[18] found five anesthetics that produce a linear, dose-dependent depression of isolated cat papillary muscle contractility (Fig. 20-6). However, the amount of depression was found to differ with enflurane > halothane > methoxyflurane > cyclopropane > diethyl ether. Iwatsuki and Shimosoto[19] in similar in vitro studies using the cat papillary muscle confirmed the dose-dependent linear depression produced by the same five anesthetics. However, these workers found that enflurane is not the most depressant drug but is similar to diethyl ether and less depressant than either halothane or methoxyflurane. Slight differences in technique (temperature, use of peer groups) may account for the different order of depression found in these two studies.

The cardiac depression seen in vitro appears to be modified in intact animals or humans. For example, neither isoflurane nor fluroxene causes myocardial depression, as indicated by the sustained amplitude of the ballistocardiogram (BCG) in volunteers anesthetized with 1.0 to 2.0 MAC of these agents (Fig. 20-7). In contrast, enflurane and halothane depress the BCG amplitude in a dose-related manner. Both 1.25 MAC methoxyflurane[20] and halothane[21] decrease right ventricular dP/dt by 15 to 20 percent of the values obtained prior to anesthesia, but this depression is less than that produced by comparable anesthetic doses in vitro. Moreover, with continuing anesthesia in humans, dP/dt returns to awake values, whereas in vitro values remain depressed.[14,16] These data imply that in vivo compensatory mechanisms counter the depressant effects of inhaled agents and, further, that the effect of these compensatory mechanisms increases with the passage of time. Echocardiography permits direct measures of contractility and afterload and demonstrates dose dependent depression of myocardial contractility by isoflurane, halothane and enflurane.[22]

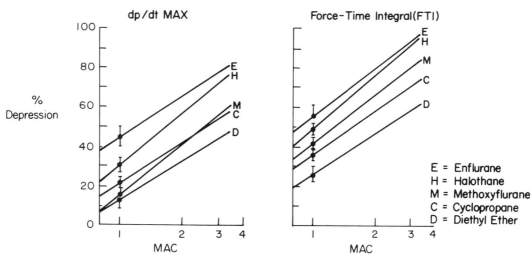

FIG. 20-6 In vitro effects of five anesthetics demonstrate a dose-dependent depression of myocardial contractility. The ordering of depression from most to least is enflurane > halothane > methoxyflurane > cyclopropane > diethyl ether. (Brown BR, Crout JR: A comparative study of the effect of five general anesthetics on myocardial contractility. Anesthesiology 34:236, 1971.)

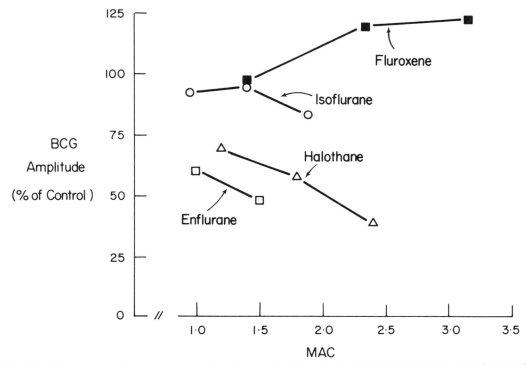

FIG. 20-7 Fluroxene and isoflurane have little effect on the IJ wave of the ballistrocardiogram. Halothane and enflurane both show dose-dependent depression.

Extensive studies of myocardial function in anesthetized patients were reported by Sonntag et al.[23] They measured left ventricular function awake and at 1.1 and 2.1 MAC halothane. As halothane increased, stroke volume, mean arterial pressure, and left ventricular dP/dt_{max} progressively decreased. Left ventricular end-diastolic pressure increased with values of 11 mm Hg in the nonanesthetized volunteers and 12 and 14 mm Hg, respectively, at 1.1 and 2.1 MAC halothane. Systemic vascular resistance remained constant. The decreased contractility at increased preload and constant systemic vascular resistance and heart rate documents the negative inotropic effect of halothane in humans.

During controlled ventilation, halothane increases left ventricular volume in dogs[24-26] and in humans[27] in a dose-related fashion despite a decrease in afterload (systemic arterial blood pressure). Both diastolic and systolic volumes increased, and in one study,[26] increases occurred despite a concomitant increase in heart rate. An increase in heart rate should increase contractility and thereby reduce ventricular volume.

Spontaneous ventilation may produce different results. In spontaneously breathing humans, 1.1. MAC halothane decreased in left ventricular diastolic dimension by 10 percent as determined with echocardiography.[28] This reduction in left ventricular dimension could be secondary to a decreased left ventricular filling pressure (see previous section on halothane effect on pulmonary artery wedge pressure), a decreased afterload, an increased heart rate, or an increased sympathetic activity associated with an elevation of $PaCO_2$.

MYOCARDIAL OXYGEN CONSUMPTION

Inhaled anesthetics reduce myocardial oxygen consumption (MVO_2) primarily by decreasing the need for oxygen. In dogs[29,30] and humans[31] 1.5 to 2.0 MAC halothane decreases myocardial oxygen consumption by 40 to 60 percent. Isoflurane causes a similar decrease in dogs.[32] In a comparative study in chronically instrumented dogs, Sybert et al.[33] found that 0.8 to 0.95 MAC isoflurane, enflurane, and halothane decreased MVO_2 to 55, 49, and 34 percent, respectively, of values obtained in awake animals.

CORONARY ARTERY BLOOD FLOW

Halothane decreases coronary blood flow (CBF). Coronary vascular resistance either increases or remains constant, depending on the effect of halothane on MVO_2 and systemic arterial pressure. Lactate extraction remains constant, suggesting adequacy of coronary artery perfusion.[30,31] If autoregulation persists during halothane anesthesia, a reduction in MVO_2 should increase coronary artery resistance (i.e., an increase in resistance does not imply that halothane is a coronary vasoconstrictor). However, halothane also lowers systemic blood arterial pressure, which should decrease coronary artery blood flow and invite a decrease in resistance. These two opposing effects, on demand and supply tend to balance. However, the balance is only partial, since coronary arteriovenous oxygen difference decreases; that is, the tendency for a decrease in resistance to occur appears to predominate and implies, in fact, that halothane is a coronary artery vasodilator.

Wolff et al.[34] demonstrated that some autoregulation exists during halothane anesthesia. They cannulated and perfused the left coronary arteries of dogs to maintain a constant coronary artery blood pressure. Administration of halothane to both the whole animal and the heart decreased coronary artery blood flow, indicating an increase in coronary artery resistance. Such an increase in resistance should occur with autoregulation, since the administration of halothane also decreased systemic pressure and hence heart work and oxygen consumption.

More recently, Sybert et al.[33] examined regional coronary artery pressure flow relationships in chronically instrumented dogs. At about 1.0 MAC, isoflurane, enflurane, and halothane all blunted the autoregulation of coronary blood flow. Isoflurane depressed autoregulation more than enflurane and halothane, whereas regulation during halothane anesthesia was closest to autoregulation determined in awake animals.

In summary, inhaled anesthetics affect coronary artery blood flow in part by affecting those variables that control oxygen supply and demand, in part by a direct effect on the coronary arteries, and in part by the "control" state. Apropos of the last of these factors, tachycardia and hypertension may accompany apprehension in an awake volunteer or a "light basal" anesthetic in an animal. Such humans or animals will demonstrate much greater decreases in CBF and MVO_2 on administration of a general anesthetic.

EFFECT OF NITROUS OXIDE

The most frequently administered inhalation anesthetic is nitrous oxide. At one time nitrous oxide was considered an impotent vehicle for the administration of more potent inhaled anesthetics. It has become clear that nitrous oxide has significant effects of its own and may appreciably alter the actions of potent agents given concomitantly.

Nitrous oxide directly depresses the myocardium. It produces a dose-dependent depression of the dog myocardium in a heart–lung preparation that is less than that produced by more potent agents.[35] Similarly, it depresses peak developed isometric tension and the maximum rate of tension development in cat heart muscle strips maintained at 37°C.[36] However, at 37°C depression is also produced by lowering oxygen partial pressure with nitrogen by an amount equal to that lowering achieved with nitrous oxide. Although this suggests that depression from nitrous oxide results from hypoxia, an experiment by Price[37] argues otherwise. Cat papillary muscle maintained at 25°C is depressed more by 50 percent nitrous oxide than by 50 percent nitrogen. The use of a lower temperature avoids the hypoxia that may develop in the deeper layers of muscle. That is, diffusion of oxygen to those deeper layers can keep pace with the lower metabolic rate at 25°C but not the higher rate at 37°C. It is noteworthy that nitrous oxide depresses the heart less than a comparable concentration of halothane.

In humans breathing 40 percent nitrous oxide, Eisele and Smith[38] found a 10 percent reduction of the amplitude of the ballistocardiogram, suggesting direct myocardial depression. To study anesthetic concentrations of nitrous oxide without concurrent hypoxia requires the use of hyperbaric pressure. Winter et al.[39] anesthetized nine normal volunteers at 1.55 and 1.10 atm of nitrous oxide. At 1.55 atm of nitrous oxide, arterial pressure and heart rate increased 6 and 10 percent, respectively, while cardiac output and systemic vascular resistance remained unchanged (Fig. 20-8). No evidence of myocardial depression was found. However, sympathetic stimulation was suggested by sweating, dilated pupils, and increased serum catecholamines and corticosteroids. This stimulation could have obscured any direct evidence of myocardial depression.

Mean arterial blood pressure and dP/dt decrease and left ventricular end-diastolic pressure increases in patients suffering from coronary artery disease who are given 40 percent nitrous oxide.[40] Similarly, cardiac output and blood pressure decrease when 60 percent nitrous oxide is added to the anesthetic regimen of patients who already have received 1 mg/kg of morphine.[41] Such studies indicate that nitrous oxide does have cardiodepressant properties.

Results from studies of the combination of

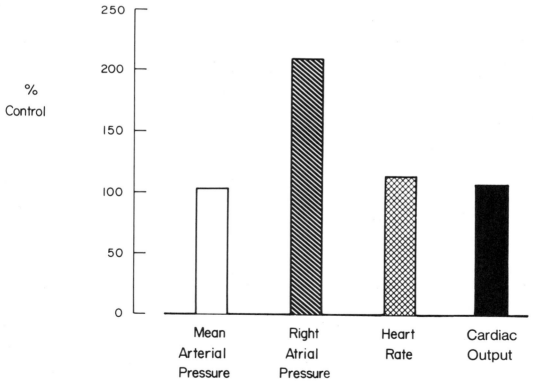

FIG. 20-8 Administration of 1.5 MAC nitrous oxide results in little change in arterial pressure, heart rate, or cardiac output. (See text for details.)

nitrous oxide with potent inhaled anesthetics also indicate that nitrous oxide is sympathomimetic and has mild cardiac depressant effects. Smith et al.[42] added 70 percent nitrous oxide to either 1 to 1.5 MAC or 2 to 2.5 MAC halothane anesthesia. In the first 10 to 20 minutes after addition of the nitrous oxide, systemic vascular resistance, arterial and right atrial pressure, and pupil diameter and plasma norepinephrine all increased, whereas heart rate, cardiac output, and the amplitude of the ballistocardiogram remained constant. Hill et al.[43] added 20, 40, and 60 percent nitrous oxide to 0.95, 1.4, and 1.9 MAC halothane. Addition of 60 percent nitrous oxide increased right atrial pressure at all concentrations of halothane. Other cardiovascular changes depended on the concentration of halothane. Subjects at 0.95, 1.4, and 1.9 MAC halothane responded to the addition of 60 percent nitrous oxide by respectively decreasing, not changing, and increasing their systemic vascular resistance. Systemic vascular

resistance changes were associated with opposite (inverse) changes in stroke volume.

Bahlman et al.[44] compared nitrous oxide plus halothane anesthesia with halothane anesthesia alone at 1.2, 1.8, and 2.4 MAC in human volunteers (Fig. 20-9). To have comparable concentrations of anesthetics, the subjects received a greater concentration of halothane when not receiving nitrous oxide. At 1.2 and 2.4 MAC anesthesia, IJ wave amplitude of the ballistocardiogram, cardiac output, right atrial pressure, and arterial pressure were higher in subjects anesthetized with halothane plus nitrous oxide. At 1.8 MAC no significant differences existed. Thus, the substitution of nitrous oxide for halothane either produced no change in or lessened the cardiovascular depression.

In a similar study with nitrous oxide and isoflurane, Dolan et al.[45] found that at 1.0 and 2.0 MAC, mean arterial blood pressure and peripheral vascular resistance were 27 and 12

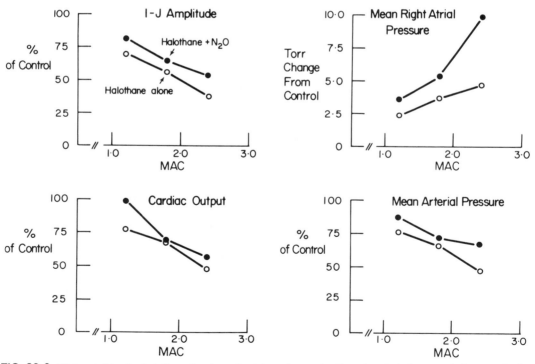

FIG. 20-9 Nitrous oxide plus halothane has less circulatory depression than does halothane at similar anesthetic concentrations. ● = Halothane + nitrous oxide; ○ = halothane alone. (Bahlman SH, Eger EI II, Smith NT, et al: The cardiovascular effects of nitrous oxide-halothane anesthesia in man. Anesthesiology 35:274, 1971.)

percent greater, respectively, in volunteers receiving nitrous oxide. No other variable differed between these two groups.

Smith et al.[46] also examined the effects of enflurane with and without nitrous oxide during controlled ventilation. The administration of nitrous oxide with enflurane at 1.5 MAC decreased cardiac output, stroke volume, IJ wave amplitude, and aortic dP/dt less than did the administration of enflurane alone.

In summary, nitrous oxide alone or combined with potent inhaled agents produces sympathetic stimulation. Such stimulation may obscure any cardiac depressant effects. The combination of nitrous oxide plus halothane or enflurane appears to produce less depression at a given MAC level than either potent agent given alone.

FACTORS THAT MAY INFLUENCE THE CIRCULATORY EFFECTS OF INHALED ANESTHETICS

DURATION OF ANESTHESIA

The cardiovascular effects of several inhaled anesthetics changes with the duration of anesthesia. In studies performed in humans, longer anesthesia is associated with an increase in β-sympathetic activity. Heart rate, cardiac output, myocardial function, and mean right atrial pressure all reflect such increased activity; function and rate increase, while atrial pressure decreases. Systemic vascular resistance falls; thus, despite an increase in cardiac output, blood pressure does not change. Cyclopropane,[8] isoflurane,[4] enflurane,[3] methoxyflurane,[20] halothane,[2] diethyl ether,[5] and fluroxene[6] each demonstrates some if not all of these temporally related changes. The largest changes are seen with diethyl ether, fluroxene, and halothane. In contrast to these in vivo

changes, in vitro depression of cat papillary muscle at a constant concentration of halothane remains unchanged over a 3-hour period, indicating that recovery with time is not based on improved intrinsic cardiac function.[47] Volunteers anesthetized with halothane do not demonstrate the temporally related stimulation if they are given propranolol prior to anesthesia.[16] These findings suggest that the effect of time is the result of an increase in sympathetic nervous activity. Recent studies demonstrate a mild increase in mean arterial pressure (14 to 18 percent) and MVO_2 (18 to 21 percent) after 3.5 hours of constant-dose halothane anesthesia.[48]

SPONTANEOUS VENTILATION

Studies of the circulatory changes produced by anesthetics during spontaneous ventilation introduce $PaCO_2$ as a variable that at equipotent anesthetic concentrations differs among anesthetics because of the different capacities of agents to depress respiration.[49-51] Carbon dioxide has three predominant actions: dilation of smooth muscle, stimulation of the sympathetic nervous system, and direct depression of the heart by acidosis. These circulatory effects of carbon dioxide may add to or oppose the action of the anesthetics.

Administration of CO_2 to awake humans stimulates the heart and decreases systemic vascular resistance.[52] Similar but attenuated results are seen during anesthesia. The attenuation is directly related to anesthetic dose[53] (Table 20-1).

In addition to affecting the circulation by altering carbon dioxide levels, the lower intrathoracic pressure associated with spontaneous as opposed to controlled ventilation favors the return of venous blood to the heart. The venoconstrictive reflex response to positive intrathoracic pressure increases peripheral venous pressure and tends to restore venous return toward normal. The inhaled anesthetics limit this compensatory venoconstriction and thereby exaggerate the depressant influence of positive pressure ventilation. During halothane anesthesia in volunteers, a change from

TABLE 20-1. Directional Change in Some Circulatory Values on Changing from Controlled to Spontaneous Ventilation

Measure	Halothane	Enflurane	Isoflurane
Cardiac output	↑	↑	↑
Arterial pressure	↑	±	±
Heart rate	↑	↑	↑
Systemic vascular resistance	↓	↓	↓
IJ wave amplitude ballistocardiogram	↑	↑	±
Mean right atrial pressure	±	↓	±

± = variable effect — mean of group unchanged; ↑ = increased; ↓ = decreased

spontaneous to controlled ventilation decreases cardiac output, heart rate, and arterial pressure.[53] Systemic vascular resistance is increased (Fig. 20-10). Similar differences are seen with other agents.[3,51]

DISEASE

The presence of heart disease increases the chance of cardiac morbidity during or following anesthesia. For example, one study reported a 0.33 percent incidence of myocardial infarction following general anesthesia in patients who had not had a prior myocardial infarct, but a 6.6 percent incidence in those who had had a prior myocardial infarction.[54] Other indices of myocardial disease may be more important than a history of infarction as a predictor of perioperative complications.[55] In any case, cardiovascular disease contributes significantly to anesthesia-surgery risk (also see Chs. 8, 9, & 10).

The quantitative estimation of cardiac disease and cardiovascular reserve is not easily accomplished. Serious ailments are often associated with normal indices of circulatory function at rest. Blood pressure, heart rate, cardiac output, myocardial contractility, filling pressures, and electrocardiogram all may be normal in the patient with coronary artery disease. Exercise stress testing frequently is used to assess coronary artery disease, but recent studies suggest this test is of limited value.[56] Since atherosclerosis is the most frequent cause of coronary artery disease, the extent of obstruction is best measured by coronary angiogram — a procedure requiring skill and not without risk.

Other cardiac diseases, such as aortic stenosis, also may present with few specific findings but may nearly eliminate the circulatory reserve needed to compensate for perioperative stress. A reduced reserve may relate both to the disease and to the treatment of that disease. For example, patients with valvular heart disease undergoing open heart surgery may be hypovolemic and may react adversely to the vasodilation produced by anesthetic agents because of this hypovolemia. The hypovolemia often is secondary to salt and water depletion induced by diuretics given to treat congestive heart failure.[57]

Diseases such as myocardial infarction and rheumatic heart disease directly affect the amount of functioning myocardium. Conditions such as ventricular hypertrophy reduce reserve by decreasing perfusion per gram of heart muscle.[58]

Right ventricular hypertrophy or congestive heart failure can be produced by partial pulmonary artery obstruction in cats. Papillary muscle from these cats has a 30 to 55 percent decrease in maximum velocity of contraction. The addition of halothane to that already compromised muscle produces proportionately the same depression as in normal muscle but the depression is greater, since the diseased muscle starts from a lower baseline.[59] These studies indicate why patients with congestive heart failure or ventricular hypertrophy may manifest undue depression in response to anesthetic concentrations that in normal patients usually are well tolerated.

The study reported by Eisele et al.[40] illustrates the interaction between disease and anesthesia. In nine patients with two-vessel coronary artery disease and reduced left ventricular ejection fractions, inhalation of 40 percent nitrous oxide significantly decreased mean arterial blood pressure and dP/dt and increased

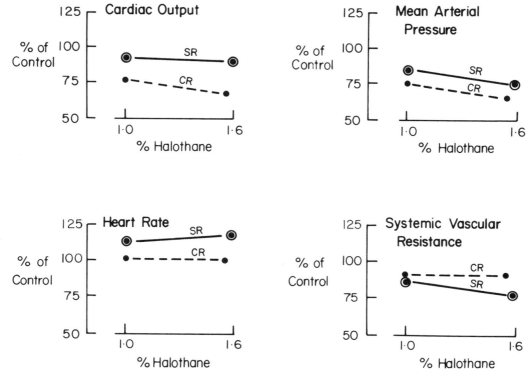

FIG. 20-10 The increase in $PaCO_2$ and reduction of mean intrathoracic pressure produced by spontaneous ventilation result in increases in cardiac output, heart rate, and mean arterial pressure and decreases in systemic vascular resistance. (Bahlman SH, Eger El II, Halsey MJ, et al: The cardiovascular effects of halothane in man during spontaneous ventilation. Anesthesiology 36: 494, 1972.)

left ventricular end-diastolic pressure. In four patients without angiographic evidence of coronary disease, breathing 40 percent nitrous oxide produced no myocardial depression. Similarly, administration of 1.5 percent halothane increased the preinjection period (PEP) and decreased left ventricular ejection time (LVET) to a greater extent in patients with heart disease than in those without heart disease.[60]

The drug therapy used to treat hypertension and ischemic heart disease (propranolol, α-methyldopa, reserpine) may attenuate the normal responses of the sympathetic nervous system. This may augment the cardiovascular depression induced by anesthesia and has led in the past to the preoperative discontinuation of these medications. One report linked the preoperative administration of propranolol with the inability to wean a patient from car-

diopulmonary bypass following open heart surgery.[61]

The interaction between propranolol and the volatile anesthetics produces effects that may depend on the specific anesthetic and on patient disease (also see Ch. 28). Anesthetics that normally stimulate the sympathetic nervous system may produce cardiac depression when β-adrenergic blockade is present. In humans anesthetized with diethyl ether, 5 mg of intravenously administered propranolol decreases heart rate, mean arterial blood pressure, cardiac output, and stroke volume and increases central venous pressure and systemic vascular resistance.[62] In dogs anesthetized with cyclopropane, 0.3 mg/kg of propranolol decreases cardiac output, stroke volume, and myocardial contractility and increases systemic vascular resistance.[63] Both ether and cyclopropane are thought to increase sympathetic activity. However, anesthetic agents that do not induce sympathetic activity also demonstrate increased circulatory depression when administered in combination with β-blocking agents. Methoxyflurane, trichloroethylene, and enflurane demonstrate mild depression in myocardial contractility, heart rate, and cardiac output at 1.0 MAC when administered to dogs in combination with β-blocking agents.[64-66] This added circulatory depression becomes more profound with increasing anesthetic concentrations.[64-66]

Circulatory depression consequent to administration of β-blockers appears to be least with halothane and isoflurane.[67-70] Similarly, the addition of stresses such as graded hemorrhage[70,71] and hypoxemia[68] appears better tolerated with these anesthetics than with enflurane, methoxyflurane, or trichloroethylene. In general, β-adrenergic blockers add to the depressant effect of any potent inhaled anesthetic. Safe anesthetic management in patients receiving β-adrenergic blockers may require both judicious selection of the specific anesthetic and/or reduction in anesthetic concentration. However, the earlier notion that β-adrenergic blockers should be discontinued prior to anesthesia largely has been discarded. Such discontinuation produces excessive complications related to the patient's underlying disease (e.g., hypertension, angina, dysrhythmias).

Valvular heart disease places narrow constraints on anesthetic choice and management (also see Chs. 9 and 41). Aortic stenosis results in ventricular hypertrophy and the potential for a reduced coronary artery perfusion pressure. Induction of peripheral vasodilation by a drug such as isoflurane, when cardiac output is limited by the stenosis, might be particularly hazardous. By contrast, this same anesthetic might prove of benefit in mitral or aortic insufficiency. With insufficiency, reduction of systemic vascular resistance favors forward cardiac flow rather than regurgitation and has been demonstrated to improve circulatory indices.[72]

Obstructive coronary artery disease presents indications for anesthetic management and choice that depend on the facets of myocardial function most affected by the coronary artery disease. For example, a patient with potential myocardial ischemia from a flow-limiting segment would theoretically benefit from a drug that reduces myocardial oxygen consumption but that does not reduce systemic vascular resistance. Halothane is such a drug, and it favorably affects electrocardiographic signs of myocardial ischemia[73] and reduces myocardial infarct size in experimental animal preparations with total coronary artery occlusion.[74] However, halothane also causes myocardial dysfunction distal to a coronary artery stenosis when administered in deep concentrations that reduces systemic pressure.[75] These results are not unexpected and demonstrate dose-related differences in drug action.

Systemic vasodilation and reduction of afterload might be sought if coronary artery disease leads to congestive heart failure. Isoflurane might then be considered the drug of choice. However, recent work by Reiz et al.[17] has suggested that this vasodilating property of isoflurane could cause myocardial ischemia. These workers measured and correlated electrocardiographic finding with systemic hemodynamics, coronary sinus blood flow, and myocardial lactate extraction in 21 patients with coronary artery disease anesthetized with 1.0 MAC isoflurane. All patients exhibited the expected isoflurane produced declines in blood pressure and MVO$_2$. Ten of the 21 patients developed either ST segment depression or T-wave inversion suggestive of myocardial ischemia. Myocardial lactate extraction remained positive but decreased in the 10 patients with ECG abnormalities. In five of the patients with ECG abnormalities, blood pressure was returned to normal values by administration of phenylephrine (Neo-Synephrine). Concurrent with the return of a normal blood pressure, two of the five patients' ECG abnormalities disappeared. Reiz and co-workers speculated that the persistent ECG abnormalities, even when blood pressure, heart rate and wedge pressure were normal, could result from a "coronary steal."[17]

Another anesthetic consideration is indicated if hypoxia or injury of myocardial muscle has led to dysrhythmias. Fifty percent of patients receiving 2.1 μg/kg of subcutaneously injected epinephrine develop ventricular extrasystoles when anesthetized with 1.25 MAC halothane. The epinephrine dose required to produce the same incidence in patients anesthetized with isoflurane is 6.4 μg/kg and is greater than 10 μg/kg when the anesthetic is enflurane.[76] In general, the halogenated alkanes (halothane, chloroform, trichloroethylene) or cyclic hydrocarbons (cyclopropane) predispose to dysrhythmias, whereas the ethers (fluroxene, enflurane, isoflurane, methoxyflurane) do not (also see Ch. 28) and are indicated in patients with significant dysrhythmias.

Disease may decrease oxygen content in arterial blood by decreasing hemoglobin or PaO_2. Hypoxemia or anemia may alter the circulatory responses to halothane. Hypoxic dogs given 1.0 to 1.25 MAC halothane have increased arterial pressure, heart rate, and cardiac output as compared with control dogs that are not hypoxic.[77] However, an increase in halothane above 1.0 to 1.25 MAC kills hypoxic animals, whereas control animals exhibit the expected increase in circulatory depression. By contrast, anemic dogs anesthetized with halothane have no difference in cardiac output, blood pressure, heart rate, left ventricular end-diastolic pressure, and arterial base excess than that of anesthetized control animals.[78] Anemia alters neither apneic or lethal concentrations of halothane.[78] Thus, a decrease of arterial oxygen content by anemia does not have the same effect on the response to halothane as does a similar decrease in content by hypoxemia.

SURGERY

Surgery modifies the circulatory effects of the volatile anesthetics. Rarely does a surgical incision not produce an increase in blood pressure and heart rate. Surgical incision is a stress that stimulates the sympathetic nervous system. Anesthesia usually opposes this response to surgical stress in a dose-dependent fashion. Roizen et al.[15] demonstrated that higher halothane or enflurane concentrations decreased or prevented surgically induced increases in serum norepinephrine levels. The anesthetic doses for blocking adrenergic responses to skin incision in 50 percent of patients studied were 1.47 MAC halothane and 1.63 MAC enflurane.

Stone et al.[72] provide an illustration of the potentially detrimental effects of surgery on

hemodynamics. These workers documented marked deterioration in hemodynamics in response to incision in patients with valvular insufficiency. Surgical incision induced an increase in systemic vascular resistance with resultant decrease in stroke volume and increase in filling pressures. Thus, surgery becomes a variable that the anesthesiologist may use and must allow for in anesthetic and anesthetic dose selection.

SUMMARY

In vitro studies demonstrate that all anesthetics produce a dose-related cardiac depression. This clear evidence of depression by all anesthetics becomes less clear in vivo wherein homeostatic mechanisms come into play. Although halothane and enflurane depress myocardial contractility, neither diethyl ether, cyclopropane, nor isoflurane reduces cardiac output, and cyclopropane actually raises arterial blood pressure. Nitrous oxide may stimulate the circulation. The circulatory actions of the inhaled anesthetics are modified by many of the variables that act on the patient in the clinical milieu. Such variables include an increase in $PaCO_2$, patient disease, surgical stress, and the presence of various drug therapies. The anesthesiologist must consider the impact of each of these factors in choosing an anesthetic and anesthetic dose. Modification of the patient's drug therapy, addition of other nonanesthetic drugs, and careful anesthetic selection may be needed to obtain the circulatory state most favorable to the patient.

Duration of anesthesia and mode of ventilation are factors in determining circulatory depression. Halothane and methoxyflurane at 1.25 MAC both depress right ventricular dP/dt in humans, but these values return to control with increasing duration of anesthesia. Controlled ventilation depresses the circulation both through mechanical impairment of venous return and by decreasing the sympathetic nervous system stimulation provided by carbon dioxide.

Patients with cardiac disease have less reserve and are less tolerant of anesthetic agents than are healthy patients. Excessive cardiac depression must be avoided, yet a high anesthetic dosage may be needed to avoid unwanted circulatory stimulation by surgery and endotracheal intubation. The severity and type of circulatory disease are major factors influencing anesthesia choice and surgical risk. For example, both congestive heart failure and asymmetrical septal hypertrophy (ASH) are heart disease. Congestive heart failure may be treated by afterload reduction and cardiac stimulation. In treatment of ASH, cardiac depressants may be administered; these patients tolerate afterload reduction poorly. Thus, two types of cardiac disease will require different drugs or anesthetics. The interrelationship between cardiovascular disease and the circulatory effects of anesthetic agents is the area in which we have only limited knowledge.

REFERENCES

1. Deutsch S, Linde HW, Dripps RD, et al: Circulatory and respiratory actions of halothane in normal man. Anesthesiology 23:631, 1962
2. Eger EI II, Smith NT, Stoelting RK, et al: Cardiovascular effects in man. Anesthesiology 32:396, 1970
3. Calverley RK, Smith NT, Prys-Roberts C, et al: Cardiovascular effects of enflurane anesthesia during controlled ventilation in man. Anesth Analg 57:619, 1978
4. Stevens WC, Cromwell TH, Halsey MJ, et al: The cardiovascular effects of a new inhalation anesthetic, Forane, in human volunteers at constant arterial carbon dioxide tension. Anesthesiology 35:8, 1971
5. Gregory GA, Eger EI II, Smith NT, et al: The cardiovascular effects of diethyl ether in man. Anesthesiology 34:19, 1971
6. Cullen BF, Eger EI II, Smith NT, et al: Cardiovascular effects of fluroxene in man. Anesthesiology 32:218, 1970
7. Jones, RE, Guldmann N, Linde HW, et al: Cyclopropane anesthesia. III. Effects of cyclopropane on respiration and circulation in normal man. Anesthesiology 21:380, 1960
8. Cullen DJ, Eger EI II, Gregory GA: The cardiovascular effects of cyclopropane in man. Anesthesiology 31:398, 1969
9. Price HL, Linde HW, Jones RE, et al: Sympathoadrenal responses to cyclopropane in man and their relation to hemodynamics. Anesthesiology 20:563, 1959
10. Price ML, Price HL: Effects of general anesthesia on contractile responses of rabbit aortic strips. Anesthesiology 23:16, 1962
11. Duke PC, Founes D, Wade JG: Halothane depresses baroreflex control of heart rate in man. Anesthesiology 46:184, 1977
12. Morton M, Duke PC, Ong B: Baroreflex control of heart rate in man awake and during enflurane and enflurane–nitrous oxide anesthesia. Anesthesiology 52:221, 1980
13. Mittler G, Wade J: The effect of methoxyflurane on baroreflex control of heart rate in man. Can Anaesth Soc J 19:60, 1972
14. Kotorly KJ, Ebert TJ, Vucins E, et al: Baroreceptor reflex control of heart rate during isoflurane anesthesia in humans. Anesthesiology 60:173, 1984
15. Roizen MF, Horrigan RW, Frazer BM: Anesthetic dose blocking adrenergic (stress) and cardiovascular responses to incision—MAC BAR. Anesthesiology 54:390, 1981
16. Reiz S, Balfors E, Gustavsson B, et al: Effects of halothane on coronary haemodynamics and myocardial metabolism in patients with ischaemic heart disease and heart failure. Acta Anaesthesiol Scand 26:133, 1982
17. Reiz S, Balfors E, Sorensen MB, et al: Isoflurane—A powerful coronary vasodilator in patients with coronary artery disease. Anesthesiology 59:91, 1983
18. Brown BR, Crout JR: A comparative study of the effects of five general anesthetics on myocardial contractility: I. Isometric conditions. Anesthesiology 34:236, 1971
19. Iwatsuki N, Shimosato S: Diethyl ether and contractility of isolated cat heart muscle. Br J Anaesth 43:420, 1971
20. Libonati M, Cooperman LH, Price HL: Time-dependent circulatory effects of methoxyflurane in man. Anesthesiology 34:439, 1971
21. Price HL, Skovsted P, Pauca AW, et al: Evidence for β-receptor activation produced by halothane in normal man. Anesthesiology 32:389, 1970
22. Beaupre PN, Cahalan MK, Kremer PF, et al: Isoflurane, halothane, and enflurane depress myocardial contractility in patients undergoing surgery. Anesthesiology 59:A59, 1983

23. Sonntag H, Donath U, Hillebrand W, et al: Left ventricular function in conscious man and during halothane anesthesia. Anesthesiology 48:320, 1978

24. Hamilton WK, Larson CP, Bristow JD, et al: Effect of cyclopropane and halothane on ventricular mechanics: A change in ventricular diastolic pressure–volume relationship. J Pharmacol Exp Ther 154:566, 1966

25. Rusy BF, Moran JE, Vongvises P, et al: The effects of halothane and cyclopropane on left ventricular volume determined by high speed biplane cineradiography in dogs. Anesthesiology 36:369, 1972

26. Vatner SF, Smith NT: Effects of halothane on left ventricular function and distribution of regional blood flow in dogs and primates. Circ Res 34:155, 1974

27. Gerson JI, Gianaris CG: Echocardiographic analysis of human left ventricular diastolic volume and cardiac performance during halothane anesthesia. Anesth Analg 58:23, 1979

28. Rathod R, Jacobs HK, Kramer NE, et al: Echocardiographic assessment of ventricular performance following induction with two anesthetics. Anesthesiology 49:86, 1978

29. Theye RA: Myocardial and total oxygen consumption with halothane. Anesthesiology 28:1042, 1967

30. Merin RG, Kumazawa T, Luka NL: Myocardial function and metabolism in the conscious dog during halothane anesthesia. Anesthesiology 44:402, 1976

31. Sonntag H, Merin RG, Donath U, et al: Myocardial metabolism and oxygenation in man awake and during halothane anesthesia. Anesthesiology 51:204, 1979

32. Theye RA, Michenfelder JD: Individual organ contributions to the decrease in whole body VO_2 with isoflurane. Anesthesiology 42:35, 1975

33. Sybert PE, Hickey RF, Hoar PF, et al: Effects of volatile anesthetics on the regulation of coronary blood flow. Anesthesiology 59:A24, 1983

34. Wolff G, Claude B, Rist M, et al: Regulation of coronary blood flow during ether and halothane anesthesia. Br J Anaesth 44:1139, 1972

35. Price HL, Helrich M: The effect of cyclopropane, diethyl ether, nitrous oxide, thiopental and hydrogen ion concentration on myocardial function of the dog heart–lung preparation. J Pharmacol Exp Ther 115:206, 1955

36. Goldberg AH, Sohn YZ, Phear WP: Direct myocardial effects of nitrous oxide. Anesthesiology 37:373, 1972

37. Price HL: Myocardial depression by nitrous oxide and its reversal by CA^{++}. Anesthesiology 44:211, 1976

38. Eisele JH, Smith NT: Cardiovascular effects of 40 percent nitrous oxide in man. Anesth Analg 51:956, 1972

39. Winter PM, Hornbein TF, Smith G: Hyperbaric nitrous oxide anesthesia in man: Determination of anesthetic potency (MAC) and cardiorespiratory effects. Abstracts of Scientific Papers, 1972 ASA meeting, p 103

40. Eisele JH, Reitan JA, Massumi RA, et al: Myocardial performance and N_2O analgesia in coronary artery disease. Anesthesiology 44:16, 1976

41. Stoelting RK, Gibbs PS: Hemodynamic effects of morphine and morphine–nitrous oxide in valvular heart disease and coronary artery disease. Anesthesiology 38:45, 1973

42. Smith NT, Eger EI II, Stoelting RK, et al: The cardiovascular and sympathomemetic responses to the addition of nitrous oxide to halothane in man. Anesthesiology 32:410, 1970

43. Hill GE, English JE, Lunn J, et al: Cardiovascular response to nitrous oxide during light, moderate and deep halothane anesthesia in man. Anesth Analg 57:84, 1978

44. Bahlman SH, Eger EI II, Smith NT, et al: The cardiovascular effects of nitrous oxide–halothane anesthesia in man. Anesthesiology 35:274, 1971

45. Dolan WM, Stevens WC, Eger EI II, et al: The cardiovascular and respiratory effects of isoflurane–nitrous oxide anesthesia. Can Anaesth Soc J 21:557, 1974

46. Smith NT, Calverley RK, Prys-Roberts C, et al: Impact of nitrous oxide on the circulation during enflurane anesthesia in man. Anesthesiology 48:345, 1978

47. Shimosato S, Yasuda I: Cardiac performance during prolonged halothane anesthesia in the cat. Br J Anaesth 50:215, 1978

48. Ritter JW, Shigezawa GY, Steven DR Sr, et al: Increased myocardial oxygen demand during prolonged halothane anesthesia in dogs. Anesth Analg 62:788, 1983

49. Munson ES, Larson CP Jr, Babad AA: The effect of halothane, fluroxene and cyclopropane on ventilation: A comparative study in man. Anesthesiology 27:716, 1966

50. Larson CP, Eger EI II, Muallenn M, et al: The effect of diethyl ether and methoxyflurane on ventilation. Anesthesiology 30:174, 1969

51. Calverley RK, Smith NT, Jones CW, et al: Ventilatory and cardiovascular effects of enflurane anesthesia during spontaneous ventilation in man. Anesth Analg 57:610, 1978

52. Cullen DJ, Eger EI II: Cardiovascular effects of carbon dioxide in man. Anesthesiology 41:345, 1974

53. Bahlman SH, Eger EI II, Halsey MJ, et al: The cardiovascular effects of halothane in man dur-

ing spontaneous ventilation. Anesthesiology 36:494, 1972

54. Tarhan S, Moffitt EA, Taylor WF, et al: Myocardial infarction after general anesthesia. JAMA 220:1451, 1972

55. Goldman L, Caldera DL, Nussbaum SR, et al: Multifactorial index of cardiac risk in noncardiac surgical procedures. N Engl J Med 297:845, 1977

56. Weiner DA, Ryan TJ, McCable CH, et al: Correlation between history and exercise ECG with coronary arteriography. N Engl J Med 301:230, 1979

57. Cohn JN, Franciosa JA: Vasodilator therapy of cardiac failure. N Engl J Med 297:27, 1977

58. Ljundquist A, Unge S: The finer intramyocardial vasculature in various forms of experimental canine hypertrophy. Acta Pathol Microbiol Scand [A] 80:329, 1972

59. Shimosato S, Yasuda I, Kemmotsu O, et al: Effect of halothane on altered contractility of isolated heart muscle obtained from cats with experimentally produced ventricular hypertrophy and failure. Br J Anaesth 45:2, 1973

60. Dauchot PJ, Rasmussen JP, Nicholson DH, et al: On-line systolic time intervals during anesthesia in patients with and without heart disease. Anesthesiology 44:472, 1976

61. Viljoen JF, Estafanous FG, Kellner GA: Propranolol and cardiac surgery. J Thorac Cardiovasc Surg 64:826, 1972

62. Jorfeldt L, Lofstromm B, Moller J, et al: Cardiovascular pharmacodynamics of propranolol during ether anaesthesia in man. Acta Anaesthesiol Scand 11:159, 1967

63. Craythorne NWB, Huffington PE: Effects of propranolol on the cardiovascular response to cyclopropane and halothane. Anesthesiology 27:580, 1966

64. Horan BF, Prys-Roberts C, Hamilton WK, et al: Haemodynamic responses to enflurane anaesthesia and hypovolemia in the dog and their modification by propranolol. Br J Anaesth 49:1189, 1977

65. Roberts JG, Foex P, Clarke TNS, et al: Haemodynamic interaction of high-dose propranolol pretreatment and anaesthesia in the dog. III. The effect of hemorrhage during halothane and trichloroethylene anaesthesia. Br J Anaesth 48:411, 1976

66. Saner CA, Foex P, Roberts JG, et al: Methoxyflurane and practalol: A dangerous combination? Br J Anaesth 47:1025, 1975

67. Roberts JG, Foex P, Clarke TNS, et al: Haemo-

dynamic interactions of high dose propranolol pretreatment and anaesthesia in the dog. I: Halothane dose-response study. Br J Anaesth 48:315, 1976

68. Roberts JG, Foex P, Clarke TNS, et al: Haemodynamic interactions of high-dose propranolol pretreatment and anaesthesia in the dog. II. The effect of acute arterial hypoxemia at increasing depth of halothane anesthesia. Br J Anaesth 48:403, 1976

69. Philbin DM, Lowenstein E: Lack of beta-adrenergic activity of isoflurane in the dog: A comparison of circulatory effects of halothane and isoflurane after propranolol administration. Br J Anaesth 48:1165, 1976

70. Weis KH, Brackenbush HD: On the cardiovascular effect of propranolol during halothane anaesthesia in normovolemic and hypovolemic dogs. Br J Anaesth 42:272, 1970

71. Horan BF, Prys-Roberts C, Roberts JG, et al: Haemodynamic responses to isoflurane anaesthesia and hypovolemia in the dog and their modification by propranolol. Br J Anaesth 49:1179, 1977

72. Stone JG, Faltas AN, Hoar PF: Sodium nitroprusside therapy for cardiac failure in anesthetized patients with valvular insufficiency. Anesthesiology 49:414, 1978

73. Bland JHL, Lowenstein E: Halothane-induced decreases in experimental myocardial ischemia in the non-failing canine heart. Anesthesiology 45:287, 1976

74. Davis RF, Deboer LW, Rude RE, et al: The effects of halothane anesthesia on myocardial necrosis, hemodynamic performance and regional myocardial blood flow in dogs following coronary artery occlusion. Anesthesiology 59:402, 1983

75. Lowenstein E, Foex P, Francis M, et al: Regional ischemic ventricular dysfunction in myocardium supplied by a narrowed coronary artery with increasing halothane concentration in the dog. Anesthesiology 55:349, 1984

76. Johnson RR, Eger EI II, Wilson C: A comparative interaction of epinephrine with enflurane, isoflurane, and halothane in man. Anesth Analg 55:709, 1976

77. Cullen DJ, Eger EI II: The effects of halothane on respiratory and cardiovascular responses to hypoxia in dogs: A dose response study. Anesthesiology 33:487, 1970

78. Loarie DJ, Wilkinson P, Tyberg J, et al: The hemodynamic effects of halothane in anemic dogs. Anesth Analg 58:195, 1979

21

Respiratory Pharmacology of Inhaled Anesthetic Agents

Edward G. Pavlin, M.D.

INTRODUCTION

Lung function may be augmented or diminished by the administration of pharmacologic agents. When choosing the appropriate therapeutic agent for treatment of pulmonary disease, systemic side effects of drugs are of major importance in determining our choice of therapy. Similarly, the choice of anesthetic agents may frequently be determined by the known side effects of these agents on various organ systems in the body. Although seldom administered primarily as pulmonary therapeutic drugs, inhaled agents may act at various sites in the CNS, airways, alveoli, and pulmonary vasculature. Knowledge of the pulmonary effects of what are primarily cerebral depressants is important in that lung function can be monitored and preserved in the face of anesthetic depression. In some circumstances, a particular pharmacologic action may determine the choice of anesthetic drug. For example, halothane is considered by many clinicians to be the most appropriate anesthetic for the asthmatic patient because of its bronchodilating qualities.

Since inhaled anesthetics pervade the whole body, pulmonary function may be affected by both direct and indirect actions. The line between "physiologic" and "pharmacologic" effects may be very thin indeed. To avoid repetition of later chapters dealing with anesthesia and the lung, this chapter describes the more direct methods by which anesthetic gases and vapors alter the activities of various anatomic components of the lung. To this end, sections deal with airway resistance, pulmonary vascular caliber, mucociliary function, and ventilatory control. Although the latter involves discussion of receptors and the nervous system anatomically removed from the lung, dose-related depression of ventilation caused by anesthesia obviously is one of the most potent and important pulmonary "side effects."

EFFECTS OF INHALED ANESTHETIC AGENTS ON BRONCHOMOTOR TONE

The increase in airway resistance observed during an acute asthmatic attack may be both frightening and potentially lethal. Although a universally accepted definition of "asthma" is difficult to enunciate, in this discussion it is considered to be a transient state of increased airway resistance caused at least in part by an increase in bronchiolar smooth muscle tone. This increased muscle tone occurs in patients who exhibit clinical manifestations of extrinsic and intrinsic asthma, as well as in those with a pharmacologically reversible component of chronic obstructive lung disease. Indeed, with the proper stimulus, bronchospasm can occur in normal subjects who have no underlying history of lung disease of any kind. A mainstay of treatment is the adminis-

tration of bronchodilating drugs. An excellent review of the mechanisms of action and clinical role of bronchodilating drugs has been published by Paterson et al.[1] Because of legitimate concerns regarding anesthesia in these patients, the pharmacology of inhaled agents with respect to their effects on bronchial smooth muscle is of great clinical importance. The effects of various anesthetics on airway resistance are summarized in Table 21-1.

PHARMACOLOGY OF BRONCHIAL MUSCLE

Some consideration must be given to the basic physiology and pharmacology of airways before the effects of inhaled agents or other types of bronchodilating agents can be predicted or evaluated. The autonomic nervous system plays a key role in the control of bron-

TABLE 21-1. Effects of Inhaled Agents on Airway Resistance (Raw)

Anesthetic Agent	Reference	Model	Measurement	Effect
Halothane	Shnider & Papper[3]	Human (retrospective)	Wheezing	++
	Waltemath & Bergman[18]	Human, normal	Raw	0
	Brakensiek & Bergman[16]	Human, bronchospasm, (aerosol)	Raw	++
	Hickey et al.[8]	Dog, bronchospasm (vagus, histamine)	Raw	++
	Coon & Kampine[9]	Dog, left lower lobe bronchoconstriction ($\downarrow CO_2$)	Raw	++
	Klide & Aviado[6]	Dog, normal	Raw	++
	Fletcher et al.[7]	Guinea pig, isolated tracheal muscle	Length	++
	Gold & Helrich[13]	Human, status asthmaticus	Raw	0
	Meloche et al.[15]	Human, cardiopulmonary bypass bronchoconstriction ($\downarrow CO_2$)	Raw	0
	Colgan[5]	Dog, normal	"Bronchial distensibility"	0
	Hirshman & Bergman[10]	Dog, bronchospasm (ascaris)	Raw	++
Diethyl ether	Shnider & Papper[3]	Human (retrospective)	Wheezing	+
Cyclopropane	Hickey et al.[8]	Dog, bronchospasm (histamine, vagus)	Raw	+
	Colgan[5]	Dog, normal	"Bronchial distensibility"	0
Enflurane	Coon & Kampine[9]	Dog, left lower lobe bronchoconstriction ($\downarrow CO_2$)	Raw	+
	Hirshman & Bergman[10]	Dog, bronchospasm (ascaris)	Raw	++
Methoxyflurane	Coon & Kampine[9]	Dog, left lower lobe bronchoconstriction ($\downarrow CO_2$)	Raw	+
Isoflurane	Hirshman et al.[12]	Dog, bronchospasm (ascaris)	Raw	++

Symbols used: ++ = pronounced bronchodilation; + = bronchodilation; 0 = no effect.

chomotor tone, both in normal airways and in those patients with bronchospastic disease (Fig. 21-1).

Airway smooth muscle, which extends as far distally as the terminal bronchioles, is under the influence of both parasympathetic and sympathetic nerves. Vagal innervation of the bronchial tree has been well documented, and sympathetic innervation, though less well defined, probably plays a role as well. The effects of the autonomic nervous sytem are thought to be mediated through their action on the stores of cyclic AMP and cyclic GMP in bronchial smooth muscle cells. Acetylcholine, or stimulation by the vagus nerve, is thought to provide an increase in the amounts of cyclic GMP relative to cyclic AMP, leading to smooth muscle contraction (Fig. 21-1). Release of histamine in the airway or various forms of mechanical or chemical stimulation can result in an increase in afferent vagal activity with subsequent reflex bronchoconstriction. This in-

crease in bronchomotor tone can be attenuated by atropine.

Adrenergic receptors in bronchial smooth muscle are classified into α and β types according to the classic desciption of Ahlquist.[2] While α receptors are in the bronchial tree in humans, their activity seems to be low and clinically unimportant. The β receptors have been further refined into β_1 and β_2 types; the latter play the most significant role in bronchial muscle, while β_1 receptors appear to be of greater importance in modifying cardiac inotropic and chronotropic activity. Stimulation of β_2 receptors in bronchial smooth muscle, either by stimulation of sympathetic nerves or by the use of circulatory or topically-applied agents possessing β_2 activity (e.g., epinephrine and isoproterenol), causes relaxation of bronchial smooth muscle. This is probably mediated by an increase within muscle cells in levels of cyclic AMP relative to cyclic GMP (also see Chs. 9 & 28). The result of these findings has been an

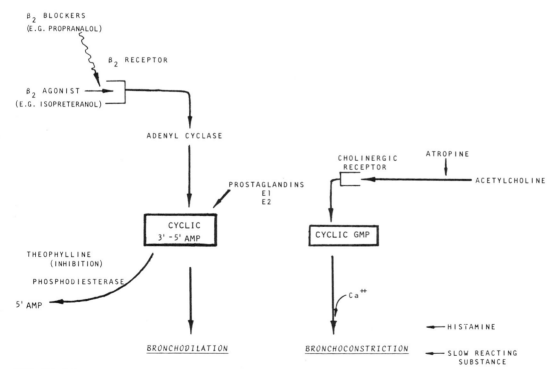

FIG. 21-1 Some aspects of sympathetic and parasympathetic control of bronchial smooth muscle tone. Not included are α-receptor mechanisms which may act by diminishing the level of cyclic 3′-5′ AMP. Interference with Ca^{++} kinetics may be an important mechanism of the bronchodilating action of some anesthetic agents.

increased interest in the formulation of β_2-specific drugs with potent bronchodilatory properties and a minimum of cardiac side effects (e.g., isoetharine, metaproterenol, terbutaline, salbutamol).

SPECIFIC INHALED ANESTHETICS

Since its clinical introduction in 1956, halothane has been recommended as the anesthetic of choice in the presence of bronchospasm because of its bronchodilating characteristics. In a retrospective study, Shnider and Papper[3] found that in 49 patients with preanesthetic wheezing, halothane was clearly superior to ether, cyclopropane, ethylene, and regional anesthesia in decreasing this audible manifestation of bronchospasm. This study suffers from its retrospective design and the fact that a clinical sign, rather than objective measurements, was used to gauge the efficacy of anesthetic agents. Nonetheless, this and other earlier clinical observations[4] established halothane as the drug of choice for patients with either a history of asthma or bronchospasm occurring during induction or maintenance of anesthesia.

The effects of inhaled agents on airway caliber have been studied in vivo. Colgan[5] noted a decrease in "bronchial distensibility" in dogs anesthetized with halothane, ether, methoxyflurane, or trichlorethylene, with halothane having the most pronounced effect. The effect of changes in functional residual capacity (FRC) during anesthesia and of unmeasured, probably varying levels of CO_2 on bronchomotor tone makes this study difficult to interpret. Subsequent to the Colgan study, it has been found that a reduction of PCO_2 in airways causes a reversible increase in airway resistance and that, conversely, increasing levels of PCO_2 have a bronchodilating effect. Klide and Aviado[6] found a dose-dependent decrease in resting airway resistance with increasing concentrations of halothane in spontaneously ventilating dogs. Again, the possibility of bronchodilation secondary to an increased resting $PaCO_2$ with deeper planes of anesthesia was not taken into account. The authors showed that this apparent effect of halothane persisted

in spite of attempts to decrease sympathetic nervous activity by sympathectomy, adrenalectomy, or treatment with reserpine, but was blocked by a β-blocking drug. The authors concluded that halothane was a pulmonary β-adrenergic agonist.

In isolated guinea pig tracheal chains, halothane, diethyl ether, and thiopental caused relaxation of resting tone.[7] These drugs also attenuated tracheal muscle constriction induced by acetylcholine, but only halothane accomplished this in clinically relevant doses. In this instance, propranolol, a β-blocking drug, did not antagonize the relaxing properties of halothane on acetylcholine-induced bronchoconstriction, leading to a conclusion different from that of Klide and Aviado[6] regarding the β-receptor-stimulating action of halothane.

Hickey et al.[8] demonstrated the importance of controlled levels of $PaCO_2$ in evaluating the effects of agents on bronchial smooth muscle tone. In anesthetized, intubated dogs whose ventilation was controlled to achieve a $PaCO_2$ of approximately 40 mm Hg, increasing concentrations of halothane and cyclopropane produced no change in resistance in the resting unstimulated airway. In the unstimulated airway, resting tone may be minimal and therefore, the bronchodilating properties of any drug may be masked because no additional relaxation of bronchial musculature can be effected. By inducing a state of increased bronchial tone by use of either histamine administration or vagal stimulation, the superior bronchodilating qualities of halothane were well demonstrated when compared to cyclopropane at 1.5 minimal alveolar concentration (MAC) levels of anesthesia (Fig. 21-2). Halothane, enflurane, and methoxyflurane were found to reverse the bronchoconstricting effects of hypocapnia in vivo in the isolated left lower (LL) lobe of the dog,[9] with halothane again proving to be the most efficacious at lower doses. This effect was not blocked by propranolol. Again, no change in unstimulated resting bronchial tone was detected after the administration of anesthetics or isoproterenol, a well-known β-agonist bronchodilator.

Bronchoconstriction produced by the methods described may not be directly comparable to that which occurs in the asthmatic patient. Recent investigations by Hirshman and Bergman[10] are exciting in that they have uti-

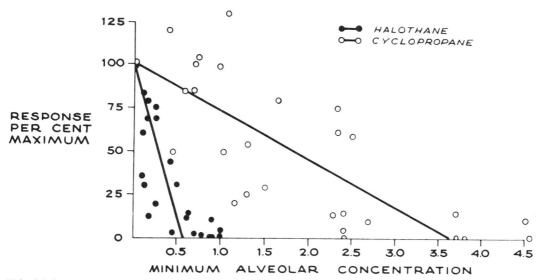

FIG. 21-2 Effects of halothane and cyclopropane on the increase in airway resistance produced by electrical stimulation of the vagus nerves of dogs. Closed circles are halothane; open circles represent cyclopropane. In the face of bronchial constriction produced by this particular stimulus, halothane appears to be a powerful bronchodilator and much more effective at equal anesthetic doses than cyclopropane. (Hickey RF, Graf PD, Nadel JA, et al: The effects of halothane and cyclopropane on total pulmonary resistance in the dog. Anesthesiology 31:334, 1969.)

lized dogs sensitized to ascaris antigen as an experimental testing model. Asthma was induced by intratracheal administration of an aerosol of ascaris antigen (a mixed reflex and direct-acting stimulus). This model is perhaps more representative of the asthmatic patient with atopic bronchospasm.[11] These authors demonstrated attentuation of antigenically induced bronchospasm[10] by concentrations of approximately 1 MAC of either halothane or enflurane with no significant difference between the two agents (Fig. 21-3). No attempt was made to describe a dose-response curve. The stimulus to bronchospasm was not continued throughout the administration of anesthetic gases, a condition that differs slightly from an "asthmatic" attack during anesthesia. Nonetheless, this is a useful model of the investigation of the bronchodilating qualities of these and other anesthetic agents.

The same experimental preparation was utilized to examine the bronchodilating effects of isoflurane. It was found that 1.5 MAC levels of both isoflurane and halothane produce a similar decrease in airway resistance in bronchospasm induced by ascaris antigen.[12] Similar results were obtained with methocholine-induced (direct-acting stimulus) airway constric-

tion. Halothane more effectively increased dynamic compliance than did isoflurane. Thus, isoflurane shares bronchodilating properties with halothane and enflurane.[10]

Because of their bronchodilating effects, anesthetics such as halothane may be an effective method of treating status asthmaticus when other more conventional treatments have failed. However, documentation of this effectiveness is lacking. Gold and Helrich[13] evaluated the effect of halothane and tracheal intubation on six patients in status asthmaticus who had been treated for at least 72 hours with bronchodilators, steroids, and antibiotics. No significant change in airway resistance was recorded in either the anesthetic or immediate postanesthetic period. Cardiac dysrhythmias proved to be of some concern during the halothane therapy. Although all six patients improved within 3 days of treatment, the lack of a similar control group makes interpretation difficult. The lack of any change in airway resistance and the appearance of ventricular dysrhythmias indicate that halothane may not be effective in this patient group.

Patterson et al.[14] measured the resistive work of breathing during cardiopulmonary bypass and found that neither airway nor sys-

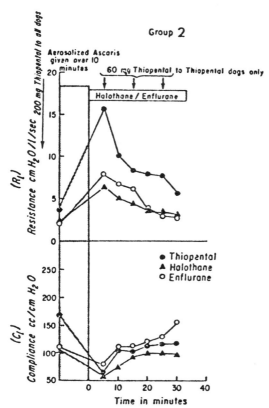

FIG. 21-3 The effect of halothane and enflurane on increased airway resistance in dogs; the airway resistance was triggered by prior administration of aerosolized ascaris. This is a model of extrinsic asthma. Although the allergic stimulus was not maintained throughout the experiment, both halothane and enflurane appear to lower airway resistance compared to the control thiopental-anesthetized animals. (Hirshman CA, Bergman NA: Halothane and enflurane protect against bronchospasm in an asthma dog model. Anesth Analg 57:629, 1978.)

temic administration of halothane caused significant changes in airway mechanics in the unstimulated state; however, the bronchoconstricting effects of low inhaled CO_2 mixtures were attenuated by inhaled halothane, but not by halothane administered via the blood. A similar experiment by Meloche et al.[15] demonstrated that administration of halothane did indeed decrease the bronchoconstriction produced by hypocapnia, although not to the same extent as did the addition of 6.5 percent CO_2 to the inhaled mixture. That systemic adminis-

tration of halothane via the bypass pump did not have similar effects suggests that halothane acts directly on the airway musculature and/ or local reflex arcs rather than via centrally controlled reflex pathways.

Measurements of resistances in normal humans have generally failed to show a bronchodilatory effect of halothane.[16] This is perhaps not surprising, since some initial smooth muscle constriction would be necessary to subsequently demonstrate reversal by any pharmacologic agent. Provoking bronchoconstriction either by hypocapnia[17] or inhalation of ultrasonic aerosols[18] has allowed the demonstration of the potential of halothane and enflurane in reversing bronchoconstriction under some circumstances (Fig. 21-4). Since different stimuli may act on bronchomotor tone through different mechanisms, either centrally or directly, it does not necessarily follow that halothane will reverse bronchoconstriction from all causes. The value and effectiveness of enflurane relative to halothane needs to be evaluated more thoroughly; the former agent offers the potential advantage of being less likely to induce cardiac dysrhythmias in patients who

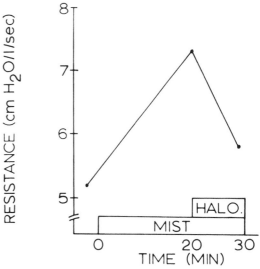

FIG. 21-4 The effect of halothane on increased respiratory resistance in man provoked by inhalation of ultrasonic mist. Halothane effectively decreased airway resistance triggered by the irritation of ultrasonic droplets. (Waltemath CL, Bergman NA: Effects of ketamine and halothane on increased respiratory resistance provoked by ultrasonic aerosols. Anesthesiology 41:473, 1974.)

frequently are receiving dysrhythmia-provoking medications. Objective data showing decreases in airway resistance in asthmatic patients during inhalational anesthesia are lacking.

The use of more conventional bronchodilators in conjunction with anesthetics has not been extensively examined. Isoetharine was found to decrease severity of wheezing and peak airway pressure in 16 patients whose tracheas were intubated and who were anesthetized with different general anesthetics.[19] However, grading of the ausculatory changes was not done in a double-blind fashion. An excellent clinical study showed that a combination of subtoxic doses of aminophylline and isoetharine yielded greater relief of bronchospasm than either agent used alone.[20] The risk of cardiac dysrhythmias following bronchodilator administration simultaneously with inhaled anesthetic agents remains unknown for most agents.

MECHANISMS OF ACTION

The mechanisms by which various general anesthetics decrease bronchial smooth muscle tone have been reviewed by Aviado.[21] By far the most extensively examined agent has been halothane. Several sites of action have been proposed; reflex bronchoconstriction in response to airway irritants may be attenuated by the anesthetic state itself, either by a reduction in afferent nerve traffic or by central medullary depression of bronchoconstriction reflexes.

Klide and Aviado[6] suggested that halothane functions as a β-agonist in bronchial smooth muscle. They demonstrated a dose-related reduction in airway resistance in dogs anesthetized with halothane that was unaffected by reserpine, guanethidine, lung denervation, or adrenalectomy. They found that a β-blocking agent, sotalol, prevented halothane-induced bronchodilation, evidence that they felt supported the claim of a β-agonist activity of halothane. Conversely, Fletcher et al.[7] found that perfusion with ether and halothane caused relaxation of guinea pig tracheal smooth muscle stimulated by acetylcholine.

Fletcher et al.[7] also found that propranolol had no effect on halothane's relaxant activity. Thus halothane appears to have a direct relaxant effect that was effective against increases in muscle tension caused by either acetylcholine- or histamine-induced constriction. In other smooth muscle preparations with β-receptor sites, relaxation by halothane has not been attributed to β-adrenergic activity. Yang et al.[22] showed that halothane or epinephrine blocked acetylcholine-induced uterine smooth muscle contraction in an in vitro preparation. While addition of propranolol blocked the effect of epinephrine, the relaxant effect of halothane was unchanged. Halothane increased the tissue concentration of cyclic AMP, a substance known to cause smooth muscle relaxation. One possible mechanism of the salutory effects of halothane is through stimulation of adenylcyclase. Conversely, Klide et al.[23] found relaxation of rabbit uterine muscle induced by halothane was prevented by a β-blocking agent, sotalol. This work provides further evidence of β-agonist activity of halothane. However, sotalol alone has been found to increase tone and motility of rabbit uterine muscle and lends some doubts to the validity of their conclusions. In a similar study, Sprague et al.[24] demonstrated that while halothane and isoflurane produced dose-dependent relaxation of rat aortic muscle strips, propranolol did not block this effect. Relaxation was associated with stimulation of cyclic AMP production in the absence of any change in phosphodiesterase activity.

Isoflurane and halothane appear to act on airway reflexes and directly on smooth muscle,[12] since airway constriction from both direct- and reflex-acting stimuli is relieved by these anesthetics. Histamine levels secondary to antigen challenge are not affected by halothane.[25] An in vitro study of dog tracheal muscle suggested that halothane may act directly on Ca^{++} stores in tracheal smooth muscle cells to interfere with the excitation-contraction coupling.[26]

In summary, inhaled anesthetics may act at several different sites in affecting bronchial smooth muscle relaxation. The direct action may involve the cyclic AMP mechanisms, although alternative actions on prostaglandins and Ca^{++} activity must be considered. While arguments for a specific β-agonist role of halothane exist, more recent data would suggest this is not the mechanism of halothane activity on smooth muscle mechanics.

CLINICAL IMPLICATIONS

The mechanisms by which increases in airway resistance may be stimulated have been summarized by Aviado.[21] Bronchospasm may occur in patients under conditions of disease other than asthma. Patients with chronic obstructive lung disease may present with elements of bronchospasm that contribute to their increased airway resistance, which may be discerned by demonstrating improvement in forced expiratory flow rates after administration of a bronchodilator. Normal healthy patients undergoing surgical stimulation of pulmonary arteries and parenchyma or trachea are known to be at risk of developing bronchospasm.[27] An isolated case report has described an episode of wheezing in a patient undergoing transurethral resection.[28] Indeed, in a lightly anesthetized patient clinically discernible bronchospasm is not an unusual event following surgical stimulation or irritation of the trachea by endotracheal tubes. In anticipating such events in patients with known reactive airway disease or in the unexpected episode of bronchospasm, the choices of preoperative medication, induction agent, muscle relaxant, and the type and dosage of anesthetic drug are important in minimizing clinical symptoms.

The variety of studies previously described strongly suggest halothane as the anesthetic of choice. Although the preponderance of data suggest halothane as the most effective bronchodilator, the work of Hirshman and colleagues[12] would suggest that isoflurane and enflurane are as effective in decreasing airway resistance in their experimental preparation. Thus, isoflurane and perhaps enflurane are good alternatives to halothane when reactive airways are concerned.

The high incidence of postanesthetic pulmonary complications in patients with chronic obstructive disease is well known. Studies of outcome with different anesthetic agents are not specific enough to evaluate the role of anes-

thetic drugs vis-à-vis effects on postoperative morbidity, airway resistance, or both. Thus more objective studies are needed to evaluate effects of various inhaled agents in patients who are at high risk of developing bronchospasm in the preoperative period.

EFFECTS OF INHALED ANESTHETIC AGENTS ON PULMONARY VASCULAR RESISTANCE

Interest in the pulmonary vasculature, sometimes referred to as "the lesser circulation," has increased geometrically over the past 15 years. Techniques for easy measurement of pulmonary blood flow (cardiac output) and pulmonary vascular pressures have become commonplace. The role of the pulmonary vasculature in various disease states and its reaction to drugs has spurred much interest.

DETERMINANTS OF PULMONARY VASCULAR RESISTANCE

The role of pharmacologic agents in determining pulmonary vascular pressures and resistances is a complicated one, since many vasoactive agents have both direct effects on pulmonary blood vessels, as well as indirect effects through alterations of cardiac output and pulmonary blood flow. Changes in pulmonary vascular resistance (PVR) and pressure may have significant effects on gas or fluid exchange in the lung. Increased PVR may give rise to an increase in pulmonary artery pressure if cardiac output is maintained constant, thereby promoting increased transudation of fluid into the interstitium of the lung. Conversely, increased resistance may cause sufficient impedance to the output of the right ventricle that cardiac output and pulmonary blood flow are reduced.

Regional changes in PVR may alter the relative distribution of blood flow within the lung, leading to altered ventilation-perfusion relationships and accompanying changes in gas exchange. Thus a localized increase in PVR in an area of atelectasis may cause a shift of blood flow away from the atelectatic segment to better ventilated regions of lung and therefore ultimately lead to improved gas exchange by decreasing blood flow to nonventilated lung.

The increase in PVR in an area of atelectasis is believed to be partially due to localized tissue hypoxia. This phenomenon, termed hypoxic vasoconstriction, has recently been of considerable interest to pulmonary physiologists because of its importance in determining the magnitude of the effects of diseased and/or nonventilated areas of lung on gas exchange and $PaCO_2$. Hypoxic vasoconstriction appears to have protective value, and drugs that interfere with this "protective" mechanism may adversely affect gas exchange. Many of the commonly used agents in anesthesia are included in the list of offenders.

Pulmonary vascular resistance can be altered by several mechanisms. Passive changes in the diameter of the pulmonary blood vessels may be induced by increased cardiac output (increased pulmonary blood flow), elevations of left atrial pressure, or both. The increased vascular distending pressure may cause an increase in the cross-sectional diameter of the pulmonary vascular bed and, hence, a fall in pulmonary vascular resistance. Similarly, changes in lung volume may alter the dimensions of the vasculature and, hence, affect resistance. Increases of lung volume above FRC caused by increased pressure in the airway are characteristically associated with passive increases in PVR; the latter are presumably caused by transmission of the higher alveolar pressures to blood vessels located in alveolar walls. On the other hand, reduction in lung volumes below normal FRC is also associated with passive increases in PVR. The latter are thought to be the result of a reduction in vascular dimensions as the lung shrinks. At low lung volumes, vessels are both shorter and narrower, apparently because of loss of a tethering effect of surrounding lung tissue. Additionally,

vessels may become tortuous and crinkled at lower lung volumes. The net effect of these changes is a rise in PVR. It is of interest that resistance in the pulmonary circuit appears to be least at normal FRC.

Active changes in pulmonary vascular tone may also contribute to the level of resistance in the lesser circulation. These may be induced by changes in sympathetic tone, local changes in PO_2 and/or PCO_2, or changes in levels of catecholamines or other vasoactive substances released locally or in blood perfusing the lung. The pulmonary vasoconstrictor response to hypoxia, hypercarbia, or both is of interest in that it is opposite to that observed in most systemic vascular beds. Many anesthetic drugs tend to reduce lung volume[29] and, therefore, may have additional effects on PVR through this mechanism as well.

A complete description of the ways in which anesthetic agents may alter PVR is well beyond the scope of this chapter. We confine ourselves to the much narrower question of how anesthetic agents may alter PVR with particular emphasis on the direct effects of anesthetic agents on hypoxic vasoconstriction. The effect of inhaled anesthetic agents on pulmonary blood flow and pulmonary artery pressure in humans without significant underlying pulmonary abnormality is small. In general, the more potent agents such as halothane and ethrane simultaneously produce a decrease in PVR and an increase in left atrial pressure.[30,31] The net effect is usually little or no change in pulmonary artery pressure and a small decrease in pulmonary blood flow. Nitrous oxide and ether have less effect on cardiac output and therefore pulmonary blood flow is relatively unaffected. Overall, changes in PVR are small, tending to rise slightly during anesthetic administration.

HYPOXIC PULMONARY VASOCONSTRICTOR RESPONSE

The hypoxic pulmonary vasoconstrictor response is believed to be mediated locally. The demonstration of this response in isolated perfused lungs reflects the local nature of this reflex. Furthermore, a similar response may be elicited in animals whose catecholamines have been depleted by reserpine or following α-adrenergic blockade. The sympathetic nervous system may, however, play a role in augmenting the response in certain circumstances, particularly in the presence of systemic hypoxemia. Sympathetic innervation of the pulmonary vasculature may play a role in mediating some types of pulmonary edema (e.g., neurogenic). Stimulation of the peripheral chemoreceptor by hypoxemia or hypercarbia produces reflex changes in the systemic circulation.[32] Increases of blood pressure and heart rate also stimulate a reflex sympathetic response. Similarly, pulmonary arterial pressure rises secondary to increased PVR, which is believed to be caused principally by increased pulmonary arteriolar tone. Pulmonary venular constriction may also occur, but this has not been well established.

Arteriolar constriction occurs in response to decreased oxygen tension in the alveolus. Hypoxic pulmonary vasoconstrictor (HPV) responses in normal lung seem to appear when PaO_2 becomes less than 100 mm Hg and maximal when PaO_2 is approximately 30 mm Hg.[33,34] Mixed venous PO_2 (PvO_2) may influence HPV in atelectatic lung, since PaO_2 in the collapsed segment approaches that of PvO_2.[35,36] Acidosis also appears to be a pulmonary vasoconstrictor, both in intact animals and in isolated perfused lungs.[37] With normal alveolar oxygen tensions, changes in PVR in response to acidosis are small, but in the presence of alveolar hypoxia they are greatly enhanced.[38] Thus vasoconstriction may be augmented by elevations in arterial hydrogen ion concentration, alveolar PCO_2, or both. The local mediator of the response to hypoxia and acidosis has not been identified.

The vasoconstrictor response of the pulmonary circulation to hypoxemia and acidosis is different from that of the systemic vasculature and appears to be suited to matching of lung perfusion to ventilation. Thus hypoxic areas of the lung, because of local pulmonary vasoconstrictor reflexes, have reduced blood flow with a shift of blood flow to the better ventilated (less hypoxic and acidotic) areas of the lung. This selective redistribution of blood away from the poorly ventilated areas has been

shown to decrease alveolar-arterial oxygen tension gradients [$P(A - a)O_2$].[39] The obliteration of this response by infusion of a pulmonary vasodilator, such as nitroprusside, has been shown to decrease arterial PO_2 and increase pulmonary shunting in dogs with oleic acid-induced pulmonary edema.[40]

INHALED AGENTS AND HYPOXIC PULMONARY VASOCONSTRICTION

A decrease in PaO_2 and an increase in $P(A - a)O_2$ has been frequently described during anesthesia. Many mechanisms exist by which this decrease in oxygenation may take place. Earlier explanations centered mostly on the effect of anesthesia on lung mechanisms. Such effects as progressive pulmonary atelectasis and diminishment of functional residual capacity relative to closing capacity of the lung have been just two of the mechanisms suggested. In 1964 Buckley et al.[41] suggested that the local pulmonary vasoconstriction in response to hypoxia might be attenuated by halothane anesthesia. Since that time the effect of numerous inhaled anesthetics on hypoxic pulmonary vasoconstriction (HPV) have been examined in a variety of animals and experimental models. Many of the studies have produced conflicting results regarding the effects of certain anesthetic agents, particularly halothane. A summary of experiments and results in this area are shown in Table 21-2.

Sykes et al.[42] examined the effects of halothane and other anesthetic agents on the HPV response in isolated perfused cat lungs. The lungs of cats were surgically isolated and perfused with oxygen-saturated blood using a nonpulsatile continuous flow technique. At constant flow rate and left atrial pressure, a rise in mean pulmonary artery pressure occurred in response to ventilation with a hypoxic gas mixture; this response was attenuated by halothane. These experiments have been criticized because the control response of pulmonary artery pressure to alveolar hypoxia decreased with time to a degree similar to that occurring during halothane anesthesia. This deterioration of hypoxic vasoconstrictive response

TABLE 21-2. Effects of Inhaled Agents on Hypoxic Pulmonary Vasoconstriction

Anesthetic Agent	Reference	Model	Effect
Halothane	Buckley et al.[41]	Dog, 5% O_2 whole lung	Inhibit
	Kaur et al.[113]	Dog, 10% O_2 whole lung	None
	Benumof & Wahrenbrock[46]	Dog, N_2 LL lobe	None
	Mathers et al.[47]	Dog, N_2 LL lobe	None
	Sykes et al.[42]	Cat, 3% O_2 isolated lung	Inhibit
	Bjertnaes et al.[44]	Rat, 2% O_2 isolated lung	Inhibit
	Loh et al.[43]	Cat, 3% O_2 innervated lung	Inhibit
	Sykes et al.[45]	Dog, whole lung	None
	Fargas-Babjak & Forrest[49]	Dog, 8% O_2 whole lung	None
	Bjertnaes[51]	Human, N_2 one lung	Inhibit
	Marshall et al.[50]	Rat, 3% O_2 isolated lung	Inhibit
Ether	Sykes et al.[42]	Cat, 3% O_2 isolated lung	Inhibit
	Sykes et al.[48]	Dog, N_2 left lung	Inhibit
	Loh et al.[43]	Cat, 3% O_2 innervated lung	Inhibit
	Bjertnaes[51]	Human, N_2 one lung	Inhibit
	Bjertnaes et al.[44]	Rat, 2% O_2 isolated lung	Inhibit
Trichloroethylene	Sykes et al.[42]	Cat, 3% O_2 isolated lung	Inhibit
	Sykes et al.[114]	Dog, N_2 one lung	Inhibit
Nitrous oxide	Buckley et al.[41]	Dog, 5% O_2 whole lung	Enhanc
	Sykes et al.[48]	Dog, N_2 one lung	Inhibit
	Hurtig et al.[58]	Cat, 3% O_2 isolated lung	Inhibit
	Mathers et al.[47]	Dog, N_2 LL lobe	Inhibit (slight)
	Benumof & Wahrenbrock[46]	Dog, N_2 LL lobe	None
	Bjertnaes et al.[44]	Rat, 2% O_2 isolated lung	None
Fluroxene	Benumof & Wahrenbrock[46]	Dog, N_2 LL lobe	Inhibit
	Mathers et al.[47]	Dog, N_2 LL lobe	Inhibit
Methoxyflurane	Sykes et al.[42]	Cat, 3% O_2 isolated lung	Inhibit
	Bjertnaes et al.[44]	Rat, 2% O_2 isolated lung	Inhibit
Isoflurane	Benumof & Wahrenbrock[46]	Dog, N_2 LL lobe	Inhibit
	Mathers et al.[47]	Dog, N_2 LL lobe	Inhibit
	Marshall et al.[50]	Rat, 3% O_2 isolated lung	Inhibit
Enflurane	Mathers et al.[47]	Dog, N_2 LL lobe	None
	Marshall et al.[50]	Rat, 3% O_2 isolated lung	Inhibit
Cyclopropane	Tait et al.[115]	Cat, 3% O_2 isolated lung	None

LL = left lower

makes quantification of the effect of inhaled anesthetics a difficult task. The apparently dose-related effect of anesthetic agents studied is also difficult to evaluate, since blood or alveolar levels of halothane, trichloroethylene, and ether were not measured. These experiments were repeated in cat lungs in which sympathetic nervous innervation was preserved.[43] Under these conditions, HPV was diminished by halothane only at inspired concentrations of 3 percent or greater. It is significant that in these latter experiments there was no evidence that the hypoxic vasopressor response deteriorated with time as had been found by the previous investigations. Again alveolar (end-expired) concentrations of

anesthetic agent were not measured and therefore the true alveolar concentration of halothane was unknown. Thus, although the effect of halothane on hypoxic pulmonary constriction appeared to be attenuated in this model as compared with the isolated denervated cat lung, it is difficult to compare equianesthetic doses of anesthetic because the alveolar concentrations were unknown. However, in studies which used isolated rat lungs halothane also attenuated the response of pulmonary artery pressure to hypoxic alveolar gas mixtures.[44] Further conflicting experimental data exist in a series of studies performed on dogs.[45] Benumof and Wahrenbrock[46] tested the hypothesis that halogenated anesthetics and nitrous oxide cause local inhibition of HPV. Their experimental design consisted of isolating the left lower lobe of a dog and selectively ventilating this lobe with hypoxic gas mixtures containing MAC multiples of inhaled anesthetics. The remainder of the lung was ventilated with 100 percent oxygen. The effect on PVR was assessed by the measurement of blood flow to the isolated lobe, the use of an electromagnetic flowmeter, and comparison with total pulmonary blood flow. With constant pulmonary blood flow (cardiac output), pulmonary artery pressure, and left atrial pressure, a significant decrease in flow to the isolated left lower lobe was found in the presence of localized alveolar hypoxia. The administration of halothane or nitrous oxide did not diminish the magnitude of the hypoxic vasoconstrictive response (Fig. 21-5), although a profound dose-related effect could be demonstrated in the presence of fluroxene and isoflurane (Fig. 21-6). The investigators then repeated these experiments[47] but administered the anesthetic agent to the whole animal as well as to the isolated lung segment. In this preparation, cardiac output was diminished by halothane, isoflurane, and enflurane but the effects on blood flow to the isolated segment were almost identical to those obtained when administration of anesthetic agent was confined to the isolated lobe alone. Halothane at levels up to 2 MAC did not significantly interfere with hypoxic vasoconstriction of the test lobe, while isoflurane, enflurane, and fluroxene did lessen the vasoconstrictive effect of hypoxemia.

Sykes et al.[45] examined the effects of alveolar hypoxia in one lung on the relative distribution of pulmonary blood flow between both lungs. Blood flow distribution was measured using xenon-133 in dogs whose tracheas were intubated with a double-lumen tube permitting independent ventilation of each lung. One lung was ventilated with nitrogen while the other lung was ventilated with 100 percent oxygen. The PaO_2 was greater than 100 mm Hg. A significant redistribution of flow to the well oxygenated lung was found, which is evidence of a brisk hypoxic vasoconstrictive response. This redistribution of pulmonary blood flow was preserved in the presence of halothane at inspired concentrations of up to 3 percent. The preparation was substantially different, of

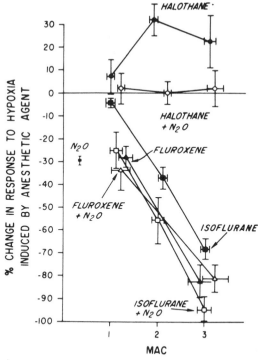

FIG. 21-5 The effect of anesthetic agents on the hypoxia-induced increase in PVR of an isolated left lower lobe of the dog. Zero on the vertical axis represents the normal distribution of pulmonary blood flow between the hypoxic left lower lobe and the remainder of the lung. A negative percentage change represents a decrease in the hypoxia-induced pulmonary vasoconstriction of the nitrogen-ventilated left lower lobe. In this preparation, halothane seems to have little effect on pulmonary vasoconstriction, but fluroxene, nitrous oxide, and isoflurane exhibit a dose-dependent decrease in hypoxic vasoconstriction. (Benumof JL, Wahrenbrock EA: Local effects of anesthetics on regional hypoxic pulmonary vasoconstriction. Anesthesiology 43:525, 1975.)

course, from the isolated cat lung experiments, and this might account for the different results observed. However, substantial reduction in hypoxic vasoconstrictive responses have been demonstrated with other anesthetic agents. Indeed, Sykes et al.[48] in the same preparation demonstrated that ether profoundly affected the redistribution of pulmonary blood flow in response to hypoxia (Fig. 21-7). Fargas-Babjak and Forrest[49] also found that the increases in PVR in a nitrogen-ventilated lung were affected by inhalation of 1.5 percent halothane. Alveolar concentrations of halothane were not

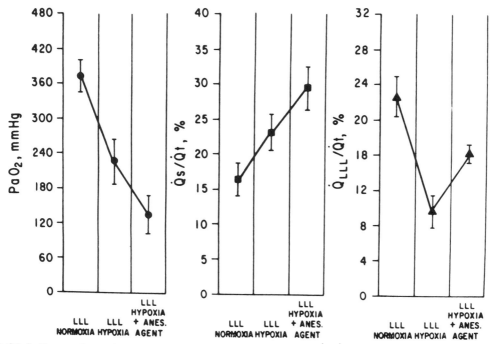

FIG. 21-6 Changes in arterial oxygen tension (PaO$_2$), physiologic shunt ($\dot{Q}s/\dot{Q}t$), and the percentage of the cardiac output perfusing the left lower lobe ($\dot{Q}_{LLL}/\dot{Q}t$) during its ventilation with nitrogen which resulted in its pulmonary artery vasoconstriction. The right-hand box of each graph illustrates the effect of adding an anesthetic agent (2 to 3 MAC fluroxene or isoflurane) to the hypoxic left lower lobe. The PaO$_2$ decreases with nitrogen ventilation of the left lower lobe, but perfusion is decreased by the hypoxic vasoconstrictive response. The addition of fluroxene and isoflurane increases the relative perfusion of the hypoxic left lower lobe, causing an increase in physiologic shunting and a further decrease in PaO$_2$. (Benumof JL, Wahrenbrock EA: Local effects of anesthetics on regional hypoxic pulmonary vasoconstriction. Anesthesiology 43:525, 1975.)

measured, however, and cardiac output was substantially reduced when compared with the unanesthetized state.

Marshall et al.[50] utilized isolated perfused rat lungs to examine the effects of halothane, enflurane, and isoflurane on HPV. Dose-response curves were carefully established for each of these anesthetics. All three anesthetics depressed HPV in a dose-related manner and the ED$_{50}$ for HPV depression occurred at similar MAC values. This in vitro preparation allowed for control of lung perfusion and negated any effect of the sympathetic nervous system.

In a study of the effects of anesthetic agents on the phenomenon in humans, Bjertnaes[51] examined the effects of diethyl ether and halothane on the distribution of pulmonary blood flow. In these human subjects, the trachea was intubated with a Carlens double-lumen tube. Each lung was then ventilated by use of a sepa-

rate anesthetic machine. Distribution of blood flow was assessed by a lung perfusion scan on two separate occasions following the injection of macroaggregated serum albumin labeled with two different radioisotopes. While one lung was ventilated with oxygen, the test lung was ventilated with nitrogen only; equal end-expiratory carbon dioxide concentrations were maintained in both lungs. Hypoxic vasoconstriction was demonstrated in the nitrogen-ventilated lung during intravenous anesthesia with barbiturates. This vasoconstrictive response disappeared with the inhalation of either halothane or diethyl ether in the N$_2$-ventilated lungs. Abolishment of the HPV response was accompanied in most patients by a decrease in PaO$_2$. The method of measurement precluded the ability to demonstrate a return of hypoxic vasoconstriction to its former level following the withdrawal of the inhaled anes-

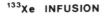

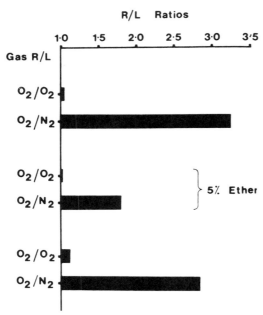

FIG. 21-7 The effect of diethyl ether anesthesia on the distribution of pulmonary blood flow between the right and left lungs of the dog. Ventilation of the left lung with nitrogen directs the blood flow to the opposite lung, thus increasing the right to left ratio of flow. This response is depressed during the administration of 5 percent diethyl ether. The hypoxic pulmonary vasoconstrictive response returns after the withdrawal of ether anesthesia. (Sykes MK, Hurtig JB, Tait AR, et al: Reduction of hypoxic pulmonary vasoconstriction during diethyl ether anesthesia in the dog. Br J Anaesth 49:293, 1977.)

thetic. In addition, pulmonary artery and left atrial pressures were not measured and it is known that changes in left atrial pressure may alter the pulmonary vascular response to hypoxia.[52]

In contrast to this study, clinical observations in humans undergoing one-lung ventilation during thoracic surgery do not seem to show changes consistent with attenuation of HPV by halothane. Comparing pulmonary gas exchange under intravenous anesthetics (ketamine) and isoflurane[53] or enflurane,[54] no significant changes in $\dot{Q}s/\dot{Q}t$ or PaO_2 were found between the two anesthetics in two separate studies. Since ketamine is said to not affect HPV, this observation would suggest that halo-

thane does not affect HPV when one lung is unventilated. However, several differences exist between these studies and others. Bjertnaes[51] ventilated one lung with O_2 and the other with nitrogen to demonstrate HPV as opposed to the clinical situation of ventilating one lung with O_2 and allowing the unventilated up lung to undergo various degrees of collapse. Thoracic surgery is carried out with an open chest and the patient on his side, altering distribution of perfusion pressures through the two lungs. The up lung may be diseased, altering pulmonary vascular responsiveness to hypoxia. It has been suggested that surgical manipulation of the lung and the pulmonary vessels may diminish HPV response, necessitating a prolonged exposure to hypoxia or possibly intermittent hypoxic exposure to reestablish HPV.[55–57] The clinical observations of Rees and Gaines[54] and Anderson and Benumof[53] should not be interpreted as suggesting inhalational agents do not alter HPV in humans. Rather, in this clinically important situation of thoracic surgery and one-lung anesthesia, HPV may be attenuated by other factors, so the effect of inhalational agents is not demonstrated.

The observed variations in response to administration of halothane may in part be due to species differences, as well as to differences in experimental protocols. While diethyl ether has been found to have a profound effect on diminishing HPV in all models tested, the pulmonary vascular response to inhalation of nitrous oxide has been as varied as that measured during the administration of halothane. Sykes and colleagues demonstrated in isolated cat lung[58] and in dog lung[48] that nitrous oxide appeared to attenuate HPV. Other investigators have shown little or no effect from the addition of nitrous oxide to inhaled gas mixtures.[46] The effects of other less commonly used anesthetic agents are summarized in Table 21-2.

The mechanism by which some anesthetic agents appear to interfere with the pulmonary vasoconstrictor responses to hypoxia remains as yet a mystery. If, in fact, pulmonary vascular smooth muscle responds to locally accumulated tissue metabolites, then anesthetic agents may be acting by interfering with the metabolic production of these vasoactive substances. It is possible that anesthetics that have a direct relaxing effect on vascular smooth muscles may counteract locally or systemically mediated vasoconstrictive responses. Interference with calcium uptake by smooth muscle has also been suggested as one possible mechanism whereby anesthetics may interfere with smooth muscle constriction. Similarly, increases in vascular tone in healthy lung caused by specific anesthetic agents or methods of ventilation might increase PVR in normal lung segments, thereby causing a redistribution of blood flow to the diseased lung.

One of the important factors involved in modulating the effects of hypoxic vasoconstriction may be the overall effect of pulmonary artery pressure. Thus high pulmonary artery pressures, by increasing vascular distending pressure, may tend to cause passive distention of constricted vascular beds and thereby tend to reverse hypoxic vasoconstriction. Similarly, reflex pulmonary and systemic vasoconstriction in response to stimuli such as hypotension may increase PVR in healthy lung segments, again leading to a shift of blood flow to the diseased or "hypoxic" areas of lung. The net effect of anesthetic agents on HPV obviously depends upon a number of other factors that commonly occur during surgery and anesthesia.

Clinically, despite some variation in experimental results, the effect of anesthetic agents on the pulmonary vasculature must be taken into account as one possible factor when considering the causes of hypoxemia under anesthesia. Although changes in distribution may account for some of these problems, attenuation of the hypoxic vasoconstrictor response may have a significant influence on PaO_2. In dogs with oleic acid-induced pulmonary edema, quite remarkable reversible increases in pulmonary shunting have been demonstrated by the administration of pulmonary vasodilators such as nitroprusside[40] and nitroglycerine.[59] Some anesthetic agents probably produce a similar response in patients with adult respiratory distress syndrome or other types of pulmonary pathology associated with large right-to-left intrapulmonary shunts. The most likely effect of the various anesthetic agents in these patients remains to be defined. The selection of the appropriate type of anesthetic drugs may be of great importance in minimizing arterial hypoxemia in patients with wide alveolar to arterial oxygen tension differ-

ences. More work needs to be done, particularly in humans, before the effect of a particular anesthetic agent can be predicted.

EFFECTS OF INHALED ANESTHETIC AGENTS ON MUCOCILIARY FUNCTION

NORMAL MUCOCILIARY FUNCTION

The clearance of mucus from the respiratory tract is an important defense mechanism of the lungs. Foreign particulate matter and the "debris" of pulmonary infection are removed by the upward and outward flow of mucus. Ciliated respiratory epithelium is located throughout the respiratory tract and extends distally as far as the terminal bronchioles,[60] although the density of such cells decreases from trachea to alveoli.[61] Mucus-producing cells (goblet and submucous glands) are similarly distributed.[62] The peculiar pattern of ciliary motion has been established for some time and is consistent through various kinds of species. A rapid stroke in a cephalad direction is followed by a slower recovery stroke in the opposite direction. The movement of cilia occurs in a coordinated fashion; movement of distal cilia are followed closely by like movements of those immediately proximal; the resulting wave of motion is referred to as metachronism.[63] The mechanism by which this coordination occurs has not been elucidated. In mammals, the sympathetic and parasympathetic nervous systems appear to play no role in the coordination of ciliary movement. The bending of individual cilia appears to be the result of an ATP-dependent sliding of two parallel fibers within the ciliary filament.

Mucus represents a mixture of water, electrolytes, and macromolecules (lipids, mucins, enzymes) secreted by goblet cells and mucosal glands. Mucous secretions appear to provide a medium for entrapping and carrying foreign material and dead cells, as well as for influencing the movement of the cilia. The "blanket" of mucus interacts with cilia and influences the rate and efficiency of ciliary movement. For instance, thicker layers of mucus appear to slow the removal of surface articles from the airway. The rheologic properties of mucus are very important and influence mucociliary function, with high elasticity and low viscosity appearing to be the characteristics required to promote the fastest transport by cilia.[64] The presence and characteristics of the mucous layer may also promote the coordination of ciliary beats.

METHODS OF MEASUREMENT OF MUCOCILIARY FUNCTION

Various methods have been used experimentally to assess mucociliary function in both normal animals and in humans and to examine the effect of airway disease and drugs (Table 21-3). Determination of the beat frequency of cilia is one such method. The movement of cilia are examined optically by the use of a microscope and high-speed photography. This has usually been accomplished in vitro, using either single cilia or tissue cultures of respiratory epithelium. In vivo techniques in animals have

made use of a tracheal window, but in vivo measurements in humans would obviously pose some difficulty. The physical and chemical characteristics of mucus have also been studied extensively by Reid.[65] Since these studies have been done on expectorated specimens, the characteristics may differ from the situation in vivo because of contamination by salivary secretions and desiccation of expectorated secretions.

Techniques more applicable to humans include the measurement of the movement of markers placed in the airway. One type of measurement, that of mucus velocity, involves the placement of radioactive markers in the airway followed by a measurement (utilizing external scintillation counters) of the velocity of these particles in a cephalad direction. This measurement is confined to the examination of mucus velocity in the trachea. Sackner et al.[66] have developed a method of determining mucus velocity through a fiberoptic bronchoscope. A second group of measurements assessing mucociliary clearance involves the deposition of radiopaque or radioactive particles throughout the lung fields followed by sequential radiographic examinations of clearance of these inhaled particles. This allows an examination of mucociliary function in both peripheral and central airways. Coughing may enhance the rate of removal, thus contributing to errors in measurements.

TABLE 21-3. Effects of Inhaled Agents on Mucociliary Function

Function	Anesthetic Agent	Reference	Model	Effect
Ciliary function	Halothane	Nunn et al.[77]	Protozoa	——
	Halothane	Manawadu et al.[78]	Dog, tracheal, culture	—
	Ether, methoxyflurane	Nunn et al.[77]	Protozoa	——
	Trichlorethylene	Nunn et al.[77]	Protozoa	——
Mucociliary flow	Halothane	Forbes[74]	Dog, intact	——
	Halothane	Forbes & Horrigan[75]	Dog, intact	——
	Halothane, nitrous oxide	Lichtiger et al.[73]	Human	——
	Enflurane	Forbes & Horrigan[75]	Dog, intact	——
	Nitrous oxide, morphine	Forbes & Horrigan[75]	Dog, intact	—
	Ether	Forbes & Horrigan[75]	Dog, intact	0
Mucociliary clearance	Halothane	Forbes & Gamsu[76]	Dog, intact	——
	Ether	Forbes & Gamsu[76]	Dog, intact	——

Symbols used:—— = pronounced depression; — = depression; 0 = no effect.

SPECIFIC EFFECTS OF ANESTHETICS

Postoperative hypoxemia and atelectasis are common findings in patients who have undergone anesthesia and surgery. Although many physiologic derangements may contribute to pulmonary complications (e.g., airway closure and decreased functional residual capacity), the role of inhibited mucociliary function has sparked some recent interest and investigation. Gamsu et al.[67] compared the rate of tantalum clearance from the lungs of two groups of postoperative patients who had received general anesthesia with that of a control group consisting of awake patients undergoing tracheography following topical application of local anesthetic to the pharynx and trachea. One group of patients, who underwent orthopedic procedures, showed no significant differences from the control group. In contrast, in patients following intra-abdominal vascular surgery, retention of tantalum was demonstrated for as long as 6 days, with an average retention time threefold greater than in the control group. Retention of tantalum was correlated with the retention of mucus demonstrated in areas of atelectasis. Disappearance of tantalum from these areas of atelectasis occurred only after reexpansion of collapsed segments of lung.

The role of anesthesia in mucus retention must be viewed with caution, because many other factors may affect and diminish mucociliary function, particularly in the mechanically ventilated patient. Extensive literature exists demonstrating the importance of maintenance of a high relative humidity of inspired gases on optimum mucociliary transport. Thus dry inspired gases may both decrease ciliary beat frequency, as well as dry out the mucous layer. In dogs, mucus flow rates measured by the rate of movement of a radioactive marker in the trachea were found to be maintained at normal rates for a 40-minute period if the inspired air temperature was greater than 32°C with an inspired water vapor content of 33 mg/L.[68] A similar study demonstrated a complete cessation of flow of tracheal mucus after 3 hours of inhalation of dry air.[69] Mucus movement could be reinstituted by restoring inspired gases to 100

percent relative humidity at 38°C. Other factors diminishing the rate of mucus movement are high inspired oxygen concentration,[70] inflation of the endotracheal tube cuff,[71] and positive pressure ventilation.[72] One must take these factors into account in assessing any study examining the effects of anesthetics per se.

In a study of tracheal mucus velocity in young anesthetized women undergoing gynecologic surgery, Lichtiger et al.[73] used a technique of placing Teflon disks on the tracheal mucosa; the disks were then observed and filmed through the lens of a fiberoptic bronchoscope. Control values in awake volunteers had revealed a tracheal mucus velocity of 20 mm/min. Induction of anesthesia with halothane (1 to 2 percent) and nitrous oxide (60 percent) decreased the rate of mucus travel to 7.7 mm/min, with little or no motion being seen by 90 minutes of anesthesia. Inspired gases were humidified, but the presence of higher than normal FIO_2, the use of a cuffed endotracheal tube, and the maintenance of ventilation by use of positive pressure could all have contributed to this dysfunction, as well as the anesthetic.

In a study in which the temperature and humidity of inspired gases and endotracheal tube cuff pressure were well controlled, Forbes[74] measured the effect of halothane anesthesia on mucociliary flow. With the use of external scintillation counters to measure the progression of radioactive droplets placed in the trachea, a dose-related depressant effect of halothane was found on this measurement of mucociliary function. Further studies showed a similar depressant effect in response to anesthesia with equipotent doses of enflurane and of nitrous oxide with halothane or nitrous oxide with narcotic anesthesia.[75] Conversely, ether anesthesia did not affect the velocity of mucus movement at concentrations of up to 2.4 MAC (Fig. 21-8).

Utilizing a different measure of mucociliary function—that of clearance of tantalum from the peripheral and central airways of anesthetized, intubated, mechanically ventilated dogs—Forbes and Gamsu[76] showed a delayed clearance of mucus both during and after 6 hours of anesthesia with halothane or ether at

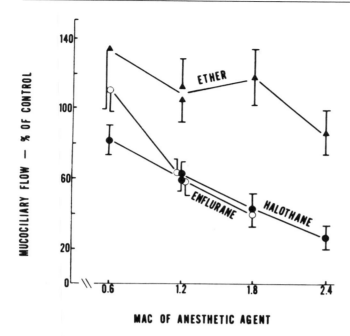

FIG. 21-8 Effects of various MAC levels of halothane, enflurane, and ether on mucociliary flow rates in dog tracheas. Each value is a mean ± SE expressed as a percentage of the thiopental control. Note the dose-dependent depression of mucus velocity with enflurane and halothane anesthesia. (Forbes AR, Horrigan RW: Mucociliary flow in the trachea during anesthesia with enflurane, ether, nitrous oxide, and morphine. Anesthesiology 46:319, 1977.)

concentrations of 1.2 MAC. The dysfunction occurred in both peripheral and central airways and persisted for 6 hours or more after the cessation of anesthesia. It is not readily apparent why ether should cause slowing of tantalum clearance whereas mucus velocity in central airways was apparently not affected.[75] These same authors[75] have recently found that controlled ventilation with O_2 in barbiturate-anesthetized dogs decreased tantalum clearance to approximately 50 percent of rates in awake spontaneously ventilating controls. Since mechanical ventilation was utilized in the previously mentioned studies, its interaction with general anesthesia is unclear. Certainly the dose-related effects of halothane speak to a primary influence of halothane, per se, on mucus velocity.

The mechanisms by which inhaled anesthetics diminish rates of mucus clearance are unknown. This could be accomplished by diminishing ciliary beat frequency or by altering the characteristics or quantity of mucus produced during the anesthetized period. Nunn et al.[77] found dose-related decreases of ciliary activity and cellular mobility of the ciliated protozoan *Tytrahymena pyriformis* by exposure to six inhalational anesthetics, including halothane. The ED_{50} for cessation of organism and

ciliary movement corresponded closely to MAC values of the various anesthetics. The mechanism by which cilia were affected was not clear, although the rapidity and reversibility of the depression suggested that metabolic depression of ATP stores was not involved. Extrapolation from the protozoan to the airway epithelia of mammals is hazardous but offers a very plausible explanation of observed slowing of mucus clearance.

In a recent study utilizing in vitro cultures of ciliated epithelium of dogs, Manawadu et al.[78] showed a depression of ciliary movement by halothane, but only at doses of 3 percent or more (Fig. 21-9); these doses were well above those of usual clinical concentrations. These sensitivities of cilia to halothane are substantially different from that found by Nunn in *T. pyriformis*. The effects of anesthetics on ciliary beat frequency in humans have not been elucidated.

Ciliary metachronism has not been studied with respect to anesthesia. Both adrenergic and cholinergic drugs involved in ciliary activity[79] have been shown to increase mucociliary clearance with the latter group of drugs affecting both ciliary frequency and volume of mucus production. The known reduction in sympathetic nervous activity caused by halo-

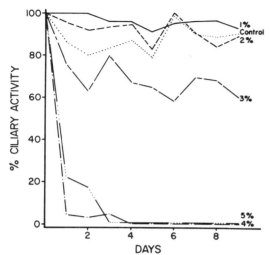

FIG. 21-9 In a culture of dog tracheal ring, ciliary activity is diminished by high doses of halothane. (Manawadu BR, Mostow ST, LaForce FM: Impairment of tracheal ring ciliary activity by halothane. Anesth Analg 58:500, 1979.)

thane and enflurane may be one mechanism by which mucus removal is compromised.

CLINICAL SIGNIFICANCE

Because many factors contribute to postoperative pulmonary complications, the role of depressed mucociliary function is not known. It would seem clear that prolonged anesthesia could lead to pooling of mucus and thus result in atelectasis and respiratory infections. The patients at greatest risk would be those with excessive or abnormal mucus production, that is, those with chronic bronchitis, asthma, respiratory tract infection, or cystic fibrosis. Some evidence exists that patients with chronic obstructive lung disease anesthetized by regional block techniques show a lesser incidence of respiratory failure than those anesthetized with general anesthetics,[80] while other studies have failed to demonstrate this advantage. Controlled studies of the effects of inhaled anesthetics on mucociliary function in these already compromised groups of patients have not been done, nor has the role of general anesthe-

sia on their rate of pulmonary complications been clearly delineated. In animals, mucus pooling appears to occur in the intra-anesthetic and postanesthetic period; this suggests a need in the immediate postoperative period for vigorous pulmonary therapy directed toward enhancing clearance of secretions from the airways.

EFFECTS OF INHALED ANESTHETIC AGENTS ON CONTROL OF VENTILATION

Of the many derangements of lung function caused by anesthetic agents, alterations of minute ventilation are the most obvious. Many different stimuli interact in a complex manner to determine the level of ventilation in humans. The traditional approach to studying anesthetic effects on ventilation has been to measure ventilatory responsiveness before and after drug administration. The index of ventilatory response may be expired minute volume, frequency of respiration, or arterial carbon dioxide tension (a measure of alveolar ventilation). All of these offer some problem in the interpretation of the effects on ventilatory control. Though an area of intense investigation, many aspects of ventilatory control are still unclear. Indeed, the precise origin of the normal respiratory pattern (the ventilatory "pacemaker") remains a mystery up to the present time. Investigations in humans are frequently hampered by being limited to measurements of expired gas volumes as an indicator of respiratory drive. Obviously, alterations in lung mechanics, such as those occurring during airway obstruction, may alter minute ventilation in the face of constant nerve traffic to the muscles of respiration. Similarly, a sufficient dose of muscle relaxant such as pancuronium will negate any ventilatory response to inhalation of carbon dioxide, but this would hardly constitute evidence of depression of ventilatory control.

A complete description of ventilatory control is beyond the scope of this chapter. Several excellent reviews of this subject already exist.[81,82] However, some understanding of normal ventilatory responses is necessary to appreciate the effects of drugs and the methods by which these effects are measured.

CONTROL OF BREATHING

The volume of gas moving in and out of the lungs is matched to the requirements of the body for oxygen delivery and carbon dioxide elimination. Oxygen consumed and carbon dioxide produced vary widely in disease, during exercise, and with alterations in the environment (including differences in the chemical composition of inspired gases). A control system that modulates ventilation is necessary, therefore, to maintain stability in blood-gas tensions and acidity (Fig. 21-10). Furthermore, changes in the environment, the mechanical properties of the lung, and the work of ventilation necessitate the presence of receptors to detect changes and provide sufficient altered "drive" to the respiratory muscles such that body homeostasis is maintained. Frequency and tidal volume are integrated in such a manner as to minimize the work of breathing in response to variations in the total ventilatory requirements.

The system responsible for receiving and integrating the many input signals and ulti-

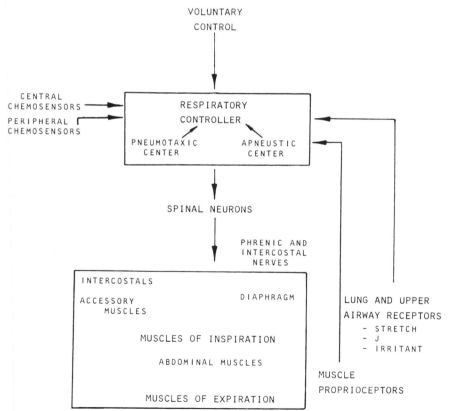

FIG. 21-10 Some aspects of the reflex control of ventilation. Inputs from many sources to alter ventilatory controller output and hence ventilation.

mately producing movement of air in and out of the lungs is composed of the following:

Sensors, which may be chemical (peripheral and central chemoreceptors) or mechanical (distortion receptors located in airways, alveoli, and respiratory muscles)

A *respiratory control system*, which integrates the signal inputs from the receptor sites, centers of consciousness, and other influences (e.g., pain) and culminates in a level and pattern of nerve traffic to the muscles of respiration)

The "*motor system*," composed of the chest wall and intercostal, diaphragmatic, and abdominal muscles, all of which respond to signals from the control center via the phrenic and spinal nerves.

For our purposes, discussion is more detailed in those areas in which the role of anesthetic agents has been most clearly delineated.

MEASUREMENT OF RESPIRATORY CONTROL CENTER OUTPUT

Detailed discussion of the respiratory control center may be found in the review of Berger et al.[81]

The "controller," located in the medulla and pons, consists of two groups of neurons: the dorsal respiratory group (DRG), composed of cells active during inspiration, and the ventral respiratory groups (VRG), containing both inspiratory and expiratory neurons. The DRG may be the source of respiratory rhythm, and the apneustic center (VRG) may determine frequency and depth of ventilation and function as the off switch for inspiration. The exact site for integration of afferent stimuli from pulmonary receptors is not clear, although the pneumotaxic center has been suggested.

The output of the respiratory control center may be assessed by measurement of cellular activity, phrenic nerve discharge, or various parameters of ventilation, of which minute ventilation ($\dot{V}E$) is most commonly used clinically. The parameter $\dot{V}E$ is a useful mea-

surement in normal humans, but becomes a doubtful indicator of respiratory drive in patients with neuromuscular or mechanical impairment of breathing. Diaphragmatic electromyography is of some interest but is distressing to the subject and sometimes not readily reproducible.

The search for a method of quantifying respiratory controller output led Whitelaw et al.[83] to develop a method measuring the pressure developed in the first 0.1 second of inspiration during the time that the airway is acutely obstructed immediately prior to inspiration. These investigators found that this parameter (P_{100}) was independent of airway resistance and well correlated with phrenic nerve discharge. It was, however, sensitive to changes in lung functional residual capacity. A study involving the measurement of respiratory drive during methoxyflurane anesthesia showed an elevation of $PaCO_2$ but no change in P_{100}.[84] One interpretation was that methoxyflurane did not decrease ventilatory drive but that the hypercapnia was caused by mechanical alterations in the lung or chest wall. Obviously, more study is required to establish such a mechanism or the validity of P_{100} as a measure of controller output under anesthesia. This is, however, a step in separating controller output ("drive") from volume of gas ventilated by the lungs. Such a separation is necessary to answer such questions as the following: Is ventilatory drive decreased in patients with chronic lung disease? Is the effect of anesthetics on such patients a decreased response to chemical stimuli or secondary to airway mechanical abnormalities?

MECHANORECEPTORS AND BREATHING

In the resting patient, the total amount of alveolar ventilation is believed to be determined by the partial pressures of oxygen and carbon dioxide, as well as by acidity in arterial blood. The pattern of ventilation by which this minute volume is attained is determined by input signals emanating from the upper airways, lungs, and chest wall and mediated by the vagus nerve.

LUNG AND AIRWAY RECEPTORS

Pulmonary receptors that may have some relevance to the effect of anesthetics include irritant receptors and pulmonary stretch receptors. Irritant receptors are believed to be situated between airway epithelial cells. Such a location may explain the rapid response of the airways to various kinds of stimuli such as chemical irritants, smoke, and dust and to sudden mechanical deformation of the bronchial tree. These receptors are involved in coughing in response to many types of stimuli, as well as in producing reflex tachypnea. They may also enhance the ventilatory response to inhaled carbon dioxide.

Pulmonary stretch receptors, located within the smooth muscle of small airways, respond to stretching or changes in lung volume. Increases in lung volume increase afferent nerve traffic via the vagus nerve to the respiratory control center, thereby inhibiting further inspiration; this phenomenon is known as the Hering–Breuer reflex. This limitation of inspiration thereby determines the relationship between tidal volume and respiratory frequency. Thus an attractive hypothesis is that although the level of alveolar ventilation is determined by chemical stimuli, the pattern of ventilation is determined by afferent mechanical signals from the lung and, to some extent, the chest wall. The pulmonary stretch receptors would therefore represent the off switch limiting tidal volume. This reflex has been demonstrated in animals at normal tidal volumes. In humans, however, tidal volumes in excess of 1 L are required to demonstrate an effect on ventilation. No change in normal breathing pattern has been observed in humans following bilateral vagal blockade, although an increase in tidal volume with no change in respiratory rate has been observed following inhalation of carbon dioxide. The data available would suggest that in awake, adult humans, many factors other than pulmonary mechanoreceptors combine to determine the pattern of breathing.

The effects of common inhaled anesthetics on breathing patterns is depicted in Figures 21-11 and 21-12. With increasing depths of anesthesia, alveolar ventilation is progressively diminished; this is effected by a decrease in tidal volume with a simultaneous dose-related increase in breathing frequency. The rate of breathing is greatest with halothane anesthesia at higher MAC concentrations.[85]

The alteration in ventilatory pattern has been attributed to sensitization of pulmonary stretch receptors leading to lower tidal volumes and tachypnea.[86] Vagal afferent activity was measured at various lung volumes in decerebrate cats with and without the intervention of various general anesthetics.[87] The presence of volatile anesthetics increased receptor discharge at any lung volume, that is, pulmonary stretch receptors did seem to be sensitized. Vagotomy in dogs produced a similar decrease in tidal volume. During ether anesthesia[88] respiratory frequency decreased in dogs, although ventilatory responses to inhaled carbon dioxide were unchanged. Little evidence exists of such a mechanism in humans. Paskin et al.[89] examined the effect of elevation of functional residual capacity in

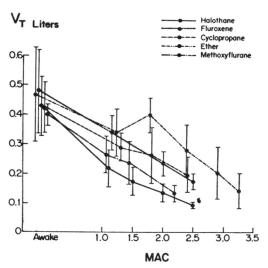

FIG. 21-11 Comparison of mean changes in tidal volume at multiples of MAC in patients anesthetized with one of five different anesthetic agents. Reduction of tidal volume was greatest for halothane and least for diethyl ether. (Larson CP, Eger EI II, Muallem M, et al: The effects of diethyl ether and methoxyflurane on ventilation. Anesthesiology 30:174, 1969.)

Respiratory
Frequency

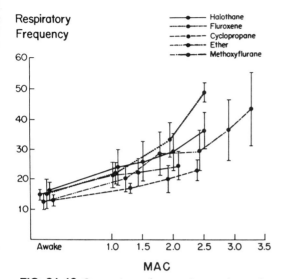

FIG. 21-12 Comparison of mean changes in respiratory frequency at multiples of MAC obtained in patients anesthetized with one of five different anesthetics. With all anesthetics, respiratory frequency increases as anesthesia is deepened. (Larson CP, Eger EI II, Muallem J, et al: The effects of diethyl ether and methoxyflurane on ventilation. Anesthesiology 30:174, 1969.)

anesthetized humans. The added volume and hence increased stimulus to pulmonary stretch receptors should have increased tachypnea; instead, respiratory frequency decreased. Thus, the mechanism of production of tachypnea with decreased tidal volume in anesthetized humans remains unclear.

MECHANORECEPTORS IN THE CHEST WALL

The force exerted by the muscles of inspiration is a function of afferent nerve traffic emanating from the control center. Although this may vary in response to chemical stimuli, mechanoreceptors in the chest wall also provide input to modify the pattern of breathing. Alteration in the position of the chest wall produces a change in efferent impulses from stretch receptors in tendons and intercostal muscle spindles. The effect of this input is to maintain tidal volume in the face of variations in inspiratory resistance. An increase in spindle discharge causes increased motor discharge to muscle

fibers until muscle shortening relieves tension in the spindles. With increased inspiratory resistance, the muscle spindles detect a failure of shortening by the appropriate amount and therefore afferent signals are increased to the motor neuron pool. Accessory muscles of inspiration may be brought into use as well. This reflex increase in inspiratory effort results in sustained tidal volume and minute ventilation with increasing inspiratory resistive loading. These and other forces explain the ability of the body to maintain normal ventilation with different body positions, inspiratory resistance, and changes in compliance.

Anesthetics diminish but do not abolish ventilatory responsiveness to inspiratory resistance.[90] During halothane anesthesia, as inspiratory loading increases minute ventilation diminishes. An exact dose-response relationship of halothane and attenuation of chest wall reflexes has not yet been established. Prolonged resistance may lead to retention of carbon dioxide. This has obvious clinical implications in anesthetized patients with partial upper airway obstruction or those breathing spontaneously through endotracheal tubes of small diameter.

During normal, quiet breathing, expiration is passively effected by the recoil characteristics of the lung. Expiratory pressures up to 10 cm H_2O do not bring abdominal muscles into play. Instead, lung volume is increased until increased lung recoil pressure offsets the elevation of expiratory resistance. In anesthetized patients[91] the ventilatory response to expiratory resistance is diminished more than to inspiratory resistance. This is curious in light of the study of Freund et al.[92] demonstrating that the onset of anesthesia immediately produced activity of abdominal muscles during expiration (i.e., active muscular as well as passive lung recoil forces acted during the expiratory phase of ventilation).

Pietak et al.[93] found that patients with chronic obstructive lung disease who did *not* retain CO_2 while awake hypoventilated to a greater degree than normal patients under halothane anesthesia. The resting $PaCO_2$ was directly proportional to the severity of the obstruction (Fig. 21-13). Thus patients with obstructive airway disease may have ventilatory responses obtunded to a greater degree by anes-

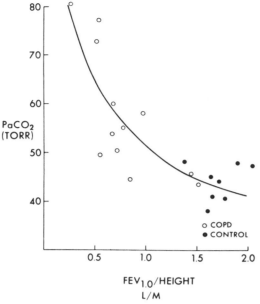

FEV$_{1.0}$/HEIGHT
L/M

FIG. 21-13 Comparison of PaCO$_2$ during anesthesia during spontaneous ventilation relative to preoperative FEV$_{1.0}$. The chronic obstructive pulmonary disease (COPD) patients did not exhibit CO$_2$ retention prior to anesthesia, yet the degree of alveolar hypoventilation is much greater in the more severely obstructed patients. (Pietak S, Weenin CS, Hickey RF, et al: Anesthetic effects on ventilation in patients with chronic obstructive lung disease. Anesthesiology 42:160, 1975.)

thesia than patients with normal pulmonary function. These data[93] clearly demonstrate the requirements for both close monitoring of alveolar ventilation and the use of mechanical ventilation in these patients.

EFFECTS OF ANESTHETICS ON VENTILATORY RESPONSE TO CHEMICAL STIMULI

Anesthetic agents and sedatives may exert potent depressant effects on the function of many organs, including those involved in the control of ventilation. Depression of ventilatory drive has been quantitated utilizing the physiologic principles of chemoreceptor function. These tests have usually involved varying a chemical stimulus (arterial carbon dioxide or

oxygen tension), measuring the ventilatory response to this variation, and then repeating this test after the administration of an anesthetic drug. The variation between the predrug and postdrug responses gives a measure of the depressant potential of the agent in question. Respiratory drive can thus be characterized by the ventilatory responsiveness to PaCO$_2$ (resting PaCO$_2$, apneic threshold, and ventilatory responses to an increase in CO$_2$ tension) or to a decrease in PaO$_2$. To obtain a more complete discussion of the basic elements of chemical ventilatory control, the reader is referred to other reviews.[81,94]

RESPONSES TO CARBON DIOXIDE

Changes in ventilation secondary to alterations in PaCO$_2$ are believed to be mediated chiefly via chemoreceptors located in the medulla. Patients whose peripheral chemoreceptor has been denervated by endarterectomy demonstrate approximately 85 percent of the increase in ventilation secondary to inhaled CO$_2$ observed prior to carotid body denervation.

RESTING PaCO$_2$

The resting PaCO$_2$ is probably the most common index of ventilatory drive used clinically. Ventilation appears to be regulated in such a manner as to maintain PaCO$_2$ very close to 40 mm Hg. Variation from this long-established normal value is interpreted as an indication of either interference with ventilatory drive or severe compromise of the mechanics of breathing. Indeed, elevation of the PaCO$_2$ is often used to define the presence of ventilatory failure. The effects of various concentrations on inhaled anesthetics on PaCO$_2$ are demonstrated in Figure 21-14.[75] Different anesthetics obviously depress resting ventilation to different degrees, with diethyl ether being least depressant and halothane being the most depressant agent. Other investigators examining the effect of enflurane on PaCO$_2$ demonstrated a PaCO$_2$ of over 60 mm Hg at 1.0 MAC enflurane.[95] These kinds of observations have estab-

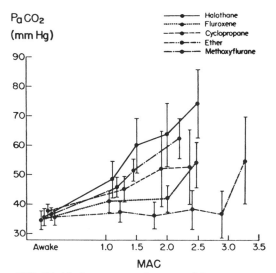

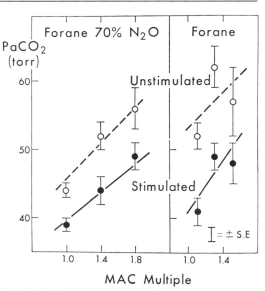

FIG. 21-14 Comparison of mean $PaCO_2$ values in patients anesthetized with one of five different agents. Patients were resting, spontaneously ventilating, and unstimulated. In this study halothane elevated $PaCO_2$ to the greatest degree at equipotent doses of anesthetic, while ether produced the least change in alveolar ventilation. (Larson CP, Eger EI II, Muallem M, et al: The effects of diethyl ether and methoxyflurane on ventilation. Anesthesiology 30:174, 1969.)

FIG. 21-15 The effect of surgical stimulation on the ventilatory depression of inhalational anesthesia with both nitrous oxide and Forane (isoflurane) or Forane alone. Surgical stimulation increased alveolar ventilation and decreased $PaCO_2$ at all depths of anesthesia examined. (Eger EI II, Dolan WM, Stevens WC, et al: Surgical stimulation antagonizes the respiratory depression produced by Forane. Anesthesiology 36:544, 1972.)

lished ether as the least depressant inhalational anesthetic agent, with little changes in $PaCO_2$ being demonstrated at concentrations as high as 3.0 MAC. An explanation of the difference between diethyl ether and other inhaled anesthetics is lacking. Resting $PaCO_2$ is unchanged in ether-anesthetized dogs following vagal denervation, high spinal anesthesia, or bilateral carotid body denervation.[88] The absence of ventilatory alterations after bilateral vagal denervation suggests that irritant receptors are not causally related to this remarkable maintenance of resting ventilation during ether anesthesia. The effects of surgical stimulation on ventilation in anesthetized patients has been noted by many clinical anesthesiologists and was documented for the anesthetic isoflurane by Eger et al. (Fig. 21-15).[96] At various multiples of MAC, these investigators demonstrated that the stimulation of surgical incision brought about a decrease in resting $PaCO_2$ of as much as 10 mm Hg. The duration of anesthesia also plays a role in the level of ventilation. For both halothane and enflurane, the

resting $PaCO_2$ after 6 hours of anesthesia was less than that measured after induction or after 3 hours of anesthesia.[97] $PaCO_2$ decreased from 63 mm Hg to 53 mm Hg over 6 hours of enflurane anesthesia. The reason for this apparent recovery of ventilatory drive is not clear.

APNEIC THRESHOLDS

Apneic threshold is defined as the highest arterial or alveolar PCO_2 at which a subject will remain apneic. It is not usually possible to demonstrate an apneic threshold in a conscious, unmedicated subject, who hyperventilates presumably because of stimuli from the cerebrum. However, one study[98] reported apneic thresholds in awake humans approximately 5 mm Hg below resting $PaCO_2$. A study by Hickey et al.[99] on the effects of ether, halothane, and isoflurane on apneic thresholds in man demonstrated a similar relationship between apnea threshold and resting $PaCO_2$ for all three anesthetics and, remarkably enough,

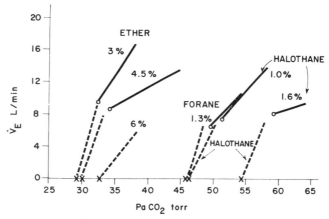

FIG. 21-16 Ventilatory responses to increased carbon dioxide and apneic thresholds during ether, Forane (isoflurane), and halothane anesthesia in patients. Note that apneic threshold in this study appeared to have a relative fixed relationship to resting $PaCO_2$. With an increase in ventilatory depression at increasing depths of anesthesia, resting $PaCO_2$ and apneic threshold increase approximately the same amount. (Hickey RF, Fourcade HE, Eger EI II, et al: The effects of ether, halothane and Forane on apneic threshold in man. Anesthesiology 35:32, 1971.)

for various concentrations of the same anesthetics (Fig. 21-16). The difference between resting $PaCO_2$ and apneic threshold bore no relationship to the slope of CO_2 response curves or to the absolute level of resting $PaCO_2$. This phenomenon suggests that assisted ventilation under the influence of anesthetics is of little use in lowering $PaCO_2$. The effectiveness would be limited to a change of approximately 5 mm Hg. Ventilation that lowered $PaCO_2$ below the apneic threshold would then in fact become "controlled" ventilation rather than "assisted" ventilation. Another clinically important aspect of this observation is in the reestablishment of spontaneous ventilation in the mechanically hyperventilated patient. On cessation of mechanical ventilation, CO_2 stores in the body must accumulate to raise the $PaCO_2$ level in the blood to the apnea threshold. The deeper the level of anesthesia, the longer the period of apnea necessary before the patient will commence spontaneous ventilation. An alternative method of management might be to decrease the anesthetic concentration by continuing mechanical ventilation with the anesthetic gases turned off. This maneuver will lower apneic threshold toward the patient's level of $PaCO_2$, thus diminishing the time of apnea required to initiate spontaneous ventilation.

CARBON DIOXIDE RESPONSE CURVES

Measuring the minute ventilation in response to varying levels of $PaCO_2$ is a common method of quantitating the effects of drugs on ventilatory drive. In the presence of a high inspired concentration of oxygen, $PaCO_2$ is elevated by the investigator, increasing concentrations of inspired carbon dioxide inhaled by the subject. This relationship of $\dot{V}E$ to $PaCO_2$ may be obtained either by the steady-state technique, in which $PaCO_2$ is elevated and maintained at various constant levels for approximately 10 minutes, or by the rebreathing method of Read,[100] in which a subject rebreathes from a 5-L bag filled with 7 percent carbon dioxide in oxygen. In the latter method, exhalation of carbon dioxide into the bag gradually increases the inspired CO_2, hence elevating $PaCO_2$ continually. This test is both faster and simpler than the steady-state method and yields approximately similar slopes of ventilation versus change in $PaCO_2$. In normal humans inspiration of CO_2 increases minute ventilation approximately 3 L/min/mm Hg $PaCO_2$, demonstrating a high gain from a central chemoreceptor in response to variations in $PaCO_2$. Within physiologic range, the response approximates a straight line. Thus the slope of the plot is an index of ventilatory drive in response to carbon dioxide stimulus.

All inhaled agents generally depress the CO_2 response curve at anesthetic levels (Fig. 21-17).[85] The degree of ventilatory depression varies both with the anesthetic agent and with the expired anesthetic concentration. Ether diminished the ventilatory response to inhaled carbon dioxide at anesthetic depths at which $PaCO_2$ is maintained at normal levels. Thus, although ether has a lesser effect on CO_2 response than other anesthetic agents, it is clear that it too is a ventilatory depressant, a conclusion that is not apparent from examination of resting $PaCO_2$ levels alone. Although sedating concentrations of halothane and enflurane have little effect on CO_2 response slopes, 1

MAC halothane is a profound depressant of this measurement. Indeed, at levels of 2.5 MAC or more, no increase in ventilation to altered inspired CO_2 is observed. Isoflurane produces a similar degree of depression.[101] The slope of the ventilatory response curve during halothane anesthesia (like the resting $PaCO_2$) returns toward normal after 6 hours of anesthesia, although ventilatory responsiveness to CO_2 is still profoundly depressed (Fig. 21-18).[97] In contrast to halothane, enflurane, and isoflurane, two other potent inhaled agents, cyclopropane and methoxyflurane, produce much more modest depression. Nitrous oxide, a relatively weak inhaled agent, did not depress the ventilatory response to CO_2 at concentrations of 50 percent. Studies by Hornbein et al.[102] showed that combined doses of nitrous oxide and halothane depressed ventilation less than an equipotent (same MAC) dose of halothane alone. It is somewhat surprising that in the only study performed at anesthetic concentrations of nitrous oxide (which took place under hyperbaric conditions), 1.5 MAC concentrations of nitrous oxide proved to be a potent respiratory depressant, lowering the CO_2 response slope to 15 percent of that of the control.[103]

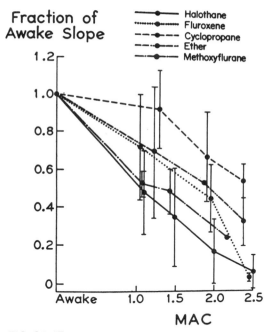

Fraction of Awake Slope

— Halothane
······ Fluroxene
—·— Cyclopropane
—··— Ether
—·— Methoxyflurane

FIG. 21-17 Comparison of mean slopes of ventilatory response to inhaled CO_2 at multiples of MAC in an anesthetized patient. Values on the ordinate are expressed as a fraction of the awake slope. In this study halothane depressed the ventilatory response to CO_2 to the greatest degree and cyclopropane was the least depressant. In all cases, increasing the depth of anesthesia diminished the ventilatory response to inhaled carbon dioxide. (Larson CP, Eger EI II, Muallem M, et al: The effects of diethyl ether and methoxyflurane on ventilation. Anesthesiology 30:174, 1969.)

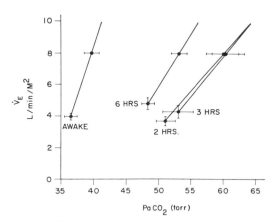

FIG. 21-18 Effects of time on the ventilatory response to inhaled carbon dioxide during constant-depth percent halothane anesthesia. The increase in arterial PCO_2 with induction of anesthesia is diminished by 6 hours, although not to the awake level of alveolar ventilation. No good explanation of this readjustment is available. (Fourcade HE, Larson CP, Hickey RF, et al: Effects of time on ventilation during halothane and cyclopropane anesthesia. Anesthesiology 36:83, 1972.)

Depression of ventilatory responsiveness to inhaled carbon dioxide has great clinical relevance. Accumulation of carbon dioxide and the ensuing arterial and tissue acidosis may cause dysfunction in several organs, including the heart, where this condition may cause potentially dangerous cardiac dysrhythmias. The attenuation of the normal ventilatory responses to elevated $PaCO_2$ (tachypnea, increased tidal volume) makes clinical diagnosis of hypercarbia difficult and necessitates the measurement of either arterial, alveolar, or end-tidal CO_2 tensions. During anesthesia, the ventilatory system will be less likely to compensate for carbon dioxide elevations secondary to rebreathing of carbon dioxide from malfunctioning anesthetic circuits or from increased metabolic production of carbon dioxide.

In their study on the effect of anesthesia on patients with chronic obstructive lung disease, Pietak et al.[93] clearly showed the decreased ability of these patients to respond to increased $PaCO_2$ (Fig. 21-19). This demonstrates the requirement for strict monitoring of arterial blood gases in these patients.

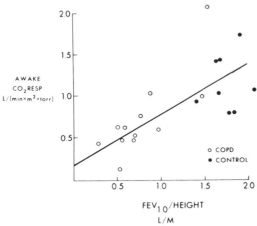

FIG. 21-19 Carbon dioxide response related to $FEV_{1.0}$ in awake patients breathing oxygen. Patients with chronic obstructive pulmonary disease (COPD) exhibit a diminished increase in ventilation to increases in inhaled carbon dioxide. The presence of airway obstruction makes the interpretation of "decreased ventilatory drive" difficult. (Pietak S, Weenig CS, Hickey RF, et al: Anesthetic effects on ventilation in patients with chronic obstructive pulmonary disease. Anesthesiology 42:160, 1975.)

VENTILATORY RESPONSES TO HYPOXEMIA

Increased ventilation in response to progressively lowered $PaCO_2$ is mediated entirely by the peripheral chemoreceptors. The hyperbolic response curve thus obtained rises most sharply at a PaO_2 of approximately 40 mm Hg. Various indices have been used to quantitate this response. Currently popular is the index A, made popular by Weil and his associates.[104] This parameter describes the curvature of the hyperbola; a low value of A is consistent with a flattened or lesser ventilatory response to progressive hypoxemia.

For some time the opinion was held that while the ventilatory responses to hypercarbia and acidosis were profoundly affected by anesthetic agents, the peripheral chemoreceptors were spared and the ventilatory response to hypoxemia preserved. It is now evident from the results of studies performed during the 1970s that this belief is erroneous. Weiskopf and colleagues[105] studied the ventilatory response to hypoxia in three dogs during halothane anesthesia (1.1 percent end-tidal halothane concentration) and at different levels of $PaCO_2$. Significant depression of ventilatory responsiveness to hypoxia was observed at 1 MAC levels of halothane. In addition, the usual synergistic effect of hypoxia and hypercarbia on ventilation was profoundly attenuated. This work has subsequently been confirmed in dogs by Hirshman et al.,[106] who extended the study to demonstrate similar ventilatory depression by both enflurane and isoflurane. Furthermore, a dose-related attentuation of the hypoxic response was demonstrated. In an important study, Knill and Gelb[107] showed a similar response to halothane anesthesia in humans; however, the peripheral chemoreceptor function was even more sensitive to the effects of anesthetic agents than in the dog. At 1.1 MAC halothane, the ventilatory response to hypoxemia was completely absent (Fig. 21-20). Furthermore, at very low anesthetic concentrations (0.1 MAC halothane) ventilatory responsiveness was severely attenuated. At the same "sedative" levels of halothane, no change was seen in the CO_2 response curve (Fig. 21-21). This profound depression of hypoxic respon-

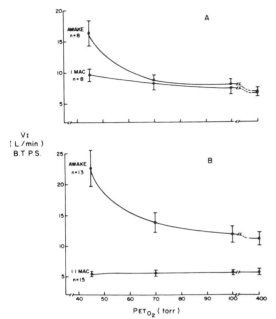

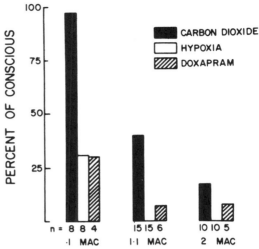

FIG. 21-21 The effect of halothane anesthesia at different doses on three different tests of ventilatory drive in human subjects. The ventilatory drive to hypoxia seems to be depressed at much lower levels of halothane anesthetic than the ventilatory increase to inhaled carbon dioxide. (Knill RL, Gelb AW: Ventilatory responses to hypoxia and hypercapnia during halothane sedation and anesthesia in man. Anesthesiology 49:244, 1978.)

FIG. 21-20 Ventilatory response to hypoxia in human volunteers and patients anesthetized with halothane. (A) The ventilatory increase to hypoxia is severely attenuated at levels of only 0.1 MAC halothane and (B) completely absent in this experiment at the 1.1 MAC halothane anesthesia. This represents a more significant depression of this measure of ventilatory drive during inhalation of anesthetics than that previously demonstrated in dogs. (Knill RL, Gelb AW: Ventilatory responses to hypoxia and hypercapnia during halothane sedation and anesthesia in man. Anesthesiology 49:244, 1978.)

siveness is clinically very important in that it suggests that patients will manifest a diminished ventilatory response to hypoxemia for some time after cessation of an anesthetic and at the arterial concentrations of halothane one would expect in a patient in the recovery room. The implications of this in patients who depend to some degree on a hypoxic drive to set their level of ventilation are obvious. The impaired function of the peripheral chemoreceptor in the presence of low levels of halothane was also demonstrated by a marked reduction in ventilatory responsiveness to doxapram or metabolic acidosis (Fig. 21-21), both of which normally have a significant stimulatory effect on the peripheral chemoreceptor. Enflurane,[108] nitrous oxide[109] and isoflurane[110] have also been shown to depress hypoxic responsiveness in humans at subanesthetic concentrations.

These studies demonstrate that, in contrast to previous beliefs, the peripheral chemoreceptor is remarkably sensitive to the depressant effects of inhaled anesthetics, as well as to many intravenous agents, such as morphine and thiopental. Is hypoxic ventilatory response diminished by depression of chemoreceptor traffic or by the effect of anesthetics on the brainstem? An earlier study[110] suggested the former mechanism. This has been supported by two recent reports. Davies et al.[111] showed that 0.5 to 1.0 percent halothane administered to decerebrate cats reduced nerve discharge in the carotid sinus nerve when the peripheral chemoreceptor was stimulated by a variety of methods. Knill and Clement[112] examined the ventilatory response to subanesthetic concentrations of halothane in normal volunteers breathing an isocapnic hypoxic gas mixture. Ventilatory response to hypoxia was depressed within 30 seconds of inhalation. The authors concluded that the peripheral chemoreceptors had to be the site of depression, since pharmacokinetic calculations appeared to preclude a buildup of halothane in the brain within 30 seconds. These studies seem to indicate anesthetic agents of subanesthetic doses depress the function of the carotid bodies by depressing their chemoreceptor response to stimuli such as hypoxia.

Greater concentrations of anesthetic depress brainstem function as well. It is clear that tachypnea and increased ventilation seen with hypoxia under normal conditions would be absent or severely decreased during even light levels of anesthesia. Lack of these clinical signs mandates the frequent assessment of arterial oxygen tensions. Patients with chronic respiratory failure in whom the level of PaO_2 may represent an important determinant of minute ventilation may be drastically affected by even low doses of inhaled anesthetics. Thus, the ability of these patients to maintain adequate ventilation while breathing spontaneously may be severely impaired.

REFERENCES

1. Paterson JW, Woolcock AJ, Shenfield GM: Bronchodilator drugs. Am Rev Respir Dis 120:1149, 1979
2. Ahlquist RP: A study of the adrenotropic receptors. Am J Physiol 153:586, 1948
3. Shnider WM, Papper EM: Anesthesia for the asthmatic patient. Anesthesiology 22:886, 1961
4. Brown D: Halothane-oxygen anesthesia for bronchoscopy, method suitable for children. Anesthesia 14:135, 1959
5. Colgan FJ: Performance of lungs and bronchi during inhalation anesthesia. Anesthesiology 26:778, 1965
6. Klide AM, Aviado DM: Mechanism for the reduction in pulmonary resistance induced by halothane. J Pharmacol Exp Ther 158:28, 1967
7. Fletcher SW, Flacke W, Alper MH: The actions of general anesthetic agents on tracheal smooth muscle. Anesthesiology 29:517, 1969
8. Hickey RF, Graf PD, Nadel JA, et al: The effects

9. of halothane and cyclopropane on total pulmonary resistance in the dog. Anesthesiology 31:334, 1969
9. Coon RL, Kampine JP: Hypocapnic bronchoconstriction and inhalation anesthetics. Anesthesiology 43:635, 1975
10. Hirshman CA, Bergman NA: Halothane and enflurane protect against bronchospasm in an asthma dog model. Anesth Analg 57:629, 1978
11. Gold WM, Kessler GF, Yu DYC, et al: Pulmonary physiologic abnormalities in experimental asthma in dogs. J Appl Physiol 33:496, 1972
12. Hirshman CA, Edelstein G, Pectz S, et al: Mechanism of action of inhalational anesthesia on airways. Anesthesiology 56:107, 1982
13. Gold MI, Helrich M: Pulmonary mechanics during general anesthesia: V, status asthmaticus. Anesthesiology 32:422, 1970
14. Patterson RW, Sullivan SF, Malm JR, et al: The effect of halothane on human airway mechanics. Anesthesiology 29:900, 1968
15. Meloche R, Norlander O, Norden I, et al: Effects of carbon dioxide and halothane on compliance and pulmonary resistance during cardiopulmonary bypass. Scand J Thorac Cardiovasc Surg 3:69, 1969
16. Brakensiek AL, Bergman JA: The effects of halothane and atropine on total respiratory resistance in anesthetized man. Anesthesiology 33:341, 1970
17. McAslan C, Mima M, Norden I, et al: Effects of halothane and methoxyflurane on pulmonary resistance to gas flow during lung bypass. Scand J Thorac Cardiovasc Surg 5:193, 1971
18. Waltemath CL, Bergman NA: Effects of ketamine and halothane on increased respiratory resistance provoked by ultrasonic aerosols. Anesthesiology 41:473, 1974
19. Sprague DH: Treatment of intraoperative bronchospasm with nebulized isoetharine. Anesthesiology 46:222, 1977
20. Wolfe JD, Tashkin DP, Calvares B, et al: Bronchodilator effects on terbutaline and aminophylline alone and in combination in asthmatic patients. N Engl J Med 298:363, 1978
21. Aviado DM: Regulation of bronchomotor tone during anesthesia. Anesthesiology 42:68, 1975
22. Yang JC, Triner L, Vulliemoz Y, et al: Effects of halothane on the cyclic 3'5'-adenosine monophosphate (cyclic AMP) system in rat uterine muscle. Anesthesiology 38:244, 1973
23. Klide AM, LPenna M, Aviado DM: Stimulation of adrenergic beta receptors by halothane and its antagonism by two new drugs. Anesth Analg 48:58, 1969
24. Sprague DH, Yang JC, Ngai SH: Effects of isoflurane and halothane on contractility and the cy-

clic 3'5'-adenosine monophosphate system in the rat aorta. Anesthesiology 40:162, 1974

25. Hermans JM, Edelstein G, Hanifen JM, et al: Inhalational anesthesia and histamine release during bronchospasm. Anesthesiology 61:69, 1984

26. Korenaga S, Tekeda K, Ho Y: Differential effects of halothane on airway nerves and muscle. Anesthesiology 60:309, 1984

27. Bennett DJ, Torda TA, Horton DA, et al: Severe bronchospasm complicating thoracotomy. Arch Surg 101:555, 1970

28. Bloch EC: Bronchospasm during anesthesia. Br J Anaesth 43:108, 1971

29. Nunn JF: Applied Respiratory Physiology. 2nd edition. Butterworth & Co. Ltd, London, 1977, p 68

30. Price HL, Cooperman LH, Warden JC, et al: Pulmonary hemodynamics during general anesthesia in man. Anesthesiology 30:629, 1969

31. Marshall BE, Cohen PJ, Klingenmaier CH, et al: Some pulmonary and cardiovascular effects of enflurane (Ethrane) anesthesia with varying $PaCO_2$ in man. Br J Anaesth 43:996, 1971

32. Bergofsky EH: Mechanisms underlying vasomotor regulation of regional pulmonary blood flow in normal and disease states. Am J Med 57:378, 1974

33. Barer GR, Howard P, Shaw JW: Stimulus-response curves for the pulmonary vascular bed to hypoxia and hypercapnia. J Physiol 211:139, 1970

34. Marshall BE, Marshal C, Benumof J, et al: Hypoxic pulmonary vasoconstriction in dogs: effect of lung segment size and oxygen tension. J Appl Physiol 51:1543, 1981

35. Benumof JL, Pirho AF, Johansen I, et al: Interaction of $P\bar{v}O_2$ with PaO_2 on hypoxic pulmonary vasoconstriction. J Appl Physiol 51:871, 1981

36. Domino KB, Wetstein L, Glasser SA, et al: Influence of mixed venous oxygen tension ($P\bar{v}O_2$) on blood flow to atelectatic lung. Anesthesiology 59:428, 1983

37. Malik AB, Kidd BSL: Independent effects of changes in H^+ and CO_2 concentrations on hypoxic pulmonary vasoconstriction. J Appl Physiol 34:318, 1973

38. Enson Y, Giuntini C, Lewis ML, et al: The influence of hydrogen ion and hypoxia on the pulmonary circulation. J Clin Invest 43:1146, 1964

39. Haas F, Bergofsky EH: Effect of pulmonary vasoconstriction on balance between alveolar ventilation and perfusion. J Appl Physiol 24:491, 1968

40. Colley PS, Chency FW Jr, Hlastala MP: Ventilation-perfusion and gas exchange effects of sodium nitroprusside in dogs with normal and edematous lungs. Anesthesiology 50:489, 1979

41. Buckley MJ, McLaughlin JS, Fort L III, et al: Effects of anesthetic agents on pulmonary vascular resistance during hypoxia. Surg Forum 15:183, 1964

42. Sykes MK, Davies DM, Chakrabarti MK, et al: The effects of halothane, trichlorethylene and ether on the hypoxic pressor response and pulmonary vascular resistance in the isolated, perfused cat lung. Br J Anaesth 45:655, 1973

43. Loh L, Sykes MK, Chakrabarti MK: The effects of halothane and ether on the pulmonary circulation in the innervated perfused cat lung. Br J Anaesth 49:309, 1977

44. Bjertnaes J, Hauge A, Nakken KF, et al: Hypoxic pulmonary vasoconstriction: inhibition due to anesthesia. Acta Physiol Scand 96:283, 1976

45. Sykes MK, Biggs JM, Loh L, et al: Preservation of the pulmonary vasoconstrictor response to alveolar hypoxia during the administration of halothane to dogs. Br J Anaesth 50:1185, 1978

46. Benumof JL, Wahrenbrock EA: Local effects of anesthetics on regional hypoxic pulmonary vasoconstriction. Anesthesiology 46:111, 1977

47. Mathers J, Benumof JL, Wahrenbrock EA: General anesthetics and regional hypoxic pulmonary vasoconstriction. Anesthesiology 46:111, 1977

48. Sykes MK, Hurtig JB, Tait AR, et al: Reduction of hypoxic pulmonary vasoconstriction during diethyl ether anesthesia in the dog. Br J Anaesth 49:293, 1977

49. Fargas-Babjak A, Forrest JB: Effect of halothane on the pulmonary vascular response to hypoxia in dogs. Can Anesth Soc J 26:6, 1979

50. Marshall C, Lindgren L, Marshall BE: Effects of halothane, enflurane and isoflurane on hypoxic pulmonary vasoconstriction in rat lungs in vitro. Anesthesiology 60:304, 1984

51. Bjertnaes LJ: Hypoxia-induced pulmonary vasoconstriction in man: inhibition due to diethyl ether and halothane anaesthesia. Acta Anaesthesiol Scand 22:570, 1978

52. Benumof JL, Wahrenbrock EA: Local effects of anesthetics on regional hypoxic pulmonary vasoconstriction. Anesthesiology 43:525, 1975

53. Anderson MW, Benumof JL: Intrapulmonary shunting during one lung ventilation and surgical manipulation. Anesthesiology 45:A377, 1981

54. Rees ID, Gaines GY: One lung anesthesia — a comparison of pulmonary gas exchange during anesthesia with ketamine or enflurane. Anesth Analg 63:521, 1984

55. Pirlo AF, Benumont JL, Trousdale FR: Potentiation of lobar hypoxic pulmonary vasoconstriction by intermittent hypoxia in dogs. Anesthesiology 55:226, 1981

56. Marshall BF: Another point of view on intermittent hypoxia. Anesthesiology 55:200, 1981

57. Benumouf JL: Intermittent hypoxia increases lobar hypoxic pulmonary vasoconstriction. Anesthesiology 58:399, 1983

58. Hurtig JB, Tait AR, Sykes MK: Reduction of hypoxic pulmonary vasoconstriction by diethyl ether in the isolated perfused cat lung: the effect of acidosis and alkalosis. Can Anaesth Soc J 24:433, 1977

59. Colley PS, Cheney FW, Hlastala MP: Ventilation-perfusion effects of nitroglycerine. Anesthesiology 51:S372, 1979

60. Delahnuty JE, Cherry J: The laryngeal saccule. J Laryngol Otol 83:803, 1969

61. Leeson TS, Leeson CR: A light and electron microscope study of developing respiratory tissue in the rat. J Anat 98:183, 1964

62. Sleigh MA: Some aspects of the comparative physiology of cilia. Am Rev Respir Dis 93:16, 1966

63. Kinosita H, Murakami A: Control of ciliary motion. Physiol Rev 47:53, 1967

64. Wanner A: Clinical aspects of mucociliary transport. Am Rev Respir Dis 116:73, 1977

65. Reid L: Natural history of mucus in the bronchial tree. Arch Environ Health 10:265, 1965

66. Sackner MA, Rosen MJ, Wanner A: Estimation of tracheal mucous velocity by bronchofiberoscopy. J Appl Physiol 34:495, 1973

67. Gamsu G, Singer MM, Vincent HH, et al: Postoperative impairment of mucous transport in the lung. Am Rev Respir Dis 114:673, 1976

68. Forbes AR: Temperature, humidity and mucous flow in the intubated trachea. Br J Anaesth 46:29, 1974

69. Hirsch JA, Tokayer JL, Robinson MJ, et al: Effects of dry air and subsequent humidification on tracheal mucous velocity in dogs. J Appl Physiol 39:242, 1975

70. Wolfe WG, Ebert PA, Sabiston DC: Effect of high oxygen tension on mucociliary function. Surgery 72:246, 1972

71. Sackner MA, Hirsch J, Epstein S: Effect of cuffed endotracheal tubes on tracheal mucous velocity. Chest 68:774, 1975

72. Forbes AR, Gamsu G: Lung mucociliary clearance after anesthesia with spontaneous and controlled ventilation. Am Rev Respir Dis 120:857, 1979

73. Lichtiger M, Landa JF, Hirsch JA: Velocity of tracheal mucus in anesthetized women undergoing gynecologic surgery. Anesthesiology 42:753, 1975

74. Forbes AR: Halothane depresses mucociliary flow in the trachea. Anesthesiology 45:59, 1976

75. Forbes AR, Horrigan RW: Mucociliary flow in the trachea during anesthesia with enflurane, ether, nitrous oxide, and morphine. Anesthesiology 46:319, 1977

76. Forbes AR, Gamsu G: Mucociliary clearance in the canine lung during and after general anesthesia. Anesthesiology 50:26, 1979

77. Nunn JF, Sturrock JE, Wills EJ, et al: The effect of inhalational anaesthetics on the swimming velocity of *Tetrahymena pyriformis*. J Cell Sci 15:537, 1974

78. Manawadu BR, Mostow SR, LaForce FM: Impairment of tracheal ring ciliary activity by halothane. Anesth Analg 58:500, 1979

79. Iravani J, Melville GN: Mucociliary function of the respiratory tract as influenced by drugs. Respiration 31:350, 1974

80. Tarhan S, Moffitt EA, Sessler AD, et al: Risk of anesthesia and surgery in patients with chronic bronchitis and chronic obstructive pulmonary disease. Surgery 74:720, 1973

81. Berger AJ, Mitchell RA, Severinghaus JW: Regulation of respiration. N Engl J Med 297:92, 138, 194, 1977

82. Hornbein TF, Sorensen SC: The chemical control of ventilation, Physiology and Biophysics. 20th edition. Edited by Ruch TC, Patton HD. Philadelphia, WB Saunders, 1974, pp 803–819

83. Whitelaw WA, Derenne JP, Milic-Emili J: Occlusion pressure as a measure of respiratory center output in conscious man. Respir Physiol 23:181, 1975

84. Dreen JP, Couture J, Iscoe S, et al: Occlusion pressures in man rebreathing CO_2 under methoxyflurane anesthesia. J Appl Physiol 40:805, 1976

85. Larson CP, Eger EI II, Muallem M, et al: The effects of diethyl ether and methoxyflurane on ventilation. Anesthesiology 30:174, 1969

86. Dundee JW, Drips RD: Effects of diethyl ether, trichloroethylene and trifluroethylvinyl ether on respiration. Anesthesiology 18:282, 1957

87. Whittenridge D, Bulbring E: Changes in the activity of pulmonary receptors in anesthesia and their influence on respiratory behavior. J Pharmacol Exp Ther 81:340, 1944

88. Muallem M, Larson CP Jr, Eger EI II: The effects of diethyl ether on $PaCO_2$ in dogs with and without vagal, somatic and sympathetic block. Anesthesiology 30:185, 1969

89. Paskin S, Skovsted P, Smith TC: Failure of the Hering-Breuer reflex to account for tachypnea in anesthetized man: a survey of halothane, fluroxene, methoxyflurane and cyclopropane. Anesthesiology 29:550, 1968

90. Freedman S, Campbell EJM: The ability of normal subjects to tolerate added inspiratory loads. Respir Physiol 10:213, 1970

91. Nunn JF, Ezi-Ashi TI: The respiratory effects of resistance to breathing in anesthetized man. Anesthesiology 22:174, 1961

92. Freund FG, Roos A, Dodd RB: Expiratory activity of the abdominal muscles in man during general anesthesia. J Appl Physiol 19:693, 1964

93. Pietak S, Weenig CS, Hickey RF, et al: Anesthetic effects on ventilation in patients with chronic obstructive pulmonary disease. Anesthesiology 42:160, 1975

94. Pavlin EG: Anesthesia and the control of ventilation, Handbook of Physiology. Bethesda, MD, American Physiologic Society (in press)

95. Caverley RK, Smith NT, Jones CW, et al: Ventilatory and cardiovascular effects of enflurane anesthesia during spontaneous ventilation in man. Anesth Analg 57:610, 1979

96. Eger EI, Dolan WM, Stevens WC, et al: Surgical stimulation antagonizes the respiratory depression produced by Forane. Anesthesiology 36:544, 1972

97. Fourcade HE, Larson CP, Hickey RF, et al: Effects of time on ventilation during halothane and cyclopropane anesthesia, Anesthesiology 36:83, 1972

98. Bainton CR, Mitchell RA: Posthyperventilation apnea in awake man. J Appl Physiol 21:411, 1966

99. Hickey RF, Fourcade HE, Eger EI II, et al: The effects of ether, halothane and Forane on apneic threshold in man. Anesthesiology 35:32, 1971

100. Read DJC: A clinical method for assessing the ventilatory response to carbon dioxide. Aust Ann Med 16:20, 1967

101. Fourcade HE, Stevens WC, Larson CP, et al: The ventilatory effects of Forane, a new inhaled anesthetic. Anesthesiology 35:26, 1971

102. Hornbein TF, Martin WE, Bonica JJ, et al: Nitrous oxide effects on the circulatory and ventilatory responses to halothane. Anesthesiology 31:250, 1969

103. Winter PM, Hornbein TF, Smith G, et al: Hyperbaric nitrous oxide anesthesia in man, Abstracts of Scientific Papers. 1972 ASA Meeting, pp 103–104

104. Weil JV, McCullough RE, Kline JS, et al: Diminished ventilatory response to hypoxia and hypercapnia after morphine. N Engl J Med 292:1103, 1975

105. Weiskopf RB, Raymond LW, Severinghaus JW: Effects of halothane on canine respiratory responses to hypoxia with and without hypercarbia. Anesthesiology 41:350, 1974

106. Hirshman CA, McCullough RE, Cohan PJ, et al: Hypoxic ventilatory drive in dogs during thiopental, ketamine, or pentobarbital anesthesia. Anesthesiology 43:628, 1975

107. Knill RL, Gelb AW: Ventilatory responses to hypoxia and hypercapnia during halothane sedation and anesthesia in man. Can Anaesth Soc J 26:5, 1979

108. Knill RL, Manninen PH, Clement JL: Ventilation and chemoreflexes during enflurane sedation and anaesthesia in man. Can Anaesth Soc J 26:5, 1979

109. Yacoub O, Doell D, Kryger MH, et al: Depression of hypoxic ventilatory response by nitrous oxide. Anesthesiology 45:385, 1976

110. Biscoe TJ, Millar RA: Effects of inhalation anesthetics on carotid body chemoreceptor activity. Br J Anaesth 40:2, 1968

111. Davies RO, Edwards MW Jr, Lahiri S: Halothane depresses the response to carotid body chemoreceptors to hypoxia and hypercapnia in the cat. Anesthesiology 57:153, 1982

112. Knill RL, Clement JL: Site of selective action of halothane on the peripheral chemoreflex pathway in humans. Anesthesiology 61:121, 1984

113. Kaur AE, Mazzic VV, Bergofski CH: Effect of anesthesia and neuromuscular blockers on pulmonary vascular responses to hypoxia and hypercapnia. Anesth Analg 51:402, 1972

114. Sykes MK, Arnot RN, Jastrzbski J, et al: Reduction of hypoxic pulmonary vasoconstriction during trichloroethylene anesthesia. J Appl Physiol 39:103, 1975

115. Tait AR, Chakrabarti MK, Sykes MK: Effect of cyclopropane on pulmonary vascular resistance and hypoxic pulmonary vasoconstriction in the isolated perfused cat lung. Br J Anaesth 50:209, 1978

22

Metabolism and Toxicity of Inhaled Anesthetics

Jeffrey M. Baden, M.B., B.S., F.F.A.R.C.S.
Susan A. Rice, Ph.D.

INTRODUCTION

The inhaled anesthetics were considered for many years to be biochemically inert drugs with therapeutic efficacy. The occasional toxicity following their administration was attributed either to direct effects of the anesthetics on susceptible tissues or organs, or to secondary effects of these agents via unwanted physiological changes. It is now clear that these views are true only in part. The inhaled anesthetics are therapeutically efficacious, but they are also metabolized in vivo. Their metabolites are responsible for the acute and chronic toxicities associated with their use. This chapter presents the current status of information on the metabolism and toxicity of the inhaled anesthetics and discusses their known and presumed associations.

METABOLISM

Early concepts of drug biotransformation assumed that metabolism existed solely for the deactivation or detoxification of drugs. Today the concepts have been expanded to acknowledge that drug metabolism may result in (1) deactivation of pharmacologic or toxic actions, (2) activation to more potent pharmacologic or toxic actions, (3) alteration of the type of pharmacologic or toxic action, or (4) production of equally active pharmacologic or toxic actions. Many factors, such as extent of drug absorption, adsorption, excretion, secretion, and metabolism, affect drug efficacy and toxicity. These factors themselves are affected by the chemical and physical properties of the drug. Because we are concerned with toxicity resulting from anesthetic metabolism to toxic products, the following sections discuss the properties of drugs and cellular membranes that influence drug availability at the cellular sites of metabolism.

PHYSICOCHEMICAL CONSIDERATIONS

PHYSICOCHEMICAL PROPERTIES OF DRUG MOLECULES

Three physicochemical properties primarily determine the distribution of a drug molecule. The drug properties that ultimately determine its availability for metabolism are ionization, lipid solubility, and molecular dimensions.[1]

The degree to which a drug is ionized depends on the pKa of the drug and the pH of the solution in which it is dissolved. Most drugs are weak bases or weak acids and have one or more functional groups that can ionize. The pKa for weak acids is high while that for weak bases is low. The relationship between the degree of ionization, the pKa and the pH of a solution is described by the Henderson-Hasselbalch equation:

$$pH = pKa + \log \frac{[\text{dissociated drug}]}{[\text{undissociated drug}]}$$

The lipid solubility of a drug is determined by the presence or absence of lipophilic (hydrophobic) or nonpolar groups in the molecule. Alkyl groups ($C_nH_{2n+1}-$), such as the methyl group (CH_3-), are nonpolar. The lipophilic property of the molecule increases as the length of the alkyl group increases. For example, the presence of an n-propyl group ($CH_3CH_2CH_2-$) makes the compound more lipophilic than the presence of a methyl group. Lipophilic properties increase any time an alkyl group is inserted in the molecule, whether the substitution occurs on a carbon,

nitrogen, oxygen, or sulfur atom. Substitution of oxygen by sulfur often increases the lipophilic properties of a drug markedly. The lipophilic properties are decreased and the hydrophilic or polar properties are increased when the molecule contains structural elements that allow hydrogen bonding to water (e.g., $-OH$, $-0-$, $-CHO$, $-COOH$, $-COOR$, $-Cl$, and $-Br$). The presence of unsaturated bonds (e.g., $-CH{=}CH-$) further promotes hydropholicity.

Molecular dimensions, size and shape also determine drug distribution. The estimated pore sizes differ for various membranes and, correspondingly, the size molecule that can pass through these membranes. For example, molecules up to about the size of albumin (MW 69,000; major axis 150 Å; minor axis 35 Å) can appear in the glomerular filtrate, but molecules larger than 4 Å radius are excluded from the erythrocyte. All three of the above physicochemical factors influence the distribution of a drug and its ability to penetrate cellular membranes.

PROPERTIES OF CELLULAR MEMBRANES

Membranes are lipoid in nature. They are thought to be a matrix consisting of a phospholipid bilayer and intercalated functional proteins.[2-4] Various cellular and subcellular membranes contain large quantities of phospholipids, cholesterol, and neutral lipids in association with proteins. Membrane phospholipids are amphoteric, that is, they have distinct polar and nonpolar regions. Nonpolar hydrocarbon chains are directed toward the center of the bilayer, while polar head groups remain in contact with the aqueous phase on the bilayer surface. The lipid structure is either completely or partially penetrated by membrane proteins that bind to interior and exterior surfaces of the bilayer. These proteins are necessary both for the maintenance of membrane integrity, and for the specialized transport of endogenous (and structurally similar exogenous) molecules. Thus, these membrane properties, in concert with drug properties, determine the ability of a drug to enter various cells.

Very small molecules and ions (e.g., K^+, Cl^-) apparently diffuse through aqueous membrane channels, while lipid-soluble molecules may diffuse freely through the membrane. Water-soluble molecules and ions of moderate size, including the ionic form of most drugs, can only enter the cell by specialized transport. The overall lipid solubility (i.e., the relative lipophilic and hydrophilic properties) of the drug molecule determines whether the drug will readily cross biologic membranes by a passive process. Membranes are generally permeable to the nonionized forms of lipid-soluble drugs. Ionized groups on the molecule (e.g., $-COO^-$, which is almost completely ionized at pH 7.4) interact strongly with water dipoles and as a result penetrate the lipoidal cell membrane poorly or not at all. For practical purposes, the diffusion rate of a drug parallels the concentration gradient for the nonionized drug form. In general the greater the lipid solubility, the greater the rate at which a drug will move through membranes.[1]

FUNCTION OF THE LIVER IN DRUG METABOLISM

The inhaled anesthetics are primarily metabolized by the liver and, to a lesser extent, by other tissues (e.g., gastrointestinal tract, kidneys, lungs, and skin). The following discussion of anesthetic metabolism is limited to the liver because of its predominant role in metabolism and because the principles of drug metabolism are similar from tissue to tissue.

Hepatic physiology is fully discussed in Chapter 34; however, a brief description is included in this discussion to aid in understanding the relationship between drug metabolism and toxicity. The liver is the largest organ in the body, weighing up to 1,500 g in humans. It is a unique organ in that it has a double blood supply: 70 percent from the portal vein and 30 percent from the hepatic artery. Blood in the portal vein comes from the alimentary canal, pancreas, and spleen. This is important because any toxic material absorbed from the alimen-

tary canal is handled by the liver before it enters the systemic circulation. The hepatic arterial blood supply presumably insures adequate oxygenation of the liver. Portal veins and hepatic arteries are distributed in such a way as to define the periphery of a roughly hexagonal zone of tissue, histologically defined as the hepatic lobule. The lobule comprises two cell types, the Kupffer cell and the liver cell (hepatocyte). The phagocytic Kupffer cell is part of the reticuloendothelial system, while the hepatocyte is primarily concerned with homeostatic synthesis and metabolism. The cuboidal hepatic cells are arranged in one-cell-thick interconnecting sheets separated by sinusoidal capillaries (sinusoids). Blood flows through these sinusoids from the periphery of the lobule, fed by portal veins and hepatic arteries, to the centrally located terminal hepatic venule (central vein). The hepatocyte has several intracellular components intimately involved in intermediary and drug metabolism. The most important is the endoplasmic reticulum. This membraneous matrix of lipoprotein is the major site of protein synthesis, electron transfer, lipid metabolism, and hormone and drug oxidation, reduction, hydroxylation, and conjugation. It is also the main center for the synthesis of cellular structural components for the endoplasmic reticulum as well as the lipid and protein components for other organelles. Microscopically, the endoplasmic reticulum appears as a series of vesicles and tubules suspended within the cytoplasm. Both the parallel arrays of rough membranes and the maze of smooth membranes, rough and smooth endoplasmic reticulum, are part of one interconnected system. This complex is the channel for the passive intracellular transport of proteins (including enzymes), lipids, and other compounds, and for the intracellular storage of some. Under normal (nonenzyme-induced) conditions, the area of rough endoplasmic reticulum is about 25,000 μm^2, while the smooth endoplasmic is about 15,000 to 20,000 μm^2. The rough endoplasmic reticulum is the site of protein synthesis identified by the presence of ribosomes (particles of ribonucleic acid [RNA]) adjacent to the tubular membrane. It is extensively developed in protein-secreting cells. The smooth endoplasmic reticulum contains no granules and is the site of drug metabolism, bilirubin conjugation, and synthesis of steroids and some enzymes. It appears extensively in steroid-secreting cells.

In hepatocytes, both smooth and rough endoplasmic reticulum are involved in drug metabolism. Many in vitro studies of endoplasmic reticulum, its components, and some types of drug metabolism have been performed with microsomes resulting from cell fractionation. Microsomes, as they are referred to in drug metabolism studies,[2] are not naturally occurring organelles but are vesicles which arise from breakage and the reformation of cisternal and tubular systems of the endoplasmic reticulum.[5]

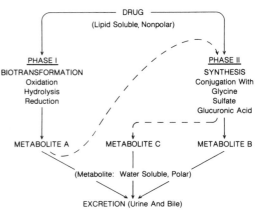

FIG. 22-1 Two phases of drug metabolism—biotransformation and synthesis—generally result in the formation of more water-soluble metabolites that are readily excreted in the urine and bile.

DRUG METABOLISM

Metabolism requires the interaction of drug (substrate) and enzyme. An enzyme-catalyzed chemical reaction proceeds at a rate approximately 10^9 times faster than a noncatalyzed reaction. The enzyme molecule and the drug molecule form a complex resulting from intermolecular forces (e.g., Van der Waals, ionic). The complex reacts and alters the substrate. The complex then decomposes, regenerating the enzyme and liberating a product (metabolite) different from the parent drug.

The major pathways of drug metabolism involve oxidation, reduction, hydrolysis, and conjugation. A drug may be of suitable chemical structure to be simultaneously biotransformed in several metabolic pathways. The enzymes of these metabolic pathways compete for the drug (substrate), and thus the ratio of end products (metabolites) depends on enzymatic reaction rates, drug concentrations near the enzyme, and physicochemical reactions between metabolites and enzymes.

The overall pattern of drug metabolism is common to all animal species; it is biphasic in nature and consists of stepwise biotransformation and synthesis reactions. Figure 22-1 shows

$$\text{enzyme} + \text{drug} \longrightarrow \text{enzyme–drug complex} \longrightarrow \text{enzyme} + \text{product}$$

The metabolism of a drug is important in determining its therapeutic activity and toxicity. Many factors affect drug biotransformation: route of administration, species, strain, sex, age, diet, temperature, season, time of day, chronic drug administration, and previous or concurrent administration of other drugs or chemicals. Unlike most drugs, the inhaled anesthetics are administered in great excess of the amount metabolized. Thus, biotransformation has little affect on pharmacologic activity but plays a significant role in determining anesthetic toxicity.

the general scheme of drug metabolism. Phase I (biotransformation) consists of oxidation (hydroxylation), hydrolysis, or reduction of a lipid-soluble or nonpolar drug. Phase II (synthesis) consists of conjugation of a drug or its metabolite with an endogenous compound (predominantly glycine, sulfate, or glucuronic acid). The net result of either phase of metabolism is the production of compounds that are more easily excreted in the bile or urine. These phases of metabolism are controlled by tissue enzymes present in plasma, cytoplasm, mitochondria, or endoplasmic reticulum. Both the quantitative and qualitative variations in metabolism seen with different species lie mainly in the nature of these enzymes.

Phase I metabolism occurs primarily in the environment of the endoplasmic reticulum, while phase II metabolism occurs generally in the more aqueous environment of the cytoplasm. Usually, but not necessarily, substrates for phase I reactions are not substrates of phase II reactions. A product of phase I metabolism, however, may be a substrate for phase II reactions.

PHASE I REACTIONS

MICROSOMAL DRUG-METABOLIZING ENZYMES

The cytochrome P-450-mediated monooxygenases are a collective example of phase I enzymes. This hydroxylating enzyme is called a mixed-function oxidase or monooxygenase because one of the two atoms of molecular oxygen (O_2) is incorporated into cellular water (H_2O). Reactions of the monooxygenase system have been extensively studied in vitro using microsomes and reconstituted systems. The overall hydroxylation reaction can be represented as follows:

contribute an electron instead of NADPH. The intermediate electron carrier for NADH is microsomal cytochrome b_5.

Figure 22-2 shows the steps in cytochrome P-450-mediated drug hydroxylation. Cytochrome P-450 is shown as Cyt P-450^{III} (the valence state of iron [Fe] in the hemoprotein is indicated), R is the drug (substrate), and RO is the hydroxylated drug metabolite. The flavoprotein NADPH–cytochrome P-450 reductase contains one flavin mononucleotide (FMN) and one flavin adenine dinucleotide (FAD). The first step of the hydroxylation reaction is assumed to be the formation of a ferric (Fe^{3+}) cytochrome P-450–substrate complex (Cyt P-450^{III}-R) by a rapid stoichiometric reaction of substrate with the oxidized hemoprotein. This complex accepts one electron (e^-) from the FADH/FMNH$_2$ complex of NADPH–cytochrome P-450 reductase to form a ferrous (Fe^{2+}) cytochrome P-450–substrate complex (Cyt P-450^{2+}-R) which rapidly combines with O_2 to yield an oxygenated complex. Upon introduction of a second electron from the flavoprotein, or possibly from cytochrome b_5, an activated iron–oxygen complex is formed ($Fe=O^{3+}$). An internal electronic rearrangement occurs, oxygen is added to the drug (RO), the complex decomposes, the hydroxylated product is liberated, and the ferric cytochrome P-450 (Cyt P-450^{3+}) is regenerated.

The cytochrome P-450-dependent mixed-function oxidases, along with other metaboli-

$$RH + NAD(P)H + H^+ + O_2 \longrightarrow ROH + NAD(P)^+ + H_2O$$

RH is the substrate, ROH is the hydroxylated product, and NADPH and NADH are the reduced forms of nicotinamide adenine dinucleotide phosphate (NADP) and nicotinamide adenine dinucleotide (NAD), respectively. The key enzyme components of this membrane-bound multicomponent enzyme system are cytochrome P-450 and the flavoprotein NADPH-cytochrome P-450 reductase. The monooxygenase system requires molecular oxygen (O_2) and NADPH.

The overall flow of electrons proceeds from NADPH to the flavoprotein (NADPH-cytochrome P-450 reductase) to molecular oxygen.[6] Under some circumstances, NADH can

cally linked enzymes, provide an important pathway whereby the cell may metabolize and thus eliminate xenobiotics. These enzyme systems are responsible not only for deactivation of toxic compounds but also for activation of drugs, chemicals, and environmental pollutants to toxic, mutagenic, and carcinogenic forms. These mixed-function oxidases of the endoplasmic membrane are distributed in a specific pattern to allow coordinated and side-directed reactions for the oxidation of a variety of substrates.

Numerous factors, predominantly genetic and environmental (including chemicals and drugs), affect the performance of the endoplas-

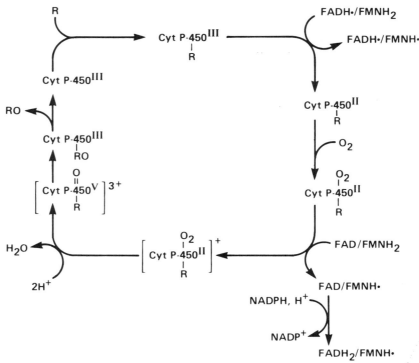

FIG. 22-2 A drug (R), which is a substrate for the hepatic mixed-function oxidase system, interacts with cytochrome P-450 and is biotransformed to a hydroxylated product (RO).

mic reticulum and its drug-metabolizing complex. The phenomena of enzyme induction and inhibition are dependent on the turnover rates, synthesis, and degradation of the various membrane and enzyme system components. Hepatic microsomal membrane proteins are heterogenous in their turnover rates, thus the microsomal membrane is not formed and degraded as a unit but is formed by the random insertion of newly synthetized protein molecules into existing membranes.[7] Various microsomal enzymes are not tightly coupled with one another. The turnover rates of cytochrome P-450 and NADPH–cytochrome P-450 reductase are different from each other, as are the turnover rates of cytochrome b_5 and NADH–cytochrome b_5 reductase.

The human liver contains less cytochrome P-450 than is found in other species (10 to 20 nmoles/g of liver tissue). Rat liver contains approximately 30 to 50 nmoles/g of liver. Likewise human liver is 2 percent of body weight,

and rat liver is approximately 4 percent. These differences in the total amount of cytochrome P-450 seem to account for the fact that humans metabolize drugs in vivo at rates that may be as much as 10 to 20 times slower than do rats.[8,9]

Microsomal cytochrome P-450 is not a single component, but rather a mixture of molecular species having different substrate specificities. Along with species and interindividual differences in the hepatic content of cytochrome P-450, differences in the cytochrome species themselves may be responsible for observed differences among human subjects and laboratory animals in rates and pathways of anesthetic metabolism in vivo and in vitro.[9,10] Experimental studies show that this may be especially true for cytochrome P-450-mediated dehalogenation and dealkylation of the inhaled anesthetics.[11-20] The differences in metabolism between humans and animals must be carefully considered when determining potential toxicity.

REACTIONS RELEVANT TO INHALED ANESTHETIC BIOTRANSFORMATION

Biotransformation reactions classified as oxidations, reductions, and hydrolyses are many and varied. They are carried out by two kinds of enzymes. The first group of enzymes is primarily involved in the metabolism of naturally occurring (endogenous) substrates. These

O-DEALKYLATION

O-Dealkylation is the result of hydroxylation of an alkyl group adjacent to the oxygen of an ether bond. The resulting hemiacetyl is a relatively unstable intermediate that rapidly decomposes to an alcohol and an aldehyde. The rate of the O-dealkylation reaction decreases as the length of the alkyl chain increases.

$$ROCH_2R' \xrightarrow{\text{[O]}} \left[ROCHR' \atop \text{OH} \right] \longrightarrow ROH + R'CHO$$

hemiacetyl

enzymes, however, will also metabolize foreign substrates. The second group of enzymes consists of the so-called drug metabolizing enzymes, including the cytochrome P-450-mediated monooxygenases, which appear to be the primary means for biotransformation of foreign compounds. These enzymes are located mainly in the endoplasmic reticulum of the hepatocyte. The inhaled anesthetics are metabolized by enzymes in this second group, primarily by oxidation reactions. Two types of oxidation—dehalogenation and O-dealkylation—are responsible for the greatest proportion of anesthetic metabolism. One ad-

DEHALOGENATION

Dehalogenation is not the result of a direct attack on the carbon–halogen bond as previously believed. It is the result of oxidation of the halogen-containing carbon, producing a chemically unstable compound that decomposes to a carboxylic acid and thus liberates any halogens. Two halogens on the terminal carbon represent the optimal condition for dehalogenation, while a terminal carbon with three halogens is oxidized to a very limited extent.[25]

$$RCHX_2 \xrightarrow{\text{[O]}} \left[RCHX_2 \atop \text{OH} \right] \longrightarrow RCOOH + 2X^-$$

ditional type of oxidation — epoxidation — is of lesser importance because few anesthetics are biotransformed via this reaction, yet it is important with respect to the toxic potential of epoxides. Only one inhaled anesthetic, halothane, is known to undergo reductive metabolism.[21-24] None is metabolized via hydrolysis because none possesses the necessary ester linkage. Examples of reactions relevant to the inhaled anesthetics are shown below.

EPOXIDATION

An epoxide is formed when oxygen is attached to adjacent unsaturated carbons of an olefin. Most epoxides are highly strained molecules and are extremely reactive because of the ease with which the ring can be opened. Some epoxides may be hydrated by the microsomal enzyme system, epoxide hydrase.[26]

$$R-CH=CH-R' \xrightarrow{\text{[O]}} R-CH-CH-R' \atop O \xrightarrow{\text{[O]}} R-CH-CH-R' \atop OH \quad OH$$

REDUCTION

The mechanisms of reductive reactions catalyzed by the cytochrome P-450 enzyme system are very different from those of oxidative reactions. Because oxygen inhibits the reduction reaction, it is thought that a substrate accepts one or more electrons directly from cytochrome P-450. Reductive metabolism involving cytochrome P-450 has been confirmed for one anesthetic, halothane.[21-24]

tially completely ionized at body pH. Many drugs that do not initially contain one or more of the chemical groups appropriate for conjugation attain one through a phase I reaction (i.e., by oxidation, reduction, or hydrolysis). Trichloroethanol, an end product of trichloroethylene metabolism, is one example of an anesthetic metabolite resulting from multiple consecutive biotransformations.[27-30] Trichloroethanol is detected in the urine both in its unchanged form and as its glucuronic acid conjugate, urochloralic acid.[30-32]

$$CF_3CHBrCl \xrightarrow{e^-} CF_2 = CHCl + F^- + Br^-$$

PHASE II REACTIONS

Phase II reactions are syntheses. They may occur when the drug contains a group suitable for combination with an endogenous compound (i.e., glycine, sulfate, and glucuronic acid). This combination of exogenous and endogenous compounds is referred to as a conjugation reaction. The chemical groups on the drug molecule usually associated with these reactions are —OH, —COOH, —NH$_2$, and —SH. The product is generally a polar, water-soluble metabolite that is readily excreted. A type of conjugation reaction is illustrated below:

ENZYME INDUCTION

Enzyme induction is the result of an increased rate of enzyme synthesis or of a decreased rate of its degradation, thus producing an increased number of molecules for that specific enzyme. The mixed-function oxidase drug-metabolizing enzyme systems are generally inducible.[33] Enzyme inducers are highly lipophilic agents and are generally metabolized by the cytochrome P-450 enzyme system that they induce. Induction is thought to be largely determined by the extent and duration of the interaction of the drug substrate (inducing agent) with the enzyme concerned. The phe-

$$UDPGA + ROH \xrightarrow{\text{glucuronyl transferase}} \text{R-O-glucuronide} + UDP$$

Conjugation of a drug (ROH) containing an appropriate chemical group, in this case an hydroxyl (—OH), to D-glucuronic acid in its "active" form, uridine diphosphate glucuronic acid (UDPGA), is catalyzed by glucuronyl transferase, located in the hepatic rough endoplasmic reticulum. The resulting glucuronide is more water soluble because of the presence of a very polar sugar moiety. The free carboxyl (—COO$^-$) in the molecule further enhances water solubility because its pKa is usually lower than that of the drug parent compound (substrate), and the carboxyl moiety is essen-

nomenon of enzyme induction is not common to all drugs. It appears to be independent of the chemical structure of the drug and unrelated to the nature of its pharmacologic or toxicologic activity.

Proliferation of the smooth endoplasmic reticulum and drug-metabolizing enzymes, as well as increased liver weight follow phenobarbital treatment.[34] NADPH–cytochrome P-450 reductase and cytochrome P-450 are preferentially increased. Available evidence indicates that induction of drug-metabolizing enzymes results from both increased synthesis and decreased degradation of hepatic enzymes in drug-treated animals. Many enzyme inducers enhance the metabolism of other drugs and chemicals as well as their own metabolism. In 1967, Conney[35] reported that more than 200 drugs and chemicals were inducers of the hepatic mixed-function oxidase system in experimental animals. Since that time the nonspecific stimulation of drug-metabolizing enzymes has been reported for numerous additional drugs, including the inhaled anesthetics.[36-38]

Enzyme activity may also be increased without a change in the amount of enzyme present. An example of this phenomenon is substrate induction observed in chronic liver disease. Generally there is a decrease in the total number of liver cells, but the amount of drug presented to any one cell is increased and thus the total amount of drug metabolized per cell is significantly increased. This observation, in part, may explain why fairly severe hepatic damage is measured before there is a noticeable alteration in drug metabolism.[39]

Several chemical and drug classes, including anticonvulsants, steroids, tranquilizers, sedatives, anesthetics, and insecticides, contain one or more compounds considered enzyme inducers. In view of the current practice of polypharmacy, enzyme induction may not be an uncommon phenomenon in patients undergoing surgery. Many case reports of drug toxicity have suggested enzyme induction as a causative factor; however, data are often unconvincing. If a drug is toxic, its enhanced metabolism may decrease toxicity; however, if the metabolite is toxic, increased metabolism may increase toxicity. Enzyme induction per se does not necessarily result in the production of toxic metabolites or in the increased metabolism of all drugs. For example, enflurane metabolism is not significantly increased in vivo following phenobarbital and phenytoin treatment in humans[18] and animals[40,41] or in vitro in animals.[15,35] Likewise, even though several anesthetic metabolites are known to be toxic to humans, studies of enzyme-induced surgical patients failed to show an increased incidence of toxic effects that could be attributed to enzyme induction.[18,43] There is some evidence to suggest enzyme induction following prolonged anesthetic exposure in humans. Duvaldestin et al.[44] demonstrated that salivary antipyrine

clearance was increased by 29 percent in anesthetists exposed to approximately 19 ppm of halothane for 4 hr/week for 2 weeks. An enzyme-inducing agent, regardless of its source, has the potential to modify both the acute and the chronic toxic effects of anesthetics.

ENZYME INHIBITION

Many compounds can inhibit the activity of the drug-metabolizing enzyme system. The consequences of enzyme inhibition for pharmacologic activity and toxicity can be just as great as the effects seen with enzyme induction. Inhibition can result in an increased duration of pharmacologic or toxic effects, an accumulation of toxic compounds not normally achieved, or decreased pharmacologic or toxic effects.

Inhibition can be of several types. One kind most frequently encountered in clinical medicine is competitive inhibition resulting from two drugs competing for the same enzymatic site. Another type of inhibition results from a decrease in the amount of cytochrome P-450 available to metabolize the drug. Two examples are inhibitors of protein synthesis (e.g., cyclohexamide) and chemicals which destroy cytochrome P-450 (e.g., 5.8 mM methoxyflurane, 13.3 mM enflurane, and 18.8 mM halothane in microsomal preparations).[45]

GENETIC-SPECIES VARIATION

Species variations in drug metabolism, both qualitative and quantitative, result from genetic differences. Differences may be observed in the metabolic pathways followed or in the ratios of metabolites formed from the same pathways. Qualitative differences among species generally result from the presence or absence of a specific enzyme in those species. Quantitative differences result from variations in the amount and localization of enzyme, the presence of a natural inhibitor, or the competition of enzymes for substrate.

In humans, genetic factors that are not readily evident under normal circumstances may play a significant role in the expression of a drug's therapeutic activity and toxicity. For example, physiologic disposition of a drug may be unusual because of a structural variation in the serum protein responsible for binding that drug. A seemingly small alteration can affect chemical equilibrium and ultimately biologic activity. Genetic factors appear to be more important than environmental factors (such as diet and pollution exposure) in determining the overall rate of drug metabolism and elimination, although enzyme induction and inhibition may account for some unusual drug responses in humans. Studies of halothane metabolism and elimination in twins have demonstrated far less variation in identical twins than in fraternal twins or in the normal population. This observation was consistent even when environmental factors were quite dissimilar.[46]

METABOLISM OF SPECIFIC ANESTHETIC AGENTS

NONHALOGENATED INHALED ANESTHETICS

DIETHYL ETHER

$$CH_3-CH_2-O-CH_2-CH_3 \xrightarrow{[O]} [?] \longrightarrow$$

$$CH_3-CHO + [?] + CH_3-CH_2OH \longrightarrow CH_3-COOH \longrightarrow CO_2 + ?-glucuronide$$

Early experiments by Haggard[47] could not demonstrate the in vivo biodegradation of diethyl ether. Subsequent studies with the ^{14}C-radiolabeled compound, however, revealed biodegradation to ^{14}CO$_2$ and nonvolatile urinary products.[48] Presumably, the ether linkage is cleaved by enzymes of the hepatic mixed-function oxidase system producing two-carbon products

such as ethanol, acetaldehyde, and acetic acid, which enter into the general metabolic pool, where they are further oxidized to CO_2.[49,50] Diethyl ether has not been studied in vitro, but in vivo metabolism is enhanced following phenobarbital treatment. Chronic exposure of rats to subanesthetic concentrations of diethyl ether results in elevated levels of hepatic microsomal enzymes[38] and increased metabolism of several drugs,[37] including diethyl ether and other inhaled anesthetics.[36]

ETHYLENE

$$H_2C=CH_2 \xrightarrow{[O]} [?] \longrightarrow CO_2 + [?]$$

Although initial experiments showed that ethylene was not metabolized, work by Van Dyke and Chenoweth[51] demonstrated ^{14}CO$_2$ and unidentified labeled nonvolatile urinary products following the administration of ^{14}C-labeled ethylene.

CYCLOPROPANE

Cyclopropane (C_3H_6) is the simplest cyclic compound that produces anesthesia. It is eliminated almost exclusively unchanged by the lungs. There are no data to suggest it is metabolized.

NITROUS OXIDE

$$N_2O \longrightarrow [N_2O^-] \longrightarrow OH + OH^- + N_2$$

Nitrous oxide (N_2O) probably is not metabolized by humans. Hong et al.[52], however, observed the in vitro reductive metabolism of a stable, heavy nitrogen isotope of N_2O to molecular nitrogen (N_2) by intestinal bacteria of rats and humans. Perhaps N_2O reduction occurs via a single electron transfer process that results in the formation of free radicals and N_2. Evidence for N_2O induction of drug metabolism is contradictory. Prolonged exposure to unspecified concentrations of N_2O produces enzyme induction in experimental animals.[53] Rats continuously exposed to 20 percent N_2O for 14 to 35 days exhibited inhibition of hepatic drug metabolism and induction of metabolism in the lung and testis.[54] Still hexobarbital sleeping times were not altered in rats exposed to 50 percent N_2O for 7 hr/day for 1 to 5 days.[37]

HALOGENATED INHALED ANESTHETICS

CHLOROFORM

tion of trichloromethanol, which spontaneously dehydrochlorinates to form phosgene ($COCl_2$).[55] Phosgene, in turn, reacts with water to form Cl^- and CO_2.[55,56] Phosgene can also react with two molecules of glutathione (GSH) to form diglutathionyl dithiocarbonate (GSCOSG).[57] GSCOSG can be rapidly metabolized via γ-glutamyl transpeptidase to N-(2-oxothiazolidine-4-carbonyl)glycine (OTZG), which is hydrolyzed to 2-oxothiazolidine-4-carboxylic acid (OTZ).[57] In two human volunteers, 50 percent of the administered $^{13}CHCl_3$ was recovered as exhaled $^{13}CO_2$.[58] In the conversion of chloroform to CO_2, a reactive intermediate, presumably phosgene, is formed that can attack nucleophilic sites on tissue macromolecules.[58-62] Metabolism and tissue binding are induced by phenobarbital[60] and 2-hexanone[62] and inhibited by disulfiram.[60] Chronic exposure to chloroform results in the enhanced

$$CHCl_3 \xrightarrow{[O]} CCl_3OH \longrightarrow Cl^- + COCl_2 \xrightarrow{HOH} CO_2 + 2Cl^-$$

$$\downarrow 2GSH$$

$$GSCOSG + 2Cl^-$$

$$\downarrow \gamma-\text{glutamyl transpeptidase}$$

$$OTZG$$

$$\downarrow HOH$$

$$OTZ$$

Initial studies by Van Dyke et al.[48] demonstrated the metabolism of $^{36}Cl-$ and $^{14}C-$labeled chloroform to $^{36}Cl^-$ and $^{14}CO_2$. Cytochrome P-450-dependent oxidation of the C-H bond of chloroform results in the forma-

in vivo metabolism of hexobarbital and presumably other anesthetics.[37]

TRICHLOROETHYLENE

$$Cl_2C{=}CHCl \xrightarrow{[O]} [?] \xrightarrow[\text{migration}]{Cl} CCl_3{-}CHO \xrightarrow{NAD} CCl_3{-}COOH$$

$$3Cl^- + CO \longleftarrow CCl_2{-}CHCl \quad \overset{O}{\diagdown\!\diagup} \quad \overset{\downarrow}{NADH}$$

$$CCl_3{-}CH_2OH$$

$$3Cl^- + CHO{-}COOH \quad [?]$$

$$\downarrow UDPG$$

$$CCl_3{-}CH_2{-}O{-}\text{glucuronide}$$

Barrett and Johnson[63] were the first to demonstrate the metabolism of an inhaled anesthetic. These workers isolated and identified trichloroacetic acid as the primary urinary metabolite of trichloroethylene in dogs. A few years later, Powell[31] quantitated the trichloroacetic acid in expired air, blood, and urine and suggested that trichloroethylene is metabolized at some site other than blood. It wasn't until 20 years later

creted unchanged in the urine; trichloroethanol, which is excreted in the urine either unchanged or as urochloralic acid, its glucuronic acid conjugate; and chloral hydrate.[65] The in vitro metabolism of trichloroethylene to chloral hydrate is increased following phenobarbital pretreatment.[64]

FLUROXENE

$$CF_3-CH_2-O-CH=CH_2 \xrightarrow{[O]} CF_3-CH_2OH + CH_2=CHO \longrightarrow [?] \longrightarrow CO_2$$

$$[CF_3-CH_2-O-CHOH-CH_2OH] \quad [CF_3-CHO]$$

$$CO_2 + CF_3-CH_2OH \qquad CF_3-COOH$$

$$\downarrow UDPG$$

$$CF_3-CH_2-O-glucuronide$$

in 1965, that Byington and Leibman[28] and subsequently Leibman and McAllister[64] demonstrated that metabolism occurs primarily by the hepatic mixed-function oxidases. Trichloroethylene was initially believed to be transformed via an epoxide and a rearrangement of chlorine atoms to chloral hydrate.[27] More recent evidence from Miller and Guengerich[30,65] suggested that chlorine migration occurs within the oxygenated trichloroethylene–cytochrome P-450 complex to form chloral hydrate. This metabolite is further transformed by oxidation to trichloroacetic acid via a soluble enzyme (requiring nicotinamide adenine dinucleotide [NAD]) or by reduction to trichloroethanol via alcohol dehydrogenase, requiring the reduced form of NAD (NADH).[28]

In vivo, the major metabolites of trichloroethylene are trichloroacetic acid, which is ex-

In humans, fluroxene is metabolized primarily in the liver to trifluoroacetic acid. Small quantities of trifluoroethanol and carbon dioxide also have been identified.[66] In mouse and dog the trifluoroethanol glucuronide has also been identified.[67] Fluroxene metabolism is increased in rats by pretreatment with the enzyme inducers phenobarbital, 3-methylcholanthrene, and 3,4-benzo[a]pyrene,[68,69] and pregnenolone-16α-carbonitrile.[70] In humans, trifluoroethanol is produced in such small quantities that there appears to be little clinical risk from this metabolite.[66] Chronic exposure to fluroxene, like many other anesthetics, results in decreased hexobarbital sleeping time in rats.[37]

HALOTHANE

$$CF_3-CHClBr \xrightarrow{[O]} [CF_3-COCl] + Br^- \xrightarrow{HOH} CF_3-COOH + Cl^-$$

$$\downarrow e^- \qquad \xrightarrow{[?]} CF_2=CBrCl + F^- \xrightarrow{[GSH?]} CH_2-S-CF_2CHClBr$$

$$[?] \qquad \qquad \qquad \qquad \qquad \qquad CH-NHCOCH_3$$

$$\downarrow \qquad \xrightarrow{e^-} CF_2=CHCl + F^- + Br^- \qquad COOH$$

$$[CF_3-\overset{\cdot}{C}HCl] + Br^- \qquad \downarrow [O]$$

$$\downarrow$$

$$CF_3-CH_2Cl \qquad [?] + F^-$$

Halothane is significantly metabolized.[48,71,72] Its major metabolite in humans and animals is trifluoroacetic acid, which is eliminated in the urine as the sodium salt.[49,71] Other urinary metabolites occurring in small amounts are Cl^-, Br^-, and F^-.[72] Although significant amounts of trifluoroethanol have been identified in urine of experimental animals, neither trifluoroethanol nor its glucuronide conjugates has been found in the urine of humans. Likewise, trifluoroacetaldehyde is a possible metabolite but thus far has not been isolated. Volatile metabolites appear as a result of reductive metabolism requiring cytochrome P-450 in the absence of oxygen.[14,23,24,73] Two reductive metabolites (difluorochloroethylene [CDE] and trifluorochloroethane [CTE]), and a metabolite-decomposition product (difluorobromochloroethylene [DBE]) were first identified by gas chromatography–mass spectrometry in the exhaled gases of patients anesthetized with halo-

matic and may only require reduced heme. In addition, suicidal inactivation of cytochrome P-450 has been demonstrated under hypoxic conditions (below 40 torr of O_2).[74] Presumably, inactivation is the result of cytochrome P-450 covalently binding the reactive intermediate of CTE.

Induction of the hepatic drug-metabolizing enzyme system in experimental animals results in increased halothane metabolism and covalent binding of reactive intermediates to tissue macromolecules following administration of inducing agents such as phenobarbital[21,22,61,74,75] and Aroclor 1254.[76,77] Prolonged exposure to subanesthetic concentrations of halothane results in increased drug metabolism in experimental animals[37,38] and humans.[44]

METHOXYFLURANE

$$CH_3-O-CF_2-CHCl_2 \xrightarrow{[O]} [CH_3-O-CF_2-CCl_2OH]$$

$$\downarrow [O]$$

$$[CH_2OH-O-CF_2-CHCl_2] \qquad\qquad [CH_3-O-CF_2-CClO] + Cl^-$$

$$\downarrow \qquad\qquad\qquad\qquad\qquad \downarrow HOH$$

$$CH_2O + [CF_2OH-CHCl_2] \qquad\qquad CH_3-O-CF_2COOH + Cl^-$$

$$\downarrow$$

$$F^- + [CFO-CHCl_2]$$

$$\downarrow HOH$$

$$F^- + COOH-CHCl_2$$

$$\downarrow [O]$$

$$2Cl^- + COOH-COOH$$

thane.[73] The formation of CDE and the release of F^- in anaerobic microsomal incubations has been proposed to result from a cytochrome P-450-mediated two-electron reduction of halothane while CTE formation and the production of free radicals results from a cytochrome P-450-mediated one-electron reduction.[24] The release of F^- and its metabolites, CDE and BDE, from halothane under anaerobic conditions can be catalyzed by reduced cytochrome P-450, hemoglobin, or hemin.[14] This finding suggests that the reaction is nonenzy-

Metabolism of methoxyflurane has been studied extensively, both in vivo and in vitro. The molecule can be oxygenated either at the methyl carbon or at the dichloromethyl carbon.[78,79] The major metabolites are F^-, dichloroacetic acid, and probably methoxydifluoroacetic acid, although it has not yet been isolated.[53,78,80] It is not known whether this latter metabolite is further metabolized in humans, although it would be expected to decompose in the acid environment of the kidneys and consequently release oxalic acid and additional F⁻. Loew et al.[25] predicted from quantum mechanical calculations that the O-

ENFLURANE

$$CHF_2-O-CF_2-CHClF \xrightarrow{[O]} [CHF_2-O-CF_2-CClFOH]$$

$$\downarrow [O] \qquad\qquad\qquad\qquad \downarrow [O]$$

$$CF_2O + [CF_2OH-CHClF] \qquad CHF_2-O-CF_2-CFO + Cl^-$$

$$\downarrow HOH \qquad \downarrow \qquad\qquad\qquad \downarrow HOH$$

$$CO_2 + 2F^- \quad CFO-CHClF + F^- \qquad CHF_2-O-CF_2-COOH + F^-$$

$$\downarrow HOH$$

$$COOH-CHClF + F^-$$

dealkylation of methoxyflurane occurs more rapidly than its dechlorination. The opposite was proposed by Holaday et al.[78] and has been supported by the experimental evidence of Ivanetich et al.[81] Recent work from Waskell's laboratory[11,73,82] has defined the stoichiometry resulting from the cytochrome P-450-dependent O-demethylation of methoxyflurane. Cytochrome b₅ is necessary as the second electron donor in the oxidative metabolism of methoxyflurane by purified cytochrome P-450.

In addition to cytochrome P-450-dependent metabolism, Warren's laboratory has demonstrated both an enzymatic non-cytochrome P-450 dependent[84,85] and a nonenzymatic[86] defluorination of methyoxyflurane. The enzymatic defluorination is glutathione-dependent with a pH optimum of about 8.5. The nonenzymatic defluorination of methoxyflurane is dependent on both glutathione and coenzyme B₁₂ and shows a pH optimum of 10. The significance of these observations is unknown and is difficult to postulate because of the relatively high pH values at which these reactions occur in vitro. Metabolism of methoxyflurane is increased in vivo and in vitro following treatment with enzyme-inducing drugs such as phenobarbital[87,88] phenytoin,[42] ethanol,[19,20] and isoniazid.[15,16] Its metabolism is subject to inhibition in vivo and in vitro by SKF-525A[81,87,89] and in vitro by metyrapone.[81] Prolonged exposure to methoxyflurane may result in the increased biotransformation of specific drugs by the decreased catabolism of NADPH–cytochrome P-450 reductase.

Enflurane is slowly metabolized by the hepatic mixed-function oxidase system. The low reaction rate has complicated metabolism studies. Biotransformation releases F⁻ presumably by one of the oxidative dehalogenation mechanisms shown above. Initial oxidation may occur at the chlorofluoromethyl carbon or at the difluoromethyl carbon. Loew et al.[25] predicted that enflurane metabolism would occur primarily at the chlorofluoromethyl carbon. Studies of deuterated enflurane-utilizing rat hepatic microsomes,[12] along with the recent isolation of difluoromethoxydifluoroacetic acid in rat liver[13] and in human urine[1,3,90] further support this early prediction. Detection of insignificant amounts of chlorofluoroacetic acid suggest very little metabolism at the difluoromethyl carbon.[13] Treatment with the classic enzyme inducers phenobarbital,[41,42] phenytoin,[42] and ethanol[19,20] only slightly increases enflurane metabolism.

Rice and Talcott[15] and Rice et al.[16] demonstrated significantly enhanced enflurane metabolism following treatment of rats with isoniazid. The reason for the fourfold enhancement of defluorination has not been fully explained. Deuteration studies[12] showed that isoniazid treatment in rats enhances metabolism only at the chlorofluoromethyl carbon. From studies with phenobarbital and two enzyme inhibitors, SKF-525A and metyrapone, Ivanetich et al.[81] suggested that only one form of phenobarbital-induced cytochrome P-450 is involved in in vitro metabolism of enflurane, while two forms are responsible for metabolism of methoxyflurane. This would partly explain the differences observed for the two anesthetics in the degree of in vitro defluorination following phenobarbital pretreatment. A study of surgical patients chronically consuming drugs such as phenobarbital, phenytoin, diazepam, and ethanol prior to anesthesia did not reveal enhanced F^- serum levels compared with untreated patients.[18] A recent study of surgical patients on chronic isoniazid therapy demonstrated significantly elevated serum F^- levels, but not of sufficient duration to induce clinical signs of nephrotoxicity.[17] Similar to methoxyflurane, defluorination of enflurane is decreased following treatment with enzyme

trifluoroacetylacylchloride, expected intermediates between isoflurane and trifluoroacetic acid, may also be produced. Although phenobarbital,[88,93] phenytoin,[42] ethanol,[19] and isoniazid[15,16] pretreatments increase the defluorination of isoflurane, enzyme induction has not produced F^- levels of clinical significance.[91,92] Isoflurane, like many of the ether anesthetics, enhances hexobarbital sleeping time following prolonged exposure of experimental animals to subanesthetic concentrations.[37]

SEVOFLURANE

$$CH_2F-O-CH-(CF_3)_2 \xrightarrow{[O]} CHOH-(CF_3)_2 + CH_2O + F^-$$

$$\downarrow$$

$$CO_2$$

inhibitors SKF-525A[81,87] and metyrapone.[81] Continuous exposure of rats to subanesthetic concentrations of enflurane significantly decreases hexobarbital sleeping time.[37]

ISOFLURANE

$$CHF_2-O-CHCl-CF_3 \xrightarrow{[O]} [CHF_2-O-CClOH-CF_3]$$

$$\downarrow [O]$$

$$CF_2O + [CHClOH-CF_3] \qquad\qquad [CHF_2-O-CO-CF_3] + Cl^-$$

$$\downarrow HOH \qquad\qquad \downarrow$$

$$CO_2 + 2F^- \qquad CHO-CF_3 + Cl^-$$

$$\downarrow$$

$$COOH-CF_3$$

Isoflurane is the most recently introduced and the most slowly metabolized of the fluorinated inhaled anesthetics.[91,92] The limited metabolism of isoflurane is mostly the result of oxidation of the alpha carbon. Similar to enflurane, the difluoromethyl carbon of isoflurane is fairly resistant to oxidation.[13] However, trifluoroacetic acid may be excreted in the urine of rats and humans. Trifluoroacetaldehyde and

The rate of sevoflurane defluorination is approximately the same as that of methoxyflurane.[94,95] The alpha carbon is the site of oxidation of sevoflurane because the trifluoromethyl carbons are unlikely sites for enzymatic attack. Holaday and Smith[96] recovered nonvolatile organic fluoride in the blood and urine of

volunteers anesthetized with sevoflurane. Hexafluoroisopropanol accounted for approximately 80 percent of the organic fluoride. It would not be subject to further degradation, although conjugation would be possible. In vivo, there is far less serum F^- found with sevoflurane than with methoxyflurane.[94,96] In the one study of human volunteers, Holaday and Smith[96] observed that most of the metabolism to F$^-$ occurred during exposure, presumably because of the very low tissue solubility and the stability of the sevoflurane metabolite. In vivo studies have shown increased sevoflurane defluorination in rat hepatic microsomes following phenobarbital treatment.[95] In vitro, sevoflurane defluorination is increased in rat hepatic miscrosomes by pretreatment with phenytoin,[42] isoniazid,[15,16] and ethanol,[20] as well as phenobarbital.[42,94]

TOXICITY

MECHANISMS OF TOXICITY

The expression of drug toxicity is a function of various factors. This section discusses mechanisms of chemical toxicity considered applicable to the inhaled anesthetics. We have focused on mechanisms of tissue injury that are experimentally reproducible and consistent from one individual to another and not on toxic responses that are the result of a rare hereditary trait (i.e., inborn metabolic error). Four general mechanisms of drug toxicity apply to tissue injury associated with the inhaled anesthetics. They are the intracellular accumulation of metabolites in toxic amounts, the formation of haptens that can initiate systemic hypersensitivity or immune responses, the production of reactive intermediates that either adduct (form covalent bonds) to tissue macromolecules or initiate destructive chain reactions, and the physicochemical reaction of nitrous oxide with vitamin B$_{12}$.

Each of the above mechanisms, except for the vitamin B$_{12}$ reaction, is dependent on the metabolism of the parent anesthetic compound. Accumulation of metabolites in toxic quantities may result in the increased production or decreased cellular secretion of either high concentrations of a metabolite with a low toxic potency or low concentrations of a highly toxic metabolite. Other chemicals or patho-

logic states may modify drug metabolism and thereby initiate metabolic accumulation. When the level of drug metabolites surpasses the intracellular "threshold" for toxicity, tissue injury results from the direct or indirect actions of the metabolite. Toxicity may directly result from the inhibition or modification of enzymatic and structural systems necessary for maintaining cellular integrity (e.g., membrane transport systems). Alternatively, toxicity may ensue following initiation of unwanted pharmacologic actions that are indirectly toxic to the "target" cell. An example is the accumulation of a metabolite possessing vasoconstrictive properties; the accumulated metabolite initiates local tissue ischemia and thus promotes cellular necrosis.

Probably the most important drug-mediated toxic mechanism is the production of reactive intermediates during drug metabolism. Intermediates are thought to initiate toxicity in two ways: they can form adducts (covalently bind) with macromolecules[97,98] or initiate aberrant free radical reactions.[99,100] Although few drugs are sufficiently reactive to form covalent bonds with cell constituents, covalent interactions between their reactive metabolites and cell macromolecules (e.g., intracellular proteins, enzymes, nucleic acid) may occur. Bioactivation of chemically nonreactive compounds, such as the inhaled anesthetics,[101] may produce phase I metabolites capable of spontaneously forming covalent complexes with cell organelles and macromolecules.

The binding of a reactive intermediate with tissue protein to produce a hapten–protein conjugate is one example of a potentially toxic covalent interaction. Such a conjugate may in turn induce the synthesis of drug- or metabolite-specific antibodies and initiate hypersensitivity or immune responses.[102] Adduction of other reactive intermediates to tissue macromolecules might produce alterations in the normal cellular operation by affecting organelles such as the endoplasmic reticulum, mitochondria, lysosomes, or the nucleus.[103] Other detrimental effects of covalent binding can result from depletion of endogenous cellular compounds necessary for normal cell function. Intracellular glutathione and other sulfhydryl-containing compounds are necessary for homeostasis. These compounds function as natural cellular antioxidants.[104] When depleted of glutathione, the cell is susceptible to oxidant effects such as those produced by cytochrome P-450-mediated monooxygenases, which continue to function in the absence of intracellular substrates by transferring electrons to cell lipids.[105] Under normal cirumstances, glutathione can terminate destructive chain reactions by forming conjugates with the radicals. In the absence of glutathione, however, destructive reactions continue and cell death can ensue.

Highly reactive metabolic intermediates such as arene oxides (a type of epoxide) may covalently bind to proteins, nucleic acids, and other cellular components.[106] Interaction between arene oxides and cellular components form chemically stable, covalent drug–protein complexes that subsequently may produce pathologic injuries such as hepatic necrosis,[104,107] mutagenesis, teratogenesis, and carcinogenesis.[26,108] Covalent binding of many classes of drug metabolites, in addition to the arene oxidases, has been suggested as responsible for organotropic and developmental carcinogenesis and teratogenesis[109] as well as for drug allergies.[102] Many drugs, such as the inhaled anesthetics, are a possible source of free radical intermediates following their phase I metabolism.

Perhaps the majority of drug effects, both therapeutic and toxic, occur through free radical mechanisms initiated by drug metabolism. Most drugs are chemically stable, but metabolism may produce a single unpaired electron in an outer molecular orbital shell. The resultant chemically reactive compound is known as a free radical. The activity of these short-lived, but highly reactive intermediates is extremely significant because they can initiate chain reactions and produce pathologic damage.[99,110]

Free radical chain reactions consist of three phases. During the initiation phase, free radicals are generated by a single reaction or series of reactions. The propagation phase consists of a sequence of reactions that conserve or increase the numbers of free radicals. The termination phase is the destruction or inactivation of the generated free radicals. Once generated, radicals react with cellular components producing polymerization or cross-linking of enzymes and proteins,[111] autooxidation of

lipids within the organelle membranes,[111] and damage to nucleic acids (e.g., main chain breaks in the nucleic acid strands or degradation of purine and pyrimidine rings).[103] Free radical reactions are generated during the normal course of cell metabolism.[105] Radical levels, however, are controlled in biologic tissues[100] such that they exist only in dilute concentrations (10^{-9} M).[110] It is only when aberrant radical reactions occur and endogenous antioxidants (e.g., glutathione) are depleted that tissue injury results.[99]

Generally, reactions of radical intermediates are assumed to be so rapid that no radicals escape the tissue in which they are formed.[103] Since the inhaled anesthetics are strongly lipophilic, damage from any reactive intermediates can be expected to occur in lipid membranes, which are especially rich in unsaturated fatty acids. These unsaturated compounds are highly susceptible to damage because the presence of a double bond weakens the carbon–hydrogen bond of the α-methylene carbon atom (i.e., the carbon atom adjacent to the carbon with an unsaturated bond). Free radicals initiate peroxidation by abstracting hydrogen from the α-methylene carbon.[100,111] This results in rearrangement of double bonds and subsequent attack by oxygen, causing cleavage of the radical. Unless terminated, the oxidative damage will be transferred to adjacent fatty acids. Several inhaled anesthetics have been implicated in the production of tissue injury via free radical initiated autooxidation of lipids (lipoperoxidation). Halothane and chloroform, at anesthetizing concentrations, stimulate lipoperoxidation in vivo in phenobarbital pretreated rats.[112]

The detrimental effects of covalent interaction on cell integrity may depend on the extent of covalent binding by free radicals and on the cellular functions that are impaired. The precise mechanism by which specific reactive intermediates initiate cellular injury is not clear. For example, although the formation of free radicals and reactive intermediates is consistent with evidence showing that metabolites bind covalently to liver microsomes, there is no strict correlation between adduction and cell damage.[113] Determination of the first cellular function to be impaired is nearly impossible to prove experimentally because adduction in nontarget cells and organs may be stronger than in those suffering injury.

ACUTE TOXICITY

EFFECTS ON THE LIVER

Clinically, drug-mediated hepatotoxicity ranges in severity from a slight increase in serum liver enzymes to jaundice. The cause of this organ-specific injury may be hepatocellular damage resulting from hepatotoxic agents or sensitizing agents, interference with bilirubin metabolism, or cholestasis. Direct hepatocellular injury, the first of three mechanisms, is probably responsible for most cases of inhaled anesthetic-mediated hepatotoxicity. Direct hepatotoxins cause dose-related, consistent, and reproducible hepatic damage in humans and animals. Two examples are carbon tetrachloride and chloroform. Sensitizing agents produce their toxic effects by hypersensitivity and immune reactions.

The extent of hepatotoxicity directly resulting from administration of inhaled anesthetics is difficult to determine. Several factors may predispose the liver to postoperative dysfunction and necrosis: chronic liver disease, viral infection (i.e., viral hepatitis and cytomegalovirus), septicemia, severe burns, pregnancy, nutritional deficiency, and previous or concomitant drug treatment. Many additional factors may be involved; for example, hypoxia, hypercarbia, and hypotension alone may cause liver damage. Strunin[114] suggests that most physiologic alterations caused by hypoxia or hypercarbia result from changes in liver blood flow, rather than from the direct effects of the anesthetics. In addition, most surgical procedures, regardless of anesthetic technique (intravenous as well as inhaled), are probably followed by adverse changes in liver function. Usually these changes are minor and directly related to the surgical procedure.[115]

All anesthetic techniques reduce the liver blood flow to some degree.[116] Although studies in healthy volunteers have demonstrated no evidence of hypoxia or anaerobic metabolism, this may not be the case for patients with preexisting liver damage or other illnesses. In general, surgical manipulation appears to be more relevant in decreasing liver blood flow than are the effects of the anesthetic agents.[117] Unfortunately, tests available to assess liver function are for the most part crude and inaccurate (i.e., not tissue specific) and only reflect abnormalities in the presence of severe disorders. Traditional measures of liver function are serum proteins, enzymes, and bilirubin. A change in serum enzymes may indicate leakage from damaged cells, failure of biliary secretion, or failure of synthesis. None of the enzymes routinely measured is entirely specific to the liver. Isoenzymes (subfractions of measurable enzymes) are occasionally used because they may be characteristic of a particular source, but only the aminotransferases and alkaline phosphatase have stood the test of time. Two aminotransferases (transaminases) routinely measured are aspartate aminotransferase (AST), formerly called glutamate-oxaloacetate transaminase (SGOT) and alanine aminotransferase, serum glutamate-pyruvate transaminase (SGPT). Aspartate aminotransferase is present in large amounts in the heart, liver, kidneys, and skeletal muscles. It is primarily a cytoplasmic enzyme and often is elevated following surgery, during liver damage and with myocardial infarction. Although alanine aminotransferase is present in the liver in quantities less than that of AST, serum increases in this enzyme are considered more specific to the liver, and significant elevations above normal levels are characteristic of hepatocellular damage.

Chloroform was discovered in 1831 and was first used in humans in 1847.[118] The first two cases of jaundice and death were observed in the same year.[119] In 1912 it was suggested by the Committee on Anesthesia of the American Medical Association to cease chloroform use for minor and major operations due to liver and cardiovascular collapse.[120] Nevertheless, chloroform continued to be used until 1957.

Several investigators have observed covalent binding of chloroform or its metabolites to hepatic tissues. Cohen and Hood[59] performed low-temperature whole-body autoradiographic studies of [14]CHCl$_3$ administered to mice by inhalation. Nonvolatile radioactivity (i.e., metabolites) were confined to the liver. Illett et al.[18] measured increased covalent binding of ^{14}C following the administration of [14]CHCl$_3$ to mice pretreated with phenobarbital, an enzyme-inducing agent. When animals were pretreated with piperonyl butoxide, an enzyme-inhibiting agent, decreased covalent binding was measured. The extent of covalent binding closely paralleled the degree of hepatocellular damage. Brown[112] demonstrated lipoperoxidation in rats pretreated with phenobarbital and subsequently treated with cloroform. When chloroform metabolism was inhibited by SKF–525A (2-diethylamino-2,2-diphenylvalerate HCl) or DPPD (N,N'-diphenyl-p-phenylendiamine), lipoperoxidation was decreased. The enhanced covalent binding and lipoperoxidation in enzyme-induced animals presented strong circumstantial evidence for the formation of a reactive chloroform metabolite which would initiate hepatotoxicity. More recent work has shown that chloroform is metabolized to phosgene (COCl$_2$) by hepatic microsomal cytochrome P-450.[55,56] COCl$_2$ probably attacks nucleophilic sites on hepatic macromolecules and produces hepatocellular damage by an unknown mechanism.[56,57]

In 1905, Bevan and Favill[121] concluded that diethyl ether is hepatotoxic on the basis of four isolated case reports. Later reviews of the cases, however, have determined that there was little solid evidence on which to base their conclusions. Studies in experimental animals have shown fatty changes and extensive degeneration in the liver but not to the extent that has been observed with the classic hepatotoxin, chloroform.[122]

To date there are no case reports of hepatic necrosis following nitrous oxide administration when asphyxia has been ruled out as a possible contributing factor.[123] Continuous exposure of rats to 20 percent nitrous oxide for as long as 35 days produced no significant changes in liver serum enzymes or in glutathione content.[54] However, nitrous oxide with intravenous barbiturate administration has resulted in several isolated reports of hepatic necrosis.[124–127] No conclusions regarding the hepatotoxic potential of nitrous oxide can be drawn from the available evidence.

Cyclopropane was considered innocuous to the liver as regards toxicity until the 1964 report of three patients in whom hepatic dysfunction developed following its use with other anesthetics.[128] Since then, there have been various case reports linking cyclopropane to hepatic damage.[125–127] The National Halothane Study reported that massive hepatic necrosis following cyclopropane administration occurred in an incidence of 1.70 in 10,000. However, in 24 of the 25 cases noted, the outcome of hepatic necrosis might have been attributed to the selection of cyclopropane for anesthetizing patients in shock. Cyclopropane might have induced liver injury as a result of splanchnic vasoconstriction produced by the anesthetic in shock patients. No other mechanism of toxicity need be elicited.

Fluroxene was introduced in 1953 and was the first volatile fluorinated anesthetic used in humans.[129] Its hepatotoxic potential was suggested in 1972, when Reynolds et al.[130] reported death following massive hepatic necrosis in a patient treated with phenobarbital and phenytoin and then anesthetized with fluroxene. Further evidence implicating fluroxene in hepatic necrosis was provided by studies of experimental animals. Enzyme-inhibited mice exposed to fluroxene exhibited no toxicity,[131] while enzyme-induced cats died of massive hepatic necrosis[132] following fluroxene administration. Necrosis after enzyme induction was presumed due to the formation of free radicals or epoxidation of the vinyl radical. Postanesthetic deaths in dogs, cats, and rabbits after long and repeated exposure to trifluoroethanol suggested that this compound or its glucuronide was responsible for liver damage.[133] Recent work with various enzyme-inducing agents in rats has conclusively shown that the rate of hepatic cytochrome P-450-dependent metabolism to trifluoroethanol determines the severity of hepatic damage.[70] Fluroxene has now been withdrawn from clinical use.

Halothane was prepared by Suckling in 1952[134] and was introduced into clinical practice in 1956.[135,136] Several clinical reports of postoperative jaundice and liver necrosis were published in 1963.[137–139] The clinical and pathologic findings resembled those classically ascribed to the hepatotoxin, chloroform. These reports prompted a number of retrospective studies that in essence concluded that there was no evidence of an increased incidence in postoperative clinical hepatic damage as compared with other anesthetics. Because some fault could be found in all the retrospective reports (i.e., lack of proper control groups or inadequate numbers), the U.S. National Halothane Study was undertaken.[140,141] The incidence of fatal massive hepatic necrosis occurring in approximately 850,000 surgical patients was reviewed retrospectively. The committee concluded that "unexplained fever and jaundice in a specific patient following halothane might reasonably be considered a contraindication to subsequent use." However, Dykes and Bunker[142] observed that "there was not a single patient in the National Halothane Study who was jaundiced after administration of halothane, and died after a second administration, and who was found at necropsy to have suffered massive or intermediate hepatic necrosis." The incidence of massive hepatic necrosis associated with halothane was 7 out of 250,000 halothane anesthetics or about 1 in 35,000, and not 1 in 10,000 as is sometimes reported.

In 1972 Strunin and Simpson[143] reviewed various reports and concluded that the data could be arranged to support or deny almost any hypothesis linking halothane anesthesia to liver damage. Much of the pre-1970s data supporting the hypothesis of liver damage due to halothane has not withstood critical examination. In rare circumstances, liver damage is associated with halothane anesthesia, often following its repeated administration.[144-147] Although halothane may be responsible for liver damage in rare circumstances, the incidence, etiology, and interaction with other factors remain obscure. Death from acute liver failure has not been reported following environmental exposure.

Determination of the precise mechanism of halothane-mediated hepatotoxicity has been severely hampered because investigators were initially unable to produce hepatoxicity in halothane-exposed experimental animals. Unlike chloroform and fluroxene, which produce fatty infiltration, centrilobular necrosis, and elevated transaminase values in experi-

mental animals, halothane did not produce hepatotoxicity in early animal studies. Even prolonged exposure of animals to halothane with or without phenobarbital pretreatment did not consistently result in hepatic lesions. Several animal models, most of which rely on increased halothane metabolism for the production of hepatic injury, have since been developed to define halothane mediated hepatoxicity. Enhanced biotransformation in humans has not been implicated in the pathogenesis of halothane hepatitis. Because jaundice does not develop immediately in patients, but develops within 1 to 16 days following anesthesia with halothane, it is difficult to determine the role of biotransformation in hepatic injury. Multiple halothane exposures are more likely to be associated with mild and severe hepatic damage. Repeated exposures, especially at short intervals, are assumed to increase risk. An immune response has been proposed to explain the increased frequency and the overall reduced latency for manifestation of hepatitis following repeated halothane exposure. The sera from 7 of 11 patients with fulminant hepatic necrosis following halothane exposure contained an antibody that reacted with the surface of hepatocytes isolated from halothane-exposed rabbits.[148] The antibody, however, was not present in the sera from the patients with mild liver dysfunction following halothane administration.[148,149] It is unclear whether this antibody initiates hepatocellular damage or is present as a result of the damage. Perhaps the covalent binding of halothane metabolites to hepatic macromolecules produces compounds suitable for inducing antibody formation. If so, the immune response occurs secondary to the hepatocellular insult and exacerbates hepatic injury.

Centrilobular necrosis following halothane exposure occurs in rats pretreated with Aroclor 1254 (polychlorinated biphenyls),[66,67] isoniazid,[150] triiodothyronine,[151,152] and phenobarbital under hypoxic conditions.[138-140] The Arocolor 1254 model has been abandoned because polychlorinated biphenyls themselves cause moderate alterations in liver ultrastructure and function. In another model, the "halothane hypoxic model," hepatic necrosis is produced in phenobarbital-pretreated rats exposed to halothane under hypoxic conditions

($FIO_2 = 7$ to 14 percent).[153-155] This "hypoxic model" is based on observation of the reductive metabolism of halothane under hypoxic conditions and the increased covalent binding of reductive metabolites in vitro to liver protein and phospholipids.[21,22] The hepatic lesion in this model is centrilobular in origin and similar to that seen in humans. This centrilobular area has the lowest oxygen concentration and the highest metabolic rate and is thus most susceptible to hypoxic injury. Lesion intensity is dependent both on the degree of enzyme induction (the amounts of reactive intermediate formed) and on the degree of hypoxia (the production of reductive metabolites). Although this model is reproducible and well defined, its clinical applicability is questionable because of the necessity of hypoxia for lesion production. The mechanism of halothane-induced hepatotoxicity remains obscure, although presumably it involves a one-electron reduction of halothane cytochrome P-450, producing Br^- and a reactive intermediate (free radical) that subsequently causes direct hepatocellular damage. Recent reports have implicated hypoxia per se in the production of hepatic necrosis.[156,161] Thus, it is difficult to resolve whether the reductive cleavage of halothane and the resultant generation of a reactive intermediate[158] or the additive effects of hypoxia[160,161] and a halothane-induced decrease in liver perfusion[159] are responsible for the hepatic necrosis observed in the halothane-hypoxic rat model.

Perhaps neither of these mechanisms is responsible for the fulminant hepatic necrosis seen in humans. Two additional rat models of hepatotoxicity further confuse the issue. The isoniazid[150] and the triiothyronine[151,152] models both produce hepatic necrosis following exposure to halothane under normoxic conditions. Neither pretreatment with isoniazid nor with triiothyronine alone produces alterations in hepatic morphology or function. These observations suggest that newer models produce hepatotoxicity by a mechanism other than the reduction of halothane.

Methoxyflurane was first synthesized in the United States in 1958 and introduced clinically in 1960.[162] Although none of the metabolites of methoxyflurane is known to be hepatotoxic, there have been a number of reports of hepatic dysfunction and death from hepatic coma following methoxyflurane exposure. A review of 24 cases of methoxyflurane associated hepatitis by Joshi and Conn[163] presented evidence for a syndrome similar to that described in 1976 by Walton et al.[147] for unexplained hepatitis following halothane administration. These workers concluded that a rare and indirect immunologic hepatic injury may occur that may have a direct effect on the liver by interfering with splanchnic circulation.[114,116,164] In humans, the adverse minor changes in liver function,[165] as well as the changes seen in isolated liver preparations,[114] appear to be reversible and may be dose related. It is still unclear whether hepatic dysfunction, as measured by bromsulfalein (BSP) retention and hepatic enzyme elevation, was the result of the depth and duration of the anesthetic exposure, the type of operation, the extent of preexisting hepatic disease, or methoxyflurane itself.

Enflurane was first used in North America in 1966.[166,167] Of the approximately 45 million enflurane anesthetics administered since that time, few isolated case reports of liver damage have been associated with its use.[168-171] Recently, Lewis et al.[172] reported 24 cases of suspected enflurane-induced hepatoxicity. Seven of the cases had been previously published. The validity of their conclusions has been questioned because critical gaps in the individual case reports raise doubts of the accuracy of the information presented. Data on the duration of anesthetic exposure and the histologic confirmation of hepatic lesions were not presented for many subjects. Thus, the accuracy of other information (i.e., previous exposure to viral hepatitis or potential hepatotoxins) is in doubt. In addition, several patients were hypotensive and in shock and underwent operations with known potential for hepatic dysfunction. Evidence from rat models of both enflurane and isoflurane hepatotoxicity suggests that liver dysfunction occurs only under conditions of severe hypoxia ($FIO_2 = 7$ to 10 percent).[141,142] These observations may solely be the result of hypoxic injury.[160]

Sevoflurane is an experimental drug that was withdrawn from clinical testing in 1980. There have been several reports regarding its metabolism[94-96] and renal toxicity,[94,95] but only one animal study of hepatic function.[96] One study of five human volunteers showed no significant changes in transaminases and hepatic function measured up to 4 weeks after exposure.[96] The one animal study in untreated, phenobarbital-treated, and Aroclor 1254-treated rats likewise showed no significant changes in serum transaminases, liver triglycerides, or glutathione levels.[173]

EFFECTS ON THE KIDNEY

Inhaled anesthetics depress renal function during their administration. They decrease urine flow, glomerular filtration rate, renal blood flow, and electrolyte excretion. These changes are usually secondary to effects on the cardiovascular, sympathetic, and endocrine systems and almost always return rapidly to normal after anesthesia and surgery have terminated. If they persist into the postoperative period, the cause is often a combination of factors such as prior existence of renal or cardiovascular disease, severe fluid and electrolyte imbalance, and the administration of mismatched blood; the choice of anesthetic is usually unimportant. Occasionally, however, fluorinated anesthetics, most noticeably methoxyflurane, may cause renal damage directly by releasing large amounts of inorganic fluoride (F^-) and possibly other nephrotoxic metabolites.

METHOXYFLURANE

In 1966, vasopressin-resistant polyuric renal insufficiency was first reported in 13 of 41 patients receiving methoxyflurane anesthesia for abdominal surgery.[174] Subsequently, the causative agent was shown to be F^-, an end product of the biotransformation of methoxyflurane. The evidence is based on three observations. First, serum F^- levels following methoxyflurane administration in humans show positive correlation with the degree of renal dysfunction.[175] Second, F^- is a potent inhibitor of many enzyme systems including that

thought to be involved in antidiuretic hormone.[176] Finally, vasopressin-resistant polyuric renal insufficiency similar to that seen in humans and rats after prolonged methoxyflurane anesthesia can be easily elicited in Fischer 344 rats injected with sodium fluoride.[177] Oxalic acid, another methoxyflurane metabolic end product, is usually associated with classic anuric renal failure and not with the type of lesion seen acutely following methoxyflurane anesthesia.[178] It is still possible, however, that oxalic acid contributes to the chronic lesion occasionally seen after methoxyflurane administration.

Fischer 344 rats provide a good animal model for methoxyflurane nephrotoxicity because they demonstrate renal changes following methoxyflurane administration similar to those seen in humans. These changes include polyuria, hypernatremia, serum hyperosmolality, increased blood urea nitrogen (BUN) and creatinine (Cr), and decreased BUN and Cr clearances. Furthermore, in this species as in humans, the serum F^- threshold for renal dysfunction is about the same.

The extent of nephrotoxicity in general surgical patients has been correlated with methoxyflurane dosage (in MAC-hours, i.e., the product of end-tidal concentration as a fraction of MAC and duration of anesthesia, in hours) and peak serum F^- levels.[179] The threshold of renal dysfunction occurs at dosages of about 2.5 to 3.0 MAC-hours methoxyflurane, which corresponds to peak serum F^- levels of 50 to 80 μM. Such patients have subclinical toxicity characterized by a delayed return to maximum preoperative urinary osmolality, elevated serum urate concentration, and decreased urate clearance. Had a vasopressin resistance test been performed on the patients, the threshold dosage and F^- values for subclinical toxicity undoubtedly would have been found to be lower. After 5 MAC-hours methoxyflurane, serum F^- levels are 90 to 120 μM, and patients have well established but mild nephrotoxicity manifested by serum hyperosmolality, hypernatremia, polyuria, and urinary hypoosmolality. Seven to 9 MAC-hours methoxyflurane leads to serum F^- levels up to 175 μM and marked nephrotoxicity.

Despite the overall correlation between nephrotoxicity and peak serum F^- levels, individual patients given the same methoxyflurane dosage vary in their nephrotoxic susceptibility. Genetic heterogeneity, drug interaction, pre-existence of renal disease, and a host of other factors could account for the differences observed among patients. One example of a drug interaction is the additive nephrotoxic effect seen in a patient receiving both methoxyflurane and the aminoglycoside antibiotic, gentamicin.[180] The same effect is seen in Fischer 344 rats in which concurrent administration of methoxyflurane and gentamicin produces greater nephrotoxicity than expected from either drug alone.[181]

Methoxyflurane is a potent anesthetic and an excellent analgesic, and thus, some anesthetists still consider it a desirable drug. Its nephrotoxic potential, however, has severely limited its clinical usefulness. In an attempt to reduce the biotransformation of methoxyflurane and the resultant production of F⁻, deuterium (D) was substituted for hydrogen in the methoxyflurane molecule. The rationale for this substitution was that the C-D bond is less chemically reactive than the C-H bond. Thus, metabolism would be slowed when cleavage of the C-H bond is the rate limiting step in a reaction. Data from both in vitro and in vivo studies indicate that when all four hydrogens are replaced by deuterium, there is a significant but small decrease in F⁻ production.[182-184] Furthermore, unlike ordinary methoxyflurane, the metabolism of completely deuterated methoxyflurane is not enhanced following enzyme induction with phenobarbital.[184] Unfortunately, the overall reduction in F⁻ production and the possible benefit to enzyme-induced patients are not sufficient to offer a significant clinical advantage.

Since it is difficult to regulate the precise alveolar concentration of methoxyflurane and thus remain below a nephrotoxic dose, Mazze[185] suggested that the practicing anesthetist limit anesthetic duration. Two hours at a gradually decreasing inspired methoxyflurane concentration would appear to be safe for most patients. However, in patients on enzyme-inducing drugs the period of exposure to methoxyflurane should probably be reduced; in patients with preexisting renal impairment, methoxyflurane should be completely avoided. These recommendations are now

somewhat moot, as methoxyflurane is seldom, if ever, used in clinical practice.

OTHER FLUORINATED ANESTHETICS

Because modern volatile inhaled anesthetics are fluorinated to reduce their flammability, they all theoretically possess nephrotoxic potential. Of the fluorinated anesthetics, halothane, enflurane, and isoflurane are in widespread clinical use, whereas sevoflurane is in the developmental stage.

Halothane is not significantly defluorinated under normal clinical conditions and thus is not nephrotoxic.[179] Defluorination occurs in phenobarbital or Aroclor 1254-pretreated rats under hypoxic conditions, but not to an extent associated with renal damage.[22] On the other hand, although defluorination for enflurane is much less than for methoxyflurane, evidence indicates that serum F⁻ levels may occasionally be high enough to produce mild renal impairment. In a study with Fischer 344 rats, 6 to 10 hours of 2.5 percent enflurane anesthesia produced mild vasopressin-resistant polyuric renal dysfunction.[40] Peak serum F⁻ levels were 40 to 57 μM, just reaching the threshold for renal toxicity; there was no increase in urinary oxalate excretion.

Surgical patients almost never show renal dysfunction following enflurane anesthesia.[186] Although serum F⁻ levels postanesthesia are significantly higher than background levels, they seldom reach the threshold for nephrotoxicity. In comparison with methoxyflurane, serum F⁻ levels following enflurane anesthesia peak earlier and fall more rapidly, emphasizing the important role that lipid solubility has in determining total F⁻ production (Fig. 22-3). In one study, peak serum F⁻ concentrations from nine surgical patients averaged 22.2 μM following enflurane exposures averaging 2.7 MAC-hours.[186] The only controlled human study to show mild renal dysfunction following enflurane anesthesia involved 11 healthy volunteers.[187] After 9.6 MAC-hours of enflurane, maximum urinary osmolality following ADH administration was reduced from approximately 1,050 to 800 mOsm/kg; mean serum F⁻

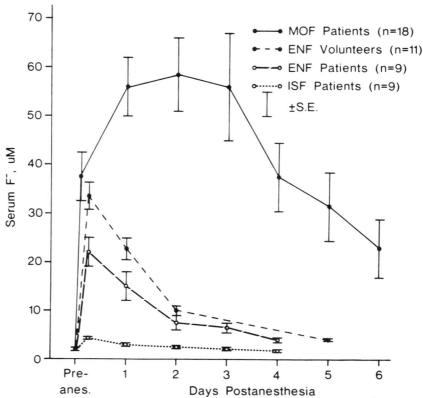

FIG. 22-3 Serum inorganic fluoride (F⁻) concentrations before and after administration of enflurane, isoflurane, and methoxyflurane anesthesia. A significant increase in F⁻ concentrations occurred immediately following enflurane anesthesia, reaching a mean peak value of $22.2 \pm 2.8\,\mu M$ 4 hours after termination of anesthesia; mean duration of anesthesia was 2.7 ± 0.3 MAC-hours.[186] F⁻ levels in volunteers receiving enflurane anesthesia peaked at 33.6 ± 2.8 μM; mean duration of exposure was 9.6 ± 0.1 MAC-hours.[187] Following 2 to 3 MAC hours of methoxyflurane,[179] mean peak serum F⁻ concentration was higher, $61 \pm 8\,\mu M$, and declined more slowly than after enflurane. There was almost no increase in F⁻ following isoflurane administration.[91] (Modified from Cousins MJ, Greenstein LR, Hitt BA, et al: Metabolism and renal effects of enflurane in man. Anesthesiology 44:44, 1976.)

concentration was 33.6 μM. The mild impairment of renal concentrating ability, however, was not associated with hypernatremia, serum hyperosmolality or increased serum creatinine or urea nitrogen and therefore was not regarded as clinically significant.

Although enflurane appears to be safe under most clinical circumstances, it does have some potential for causing renal dysfunction. It has therefore been speculated that enflurane administered to patients with significant preexisting renal disease could produce additional renal dysfunction. Such fears have not been borne out in studies of Fischer 344 rats with surgically induced chronic renal insufficiency.[188,189] Furthermore, results of a recent study of patients with mild to moderate renal insufficiency showed no clinically significant difference between pre- and postoperative renal function following either enflurane or halothane administration.[190] Whether there are any circumstances in which enflurane may cause a clinically significant deterioration in renal function, remains to be seen.

Isoflurane, an isomer of enflurane, is defluorinated much less than enflurane. In nine surgical patients, mean peak serum F⁻ concentration measured 6 hours after anesthesia was only 4.4 μM.[93] Thus, isoflurane is not associated with F⁻ nephrotoxicity.

Sevoflurane is a new fluorinated ether anesthetic with a low blood–gas partition coefficient of approximately 0.6. Results of in vitro studies indicate that it is defluorinated more than enflurane but less than methoxyflurane. In a study of six healthy volunteers, serum F^- levels averaged 22 μM by the end of a 1 hour exposure to 3 percent sevoflurane and had fallen to low levels by 24 hours after anesthesia.[96] Peak serum F^- levels, however, were not measured and anesthesia for longer than 1 hour was not performed. Thus, the clinical safety of this drug has yet to be established in more extensive human studies.

ROLE OF ENZYME INDUCTION IN ANESTHETIC NEPHROTOXICITY

Because the volatile inhaled anesthetics are defluorinated by the mixed-function oxidase system (cytochrome P-450), drugs that induce the enzymes of this system may lead to increased F^- production and nephrotoxicity. This effect has been clearly demonstrated with methoxyflurane; both Fischer 344 rats[191] and human volunteers[179] pretreated with the classic enzyme inducers, phenobarbital or pentobarbital, show increased defluorination and nephrotoxicity. Another enzyme inducer, phenytoin, also increases methoxyflurane defluorination in rats.[42]

The effects of phenobarbital and phenytoin on metabolism of other fluorinated anesthetics are less certain. Phenobarbital pretreatment increases in vitro defluorination of sevoflurane[95] while only slightly increasing that of isoflurane.[41] Enflurane defluorination is not significantly increased.[41] The result with enflurane is surprising, but consistent with data obtained from a human study.[18] A series of 102 surgical patients were divided into the following four groups according to their drug intake histories: control (on no drug), 26 patients; chronic ethanol, 31 patients; chronic phenobarbital and/or phenytoin, 12 patients; and miscellaneous drugs, 33 patients. Regression lines of average peak serum F^- levels on enflurane dosage were not significantly different among the groups. Thus, in this study, prior treatment of surgical patients with enzyme inducing drugs did not increase serum F^- levels following enflurane anesthesia. Presumably, there is little or no increase in the rate of enflurane metabolism in vivo. In contrast with phenobarbital- and phenytoin-pretreated patients, several isoniazid-pretreated patients had high serum F^- levels and a transient urinary concentrating defect following enflurane anesthesia. Work with Fischer 344 rats has confirmed that unlike phenobarbital and phenytoin, isoniazid significantly increases enflurane defluorination.[16] In addition, a study of surgical patients has shown that approximately one-half those chronically treated with isoniazid prior to enflurane anesthesia had significantly higher serum F^- levels than predicted[17] but not high enough to produce clinically significant renal impairment.

EFFECTS ON THE GONADS

Concern that inhaled anesthetics or their metabolites may cause damage to germ cells has led to a number of studies. In one of the earliest, male LEW/Mai rats were exposed to 20 percent nitrous oxide either continuously or for 8 hr/day for up to 35 days.[192] After only 2 days, minor damage to seminiferous tubules was noted, and after longer periods atrophy of the seminiferous tubules, decreased sperm count, and decreased testicular weight were seen. In another study, effects on spermatogonial cells of chronic exposure to a low-dose N_2O/halothane mixture were assessed.[193] Exposure was either to air, 50 ppm N_2O/1 ppm halothane or 500 ppm N_2O/10 ppm halothane and was for 7 hr/day, 5 days/week for 52 weeks. The investigators reported that this chronic exposure to low-dose N_2O/halothane resulted in dose-dependent chromosomal damage in spermatogonial cells. In a study that examined mouse sperm morphology following exposure to anesthetics during early spermatogenesis, chloroform (0.08 percent and 0.04 percent), trichloroethylene (0.2 percent), and enflurane (1.2 percent) all slightly but significantly increased the number of sperm abnormalities above normal; other inhaled anesthetics studied gave negative results.[194]

In contrast to these positive studies, two studies have given negative results. In the first, Swiss/ICR mice were exposed to 0.3 percent enflurane, 4 hr/day, 5 days/week for 52 weeks; no increase in the rate of abnormal sperm or chromosomal aberrations in spermatogonal cells was observed.[195] In the second study, male and female Swiss Webster mice were exposed to a maximum of 50 percent nitrous oxide for 4 hr/day, 5 days/week for 14 weeks; no change in the percentage of abnormal sperm or the number of oocytes was seen as compared with control mice exposed only to air.[196]

In the only study in humans, semen was collected from 46 anesthesiologists who had worked for a minimum of 1 year in a scavenged

in 1956 in six patients with tetanus who received 50 percent nitrous oxide over several days for sedation.[198] Their bone marrow became hypoplastic and grossly megaloblastic; one patient developed fatal marrow failure. Subsequently, many patients have been shown to have megaloblastic hemopoiesis following surgery and postoperative sedation with nitrous oxide.[199,200] The biochemical consequences of vitamin B_{12} inactivation by nitrous oxide are reasonably well understood. In experimental animals, the activity of methionine synthetase, which has vitamin B_{12} as a coenzyme, is progressively decreased by 50 percent nitrous oxide and is virtually zero after 6 hours.[201] Methionine synthetase is involved in the following reaction:

$$\text{Homocysteine} + \text{methyltetrahydrofolate} \xrightarrow[\text{synthetase}]{\text{methionine}} \text{methionine} + \text{tetrahydrofolate}$$

operating suite.[197] Semen from 26 residents beginning an anesthesia training program were used as controls. The concentration of sperm and the percentage of abnormally shaped sperm in semen of working anesthesiologists were not different from those of beginning residents. Furthermore, after collecting a second sample of semen from 13 of the 26 residents after they had been working for 1 year and comparing them with the first sample, no significant differences in the sperm were found.

Thus, despite some suggestive animal data, inhaled anesthetics do not have any significant effect on germ cells in humans. However, until studies are performed on patients exposed to high concentrations of anesthetics or on personnel working in unscavenged operating suites, damage to germ cells of man cannot be discounted entirely.

HEMATOPOIETIC SYSTEM

Nitrous oxide irreversibly oxidizes vitamin B_{12}, rendering it inactive in certain biochemical reactions. In humans, megaloblastic anemia may follow. This was first recognized

Recovery of methionine synthetase activity after withdrawal of nitrous oxide is slow, often taking 4 days or more.

A manifestation of chronic exposure to nitrous oxide in humans is a neuropathy similar if not identical to subacute combined degeneration of the spinal cord seen in patients with pernicious anemia. Most likely, this is due to chronic methionine deficiency, because in experimental animals the neuropathy can be alleviated by supplementing the animal's diet with methionine.[202,203]

CHRONIC TOXICITY

From the time that chloroform hepatotoxicity was first recognized more than 100 years ago, great emphasis has been placed on anesthetic-induced acute organ toxicity. In recent years, proof that methoxyflurane can cause nephrotoxicity and suspicion that halothane may produce hepatotoxicity have enhanced interest in this topic. Historically, however, little thought has been given to possible long-term adverse effects on health from occupational exposure to trace concentrations of waste anesthetic gases.

Even if anesthetics have low potential for causing long-term toxicity, exposure of a large population of individuals may represent a considerable public health hazard. In the United States, about 50,000 hospital operating room personnel, including anesthesiologists, nurse-anesthetists, and operating room nurses and technicians, are exposed daily to waste anesthetic gases.[204] In addition, surgeons, dental personnel, and veterinarians and their technical assistants have a variable but sometimes heavy exposure to anesthetics. For example, peak levels of at least 50 ppm halothane and 5,000 ppm nitrous oxide have occasionally been recorded in operating room and dental operatory atmospheres.[205,206] The total number of exposed or potentially exposed personnel in the United States each year is about 225,000.[204] Of particular concern are reports that inhaled anesthetics possess mutagenic, carcinogenic, or teratogenic potential.

MUTAGENICITY

In recent years, investigators have become increasingly interested in the mutagenic potential of inhaled anesthetics for several reasons. First, chemical mutagenicity and carcinogenicity are closely correlated. Thus, finding that a particular anesthetic is a mutagen also implies that it is a potential carcinogen and should be studied in an animal test system. Because in vitro assays for mutagenicity require much less time and expense than in vivo assays for carcinogenicity, they have become popular screening methods for detection of carcinogens. A second reason for identifying mutagens present in the environment is that they may pose a threat to the integrity of the human genome (the totality of genes and chromosomes) and thus to future generations of humans.

To interpret results of in vitro mutagenicity tests with anesthetics, we must understand the mutation process. In a broad sense, muta-

tion refers to heritable change in genetic information. Four types are generally recognized:

1. Base-pair mutation in which one of the four DNA bases (adenine, guanine, thymine, or cytosine) is replaced by one of the others
2. Frame-shift mutation in which a base pair is added or deleted (In this case, all bases distal to the point of addition or deletion will be out of register, a potentially more serious mutation than the base-pair kind.)
3. Large deletions or rearrangements of DNA segments
4. Nondisjunction in which unequal partition of chromosomes occur between daughter cells

A wide variety of test systems has been used to examine the mutagenicity of inhaled anesthetics including assays with bacteria, yeast, mammalian cells in culture and intact mammals. Most of these have been reviewed elsewhere and will only be summarized here.[207,208]

Extensive work has been done with the Ames *Salmonella*/mammalian microsome system, which uses several strains of histidine-dependent *S. typhimurium* as the tester organism. This system is a well-validated assay for mutagenicity and often is regarded as the standard against which other systems are compared. It has been used to test most current and former anesthetics. Only divinyl ether and fluroxene give unequivocally positive responses (Fig. 22-4), whereas trichlorethylene gives a weak mutagenic response. Other anesthetics including nitrous oxide, halothane, and enflurane are not mutagenic when tested under a wide variety of experimental conditions and anesthetic concentrations. The general finding that anesthetics containing a double-bonded structure are mutagenic is consistent with knowledge about the high reactivity and mutagenicity of this class of chemicals.[209] Similarly, of all metabolites of inhaled anesthetics tested in the *Salmonella* assay, only 1,1-difluoro-2-bromo-2-chloroethylene (CF_2CBrCl) and 1,1-difluoro-2-chloroethylene (CF_2CHCl), which contain a double-bonded structure, have been found to be even weakly mutagenic.

In general, results from numerous studies

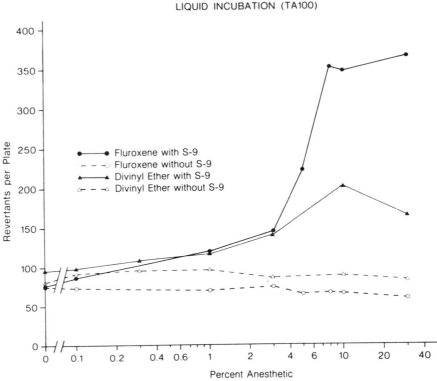

FIG. 22-4 Number of revertant colonies per plate of *Salmonella typhimurium,* TA100, after liquid suspension with fluroxene or divinyl ether, with or without S-9. Both fluroxene and divinyl ether showed a dose-dependent mutagenic response at concentrations greater than 1 percent in the presence of S-9.

with other test systems have confirmed those from studies with *Salmonella* (Table 22-1). Some anomalous results do exist, most notably the findings that nitrous oxide and halothane are weakly mutagenic in *Drosophila*[210-212] and nitrous oxide is weakly mutagenic in *Tradescantia.*[213] Nonetheless, the overwhelming evidence from in vitro tests indicates that all currently used and most previously used anesthetics are not mutagens and therefore are probably not carcinogens. By contrast, anesthetics that contain a double-bonded structure are mutagens and potential carcinogens.

Mutagenicity studies in humans exposed to inhaled anesthetics have been uniformly negative. In an early study, no significant difference in the number of chromosomal aberrations could be detected between lymphocytes obtained from operating room nurses and those obtained from surgical outpatient nurses.[214] In another study, no mutagenic activity could be

TABLE 22-1. Tests of Mutagenicity

Anesthetic	Positive	Negative
Halothane	D	A,8-AzG,D,SCE,L,C
Nitrous oxide	D, T	A,8-AzG, SCE
Chloroform	—	A,8-AzG, SCE
Enflurane	—	A,8-AzG, D, SCE
Methoxyflurane	—	A, SCE
Isoflurane	—	A, D, SCE
Cyclopropane	—	A
Diethyl ether	—	D, SCE
Sevoflurane	—	A
Synthane	—	A
Dioxychlorane	—	A
Dioxyflurane	—	A
Trichloroethylene	A, M, S	A, SCE
Fluroxene	A, D, SCE	—
Divinyl ether	A, SCE	—

Abbreviations used: A = Ames *Salmonella* or *Escherichia*/mammalian microsome, C = chromosomal mutations in mice, 8-AzG = 8-azaguanine–Chinese hamster lung fibroblasts, D = *Drosophila,* L = mouse dominant lethal test, M = mouse spot test, S = *Saccharomyces,* SCE = sister chromatid exchange–Chinese hamster ovary cells, and T = *Tradescantia.*

detected by *Salmonella* assay in urine of operating room personnel working in scavenged or unscavenged operating rooms, or in urine of anesthesiologists up to 15 months after the start of training.[215] Finally, lymphocytes from personnel exposed to waste anesthetic gases for durations up to 312 months had no higher incidence of chromosomal aberrations or sister chromatid exchange, as compared with those from unexposed individuals.[216] The study was an extension of previous negative studies of sister chromatid exchanges in lymphocytes of operating room personnel exposed to waste anesthetic gases and patients anesthetized with halothane, enflurane or fluroxene.[217-219] Thus, to date, no mutagenic effect of long-term or short-term exposure to inhaled anesthetics has been demonstrated in humans.

CARCINOGENICITY

The development of chemically induced tumors (chemical carcinogenesis) has three broad phases (Fig. 22-5). The first involves metabolic activation of the administered chemical to a positively charged reactive intermediate or electrophile. The second is covalent binding of the electrophile to some critical tissue macromolecule. Although chemicals and metabolites bind to lipid, protein, RNA, and DNA, the latter is thought to be the target molecule for chemical carcinogenesis. After covalent binding has occurred, cells may be re-paired, remain dormant or progress to the third phase which involves cellular proliferation and development of clinically apparent tumors. This final phase which occurs over a long time period and involves a multiplicity of mechanisms is little understood.

Covalent binding of reactive intermediates to tissue macromolecules is presumed to be necessary but not to be the only requirement for chemical carcinogenesis. As indicated in the section on specific organ toxicity, covalent binding of anesthetic metabolites has been recognized for many years. Low-temperature whole-body autoradiography in mice has shown that both chloroform and halothane fragments bind covalently to liver and other body tissues.[59,220] Thus, some anesthetics satisfy at least one criterion for chemical carcinogenicity.

Structural similarity provides further circumstantial evidence of an association between anesthetics and chemical carcinogens (Fig. 22-6). Methoxyflurane, enflurane, and isoflurane arel α-haloethers as are the non-anesthetic but carcinogenic chemicals bis(chloromethyl)ether, chloromethyl methyl ether, and bis(α-chloroethyl)ether.[221,222] Halothane and chloroform are alkyl halides; methyl iodide, butyl bromide, and butyl chloride are from the same chemical group and are animal carcinogens.[223] Finally, the anesthetic agent and industrial solvent, trichloroethylene, is a halogenated alkene similar to the human[224] and animal carcinogen,[225] vinyl chloride. Fluroxene and divinyl ether also contain the vinyl moiety. Although these observations on structure are

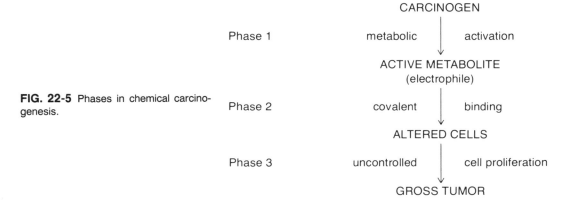

FIG. 22-5 Phases in chemical carcinogenesis.

CARCINOGEN

Phase 1   metabolic | activation

ACTIVE METABOLITE
(electrophile)

Phase 2   covalent | binding

ALTERED CELLS

Phase 3   uncontrolled | cell proliferation

GROSS TUMOR

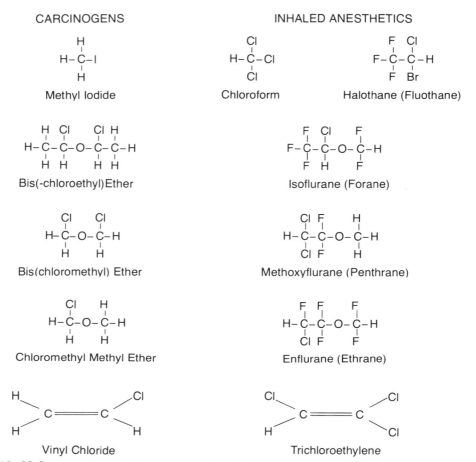

CARCINOGENS

Methyl Iodide

Bis(-chloroethyl)Ether

Bis(chloromethyl) Ether

Chloromethyl Methyl Ether

Vinyl Chloride

INHALED ANESTHETICS

Chloroform

Halothane (Fluothane)

Isoflurane (Forane)

Methoxyflurane (Penthrane)

Enflurane (Ethrane)

Trichloroethylene

FIG. 22-6 Structural formulas of several known human carcinogens and the inhaled anesthetic agents.

suggestive, they are by no means proof that anesthetics have carcinogenic potential. Minor structural differences often impart major changes in function, as has been clearly shown with aromatic hydrocarbons.[226] Epidemiologic surveys, animal studies, and in vitro carcinogenicity assays provide more definitive evidence.

Despite the obvious advantage of surveying human populations to determine the carcinogenic risk of exposure to anesthetics, such surveys have provided little information on the carcinogenicity of specific anesthetics. The primary reason is that levels of anesthetics to which surveyed individuals have been exposed either have not been measured or at best have only been estimated. Nonetheless, the studies so far performed should indicate whether working in a surgical or dental suite is associated with a higher incidence of cancer, regardless of the cause.

There have been several surveys of cancer incidence among exposed workers (Table 22-2). In the largest, the American Society of Anesthesiologists (ASA) conducted a retrospective survey of 49,595 operating room personnel working throughout the United States.[229] A 1.3- to 2.0-fold increase in cancer incidence was noted among female members of the ASA and the American Association of Nurse Anesthetists compared with unexposed control groups. No increase in cancer incidence was seen among surveyed males. In an earlier study, the incidence of cancer among 525 nurse anesthetists in Michigan was compared with that of

TABLE 22-2. Epidemiologic Surveys for Cancer Incidence or Deaths Among Personnel Exposed to Waste Anesthetic Gases

Studied	Population*	Results	Investigators†
Deaths	ASA members	Negative	Bruce et al. (1968)[227]
Incidence	Nurse anesthetists	3.3-fold increase for 1971	Corbett et al. (1973)[228]
Incidence	ASA members	1.3- to 1.9-fold increase for women; negative for men	American Society of Anesthesiologists (1974)[229]
Deaths	ASA members	Negative	Bruce et al. (1974)[230]
Deaths	Anesthetists	Negative	Doll and Peto (1977)[231]
Deaths	ASA members	Negative	Lew (1979)[232]
Incidence	Anesthetists and offspring	Negative	Tomlin (1979)[233]
Incidence	Dental personnel	1.5-fold increase for women; negative for men	Cohen et al. (1980)[234]

* ASA = American Society of Anesthesiologists.
† References are given as superscripts

women participating in the Connecticut Tumor Registry.[228] The nurse anesthetists had a higher incidence of malignancies diagnosed during 1971 than did all the women of Connecticut during 1966–1969. Most recently, a national survey of health among dental personnel was reported.[234] The study population consisted of 30,650 dentists and 30,547 chairside assistants and was readily divided into those who used or did not use inhaled anesthetics to provide pain relief and sedation. Otherwise, both groups did similar work under similar conditions. An estimate of anesthetic exposure was made by noting the number of hours per week spent by each respondent in the dental operatory. About 80 percent of users of inhaled anesthetics were exposed to nitrous alone, while the remainder were exposed to potent volatile anesthetics in addition. The cancer incidence among female chairside assistants exposed to waste anesthetics for more than 8 hours per week was 50% greater than among those not exposed, although the increase was not statistically significant ($P = 0.056$). Analysis of various types of cancer showed that only cancer of the cervix occurred more frequently ($P = 0.06$) in exposed women than in unexposed women.

Collectively, the above studies of cancer incidence appear to show a small risk to females directly exposed to waste anesthetic gases. However, because of problems with study design and the low increase in cancer incidence observed, reviewers have generally been unconvinced of the existence of a hazard to humans.[235–238] Their lack of conviction is

strengthened by results of surveys (Table 22-3) of deaths from cancer, which have all been negative.

Because of the problems of interpreting epidemiologic surveys, many investigators have turned to animal studies to provide information on the carcinogenic potential of specific anesthetics. When administered in extremely large dosages by oral gavage, chloroform[239] produced liver cancer in B6C3F1 mice and renal tumors in male or female Osborne-Mendel rats, whereas trichloroethylene[240] caused liver tumors in mice but not in rats. Fifty animals were used in both studies for each treatment and control group. Although oral gavage may be appropriate for studying dietary and therapeutic intake of chloroform or trichloroethylene, this route of administration probably is not relevant to inhaled exposure of patients or operating room personnel. Indeed, administering a drug by an unusual route often leads to confounding carcinogenicity data.[241] Furthermore, when trichloroethylene was studied, the agent tested contained 0.19 per-

TABLE 22-3. Teratogenic Mechanisms

Mutation*
Interference with cell division
Alteration of nucleic acid function
Removal of cell precursors and substrates
Lack of energy source
Enzyme inhibition
Change in cell membrane characteristics

* Four types — see text.
(Based on data in Wilson JE (editor): Environment and Birth Defects. New York, Academic Press, 1973.)

cent 1,2-epoxybutane and 0.09 percent epichlorohydrin, both known mutagens.[242,243] Epichlorohydrin is also a rodent carcinogen.[244] The presence of these contaminants, although in trace amounts, casts doubt on the significance of data gathered on trichlorethylene carcinogenicity.

In the only positive study of an anesthetic administered via inhalation, isoflurane led to an increased incidence of liver tumors in male, but not female, Swiss/ICR mice exposed in utero and for a short period postnatally.[245] Several factors, however, confound the interpretation of this finding, including the presence of high levels of polybrominated biphenyls in the livers of isoflurane-treated mice. In a more complete study, in which a similar exposure regimen was used, no increased incidence of liver or other tumors could be demonstrated in Swiss/ICR mice exposed to either isoflurane, halothane, enflurane, methoxyflurane, or nitrous oxide.[246] Halothane and enflurane have also been tested at their maximum tolerated dose in two lifetime carcinogenicity studies in Swiss/ICR mice.[247,248] In the first, 161 mice were exposed to 500 ppm halothane for 2 hr/day both in utero and for 78 weeks after birth. In the second study, 250 weanling mice were exposed to 3,000 ppm enflurane, 4 hr/day for 78 weeks. Despite lifetime exposure to maximum tolerated doses, neither anesthetic was carcinogenic. In a further study, groups of 50 Fischer 344 rats exposed for life to a nitrous oxide/halothane mixture at concentrations of 50 ppm/1 ppm or 500 ppm/10 ppm showed no higher incidence of tumors than rats exposed to air alone.[249]

The overhelming conclusion from both animal and human studies is that there is no carcinogenic risk either from working in the operating or dental suite or from exposure to anesthetics.

TERATOGENICITY

Embryogenesis is an extremely complex process involving a number of interrelated events such as cell proliferation and death, differentiation, migration, and organization into organ systems. Disruption at any stage can have serious consequences for the developing embryo and fetus. Although the developmental process is remarkably consistent, embryogenesis is not always perfect; congenital malformations, both severe and trivial, are found in about 2 to 4 percent of all births in countries in which records are kept.[250]

The term teratogenesis refers to adverse effects on developing biologic systems, namely, germ cells, embryos, fetuses, and immature postnatal individuals. Possible mechanisms that produce abnormal development (Table 22-3) are only partially understood. Mutations, especially those resulting in specific biochemical abnormalities and chromosomal nondisjunction, are well established mechanisms of human congenital anomalies. Cellular effects such as interference with cell division and alterations of cell membrane are less certain mechanisms of teratogenicity but have been observed with inhaled anesthetics at clinical concentrations.[251,252] Although the cause of most defects remains unknown, chemical teratogenesis in humans is well established (Table 22-4).

When discussing the potential carcinogenicity of anesthetics, we were most concerned about personnel chronically exposed to low concentrations rather than patients acutely exposed to high concentrations. In contrast, both patients administered anesthetics during pregnancy and personnel exposed chronically to waste anesthetic gases may be at increased risk of having an adverse reproductive outcome. Thus, in the following section we will consider the possible hazard to both groups.

Most surveys that have examined the reproductive performance of operating room and

TABLE 22-4. Known Human Chemical Teratogens*

Androgenic hormones
Folic antagonists
Thalidomide
Organic mercury
Some hypoglycemics (?)
Some anticonvulsants (?)

* Account for only 2 to 3 percent of known causes of developmental defects in humans.

(Based on data in Askrog V, Harvald B: Teratogen effect of inhalation anesthetics. Nord Med 83:498, 1970.)

TABLE 22-5. Results of Controlled Epidemiologic Surveys of Adverse Reproductive Effects Among Personnel Exposed to Waste Anesthetic Gases, and Their Spouses*

	Results			
	Exposed Women		Wives of Exposed Men	
Investigators	Spontaneous Abortion	Major Anomaly in Offspring	Spontaneous Abortion	Major Anomaly in Offspring
Askrog and Harvald (1970)[254]	65%	Negative	170%	Negative
Cohen et al. (1971)[255]	270%	—	—	—
Knill-Jones et al. (1972)[256]	30%	160%	—	—
Rosenberg and Kirves (1973)[257]	70%	Negative	—	—
Corbett et al. (1974)[258]	—	190%	—	—
American Society of Anesthesiologists (1974)[229]	30%	60%	Negative	30%
Knill-Jones et al. (1975)[259]	40%	Negative	Negative	Negative
Cohen et al. (1975)[260]	—	—	80%	Negative
Pharoah et al. (1977)[261]	Negative	Negative	—	—
Ericson and Kallen (1979)[262]	Negative	Negative	—	—
Cohen et al. (1980)[234]	160%	60%	50%	Negative
Axelsson and Rylander (1982)[263]	Negative	—	—	—

* Approximate percentage increase above control.

dental personnel are listed in Table 22-5. In a recent review of many of these studies, an estimate was made of the overall percentage increase for particular health hazards.[238] Relative risk for each hazard (rate of hazard among those exposed to anesthetics over rate among those not exposed) was calculated for each study. An overall relative risk with 95 percent confidence limits was then calculated by pooling the individual relative risks such that more weight was given to studies with larger sample sizes. The magnitude of the relative risk for spontaneous abortion among exposed women was approximately 1.3, representing a 30 percent increase for this hazard. The increase was both consistent and statistically significant. For congenital abnormalities among offspring of exposed women, the relative risk was approximately 1.2. The overall data were less consistent than for spontaneous abortion, with physicians having a 52% increase, which was significant, and nurses having an 11% increase, which was not significant. There was no consistent increase in incidence of spontaneous abortion among wives of exposed males or of congenital abnormalities among those offspring. Colton et al. commented that the increases observed were small and could not be attributed to a specific cause. Exposure to waste anesthetic gases, viruses, roentgeno-

grams, a variety of chemicals other than anesthetics, or a combination of these factors could have accounted for the positive results. Furthermore, most surveys had serious methodologic faults, including failure to verify the medical data supplied by respondents. Interestingly, in the only two studies in which medical records were used to confirm medical data, negative results were obtained for a number of adverse reproductive hazards including spontaneous abortion. The implication is that responder bias may be a factor in studies in which positive results have been reported.

Although some doubt remains concerning the adverse reproductive effects of waste anesthetic gases, there is no doubt about the detrimental effects of surgery and anesthesia on the pregnant patient. In the United States, at least 50,000 pregnant women (about 1.6 percent) undergo anesthesia and surgery during gestation for indications unrelated to pregnancy.[264] Operations for ovarian cysts, acute appendicitis, mammary tumors and repair of incompetent cervix are most common. The risk of unexpected abortion or premature labor clearly is higher following an anesthetic. What is not immediately obvious is whether the patient's disease, surgery, anesthesia, or a combination of these is the precipitating cause. Another concern, although not yet substantiated, is that anesthesia during pregnancy leads to an increased incidence of congenital abnormalities.

To assess the exact incidence of various anesthetic and surgery related hazards occurring during pregnancy, at least three studies have been performed.[264-266] In the first, all obstetric records in the U.S. Naval Hospital in Portsmouth, Virginia, were examined for the period 1957–1961.[265] During this period, 18,248 live births and 255 stillbirths were recorded; 67 patients had surgery during pregnancy, 24 having general and 43 having regional anesthesia. Nine stillbirths or abortions occurred after anesthesia, but no congenital anomalies were noted. Of the nine fetal losses, four were associated with appendiceal abscesses and four with Shirodkar procedures for incompetent cervical os. All nine cases resulting in fetal loss received spinal anesthesia although the investigator attributed this to sampling bias. In the second and larger study, two sources of data were analyzed.[264] The first was records of 9,073 obstetric patients delivered at the University of California Medical Center, San Francisco, between July 1959 and August 1964. The second source was records of 60,912 obstetric patients from 17 hospitals taking part in an Obstetrical Statistical Cooperative. Of the first group, 147 women (1.6 percent) had operations during their pregnancies. In the second group, 50 appendectomies and 71 Shirodkar procedures were recorded. Premature delivery after operation occurred in 8.8 percent; perinatal mortality was 7.5 percent compared with 2 percent in the nonsurgical group. On the basis of a detailed analysis of data obtained from these records, the authors concluded that premature labor after operation is mainly the result of the patient's surgical disease rather than the surgical or anesthetic technique, per se. In fact, no specific anesthetic technique, general or regional, had advantage in lowering the incidence of premature labor, perinatal mortality, or congenital anomalies. As expected, there is a particularly high incidence of premature labor and perinatal mortality associated with operations for incompetent surgical os. The authors also noted that although the expected incidence of congenital anomalies was normal following operation, the number of cases was too small to give conclusive results. They therefore recommended that if possible, anesthesia not be administered during pregnancy or at least that it be delayed until after the period of maximum organogenesis (first trimester). Naturally, whether this advice can be heeded depends on the precise circumstances of each case. In the final study, Brodsky et al.[266] used the results of the questionnaire survey of health among dental personnel[234] to determine fetal outcomes among 287 wives of dentists or dental assistants who underwent surgery during the first or second trimester of pregnancy. Anesthesia for surgery during the first trimester in those not occupationally exposed to waste anesthetic gases was associated with a significantly increased rate of spontaneous abortion from 5.1 to 8.0 percent; during the second trimester, the rate increased from 1.4 to 6.9 percent. There was no significant increase noted, however, in the number of congenital abnormalities in children born to these women.

In 1961, the disastrous effects of thalidomide ingested during pregnancy were first recognized.[267] Since then, sophisticated animal studies have gradually been developed for examining potential teratogenicity of chemicals. Complete testing now involves assessing the effect of a chemical on many aspects of reproductive function, such as fertility, mating behavior, in utero embryonic and fetal wastage, congenital anomalies, and postnatal survival and behavior. Despite their apparent thoroughness, animal studies remain far from perfect. Apart from the difficulty extrapolating animal data to humans, the number of animals exposed in any experiment is small compared with the number of humans exposed; thus, there is usually insufficient statistical power to evaluate the presence of a weak teratogen. Nonetheless, because direct human experimentation is obviously not possible, animal studies are still necessary and continue to provide useful information.

Effects of inhaled anesthetics on reproductive processes of experimental animals have been the subject of many reports. In an effort to simulate occupational exposure, experimental animals have received trace or subanesthetic concentrations of anesthetics by inhalation. The large number of such studies precludes a complete discussion in the present chapter. The interested reader is referred to three more comprehensive reviews.[204,208,268]

In general, nitrous oxide is the only inhaled anesthetic which has been convincingly shown to be directly teratogenic to experimental animals. High concentrations (50 to 75 percent) delivered to rats for 24-hour periods during organogenesis and low concentrations (0.1 percent) delivered throughout pregnancy result in an increased incidence of fetal resorptions and visceral and skeletal abnormalities.[269,270]

The mechanisms that produce these teratogenic effects are unknown but are likely to involve the biochemical and cellular effects of nitrous oxide noted above in the section on the hematopoietic system. Although effects in rodents are seen only after long periods of continuous exposure, is not known whether humans are more sensitive than rodents and would therefore show effects after shorter periods of exposure.

The other currently used inhaled anesthetics, halothane, enflurane and isoflurane, are also teratogenic to rodents but only when administered at anesthetizing concentrations for many hours on several days during pregnancy. The concensus is that unlike the case with nitrous oxide, the teratogenic effects observed are caused by the physiologic changes associated with the administration of these anesthetics rather than by the anesthetics themselves. Nonetheless, such findings emphasize the potential for anesthetics to cause teratogenic changes regardless of whether the mechanism is physiologic alteration or direct toxicity.

Attention has recently focused on another aspect of teratogenesis, enduring behavioral deficits without any observable morphologic changes. While many organ systems are most sensitive to chemical teratogens during organogenesis, the central nervous system may be particularly vulnerable during myelination. In humans this period is from the fourth intrauterine month through the second postnatal year. Thus, a chemical may produce behavioral teratogenesis if administered late in gestation or even after birth. Anesthetics have not escaped scrutiny as possible behavioral teratogens.

Rats exposed chronically to halothane (10 ppm) from conception to 60 days of age have been reported to have enduring learning deficits when tested on a shock-motivated light–dark discrimination task and a food-motivated symmetrical maze.[271,272] Tissue sampling of cerebral cortex showed electron microscopic evidence of neuronal degeneration and malformed synaptic membranes. In a more complete study, electron microscopic examination of cerebral cortical sections from rats exposed to halothane in utero showed central nervous system (CNS) damage such as synaptic malformation, disruption of the nuclear envelope and cell death.[273] Sensitive periods during gestation have been demonstrated in which halothane administration to the mother produces behavioral deficits in the offspring.[274] On days 3, 10, or 17 of pregnancy (roughly corresponding to the middle of first, second, or third trimester of pregnancy in humans), rats were anesthetized with 1.2 percent halothane for 120 minutes. Activity of adult males and offspring as well as body weights and water intake were not different among groups. At 75 days of age, male offspring were tested on the shock-motivated Y-maze discrimination task. Rats exposed on the days 3 and 10 performed statistically less well than those exposed on day 17 or those not exposed (control animals). These same animals were also significantly more sensitive to footshock than were rats exposed on day 17 or not exposed.

Offspring of Fischer 344 rats exposed to air or 1,500 ppm (0.15 percent) enflurane for 6 hr/day from conception to delivery have also been studied from 2 days to 90 weeks of age.[275] No significant treatment effects were observed.

Human studies have generally focused on long-term behavioral effects of maternal obstetric medication, including epidural anesthesia. Claims have been made that if the mother is given medication at delivery, the result will be depressed cognition, motor skills, and language ability of offspring for at least the first 7 years of life. Such claims, however, are extremely controversial. Behavioral abnormalities of offspring whose mothers received inhaled anesthetics at any time during delivery have not been well studied. Furthermore, studies have not been done to assess neurobehavior of children of operating room personnel who have been exposed to waste anesthetic gases. Firm conclusions about the risk of behavioral teratogenesis to the offspring of exposed personnel or to patients therefore await further investigation.

REFERENCES

1. Daniels TC, Jorgensen EC: Physiochemical properties in relation to biologic action, Textbook of Organic Medicinal and Pharmaceutical Chemistry. 7th Ed. Edited by Wilson CO, Gisvold O, Doerge RF. Philadelphia, Lippincott, 1977, pp 5–67
2. Singer SJ: The molecular organization of biological membranes, Structure and Function of Biological Membranes. Edited by Rothfield L. New York, Academic Press, 1971, pp 146–222
3. Singer SJ, Nicolson GL: The fluid mosaic model of the structure of cell membranes. Science 175:720, 1972
4. Guidotti G: The structure of intrinsic membrane proteins. J Supramol Struct 7:489, 1977
5. DePierre JW, Dallner G: Structural aspects of the membrane of the endoplasmic reticulum. Biochim Biophys Acta 415:411, 1975
6. Guengerich FP, Macdonald TL: Chemical mechanisms of catalysis by cytochromes P-450: A unified view. Acc Chem Res 17:9, 1984
7. Omura T, Siekevitz P, Palade GE: Turnover of constituents of the endoplasmic reticulum membrane of rat hepatocytes. J Biol Chem 242:2389, 1967
8. Quinn GP, Azelrod J, Brodie BB: Species, strain and sex differences in metabolism of hexobarbitone, amidopyrine, antipyrine and aniline. Biochem Pharmacol 1:152, 1958
9. Boobis AR, Davis DS: Human cytochromes P-450. Xenobiotica 14:151, 1984
10. Lu AYH, West SB: Multiplicity of mammalian microsomal cytochromes P-450. Pharm Rev 31:277, 1980
11. Waskell L, Gonzales J: Dependence of microsomal methoxyflurane O-demethylation on cytochrome P-450 reductase and the stoichiometry of fluoride ion and formaldehyde release. Anesth Analg 61:609, 1982
12. Burke TR Jr, Martin JL, George JW, et al: Investigation of the mechanisms of defluorination of enflurane in rat liver microsomes with specifically deuterated derivatives. Biochem Pharmacol 29:1623, 1980
13. Burke TR, Branchflower RV, Lees DE, et al: Mechanism of defluorination of enflurane. Identification of an organic metabolite in rat and man. Drug Metab Dispos 9:19, 1981
14. Baker MT, Nelson RM, Van Dyke RA: The release of inorganic fluoride from halothane and halothane metabolites by cytochrome P-450, hemin, and hemoglobin. Drug Metab Dispos 1:308, 1983
15. Rice SA, Talcott RE: Effects of isoniazid treatment on selected hepatic mixed function oxidases. Drug Metab Dispos 7:260, 1979
16. Rice SA, Sbordone L, Mazze RI: Metabolism by rat hepatic microsomes of fluorinated ether anesthetics following isoniazid administration. Anesthesiology 53:489, 1980
17. Mazze RI, Woodruff RE, Heerdt ME: Isoniazid-induced enflurane defluorination in humans. Anesthesiology 57:5, 1982
18. Dooley JR, Mazze RI, Rice SA, et al: Is enflurane defluorination inducible in man? Anesthesiology 50:213, 1979
19. Van Dyke RA: Enflurane, isoflurane, and methoxyflurane metabolism in rat hepatic microsomes from ethanol-treated animals. Anesthesiology 58:22, 1983
20. Rice SA, Dooley JR, Mazze RI: Metabolism by rat hepatic microsomes of fluorinated ether anesthetics following ethanol consumption. Anesthesiology 58:237, 1983
21. Van Dyke RA, Gandolfi AJ: Anaerobic release of fluoride from halothane. Relationship to the binding of halothane metabolites to hepatic cellular constituents. Drug Metab Dispos 4:40, 1976
22. Widger LA, Gandolfi AJ, Van Dyke RA: Hypoxia and halothane metabolism in vivo: Release of inorganic fluoride and halothane metabolite binding to cellular constituents. Anesthesiology 44:197, 1976
23. Maiorino RM, Sipes IG, Gandolfi AJ, et al: Factors affecting the formation of chlorotrifluoroethane and chlorodifluoroethylene from halothane. Anesthesiology 53:383, 1981
24. Ahr HJ, King LJ, Nastainczk W, et al: The mechanism of reproductive dehalogenation of halothane by liver cytochrome P-450. Biochem Pharmacol 31:383, 1982
25. Loew G, Motulsky H, Trudell J, et al: Quantum chemical studies of the metabolism of the inhalation anesthetics methoxyflurane, enflurane, and isoflurane. Mol Pharmacol 10:406, 1974
26. Oesch F: Mammalian epoxide hydrases: Inducible enzymes catalyzing the inactivation of carcinogenic and cytotoxic metabolites derived from aromatic and olefinic compounds. Xenobiotica 3:305, 1973

27. Daniel JW: The metabolism of [36]Cl-labeled trichloroethylene and tetrachloroethylene in the rat. Biochem Pharmacol 12:795, 1963

28. Leibman KC, McAllister WJ: Metabolism of trichloroethylene in liver microsomes: I. Characteristics of the reaction. Mol Pharmacol 1:239, 1965

29. Byington KH, Leibman KC: Metabolism of trichloroethylene in liver microsomes: II. Identification of the reaction product as chloral hydrate. Mol Pharmacol 1:247, 1965

30. Miller RE, Guengerich FP: Metabolism of trichloroethylene in isolated hepatocytes, microsomes and reconstituted enzyme systems containing cytochrome P-450. Cancer Res 43:1145, 1983

31. Powell JF: Trichloroethylene: Absorption, elimination and metabolism. Br J Ind Med 2:142, 1945

32. Soucek B, Vlachova D: Excretion of trichloroethylene metabolites in human urine. Br J Med 17:60, 1960

33. Parke DV: Mechanisms and consequences of the induction of microsomal enzymes of mammalian liver. Biochem J 130:53P, 1972

34. Remmer H, Merker HJ: Drug-induced changes in the liver endoplasmic reticulum. Association with drug-metabolizing enzymes. Science 142:1657, 1963

35. Conney AH: Pharmacological implications of microsomal enzyme induction. Pharm Rev 19:317, 1967

36. Brown BR Jr, Sagalyn AM: Hepatic microsomal enzyme induction by inhalation anesthetics: Mechanism in the rat. Anesthesiology 40:152, 1974

37. Linde HW, Berman ML: Nonspecific stimulation of drug-metabolizing enzymes by inhalation anesthetic agents. Anesth Analg 50:656, 1971

38. Ross WT, Cardell RR: Proliferation of smooth endoplasmic reticulum and induction of microsomal drug-metabolizing enzymes after ether or halothane. Anesthesiology 8:325, 1978

39. Shideman FE, Kelly AR, Adams BJ: The role of the liver in the detoxification of thiopental (Pentothal) and two other thiobarbiturates. J Pharmacol Exp Ther 91:331, 1947

40. Barr GA, Cousins MJ, Mazze RI, et al: A comparison of the renal effects and metabolism of enflurane and methoxyflurane in Fischer 344 rats. J Pharmacol Exp Ther 190:530, 1974

41. Hitt BA, Mazze RI: Effect of enzyme induction on nephrotoxicity of halothane related compounds. Environ Health Perspect 21:179, 1977

42. Caughey GH, Rice SA, Kosek JC, et al.: Effect of phenytoin (DPH) treatment on methoxyflurane

metabolism in rats. J Pharmacol Exp Ther 210:180, 1979

43. Greene NM: Halothane anesthesia and hepatitis in a high risk population. N Engl J Med 289:304, 1973

44. Duvaldestin P, Mazze RI, Nivoche Y, et al: Occupational exposures to halothane results in enzyme induction in anesthetists. Anesthesiology 54:57, 1981

45. Ivanetich KM, Lucas S, Marsh JA, et al: Organic compounds, their interaction with and degradation of hepatic microsomal drug-metabolizing enzymes in vitro. Drug Metab Dispos 6:218, 1978

46. Cascorbi HF, Vessel ES, Blake DA: Genetic and environmental influence on halothane metabolism in twins. Clin Pharmacol Ther 12:50, 1971

47. Haggard HW: The absorption, distribution, and elimination of ethyl ether. J Biol Chem 59:737, 1924

48. Van Dyke RA, Chenoweth MB, Van Poznak A: Metabolism of volatile anesthetics. I. Conversion in vivo of several anesthetics to [14]CO_2 and chloride. Biochem Pharmacol 13:1239, 1964

49. Cohen EN: Metabolism of the volatile anesthetics. Anesthesiology 35:193, 1971

50. Green K, Cohen EN: On the metabolism of ^{14}C-diethyl ether in the mouse. Biochem Pharmacol 20:393, 1971

51. Van Dyke RA, Chenoweth MB: Metabolism of volatile anesthetics. Anesthesiology 26:348, 1965

52. Hong K, Trudell JR, O'Neill Jr, et al: Metabolism of nitrous oxide by human and rat intestinal contents. Anesthesiology 52:16, 1980

53. Van Dyke RA: Biotransformation, Handbook of Experimental Pharmacology. Edited by Chenoweth MB. New York, Springer-Verlag, 1972, p 345

54. Rao GS, Meridian DJ, Tong YS, et al: Biochemical toxicology of chronic nitrous oxide exposures. Pharmacologist 21:216, 1979

55. Pohl LR, Bhooshan B, Whittaker NE, et al: Phosgene: A metabolite of chloroform. Biochem Biophys Res Commun 79:684, 1977

56. Pohl LR, Martin JL, George JW: Metabolic activation of chloroform by rat liver microsomes. Biochem Pharmacol 29:3271, 1980

57. Pohl LR, Branchflower RV, Highet RJ, et al: The formation of digluthathionyl dithiocarbonate as a metabolite of chloroform, bromotrichloromethane and carbon tetrachloride. Drug Metab Dispos 9:334, 1981

58. Charlesworth FA: Patterns of chloroform metabolism. Fed Cosmet Toxicol 14:59, 1976

59. Cohen EN, Hood N: Application of low-temperature autoradiography to studies of the uptake and metabolism of volatile anesthetics in the

mouse. I. Chloroform. Anesthesiology 30:306, 1969

60. Illett KF, Reid WD, Sipes GI, et al: Chloroform toxicity in mice: Correlation of renal and hepatic necrosis with covalent binding of metabolites to tissue macromolecules. Exp Mol Pathol 19:25, 1973

61. Scholler KL: Electron-microscopic and autoradiographic studies on the effect of halothane and chloroform on liver cells. Acta Anaesthesiol Scand (suppl) 32:5, 1968

62. Cowlen MS, Hewitt WR, Schroeder F: 2-Hexanone potentiation of [¹⁴C]chloroform hepatoxicity: Covalent interaction of a reactive intermediate with rat liver phospholipid. Toxicol Appl Pharmacol 73:478, 1984

63. Barrett HM, Johnston JH: The fate of trichloroethylene in the organism. J Biol Chem 127:765, 1939

64. Leibman KC, McAllister WJ: Metabolism of trichloroethylene in liver microsomes. III. Induction of the excretion of metabolites. J Pharmacol Exp Ther 157:574, 1967

65. Miller RE, Guengerich FP: Oxidation of trichloroethylene by liver microsomal cytochrome P-450: Evidence for chlorine migration in a transition state not involving trichloroethylene oxide. Biochemistry 21:1090, 1982

66. Gion H, Yoshimura N, Holaday DA, et al: Biotransformation of fluroxene in man. Anesthesiology 40:553, 1974

67. Blake DA, Rozman RS, Cascorbi HF, et al: Anesthesia LXXIV: Biotransformation of fluroxene. I. Metabolism in mice and dogs in vivo. Biochem Pharmacol 16:1237, 1967

68. Ivanetich KM, Bradshaw JJ, Marsh JA, et al: The role of cytochrome P-450 in the toxicity of fluroxene (2,2,2-trifluoroethyl vinyl ether) anesthesia in vivo. Biochem Pharm 25:773, 1976

69. Ivanetich KM, Bradshaw JJ, Marsh JA, et al: The interactions of hepatic microsomal cytochrome P-450 with fluroxene (2,2,2-trifluoroethyl vinyl ether) in vitro. Biochem Pharm 25:779, 1976

70. Murphy MJ, Dunbar DA, Kaminsky LS: Acute toxicity of fluorinated ether anesthetics: Role of 2,2,2-trifluroethanol and other metabolites. Toxicol Appl Pharmacol 71:84, 1983

71. Stier A: Trifluoroacetic acid as a metabolite of halothane. Biochem Pharmacol 12:544, 1964

72. Stier A, Alter H, Hessler O, et al: Urinary excretion of bromide in halothane anesthesia. Anesth Analg 43:723, 1964

73. Sharp JH, Trudell JR, Cohen EN: Volatile metabolites and decomposition products of halothane in man. Anesthesiology 50:2, 1979

74. de Groot H, Harnisch U, Noll T: Suicidal activation of microsomal cytochrome P-450 by halo-thane under hypoxic conditions. Biochem Biophys Res Commun 107:885, 1982

75. Clauberg G: Untersuchungen über den Einfluss von Inhalationsnarkose und Operation auf die Leberfunktion unter besonderer Berücksichtigung des Halothans. Anaesthesist 19:324, 1970

76. Reynolds ES, Moslen MT: Halothane hepatotoxicity: Enhancement by polychlorinated biphenyl pretreatment. Anesthesiology 47:19, 1977

77. Sipes IG, Brown BR Jr: An animal model of hepatotoxicity associated with halothane anesthesia. Anesthesiology 45:622, 1976

78. Holaday DA, Rudofsky S, Treuhaft PS: Metabolic degradation of methoxyflurane in man. Anesthesiology 33:579, 1970

79. Van Dyke RA, Wood CL: Metabolism of methoxyflurane: Release of inorganic fluoride in human and rat hepatic microsomes. Anesthesiology 39:613, 1973

80. Yoshimura N, Holaday DA, Fiserova-Bergerova V: Metabolism of methoxyflurane in man. Anesthesiology 44:372, 1976

81. Ivanetich KM, Lucas SA, Marsh JA: Enflurane and methoxyflurane. Their interaction with hepatic cytochrome P-450 in vitro. Biochem Pharm 28:785, 1979

82. Canova-Davis E, Waskell L: The enhancement of cytochrome P-450 catalyzed methoxyflurane metabolism by a heat-stable microsomal protein. Biochem Biophys Res Commun 108:1264, 1982

83. Canova-Davis E, Waskell L: The identification of the heat-stable microsomal protein required for methoxyflurane metabolism as cytochrome b_5. J Biol Chem 259:2541, 1984

84. Warren WA, Baker FD, Bellatoni J: Enzymatic defluorination of methoxyflurane. Biochem Pharmacol 25:723, 1976

85. Madelian V, Warren WA: Defluorination of methoxyflurane by a glutathione-dependent enzyme. Res Commun Chem Pathol Pharmacol 16:385, 1977

86. Warren W, Madelian V: Defluorination of methoxyflurane by glutathione and coenzyme B_{12}. Res Commun Chem Pathol Pharmacol 35:515, 1982

87. Berman ML, Lowe HJ, Bochantin JS, et al: Uptake and elimination of methoxyflurane as influenced by enzyme induction in the rat. Anesthesiology 38:352, 1973

88. Mazze RI, Hitt BA, Cousins MJ: Effect of enzyme induction with phenobarbital on the in vivo and in vitro defluorination of isoflurane and methoxyflurane. J Pharmacol Exp Ther 190:523, 1974

89. Fiserova-Bergerova V: Changes of fluoride con-

tent in bone: An index of drug defluorination *in vivo*. Anesthesiology 38:345, 1973

90. Miller MS, Gandolfi AJ: Enflurane biotransformation in humans. Life Sci 27:1465, 1980

91. Mazze RI, Cousins MJ, Barr GA: Renal effects and metabolism of isoflurane in man. Anesthesiology 40:536, 1974

92. Holaday DA, Fiserova-Bergerova V, Latto IP, et al: Resistance of isoflurane to biotransformation in man. Anesthesiology 54:383, 1981

93. Hitt BA, Mazze RI, Cousins MJ: Metabolism of isoflurane in Fischer 344 rats and man. Anesthesiology 40:62, 1974

94. Cook TL, Beppu WJ, Hitt BA, et al: Renal effects and metabolism of sevoflurane in Fischer 344 rats. An *in vivo* and *in vitro* comparison with methoxyflurane. Anesthesiology 43:70, 1975

95. Cook TL, Beppu WJ, Hitt BA, et al: A comparison of renal effects and metabolism of sevoflurane and methoxyflurane in enzyme induced rats. Anesth Analg 54:829, 1975

96. Holaday DA, Smith FR: Clinical characteristics and biotransformation of sevoflurane in healthy human volunteers. Anesthesiology 54:100, 1981

97. Miller EC, Miller JA: Mechanisms of chemical carcinogenesis: Nature of proximate carcinogens and interactions with macromolecules. Pharmacol Rev 18:805, 1966

98. Mitchell JR, Jollows DJ: Metabolic activation of drugs to toxic substances. Gastroenterology 68:392, 1975

99. Demopoulos HB: The basis of free radical pathology. Fed Proc 32:1859, 1973

100. Demopoulos HB: Control of free radicals in biological systems. Fed Proc 32:1903, 1973

101. Brown BR, Jr, Sagalyn AM: Reactive intermediates of anesthetic biotransformation and hepatotoxicity, Molecular Mechanisms of Anesthesia, Progress in Anesthesiology. Vol. 1. Edited by Fink BR. New York, Raven Press, 1975

102. Levine BB: Immunochemical aspects of drug allergy. Br Rev Med 17:23, 1966

103. Myers LS JR: Free radical damage of nucleic acids and their components by ionizing radiation. Fed Proc 32:1882, 1973

104. DiLuzio NR: Antioxidants, lipid peroxidation and chemical-induced liver injury. Fed Proc 32:1875, 1973

105. King MM, Lai EK, McCay PB: Singlet oxygen production associated with enzyme-catalyzed lipid peroxidation in liver microsomes. J Biol Chem 250:6496, 1975

106. Udenfriend S: Arene oxide intermediates in enzymatic hydroxylation and their significance with respect to drug toxicity, Edited by Vessell ES. Ann NY Acad Sci 179:295, 1971

107. Recknagel RO: Alterations produced in the endoplasmic reticulum by carbon tetrachloride. Minerva Med 69:455, 1978

108. Udenfriend S, Bartl P: Symposium on the Biochemistry and Metabolism of Arene Oxides. Roche Institute of Molecular Biology, Nutley, NJ, 1972

109. Druckrey H: Specific carcinogenic and teratogenic effects of "indirect" alkylating methyl and ethyl compounds and their dependency on stages of ontogenic development. Xenobiotica 3:271, 1973

110. Pryor WA: Free radical reactions and their importance in biochemical systems. Fed Proc 32:1862, 1973

111. Tappel AL: Lipid peroxidation damage to cell components. Fed Proc 32:1870, 1973

112. Brown BR Jr: Hepatic microsomal lipoperoxidation and inhalational anesthetics: A biochemical and morphologic study in the rat. Anesthesiology 36:458, 1972

113. Weinstein IB, Yamaguchi R, Gebert R, et al: Use of epithelial cell cultures for studies on the mechanism of transformation by chemical carcinogens. In Vitro 11:130, 1975

114. Strunin L: The liver and anaesthesia, Major Problems in Anaesthesia. Vol 3. Edited by Mushin WW. London, WB Saunders, 1977, pp 144–146

115. Clarke RSJ, Doggart JR, Lavery T: Changes in liver function after different types of surgery. Br J Anaesth 48:119, 1976

116. Libonati M, Malsch E, Price HL, et al: Splanchnic circulation in man during methoxyflurane anesthesia. Anesthesiology 38:366, 1973

117. Gelman SI: Disturbances in hepatic blood flow during anaesthesia and surgery. Arch Surg 111:881, 1976

118. Simpson JY: On a new anaesthetic agent, more efficient than sulphuric ether. Lancet 2:549, 1847

119. Defalque RJ: The first delayed chloroform poisoning. Anesth Analg 47:374, 1968

120. Henderson Y, Cullen TS, Martin ED, et al: Report of the Committee on Anesthesia of the American Medical Association. JAMA 58:1908, 1912

121. Bevan AD, Favill HB: Acid intoxication, and late poisonous effects of anesthetics. Hepatic toxemia. Acute fatty degeneration of the liver following chloroform and ether anesthesia. JAMA 45:691, 754, 1905

122. Goldschmidt S, Ravdin IS, Lucke B: Anesthesia and liver damage. 1. The protective action of oxygen against the necrotizing effect of certain anesthetics on the liver. J Pharmacol Exp Ther 59:1, 1937

123. Cavalieri E, Calvin M: Molecular characteris-

tics of some carcinogenic hydrocarbons. Proc Natl Acad Sci USA 68:1251, 1971

124. Caravati CM, Wootton P: Acute massive hepatic necrosis with fatal liver failure. South Med J 55:1268, 1962

125. Gingrich TF, Virtue RW: Postoperative liver damage. Is anesthesia involved? Surgery 57:241, 1965

126. Herber R, Specht NW: Liver necrosis following anesthesia. Arch Intern Med 115:266, 1965

127. Slater EM, Gibson JM, Dykes MHM, et al: Postoperative hepatic necrosis. Its incidence and diagnostic value in association with the administration of halothane. N Engl J Med 270:983, 1964

128. Bennike KW, Hagelsten JO: Cyclopropane hepatitis. A Danish disease? Lancet 2:255, 1964

129. Krantz JC, Carr CJ, Lu G, et al: Anesthesia XL. The anesthetic action of trifluoroethyl vinyl ether. J Pharmacol Exp Ther 108:488, 1953

130. Reynolds ES, Brown BR Jr, Vandam LD: Massive hepatic necrosis after fluroxene anesthesia —A case of drug interaction. N Engl J Med 286:530, 1972

131. Cascorbi HF, Singh-Amaranath AV: Fluroxene toxicity in mice. Anesthesiology 37:480, 1972

132. Harrison GG, Smith JS: Massive lethal hepatic necrosis in rats anesthetized with fluroxene after microsomal enzyme induction. Anesthesiology 39:619, 1973

133. Johnston RR, Cromwell TH, Eger EI, et al: The toxicity of fluroxene in animals and man. Anesthesiology 38:313, 1973

134. Suckling CW: Some chemical and physical factors in the development of Fluothane. Br J Anaesth 29:466, 1957

135. Brennan RW, Hunter AR, Johnstone M: Halothane—A clinical assessment. Lancet 2:453, 1957

136. Johnstone M: The human cardiovascular response to Fluothane anaesthesia. Br J Anaesth 28:392, 1956

137. Brody GL, Sweet RB: Halothane anesthesia as a possible cause of massive hepatic necrosis. Anesthesiology 24:29, 1963

138. Bunker JP, Blumenfeld CM: Liver necrosis after halothane anesthesia. Cause or coincidence? N Engl J Med 268:531, 1963

139. Lindenbaum J, Leifer E: Hepatic necrosis associated with halothane anesthesia. N Engl J Med 268:525, 1963

140. Bunker JP, Forrest WH, Mostseller F, et al: A Study of the Possible Association between Halothane Anesthesia and Postoperative Hepatic Necrosis. National Halothane Study. Washington DC, US Government Printing Office, 1969

141. Subcommittee on the National Halothane Study of the Committee on Anesthesia. National Academy of Sciences–National Research Council. Summary of the National Halothane Study. Possible association between halothane anesthesia and postoperative necrosis. JAMA 197:775, 1966

142. Dykes MHM, Bunker JP: Hepatotoxicity and anesthetics. Pharmacol Physicians 4:15, 1970

143. Strunin L, Simpson BR: Halothane in Britain today. Br J Anaesth 44:919, 1972

144. Bottinger LE, Dalen E, Hallen B: Halothane-induced liver damage: An analysis of the material reported to the Swedish Adverse Drug Reaction Committee 1966–1973. Acta Anaesth Scand 20:40, 1976

145. Druckrey H: Specific carcinogenic and teratogenic effects of "indirect" akylating methyl and ethyl compounds and their dependency on stages of ontogenic development. Xenobiotica 3:271, 1973

146. Moult PJA, Sherlock S: Halothane related hepatitis. A clinical study of twenty-six cases. Q J Med (new series XLIV) 173:99, 1975

147. Walton B, Simpson BR, Strunin L, et al: Unexplained hepatitis following halothane. Br Med J 1:1171, 1976

148. Vergani D, Mieli-Vergani G, Alberti A, et al: Antibodies to the surface of halothane-altered rabbit hepatocytes in patients with severe halothane-associated hepatitis. N Engl J Med 303:66, 1980

149. Davis M, Eddleston ALWF, Neuberger JM, et al: Halothane hepatitis. N Engl J Med 303:1123, 1980

150. Rice SA, Maze M, Mazze RI, et al: Hepatotoxicity following halothane anesthesia in isoniazid treated rats. Fed Proc 38:683, 1979

151. Wood M, Berman ML, Harbison RD, et al: Halothane-induced hepatic necrosis in triiodothyronine-pretreated rats. Anesthesiology 52:470, 1980

152. Uetrecht J, Wood AJJ, Phythyon JM, et al: Contrasting effects on halothane hepatotoxicity in the phenobarbital-hypoxia and triiodothyronine model: Mechanistic implications. Anesthesiology 59:196, 1983

153. Jee R, Sipes IG, Gandolfi AJ, et al: Factors influencing an animal model of halothane hepatotoxicity. Toxicol Appl Pharmacol 52:267, 1980

154. McLain GE, Sipes IG, Brown BR Jr: An animal model of halothane hepatotoxicity. Anesthesiology 51:321, 1979

155. Ross WT Jr, Daggy BP, Cardell RR: Hepatic necrosis caused by halothane and hypoxia in phenobarbital-treated rats. Anesthesiology 51:327, 1979

156. Van Dyke RA: Hepatic centrilobular necrosis in rats after exposure to halothane, enflurane, or isoflurane. Anesth Analg 61:812, 1982

157. Harper MH, Collins P, Johnson B, et al: Hepatic injury following halothane, enflurane, and isoflurane in rats. Anesthesiology 56:14, 1982

158. Plummer JL, Beckwith ALJ, Bastin FN, et al: Free radical formation *in vivo* and hepatotoxicity due to anesthesia with halothane. Anesthesiology 57:160, 1982

159. Ross WT Jr, Daggy BP: Hepatic blood flow in phenobarbital-pretreated rats during halothane anesthesia and hypoxia. Anesth Analg 60:306, 1981

160. Shingu K, Eger EI II, Johnson BH: Hypoxia *per se* can produce hepatic damage without death in rats. Anesth Analg 61:820, 1982

161. Shingu K, Eger EI II, Johnson BH: Hypoxia may be more important than reproductive metabolism in halothane-induced hepatic injury. Anesth Analg 61:824, 1982

162. Artusio JF Jr, Van Poznack A, Hunt RE, et al: A clinical evaluation of methoxyflurane in man. Anesthesiology 21:512, 1960

163. Joshi PH, Conn HO: The syndrome of methoxyflurane associated hepatitis. Ann Intern Med 80:395, 1974

164. Cale JO, Parks CR, Jenkins MT: Hepatic and renal effects of methoxyflurane in dogs. Anesthesiology 23:248, 1962

165. Dahlgren BE, Goodrich BH: Changes in kidney and liver function after methoxyflurane (Penthrane) anesthesia. Br J Anaesth 48:145, 1976

166. Botty C, Brown B, Stanley V, et al: Clinical experiences with compound 347—a halogenated anesthetic. Anesth Analg 47:499, 1968

167. Dobkin HB, Heinrich RG, Israel JS, et al: Clinical and laboratory evaluation of a new inhalation agent: Compound 347 (CHF$_2$-O-CF$_2$-CHFCl). Anesthesiology 29:275, 1968

168. Denlinger KJ, Lecky JH, Nahrwold ML: Hepatocellular dysfunction without jaundice after enflurane anesthesia. Anesthesiology 41:86, 1974

169. Sadove MS, Kim SI: Hepatitis after use of two different fluorinated anesthetic agents. Anesth Analg 53:336, 1974

170. Van der Reis L, Askin SH, Freckner GN, et al: Hepatic necrosis after enflurane anesthesia. JAMA 227:76, 1974

171. Ona FV, Paranella H, Ayub A: Hepatitis associated with enflurane anesthesia. Anesth Analg 59:146, 1980

172. Lewis JH, Zimmerman HJ, Ishak KG, et al: Enflurane hepatoxicity. A clinico-pathologic study of 24 cases. Ann Intern Med 98:984, 1983

173. Lynch S, Martis L, Woods E: Evaluation of hepatotoxic potential of sevoflurane in rats. Pharmacologist 21:221, 1979

174. Crandell WB, Pappas SG, MacDonald A: Nephrotoxicity associated with methoxyflurane anesthesia. Anesthesiology 27:591, 1966

175. Mazze RI, Shue GL, Jackson SH: Renal dysfunction associated with methoxyflurane anesthesia. A randomized prospective clinical evaluation. JAMA 216:278, 1971

176. Smith FA (editor) Handbook of Experimental Pharmacology. Pharmacology of Fluorides. New York, Springer-Verlag, 1970

177. Mazze RI, Cousins MJ, Kosek JC: Dose-related methoxyflurane nephrotoxicity in rats: A biochemical and pathologic correlation. Anesthesiology 36:571, 1972

178. Jeghers H, Murphy R: Medical progress, practical aspects of oxalate metabolism. N Engl J Med 233:208, 1945

179. Cousins MJ, Mazze RI: Methoxyflurane nephrotoxicity: A study of dose response in man. JAMA 225:1611, 1973

180. Mazze RI, Cousins MJ: Combined nephrotoxicity of gentamicin and methoxyflurane anesthesia in man. A case report. Br J Anaesth 45:394, 1973

181. Barr GA, Mazze RI, Cousins MJ, et al: An animal model for combined methoxyflurane and gentamicin nephrotoxicity. Br J Anaesth 45:306, 1973

182. Hitt BA, Mazze RI, Denson DD: Isotopic probe of the mechanisms of methoxyflurane defluorination. Drug Metab Disp 7:446, 1979

183. McCarty LP, Malek RS, Larsen ER: The effects of deuteration on the metabolism of halogenated anesthetics in the rat. Anesthesiology 51:106, 1979

184. Baden JM, Rice SA, Mazze RI: Effects of deuterated methoxyflurane (d$_4$-MOF) on renal function in Fischer 344 rats. Anesthesiology 56:203, 1982

185. Mazze RI: The kidney: Anesthesia induced malfunction. Twenty-Seventh Annual Refresher Course Lectures of the American Society of Anesthesiologists, San Francisco, 1976, p 229

186. Cousins MJ, Greenstein LR, Hitt BA, et al: Metabolism and renal effects of enflurane in man. Anesthesiology 44:44, 1976

187. Mazze RI, Calverley RK, Smith NT: Inorganic fluoride nephrotoxicity: Prolonged enflurane and halothane anesthesia in volunteers. Anesthesiology 46:265, 1977

188. Sievenpiper TS, Rice SA, McClendon F, et al: Renal effects of enflurane anesthetics in Fischer 344 rats with pre-existing renal insufficiency. J Pharmacol Exp Ther 211:36, 1979

189. Fish K, Sievenpiper TS, Rice SA, et al: Renal

function in Fischer 344 rats with chronic renal impairment after the administration of enflurane and gentamicin. Anesthesiology 53:481, 1980

190. Mazze RI, Sievenpiper TS, Stevenson J: Renal effects of enflurane and halothane in patients with abnormal renal function. Anesthesiology 60:161, 1984

191. Cousins MJ, Mazze RI, Kosek JC, et al: The etiology of methoxyflurane nephrotoxicity. J Pharmacol Exp Ther 190:530, 1974

192. Kripke BJ, Kelman AD, Shah NK, et al: Testicular reaction to prolonged exposure to nitrous oxide. Anesthesiology 44:104, 1976

193. Coate WB, Kapp RW, Lewis TR: Chronic exposure to low concentrations of halothane-nitrous oxide: Reproductive and cytogenetic effects in the rat. Anesthesiology 50:310, 1979

194. Land PC, Owen EL, Linde HW: Mouse sperm morphology following exposure to anesthetics during early spermatogenesis. Anesthesiology 51:S259, 1979

195. Baden JM, Land PC, Egbert B, et al: Lack of toxicity of enflurane on male reproductive organs in mice. Anesth Analg 61:19, 1980

196. Mazze RI, Rice SA, Wyrobeck AJ, et al: Germ cell studies in mice after prolonged exposure to nitrous oxide. Toxicol Appl Pharmacol 67:370, 1983

197. Wyrobek AJ, Brodsky J, Gordon L, et al: Sperm studies in anesthesiologists. Anesthesiology 55:527, 1981

198. Lassen HCA, Henriksen E, Neukirch F, et al: Treatment of tetanus. Severe bone-marrow depression after prolonged nitrous-oxide anesthesia. Lancet 1:527, 1956

199. Amess JAL, Burman JF, Rees GM, et al: Megaloblastic haemopoiesis in patients receiving nitrous oxide. Lancet 2:239, 1978

200. Skacel PO, Hewlett AM, Lewis JD, et al: Studies on the haemopoietic toxicity of nitrous oxide in man. Br J Haematol 53:189, 1983

201. Deacon R, Lumb M, Perry J, et al: Inactivation of methionine synthase by nitrous oxide. Eur J Biochem 104:419, 1980

202. Scott JM, Wilson P, Dinn JJ, et al: Pathogenesis of subacute combined degeneration: A result of methyl group deficiency. Lancet 1:334, 1981

203. Van der Westhuyzen J, Fernandes-Costa F, Metz J: Cobalamin inactivation by nitrous oxide produces severe neurological impairment in fruit bats: Protection by methionine and aggravation by folates. Life Sci 31:2001, 1982

204. NIOSH: Criteria for a recommended standard . . . occupational exposure to waste anesthetic gases and vapors. DHEW (NIOSH) Publ No 77-140, 1977

205. Millard RI, Corbett TH: Nitrous oxide concentration in the dental operatory. J Oral Surg 32:593, 1974

206. Pfaffli P, Nikki P, Ahlman K: Halothane and nitrous oxide in end-tidal air and venous blood of surgical personnel. Ann Clin Res 4:273, 1972

207. Baden JM, Simmon VF: Mutagenic effects of inhalation anesthetics. Mutat Res 75:169, 1980

208. Baden JM: Chronic toxicity of inhalation anaesthetics, Clinics in Anaesthesiology, vol 1. Edited by Mazze, RI. pp 441–456, 1983

209. Simmon VF, Baden JM: Mutagenic activity of vinyl compounds and derived epoxides. Mutat Res 78:227, 1980

210. Garrett S, Fuerst R: Sex-linked mutations in *Drosophila* after exposure to various mixtures of gas atmospheres. Environ Res 7:286, 1974

211. Kramers JC, Burm GL: Mutagenicity studies with halothane in *Drosophila melanogaster*. Anesthesiology 50:510, 1979

212. Kundomal Y, Baden JM: Mutagenicity of inhaled anesthetics in *Drosophilia melanogaster*. Anesthesiology 62:305, 1985

213. Sparrow AH, Schairer LA: Mutagenic response of *Tradescantia* to treatment with x-rays, EMS, DBE, ozone, SO_2, N_2O and several insecticides. Mutat Res 26:445, 1974

214. Rosenberg PH, Kallio H: Operating-theatre gas pollution and chromosomes. Lancet 2:452, 1977

215. Baden JM, Kelly MJ, Cheung A, et al: Lack of mutagens in urine of operating personnel. Anesthesiology 53:195, 1980

216. Husum B, Niebuhr E, Wulf HC, et al: Sister chromatid exchanges and structural chromosome aberrations in lymphocytes in operating room personnel. Acta Anaesth Scand 27:262, 1983

217. Husum B, Wulf HC: Sister chromatid exchanges in lymphocytes in operating room personnel. Acta Anaesth Scand 24:22, 1980

218. Husum B, Wulf HC, Niebuhr E: Sister chromatid exchanges in lymphocytes after anesthesia with halothane or enflurane. Acta Anaesth Scand 25:97, 1981

219. Husum B, Wulf HC, Niebuhr E: Sister chromatid exchanges and structural chromosome aberrations in human lymphocytes after anaesthesia with fluroxene. Br J Anaesth 54:987, 1982

220. Cohen EN, Hood N: Application of low-temperature autoradiography to studies of the uptake and metabolism of volatile anesthetics in the mouse. III. Halothane. Anesthesiology 31:553, 1969

221. Leong BKJ, MacFarland HN, Reese WH: Induction of lung adenomas by chronic inhalation of bis (chloromethyl) ether. Arch Environ Health 22:663, 1976

222. Van Duuren BL, Goldschmidt BM, Katz C, et al:

Alphahaloethers: A new type of alkylating carcinogen. Arch Environ Health 16:472, 1968

223. Poirier LA, Stober GD, Shimkin MB: Bioassay of alkyl halides and nucleotide base analogs by pulmonary tumor response in strain A mice. Cancer Res 35:1411, 1975

224. Creech JL, Johnson MN: Angiosarcoma of the liver in the manufacture of polyvinylchloride. J Occup Med 16:150, 1974

225. Viola PL, Bigotti A, Caputo A: Oncogenic response of rat skin, lungs, and bone to vinyl chloride. Cancer Res 31:516, 1971

226. Cavalieri E, Calvin M: Molecular characteristics of some carcinogenic hydrocarbons. Proc Natl Acad Sci USA 68:1251, 1971

227. Bruce DL, Eide KA, Linde HW, et al: Causes of death among anesthesiologists: A 20-year survey. Anesthesiology 29:565, 1968

228. Corbett TH, Cornell RG, Lieding K, et al: Incidence of cancer among Michigan nurse anesthetists. Anesthesiology 38:260, 1973

229. American Society of Anesthesiologists. Report of an ad hoc committee on the effect of trace anesthetics on the health of operating room personnel. Occupational Disease Among Operating Room Personnel: A National Study. Anesthesiology 41:321, 1974

230. Bruce DL, Eide KA, Smith NJ, et al: A prospective survey of anesthesiologist mortality, 1967–1971. Anesthesiology 41:71, 1974

231. Doll R, Peto R: Mortality among doctors in different occupations. Br Med J 1:1433, 1977

232. Lew EA: Mortality experience among anesthesiologists, 1954–1976. Anesthesiology 51:195, 1979

233. Tomlin PJ: Health problems of anaesthetists and their families in the West Midlands. Br J Med 1:779, 1979

234. Cohen EN, Brown BW, Wu M: Occupational disease in dentistry and chronic exposure to trace anesthetic gases. J Am Dent Assoc 101:21, 1980

235. Walts LF, Forsythe AB, Moore JG: Critique: Occupational disease among operating room personnel. Anesthesiology 42:608, 1975

236. Fink BR, Cullen BF: Anesthetic pollution: What is happening to us? Anesthesiology 45:79, 1976

237. Vessey MP: Epidemiological studies of the occupational hazards of anesthesia — A review. Anaesthesia 33:430, 1978

238. Buring JE, Hennekens CH, Mayrent SL, et al: Health experiences of operating room personnel. Anesthesiology 62:325, 1985

239. Department of Health, Education and Welfare, FDA: Chloroform as an ingredient of human drug and cosmetic products. Fed Reg 14:15026, 1976

240. National Cancer Institute: Carcinogenesis technical report series, No 2, Carcinogenesis bioassay of trichloroethylene, CAS No. 79-01-6, 1976

241. Oppenheimer BS, Oppenheimer ET, Danishefsky I, et al: Carcinogenic effect of metals in rodents. Cancer Res 16:439, 1956

242. Kucerova M, Zhurkov VS, Polivkova Z, et al: Mutagenic effect of epichlorohydrin, II. Analysis of chromosomal aberrations in lymphocytes of persons occupationally exposed to epichlorohydrin. Mutat Res 48:355, 1971

243. McCann J, Choi E, Yamasaki E, et al: The detection of carcinogens as mutagens in the *Salmonella*/microsome test: Assay of 300 chemicals, Part 1. Proc Natl Acad Sci USA 72:5135, 1975

244. Van Duuren BL, Goldschmidt BM, Katz C, et al: Carcinogenic activity of alkylating agents. J Natl Cancer Inst 53:695, 1974

245. Corbett TH: Cancer and congenital anomalies associated with anesthesia. Ann NY Acad Sci 271:58, 1976

246. Eger EI II, White AE, Brown CL, et al: A test of the carcinogenicity of enflurane, isoflurane, halothane, methoxyflurane and nitrous oxide in mice. Anesth Analg 57:678, 1978

247. Baden JM, Mazze RI, Wharton RS, et al: Carcinogenicity of halothane in Swiss/ICR mice. Anesthesiology 51:20, 1979

248. Baden JM, Egbert B, Mazze RI: Carcinogen bioassay of enflurane in mice. Anesthesiology, 56:9, 1982

249. Coate WB, Ulland BM, Lewis TR: Chronic exposure to low concentrations of halothane–nitrous oxide: Lack of carcinogenic effect in the rat. Anesthesiology 50:306, 1979

250. Klingberg MA, Weatherall JA (editors): Epidemiologic Methods for Detection of Teratogens. Basel, S Karger, 1979

251. Sturrock JE, Nunn JF: Mitosis in mammalian cells during exposure to anesthetics. Anesthesiology 43:21, 1975

252. Trudell JR: A unitary theory of anesthesia based on lateral phase separations in nerve membranes. Anesthesiology 46:5, 1977

253. Wilson JE (editor): Environment and Birth Defects. New York, Academic Press, 1973

254. Askrog V, Harvald B: Teratogen effect of inhalation anesthetics. Nord Med 83:498, 1970

255. Cohen EN, Bellville JW, Brown BW: Anesthesia, pregnancy and miscarriage: A study of operating room nurses and anesthetists. Anesthesiology 35:343, 1971

256. Knill-Jones RP, Moir DB, Rodrigues LV, et al: Anaesthetic practice and pregnancy: A controlled study of women anesthetists in the United Kingdom. Lancet 1:1326, 1972

257. Rosenberg P, Kirves A: Miscarriages among operating theatre staff. Acta Anaesthesiol Scand 53:37, 1973

258. Corbett TH, Cornell RG, Endres JL, et al: Birth defects among children of nurse anesthetists. Anesthesiology 41:341, 1974

259. Knill-Jones RP, Newman BJ, Spence AA: Anaesthetic practice and pregnancy: Controlled survey of male anaesthetists in the United Kingdom. Lancet 2:807, 1975

260. Cohen EN, Brown BW, Bruce DL, et al: A survey of anesthetic health hazards among dentists. J Am Dent Assoc 90:1291, 1975

261. Pharoah PO, Alberman E, Doyle P: Outcome of pregnancy among women in anaesthetic practice. Lancet 1:34, 1977

262. Ericson A, Kallen B: Survey of infants born in 1973 or 1975 to Swedish women working in operating rooms during their pregnancies. Anesth Analg 58:302, 1979

263. Axelsson G, Rylander R: Exposure to anesthetic gases and spontaneous abortion: Response in a postal questionnaire study. Int J Epidemiol 11:250, 1982

264. Shnider SM, Webster GM: Maternal and fetal hazards of surgery during pregnancy. Am J Obstet Gynecol 92:891, 1965

265. Smith BE: Fetal prognosis after anesthesia during gestation. Anesth Analg 42:521, 1963

266. Brodsky JB, Cohen EN, Brown BW, et al: Surgery during pregnancy and fetal outcome. Am J Obstet Gynecol 8:1165, 1980

267. McBride WG: Thalidomide and congenital anomalies. Lancet 2:1358, 1961

268. Ferstandig LL: Trace concentrations of anesthetic gases: A critical review of their disease potential. Anesth Analg 57:328, 1978

269. Shepard TH, Fink BR: Teratogenic activity of nitrous oxide in rats, Toxicity of Anesthetics. Edited by Fink BR. Baltimore, Williams & Wilkins, 1968, pp 308–323

270. Vieia E, Cleaton-Jones P, Austin JC, et al: Effects of low concentration of nitrous oxide on rat fetuses. Anesth Analg 59:175, 1980

271. Quimby KL, Katz J, Bowman RE: Behavioral consequences in rats from chronic exposure to 10 ppm halothane during early development. Anesth Analg 54:628, 1975

272. Quimby KL, Aschkanase LJ, Bowman RE, et al: Enduring learning deficits and cerebral synaptic malformation from exposure to 10 parts of halothane per million. Science 185:625, 1974

273. Chang LW, Dudley AWJ, Katz J: Pathological changes in the nervous system following exposure to halothane. Environ Res 11:40, 1976

274. Smith RF, Bowman RE, Katz J: Behavioral effects of exposure to halothane during pregnancy. Anesthesiology 49:319, 1978

275. Peters MA, Hudson AM: Postnatal development and behavior in offspring of enflurane exposed pregnant rats. Arch Int Pharmacol Ther 256:134, 1982

23

Pharmacology of Intravenous Narcotic Anesthetics

Peter L. Bailey, M.D.
Theodore H. Stanley, M.D.

INTRODUCTION

Opioids have been administered for hundreds of years to allay anxiety and reduce the pain associated with surgery.[1] Many of these compounds are not only used as intravenous analgesic supplements but also as primary or sole intravenous anesthetics. Some investigators have recently suggested that, with minor modifications, a number of new synthetic opioids may qualify as the "ideal intravenous anesthetic."[2-6] Others state that it is unrealistic to expect newer opioids to be markedly different from, or more efficacious as, analgesic/anesthetic agents than older compounds.[7] In this chapter, we discuss the pharmacology and use of naturally occurring and synthetic intravenous opioids in contemporary anesthetic practice. The terms "opioid," "narcotic analgesic," and "narcotic anesthetic" are used to describe drugs that specifically bind to any of several subspecies of opioid receptors and produce some opioid agonist effects.

HISTORY

The isolation of morphine from opium by Serturner in 1803 and the introduction of the syringe and hollow needle to clinical practice by Wood in 1853 finally permitted opioids to be administered in carefully measured doses.[1] Morphine then was frequently used intramuscularly for preoperative medication as a supplement during ether or chloroform anesthesia, and postoperatively for analgesia. Late in the nineteenth century, large amounts of morphine (1 to 2 mg/kg) plus scopolamine (1 to 3 mg/70 kg) were administered in divided doses intravenously, intramuscularly, or both, as a complete anesthetic.[8,9] Although initially popular, this technique rapidly fell into disfavor because of an alarming increase in operative morbidity and mortality.[1,10] For the next 30 to 40 years, anesthesiologists rarely used narcotic analgesics intraoperatively (also see Ch. 1).

Introduction of the ultra-short-acting barbiturates as intravenous anesthetics and popularization of the concept of "balanced anesthesia"[11] led to renewed enthusiasm for the intraoperative use of opioids. Two important events in this development were the synthesis of meperidine in 1939 and its use for anesthesia with nitrous oxide (N_2O) with or without d-tubocurarine.[12] Many variations of the "nitrous oxide-narcotic" technique became popular. At first, thiopental (as an induction agent and/or as an additional supplement during maintenance), d-tubocurarine (for muscular relaxation), and opioids such as morphine, meperidine, or α-prodine were used for nitrous oxide-narcotic anesthesia. After the introduction of Innovar-nitrous oxide anesthesia[13] (Innovar consists of droperidol, a tranquilizer, and fentanyl, a short-acting narcotic), a variety of intravenous supplements were employed (including hypnotics, sedatives, tranquilizers, and additional analgesics).[14-18] These techniques were often termed balanced anesthesia, presumably because each intravenously administered compound was selected and used for a specific purpose, such as analgesia, amnesia, muscle relaxation, or abolition of autonomic reflexes. More recently, opioids, as well as other analgesics (synthetic agonist/antagonists) and hypnotics, are being administered intravenously during anesthesia with potent inhaled anesthetics.[19] This practice is based on the belief that many of these drugs reduce the concentrations of inhaled anesthetics required for anesthesia and thus result in less depression of the cardiovascular and other organ systems.[20,21]

DeCastro[22] and Lowenstein et al.[23] reintroduced the concept that high doses of opioids could produce "complete" anesthesia. They administered fentanyl or morphine intravenously until consciousness was lost and then controlled ventilation with a high inspired concentration of oxygen. Morphine, 0.5 to 1.0 mg/kg, administered intravenously to patients while they breathed 100 percent oxygen did not alter the cardiovascular dynamics in those patients who did not have cardiac disease and in many cases improved the cardiovascular status of those with significant valvular disease. These reports led to many additional studies evaluating morphine and other opioids as the sole anesthetic for patients with poor cardiovascular reserve undergoing a major operative procedure.[24-27] Unfortunately, problems with incomplete amnesia,[28,29] histamine release,[29,30] prolonged postoperative respiratory depression,[31,32] increased blood volume requirements secondary to marked venovasodilation,[26] and hypertension[25] decreased the popularity of morphine as a "complete" anesthetic.

In contrast, the synthetic opioid fentanyl, has become popular as a component of balanced (nitrous oxide-narcotic) anesthesia,[13,27] as a supplement when using an inhaled anesthetic,[19] but also in larger (anesthetic) doses (50 to 150 μg/kg) as a primary or complete anesthetic.[2,3,29] Unfortunately, large doses of fentanyl also cause significant postoperative respiratory depression,[2,3] generally mitigating against their use in healthy patients undergoing more routine operative procedures. Nevertheless, as with anesthetic doses of morphine, large intravenous doses of fentanyl can produce complete anesthesia without depressing cardiovascular function and are ideal for patients who have little or no cardiovascular reserve. In addition, fentanyl-oxygen anesthesia produces less prolonged postoperative respiratory depression, greater cardiovascular stability, little or no histamine release, and no venovasodilation, as compared with morphine.[2,3,29-33]

Despite some problems (e.g., muscle rigidity, incomplete anesthesia), opioids will probably remain popular as anesthetic supplements and as complete anesthetics in the future because of their minimal effect on most organ systems.[2-6]

CLASSIFICATION

Opioids are usually classified as naturally occurring, semisynthetic, and synthetic (Table 23-1). Morphine, codeine, and papaverine, the only naturally occurring opioids of clinical significance, are obtained from the poppy plant, *Papaver somniferum*. These compounds can be divided into two chemical classes, the phenanthrenes (morphine and codeine) and the benzylisoquinoline derivatives (papaverine). Of the naturally occurring opioids, only morphine is of importance as an intravenous analgesic or anesthetic.

The semisynthetic opioids are derivatives of morphine in which any one of several changes has been made, such as etherification of one hydroxyl group (codeine), esterification of both hydroxyl groups (heroin), oxidation of the alcoholic hydroxyl to a ketone, or reduction of a double bond on the benzene ring (*d*-hydromorphone hydrochloride (Dilaudid). Thebaine derivatives used clinically to provide analgesia include oxymorphone and oxycodone. Etorphine (M99), another thebaine derivative, is several thousand times more potent than morphine; this compound has been used successfully for immobilization and anesthesia in wildlife management.[34]

The synthetic compounds resemble morphine but are usually entirely synthesized. They are divided into four groups: the mor-phinan derivatives (levorphanol), the diphenyl or methadone derivatives (methadone, *d*-propoxyphene), the benzomorphans (phenazocine, pentazocine), and the phenylpiperidine derivatives (meperidine, fentanyl) (Fig. 23-1). Important opiate receptor research compounds (ketocyclazocine and SKF 10,047) also belong to this group. Although many of these opioids have been used intravenously for analgesia or anesthesia experimentally, only the phenylpiperidine derivatives currently play an important role in anesthesia.

MECHANISM

The mechanism of action of opioid compounds can be explained in terms of their structure, site of action, and their interaction with endogenous CNS peptides.

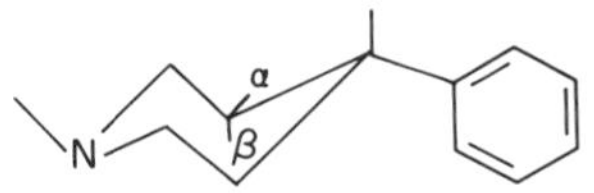

TABLE 23-1. Classification of Opioid Compounds

Naturally occurring
  Morphine
  Codeine
  Papaverine
  Thebaine

Semisynthetic
  Heroin
  Dihydromorphone/morphinone
  Thebaine derivatives (e.g., etorphine)

Synthetic
  Morphinan series (e.g., levorphanol)
  Diphenylpropylamine series (e.g., methadone)
  Benzomorphinan series (e.g., pentazocine)
  Phenylpiperidine series (e.g., fentanyl, sufentanil)

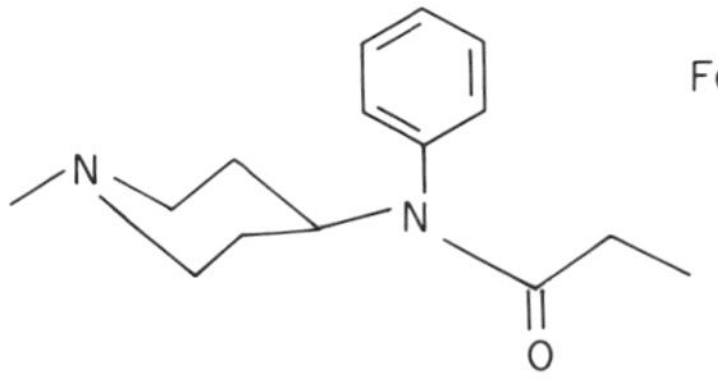

FIG. 23-1 The phenylpiperidine skeleton structure and synthetic phenylpiperidine opioids, meperidine and fentanyl.

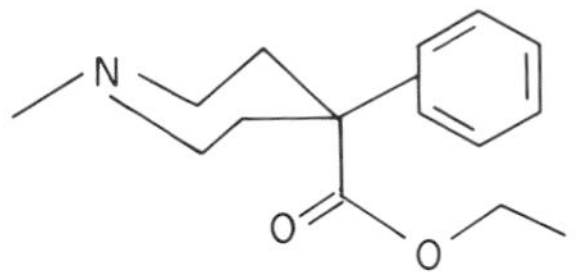

STRUCTURE – ACTIVITY RELATIONSHIP

The structural dissimilarities among compounds displaying opiate activity almost defy a common mechanism as the basis for opioid structure–activity relationships. However, a detailed analysis of opioid stereospecificity has been used to describe a hypothetical three-dimensional model of the opiate receptor responsible for opioid activity.[35] Structurally, opioids are complex, three-dimensional compounds that usually exist as two optical isomers, that is, molecules that are mirror images of each other and identical in chemical composition but that cannot be superimposed.[36] Usually only the *l*-rotatory isomer is capable of producing analgesia.

A close relationship exists between the stereochemical structure of an opioid compound and the presence or absence of analgesic activity.[37,38] Indeed, relatively minor molecular changes such as the degree of ionization produced by variations in pH may cause significant alteration in pharmacologic activity of opioid compounds.[38]

The prototype opioid is morphine. Its rigid pentacyclic structure conforms to a **T** shape[35] (Fig. 23-2). Morphine demonstrates several other structural characteristics common to most opioids: a tertiary positively charged basic nitrogen, a quaternary carbon (C-13 in morphine) that is separated from the basic nitrogen by an ethane chain ($—CH_2—CH_2—$) and attached to a phenyl group, a phenolic hydroxyl group (in morphine derivatives) or ketone group (meperidine, methadone), and the presence of an aromatic ring whose center is 4.55 angstroms from the nitrogen atom.[35,39,40]

The morphine molecule also contains a phenylpiperidine structure (an aromatic ring attached to a six-membered ring containing five carbons and one nitrogen). This moiety is seen in opioids that otherwise seem unrelated to morphine.[35] Short-chain alkyl group substitution at the basic amino group (the group essential for opioid activity) results in mixed opioid agonist/antagonists.[47] Additional hydroxylation of C-14 produces opioids with antagonist and no agonist properties.[41] Phenylalanine and tyrosine may be important structural elements of the endogenous opioids (enkephalins and endorphins) and other endogenous opioidlike neural transmitters and modulators.[42,43] A more detailed description of additional structure–activity relationships and their stereochemical implications is beyond the scope of this chapter but has recently been reviewed.[35]

SITE OF ACTION: OPIATE RECEPTORS

In 1973 three independent investigators described the presence of an "opioid receptor" in nervous tissue and hypothesized that endogenous substances probably stimulate this structure.[44–46] A few years later, the endogenous opiates were discovered.

The lock-and-key analogy for the recep-

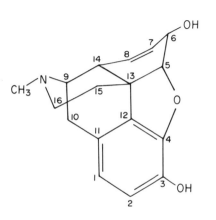

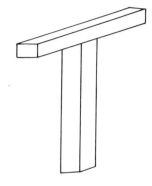

FIG. 23-2 The T-shaped molecule of morphine.

tor–agonist opioid interactions, although surely an oversimplification, appears to be reasonably accurate. While agonist and antagonist opioids have both been described as "fitting" into the lock, only the agonist is able to "turn in the lock." Thus, pure antagonist opioids have intrinsic activities or efficacies of 0, while pure agonist opioids have intrinsic activities of 1. Some opioids (i.e., mixed agonist-antagonists) exhibit intermediate intrinsic activities.

The individual profile of a receptor is derived from the potency and the physiologic effects of a variety of agonists and agonist-antagonists, agonist–antagonist interactions, the results of various bioassay and binding studies, structure–activity relationship data, and numerous other screening evaluations. For example, potency usually correlates well with receptor affinity and is described by the IC_{50} value (the concentration of an agent that lowers the specific binding of ^3H-naloxone by 50 percent). The greater the affinity of a drug for the receptor, the lower the IC_{50}.[47]

Agonist and antagonist interactions can be quantified by the pA_2 (the negative log of the concentration of antagonist that doubles the concentration of agonist necessary to produce a particular response).[48] Numerous studies have shown that the pA_2 of naloxone for a variety of pure agonist opioids is 7. This suggests a common receptor mechanism.[49,50] In contrast, a pA_2 of 6 for [d-Ala^2-d-Leu^5]enkephalin implies that this particular opioid acts on a different receptor.[51] Bioassay systems are used to help evaluate potency. The two most important of these systems are the guinea pig ileum (GPI) and mouse vas deferens (MVD) (morphine inhibits electrically induced contraction of the isolated guinea pig ileum). Data from these systems correlate well with opioid analgesic potency[52] as determined via numerous intact animal and clinical evaluations. Biochemical characterization of the opiate receptor (synaptosomal protein and lipid), binding assays, and biochemical treatments are other tools that have been used in receptor research.[47]

Soon after the structures of some of the endogenous opioids were determined, differences were noted in their activity, particularly when they were compared with morphine in bioassay systems. As a result, investigators suggested that separate and/or different receptors of these compounds exist, such as a μ-receptor for morphine and a δ-receptor or enkephalin. These proposals were supported by CNS binding and autoradiographic studies[53,54]; for example, the IC_{50} for morphine is 70 times greater at the Δ-receptor than at the μ-receptor. The picture soon became even more complex. Although enkephalins and morphine do not show cross-tolerance in bioassay systems, that is, guinea pig ileum and mouse vas deferens evaluations, they do in analgesic studies. Thus, it appears that analgesia is probably mediated through a number of receptors, some with high affinity for narcotic analgesics, the μ_1-receptors, and some with low affinity, the μ_2- and δ-receptors.[55,56] Furthermore, the concentration and proportion of the receptor subtypes seem to change with time and body location; for example, μ_1-receptors increase in number and concentration as mice grow older and thus provide more analgesia after a similar dose of an opioid agonist.[57] μ_1-Receptors also appear more prominent in supraspinal analgesia, whereas δ-receptors may be more important for spinal analgesia.[58] Numerous other opioid receptor subtypes seem to play a role in endogenous opioid neurotransmission and as modulators of other receptor–transmitter systems (Table 23-2). For example, the κ-receptor agonist ethylketocyclazocine (EKC) produces sedation and analgesia without causing appreciable respiratory depression.[59] κ-Receptor activation may explain in part some of the effects

TABLE 23-2. Tentative Classification of Opioid-Binding Sites

Class of Site	Prototypic Compound
μ	Morphine
$\quad\mu_1$	
$\quad\mu_2$	
κ	Ketocyclazocine
σ	N-Allylnormetazocine (SKF 10,047)
$\quad\sigma_1$	
$\quad\sigma_2$	
δ	Enkephalin
ϵ	β-Endorphin

Pasternak GW, Childers SR: Opiates, opioid peptides and their receptors, Critical Care: State of the Art. Vol. V. Edited by Shoemaker WM. Society of Critical Care Medicine, Fullerton, CA 1984, pp (F)1–60.

TABLE 23-3. Opiate Actions in the Chronic Spinal Dog

	μ Morphine	κ Ketocyclazocine	σ SKF 10,047
Pupil	Miosis	Miosis	Mydriasis
Respiratory rate	Stimulation, then depression	No change	Stimulation
Heart rate	Bradycardia	No change	Tachycardia
Body temperature	Hypothermia	No change	No change
Affect	Indifference	Sedation	Delirium
Nociceptive reflexes			
Flexor	Decrease	Decrease	Moderate decrease
Skin twitch	Decrease	No effect	No effect

(Iwamato ET, Martin WR: Multiple opioid receptors. Med Res Rev 1:411, 1981.)

(analgesia with limited respiratory depression) of some mixed agonist-antagonists such as nalbuphine[60] (Table 23-3).

Opiate receptors are found in many areas in the CNS, including the cerebral cortex, the limbic cortex (anterior and posterior amygdala and hippocampus), hypothalamus, medial thalamus, midbrain (periaqueductal gray), extrapyramidal area (caudate, striatum, and putamen), substantia gelatinosa, and sympathetic preganglionic neurons.[59,61] Gray matter has more receptors than does white matter (Table 23-4). Structures and pathways involved with pain usually contain the highest concentrations of opiate receptors[62]; however, the presence of opioid receptors in other areas of the CNS (e.g., basal ganglia, limbic area, cerebral cortex) suggests other roles for the endogenous opiates and their receptors.

The periaqueductal gray area is one of the few regions in the CNS in which microinjections of morphine or direct electrical stimulation produce analgesia that can be blocked with naloxone.[63-65] Stimulation of periaqueductal gray receptors with morphine, electric-ity, or the endogenous opiate-like peptides may result in a barrage of impulses that move down the CNS and inhibit the transmission of nociceptive information from peripheral nerves into the spinal cord.[65] The integrity of certain neurotransmitter systems connecting the pain-inhibiting system in the brain to the spinal cord is necessary for morphine to exert its full analgesic action. Satoh and Takagi[66] found that morphine blockade of transmission of spinal cord potentials evoked by painful stimulation is inhibited by high spinal cord transection.

Unfortunately, this theory of descending inhibition does not entirely explain the analgesic action of morphine. The substantia gelatinosa of the spinal cord also possesses a dense collection of opiate receptors.[36,67,68] Direct application of narcotics to these receptors creates intense analgesia. Undoubtedly, narcotics produce analgesia by acting at receptors both in the spinal cord and in higher centers. Opiate receptors are also localized in the substantia gelatinosa of the caudal spinal trigeminal nucleus, the nucleus receiving pain fibers from the face and hands via branches of the 5th, 7th,

TABLE 23-4. μ and δ Opiate Receptors in Rat Brain Regions

Predominantly μ	Predominantly δ	μ and δ
Laminae I and IV of cerebral cortex	Laminae II, III, and V of cerebral cortex	Laminae VI of cerebral cortex
Streaks and clusters in corpus striatum	Diffuse grains in corpus striatum	Nucleus tractus solitarius
Thalamus (dorsomedial, ventral)	Amygdala	Vagal fibers
Hypothalamus	Nucleus accumbens	Nucleus ambiquus
Hippocampus (pyramidal cell layer)	Olfactory tubercle	Substantia gelatinosa of spinal cord
Periaqueductal gray	Pontine nuclei	Trigerminal nucleus
Interpenduncular nucleus		
Inferior colliculus		
Midbrain median raphe		

(Goodman RR, Snyder SH, Kuhar MJ, et al: Differentiation of delta and mu opiate receptor localizations by light microscopic autoradiography. Proc Natl Acad Sci USA 77:6239, 1980.)

9th, and 10th cranial nerves.[63] Within the brain stem, opiate receptors are highly concentrated in the solitary nuclei that receive visceral sensory fibers from the 9th and 10th cranial nerves and the area postrema. Stimulation of the solitary nuclei depresses gastric secretion and the cough reflex and causes orthostatic hypotension. Stimulation of the area postrema with its chemoreceptor trigger zone results in nausea and vomiting.

The clinical implications of opiate receptor physiology are just beginning to be understood. Morphine and most opioids are effective in relieving dull, boring, poorly localized, visceral-type pain but are not nearly as effective in influencing highly localized somatic pain.[63] The lateral thalamic nuclei are involved with highly localized pain, whereas the medial thalamic nuclei mediate poorly localized and emotionally influenced pain. As might be expected, higher concentrations of opiate receptors are found in medial than in lateral thalamic nuclei.

Opioid receptor occupancy is highly correlated with analgesia and anesthesia in rats.[69] Increasing doses of the highly potent synthetic μ-receptor-stimulating opioid, lofentanil, produce increasing analgesia and finally, at 25 to 30 percent receptor occupancy, anesthesia.[69]

ENDOGENOUS OPIATES

The discovery of opioid receptors in the CNS led to the hypothesis, and later the discovery, of endogenous opiate-like substances. Hughes et al.[70] first described two brain pentapeptides, methionine-enkephalin and leucine-enkephalin, that shared a four-amino acid sequence (Tyr-Gly-Gly-Phe), had potent affinities for opiate binding sites, and whose opiate effects were reversed by naloxone. Larger endogenous opioid peptides, β-endorphin[71] and dynorphin,[72] were also described.

The biosynthesis of all these endogenous opiates is complex. It is now known that pro-opiocortin, a prohormone with a molecular weight of 30,000, is cleaved to form adrenocorticotropic hormone (ACTH) and a substance called β-lipotropin (β-LPH).[47] β-LPH is devoid

of opioid activity and in turn is cleaved to yield β-endorphin.[73]

The enkephalins have different precursors than those of β-endorphin, although the amino acid sequence for methionine-enkephalin is contained in β-LPH (amino acid sequence 61–65). Proenkephalin, a peptide with a molecular weight of 30,000, is the precursor for Met-enkephalin and several other enkephalins.[74] Dynorphin, one of the more recently described endogenous opioids, is derived from a third precursor, called prodynorphin. Thus, differential biochemical processing of endogenous opiates parallels regional differences in endogenous opiate structure, distribution, and concentration.[47] In spite of their differences, all three families of endogenous opioids possess the common amino acid sequence, Tyr-Gly-Gly-Phe.

The endogenous opiates exist in virtually all vertebrate species and in many invertebrates as well.[75] The highest concentrations of β-endorphin occur in the pituitary gland (anterior and intermediate lobes greater than posterior lobe) and in the medial basal and arcuate region of the hypothalamus.[76] Some long-axoned endorphin-releasing neurons synapse at upper brain stem locations including diencephalic, telencephalic, medullary, and spinal cord nuclei.[77] β-Endorphin also exists outside the CNS, in the small intestine, placenta, and plasma.[78,79] By contrast, enkephalins are widely distributed in many areas of the CNS (amygdala, globus pallidus, striatum, hypothalamus, thalamus, brainstem, spinal cord dorsal horn laminae I and II, and in the peripheral nervous system (peripheral ganglia, autonomic nervous system, adrenal medulla), as well as the gastrointestinal tract and plasma.[47] The distribution of dynorphins is less well described, but high concentrations are found in the hypothalamus.[47] Although the physiologic functions and roles of the endogeneous opiates are not precisely defined, they appear to have a role in neurotransmission and its regulation.

Many of the endogenous opiates interact with opioid receptors to modulate pain perception and produce analgesia. Most of these peptides are indistinguishable from morphine in their activity in synaptosomal opiate-binding assays.[80] The enkephalins and most of the endorphins are, on a molar basis, about as active as morphine.[80] By contrast, β-endorphin is 5 to 10 times more potent than morphine. Unfortunately, the analgesic potency of the enkephalins is difficult to evaluate in vivo, because they are rapidly degraded when injected intravenously or directly into cerebral ventricles. Endorphins, however, have been shown to produce analgesia for as long as 15 to 60 minutes. Interestingly, some endorphins appear to produce analgesia in specific body areas (i.e., the face and neck), whereas β-endorphin produces analgesia of the entire body.

It is unknown where and how the endogenous opiates interact and affect pain perception or physiologic responses following recognition of pain. Enkephalin fibers and terminals exist in high density in the marginal zone, substantia gelatinosa, and lateral region of the nucleus proprius of the spinal cord dorsal horn and trigeminal caudalis. These areas receive primary afferent nociceptors and give rise to spinothalamic or trigeminothalamic projections.[77] Just how the many substances located within the dorsal horn, such as substance P, 5-hydroxytryptamine (5-HT), enkephalin, and γ-aminobutyric acid (GABA), interact with endogenous opiates, opioid receptors, and pain pathways is complex and incompletely understood. Similarly, the periaqueductal gray, rich in enkephalins, sends fibers to the raphe nuclei of the brainstem. The raphe nuclei are serotonergic and project to the spinal cord gray via the dorsolateral funiculus. This descending pathway can suppress the response of spinothalamic cells to nociception.[81] It is unclear whether and how the endogenous opioids and opioid receptors are involved in this pathway.

ANALGESIA-AMNESIA-ANESTHESIA

The reintroduction in 1969 of morphine plus oxygen as an anesthetic technique for patients with heart disease was based on the premise that large doses of morphine could produce anesthesia without significant changes in cardiovascular dynamics. Unfortunately, problems such as occasional bronchospasm and severe hypotension during induction of anesthesia, as well as hypertension and tachycardia with surgical stimulation, increased blood requirements during and after operation, prolonged postoperative respiratory depression, and other complications resulted in disenchantment with "morphine anesthesia."[7] These problems also stimulated the evaluation of other more potent opioids such as fentanyl, sufentanil, and alfentanil and other synthetic opioids as anesthetics or principal components of the narcotic-based anesthetic state. Many of these studies demonstrated that as potency increased, undesirable side effects of narcotic analgesics decreased. Opioids, particularly pure μ-receptor stimulating agonists, produce unconsciousness and anesthesia in humans when given in high enough doses. Yet some investigators still believe that opioids—all of them—should not be expected to produce unconsciousness and anesthesia.[7,82] Reports demonstrating that fentanyl is only able to decrease the minimal alveolar concentration (MAC) of isoflurane approximately 65 percent in dogs, and similar studies in rats and experimental animals, are often submitted as evidence in support of this position.[164] Unfortunately, equieffective doses of narcotic analgesics and many other intravenous sedative-hypnotics and anesthetics vary enormously in different species.[84] Thus, dosage requirements for some opioids (fentanyl) are 30 times higher in dogs than in humans. Furthermore, metabolic processing of opioids is often dramatically different in the dog and other animals than in humans. Clearly, data obtained from animals using doses of opioids and infusion schemes similar to those used in the clinical setting are of questionable relevance when applied to humans.

Still, incomplete amnesia remains an occasional problem with low and high doses of opioid-based anesthesia. In virtually all cases, recall of pain is rare. A most likely reason for awareness and/or inadequate anesthesia during narcotic analgesic-based anesthesia is the difficulty of reliably predicting the appropriate dose of an opioid in any individual patient. Generally, healthier patients, that is, American Society of Anesthesiologists (ASA) class I or II, with normal or high cardiac outputs prior to anesthesia require larger doses of narcotics for anesthesia than do patients who have serious metabolic disease, cardiovascular limitations, or reduced cardiac output.[2,3,32,86] Older patients experience higher blood and presumably brain concentrations of opioids than do younger patients. Most likely this explains the ease with which they are rendered anesthetic with opioids[86] (Table 23-5). Patients' habits (e.g., smoking, alcohol consumption) may also influence anesthetic requirements.[87] Undoubtedly, differences in plasma protein binding, fat solubility, hepatic metabolism, renal excretion, and regional perfusion influence requirements for opioids as well. How and why all these factors influence opioid and analgesic and anesthetic requirements in humans is unknown. However, if data obtained in rat receptor-binding studies are applicable, the answer may lie in determining and ensuring that the percentage of CNS opioid-receptor occupation necessary for anesthesia is achieved in every patient.[69] This will undoubtedly be difficult for many reasons, not the least of which relates to variability of opioid requirements in the same individual. Indeed, acute tolerance, as seen with barbiturates, may occur with opioids. Awakening or absence of analgesia can take place at higher plasma opioid levels than are associated with initial loss of consciousness or onset of analgesia.[88]

When an opioid is used in large doses as a complete anesthetic or with supplements, such as nitrous oxide or other intravenous compounds, there are few reliable, measurable clinical indications of amnesia. This too contributes to the problem of inadequate anesthesia. Profound analgesia and apnea can easily be achieved with opioids without producing anesthesia.[26] While administration of supplements (nitrous oxide, diazepam, droperidol) or of larger doses of narcotic anesthetics will increase the likelihood of amnesia, they do not guarantee it.[86] Furthermore, undesirable side effects such as prolonged postoperative respiratory depression and cardiovascular depression are frequent after administration of some supplements.[14,15,89]

The reported frequency of awareness with fentanyl anesthesia in human subjects is comparable to that with inhaled anesthetics.[90-95] Nonetheless, concern about the occurrence of awareness remains legitimate. Hypertension and traumatic neurosis (consisting of repetitive nightmares, anxiety, preoccupation with death, and patient resistance to talking about recall) can occur.[93,96] Awareness associated with anesthesia is best dealt with by preoperatively informing patients of its possibility and by frank and open discussion of such an episode postoperatively. Direct explanation may be most helpful to a reluctant and fearful patient.[96]

TABLE 23-5. Unconsciousness As a Function of Age in 72 Patients Given Fentanyl (30 μg/kg) for Induction of Anesthesia*

Age (years)	Rendered Unconscious (%)
18–30	57
31–45	77
46–60	53
>60	100

*Chi^2 = 4.787; P = 0.0287.
(Bailey PL, Wilbrink J, Zwanikken P, et al: Anesthetic induction with fentanyl. Anesth Analg 64:48, 1985.)

CARDIOVASCULAR ACTIONS

The discussion of the cardiovascular effects of narcotic analgesics concentrates on morphine and fentanyl (Sublimaze) and to a lesser extent meperidine (Demerol). The new opioids, alfentanil and sufentanil, are also discussed but in less detail, as less information is available at this time. Although hypotension, hypertension, bradycardia, and numerous other cardiovascular problems were reported after morphine administration, those side effects seem to occur less frequently when fentanyl is used.[2,23] The newer, more potent opioid, sufentanil, also usually produces minimal changes in cardiovascular dynamics.[97,98] In fact, administration of morphine, 1 mg/kg IV, usually does not cause significant circulatory changes in patients with or without cardiac disease.[23] In patients with aortic valvular disease, stroke volume and cardiac output may be increased after morphine administration, probably because the compound does not result in myocardial depression but does decrease systemic vascular resistance, at least transiently.[23,99,100] Vasko and co-workers[101] found that morphine has a significant positive inotropic effect that is dependent on endogenous catecholamine release in dogs. This action is inhibited by β-adrenergic blocking agents or by previous adrenalectomy. Morphine has also been found to increase blood and urine catecholamine concentrations in a dose-dependent manner in patients with cardiac disease.[102–104]

Although large doses (0.5 to 30 mg/kg) of fentanyl produce significant increases in plasma catecholamines in dogs,[105] anesthetic doses of fentanyl (24 to 75 μg/kg) decrease rather than increase plasma catecholamine and cortisol concentrations in humans.[106] The effect of fentanyl on plasma catecholamines may be dose dependent. Hicks et al.[107] noted elevated plasma norepinephrine levels after 15 μg/kg of fentanyl, but normal (baseline) values after 50 μg/kg in human subjects. Anesthetic doses of sufentanil also do not change circulating catecholamine concentrations. Most investigators have reported that fentanyl has no effect on myocardial contractility or cardiac output.[2,108,109] However, others have reported negative[107] or positive[20] inotropic effects, and still others a myocardial depression-sparing action of fentanyl during halothane and enflurane anesthesia.[20,21]

Despite these minimal cardiovascular effects of opioids, significant hypotension, hypertension, and cardiac dysrhythmias have been reported after the administration of virtually all opioid compounds in some patients. Therefore, certain precautions should be observed during the induction and maintenance of anesthesia with morphine and other opioids.

HYPOTENSION

MORPHINE

Hypotension can occur during and after administration of even small doses of morphine (5 to 10 mg IV).[110] With anesthetic doses (1 to 4 mg/kg IV), profound hypotension can occur.[28,111] Indeed, Conahan et al.[111] found an incidence of hypotension (systolic blood pressure <70 mm Hg) of 10 percent during anesthetic induction with morphine in patients about to undergo cardiac valvular surgery.

Several mechanisms, including vagal-induced bradycardia, venous and arterial vasodilation, and splanchnic sequestration of blood, may explain some of the hypotension observed after morphine anesthesia. Rate of morphine infusion also appears to be important in producing and/or avoiding hypotension. Hypotension is not uncommon when the infusion rate is 10 mg/min but is rare when it is ≤5 mg/min.[112] Rate of infusion seems to have less of an effect on blood pressure after fentanyl and sufentanil but may be important with alfentanil.

Morphine, 1 mg/kg, produces marked increases in plasma histamine in some patients (Table 23-6). These changes usually result in an increase in cardiac index and in decreased arterial blood pressure and systemic vascular resistance.[113] Similar cardiovascular changes occur when patients are pretreated with diphenhydramine (a histamine H_1-antagonist) or cimetidine (a histamine H_2-antagonist) before morphine. However, in patients pretreated with both H_1- and H_2-antagonists, the cardiovascular responses are significantly attenuated despite comparable increases in plasma histamine concentrations. These data and other reports[114–116] strongly suggest that many of the hemodynamic effects of morphine may be caused by histamine and indicate a possible means of preventing these changes. Significant hypotension rarely occurs with high-dose fentanyl anesthesia, possibly because, unlike morphine, fentanyl does not produce increases in plasma histamine.[113] Sufentanil and alfentanil do not produce changes in plasma histamine.[33]

Morphine has been shown to reduce venous and arterial tone both in experimental animals and in human subjects, which results in a decrease in venous return to the heart and may contribute to hypotension.[23,26,117–122] Arterial dilation occurs sooner and is of shorter duration than venodilation after morphine.[120,123] The degree of venodilation is dose related and necessitates an increase in the volume of blood and/or crystalloid fluids to maintain adequate

TABLE 23-6.   Correlations of Histamine Release and Cardiac Index, Heart Rate, Blood Pressure, and System Vascular Resistance During Administration of Morphine (1 mg/kg)

Period	BP (mm Hg)	Diastolic BP (mm Hg)	CI (l/min/m²)	HR (beats/min)	SVR (mm Hg/L min)	Venous Histamine (pg/ml)
I Control	88 ± 4	71 ± 3	2.4 ± 0.2	57 + 2	15.5 ± 1	880 ± 163
II Placebo	85 ± 3	67 ± 2	2.6 ± 0.1	57 = 2	14.8 ± 1	657 ± 98
III One-third in	79 ± 5	61 ± 4*	2.8 ± 0.1	58 = 2	12.2 ± 1*	2.467 ± 1.208*
IV 2 min after	61 ± 4*	45 ± 4*	3.0 ± 0.2	59 = 3	9.0 ± 1*	7.437 ± 2.684*
V 5 min after	73 ± 8	59 ± 7*	2.9 ± 0.3	64 = 4	11.5 ± 1*	4.980 ± 1.681*
VI 10 min after	74 ± 5	57 ± 5*	2.7 ± 0.2	59 = 4	12.7 ± 1*	3.307 ± 1.090*

* $P < 0.05$ compared with control.
Abbreviations used: BP = blood pressure; CI = cardiac index; HR = heart rate; SVR = systemic vascular resistance.
(Moss J, Rosow CE: Histamine release by narcotics and muscle relaxants in humans. Anesthesiology 59:330, 1983.)

ventricular filling pressure.[26,120] Patients anesthetized with halothane as compared with those anesthesized with morphine have increased blood requirements during and after operation (see Table 23-7). Venodilation and increased blood requirements apparently do not occur with lower doses of morphine (<0.5 mg/kg) plus N_2O.

Although morphine reduces venous return to the heart in the dog by causing hepatic sequestration of plasma,[121,122] there is no evidence that this mechanism is of any significance in humans. Others have suggested that venous vasodilation after large doses of morphine is the primary cause for decreased venous return.[26,120,123] This is not caused by the preservatives present in commercial preparations of the drug[123] but may be related to a reflex mechanism(s). Zelis and co-workers[124]

found that morphine selectively impairs certain sympathetic reflexes involving peripheral veins. Their data suggested that this response was due to a CNS action of the drug. Vasodilation after morphine may also be due to a direct effect of morphine on vascular smooth muscle.[113,117,123] Venoconstriction in response to tilting or inhalation of carbon dioxide is also impaired by morphine.[125] In dogs, hypotension after large doses of morphine (1 mg/kg) has been attributed to changes in distribution of blood flow.[126] Although not associated with sustained decreases in cardiac output, blood pressure, or total peripheral resistance, Priano and Vatner[126] found 1 and 3 mg/kg of morphine to produce significant decreases in mesenteric and renal blood flow in dogs.

The hypotension that occurs after morphine does not cause significant myocardial

TABLE 23-7.   Blood Requirements During Operation and for the First Postoperative Day in 61 Patients Anesthetized with Morphine (1-4 mg/kg) plus Oxygen or Halothane (0.1-1.5%) Plus 30% Nitrous Oxide and Oxygen and Undergoing Aortic Valve Replacement or Coronary Artery Bypass Operation

Pathology	Anesthetic	Mean blood Requirements (ml) Intraoperative	Postoperative
Aortic valvular disease	Morphine	2,800*	1,652*
	Halothane	1,010	757
Coronary artery disease	Morphine	2,705*	1,417*
	Halothane	1,750	722

* $P < 0.05$. Student's paired *t*-test when compared to halothane values.
(Modified from Stanley TH, Gray NH, Isern-Amaral JH, et al: Comparison of blood requirements during morphine and halothane anesthesia for open-heart surgery. Anesthesiology 41:34, 1974.)

depression, although in healthy volunteers morphine (2 mg/kg) does cause a prolongation of the preejection period, an estimate of isovolumetric cardiac contractility.[127,128] High doses of morphine (3 mg/kg) acutely activate the sympathoadrenal system (while producing peripheral vasodilation).[129] These changes could counteract any myocardial depressant effects of the opioid. On the other hand, increases in sympathetic activity could be detrimental in some patients. Indeed, Moffitt et al.[100] showed that 1 mg/kg of morphine may not inhibit lactate production and can produce ischemia with surgical stimulation in patients undergoing coronary artery bypass operations. In summary, hypotension from morphine can be minimized or eliminated by pretreatment with H_1- and H_2-histamine antagonists, use of a slow drug-infusion rate, volume loading, and/or placement of patients in a Trendelenburg (head-down) position.

MEPERIDINE

Hypotension also occurs after the intravenous administration of meperidine. Indeed, meperidine has been studied in isolated cardiac preparations, intact dogs, and human subjects in a variety of experimental conditions by several investigators.[130-136] Meperidine also causes significant increases of plasma histamine.[115] Most investigations indicate that meperidine decreases myocardial contractility[136] and that, even in low doses (2 to 2.5 mg/kg), causes a significant drop in arterial blood pressure, peripheral resistance, and cardiac output. The latter are often accompanied by tachycardia in intact animals[130-132,135] and man.[133,134]

Anesthetic doses of meperidine (10 mg/kg IV) are associated with marked decreases in cardiac output and frequently cause cardiac arrest in dogs[130] (Fig. 23-3). The cardiovascular depression seen with meperidine in animal experiments appears to be due to peripheral vasodilation and to a decrease in myocardial contractility.[130,132,135,136] When equianalgesic doses of meperidine were compared with morphine, meperidine was found to be 20 times more depressant to the contractile element of the isolated cat papillary muscle than was observed

with morphine.[136] In contrast to morphine, meperidine rarely results in bradycardia but can cause tachycardia. This may be due to its structural similarity to atropine. Because of its more significant cardiovascular actions, meperidine has little value as a "complete anesthetic" and may be a detriment to patients who have little cardiovascular reserve, even in small doses.

α-PRODINE

α-Prodine, which is structurally similar to meperidine, has had limited use as an analgesic supplement in patients in the operating room and delivery suite. Despite the fact that α-prodine is somewhat shorter acting than meperidine, it possesses all of the latter's cardiovascular depressant qualities.[137]

FENTANYL

Fentanyl, in analgesic (2 to 10 μg/kg) or anesthetic (30 to 100 μg/kg) doses, rarely causes decreases in blood pressure, even in pa-

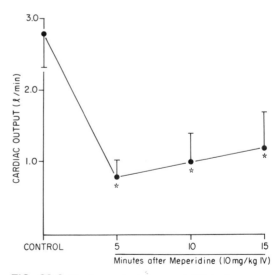

FIG. 23-3 Cardiac output (mean ±SD) before and after meperidine (10 mg/kg IV) in nine basally anesthetized (sodium thiopental) mongrel dogs. *$P < 0.0.01$, one-way analysis of variance. (T.H. Stanley, unpublished data.)

tients with poor left ventricular (LV) function.[2,27,107,108,136,138,139] Some investigators believe that absence of hypotension after fentanyl is related to this opioid's lack of effect on plasma histamine concentrations.

Most evidence indicates that fentanyl produces little or no change in myocardial contractility,[2,20,108,109,140] although a few workers have reported a negative inotropic effect.[107,113,141] Virtually all hemodynamic variables, including heart rate, arterial blood pressure, cardiac output, systemic and pulmonary vascular resistance, and pulmonary artery occlusion or wedge pressure, remain unchanged during anesthetic induction with fentanyl.[2,108,113,138,139,141] Hypotension does occasionally occur (usually due to bradycardia) but can be either prevented or attenuated by prophylactic premedication with atropine or glycopyrrolate or antagonized with ephedrine or pancuronium.[143,144] The use of adjuvants to supplement opioid anesthesia results in a higher incidence of hypotension (see below).

SUFENTANIL

Sufentanil is a new synthetic opioid that is approximately 5 to 10 times more potent than fentanyl, with a therapeutic index (LD_{50}/ED_{50}) approximately 100 times greater than that of the latter (25,000 versus 277) in rats.[145] Sufentanil was approved for clinical use by the Federal Drug Administration (FDA) in 1984 as an anesthetic supplement and complete anesthetic. The cardiovascular actions of sufentanil are similar to those of fentanyl. However, sufentanil may be more effective in blocking sympathetic activation during surgical stimulation, especially in patients more susceptible to intraoperative hypertension. Like fentanyl, sufentanil results in no change in plasma histamine concentrations.[33]

ALFENTANIL

Alfentanil is one-fourth as potent as fentanyl. This particularly short-acting agent also has a high therapeutic index (1,080) in rats.[146]

These actions have indicated that the drug may have use as an anesthetic induction agent or analgesic supplement, especially in patients undergoing short operative procedures. Studies in dogs demonstrated little change in hemodynamics with moderate doses (160 μg/kg) of alfentanil, while very large doses (5 mg/kg) resulted in transient cardiac stimulation (increases in LV contractility, aortic blood flow velocity, and acceleration).[132] Heart rate, cardiac output, and pulmonary and systemic vascular resistance also increased following 5 mg/kg of alfentanil. Others have reported transient increases in myocardial contractility, mean aortic, pulmonary artery, left and right atrial pressures, and increased systemic vascular resistance[147] with lower doses (200 μg/kg) of alfentanil in dogs.[148] Although induction of anesthesia with alfentanil (35 to 150 μg/kg) in patients with and in patients without cardiac disease has been reported to be fast (45 to 140 seconds) and associated with little change in cardiovascular dynamics even after endotracheal intubation,[149] some workers have suggested this may not always be the case. Indeed, hypotension can occur during induction of anesthesia with alfentanil in ASA class II to IV patients.[150,151] Modest increases in heart rate and arterial blood pressure have also been reported following anesthesia with alfentanil in young unpremedicated adults. It appears that more experience is necessary before conclusions can be drawn about the value of alfentanil as an induction agent or analgesic supplement.

HYPERTENSION

MORPHINE

Hypertension during cardiovascular surgery was also a problem in patients anesthetized with morphine.[25,111,152] Arens et al.[25] reported a 36 percent incidence of hypertension, defined as a rise in systolic blood pressure to >200 mm Hg or an increase of 60 mm Hg above preoperative pressure, in patients undergoing coronary artery surgery with 2 mg/kg of morphine. Hypertension during morphine anesthesia has been variously attributed to light or inadequate anesthesia,[28] reflex mechanisms,[28] stimulation of the renin-angiotensin mechanism,[153] and sympathoadrenal activation.[129]

FENTANYL

With the exception of inadequate anesthesia,[154] the above explanations do not appear to be valid in the case of fentanyl and, to date, the mechanism responsible for hypertension with fentanyl anesthesia remains unclear despite various suggested explanations.[142] Although hypertension is rare before endotracheal intubation or surgical stimulation with high-dose fentanyl anesthesia for cardiac surgery, it is the most common cardiovascular disturbance during or after sternotomy and aortic root manipulation.[138,155-157] The reported incidence of hypertension with fentanyl-based anesthesia varies widely. Stanley et al.[2,3] reported no change in cardiovascular variables following surgical stimulation. Other investigators have reported incidences of hypertension specifically related to sternotomy from 0 to 100 percent in patients given fentanyl 50 to 100 μg/kg.[87,138,142,154-158] The reason for this variability between investigators is not clear. Possible explanations include the rate of fentanyl administration, the induction and subsequent dose and their time of administration, and the type of muscle relaxant used for endotracheal intubation and the rate of its administration. Other possible factors include the kind and dose of maintenance muscle relaxant, the degree of β-adrenergic and/or calcium channel blockade present at the time of surgery, preoperative ventricular function, patient habits, presence or absence of awareness.[87,93,154,156-158] In an investigation comparing fentanyl requirements in patients undergoing coronary artery surgery in Salt Lake City, Utah, and Leiden (The Netherlands), it was found that poststernotomy hypertension occurred in only 10 percent of patients in Salt Lake City with fentanyl (75 μg/kg) but was present in 80 percent of Dutch patients in spite of 121 μg/kg of fentanyl.[154] Higher doses of fentanyl (130 to 140 μg/kg) reduced this incidence of hypertension in Dutch patients. A recent study suggests that these differences in fentanyl requirements between populations may be related to different patient habits.[87] Apparently, a history of smoking plus alcohol and caffeine consumption increases fentanyl requirements for anesthesia.

Although satisfactory control of hemodynamics can be achieved by increasing the dose of fentanyl,[154,156] the use of such extremely high doses is inappropriate considering associated problems and the availability of alternative techniques. Doses of fentanyl of 140 μg/kg are likely to result in prolonged respiratory depression during the postoperative period.[154] Satisfactory blood pressure control can be achieved with fentanyl (50 to 120 μg/kg) plus vasodilator therapy.[142,154-156,159] However, with lower doses of fentanyl ($\leq$ 50 μg/kg), and no supplements, there may be an increased risk of intraoperative awareness that has never been reported with doses of > 120 μg/kg but has occasionally been reported with lower doses.[93-95]

The total amount of fentanyl used is often limited to 100 μg/kg. When hemodynamic control is not achieved with this dose, vasodilator therapy is begun with sodium nitroprusside. Other clinicians may supplement anesthesia with a potent inhaled anesthetic and/or an intravenous sedative-hypnotic[2,93] to control episodes of hypertension. Mixing opioids with inhaled anesthetics decreases stroke volume, cardiac output, and mean arterial blood pressure (MABP) and increases ventricular filling pressure.[19,160] Yet fentanyl and potent inhaled anesthetics (enflurane or halothane) can be given together without decreasing myocardial contractility or blood pressure, cardiac output, and stroke volume.[20,21] Furthermore, some inhaled anesthetics (halothane or isoflurane) may be protective to the myocardium during periods of ischemia.[161,162] Nonetheless, the effects of adding inhaled anesthetics to large doses of fentanyl or other opioids on the myocardial oxygen supply–demand ratio in patients with coronary artery disease are uncertain.

SUFENTANIL

Sufentanil may result in a lower incidence of hypertension when used in anesthetic doses (10 to 20 μg/kg) with oxygen for myocardial revascularization. Sufentanil also decreases the MAC of potent inhaled anesthetics to a greater degree than has been found with fentanyl in animal studies.[163,164] Whether these data have relevance to humans remains to be proved. Nonetheless, significantly lower incidences of hypertension (requiring vasodilation therapy) have been reported with sufentanil as compared with equipotent doses of fentanyl.[98,142] Sufentanil also provides as much[165,166] cardiovascular stability as fentanyl (or possibly greater) when employed in a balanced anesthetic technique.[97,167]

ALFENTANIL

More experience is necessary before conclusions can be drawn concerning hypertension in association with alfentanil. However, it is already apparent that hypertension during induction with an alfentanil-based anesthetic is not uncommon.[168]

HEART RATE AND RHYTHM

With the exception of meperidine, all μ-receptor stimulating opioid analgesics usually produce decreases in heart rate. These changes are due to stimulation of the central vagal nucleus in the medulla, since they can be blocked with bilateral vagal ligation or the use of atropine or similar belladonna-like drugs in experimental animals.[169]

Fentanyl-induced bradycardia is more marked in anesthetized than in conscious dogs or human subjects.[169,170] When used for induction of anesthesia, there is a higher incidence of bradycardia when patients or dogs breathe pure oxygen than when nitrous oxide is used with oxygen.[171,172] This may be due to the increase in sympathetic nervous system activity associated with nitrous oxide anesthesia.[173,174] Second and subsequent doses of fentanyl cause less bradycardia than do initial doses.[105,171] Infusions in dogs decrease heart rate within the first 50 μg/kg of fentanyl.[171] Administration of

additional fentanyl (up to 2 mg/kg) is required to duplicate the initial percentage decrease in heart rate in dogs.[105] The degree of bradycardia after infusion of opioids may, to some extent, be dose related,[105,169,175] although an equally important factor is the speed of injection. While a well-controlled experimental investigation has not been published, clinical experience in human subjects and animals studies with numerous species[171,175-178] suggest that bradycardia can be minimized by slow administration of potent opioids. Premedication with atropine or glycopyrrolate can minimize bradycardia induced by morphine, fentanyl, or other highly potent opioids but does not always eliminate it.[2,3,86,105,171,176] Atropine is also usually effective in treating opioid-induced bradycardia, but anecdotal reports suggest that even large doses (1 to 2 mg) are occassionally ineffective. Prior administration of small to moderate doses of intravenous pancuronium (0.5 to 2.0 mg) before induction of anesthesia with fentanyl or other potent narcotics attenuates bradycardia.[142,179,180]

The mechanism of fentanyl-induced bradycardia is not completely understood, although stimulation of the central vagal nucleus is likely.[169] Bradycardia is almost totally prevented by bilateral vagatomy[169] or pharmacologic vagal block with atropine.[171] Blockade of sympathetic chronotropic action may also have a minor role.[169] Similar mechanisms have been proposed for morphine.[181,182] Morphine is also thought to have a direct effect on the sino-atrial (SA) node[183-186] and to depress atrioventricular (AV) conduction.[186] It is likely that fentanyl has a similar action. The latter properties may play a role in the antidysrhythmic actions of morphine[184-186] and fentanyl.[187,188]

Although theoretically these effects could also lead to the development of reentry-type dysrhythmias, in practice this rarely occurs. Doses of epinephrine sufficient to induce dysrhythmias in dogs were recently found to be no greater during narcotic-nitrous oxide anesthesia than during halothane, enflurane, or nitrous oxide anesthesia.[189] However, the incidence of malignant dysrhythmias (ventricular tachycardia and ventricular fibrillation) was less with narcotics plus nitrous oxide than with most potent inhaled anesthetics.[189]

The most common dysrhythmia, other than bradycardia, noted during narcotic anesthetic techniques is supraventricular tachycardia,[190] which usually occurs during or immediately after endotracheal intubation or surgical stimulation. This suggests that inadequate anesthesia rather than a direct effect of the narcotic is probably responsible for these abnormalities.

SUPPLEMENTS

A variety of adjuvant drugs have been used as supplements in combination with opioids. Rationales for this approach include attempts to reduce awareness, control hypertension, and decrease the total dose of opioid to minimize postoperative respiratory depression. Unfortunately, with few exceptions, supplements in combination with opioids usually result in loss of cardiovascular stability.

NITROUS OXIDE

The most common supplement used with intravenous opioids is nitrous oxide. Nitrous oxide has minimal effects on cardiovascular dynamics when administered by itself in dogs,[191] but it can depress myocardial contractility in humans.[192] On the other hand, its use in combination with opioids is associated with significant cardiovascular depression (Table 23-8). After administration of morphine (2 mg/kg), McDermott and Stanley[193] found that nitrous oxide produced concentration-dependent decreases in stroke volume, cardiac out-

TABLE 23-8. Cardiovascular Effects of Supplements During Narcotic Anesthesia

1. Addition of N_2O to most narcotics produces cardiovascular depression.
2. Impairment of blood pressure during N_2O-narcotic anesthesia is usually much less than reduction of cardiac output.
3. Most supplements depress cardiac output when added during narcotic anesthesia.
4. Narcotics are added during potent inhalational anesthesia to decrease the concentration of the inhaled agent and to decrease cardiovascular depression.
5. Combinations of narcotics and inhaled compounds can result in severe cardiovascular depression.

put, and arterial blood pressure and increases in systemic vascular resistance (Table 23-9). These have been consistent findings in humans and animals with all opioids studied, including morphine[24,131,133,193] and fentanyl.[27,65,171,194,195] Myocardial ischemia may occur as coronary flow decreases from hypotension and coronary vascular resistance increases.[195] While fentanyl alone produces no ventricular dysfunction in the presence of significant coronary artery stenosis, the addition of nitrous oxide can yield significant cardiovascular depression.[27] The mechanism(s) producing cardiovascular depression when nitrous oxide is used along with opioids is unknown and may not be related to the plasma concentration of the opioid.

DIAZEPAM

Diazepam produces few effects on cardiovascular dynamics when used alone. Unfortunately, the same is not true when it is combined with an opioid, usually for its amnestic properties. In combination with fentanyl, diazepam produces significant cardiovascular depression, including decreases in myocardial contractility, arterial blood pressure, systemic vascular resistance, heart rate, and cardiac output[2,86,196] (see Fig. 23-4). The mechanism(s) producing these changes are not clear but may be related to the sympatholytic actions of the combination (i.e., decreases in plasma epinephrine and norepinephrine or decreased peripheral sympathetic nervous activity with resultant vasodilation). Diazepam will also result in cardiovascular depression (hypotension, decreased cardiac output) when combined with morphine.[197] Similar interactions will probably also occur with combinations of other opioids and benzodiazepines.

OTHER SUPPLEMENTS

Cardiovascular depression also occurs when other intravenous supplements are combined with narcotics during anesthesia. When thiamylal (a barbiturate) is given (4 mg/kg IV) after morphine (1 mg/kg IV), cardiac output and stroke volume are decreased 30 to 40 percent and arterial blood pressure by 16 percent.

TABLE 23-9. Cardiovascular Effects of 0-50% Nitrous Oxide During Morphine Anesthesia (Means)

Parameter	Percent N_2O					
	0	10	20	30	40	50
Stroke volume (ml)	57.0	51.0*	50.0*	46.0*	42.0*	36.0*
Cardiac output (L/min)	5.2	4.6*	4.3*	4.0*	3.7*	2.9*
Systolic arterial blood pressure (mm Hg)	124.0	119.0*	117.0*	109.0*	104.0*	94.0*
Peripheral resistance (PRU)	159.0	176.0*	183.0*	204.0*	259.0*	312.0*

$* P < 0.05$. Student's paired t-test when compared to control values.
(McDermott R, Stanley TH: The cardiovascular effects of low concentrations of nitrous oxide during anesthesia. Anesthesiology 41:89, 1974.)

Systemic vascular resistance is increased 35 percent.[14] Of other intravenous supplements that have been studied, only scopolamine and droperidol do not produce significant myocardial depression or marked changes in cardiovascular dynamics when combined with opioids.[16,27,155] However, droperidol may result in decreased systemic vascular resistance and arterial blood pressure[27,197] and increased requirements for crystalloid infusion after opioids.[198]

Opioids have also been combined with potent inhaled anesthetics. Fentanyl and some of the other opioids are often used in low doses during halothane, enflurane, or isoflurane anesthesia to decrease heart rate, especially after surgical stimulation.[199] Unfortunately, the addition of low to moderate concentrations of halothane after large doses of morphine can produce marked cardiovascular depression in patients with coronary artery disease.[160] Similar results have been found with all but very small doses of fentanyl ($\leq 100\ \mu g$) during enflurane anesthesia.

Neuromuscular relaxants may also alter hemodynamics during opioid-based anesthesia. For example, after 75 $\mu g/kg$ of fentanyl, 0.1 mg/kg of pancuronium usually increases heart rate and cardiac index,[200] while d-tubocurarine may cause decreases in arterial blood pressure.

RESPIRATORY ACTIONS

All μ-receptor-stimulating opioids result in a dose-dependent depression of respiration,[201] primarily through a direct action on the

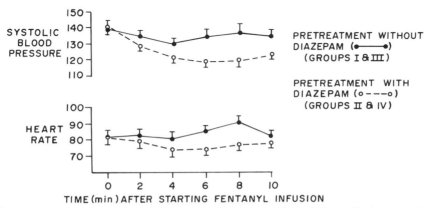

FIG. 23-4 Diazepam pretreatment (groups II and IV) before fentanyl (30 $\mu g/kg$) over 5 minutes produced significantly lower systolic blood pressures ($F(1,67) = 4.37$; $P = 0.04$) and heart rates ($F(1,67) = 3.95$; $P = 0.05$) when compared to groups I and III without diazepam pretreatment. (Bailey PL, Wilbrink J, Zwanikken P, et al: Anesthetic induction with fentanyl. Anesth Analg 64:48, 1984.)

brainstem respiratory center.[202,203] The responsiveness of the brain-stem respiratory centers to CO_2 is significantly reduced by opioids. Thus, the slopes of the ventilatory and occlusion pressure responses to CO_2 are decreased, and minute ventilatory responses to increases in $PaCO_2$ are shifted to the right (Fig. 23-5). In addition, the apneic threshold ($PaCO_2$ below which spontaneous ventilation is not initiated without hypoxia) and resting end-tidal CO_2 are increased by opioids. Opioids also decrease hypoxic ventilatory drive.[204,205] Opioids also blunt the increase in respiratory drive normally associated with increased airway resistance.[205]

Opioids interfere with pontine and medullary respiratory centers that regulate respiratory rhythmicity. These changes can increase respiratory pauses, delay expiration, and result in irregular and/or periodic breathing with slow respiratory rates and decreased, normal, or increased tidal volumes. Marked depression of the rib cage response and relative stability of abdominodiaphragmatic motion occur after administration of narcotic analgesic compounds.[206] Carefully performed comparisons of the effects of opioids and other anesthetics on respiration have not been frequently performed; however, fentanyl may produce a greater depressant effect on respiration than that produced with enflurane.[207] Fentanyl depresses respiratory drive, phase timing, and activation of respiratory muscles, whereas enflurane decreases only respiratory drive.[207] High doses of opioids totally block spontaneous respirations.[3,26] They can do this without necessarily producing unconsciousness. These patients are often still responsive to verbal command and will breathe when directed to do so.

Peak onset of respiratory depression after an analgesic dose of morphine is slower than that of fentanyl, 30 ± 15 minutes versus 5 to 10 minutes.[201] This is due in part to the lower lipid solubility of morphine (see section on pharmacokinetics). Respiratory depression induced by small doses of morphine usually lasts longer than equipotent doses of fentanyl for the same reason.[208] Downes et al.[209] found intravenous fentanyl (100 and 200 μg/70 kg) to result in a somewhat shorter period of respiratory depression than an equipotent dose of meperidine (65 to 75 mg/70 kg). These workers also noted a faster onset and peak effect with fentanyl than with meperidine.[209] Even though fentanyl has a shorter onset and recovery than that of morphine and meperidine, small doses (2 μg/kg) produce respiratory depression for longer than is generally appreciated (at least an hour) in contrast to analgesia (20 to 30 minutes).[210-212] Shorter duration of analgesia than respiratory depression may only reflect the insensitivity of current methods of measuring these variables. Although fentanyl (10 μg/kg) given during induction of anesthesia does not usually produce significant respiratory depression, some investigators have found that 5 hours later (during the postoperative period),[213] its respiratory depressant effects are often prolonged, that is, they are not very different from those of morphine.[198,214,215] The important point is that substantial blood levels of fentanyl (enough to result in significant respiratory depression) persist for hours, even after small doses.

With the higher (anesthetic) doses of fentanyl ($\geq$ 50 to 100 or more μg/kg), respiratory depression can persist for many hours. Indeed, ventilation may need to be controlled for 12 to 18 hours after induction of anesthesia. Interestingly, some patients recover respiratory function more rapidly than do others (for unexplained reasons) and can tolerate extubation of

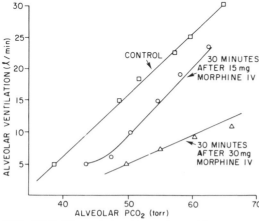

FIG. 23-5 Effect of morphine (15 and 30 mg IV) on alveolar ventilation and alveolar PCO_2 ($PACO_2$).

the trachea within 6 to 8 hours of drug administration with minimal or no elevation in $PaCO_2$.[108,154] Nonetheless, when moderate (20 to 50 μg/kg) or larger doses of fentanyl are used for any kind of operation, facilities should exist for postoperative mechanical ventilation, if necessary.

Many factors can change both the magnitude and duration of respiratory depression after opioid administration. Patients who are sleeping are usually more sensitive to the respiratory depressant effects of narcotics.[216] This can be worrisome when patients have a narcotic-based anesthetic and an operation that results in little or no postoperative pain. In these patients normal breathing and even a normal or near-normal end-tidal $PaCO_2$ can change to inadequate respiration and a high $PaCO_2$ when allowed to fall asleep. It appears that even small doses of narcotics markedly potentiate the normal right shift of the $PaCO_2$–alveolar ventilation curve that occurs during natural sleep.[217,218]

Recurrence of respiratory depression has been observed during recovery from anesthesia when narcotic analgesics were employed. The reason for this is not clear, but one explanation, aside from natural sleep, that is often advanced is that a second increase in plasma opioid concentration occurs due to sequestration of the compound in the acid medium of the stomach with subsequent reabsorption into plasma via the alkaline medium of the small intestine.[219,220] This sequence of events can result in slight increases in plasma concentrations of opioids and some degree of recurrent respiratory depression in a few patients in the recovery room.[215,221,222] However, whether these changes in plasma concentration are sufficient by themselves to produce profound respiratory effects (respiratory arrest or apnea) has not been confirmed and is probably unlikely, unless other factors (e.g., coadministration of other drugs, change in temperature, stimulation) are also operational.

Older patients (over 60 years of age) are more sensitive to the anesthetic[86] and respiratory depressant effects of opioids.[216] Furthermore, older patients have higher concentrations of plasma and probably of brain opioid than those of younger patients when opioids are administered on a weight basis.[223] Although older patients tend to have lower blood volumes than those of younger patients (also see Ch. 50), the precise reason for higher plasma concentrations after similar dosage administration is unknown. The respiratory depressant effects of opioids are increased and/or prolonged when administered with other CNS depressants, including the potent inhaled anesthetics,[224] alcohol,[216] the barbiturates,[216] the benzodiazepines,[211] and most of the intravenous sedatives and hypnotics. One exception to this rule is droperidol, which does not enhance the respiratory depressant effects of fentanyl and probably of other narcotics.[221,225] Pain, particularly surgically induced pain, counteracts the respiratory depressant effects of narcotic compounds.[224,226]

Although opioid action is usually dissipated via hepatic metabolism, rather than via urinary excretion (see section on pharmacokinetics), adequacy of renal function may influence duration of narcotic activity.[32] After being anesthetized with large doses of morphine for open-heart surgery, patients having higher intraoperative and postoperative urine outputs excrete more morphine in their urine and are able to sustain adequate spontaneous ventilation sooner than are patients with lower urine outputs.[32]

Hypocapnic hyperventilation has been shown to enhance and prolong postoperative respiratory depression after fentanyl (10 and 25 μg/kg).[213] Decreased liver clearance via decreased cardiac output and hepatic blood flow may explain this phenomenon. Conversely, intraoperative hypocapnia was not found to decrease fentanyl requirements for pain in the postoperative period.

Opioids have differing effects on the distal respiratory tract. When $PaCO_2$ is kept normal after administration of morphine, pulmonary deadspace decreases. When $PaCO_2$ is allowed to increase, pulmonary deadspace remains unchanged by morphine.[227] High doses of morphine (and probably many of the other opioids) decrease bronchial ciliary motion.[228] Fentanyl has antimuscarinic, antihistaminergic, and antiserotonergic actions and may be superior to morphine for use in patients with asthmatic or bronchospastic disease processes.[229]

NEUROPHYSIOLOGIC ACTIONS

The neurophysiologic state obtained by use of large doses of opioid analgesics is not the same as the "general anesthetic" state resulting from inhaled anesthetics[230] (also see Ch. 18). "General anesthetics" produce a dose-related generalized depression of the CNS, while opioid analgesics are more selective in action. Perhaps opioids produce anesthesia by blocking afferent input into the CNS rather than by generalized CNS depression.[230,231] High-dose fentanyl anesthesia produces a reproducible electroencephalographic (EEG) response characterized by high-voltage slow Δ waves.[230] A similar EEG pattern has been reported after the administration of meperidine, 400 mg.[232] The EEG appearance with fentanyl does not change with the addition of N_2O or surgical stimulus and is consistent with surgical anesthesia.[230] As the "anesthetic" effects of a high dose of an opioid decrease, the EEG waves become more frequent and of lower amplitude, suggesting recovery from anesthesia.[223] However, a strong cause-and-effect relationship between EEG changes and depth of anesthesia is yet to be established. Increasing dosage with inhaled anesthetics produces a continuum of EEG changes, resulting in burst suppression and a flat EEG with overdosage. In contrast, a "ceiling effect" is reached with fentanyl, morphine, sufentanil, and other opioids. Increasing the fentanyl dosage from 50 to 150 μg/kg does not further effect the EEG (P.S. Sebel and J.G. Bovil, unpublished data).[231] Furthermore, the EEG recordings of some patients only slowly return toward "control" even though plasma and presumably brain concentrations are rapidly decreasing. Despite these problems, recent work by Scott et al.[231] and Smith et al.[233] suggest that computer-assisted analysis of the EEG during high-dose fentanyl or other opioid anesthesia may be of value in determining depth of anesthesia.

Morphine (1 and 3 mg/kg) with 70 percent N_2O causes nonsignificant changes in cerebral blood flow (CBF) and cerebral metabolic rates (CMR) for oxygen, glucose, and lactate in humans.[234] Fentanyl, with or without droperidol, results in small decreases in both CMR and CBF. Decreases in CBF are somewhat greater than CMR in dogs.[235] Reductions in CBF may be of benefit in patients with elevated intracranial pressure.

MUSCLE RIGIDITY

Opioids can increase muscle tone, leading to severe rigidity.[236] Problems with muscular rigidity associated with the use of opioids during anesthesia have been known for years.[236-239,271] Corrsen et al.[236] reported an 80 percent incidence of some rigidity in patients receiving droperidol and fentanyl. Grell et al.[240] found that single intravenous doses of fentanyl (0.5 to 0.8 mg) consistently produced chest wall rigidity within 60 to 90 seconds of administration. Since the advent of opioid anesthetic techniques, the reported incidence of rigidity has varied from 0 to 100 percent.[86,108,144,149,236,238,240-242]

Opioid-induced rigidity is characterized by increased muscle tone progressing to severe stiffness, particularly in the thoracic and abdominal muscles. Rigidity usually begins just as the patient is losing consciousness; however, it is occasionally present in conscious patients.[138,149] Rigidity of the thoracic muscles (wooden chest syndrome), can impair ventilation in the nonparalyzed anesthetized patient.[241] Glottic closure has also been suggested to cause the difficulties with controlled ventilation associated with rigidity.[242] While a well-controlled study evaluating numerous rates of infusion of fentanyl or of any other opioid on the incidence of chest wall (truncal) rigidity has not been performed, rapid or bolus injection increases the severity of rigidity.[13,144,149,243] Rigidity is also more common the older the patient, when dosage is high, and when N_2O is used together with narcotic analgesic compounds.[13,86,243-246]

Abnormal muscle movements ranging from extremity flexion and/or single or multiple extremity tonic–clonic movements to global tonic–clonic motions can also occur after the use of opioids.[86] Whether these additional movements are part of a spectrum of neuromuscular activity associated with opioids, represent an "excited stage" during opioid anesthetic induction, or represent subcortical seizure activity is unclear (see the Section Neuroexcitatory Phenomena below).

The precise mechanism by which opioids cause muscle rigidity is not clearly understood. Muscle rigidity is not due to a direct action on muscle fibers, since it can be decreased or prevented by pretreatment with muscle relaxants.[86,144,247] Also, opioid-induced muscle rigidity is not associated with increases in creatine kinase,[244] suggesting that little or no muscle damage occurs during this period. Opioids do not have significant effects on nerve conduction and result in only minimal depression of monosynaptic reflexes associated with muscle stretch receptors.[244,246] Opioid-induced rigidity is probably related to the catatonic state, which can be induced by all narcotic analgesics.[248] Although some investigators have suggested that opioids produce rigidity by increasing dopamine concentrations within the striatum of the brain,[249,250] the mechanism is probably more complex. Rigidity may be the result of stimulation of μ-receptors located on GABA-ergic interneurons, which can be blocked by lesions in the striatum. Also, striatonigral GABA pathways involved with rigidity can be affected by GABA agonists.[251-253] Some aspects of opioid-induced catatonia and rigidity (increased incidence with age, extrapyramidal side effects) are similar to Parkinson's disease and suggest a common neurochemical mechanism.

Rigidity can diminish or preclude adequate ventilation and cause hypercarbia,[144,241] hypoxia, and disturbing cardiovascular changes (e.g., increases in pulmonary vascular resistance).[241] Although succinylcholine will reliably and rapidly terminate rigidity (provided the intravenous infusion is not impaired by a rigid flexed extremity) as well as permit adequate ventilation and minimize physiologic perturbations, the unpleasant esthetics and potential risk of rigidity episodes have motivated the search for prophylactic preventive measures. Pretreatment or concomitant use of nondepolarizing muscle relaxants can decrease the incidence and severity of rigidity (Table 23-10).[86,144,247] Interestingly, small doses of diazepam (0.15 mg/kg) have no effect by themselves but potentiate the effects of small (pretreatment) doses of pancuronium (0.022 mg/kg) as an inhibitor of opioid-induced chest wall rigidity.[86] A recent study demonstrated that equipotent doses of metocurine were more effective than pancuronium in both attenuating and abating rigidity, suggesting that neuromuscular blocking agents that act on prejunctional receptors should be more effective in minimizing rigidity than those acting on postjunctional receptors.[247] Sodium thiopental neither blunts nor terminates opioid-induced rigidity. Chest wall rigidity has also been reported after emergence (during recovery) from anesthesia.[254] The mechanism for its occurrence may be related to a second peak in plasma fentanyl concentrations, as discussed above, or may be due to muscle movements or renewed muscle perfusion after rewarming.

TABLE 23-10. Incidence (Percent) and Degrees of Rigidity After 30 μg/kg of Fentanyl in 72 Patients

Pretreatment Drug	Number of Subjects	Degree of Rigidity* (%)			
		0	1	2	3
Pancuronium					
No	37	14	3	32	51
Yes	35	54	6	20	20
Diazepam					
No	38	32	8	23	37
Yes	34	35	0	30	35

* 0 = no rigidity; 1 = mild rigidity; 2 = moderate rigidity; 3 = severe rigidity.

(Bailey PL, Wilbrink J, Zwanikken P, et al: Anesthetic induction with fentanyl. Anesth Analg 64:48, 1984.)

NEUROEXCITATORY PHENOMENA

Narcotic analgesics and other anesthetic agents can cause neuroexcitatory phenomena.[239,249,250,255-260] Fentanyl causes EEG seizure activity in cats (20 to 80 μg/kg),[239] rats (200 to 400 μg/kg),[248] and dogs ($>$1,250 μg/kg).[258]

Several investigators have reported grand mal seizure-like motor behavior in patients given fentanyl.[86,261,262] However, cortical electroencephalography has failed to document epileptic spike waves or any abnormal patterns except for nonelliptoid isolated sharp waves during induction or maintenance of anesthesia with fentanyl[230,264] or sufentanil[263] in spite of high plasma concentrations of the opioids (e.g., 175 ng/ml fentanyl). The spike wave activity has been attributed to subcortical (limbic area) excitation, but whether the waves arise from this area or are of any clinical importance has not been confirmed. Nonetheless, the limbic area is rich in opioid receptors that are probably normally stimulated by endogenous peptides.[47] Other purported mechanisms of opioid-associated neuroexcitation and/or seizure activity include disinhibition of pyramidal cells of the hippocampus[265] and increased release of excitatory neurotransmitters, such as Met- and Leu-enkephalin, which possess epileptogenic properties.[256]

Although a large clinical and reported experience with fentanyl has documented both its safety and efficacy, concern about the potential for seizures is legitimate. Aside from focal neuroexcitation producing possible local increases in CBF[266] and metabolism,[267] prolonged seizure activity, even if focal, can lead to neuronal injury and/or cellular death.[257,268,269] No neurologic deficit has yet been attributed to the neuroexcitatory effects of opioids.

EFFECTS ON THE KIDNEY

The effects of morphine (10 to 30 mg/70 kg) on the kidney have been extensively studied in humans and animals.[270,271] Most investigators agree that morphine can have significant antidiuretic properties, which may be due to a release of antidiuretic hormone (ADH).[270] However, in humans this morphine-induced release of ADH does not occur except in unusual circumstances (i.e., when nausea and vomiting occur) or during surgical stimulation in lightly anesthetized patients.[287,289] Antidiuresis after morphine administration has therefore been related to a decrease in renal dynamics, that is, decreases in renal blood flow and glomerular filtration rate (GFR).[270,271] In a comparison of anesthetics, our group found that intraoperative and postoperative urine outputs of 61 patients undergoing similar open-heart operations with high-dose morphine or halothane anesthesia did not differ.[120]

The effects of morphine, 2 mg/kg IV, were studied in volunteers whose ventilation was controlled to keep $PaCO_2$ within normal levels.[273] Morphine was given slowly with intravenous fluids in adequate amounts so that cardiovascular dynamics were unchanged. Under these conditions, morphine had no effect on GFR, urine osmolarity, or urine output. However, addition of 60 percent N_2O or a more rapid administration of morphine, so that arterial blood pressure and cardiac output were reduced, markedly diminished all those tests of renal function. Other work has confirmed that large doses of morphine and fentanyl probably do not stimulate ADH release in humans.[3,13]

On the other hand, in supine normovolemic, normocapnic dogs, morphine reduces urine output and increases urine osmolarity despite its minimal effects on cardiovascular dynamics.[274] These data suggest that morphine may increase blood levels of ADH in the dog. It appears that morphine is not an antidiuretic in supine normovolemic, normocarbic humans, whereas it is in the dog. In the absence of surgery, morphine does not stimulate release of ADH in humans. If renal function does change during opioid anesthesia and surgery, it is probably due to secondary changes in systemic and renal hemodynamics. Also, giving morphine to patients whose bladders are not catheterized may cause a decrease in urine output by an increase in detrusor and urethral sphincter tone, resulting in retention of urine in the bladder.

Increases in urine volume and decreases in urinary sodium excretion and urine osmolality have been reported during fentanyl-O_2 anesthesia. The absence of increases in plasma ADH, renin, or aldosterone indicates that fentanyl as well as sufentanil and alfentanil anesthesia preserves renal function.[275,280]

EFFECTS ON THE GASTROINTESTINAL TRACT

Analgesic doses of opioids are significant emetics due to stimulation of the chemoreceptor trigger zone in the area postrema of the medulla.[276] Emesis with opioids may also be related to increased volume of secretions in the gastrointestinal (GI) tract[294] or to decreased GI tract activity and prolonged emptying times.[277] Morphine increases the tone of smooth muscle in the GI tract and tightens various sphincters such as the sphincter of Oddi and the choledochoduodenal sphincter. Whether agonist-antagonist agents such as pentazocine, butorphanol, and nalbuphine cause as much, less, or no sphincter spasm, as compared in equianalgesic doses with agonists such as fentanyl, meperidine, or morphine is controversial.[279] Some reports indicate that biliary tract pressure is increased by all pure μ-receptor agonists but significantly less by agonist-antagonist compounds.[281] However, even the largest increases in biliary tract pressure are either rare or not marked and therefore of little clinical significance.[279] Increases in biliary tract pressure are easily antagonized by naloxone.[282,283]

ADDICTION

EPIDEMIOLOGY AND SIGNS

Addiction to any addictive substance is a complex and difficult problem to define. Addicts usually suffer from chronic physical, psychological, and social disorders characterized by compulsion and loss of control concerning drug intake in spite of adverse consequences. Opioid addiction usually leads to disability and death or to a severe withdrawal syndrome. Early recognition and proper treatment can lead to cure or successful rehabilitation, or both.[284,285]

Physicians, and particularly anesthesiologists, are frequent abusers of narcotic analgesics. Although only 4 percent of physicians are anesthesiologists, 10 to 14 percent of physicians treated for drug-related problems are anesthesiologists.[284] Many risk factors are identifiable in the susceptible individual, including self-medication and prescription writing, stress-related problems, personal health sacrifices and/or inattention, drug availability, and lack of adequate control procedures minimizing drug availability.

Signs of addiction include irritability, domestic turmoil, multiple legal and/or health problems, decreased professional performance, and complex behavioral problems. Denial is a primary concern because recognition and intervention are essential to successful management, that is, 60 to 80 percent recovery with treatment. Direct constructive assistance from colleagues and others is usually necessary.[284,285]

MECHANISM

The biochemical and physiologic mechanisms that lead to addiction and withdrawal are many and beyond the scope of this chapter.[285] Briefly, dependence has been attributed to altered metabolic function, cellular adaptation, disuse sensitization, and altered neuroregulatory functions. Early symptoms (first 10 hours) of withdrawal include anxiety, sweating, tachypnea, rhinorrhea, and dilated reactive pupils. Later signs (10 hours to 10 days) include marked lacrimation and rhinorrhea, tachycardia and hypertension, tremor, piloerection, nausea, vomiting, abdominal pain, and fever. Symptoms can last up to 5 months. Interestingly, although clonidine does not exhibit opiate receptor activity, it is an effective treatment for many of the heightened sympathetic symptoms associated with withdrawal. The effectiveness of clonidine is attributed to its ability to depress adenylate cyclase activity and cyclic AMP levels in the locus ceruleus (a major CNS noradrenergic center), sympathetic preganglionic neurons, and probably other CNS sites.[286]

Patients suffering from postoperative pain are often inadequately treated with opioid analgesics because the medical and paramedical personnel fear that such treatment might lead to addiction.[287,288] This approach is totally unjustified because such patients do not have the compulsion and behavioral complex essential for addiction.[284,285,289]

ANESTHESIA AND THE ADDICTED PATIENT

The anesthetic management of the opioid-addicted patient should be tailored to the patient's specific complex of problems. Common cardiopulmonary problems include bacterial endocarditis (particularly of the tricuspid valve), cardiac tamponade, cardiac dysrhythmias, thrombophlebitis, mycotic aneurysm, septic pulmonary and systemic emboli, sepsis, pulmonary edema, bacterial pneumonia, pulmonary aspiration and abscesses, pulmonary hypertension, and talc granulomata. Restrictive lung disease and increased alveolar-arterial oxygen gradients are also not uncommon in addicted patients.[290-292] Renal disease, especially the nephrotic syndrome, is seven times more prevalent in addicted than in nonaddicted patients. Likewise, addicted patients have a higher incidence of other genitourinary problems,[290] as well as decreased erythrocyte counts and hemoglobin concentrations. Chronic morphine administration causes adrenal hypertrophy and impairs corticosteroid secretion.[1] Other problems that occur with increased incidence in opioid abusers are viral and nonviral hepatitis, osteomyelitis, muscle weakness associated with rhabdomyolysis and myoglobinuria, and neurologic complications such as transverse myelitis, encephalitis, and cerebral abscess.

Planning anesthetic management for the addicted patient is difficult. Adequate premedication is advisable, and narcotic analgesics should not be avoided. There is no ideal anesthetic agent or technique to employ in the chronic addict or in the patient with an acute opiate overdose. The patient with an acute opiate overdose comes to the operating room with hypotension, bradycardia, hypoventilation, relative hypovolemia, and a GI tract that must be considered arrested and full of recently ingested material. The cardiovascular changes can be reversed with increments of naloxone (0.2 mg every 5 minutes IV) until respiration is adequate. Support of the circulatory system with fluids and monitoring of arterial oxygen tension and the pulmonary shunt fraction are also important. It should be remembered that complete opioid reversal may turn the patient into an uncontrollable menace. Furthermore, virtually all opioid antagonists have a shorter duration of action than the narcotic effect being treated. Therefore, renarcotization is a potential hazard during surgery or the postoperative period.

Although some opiate addicts may be managed with local or regional anesthesia, associated psychological problems make general anesthesia easier and frequently safer. Management during surgery requires normal fluid replacement, a high oxygen concentration, frequent arterial blood gas monitoring and, on occasion, positive end-expiratory pressure (PEEP). Mechanical difficulties encountered in attempting venous cannulations may occasionally necessitate femoral vein catheterization.

Pain relief during the postoperative period should be appropriate for the degree of pain and terminated with the resolution of the acute surgical condition. Methadone maintenance can be instituted for more gradual opiate withdrawal. Complete reviews of the anesthetic management of addicted patients are available.[293-295]

ANESTHETIC TECHNIQUES

BALANCED ANESTHESIA

The concept of balanced anesthesia dates back to 1910, when George W. Crile introduced his theory of anoci association.[296] Crile taught that psychic stimuli associated with operations could be prevented by light general anesthesia, while painful stimuli could be blocked by local analgesia. The term "balanced anesthesia" was introduced by Lundy in 1926.[11] Lundy suggested that a balance of agents and techniques (e.g., premedication, regional anesthesia, general anesthesia with one or more agents) be used to produce the different components of anesthesia (i.e., analgesia, amnesia, muscle relaxation, and abolition of autonomic reflexes with maintenance of homeostatis)[297,298] (Fig. 23-6).

The introduction of d-tubocurarine in 1942 enabled anesthesiologists to obtain relatively controllable muscle relaxation without the need for very deep levels of anesthesia.[299] Several techniques of balanced anesthesia were described involving anesthetic induction with sodium thiopental, maintenance with nitrous oxide and oxygen supplemented with small additional doses of thiopental, and mus-

cle relaxation with d-tubocurarine.[300,301] However, the combination of thiopental and N_2O provided insufficient analgesia for reliable prevention of unwanted sympathetic stimulation during surgery. In other words, not all the elements of proper balanced anesthesia were being achieved. In order to achieve additional analgesia, Neff et al.[12] introduced meperidine as a supplement during nitrous oxide anesthesia in the United States in 1947. Two years later, a similar technique was introduced in Great Britain by Mushin and Rendell-Baker.[302] These techniques rapidly achieved widespread popularity, and many inidividual variations using meperidine[302,305] and other opioids were described.[306,307] More recently, fentanyl has become popular as an intravenous supplement during general anesthesia with nitrous oxide, other inhaled and intravenous anesthetics, and combinations of intravenous and inhaled anesthetics.[19,210,211,308] In a double-blind comparison of fentanyl, phenoperidine, and morphine in combination with nitrous oxide for general anesthesia, little difference could be discerned among the drugs.[210] A characteristic of all opioid compounds when combined with other anesthetics is that differences between them with respect to their cardiovascular and other organ system effects tend to be obscured.

The inclusion of an opioid as a component of balanced anesthesia offers several advantages.[19,309] The course of anesthesia tends to be associated with less fluctuation in cardiovascular dynamics.[21] In addition, opioids decrease requirements for inhaled anesthetics[310] and provide increased postoperative analgesia. The use of opioids is particularly advantageous in operations involving sudden painful manipulations, such as pulling on visceral organs during intraabdominal surgery. Anticipation of these events and prior supplementation with a small dose of an opioid (e.g., 50 to 100 μg fentanyl IV) will often be sufficient to prevent increases in arterial blood pressure and heart rate associated with these manipulations. However, it is important that the timing and the dose of supplemental opioid be tailored to the specific pathology of the patient and the expected duration of the operation in order to avoid postoperative problems. In addition, the duration of action of an opioid is determined not only by its pharmacokinetic properties but by

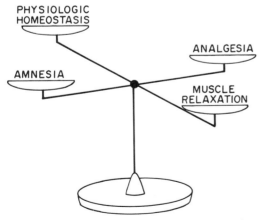

FIG. 23-6 Balanced anesthesia. Addressing the four components of anesthesia.

the timing, dosage, and interaction of the drug with other compounds being used as well. Giving a large dose of any opioid shortly before the end of surgery is very likely to result in postoperative respiratory depression and may potentiate and prolong respiratory depression.

NEUROLEPTANALGESIA-ANESTHESIA

In 1949, Laborit and Huygenard[311] introduced the concept of an anesthetic technique that blocked not only cerebrocortical responses but also some cellular, endocrine, and autonomic mechanisms usually activated by surgical stimulation. This state was called "ganglioplegia" or "neuroplegia" (artificial hibernation) and was achieved by the use of a lytic cocktail consisting of chlorpromazine, promethazine, and meperidine. From this idea, De Castro and Mundeleer[309] derived the concept of neuroleptanalgesia, which involved the combination of a major tranquilizer (usually the butyrophenone droperidol) and a potent opioid analgesic (fentanyl or phenoperidine) to produce a detached, pain-free state of immobility and insensitivity to pain. Neuroleptanalgesia is characterized by analgesia, absence of clinically apparent motor activity, suppression of autonomic reflexes, maintenance of cardiovascular stability, and amnesia in some but not all patients.

Combinations of drugs such as droperidol, which may have a duration of action of up to 24 hours, with fentanyl, which at least in the doses usually used in neuroleptanalgesia (3 to 5 μg/kg) lasts for a few hours, are not generally considered desirable.[310] This is because the effects of the tranquilizer may last much longer than the analgesic and result in a patient who is apparently calm yet may be suffering from pain and mental agitation.[310] In addition, droperidol in doses of ≥0.1 mg/kg occasionally results in prolonged postoperative somnolence. Nonetheless, the commercial preparation of droperidol-fentanyl (Innovar) has gained widespread popularity, both in the United States and in Europe, as the principal component of a balanced anesthetic technique that also usually employs N_2O. The most important reason for the contin-

ued popularity of Innovar is probably related to the associated intraoperative cardiovascular stability and relatively event-free recovery from anesthesia. Morgan and colleagues[312] found doses of droperidol of 5 to 20 mg and of fentanyl of 0.1 to 0.8 mg necessary for induction of anesthesia using neuroleptanalgesia in combination with muscle relaxants for major surgery. Nitrous oxide-oxygen was used during controlled ventilation and fentanyl (mean dose 0.1 mg/hr) administered for maintenance of anesthesia. The advantages of the technique were cardiovascular stability (with the exception of occasional hypotension on induction of anesthesia) and an awake and cooperative patient at the end of the procedure. Other workers found similar results using neuroleptanalgesia for cardiovascular and other major surgical procedures.[313] Neuroleptanalgesia has also been effectively used in neurosurgery for its ability to reduce CSF pressure in patients with and without space-occupying lesions[314] (also see Ch. 36).

TECHNIQUES OF HIGH-DOSE OPIOID ANESTHESIA

MORPHINE

To minimize the risk of hypotension during anesthesia induction, morphine is often administered slowly over a minimum of 10 to 15 minutes. This is most easily accomplished using a 0.1 percent solution of morphine in either dextrose (5 percent) or dextrose-saline at a rate of 5 to 10 mg/min with the patient breathing 100 percent oxygen or oxygen plus N_2O until a satisfactory level of anesthesia is achieved.[24-26,28,315] The incidence of hypotension during induction may also be minimized by concurrent administration of a rapid infusion of intravenous fluids,[26] by placing the patient in a modified Trendelenburg position[26] and/or by pretreatment with histamine (H_1 and H_2) receptor blockers.[315]

Induction of anesthesia usually requires 1 to 3 mg/kg of morphine,[23,24,26,28,152] depending on the patient's clinical condition but may require larger amounts, especially in patients who have reasonable cardiac reserve.[26] Since significant respiratory depression will occur before loss of consciousness in most patients, ventilatory assistance and then controlled ventilation are usually required. Often sedative-hypnotic compounds are added before or during administration of morphine to reduce opioid dosage and ensure amnesia.[28] Once unconsciousness has been achieved, a muscle relaxant is given, the trachea is intubated, and ventilation continued with either oxygen, an air-oxygen mixture, or nitrous oxide in oxygen.[23,24] Careful observation of the patient's response to laryngoscopy and intubation can provide useful information as to the adequacy of anesthesia. Increases in arterial blood pressure and heart rate, muscle or eyelid movement, and furrowing of the forehead all suggest an inadequate depth of anesthesia and are indications for additional morphine and/or intravenous or inhalation anesthetic supplementation before surgery commences. Likewise, reactions to surgical stimuli can usually be treated by similar therapies or, if the patient is considered to be adequately anesthetized, with an intravenous (nitroglycerin or sodium nitroprusside) or inhalation (low concentrations of enflurane or isoflurane) vasodilator.[16]

FENTANYL

Similar infusion techniques have been used by many clinicians and investigators to achieve anesthesia with fentanyl.[2,105,259,262,268] Induction of anesthesia via slow infusion of fentanyl, in contrast to infusion of morphine, is usually begun after a small dose of nondepolarizing muscle relaxant (pancuronium, 1 to 1.5 mg; *d*-tubocurarine, 3 to 4.5 mg; or metocurine, 1.0 to 3.5 mg) to minimize or prevent muscle rigidity. Infusion rates of fentanyl have generally ranged from 200 to 400 μg/min, but the rationale for, and techniques of, preoperative patient preparation, premedication, anesthetic supplementation during induction and maintenance periods, determination of unconsciousness (anesthesia), use of muscle relaxants and doses of fentanyl for endotracheal intubation, the remainder of the operation, and

total doses of fentanyl have varied enormously.[2,7,27,82,154,247] Many of these differences may be attributed to the debate as to whether fentanyl should be considered an anesthetic.[7,82,316,317] Similar questions were raised more than a decade ago, when high doses of morphine were popular.[28] Unfortunately, these questions are, as yet, incompletely answered, and it is likely that the debate and enormous variety of methods of using fentanyl for complete anesthesia or as an analgesic supplement will continue.

Some clinicians believe it is quicker, easier, and more efficacious to infuse a single large, precalculated bolus of fentanyl (50 to 100 μg/kg), usually with a large dose of pancuronium (0.1 to 0.12 mg/kg, to minimize fentanyl-induced bradycardia), for both induction and maintenance of anesthesia.[93-95,109,142,144,155,318,319] Following this approach, ventilation is controlled, the trachea is intubated and, within moments, the patient is ready for surgical preparation. Variations on the bolus technique are as numerous as the slower infusion approach of using fentanyl, undoubtedly for the same reasons.

HORMONAL RESPONSES WITH OPIOID ANESTHESIA

Considerable interest has been expressed in recent years in possible anesthetic modification of the hormonal and associated metabolic responses to surgical trauma. The so-called surgical "stress response" consists of increases in plasma concentrations of the catecholamines, cortisol, ADH, human growth hormone, glucose, lactate, pyruvate, and sometimes other hormones and metabolites. Plasma concentrations of the stress hormones increase during general anesthesia with most inhalation and intravenous agents and are further increased with operation.[106,320-322] Surgically induced increases in most stress hormones are related to the severity of the operative trauma,[320] being much greater during intraabdominal surgery than during body surface procedures.[321,322] These increased levels of stress hormones are considered undesirable because they promote hemodynamic instability and intraoperative and postoperative metabolic catabolism. For example, cardiac surgery with cardiopulmonary bypass produces profound endocrine and metabolic changes.[106]

MORPHINE

Analysis of hormonal data from a number of studies suggests that morphine modifies hormonal responses to surgical trauma in a dose-related fashion.[323-328] Morphine, even in small doses, inhibits the release of ACTH and blocks at least part of the pituitary-adrenal response to surgical stress.[324] After morphine (0.33 mg/kg) anesthesia, significant decreases in blood lactate occur; however, pyruvate concentrations remain unchanged.[325] Morphine (1 mg/kg) anesthesia suppresses surgically induced increases in plasma cortisol, but not human growth hormone, during major abdominal operations.[326] During cardiac surgery with morphine (4 mg/kg) anesthesia, plasma concentrations of both cortisol and human growth hormone are not increased in the pre-bypass period but are increased during bypass.[326-328] Increases in plasma concentrations of these hormones continue after bypass as well as postoperatively.[327]

Morphine has also been shown to increase some stress-response hormones.[328,329] Plasma catecholamine levels are increased after morphine anesthesia in dogs.[329] While the reasons for these changes are not clear, it has been suggested that morphine alters adrenal medullary release mechanisms[329,330] and to a lesser extent stimulates catecholamine release from sympathetic nerve endings.[331] Other possibilities include reflex responses to increased CO_2 or hypotension (secondary to morphine-induced ventilatory depression and/or vasodilation). Increases in plasma catecholamine concentrations appear to be responsible for the positive inotropic effect of morphine in dogs, since they are blocked by β-adrenergic blocking drugs or previous surgical adrenalectomy.[101] Morphine can also increase concentrations of catecholamines in both blood and urine in humans.[102-104] Secretion of catecholamines in humans may

be related to inadequate analgesia (anesthesia) but may also be dependent on the functional state of the sympathetic nervous system and the plasma concentration of morphine. For example, patients with hypertension and other evidence of increased sympathetic activity and patients with low morphine blood levels have higher urine norepinephrine excretion rates than those of similar normotensive patients or those with high morphine blood levels.[102,103] There is also evidence that the change in plasma norepinephrine concentration with anesthesic induction with morphine is related to the preinduction plasma norepinephrine concentrations; patients with low preoperative plasma norepinephrine concentrations experience a small rise in these amines, whereas patients with higher preoperative plasma norepinephrine concentrations experience no change or decreases in these concentrations after anesthetic induction.[102,103] Similar changes are also observed after induction of anesthesia with inhalational agents.[332]

Although morphine is known to stimulate ADH secretion in dogs and rats,[333,334] it does not appear to do so in the absence of surgical stimulus in humans.[272] Plasma ADH rises significantly during morphine (1 mg/kg) plus nitrous oxide anesthesia in humans during surgery before cardiopulmonary bypass and increases further during bypass.[272] Plasma renin activity also increases markedly in patients anesthetized with morphine (1 to 3 mg/kg) and nitrous oxide during cardiac surgery.[153] Increases in plasma renin are frequently but not always correlated with simultaneous increases in arterial pressure in these patients.[153]

FENTANYL

Fentanyl and some of its newer congeners seem to be even more effective than morphine in modifying hormonal responses to surgery. In a study of healthy women undergoing prolonged gynecologic surgery, anesthesia with nitrous oxide supplemented with fentanyl (50 μg/kg) was compared with halothane and nitrous oxide.[335] Fentanyl abolished the hyperglycemic response to surgery and reduced cortisol and growth hormone responses as compared with halothane. Similar results have also been reported with large doses of fentanyl in patients undergoing gastric surgery.[336]

The catecholamine response to induction of anesthesia with fentanyl infusion in patients about to undergo coronary artery surgery was recently investigated.[107] Plasma norepinephrine levels were significantly elevated after fentanyl, 15 μg/kg, was administered (probably secondary to inadequate analgesia) and remained elevated after 30 μg/kg but returned to control values after 50 μg/kg. No significant changes occurred in plasma epinephrine or dopamine. Other investigations have found that fentanyl in doses of $\geq$50 μg/kg prevents increases in plasma catecholamine concentrations during cardiac surgery,[106,159,275] although marked increases have occurred during cardiopulmonary bypass.[106,159] The hormonal changes associated with fentanyl (60 μg/kg) anesthesia during cardiac surgery are summarized in Figure 23-7. Marked increases in catecholamine concentrations measured during cardiopulmonary bypass that are not blocked by maintaining plasma concentrations close to prebypass levels[159] or by increasing these concentrations above prebypass levels (T.H. Stanley, unpublished data) are presumably a response to the significant abnormal physiologic state during this period (i.e., hemodilution, hypothermia, and nonpulsatile flow). Indeed, there is some evidence that vasopressin and catecholamine responses to cardiopulmonary bypass can be significantly attenuated by the use of pulsatile flow,[337] although this has not been confirmed by all investigators.[338]

Anesthesia with fentanyl, 60 to 100 μg/kg, prevents rises in plasma ADH, renin, and aldosterone during the period before cardiopulmonary bypass.[3,275] This is in contrast to the significant increases of these hormones observed in similar patients anesthetized with morphine.[272] However, during bypass, plasma ADH rises significantly in spite of high doses (100 μg/kg) of fentanyl.[3] High-dose fentanyl anesthesia usually prevents increases in blood glucose, plasma cortisol, and plasma growth hormone concentrations in most patients throughout open-heart operations.[106,159,275,339] However, this reduction in the stress response is not consistently found in all patients, espe-

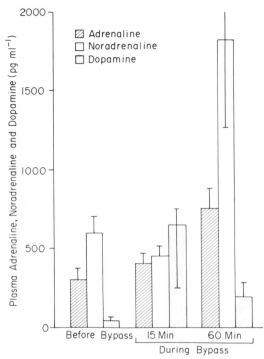

FIG. 23-7 Change in plasma catecholamine concentration (pg/ml) during cardiopulmonary bypass (mean $\pm$ SEM). (Sebel PS, Bovill JG, Schellekins APM, et al: Br J Anaesth 53:941, 1981)

cially during and after cardiopulmonary bypass and during the postoperative period, even when fentanyl administration is continued for 12 to 18 hours after surgery.[339]

In summary, fentanyl appears to be somewhat more effective than morphine in reducing the endocrine and metabolic responses to surgery. Although this may be due to pharmacologic differences between the drugs, it may also be the result of differences in potency (as sufentanil, which is 5 to 10 times as potent as fentanyl, appears more effective as a inhibitor of stress hormonal responses than the latter[280]), increased dosage,[106,275,337] anesthetic technique,[106] or increased speed of onset of action (as has been suggested with alfentanil in clinical studies[180] and with carfentanil in investigations with wild animals).[175] The effects of other opioids on the stress response to surgery have received little attention. Papaverine (extract of opium) is significantly less effective than fentanyl in attenuating the changes associated with cardiac surgery.[339] However, the new narcotics, alfentanil and sufentanil, seem to be more effective than fentanyl in cardiac and noncardiac operations,[167,280] although only a few carefully controlled clinical studies have been completed.[167]

MECHANISM

The mechanism by which large doses of opioids inhibit the stress response to surgical trauma is unknown. Whatever the mechanism, it probably involves pituitary release of ACTH and perhaps other stress hormone precursors, as ACTH secretion is reduced by high doses of opioids. It is interesting that decreases in plasma human growth hormone concentrations produced by morphine (4 mg/kg) are totally reversible after ACTH administration.[328] It is known that the endogenous opioid-like peptides play an important regulatory role in the secretion of several pituitary hormones,[340] possibly via alteration in the release of neurotransmitters (e.g., dopamine) that regulate secretion of pituitary hormone-releasing or release-inhibiting factors.[341,342] Perhaps exogenous opiates have similar inhibiting or stimulating actions.

Thus, techniques of opioid analgesia, particularly techniques of high-dose fentanyl anesthesia, diminish the hormonal "stress" response to surgery. This metabolic response is appropriate when "fight or flight" is required, for it ensures an increase in metabolism and energy availability necessary for the increased work associated with these states. However, such responses may be totally inappropriate in patients undergoing some forms of cardiovascular surgery, such as patients with ischemic coronary artery disease undergoing coronary artery bypass grafting. Increases in plasma catecholamine concentrations in these patients will lead to increased myocardial work and may further compromise an already damaged myocardium. Elevated plasma levels of the stress hormones in the period after surgery increase protein catabolism and may delay re-

covery. If these metabolic responses are modified, morbidity and mortality should be reduced. However, there is as yet no evidence to support this theoretical benefit. "Stress-free anesthesia" is at best an attractive biochemical concept. Whether it is of clinical benefit is uncertain. Certainly any reduction in the metabolic responses to anesthesia and surgery is short lived.[159,336,339] With morphine, at least, there is no improvement in postoperative nitrogen balance.[327] Whether the same is true following high doses of fentanyl or the newer synthetic opioids remains to be documented.

OPIOID ANTAGONISTS AND AGONIST-ANTAGONISTS

NALOXONE

Opioid effects can be reversed by opioid antagonists such as naloxone. Reversal of opioid effects is, and will probably continue to be, complex. As different opiate-receptor populations become defined, substances once thought to be pure antagonists (e.g., naloxone) will undoubtedly be shown to have actions at different receptor sites, especially when interacting with other drugs. With a few changes (see early section, on structure–activity relationships), opioid agonists can be rendered antagonistic at one or more receptor subtypes. Naloxone is considered the "purest" of opioid antagonists and is therefore used most frequently. It antagonizes opioid effects mediated by all receptor subtypes (but to differing degrees).

While naloxone is primarily used to reverse postoperative respiratory depression, other, less frequent applications of the drug are wakeup testing during narcotic-anesthesia, resuscitation of patients in shock,[343,344] and treatment of postoperative rigidity. The usual dose of naloxone is a bolus of 1 μg/kg or 0.04 to 0.08 mg IV titrated to a desired effect in a 70-kg adult. Repeat doses may be administered every 5 to 10 minutes. It is not clear whether careful titration can reverse respiratory depression without antagonizing analgesia, but opiate receptor subpopulation characteristics and animal (rat) studies[345] suggest that this should be possible. However, whatever the objective, ample clinical reports indicate that caution should always be exercised with naloxone administration.

Although in the past naloxone (presumably a "pure antagonist") was thought to have little effect of its own, this belief is no longer tenable. There are many reports indicating that naloxone has significant effects on cardiovascular function with or without prior narcotic-analgesic administration.[346-351] Complications have included systemic arterial hypertension, pulmonary edema, ruptured cerebral aneurysm, dysrhythmias (atrial and ventricular), cardiac arrest, and sudden death. These problems are not restricted to patients with cardiovascular disease.[351] Pain is the most frequently quoted cause of opioid reversal problems. Other mechanisms include a general analeptic effect,[352] "unmasking" of acute physical dependence,[353] and an increase in circulating catecholamines. Some investigators believe that naloxone can produce marked changes in plasma catecholamines in some patients.[354] Others do not agree.[355] Nevertheless, overlap of opioid and adrenergic effects in preganglionic sympathetic neurons is well documented.[286] Furthermore, recent studies document that naloxone with or without opioid pretreatment increases preganglionic sympathetic neuron activity (B. Hare, personal communication).

Small intravenous doses of naloxone rapidly antagonize opioid-induced respiratory depression, analgesia, and euphoria. The duration of action of naloxone is short in comparison with usual doses of fentanyl or other opioids employed during anesthesia. Therefore, renarcotization with recurrence of significant respiratory depression occurs not infrequently.[86,356] Intramuscular or subcutaneous injections provide increased protection against opioid renarcotization but are not foolproof.

Interest has been shown in the possibility of antagonizing opioids with the tertiary anticholinesterase physostigmine. Although an advantage of this technique might be persistent analgesia,[357] the duration of action of physostigmine is too short (35 to 45 minutes) to be of practical value. Furthermore, the drug results in impressive side effects (e.g., nausea, vomiting, bradycardia), and its action is unpredictable, especially when $PaCO_2$ is elevated.[358,359] Therefore, our current recommendation would be to rely on more predictable and/or specific opioid antagonists.

NEW AGONIST-ANTAGONIST ANALGESICS

The first recorded specific opioid antagonist was developed by Pohl in 1914 who, in an attempt to improve the analgesic properties of codeine, synthesized N-allylnorcodeine.[360] He observed that this compound mildly antagonized the respiratory depression and sleep produced by morphine. However, this discovery was unnoticed for 26 years until McCawley et al.,[361] in a search for a strong analgesic with "built-in" antagonistic action, attempted to prepare N-allylmorphine in 1940. This compound, nalorphine, was successfully synthesized by Weijland and Erickson in 1942[362] and was found to be strongly antagonistic to almost all the properties of morphine.[363,364] It was also found to possess fairly strong analgesic properties in humans[365] and animals.[366,367] Unfortunately, doses of nalorphine sufficient to produce analgesia were accompanied by severe psychomimetic effects rendering it unsuitable for clincal use as an analgesic. It was, however, very widely used in lower doses as an effective opioid antagonist.

The discovery of nalorphine provided the stimulus to search for other drugs with combined agonist and antagonist properties. Considerable progress has been made since 1955 toward the development of potent pain-relieving drugs without the depressant and, perhaps more important, addictive potential of morphine. Most of these represent only minor molecular modifications of an existing opioid, most commonly alkylation of the piperidine nitrogen in morphine with a three-carbon side chain such as propyl, allyl, or methylallyl.[368] Changing the side chain to an amyl group restores agonist activity.

PENTAZOCINE

The first opioid agonist-antagonist to be widely used in humans was pentazocine, a benzomorphan derivative.[369,370] Pentazocine has one-half to one-fourth the analgesic properties of morphine but, unfortunately, in equipotent doses produces similar degrees of respiratory depression. Although its potential for abuse is less than with morphine,[370] prolonged use can lead to physical dependence.[369] In addition, nalorphine-like dysphoric side effects are common, especially in the elderly, or at doses exceeding 60 mg. These can be reversed with naloxone. Effects on the GI tract are similar to those of other opioids (see section on gastrointestinal effects). Unlike morphine, the hemodynamic effects of which make it a useful analgesic in the treatment of patients with myocardial infarction,[371] the cardiovascular effects of pentazocine are such that it is commonly thought to be contraindicated in such circumstances.[372] Pentazocine depresses myocardial contractility[373] and increases peripheral resistance, arterial blood pressure, pulmonary artery pressure,[374,375] and the LV work index.[372,374,375] Pentazocine also increases the concentration of catecholamines in plasma. All these changes result in an increase in myocardial oxygen demand and can lead to extension of an area of ischemia after myocardial infarction.

Pentazocine, despite initial enthusiasm, does have significant abuse and addictive potential.[376-378] It has weak antagonist properties and, although not very useful in reversing the respiratory depressant effects of fentanyl,[379] can precipitate opioid withdrawal symptoms.[380-381]

Orally administered pentazocine is one-fourth as potent as a parenteral dose, which is one-fourth as potent as morphine. The plasma half-life of pentazocine is 2 to 3 hours with biotransformation terminating biologic effect and urinary excretion eliminating metabolites. Significant first past effect (uptake by the liver) exists. This, in combination with considerable variability in hepatic metabolism, leads to variable duration of action.

BUTORPHANOL

More recently, two totally different synthetic agonist-antagonist analgesics, butorphanol and nalbuphine, have become available. The synthesis of butorphanol (BC-2627) was reported in 1973.[382] In humans its analgesic potency is five to eight times that of morphine[383-385] and 30 to 50 times that of meperidine.[386,387] Its duration of action is similar to that of morphine.[383,388] The degree of respiratory depression produced by butorphanol (2 mg) is similar to that of morphine (10 mg). In patients undergoing cardiac catheterization, analgesic doses of butorphanol were found to produce similar degrees of respiratory depression as that produced by an equianalgesic dose of morphine.[389] However, unlike morphine, the degree of respiratory depression does not increase in a dose-related fashion with increasing doses of butorphanol.[390] Major side effects include drowsiness, sweating, nausea, and psychomimetic effects. The latter are qualitatively similar but occur less frequently than after pentazocine. Weaker μ than κ or σ receptor effects may account for these findings after butorphanol.

In healthy volunteers, butorphanol, 0.03 or 0.06 mg/kg IV, produced no significant cardiovascular changes.[390] However, in patients with cardiac disease, butorphanol caused progressive and significant increases in cardiac index and pulmonary artery pressure. Left ventricular end-diastolic pressure was also increased by a small amount.[389] These cardiovascular changes are quite similar to those observed in a similar patient population given pentazocine.[374] These studies indicate that butorphanol is less useful than morphine in patients with congestive heart failure or with a history of previous myocardial infarction.

Butorphanol has been reported to provide adequate analgesia when used as a supplement in nitrous oxide-opioid-oxygen anesthetic techniques.[391,392] The possibility that higher doses of butorphanol used alone with oxygen might be capable of producing surgical anesthesia with less postoperative respiratory depression than occurs with equivalent doses of morphine or fentanyl has been investigated.[393] The cardiovascular and anesthetic effects of two intravenous infusions of butorphanol (0.1 and 0.2 mg/kg/min) were studied in dogs under basal anesthesia with sodium thiopental. Seventy-five percent of dogs receiving the lower infusion rate and 25 percent of those receiving the higher rate moved in response to a tail-clamp stimulus after 45 minutes of infusion. Higher doses of butorphanol are not, unfortunately, more effective in preventing movement after surgical stimulus. More importantly, significant cardiovascular depression occurred with both infusion rates. Addition of nitrous oxide resulted in further cardiac depression. These data and other anecdotal reports from clinicians using high doses of butorphanol in humans suggest that butorphanol is not an attractive alternative to morphine or fentanyl as an opioid "anesthetic."

As a component of N_2O-opioid balanced anesthesia, butorphanol appears to be unable to block tachycardia and hypertension (irrespective of dosage) with surgical stimulation.[394] Addition of diazepam or use of inhalation agents (e.g., enflurane) can prevent these changes, but they produce increasing postoperative CNS depression, including prolonged and marked respiratory depression. Butorphanol is subject to abuse and has addictive potential.[395] Withdrawal symptoms can occur after prolonged use[396] and usually increase in severity for up to 2 days. Butorphanol is only available in parenteral form. After intramuscular injection, peak analgesia occurs within 1 hour. Hepatic metabolism and urinary and a small amount of biliary excretion account for drug elimination.

NALBUPHINE

Nalbuphine (EN-2234A) is an agonist-antagonist opioid analgesic structurally related to oxymorphone and the opioid antagonist naloxone. Nalbuphine has an analgesic potency and duration of action similar to that of morphine.[397] However, in a study comparing equal doses (0.1 mg/kg) of nalbuphine and morphine as intravenous premedicants prior to minor gynecologic operations, patients receiving morphine required significantly less analgesic therapy postoperatively than did those given nalbuphine.[398] This suggests either that nalbuphine is less potent than morphine or that it has a shorter duration of analgesic action. When used as an analgesic supplement to nitrous oxide for balanced anesthesia, relatively large doses (up to 3 mg/kg) of nalbuphine are required.[399] Both nalbuphine and butorphanol produce significant but limited (approximately 10 percent) reductions in the MAC of enflurane.[400] Up to 3 mg/kg of nalbuphine produces moderate analgesia and moderate sedation with little or no respiratory depression in awake volunteers. Volunteers can still ambulate after receiving these doses of nalbuphine (P. Bailey, unpublished data). Nalbuphine, 2 to 3 mg/kg, results in only small changes in cardiovascular dynamics when used alone or in combination with N_2O.[401-403] Some studies indicate that the analgesic effect of nalbuphine results from an action on κ-opioid receptors.[404] These data suggest that nalbuphine binds with, but does not activate, μ-receptors to the same extent as morphine or other pure agonist opioids.[404] Nalbuphine, like butorphanol, results in respiratory depression, but this effect plateaus with higher doses. This response seems to be characteristic of all the agonist-antagonist opioids.

Nalbuphine has been reported to be a satisfactory antagonist of respiratory depression associated with opioid anesthesia.[86,405-409] However, sedation is usually unchanged or increased, and respiratory depression induced by analgesic doses of morphine (10 to 15 mg/70 kg) is not reversed by nalbuphine (P. Bailey, unpublished data). Although purported advantages of nalbuphine opioid reversal (as compared with naloxone) are longer duration of action, little (less) effect on analgesia, and decreased side effects (e.g., hypertension), a well-controlled study documenting such is lacking.

Nalbuphine is only available for parenteral therapy. In low doses (0.1 to 0.3 mg/kg), the drug is approximately equianalgesic to a similar dose of morphine. Onset of analgesia is fast (10 to 20 minutes) and duration 3 to 6 hours. Hepatic metabolism and fecal excretion account for most elimination. Abuse and addiction potential are unconfirmed but likely to be similar to that with other opioids.

In summary, the mixed agonist-antagonists may provide advantages as premedicants and analgesics because of less (unproved) addiction liability and "ceiling" effects with respect to respiratory depression. In the operating room, the agonist-antagonist drugs can serve as analgesic adjuvants (optimal dosages are not clear) but cannot produce anesthesia.[402] The place and advantage of drugs such as nalbuphine as an alternative to naloxone (as a narcotic antagonist after narcotic analgesia and/or anesthesia) is inadequately defined at this time.

the body) and pharmacokinetics (i.e., the factors determining concentrations of a drug after a given dose, over time).

Most clinicians administer inhalational anesthetics "to a desired effect" rather than to any predetermined or "magic" concentration. Likewise, and in spite of recent publications of the pharmacokinetic profiles of numerous narcotic analgesics, it should not be anticipated that mathematical formulas derived from our increased understanding of opioid pharmacology permit empiric delivery of narcotic anesthesia. Rather, titration to a desired clinical effect remains the principle that should govern the use of analgesic or anesthetic doses of opioids.

PHARMACOKINETICS

MORPHINE

Pharmacokinetics is the quantitative study of the disposition of drugs in the body and includes the processes of absorption, distribution, biotransformation, and excretion. (These pharmacologic principles are discussed in depth in Ch. 3.) This section is restricted to the pharmacokinetics of the commonly used narcotic analgesics and anesthetics, morphine, meperidine, and fentanyl, along with the newer opioids, alfentanil and sufentanil (Table 23-11). The considerable variability in patient responses to narcotic anesthetics is probably due to variations in pharmacodynamics (i.e., the effects of a given concentration of a drug on

Biexponential or triexponential equations describe the distribution of morphine to one or two peripheral compartments in the body, after intravenous injection. Several reports have documented a rapid distribution half-life ($t\frac{1}{2}\pi$) of between 0.9 and 2.4 minutes and/or a slow distribution half-life ($t\frac{1}{2}\alpha$) of 10 to 20 minutes.[410-414] Thus, free morphine rapidly leaves the blood and is taken up by the parenchymatous tissues and skeletal muscle. At a pH of 7.4, morphine is about 25 percent un-ionized and one-third bound to plasma proteins—mostly serum albumin. Morphine is not lipid soluble. Its octanol : water partition coefficient

TABLE 23-11. Averaged Pharmacokinetic Data for Five Opioids*

	Morphine	Meperidine	Fentanyl	Alfentanil	Sufentanil
pKa	8.0	8.5	8.4	6.5	8.0
% un-ionized at pH 7.4	23	<10	<10	90	20
Octanal: water partition coefficient (apparent at pH 7.4)	1.4	39	813	145	1,778
Percentage bound to plasma proteins	30	70	84	92	93
$t\frac{1}{2}\pi$ (min)	0.9–2.4	—	1–3	1–3	0.5–2
$t\frac{1}{2}\alpha$ (min)	10–20	5–15	5–20	5–20	5–15
$t\frac{1}{2}\beta$ (hr)	2–4	3–5	2–4	1–2	2–3
Vd$_{cc}$ (L/kg)	0.1–0.4	1–2	0.5–1.0	0.1–0.3	0.1
Vd$_{ss}$ (L/kg)	3–5	3–5	3–5	0.5–1.0	2.5
Clearance (ml/min)	10–20	8–18	10–20	3–8	10–12

Abbreviations used: $t\frac{1}{2}\pi$ = rapid distribution half-life; $t\frac{1}{2}\alpha$ = slow distribution half-life; $t\frac{1}{2}\beta$ = elimination half-life; Vd$_{cc}$ = volume of distribution (central compartment); Vd$_{ss}$ = volume of distribution (steady state).
* Data obtained from multiple references (see text).

is 6 when un-ionized, compared with 11,000 for fentanyl. As a result, the penetration of morphine into the CNS is delayed and does not parallel its disappearance from plasma.[415] Exit from the CNS is also delayed. This is probably the most important reason for the long duration of action of the drug. Despite a much smaller fat:plasma protein partition coefficient (0.8:1) than that of fentanyl (35:1), the volume of distribution of morphine at steady state is large (approximately 4 ± 1.0 L/kg).[410-414] This indicates that other tissues besides fat are responsible for the extensive uptake of morphine.

Clearance of morphine from the body is largely dependent on hepatic biotransformation (mostly glucuronidation, some N-demethylation, and possibly some oxidation to pseudomorphine or methylation to codeine) and renal excretion. Only 5 to 10 percent of morphine and its metabolites is excreted in feces.[416,417] The high clearance rate (10 to 20 ml/kg/min)[410-414] of morphine is consistent with a high hepatic extraction ratio. Thus, clearance of morphine is hepatic blood flow dependent. Reuptake from peripheral depots by the blood is another important limiting factor in the metabolism of morphine. Only about 10 percent of morphine is excreted unchanged in the urine.[418,419] Although usually inactive, the metabolite morphine-3-glucuronide may exercise some opioid effect in certain pathophysiologic states (e.g., renal failure).[420] The elimination half-life of morphine (t$\frac{1}{2}$ β) is 2 to 4 hours.[410-414] The physiologic and pathophysiologic factors that influence pharmacokinetics are simultaneously discussed for morphine, meperidine, and fentanyl in this section.

MEPERIDINE

The plasma concentration versus time decay curve of meperidine is characterized by a biexponential equation with reported distribution half-lives (t$\frac{1}{2}$ α) varying from 5 to 15 minutes.[421-425] Meperidine is more plasma protein bound than morphine. About 70 percent of meperidine is bound to α_1-acid glycoprotein. Meperidine binds only to a minor extent to plasma albumin. Meperidine is even less un-ionized (less than 10 percent) than morphine at physiologic pH but is significantly more lipid soluble. The volume of distribution of meperidine is quite similar to that of morphine (about 4 ± 1 L/kg),[421-425] as is its clearance (about 8 to 18 mg/kg/min).[421-425] Like morphine, a high hepatic extraction ratio results in biotransformation that is hepatic blood flow dependent. Principal metabolic pathways of meperidine include N-demethylation and deesterification producing normeperidine, meperidinic acid, and normeperidinic acid as the major metabolites. Normeperidine has some opioid action and is roughly twice as potent as its parent compound in producing seizures in animals,[426] a major side effect of meperidine that causes its therapeutic index to be more than 10-fold lower than that of morphine (5 versus 70). The elimination half-life (t$\frac{1}{2}$ β) for meperidine is approximately 4 ± 1 hours,[421-425] and excretion of metabolites occurs predominantly via the kidney. The elimination half-life of normeperidine is considerably greater than that of meperidine and cumulative doses, paired with renal and hepatic disease, can easily produce overdosage and toxicity.[427]

FENTANYL

After bolus administration, the plasma fentanyl concentration declines in a triexponential fashion. Like morphine, the rapid distribution half-life (t$\frac{1}{2}$ π) of fentanyl is only 1 to 3 minutes, while its slower distribution half-life varies between 5 to 20 minutes.[428-430] Fentanyl is significantly bound (about 80 percent) to plasma proteins, and less than 10 percent is un-ionized at physiologic pH. However, penetration of fentanyl into CNS is greater than that of morphine due to a markedly greater lipid solubility. This characteristic is clearly the most important reason for the rapid onset and shorter duration of action of the drug. The volume of distribution at steady state (about 4 L/kg) of fentanyl is quite similar to that of morphine and meperidine, as is its clearance.[428-430] Clearance of fentanyl is predominantly dependent on hepatic metabolism, although other sites of metabolism do exist (e.g., lung).[431] Less than 10 percent of fentanyl is excreted unchanged in the urine.[428] Again, hepatic blood flow and peripheral perfusion and reuptake of fentanyl are important biotransformation rate-limiting factors. Slow reuptake from fat depots yields an elimination half-life ($t\frac{1}{2} \beta$) similar to those of meperidine and morphine (about $2\frac{1}{2}$ to $3\frac{1}{2}$ hours).[428,432,433] The metabolism of fentanyl is complex[434,435]; however, none of the metabolites exerts significant opioid action.

PHYSIOLOGIC AND PATHOPHYSIOLOGIC FACTORS INFLUENCING OPIOID PHARMACOLOGY

ACID–BASE

The pharmacokinetic profile of opioids is easily altered by numerous normal or pathologic processes that ultimately change opioid drug disposition and thus the pharmacodynamics of the compound. Variations in arterial pH can affect drug ionization, plasma protein binding, and drug disposition in a variety of tissues. Morphine, meperidine, and fentanyl are all weak bases. As demonstrated by the Henderson-Hasselbalch equation

$$pH = pKa + \log \frac{\text{proton acceptor (B)}}{\text{proton donor (BH}^+)}$$

weak bases (ionized as a proton donor) become less ionized as the pH rises. Thus, an increase in arterial pH should increase the penetration of morphine into the brain.[436–438] However, protein binding will also be enhanced and cerebral blood flow decreased by respiratory alkalosis, although the sum of effects may not be readily apparent. Interestingly, respiratory alkalosis has been shown to be associated with increased brain levels of fentanyl.[439] Increased duration of respiratory depression due to increased tissue binding and slower CNS removal has also been associated with respiratory alkalosis.[213,439] Respiratory acidosis should result in opposite effects (i.e., increased plasma ionization, decreased plasma protein binding, and increased cerebral blood flow). Hypercarbia usually results in higher plasma and brain concentrations of morphine than are found in normocarbia.[437] The complex nature of the effects of changes in pH guarantees conflicting reports[440] as well as difficulties in defining the sum of separate effects and their clinical significance.

Biphasic respiratory depression and secondary peaks in fentanyl plasma concentrations have been described.[215,221,222] The role played by acid–base equilibria and stomach sequestration[219,220] in contributing to this phenomenon is uncertain and deserves further detailed study.

AGE

Age is an important factor that profoundly affects opioid action. Several reports indicate older patients sustain higher plasma concentrations after opioid administration on the basis of weight.[228,441] A strong positive correlation between age and the incidence of unconsciousness after 30 μg/kg of fentanyl IV has recently been described. In this study all patients over 60 years of age but only one-half less than 40 years of age lost consciousness whether or not they were premedicated with diazepam.[86] Unfortunately, changes in volumes of distribution and clearance do not consistently explain these results. Whether infants and children have significantly different pharmacokinetics for morphine, meperidine, or any of the other opioids is unclear. Neonates do eliminate meperidine more slowly than do adults.[442]

DOSE

Dose generally does not alter pharmacokinetic variables.[433,443] This suggests that biotransformation and excretion mechanisms are not easily saturated by clinical doses of opioids and that kinetics usually remain first order (drug concentration dependent).

LIVER DISEASE

Acute (hepatitis) and chronic (cirrhosis) liver disease prolong the elimination half-life and clearance of meperidine[422,444-446] and probably of other opioids as well. Interestingly, cirrhosis does not alter hepatic clearance or duration of action of fentanyl. The volume of distribution of meperidine is only slightly increased[422] and protein binding unaffected by hepatitis and cirrhosis. These data suggest that although initial doses may have an approximately normal duration, subsequent administration will result in more prolonged effects.[434]

RENAL DISEASE

Active metabolites of opioids are usually only of clinical importance during renal failure. While fentanyl has no or few active metabolites,[447] both morphine-3-glucuronide and normeperidine may play a role in the prolonged effect (or toxicity) observed with morphine or meperidine in renal failure patients.[436] Although acute and chronic renal disease produces changes in protein binding (e.g., decreases with morphine), this is probably of no clinical importance.[448]

CARDIOPULMONARY BYPASS

A cardiopulmonary bypass produces marked changes in drug pharmacokinetics. Elimination half-life is prolonged due to a larger volume of distribution and decreased hepatic blood flow.[318,449-451] Plasma protein binding is decreased (due to dilution) and, although total plasma drug concentration is reduced, decreases in free concentration will be buffered by large peripheral compartment stores. Decreased tissue (skeletal muscle) perfusion during bypass or bypassed tissue (lung) will affect drug kinetics, and decreases in hepatic perfusion and body temperature will slow hepatic drug clearance and metabolism. The bypass apparatus also absorbs significant amounts of fentanyl.[452]

SUFENTANIL

Sufentanil (Fig. 23-8) is a recently released potent synthetic opioid agonist that is 5 to 10 times more potent than fentanyl. The plasma decay curve of sufentanil fits a three-compartment model with a rapid ($t\frac{1}{2}\ \pi$) distribution half-life of 0.72 minutes and a $t\frac{1}{2}\ \alpha$ of 13.7 minutes.[453] Sufentanil is highly protein bound (92.5 percent),[454] predominantly to α_1-acid glycoprotein, is quite lipophilic, and has a faster onset of action than that of fentanyl.[158,455,456] At steady state, the volume of distribution of sufentanil is 2.48 L/kg, somewhat less than that of fentanyl. This, coupled with a shorter elimination half-life ($t\frac{1}{2}\ \beta$) of 148 minutes may explain the reported shorter duration of postoperative respiratory depression and time to endotracheal extubation with sufentanil.[455] The clearance (11.8 mg/min/kg) and hepatic extraction ratio (0.72) of sufentanil are similar to those of fentanyl. As with fentanyl, the effect of small doses is likely to be terminated by redistribution to the peripheral compartment. With larger doses, plasma concentrations of sufentanil are not rendered subtherapeutic by redistribution, due to relative saturation of the peripheral compartment. In this instance, hepatic biotransformation is responsible for termination of clinical effect.

ALFENTANIL

Alfentanil (Fig. 23-8) is another new fentanyl derivative. Alfentanil is approximately one-third to one-fifth as potent as fentanyl, but has a faster onset and shorter duration of action than that of the former. At doses of 50 to 260 mg/kg, $t\frac{1}{2}\ \pi$ and $t\frac{1}{2}\ \alpha$ have been reported to be about 2 to 3 minutes and 10 to 20 minutes, respectively.[457,458] Alfentanil is significantly less lipophilic than fentanyl and has a smaller (0.5 to 1.0 L/kg) volume of distribution at steady state. Alfentanil is approximately 10 percent ionized at pH 7.4 but is highly bound to plasma proteins (92 percent). Although rapidly metabolized by the liver, the clearance of alfentanil is less than that of fentanyl (4 to 8 vs 10 to 20

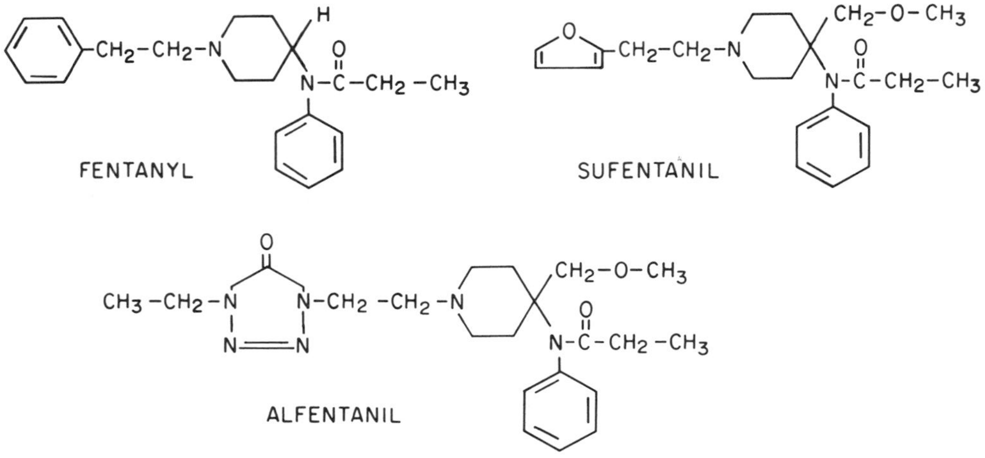

FIG. 23-8 Structural formulas of fentanyl, sufentanil, and alfentanil.

ml/kg/min). However, the small volume of distribution of alfentanil at steady state results in an elimination half-life (t$\frac{1}{2}$ β) considerably less than that of fentanyl (1.5 vs 3.5 hours). The markedly different pharmacokinetic profile of alfentanil explains the more rapid onset of action and shorter duration of effect of the drug. It may be most suitably applied by infusion techniques.[459]

PHARMACOKINETICS AND THE CLINICAL USE OF INTRAVENOUS NARCOTIC ANESTHETICS

The nature of narcotic anesthesia (i.e., "light anesthesia") and of most popular techniques used in the past (i.e., bolus injection producing initially supratherapeutic blood levels and relative albeit safe overdose) has often led to prolonged effects during the postoperative period. Investigators interested in minimizing this "side effect" have searched for ways of more accurately delivering opioids yet ensuring that plasma concentrations are "anesthetic." Use of pharmacokinetic principles and the theoretic ability to produce known plasma concentrations of drugs[460] has led to a more sci-

entific approach in an attempt to refine the administration of opioid anesthesia.

Alfentanil is relatively more predictable than fentanyl in that its elimination is less variable. Its smaller volume of distribution reduces the contribution of redistribution to termination of drug effect, and its lower hepatic clearance renders that clearance less dependent on hepatic blood flow.[461,462] However, these are modest gains when one considers the gaps in our knowledge. Fundamental principles such as the relationship between pharmacokinetics and dynamics and factors producing variations in that relationship remain largely unanswered.

The role and importance of pharmacokinetics will continue to be defined; for example, obesity increases the elimination half-life of alfentanil due to decreased clearance[463] and cardiopulmonary bypass increases the volume of distribution for alfentanil and fentanyl.[464] This science is at least valuable food for thought. Whether it will help the clinician provide a clinically safer and better anesthetic remains to be seen. How much, at what rate, to produce what concentration (measured or assumed), so as to yield certain effects, and what clinical factors one must consider to calculate a patient's anesthetic requirements accurately are basic questions that now appear overwhelming but may one day be straightforward.

REFERENCES

1. Foldes FF, Swerdlow M, Siker ES: Narcotics and Narcotic Antagonists. Springfield, IL, Charles C Thomas, 1964, pp 3–9
2. Stanley TH, Webster LR: Anesthetic requirements and cardiovascular effects of fentanyl-oxygen and fentanyl-diazepam-oxygen anesthesia in man. Anesth Analg 57:411, 1978
3. Stanley TH, Philbin DM, Coggins CH: Fentanyl-oxygen anaesthesia for coronary artery surgery: Cardiovascular and antidiuretic hormone responses. Can Anaesth Soc J 26:168, 1979
4. Hall GM: Analgesia and the metabolic response to surgery. Proc R Soc Med 3:19, 1978
5. Florence A: Attenuation of stress and haemodynamic stability. Proc R Soc Med 3:23, 1978
6. Hug CC, Murphy MR: Fentanyl disposition in cerebrospinal fluid and plasma and its relationship to ventilatory depression in the dog. Anesthesiology 50:342, 1979
7. Lowenstein E, Philbin D: Narcotic "anesthesia" in the eighties (editorial). Anesthesiology 55:195, 1981
8. Van Hoosen B: Scopolamine-Morphine Anaesthesia. Chicago, House of Manz, 1915
9. Smith RR: Scopolamine-morphine anaesthesia, with report of two hundred and twenty-nine cases. Surg Gynecol Obstet 7:414, 1908
10. Sexton JC: Death following scopolamine-morphine injection. Lancet Clin 55:582, 1905
11. Lundy JS: Balanced anesthesia. Minn Med 9:399, 1926
12. Neff W, Mayer EC, de la Luz Perales M: Nitrous oxide and oxygen anesthesia with curare relaxation. Calif Med 66:67, 1947
13. Holderness MC, Chase PE, Dripps RD: A narcotic analgesic and a butyrophenone with nitrous oxide for general anesthesia. Anesthesiology 24:336, 1963
14. Stoelting RK: Influence of barbiturate anesthetic induction on circulatory responses to morphine. Anesth Analg 56:615, 1977
15. Stanley TH, Bennett GM, Loeser EA, et al: Cardiovascular effects of diazepam and droperidol during morphine anesthesia. Anesthesiology 44:255, 1976
16. Bennett GM, Loeser EA, Stanley TH: Cardiovascular effects of scopolamine during morphine-oxygen and morphine-nitrous oxide-oxygen anesthesia in man. Anesthesiology 46:255, 1977
17. Mannheimer WH: The use of morphine and intravenous alcohol in the anesthetic management of open heart surgery. South Med J 64:1125, 1971
18. Stanley TH: Blood pressure and pulse rate responses to ketamine during general anesthesia. Anesthesiology 39:648, 1973
19. Bennett GM, Stanley TH: Cardiovascular effects of fentanyl during enflurane anesthesia in man. Anesth Analg 58:179, 1979
20. Hamm D, Freedman, B, Pellom G, et al: The maintenance of myocardial contractility by fentanyl during enflurane administration. Anesthesiology 59:A86, 1983
21. Freedman B, Ham D, Pellom G, et al: Fentanyl-halothane anesthesia maintains myocardial contractility. Anesthesiology 59:A35, 1983
22. De Castro J: Analgesic anesthesia based on the use of fentanyl in high doses. Anesth Vigil Subvigile 1:87, 1970
23. Lowenstein E, Hallowell P, Levine FH, et al: Cardiovascular response to large doses of intravenous morphine in man. N Engl J Med 281:1389, 1969
24. Stoelting RK, Gibbs, PS: Hemodynamic effects of morphine and morphine-nitrous oxide in valvular heart disease and coronary artery disease. Anesthesiology 38:45, 1973
25. Arens JF, Benbow BP, Ochsner JL, et al: Morphine anesthesia for aorto-coronary bypass procedures. Anesth Analg 51:901, 1972
26. Stanley TH, Gray NH, Stanford W, Armstrong R: The effects of high-dose morphine on fluid and blood requirements in open-heart operations. Anesthesiology 38:536, 1973
27. Stoelting RK, Gibbs PS, Creasser CW, et al: Hemodynamic and ventilatory responses to fentanyl, fentanyl-droperidol, and nitrous oxide in patients with acquired valvular heart disease. Anesthesiology 42:319, 1975
28. Lowenstein, E: Morphine "anesthesia" — A perspective. Anesthesiology 35:563, 1971
29. Hug CC: Pharmacology — Anesthetic drugs, Cardiac Anesthesia. Edited by Kaplan JA. New York, Grune & Stratton, 1979, pp 3–37
30. Thompson WL, Walton RP: Elevation of plasma histamine levels in the dog following administration of muscle relaxants, opiates and macromolecular polymers. J Pharmacol Exp Ther 143:131, 1964
31. Bedford RF, Wollman H: Postoperative respiratory effects of morphine and halothane anesthesia: A study in patients undergoing cardiac surgery. Anesthesiology 43:1, 1975
32. Stanley TH, Lathrop GD: Urinary excretion of morphine during and after valvular and coronary-artery surgery. Anesthesiology 46:166, 1977
33. Rosow CE, Philbin DM, Keegan CR, et al: Hemodynamics and histamine release during induc-

tion with sufentanil or fentanyl. Anesthesiology 60:489, 1984

34. Woolf A: Immobilization of captive and free ranging white-tailed deer with etorphine hydrochloride. J Am Vet Med Assoc 156:636, 1970

35. Thorpe AH: Opiate structure and activity: A guide to understanding the receptor. Anesth Analg 63:143, 1984

36. Snyder SH: Opiate receptors and internal opiates. Sci Am 236:44, 1977

37. Beckett AH, Casey AF: Synthetic analgesics, stereochemical considerations. J Pharm Pharmacol 6:986, 1954

38. Beckett AH: Analgesics and their antagonists: Some steric and chemical considerations. Part I. The dissociation constants of some tertiary amines and synthetic analgesics, the conformations of methadone-type compounds. J Pharm Pharmacol 8:848, 1956

39. Braenden OJ, Eddy NB, Halback H: Synthetic substances with morphine-like effect: Relationship between chemical structure and analgesic action. Bull WHO 13:937, 1955

40. Reynolds AK, Randall LO: Morphine and Allied Drugs. Toronto, University of Toronto Press, 1957, pp 151–160, 365–377

41. Osei-Gyimah P, Archer S: Some 14-beta-substituted analogues of N-(cyclopropylmethyl)normorphine. J Med Chem 24:212, 1981

42. Portoghese PS, Alreja BD, Larson DL: Allylprodine analogues as receptor probes. Evidence that phenolic and nonphenolic ligands interact with different subsites on identical opioid receptors. J Med Chem 24:782, 1981

43. Gorin FA, Balasubramanian TM, Cicero TJ, et al: Novel analogues of enkephalin: Identification of functional groups required for biological activity. J Med Chem 23:1113, 1980

44. Pert CB, Snyder SH: Opiate receptor: Demonstration in nervous tissue. Science 179:1011, 1973

45. Terenius L: Characteristics of the "receptor" for narcotic analgesics in synaptic plasma membrane fractions from rat brain. Acta Pharmacol Toxicol (Copenh) 13:377, 1973

46. Simon EJ, Hiller JM, Edelman I: Stereospecific binding of the potent narcotic analgesic [³H]-etorphine to rat-brain homogenate. Proc Natl Acad Sci USA 70:1947, 1973

47. Pasternak GW, Childers SR: Opiates, opioid peptides and their receptors, Critical Care: State of the Art. Vol. V. Edited by Shoemaker WM. Society of Critical Care Medicine, Fullerton, CA, 1984, pp (F)1-60

48. Yaksh TL, Howe JR: Opiate receptors and their definition by antagonists. Anesthesiology 56:246, 1982

49. Takemori A: Determination of pharmacological constants: Use of narcotic antagonists to characterize analgesic receptors. Adv Biochem Psychopharmacol 8:335, 1974

50. Yaksh TL: Spinal opiate analgesia: Characteristics and principles of action. Pain 11:293, 1981

51. Tung AS, Yaksh TL: In vivo evidence for multiple opiate receptors mediating analgesia in the rat spinal cord. Brain Res 247:75, 1982

52. Creese I, Snyder, SH: Receptor binding and pharmacological activity of opiates in the guinea pig ileum intestine. J Pharmacol Exp Ther 194:205, 1975

53. Chanag KJ, Cuatrecasas P: Multiple opiate receptors: Enkephalins and morphine bind to receptors of difference specificity. J Biol Chem 254:2610, 1979

54. Goodman RR, Snyder, SH, Kuhar MJ, et al: Differentiation of delta and mu opiate receptor localizations by light microscopic autoradiography. Proc Natl Acad Sci USA 77:6239, 1980

55. Pasternak GW, Snyder SH: Identification of novel high affinity opiate receptor binding in rat brain. Nature 253:563, 1975

56. Wolozin BL, Pasternak GW: Classification of multiple morphine and enkephalin binding sites in the central nervous system. Proc Natl Acad Sci USA 78:6181, 1981

57. Pasternak GW, Zhang AZ, Tecott L: Developmental differences between high and low affinity opiate binding sites: Their relationship to analgesia and respiratory depression. Life Sci 27:1185, 1980

58. Ling GSF, Pasternak GW: Spinal and supraspinal analgesia in the mouse: The role of subpopulations of opioid binding sites. Brain Res 271:152, 1983

59. Kuhar MJ, Pert CB, Snyder SH: Regional distribution of opiate receptor binding in monkey and human brain. Nature 245:447, 1973

60. Martin WR, Eades CG, Thompson JA, et al: The effects of morphine- and nalorphine-like drugs in the nondependent and morphine-dependent chronic spinal dog. J Pharmacol Exp Ther 197:517, 1976

61. Franz DN, Hare BD, McCloskey KL: Spinal sympathetic neurons: Possible sites of opiate withdrawal suppression by clonidine. Science 215:1643, 1982

62. Pert A, Yaksh T: Sites of morphine-induced analgesia in the primate brain: Relation to pain pathways. Brain Res 80:135, 1974

63. Goldstein A: Opiate receptors. Life Sci 14:615, 1974

64. Snyder SH: Opiate receptors in the brain. N Engl J Med 296:266, 1977

65. Mayer DJ, Wolfle TL, Akil H, et al: Analgesia

from electrical stimulation in the brainstem of the rat. Science 174:1351, 1971

66. Satoh M, Takagi H: Enhancement by morphine of the central descending inhibitory influence on spinal sensory transmission. Eur J Pharmacol 14:60, 1971

67. Yaksh TL, Rudy TA: Studies on the direct spinal action of narcotics in the production of analgesia in the rat. J Pharmacol Exp Ther 202:411, 1977

68. Yaksh TL, Frederickson RCA, Huang SP, et al: In vivo comparison of the receptor populations acted upon in the spinal cord by morphine and pentapeptides in the production of analgesia. Brain Res 148:516, 1978

69. Stanley TH, Leysen J, Niemegeers JE, et al: Narcotic dosage and central nervous system opiate receptor binding. Anesth Analg 62:705, 1983

70. Hughes J, Smith TW, Kosterlitz HW, et al: Identification of two related pentapeptides from the brain with potent opiate agonist activity. Nature 258:577, 1975

71. Cox BM, Opheim KE, Teschemaker H, et al: A peptide-like substance from pituitary that acts like morphine. Purification and properties. Life Sci 16:1777, 1975

72. Goldstein A, Fischli W, Lowney LI, et al: Porcine pituitary dynorphin: Complete amino acid sequence of the biologically active heptadecapeptide. Proc Natl Acad Sci USA 78:7219, 1981

73. Mains RE, Eipper BA, Ling N: Common precursor to corticotropins and endorphins. Proc Natl Acad Sci USA 74:3014, 1977

74. Gubler U, Kilpatrick DL, Seeburg PH, et al: Detection and partial characterization of proenkephalin in mRNA. Proc Natl Acad Sci USA 78:5484, 1981

75. Olson GA, Olson RD, Kastin AJ, et al: Endogenous opiates: 1980. Peptides 2:349, 1981

76. Rossier J, Vargo TM, Minick S, et al: Regional dissociation of beta-endorphin and enkephalin contents in rat brain and pituitary. Proc Natl Acad Sci USA 74:5162, 1977

77. LaMotte CC, Collins JG, Robinson CJ: Endogenous opiate systems and opiate receptors, Narcotic Analgesics in Anesthesiology. Edited by Kitahata LM, Collins JG. Waverly Press, Baltimore/London 1982, pp 43–52

78. Orwall ES, Kendall JW: B-endorphin and ACTH in extra-adrenocorticotropin pituitary sites: Gastrointestinal tract. Endocrinology 107:438, 1980

79. Houck JC, Kimball C, Chang C, et al: Placental beta-endorphin-like peptides. Science 207:78, 1980

80. Goldstein AL: Opioid peptides (endorphins) in pituitary and brain. Science 193:1981, 1976

81. Fields HL, Anderson SD: Evidence that raphe-spinal neurons mediate opiate and midbrain stimulation-produced analgesia. Pain 5:333, 1978

82. Wong KC: Narcotics are not expected to produce unconsciousness and amnesia (editorial). Anesth Analg 62:625, 1983

83. Murphy MR, Hug CC: Efficacy of fentanyl in reducing isoflurane MAC; Antagonism by naloxone and nalbuphine. Anesthesiology 59: A338, 1983

84. Port JD, Stanley TH, Steffey EP, et al: Intravenous carfentanil in the dog and rhesus monkey. Anesthesiology 61:A378, 1984

85. Stanley TH, Liu WS, Lathrop GD: The effects of morphine and halothane anaesthesia on urine norepinephrine during surgery for congenital heart disease. Can Anaesth Soc J 23:58, 1976

86. Bailey PL, Wilbrink J, Zwanikken P, et al: Anesthetic induction with fentanyl. Anesth Analg 64:48, 1985

87. Stanley TH, deLange S: The influence of patient habits on dosage requirements during high dose fentanyl anesthesia. Can Anaesth Soc J 31:368, 1985

88. Shafter A, White PG, Schuttler J, et al: Use of a fentanyl infusion in the intensive care unit: Tolerance to its anesthetic effect. Anesthesiology 59:245, 1983

89. Tomichek RC, Rosow CE, Philbin DM, et al: Diazepam–fentanyl interaction—Hemodynamic and hormonal effects in coronary artery surgery. Anesth Analg 62:881, 1983

90. Sebel PS, Bovill JG: Opioid anaesthesia—Fact or fallacy? (editorial). Br J Anaesth 54:1149, 1982

91. Wilson SL, Vaughan RW, Stephen CR: Awareness, dreams and hallucinations associated with general anesthesia. Anesth Analg 54:609, 1975.

92. Saucier N, Walts LF, Moreland JR: Patient awareness during nitrous oxide, oxygen and halothane anesthesia. Anesth Analg 62:239, 1983

93. Mark JB, Greenberg LM: Intraoperative awareness and hypertensive crisis during high-dose fentanyl-diazepam-oxygen anesthesia. Anesth Analg 62:698, 1983

94. Hilgenberg JC: Intraoperative awareness during high-dose fentanyl-oxygen anesthesia. Anesthesiology 54:341, 1981

95. Mummanemi N, Rao T, Montoya A: Awareness and recall with high-dose fentanyl oxygen anesthesia. Anesth Analg 59:943, 1980

96. Blacher RS: On awakening paralyzed during surgery. A syndrome of traumatic neurosis. JAMA 234:67, 1975

97. Van De Walle J, Lauwers P, Adriaensen H: Dou-

ble blind comparison of fentanyl and sufentanil in anesthesia. Acta Anaesthesiol Belg 27:129, 1976

98. Sebel PS, Bovill JG: Cardiovascular effects of sufentanil anesthesia: A study in patients undergoing cardiac surgery. Anesth Analg 61:115, 1982

99. Schmidt CF, Livingston AE: The action of morphine on the mammalian circulation. J Pharmacol Exp Ther 47:411, 1933

100. Moffitt EA, Sethna DH, Bussell JA, et al: Myocardial metabolism and hemodynamic responses to halothane or morphine anesthesia for coronary artery surgery. Anesth Analg 61:979, 1982

101. Vasko JS, Henney RP, Brawley RK, et al: Effects of morphine on ventricular function and myocardial contractile force. Am J Physiol 210:329, 1966

102. Stanley TH, Isern-Amaral J, Lathrop GD: Effects of morphine and halothane anaesthesia on urine norepinephrine during and after coronary artery surgery. Can Anaesth Soc J 22:478, 1975

103. Stanley TH, Isern-Amaral J, Lathrop GD: Urine norepinephrine excretion in patients undergoing mitral or aortic valve replacement with morphine anesthesia. Anesth Analg 54:509, 1975

104. Balasariswathi K, Glisson SN, El-Etr AA, et al: Serum epinephrine and norepinephrine during valve replacement and aortocoronary bypass. Can Anaesth Soc J 25:198, 1978

105. Liu WS, Bidwai AV, Lunn JK, et al: Urine catecholamine excretion after large doses of fentanyl, fentanyl and diazepam and fentanyl, diazepam and pancuronium. Can Anaesth Soc J 24:371, 1977

106. Stanley TH, Berman L, Green O, et al: Plasma catecholamine and cortisol responses to fentanyl-oxygen anesthesia for coronary-artery operations. Anesthesiology 53:250, 1980

107. Hicks HC, Mowbray AG, Yhap EO: Cardiovascular effects of and catecholamine responses to high dose fentanyl-O$_2$ for induction of anesthesia in patients with ischemic coronary artery disease. Anesth Analg 60:563, 1981

108. Lunn JK, Stanley TH, Webster LR, et al: High dose fentanyl anesthesia for coronary artery surgery: Plasma fentanyl concentration and influence of nitrous oxide on cardiovascular responses. Anesth Analg 58:390, 1979

109. Kentor ML, Schwalb AJ, Lieberman RW: Rapid high dose fentanyl induction for CABG. Anesthesiology 53:S95, 1980

110. Drew JH, Dripps RD, Comroe JH: Clinical studies on morphine. II. The effect of morphine upon the circulation of man and upon the circulatory

and respiratory responses to tilting. Anesthesiology 7:44, 1946

111. Conahan TJ, Ominsky AJ, Wollman H, et al: A prospective random comparison of halothane and morphine for open-heart anesthesia: One year's experience. Anesthesiology 38:528, 1973

112. Lappas DG, Geha D, Fischer JE, et al: Filling pressures of the heart and pulmonary circulation of the patient with coronary-artery disease after large intravenous doses of morphine. Anesthesiology 42:153, 1975

113. Rosow CE, Moss J, Philbin DM, et al: Histamine release during morphine and fentanyl anesthesia. Anesthesiology 56:93, 1982

114. Falmy NR, Sunder N, Soter NA: Role of histamine in the hemodynamic and plasma catecholamine responses to morphine. Clin Pharmacol Ther 33:615, 1983

115. Flacke, JW, Van Etten A, Flake WE: Greatest histamine release from meperidine among four narcotics: Double-blind study in man. Anesthesiology 59:A51, 1983

116. Moss J, Rosow CE: Histamine release by narcotics and muscle relaxants in humans. Anesthesiology 59:330, 1983

117. Lowenstein E, Whiting RB, Bittar DA, et al: Local and neurally mediated effects of morphine on skeletal muscle vascular resistance. J Pharmacol Exp Ther 180:359, 1972

118. Henney RP, Vasko JS, Brawley RK, et al: The effects of morphine on the resistance and capacitance vessels of the peripheral circulation. Am Heart J 72:242, 1966

119. Ward JM, McGrath RC, Weil JL: Effect of morphine on the peripheral vascular response to sympathetic stimulation. Am J Cardiol 29:659, 1972

120. Stanley TH, Gray NH, Isern-Amaral J, et al: Comparison of blood requirements during morphine and halothane anesthesia for open-heart surgery. Anesthesiology 41:34, 1974

121. Greene JF, Jackman AP, Krohn KA: Mechanism of morphine induced shifts in blood volume between extracorporeal reservoir and the systemic circulation of the dog under conditions of constant blood flow and vena caval pressures. Circ Res 42:479, 1978

122. Greene JF, Jackman AP, Parsons G: The effects of morphine on the mechanical properties of the systemic circulation in the dog. Circ Res 42:474, 1978

123. Hsu HO, Hickey RF, Forbes AR: Morphine decreases peripheral vascular resistance and increases capacitance in man. Anesthesiology 50:98, 1979

124. Zelis R, Mansour EJ, Capone RJ, et al: The cardiovascular effects of morphine: The peripheral

capacitance and resistance vessels in human subjects. J Clin Invest 54:1247, 1974

125. Zelis R, Flaim SF, Eisele JH: Effects of morphine on reflex arteriolar constriction induced in man by hypercapnia. Clin Pharmacol Ther 22:172, 1977

126. Priano LL, Vatner SF: Morphine effects on cardiac output and regional blood flow distribution in conscious dogs. Anesthesiology 55:236, 1981

127. Wong KC, Martin WE, Hornbein TF, et al: The cardiovascular effects of morphine sulfate with oxygen and with nitrous oxide in man. Anesthesiology 38:542, 1973

128. Moores WY, Weiskopf RB, Baysinger M, et al: Effects of halothane and morphine sulfate on myocardial compliance following total cardiopulmonary bypass. J Thorac Cardiovasc Surg 81:163, 1981

129. Hoar PF, Nelson NT, Mangano DT, et al: Adrenergic response to morphine-diazepam anesthesia for myocardial revascularization. Anesth Analg 60:406, 1981

130. Freye E: Cardiovascular effects of high dosages of fentanyl, meperidine and naloxone in dogs. Anesth Analg 53:40, 1974

131. Stanley TH, Bidwai AV, Lunn JK, et al: Cardiovascular effects of nitrous oxide during meperidine infusion in the dog. Anesth Analg 56:836, 1977

132. DeCastro J, Van de Water A, Wouters L, et al: Comparative study of cardiovascular, neurological and metabolic side effects of eight narcotics in dogs. Acta Anaesthesiol Belg 30:5, 1979

133. Stanley TH, Liu WS: Cardiovascular effects of meperidine-N_2O anesthesia before and after pancuronium. Anesth Analg 56:669, 1977

134. King BD, Elder JD, Dripps RD: The effect of the intravenous administration of meperidine upon the circulation of man and upon the circulatory response to tilt. Surg Gynecol Obstet 94:591, 1952

135. Sugioka K, Boniface KJ, Davis DA: The influence of meperidine on myocardial contractility in the intact dog. Anesthesiology 18:623, 1957

136. Strauer BE: Contractile responses to morphine, piritramide, meperidine and fentanyl: A comparative study of effects on the isolated ventricular myocardium. Anesthesiology 37:304, 1972

137. Reddy P, Liu WS, Stanley TH, et al: Hemodynamic effects of anesthetic doses of alpha-prodine and sufentanil in dogs. Anesthesiology 51:S102, 1979

138. Waller JL, Hug CC, Nagle DM, et al: Hemodynamic changes during fentanyl-oxygen anesthesia for aortocoronary bypass operations. Anesthesiology 55:212, 1981

139. Wynands JE, Wong P, Whalley DG, et al: Oxygen-fentanyl anesthesia in patients with poor left ventricular function, hemodynamics and plasma fentanyl concentrations. Anesth Analg 62:476, 1983

140. Hamm D, Freedman B, Pellom G, et al: The effect of fentanyl on left ventricular function. Anesthesiology 59:A37, 1983

141. Motomura S, Kissin I, Aultman D, et al: Effects of fentanyl and nitrous oxide on contractility of blood-perfused papillary muscle of the dog. Anesth Analg 63:47, 1984

142. Sebel PS, Bovel JG, Boekhorst RAA, et al: Cardiovascular effects of high dose fentanyl anesthesia. Acta Anaesthesiol Scand 26:308, 1982

143. Liu WS, Bidwai AV, Stanley TH, et al: The cardiovascular effects of diazepam and of diazepam and pancuronium during fentanyl and oxygen anaesthesia. Can Anaesth Soc J 23:395, 1976

144. Hill AB, Nahrwold ML, de Rosayro M, et al: Prevention of rigidity during fentanyl-oxygen induction of anesthesia. Anesthesiology 55:452, 1981

145. Van Bever WFM, Niemegeers CJE, Schellekens KHL, et al: Sufentanil: A potent and extremely safe intravenous morphine-like compound in mice, rats and dogs. Arzneimittelforsch 26:1551, 1976

146. Niemegeers CJE, Janssen PAJ: Alfentanil, a particularly short-acting intravenous narcotic analgesic. Drug Dev Res 1:83, 1981

147. Schauble JF, Chen BB, Murray PA: Marked hemodynamic effects of bolus administration of alfentanil in conscious dogs. Anesthesiology 59:A85, 1983

148. de Bruijn ND, Christian C, Fagraeus L, et al: The effects of alfentanil on global ventricular mechanics. Anesthesiology 59:A33, 1983

149. Nauta J, de Lange S, Koopman D, et al: Anesthetic induction with alfentanil: A new short acting narcotic analgesic. Anesth Analg 61:267, 1982

150. Moldenhauer CC, Griesemer RW, Hug CC, et al: Hemodynamic changes during rapid induction of anesthesia with alfentanil. Anesth Analg 62:276, 1983

151. Bartkowski RR, McDonnell TE: Alfentanil as an anesthetic induction agent: A comparison with thiopental-lidocaine. Anesth Analg 63:330, 1984

152. Hasbrouck JD: Morphine anesthesia for open heart surgery. Ann Thorac Surg 10:364, 1970

153. Bailey DR, Miller ED, Kaplan JA, et al: The renin-angiotensin-aldosterone system during cardiac surgery with morphine-nitrous oxide anesthesia. Anesthesiology 42:538, 1975

154. de Lange S, Stanley TH, Boscoe M: Fentanyl-ox-

ygen anesthesia: Comparison of anesthetic requirements and cardiovascular responses in Salt Lake City and Leiden, Holland, Proceedings of the Seventh World Congress of Anaesthesiology. Edited by Zindler M, Rugheimer E. Amsterdam, Excerpta Medica, 1980, p 313

155. Quinton L, Whalley DG, Wynands JE, et al: Oxygen-high dose fentanyl-droperidol anesthesia for aortocoronary bypass surgery. Anesth Analg 60:412, 1981

156. Wynands JE, Townsend GE, Wong P, et al: Blood pressure response and plasma fentanyl concentrations during high- and very high-dose fentanyl anesthesia for coronary artery surgery. Anesth Analg 62:661, 1983

157. Edde RR: Hemodynamic changes prior to and after sternotomy in patients anesthetized with high-dose fentanyl. Anesthesiology 55:444, 1981

158. de Lange S, Stanley TH, Boscoe MJ, et al: Comparison of sufentanil-O$_2$ and fentanyl-O$_2$ for coronary artery surgery. Anesthesiology 56:112, 1982

159. Sebel PS, Bovill JG, Schellekens APM, et al: Hormonal responses of high-dose fentanyl anaesthesia: A study in patients underoing cardiac surgery. Br J Anaesth 53:941, 1981

160. Stoelting RK, Creasser CW, Gibbs PS, et al: Circulatory effects of halothane added to morphine anesthesia in patients with coronary-artery disease. Anesth Analg 53:449, 1974

161. Bland JHL, Chir B, Lowenstein E: Halothane-induced decrease in experimental myocardial ischemia in the non-failing canine heart. Anesthesiology 45:287, 1976

162. Freedman B, Christian C, Hamm D, et al: Isoflurane and myocardial protection. Anesthesiology 59:A25, 1983

163. Hecker BR, Lake CL, DiFazio CA, et al: The decrease of the minimum alveolar anesthetic concentration produced by sufentanil in rats. Anesth Analg 62:987, 1983

164. Murphy MR, Hug CC: The anesthetic potency of fentanyl in terms of its reduction of enflurane MAC. Anesthesiology 57:485, 1982

165. Rolly G, Kay B, Cocks F: A double blind comparison of high doses of fentanyl and sufentanil in man. Influence on cardiovascular, respiratory and metabolic parameters. Acta Anaesthesiol Belg 30:247, 1979

166. Larsen R, Sonntag H, Schenk HD, et al: Die Wirkungen von Sufentanil und Fentanyl auf Hamodynamik, Coronardurchblutung und Myocardialen Metabolismus des Menschen. Anaesthesist 29:277, 1980

167. Flacke JW, Kripke BK, Bloor BC, et al: Intraoperative effectiveness of sufentanil, fentanyl, me-

peridine or morphine in balanced anesthesia: A double blind study. Anesth Analg 62:259, 1983

168. de Lange S, Stanley TH, Boscoe MJ: Alfentanil-oxygen anaesthesia for coronary artery surgery. Br J Anaesth 53:1291, 1981

169. Reitan JA, Stengert KB, Wymore ML, et al: Central vagal control of fentanyl induced bradycardia during halothane anesthesia. Anesth Analg 57:31, 1978

170. Tammisto T, Takki S, Toikka P: A comparison of the circulatory effects in man of the analgesics fentanyl, pentazocine and pethidine. Br j Anaesth 42:317, 1970

171. Liu WS, Bidwai AV, Stanley TH, et al: Cardiovascular dynamics after large doses of fentanyl and fentanyl plus N$_2$O in the dog. Anesth Analg 55:168, 1976

172. Prakash O, Verdouw PD, De Jong JW, et al: Haemodynamic and biochemical variables after induction of anaesthesia in patients undergoing coronary artery bypass surgery. Can Anaesth Soc J 27:223, 1980

173. Hornbein TF, Martin WE, Bonica JJ, et al: Nitrous oxide effects on the circulatory and ventilatory responses to halothane. Anesthesiology 31:250, 1969

174. Smith NT, Eger EI, Stoelting RK, et al: The cardiovascular and sympathomimetic responses to the addition of nitrous oxide to halothane in man. Anesthesiology 32:410, 1970

175. Meuleman T, Port JD, Stanley TH, et al: Immobilization of elk and moose with carfentanil. J Wildl Mgmt 48:258, 1984.

176. Reddy P, Liu WS, Port D, et al: Comparison of haemodynamic effects of anaesthetic doses of alphaprodine and sufentanil in the dog. Can Anaesth Soc J 27:345, 1980

177. Williard KF, Port JD, Stanley TH: Narcotic-oxygen anesthesia without respiratory support in the basally anesthetized dog. Anesthesiology 59:A321, 1983

178. Port JD, Stanley TH, McJames S: Topical narcotic anesthesia. Anesthesiology 59:A325, 1983

179. de Lange S, Boscoe MJ, Stanley TH, et al: Antidiuretic and growth hormone responses during coronary artery surgery with sufentanil-oxygen and alfentanil-oxygen anesthesia in man. Anesth Analg 61:434, 1982

180. de Lange S, de Bruijn N: Alfentanil-oxygen anesthesia: Plasma concentration and clinical effects during variable rate continuous infusion for coronary artery surgery. Br J Anaesth 55:S183, 1983

181. Cohn AE: The effect of morphine on the mechanism of the dog's heart after removal of one vagus nerve. Proc Soc Exp Biol Med 10:93, 1913

182. Robbins BH, Fitzhugh OG, Baxter JH Jr: The ac-

tion of morphine in slowing the pulse. J Pharmacol Exp Ther 66:216, 1939

183. Kennedy BL, West TC: Effect of morphine on electrically-induced release of autonomic mediators in the rabbit sinoatrial node. J Pharmacol Exp Ther 157:149, 1967

184. Urthaler F, Isobe JH, Gilmour KE, et al: Morphine and autonomic control of the sinus node. Chest 64:203, 1973

185. Urthaler F, Isobe JH, James TN: Direct and vagally mediated chronotropic effects of morphine studied by selective perfusion of the sinus node of awake dogs. Chest 68:222, 1975

186. De Silva RA, Verrier RL, Lown B: Protective effect of vagotonic action of morphine sulfate on ventricular vulnerability. Cardiovasc Res 12:167, 1978

187. Freye E: Effects of high doses of fentanyl on myocardial infarction and cardiogenic shock in the dog. Resuscitation 3:105, 1974

188. Eisele JH, Reitan JA, Torten M, et al: Myocardial sparing effect of fentanyl during halothane anaesthesia in dogs. Br J Anaesth 47:937, 1975

189. Puerto BA, Wong KC, Puerto AX, et al: Epinephrine-induced dysrhythmias: Comparison during anaesthesia with narcotics and with halogenated agents in dogs. Can Anaesth Soc J 26:263, 1979

190. Bennett GM, Stanley TH: Comparison of the cardiovascular effects of morphine-N_2O and fentanyl-N_2O balanced anesthesia before and after pancuronium in man. Anesthesiology 51:S138, 1979

191. Craythorne NWB, Darby TD: The cardiovascular effects of nitrous oxide in the dog. Br J Anaesth 37:560, 1965

192. Eisele JH, Smith NT: Cardiovascular effects of 40 percent nitrous oxide in man. Anesth Analg 51:956, 1972

193. McDermott RW, Stanley TH: Cardiovascular effects of low concentrations of nitrous oxide during morphine anesthesia. Anesthesiology 41:89, 1974

194. Bennett GM, Ready P, Liu WS, et al: Hemodynamic effects of anesthetic doses of alpha-prodine and sufentanil in dogs. Anesthesiology 51:S102, 1979

195. Moffitt EA, Scovil JE, Barker RA, et al: Myocardial metabolism and hemodynamics of nitrous oxide in fentanyl or enflurane anesthesia in coronary patients. Anesthesiology 59:A31, 1983

196. Tomichek RC, Rosow CE, Schneider RC, et al: Cardiovascular effects of diazepam-fentanyl anesthesia in patients with coronary artery disease. Anesth Analg 61:217, 1982

197. Stanley TH, Bennett GM, Loeser EA, et al: Cardiovascular effects of diazepam and droperidol during morphine anesthesia. Anesthesiology 44:255, 1975

198. Holmes CM: Supplementation of general anaesthesia with narcotic analgesics. Br J Anaesth 48:907, 1976

199. Cahalan MK, Lurz FW, Beaupre PN, et al: Narcotics alter the heart rate and blood pressure response to inhalational anesthetics. Anesthesiology 59:A26, 1983

200. Salmenpera M, Peltola K, Takkunen G, et al: Cardiovascular effects of pancuronium and vecuronium during high-dose fentanyl anesthesia. Anesth Analg 62:1059, 1983

201. Hickey RF, Severinghaus JW: Regulation of breathing: Drug effects, Lung Biology in Health and Disease. Vol. 17, Part II: Regulation of Breathing. Edited by Hornbein TF. Marcel Dekker, Inc., New York, 1981, pp 1251–1298

202. Ngai SH: Effects of morphine and meperidine on the central respiratory mechanisms in the cat, the action of levallorphan in antagonizing these effects. J Pharmacol Exp Ther 131:91, 1961

203. Tabatabai M, Collins JG, Kitabata LM: Disruption of the activity of the medullary inspiratory neurons by high-dose fentanyl and reversal with nalbuphine. Anesthesiology 59:A485, 1983

204. Weil JV, McCullough RE, Kline JS, et al: Diminished ventilatory response to hypoxia and hypercapnia after morphine in normal man. N Engl J Med 292:1103, 1975

205. Kryger MH, Yacoub O, Dosman J, et al: Effect of meperidine on occlusion pressure responses to hypercapnia and hypoxia with and without external inspiratory resistance. Am Rev Respir Dis 114:333, 1976

206. Rigg RAJ, Rondi P: Changes in rib cage and diaphragm contribution to ventilation after morphine. Anesthesiology 55:507, 1981

207. Drummond GB: Comparison of decreases in ventilation caused by enflurane and fentanyl during anesthesia. Br J Anaesth 55:825, 1983

208. Nielsen CH, Camporesi EM, Bromage PR, et al: CO_2 sensitivity after epidural and I.V. morphine. Anesthesiology 55:A372, 1981

209. Downes JJ, Kemp RA, Lambertsen CJ: The magnitude and duration of respiratory depression due to fentanyl and meperidine in man. J Pharmacol Exp Ther 158:416, 1967

210. Holmes CM: Supplementation of general anaesthesia with narcotic analgesics. Br J Anaesth 48:907, 1976

211. Bailey PL, Andriano KP, Pace NL, et al: Small doses of fentanyl potentiate and prolong diazepam induced respiratory depression. Anesth Analg 63:183, 1984

212. Kay B, Rolly G: Duration of action of analgesic

supplement to anesthesia. Acta Anaesthesiol Belg 28:25, 1977

213. Cartwright P, Prys-Roberts C, Gill K, et al: Ventilatory depression related to plasma fentanyl concentrations during and after anesthesia in humans. Anesth Analg 62:966, 1983

214. Rigg JRA, Goldsmith CH: Recovery of ventilatory response to carbon dioxide after thiopentone, morphine and fentanyl in man. Can Anaesth Soc J 23:370, 1976

215. Adams AP, Pybus DA: Delayed respiratory depression after use of fentanyl during anaesthesia. Br Med J 1:278, 1978

216. Foldes FF, Swerdlow M, Siker SS: Narcotics and Narcotic Antagonists. Springfield, IL, Charles C Thomas, 1964, pp 55–56

217. Reed DJ, Kellog RH: Changes in respiratory response to CO_2 during natural sleep at sea level and at altitude. J Appl Physiol 13:325, 1958

218. Forrest WH, Bellville JW: The effect of sleep plus morphine on the respiratory response to carbon dioxide. Anesthesiology 25:137, 1964

219. Stoeclkel H, Hengstmann JH, Schutter J: Pharmacokinetics of fentanyl as a possible explanation of recurrence of respiratory depression. Br J Anaesth 51:741, 1979

220. Trudowski RJ, Gessner T: Gastric sequestration of meperidine following intravenous administration. Abstracts of Scientific Papers, ASA Meeting, 1975, pp 327–328

221. Becker LD, Paulson BA, Miller RD, et al: Biphasic respiratory depression after fentanyl-droperidol or fentanyl alone used to supplement nitrous oxide anesthesia. Anesthesiology 44: 291, 1976

222. Stoeckel H, Schuttler J, Magnussen H, et al: Plasma fentanyl concentrations and occurrence of respiration depression in volunteers. Br J Anaesth 54:1087, 1982

223. Berkowitz BA, Ngai SH, Yang JC, et al: The disposition of morphine in surgical patients. Clin Pharmacol Ther 17:629, 1975

224. Eckenhoff JE, Oech SR: The effects of narcotics and antagonists upon respiration and circulation in man. Clin Pharmacol Ther 1:483, 1960

225. Harper MH, Hickey RF, Cromwell TH, et al: The magnitude and duration of respiratory depression produced by fentanyl and fentanyl plus droperidol in man. J Pharmacol Exp Ther 199:464, 1976

226. Keats AS, Girgis KZ: Respiratory depression associated with relief of pain by narcotics. Anesthesiology 29:1006, 1968

227. Cooper DY, Lambertson CJ: Effect of changes in tidal volume and alveolar carbon dioxide on physiological dead space. Anesthesiology 18: 160, 1957

228. Van Dongen K, Leusink H: The action of opium-alkaloids and expectorants on the ciliary movements in the air passages. Arch Int Pharmacodyn Ther 93:261, 1953

229. Toda N, Hatano Y: Contractile responses of canine tracheal muscle during exposure to fentanyl and morphine. Anesthesiology 53:93, 1980

230. Sebel PS, Bovill JG, Wauquier A, et al: Effects of high dose fentanyl anesthesia on the electroencephalogram. Anesthesiology 55:203, 1981

231. Scott JC, Stanski DR, Ponganis KV: Quantitation of fentanyl's effect on the brain using the EEG. Anesthesiology 59:A370, 1983

232. Pearcy WC, Knott JR, Bjurstrom RO: Studies on nitrous oxide, meperidine and levallorphan with unipolar electroencephalography. Anesthesiology 18:310, 1957

233. Smith NT, Quinn M, Dec-Silver H, et al: Aperiodic analysis of EEG response to fentanyl and sufentanil anesthesia during open heart surgery. Anesth Analg 62:284, 1983

234. Jober DR, Kennell EM, Bush GL, et al: Cerebral blood flow and metabolism during morphine-nitrous oxide anesthesia in man. Anesthesiology 47:16, 1977

235. Mehenfelder JD, Theye RA: Effects of fentanyl, droperidol, and Innovar on canine cerebral metabolism and blood flow. Br J Anaesth 43:630, 1971

236. Corssen G, Domino EF, Sweet RB: Neuroleptanalgesia and anesthesia. Anesth Analg 43:748, 1964

237. Hamilton WK, Cullen SC: Effect of levallorphan tartrate upon opiate induced respiratory depression. Anesthesiology 14:550, 1953

238. Janis KM: Acute rigidity with small intravenous doses of innovar: A case report. Anesth Analg 51:375, 1972

239. Freman J, Ingvar DH: Effects of fentanyl on cerebral cortical blood flow and EEG in the cat. Acta Anaesthesiol Scand 11:381, 1967

240. Grell FL, Koons DA, Denson JS: Fentanyl in anesthesia: A report of 500 cases. Anesth Analg 49:523, 1970

241. Comstock MK, Carter JG, Moyers JR, et al: Rigidity and hypercarbia associated with high-dose fentanyl induction of anesthesia. Anesth Analg 60:362, 1981

242. Scamman FL: Fentanyl-O_2-N_2O rigidity and pulmonary compliance. Anesth Analg 62:332, 1983

243. Coe V, Shafer A, White PF: Techniques for administering alfentanil during outpatient anesthesia—A comparison with fentanyl. Anesthesiology 59:A347, 1983

244. Gergis SD, Hoyt JL, Sokoll MD: Effects of Innovar and Innovar plus nitrous oxide on muscle tone and "H" reflex. Anesth Analg 50:743, 1971

245. Freund FG, Martin WE, Wong KC, et al: Abdom-

inal muscle rigidity induced by morphine and nitrous oxide. Anesthesiology 38:358, 1973

246. Sokoll MD, Hoyt JL, Gergis SD: Studies in muscle rigidity, nitrous oxide, and narcotic analgesic agents. Anesth Analg 51:16, 1972

247. Jaffe TB, Ramsey FM: Attenuation of fentanyl-induced truncal rigidity. Anesthesiology 58:562, 1983

248. Mavrojammis M: L'action cataleptique de la morphine chez les rats. Contribution à la théorie toxique de la catalepsie. C R Soc Biol (Paris) 55:1092, 1903

249. Jurna I, Ruzdic N, Nell T, et al: The effect of alpha-methyl-p-tyrosine and substantia nigra lesions on spinal motor activity in the rat. Eur J Pharmacol 20:341, 1972

250. Freye E, Kuschinsky K: Effects of fentanyl and droperidol on the dopamine metabolism of the rat striatum. Pharmacology 14:1, 1976

251. Havemann U, Winkler M, Kuschinsky K: Opioid receptors in the caudate nucleus can mediate EMG recorded rigidity in rats. Naunyn Schmiedebergs Arch Pharmacol 313:139, 1980

252. Havemann U, Winkler M, Gene E, et al: Effects of striatal lesions with kainic acid on morphine-induced "catatonia" and increase of striatal dopamine turnover. Naunyn Schmiedebergs Arch Pharmacol 317:44, 1981

253. Havemann U, Kuschinsky K: Further characterization of opioid receptors in the striatum mediating muscular rigidity in rats. Naunyn Schmiedebergs Arch Pharmacol 317:321, 1981

254. Christian CM, Waller JL, Moldenhauer CC: Postoperative rigidity following fentanyl anesthesia. Anesthesiology 58:275, 1983

255. Carlson C, Smith DS, Keykah MM, et al: The effects of high-dose fentanyl in cerebral circulation and metabolism in rats. Anesthesiology 57:375, 1982

256. Frenk H, Urca G, Liebeskind JC: Epileptic properties of leucine and methionine-enkephalin: Comparison with morphine and reversibility by naloxone. Brain Res 147:327, 1978

257. Ingvar MK, Shapiro HM: Selective metabolic activation of the hippocampus during lidocaine-induced pre-seizure activity. Anesthesiology 54:33, 1981

258. DeCastro J, Van de Water A, Wouters L, et al: Comparative study of cardiovascular, neurological and metabolic side effects of eight narcotics in dogs. Acta Anaesthesiol Belg 30:5, 1979

259. Myers RR, Shapiro HM: Local cerebral metabolism during enflurane anesthesia: Identification of epileptogenic foci. Electroencephalogr Clin Neurophysiol 47:153, 1979

260. Crosby G, Crane AM, Sokoloff L: Local changes in cerebral glucose utilization during ketamine anesthesia. Anesthesiology 56:437, 1982

261. Rao TLK, Mummaneni N, El-Etr AA: Convulsions: An unusual response to intravenous fentanyl administration. Anesth Analg 61:1020, 1982

262. Safwat AM, Daniel D: Grand-mal seizure after fentanyl administration. Anesthesiology 59:78, 1983

263. Bovill JG, Sebel PS, Wauquier A, et al: Electro-encephalographic effects of sufentanil anaesthesia in man. Br J Anaesth 54:45, 1982

264. Murkin JM, Moldenhauer CC, Hug CC, et al: Absence of seizures during induction of anesthesia with high-dose fentanyl. Anesth Analg 63:489, 1984

265. Gloor P, Vera CL, Sperti L, et al: Investigations on the mechanism of epileptic discharges in the hippocampus. Epilepsia 2:42, 1961

266. Safo Y, Greenberg J, Young M, et al: Effects of high dose fentanyl on regional cerebral blood flow. Anesthesiology 59:A306, 1983

267. Tommasino C, Mackawa T, Shapiro HM: Fentanyl-induced seizures activate subcortical brain metabolism. Anesthesiology 60:283, 1984

268. Siesjo BK: Brain Energy Metabolism. New York, Wiley, 1978, pp 378–379

269. Dam AM: Hippocampal neuron loss in epilepsy and after experimental seizures. Acta Neurol Scand 66:601, 1982

270. Papper S, Papper EM: The effects of pre-anesthetic, anesthetic, and postoperative drugs on renal function. Clin Pharmacol Ther 5:205, 1964

271. Deutch S, Bastron RD, Pierce EC, et al: The effects of anaesthesia with thiopentone, nitrous oxide, narcotics and neuromuscular blocking drugs on renal function in normal man. Br J Anaesth 41:807, 1969

272. Philbin DM, Wilson NE, Sokoloski J, et al: Radioimmunoassay of antidiuretic hormone during morphine anaesthesia. Can Anaesth Soc J 23:290, 1976

273. Stanley TH, Gray NH, Bidwai AV, et al: The effects of high dose morphine and morphine plus nitrous oxide on urinary output in man. Can Anaesth Soc J 21:379, 1974

274. Bidwai AV, Stanley TH, Bloomer HA: Effects of anesthetic doses of morphine on renal function in the dog. Anesth Analg 54:357, 1975

275. Kono K, Philbin DM, Coggins CH, et al: Renal function and stress response during halothane or fentanyl anesthesia. Anesth Analg 60:552, 1981

276. Wang SC, Glaviano VV: Locus of emetic action of morphine and hydergine in dogs. J Pharmacol Exp Ther 111:329, 1954

277. Reynolds AK, Randall LO: Morphine and Allied Drugs. Toronto, University of Toronto Press, 1957

278. Chapman WP, Rowland EN, Jones CM: Multi-

ple-balloon kymographic recording of the comparative action of demerol, morphine and placebos on the motility of the upper small intestine in man. N Engl J Med 243:171, 1950

279. Martin DE, Joehl RJ: Butorphanol and nalbuphine cause human bile duct obstruction. Anesthesiology 59:A324, 1983

280. de Lange S, Boscoe MJ, Stanley TH, et al: Antidiuretic and growth hormone responses during coronary artery surgery with sufentanil-oxygen and alfentanil-oxygen anesthesia in man. Anesth Analg 61:434, 1982

281. McCammon RL, Stoelting RK, Madura JA: Effects of butorphanol, nalbuphine and fentanyl on intrabiliary tract dynamics. Anesth Analg 63:139, 1984

282. Radnay PA, Duncalf D, Novakoric M, et al: Common bile duct pressure changes after fentanyl morphine, meperidine, butorphanol and naloxone. Anesth Analg 63:441, 1984

283. McCammon RL, et al: Naloxone reversal of choledochoduodenal sphincter spasm associated with narcotic administration. Anesthesiology 48:437, 1978

284. Spiegelman WG, Saunders L, Mazze RI: Addiction and anesthesiology. Anesthesiology 60:335, 1984

285. Stimmel B: Pain, analgesia and addiction, The Pharmacologic Treatment of Pain. New York, Raven Press, 1983, pp 39–55, 119–132

286. Franz DN, Hare BD, McCloskey KL: Spinal sympathetic neurons: Possible sites of opiate withdrawal suppression by clonidine. Science 215:1643, 1982

287. Marks RM, Sachar EJ: Undertreatment of medical inpatients with narcotic analgesics. Ann Intern Med 78:173, 1973

288. Miller RR, Jick H: Clinical effects of meperidine in hospitalized medical patients. J Clin Pharmacol 18:180, 1978

289. Porter J, Jick H: Addiction rare in patients treated with narcotics. N Engl J Med 203:123, 1980

290. Thornton WE, Thornton BP: Narcotic poisoning: A review of the literature. Am J Psychiatry 131:867, 1974

291. Cherubin CE: The medical sequelae of narcotics addiction. Ann Intern Med 67:23, 1967

292. Fracchia C: Medical complications of heroin use. Anesthetic considerations. Anesth Rev 4:45, 1977

293. Caldwell TB III: Anesthesia for patients with behavioral and environmental disorders. Anesthetic management of the narcotic addict, Anesthesia and Uncommon Diseases. Edited by Katz J, Benumof JJ, Kadis LB. Philadelphia, WB Saunders, 1981, pp 681–689

294. Giuffrida JG, Bizzarri DV, Saure AC, et al: Anes-

thetic management of drug abusers. Anesth Analg 49:272, 1970

295. Jenkins LC: Anaesthetic problems due to drug abuse and dependence. Can Anaesth Soc J 19:461, 1972

296. Crile GW: Phylogenetic association in relation to certain medical problems. Boston Med Surg J 163:893, 1910

297. Gray TC, Rees GJ: The role of apnoea in anaesthesia for major surgery. Br Med J 2:891, 1952

298. Woodbridge PD: Changing concepts concerning depth of anesthesia. Anesthesiology 18:536, 1957

299. Griffith HR, Johnson GE: The use of curare in general anesthesia. Anesthesiology 3:418, 1942

300. Chadwick TH, Swerdlow M: Thiopentone-curare in abdominal surgery. Anaesthesia 4:76, 1949

301. Paulson JA: Thiopental sodium and ether anesthesia. JAMA 150:983, 1952

302. Mushin WW, Rendell-Baker L: Pethidine as a supplement to nitrous oxide anaesthesia. Br Med J 2:472, 1949

303. Randall HS, Belton MK, Leigh MD: Continuous infusion of demerol during anaesthesia. Can Med Assoc J 67:311, 1952

304. Auld W: Pethidine, curare, nitrous oxide-oxygen anaesthesia in children. Anaesthesia 7:161, 1952

305. Brotman M, Cullen SC: Supplementation with demerol during nitrous oxide anesthesia. Anesthesiology 10:696, 1949

306. Siker ES, Foldes FF, Pahk NM, et al: Nisentil (1,3, dimethyl-4-phenyl-4-propionoxy piperidine): A new supplement for nitrous oxide oxygen thiopentone (pentothal sodium) anaesthesia. Br J Anaesth 26:405, 1954

307. Dundee JW, Brown SS, Hamilton RC, et al: Analgesic supplementation of light general anesthesia. A study of its advantages using sequential analysis. Anaesthesia 24:52, 1969

308. Goroszeniuk T, Whitwam JG, Morgan M: Uses of methohexitone, fentanyl and nitrous oxide for short surgical procedures. Anaesthesia 32:209, 1977

309. De Castro J, Mundeleer R: Anesthesie sans barbituratiques: La neuroleptanalgésie. Anaesth Analg 16:1022, 1959

310. Edmonds-Seal J, Prys-Roberts C: Pharmacology of drugs used in neuroleptanalgesia. Br J Anaesth 42:207, 1970

311. Laborit H, Huygenard P: Practique, de l'Hibernotherapie en chirurgie et en médécine. Paris, Masson, 1954

312. Morgan M, Lumley J, Gillies IDS: Neuroleptanaesthesia for major surgery: Experience with 500 cases. Br J Anaesth 46:288, 1974

313. Corssen G, Chodoff P, Domino EF, et al: Neuro-

leptanalgesia and anesthesia for open-heart surgery. J Thorac Cardiovasc Surg 49:901, 1965

314. Fitch W, Barker J, Jennett WB, et al: The influence of neuroleptanalgesic drugs on cerebrospinal fluid pressure. Br J Anaesth 41:800, 1969

315. Philbin DM, Moss J, Akins CW, et al: The use of H_1 and H_2 histamine antagonists with morphine anesthesia: A double-blind study. Anesthesiology 55:292, 1981

316. Stanley TH: High dose narcotic anesthesia. Semin Anesth 1:21, 1982

317. Stanley TH: Narcotics as complete anesthetics, Trends in Intravenous Anesthesia. Edited by Aldrete JA, Stanley TH. Chicago, Year Book, 1980, pp 367–384

318. Bovill JG, Sebel PS: Pharmacokinetics in high-dose fentanyl: A study in patients undergoing cardiac surgery. Br J Anaesth 52:795, 1980

319. Wynands JE, Townsend GE, Wong P, et al: Blood pressure response and plasma fentanyl concentration during high- and very high-dose fentanyl anesthesia for coronary artery surgery. Anesth Analg 62:661, 1983

320. Madsen SN, Engquist A, Badawi I, et al: Cyclic AMP, glucose and cortisol in plasma during surgery. Horm Metab Res 8:483, 1976

321. Clarke RSJ: The hyperglycaemic response to different types of surgery and anaesthesia. Br J Anaesth 42:45, 1970

322. Clarke RSJ, Johnston H, Sheridan B: The influence of anaesthesia and surgery on plasma cortisol, insulin and free fatty acids. Br J Anaesth 42:295, 1970

323. McDonald RK, Evans FT, Weise VK, et al: Effects of morphine and nalorphine on plasma hydrocortisone levels in man. J Pharmacol Exp Ther 125:241, 1959

324. Briggs FN, Munson PL: Studies on the mechanism of stimulation of ACTH secretion with the aid of morphine as a blocking agent. Endocrinology 57:205, 1955

325. Di Fazio CA, Chen P: The influence of morphine on excess lactate production. Anesth Analg 50:211, 1971

326. George JM, Reier CE, Lanese RR, et al: Morphine anesthesia blocks cortisol and growth hormone response to surgical stress in humans. J Clin Endocrinol Metab 38:736, 1974

327. Brandt MR, Korshin J, Prange Hansen A, et al: Influence of morphine anesthesia on the endocrine-metabolic response to open heart surgery. Acta Anaesthesiol Scand 22:400, 1978

328. Reier CE, George JM, Kilman JW: Cortisol and growth hormone response to surgical stress during morphine anesthesia. Anesth Analg 52:1003, 1973

329. Kayaalp SO, Kaymakcalan S: Studies on the morphine-induced release of catecholamines

from the adrenal glands in the dog. Arch Int Pharmacodyn Ther 172:139, 1968

330. Fennessey MR, Ortiz A: The behavioral and cardiovascular actions of intravenously administered morphine in the conscious dog. Eur J Pharmacol 3:177, 1968

331. Klingman GI, Maynert EW: Tolerance to morphine. III. Effects on catecholamines in the heart, intestine and spleen. J Pharmacol Exp Ther 135:300, 1962

332. Roizen MF, Horrigan RW, Frazer BM: Anesthetic doses blocking adrenergic (stress) and cardiovascular responses to incision—MAC BAR. Anesthesiology 54:390, 1981

333. Giarmann NJ, Mattie LR, Stephenson WF: Studies on the antidiuretic action of morphine. Science 117:225, 1953

334. De Bodo RC: The antidiuretic action of morphine, and its mechanisms. J Pharmacol Exp Ther 82:74, 1944

335. Hall GM, Young C, Holdcroft A, et al: Substrate mobilisation during surgery: A comparison between halothane and fentanyl anaesthesia. Anaesthesia 33:924, 1978

336. Cooper GM, Paterson JL, Ward ID, et al: Fentanyl and metabolic response to gastric surgery. Anaesthesia 36:667, 1981

337. Philbin DM, Levine FH, Kono K, et al: Attenuation of the stress response to cardiopulmonary bypass by the addition of pulsatile flow. Circulation 64:808, 1981

338. Frater RWM, Wakayama S, Oka Y, et al: Pulsatile cardiopulmonary bypass: Failure to influence hemodynamics or hormones. Circulation 62 (suppl 1):19, 1980

339. Walsh ES, Patterson JL, O'Riordan JBA, et al: Effects of high dose fentanyl anaesthesia on the metabolic and endocrine response to cardiac surgery. Br J Anaesth 53:1155, 1981

340. Bruni JF, Van Vugt D, Marshall S, et al: Effects of naloxone, morphine and methionine enkephalin on serum prolactin, leuteinizing hormone, follicle stimulating hormone, thyroid stimulating hormone and growth hormone. Life Sci 21:461, 1977

341. Fishman J: The opiate and the endocrine system, The Basis of Addiction. Edited by Fishman J. Berlin, Dahlern Konferenzen, Abakon Verlagsgesellschaft, 1978, pp 257–279

342. Beaumont A, Hughes J: Biology of opioid peptides. Annu Rev Pharmacol Toxicol 19:245, 1979

343. Higgins TL, Sirak ED, O'Neil DM, et al: Reversal of hypotension by continuous naloxone infusion in a ventilator dependent patient. Ann Intern Med 98:47, 1983

344. Gurll NJ, Reynolds DG, Vargish T, et al: Naloxone without transfusion prolongs survival and

enhances cardiovascular function in hypovolemic shock. J Pharmacol Exp Ther 220:621, 1982

345. Hensel JI, Albrecht RF, Miletich DJ: The reversal of morphine mediated respiratory depression but not analgesia in rats. Anesthesiology 59:A195, 1983

346. Patschke D, Eberlein HJ, Hess W, et al: Antagonism of morphine with naloxone in dogs. Cardiovascular effects with special reference to the coronary circulation. Br J Anaesth 49:525, 1977

347. Tanaka GY: Hypertensive reaction to naloxone. JAMA 228:25, 1974

348. Azar I, Turndorf H: Severe hypertension and multiple atrial premature contractions following naloxone administration. Anesth Analg 58:524, 1979

349. Michaelis LL, Hickey PR, Clark TA, et al: Ventricular irritability associated with the use of naloxone hydrochloride. Ann Thorac Surg 18:608, 1974

350. Azar I, Patel AK, Phau CQ: Cardiovascular responses following naloxone administration during enflurane anesthesia. Anesth Analg 60:237, 1981

351. Taff RH: Pulmonary edema following naloxone administration in a patient without heart disease. Anesthesiology 59:576, 1983

352. Kraynack BJ, Gintautas JG: Naloxone: Analeptic action unrelated to opiate receptor antagonism? Anesthesiology 56:251, 1982

353. Jaffe JH, Martin WR: Opioid analgesics and antagonists, Goodman and Gilman's The Pharmacological Basis of Therapeutics. 6th Ed. Edited by Gilman AG, Goodman LS, Gilman A. New York, Macmillan, 1980, pp 494–534

354. Mannelli M, Maggi M, De Feo ML, et al: Naloxone administration releases catecholamines. N Engl J Med 308:654, 1983

355. Estilo AE, Cottrell JE: Hemodynamic and catecholamine changes after administration of naloxone. Anesth Analg 61:349, 1982

356. Purdell-Lewis J: Studies of fentanyl-supplemented anaesthesia: Effect of naloxone on circulation and respiration. Can Anaesth Soc J 27:323, 1980

357. Weinstock M, Davidson JT, Rosin AJ, et al: Effect of physostigmine on morphine-induced postoperative pain and somnolence. Br J Anaesth 54:429, 1982

358. Snir-Mor I, Weinstock M, Davidson JT, et al: Physostigmine antagonizes morphine-induced respiratory depression in human subjects. Anesthesiology 59:6, 1983

359. Smith M, Ketcham TR, Nahrwold ML: Morphine, physostigmine and respiratory depression. Anesthesiology 55:A374, 1981

360. Pohl J: Uber das N-allylnorcodeine, einen Anta-gonisten des Morphins. J Exp Pathol Ther 17:370, 1915

361. McCawley WL, Hart ER, Marsh DF: The preparation of N-allylnormorphine. J Am Chem Soc 63:314, 1941

362. Weijland J, Erickson AE: N-allyormorphine. J Am Chem Soc 64:870, 1942

363. Unna K: Antagonistic effect of N-allylnormorphine upon morphine. J Pharmacol Exp Ther 79:27, 1943

364. Hart ER, McCawley EL: The pharmacology of N-allynormorphine as compared with morphine. J Pharmacol Exp Ther 82:339, 1944

365. Schnider O, Hellerback J: Synthese von Morphinan. Helv Chem Acta 33:1437, 1950

366. Pearl J, Stander H, McKean DB: Effects of analgesics and other drugs on mice in phenylquinone and rotarod test. J Pharmacol Exp Ther 167:9, 1969

367. Perrin TD, Atwell L, Tice IB, et al: Analgesic activity as determined by the Nilsen method. J Pharm Sci 61:86, 1972

368. Clark RL, Pessolano AA, Weijlard J: N-substituted eponymorphinans. J Am Chem Soc 75:4974, 1953

369. Jasinski DR, Martin WR, Hoeldtke RD: Effects of short- and long-term administration of pentazocine in man. Clin Pharmacol Ther 11:385, 1970

370. Fraser HF, Rosenberg DE: Studies on the human addiction liability of 2-hydroxy-5,9-dimethyl-2-(3,3-dimethylallyl)-6,7-benzomorphan (Win 20,228): A weak narcotic antagonist. J Pharmacol Exp Ther 143:149, 1964

371. Leaman DM, Nellis SH, Zelis R, et al: Effects of morphine sulfate on human coronary blood flow. Am J Cardiol 41:324, 1978

372. Lee G, De Maria AN, Amsterdam EA, et al: Comparative effects of morphine, meperidine and pentazocine on cardiocirculatory dynamics in patients with acute myocardial infarction. Am J Med 60:949, 1976

373. Jewitt DE, Maurer BJ, Sonnenblick EJ, et al: Pentazocine: Effect on ventricular muscle and hemodynamic changes in ischemic heart disease. Circulation 44(suppl II):118, 1971

374. Alderman EL, Barry WH, Graham AF, et al: Hemodynamic effects of morphine and pentazocine differ in cardiac patients. N Engl J Med 287:623, 1972

375. Jewitt DE, Maurer BJ, Hubner PJB: Increased pulmonary arterial pressures after pentazocine in myocardial infarction. Br Med J 1:795, 1970

376. Alarcon RD, Gelfond SD, Alarcon GS: Parenteral and oral pentazocine abuse. Johns Hopkins Med J 129:311, 1971

377. Parwatikar S, Gomez H, Knowles RR: Pentazocine dependency. Int J Addict 8:87, 1973

378. Sandoval RG, Wang RIH: Tolerance and dependence on pentazocine. N Engl J Med 280:1391, 1969

379. Kaukinen L, Kaukinen S, Eerola R, et al: The antagonistic effect of pentazocine on fentanyl induced respiratory depression compared with nalorphine and naloxone. Ann Clin Res 13:396, 1981

380. Beaver WT, Wallenstein SL, Houde RW, et al: A comparison of the analgesic effects of pentazocine and morphine in patients with cancer. Clin Pharmacol Ther 7:740, 1966

381. Goetz RL, Bain RV: Neonatal withdrawal symptoms associated with maternal use of pentazocine. J Pediatr 84:887, 1974

382. Monkovic I, Conway TT, Wang H, et al: Total synthesis and pharmacological activities of N-substituted 3,14-dihydroxymorphinans. J Am Chem Soc 95:7910, 1973

383. Dobkin AB, Eamkaow S, Zak S, et al: Butorphanol: A double-blind evaluation in postoperative patients with moderate or severe pain. Can Anaesth Soc J 21:600, 1974.

384. Tavakoli M, Corrsen G, Caruso FS: Butorphanol and morphine: A double-blind comparison of their parenteral analgesic activity. Anesth Analg 55:394, 1976

385. DelPizzo A: Butorphanol, a new intravenous analgesic: Double-blind comparison with morphine sulfate in postoperative patients with moderate or severe pain. Curr Ther Res 20:221, 1976

386. Gilbert MS, Hanover RM, Moylan DS, et al: Intramuscular butorphanol and meperidine in postoperative pain. Clin Pharmacol Ther 20:359, 1976

387. Galloway FM, Hrdlicka J, Losada M, et al: Comparison of analgesia by intravenous butorphanol and meperidine with postoperative pain. Can Anaesth Soc J 24:90, 1977

388. Corssen G, Tavakoli M, Caruso FS: Butorphanol and morphine: A double-blind comparison of the parenteral analgesic activity. Anesth Analg 55:394, 1976

389. Popio KA, Jackson DH, Ross AM, et al: Hemodynamic and respiratory effects of morphine and butorphanol. Clin Pharmacol Ther 23:281, 1978

390. Nagashima H, Karamanian A, Malovany R, et al: Respiratory and circulatory effects of intravenous butorphanol and morphine. Clin Pharmacol Ther 19:738, 1976

391. Del Pizzo A: A double-blind study of the effects of butorphanol compared with morphine in balanced anaesthesia. Can Anaesth Soc J 25:392, 1978

392. Zauder HL: Butorphanol, a new non-narcotic analgesic, Trends in Intravenous Anesthesia.

Edited by Aldrete JA, Stanley TH. Chicago, Year Book, 1980, pp 367–383

393. Sederberg J, Stanley TH, Reddy P, et al: Hemodynamic effects of butorphanol-oxygen anesthesia in dogs. Anesth Analg 60:715, 1981

394. Stanley TH, Reddy P, Tilmore S, et al: The cardiovascular effects of high-dose butorphanol-nitrous oxide anaesthesia before and during operation. Can Anaesth Soc J 30:337, 1983

395. Vandam LD: Drug therapy: Butorphanol. N Engl J Med 302:381, 1980

396. Heel RC, Brogden RN, Speight TM, et al: Butorphanol: A review of its pharmacological properties and therapeutic efficacy. Drugs 16:473, 1978

397. Beaver WT, Feise GA: A comparison of the analgesic effect of intramuscular nalbuphine and morphine in patients with postoperative pain. J Pharmacol Exp Ther 204:487, 1978

398. Fragen RJ, Caldwell N: Acute intravenous premedication with nalbuphine. Anesth Analg 56:808, 1977

399. Magruder MR, Christoforetti R, Di Fazio CA: Balanced anesthesia with nalbuphine hydrochloride. Anesthesiol Rev 9:25, 1980

400. Murphy MR, Hug CC: The enflurane sparing effect of morphine, butorphanol and nalbuphine. Anesthesiology 57:489, 1982

401. Fahmy NR, Sunder N, Roberts JT: Nalbuphine: Hemodynamic effects and efficacy in suppressing reflex activity in "balanced" anesthesia. Anesth Analg 61:184, 1982

402. Lake CL, Duckworth EN, Difazio CA, et al: Cardiovascular effects of nalbuphine in patients with coronary or valvular heart disease. Anesthesiology 57:498, 1982

403. Romagnoli A, Keats AS: Comparative hemodynamic effects of nalbuphine and morphine in patients with coronary artery disease. Bull Tex Heart Inst 5:19, 1978

404. DiFazio CA, Moscicki JC, Magruder MR: Anesthetic potency of nalbuphine and interaction with morphine in rats. Anesth Analg 60:629, 1981

405. Gilbert PE, Martin WR: The effects of morphine and nalorphine-like drugs in the nondependent, morphine-dependent and cyclazocine-dependent chronic spinal dog. J Pharmacol Exp Ther 198:66, 1976

406. Roach GW, Hug CC Jr: Nalbuphine reversal of respiratory depression following high dose fentanyl anesthesia. Abstract presented at Society of Cardiovascular Anesthesiologists, San Diego, 1983

407. Magruder MR, Delaney RD, Difazio CA: Reversal of narcotic-induced respiratory depression with nalbuphine hydrochloride. Anesthesiol Rev 9:34, 1982

408. Julien RM: Effects of nalbuphine on normal and oxymorphine-depressed ventilatory responses to carbon dioxide challenges. Anesthesiology 57:A320, 1982

409. Tabatabai M, Javadi P, Tadjziechy M, et al: Effect of nalbuphine, hydrochloride on fentanyl induced respiratory depression and analgesia. Anesthesiology 61:A475, 1984

410. Stanski DR, Greenblatt DJ, Lowenstein E: Kinetics of intravenous and intramuscular morphine. Clin Pharmacol Ther 24:52, 1978

411. Dahlstrom B, Bolme P, Feychting H, et al: Morphine kinetics in children. Clin Pharmacol Ther 26:354, 1979

412. Stanski DR, Paalzow L, Edlund PO: Morphine pharmacokinetics: GLC assay versus radio immunoassay. J Pharm Sci 71:314, 1982

413. Murphy MR, Hug CC Jr: Pharmacokinetics of intravenous morphine in patients anesthetized with enflurane-nitrous oxide. Anesthesiology 54:187, 1981

414. Dahlstrom B, Tamsen A, Paalzow L, et al: Patient controlled analgesia therapy IV: Pharmacokinetics and analgesic plasma concentrations of morphine. Clin Pharmacokinet 7(3):266, 1982

415. Hug CC, Jr., Murphy MR, Rigel EP, et al: Pharmacokinetics of morphine injected intravenously into the anesthetized dog. Anesthesiology 54:38, 1981

416. Way EL, Adler TK: The biological disposition of morphine and its surrogates. 1. Bull WHO 25:227, 1961

417. Wolff WA, Riegel C, Fry EG: The excretion of morphine by normal and tolerant dogs. J Pharmacol Exp Ther 47:391, 1933

418. Yeh SY: Urinary excretion of morphine and its metabolites in morphine dependent subjects. J Pharmacol Exp Ther 192:201, 1975

419. Brunk SF, Della M: Morphine metabolism in man. Clin Pharmacol Ther 16:51, 1974

420. Sasajima M: Analgesic effect of morphine-3-glucuronide. Keio J Med 47:421, 1970

421. Mather LE, Tucker GT, Pflug AE, et al: Meperidine kinetics in man: Intravenous injection in surgical patients and volunteers. Clin Pharmacol Ther 17:21, 1975

422. Klotz U, McHorse TS, Wilkinson GR, et al: The effect of cirrhosis on the disposition and elimination of meperidine in man. Clin Pharmacol Ther 16:667, 1974

423. Verbeeck RK, Branch RA, Wilkinson GR: Meperidine disposition in man: Influence of urinary pH and route of administration. Clin Pharmacol Ther 30:619, 1981

424. Stambaugh JE, Wainer IW, Sanstead JK, et al: The clinical pharmacology of meperidine: Comparison of routes of administration. J Clin Pharmacol 16:245, 1976

425. Austin KL, Stapleton JV, Mather LE: Multiple intramuscular injection: A major source of variability in analgesic response to meperidine. Pain 8:47, 1980

426. Miller JW, Anderson HH: The effect of N-demethylation on certain pharmacologic actions of morphine, codeine and meperidine in the mouse. J Pharmacol Exp Ther 112:191, 1954

427. Szeto HH, Inturrisi CE, Houde R, et al: Accumulation of normeperidine, an active metabolite of meperidine, in patients with renal failure or cancer. Ann Intern Med 86:738, 1977

428. McClain DA, Hug CC Jr: Intravenous fentanyl kinetics. Clin Pharmacol Ther 28:106, 1980

429. Fung DL, Eisele JH: Fentanyl pharmacokinetics in awake volunteers. J Clin Pharmacol 20:652, 1980

430. Schleimer R, Benjamini E, Eisele J, et al: Pharmacokinetics of fentanyl as determined by radioimmunoassay. Clin Pharmacol Ther 23:188, 1978

431. Hug CC, Jr., Murphy MR, Sampson JF, et al: Biotransformation of morphine and fentanyl in anhepatic dogs. Anesthesiology 55:A261, 1981

432. Bower S, Hull CJ: The comparative pharmacokinetics of fentanyl and alfentanil. Br J Anaesth 54:871, 1982

433. Koska AJ, Kramer WG, Romagnoli A, et al: Pharmacokinetics of high-dose meperidine in surgical patients. Anesth Analg 60:8, 1981

434. Hug CC, Murphy MR: Tissue redistribution of fentanyl and termination of its effects in rats. Anesthesiology 55:369, 1981

435. Goromaru T, Furuta T, Baba S, et al: Metabolism of fentanyl in rats and man. Anesthesiology 55:A173, 1981

436. Benson DW, Kaufman JJ, Koski WS: Theoretic significance of pH dependence of narcotics and narcotic antagonists in clinical anesthesia. Anesth Analg 55:253, 1976

437. Finck AD, Berkowitz BA, Hempstead J, et al: Pharmacokinetics of morphine: Effects of hypercarbia on serum and brain morphine concentrations in the dog. Anesthesiology 47:407, 1977

438. Nishitateno K, Ngai SH, Finck AD, et al: Pharmacokinetics of morphine: Concentrations in the serum and brain of the dog during hyperventilation. Anesthesiology 50:520, 1979

439. Ainslie SG, Eisele JH, Corkill G: Fentanyl concentrations in brain and serum during respiratory acid–base changes in the dog. Anesthesiology 51:293, 1979

440. Gill KJ, Cartwright DP, Scoggins A, et al: Ventilatory depression related to plasma fentanyl concentrations during and after anaesthesia. Br J Anaesth 52:632P, 1980

441. Chan K, Vaughan DP, Mitchard M: Plasma con-

centrations and urinary excretion of pethidine and metabolites. Abstracts of the Symposium on the Assessment of Drug Metabolism in Man — Methods and Clinical Applications, University of Dundee, 1974

442. Cooper LV, Stephen GW, Aggett PJA: Elimination of pethidine and bupivicaine in the newborn. Arch Dis Child 52:638, 1977

443. Murphy MR, Hug CC: Dose independent pharmacokinetics of fentanyl. Anesthesiology 57: A347, 1982

444. Neal EA, Meffin PJ, Gregory PB, et al: Enhanced bioavailability and decreased clearance of analgesics in patients with cirrhosis. Gastroenterology 77:96, 1979

445. Pond SM, Tong T, Benowitz NL, et al: Presystemic metabolism of meperidine to normeperidine in normal and cirrhotic subjects. Clin Pharmacol Ther 30:183, 1981

446. McHorse TS, Wilkinson GR, Johnson RF, et al: Effect of acute viral hepatitis in man on the disposition and elimination of meperidine. Gastroenterology 68:775, 1975

447. Coral IM, Moore AR, Strunin L: Plasma concentrations of fentanyl in normal surgical patients and those with severe renal and hepatic disease. Br J Anaesth 52:101P, 1980

448. Don HF, Dieppa RA, Taylor P: Narcotic analgesics in anuric patients. Anesthesiology 42:745, 1975

449. Hug CC Jr., DeLange S, Burm AGL: Alfentanil pharmacokinetics in cardia surgical patients before and after cardiopulmonary bypass (CPB). Anesth Analg 62:266, 1983

450. Hug CC Jr, Moldenhauer CC: Pharmacokinetics and dynamics of fentanyl infusions in cardiac surgical patients. Anesthesiology 54:A45, 1982

451. Koska AJ, Romagnoli A, Kramer WG: Effect of cardiopulmonary bypass on fentanyl distribution and elimination. Clin Pharmacol Ther 29:100, 1981

452. Koren G, Crean P, Goresky G, et al: Irreversible binding of fentanyl to the cardiopulmonary bypass. Anesth Analg 63:175, 1984

453. Bovill JG, Sebel PS, Blackburn CL, et al: Kinetics of alfentanil and sufentanil: A comparison. Anesthesiology 55:A174, 1981

454. Meuldermans WEG, Hurkmans RMA, Heykants JJP: Plasma protein binding and distribution of fentanyl, sufentanil, alfentanil and lofentanil in blood. Arch Int Pharmacodyn Ther 257:4, 1982

455. Smith NT, Dec-Silber H, Harrison WK, et al: A comparison among morphine, fentanyl and sufentanil anesthesia for open-heart surgery: Induction, emergence and extubation. Anesthesiology 57(3S):A291, 1982

456. Kay B, Rolly G: Duration of action of analgesic supplements to anesthesia. A double-blind comparison between morphine, fentanyl and sufentanil. Acta Anaesthesiol Belg 28:25, 1977

457. Bovill JG, Sebel PS, Blackburn CL, et al: The pharmacokinetics of alfentanil (R 39209): A new opioid analgesic. Anesthesiology 57:439, 1982

458. Camu F, Gepts E, Rucquio M, et al: Pharmacokinetics of alfentanil in man. Anesth Analg 61:657, 1982

459. de Lange S, de Bruijin N: Alfentanil-oxygen anaesthesia: Plasma concentration and clinical effects during variable rate continuous infusion for coronary artery surgery. Br J Anaesth 55:S183, 1983

460. Wagner JG: A safe method for rapidly achieving plasma concentration plateaus. Clin Pharmacol Ther 16:691, 1974

461. Hug CC Jr, Stanski DR: Editorial: Alfentanil — A kinetically predictable narcotic analgesic. Anesthesiology 57:435, 1982

462. Hug CC Jr, Stanski DR: In reply. Anesthesiology 59:257, 1983

463. Bentley JB, Finely JH, Humphrey LR, et al: Obesity and alfentanil pharmacokinetics. Anesth Analg 62:251, 1983

464. Hug CC, de Lange S, Burn AGL: Alfentanil pharmacokinetics in patients before and after cardiopulmonary bypass. Anesth Analg 62:266, 1983

Index

Note: Page numbers followed by f denote figures; those followed by t denote tables.